Building
a Medical
Vocabulary
with Spanish Translations

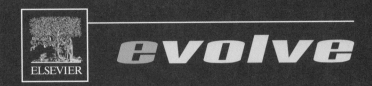

Seventh Edition

Building
a Medical
Vocabulary

with Spanish Translations

Peggy C. Leonard, MT, MEd

St. Louis County, Missouri

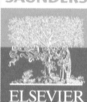

SAUNDERS

ELSEVIER

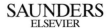

SAUNDERS
ELSEVIER

11830 Westline Industrial Drive
St. Louis, Missouri 63146

Notice

Neither the Publisher nor the Author assumes any responsibility for any loss or injury and/or damage to persons or property arising out of or related to any use of the material contained in this book. It is the responsibility of the treating practitioner, relying on independent expertise and knowledge of the patient, to determine the best treatment and method of application for the patient.

The Publisher

Library of Congress Cataloging-in-Publication Data
Leonard, Peggy C.
Building a medical vocabulary: with Spanish translations / Peggy C. Leonard.—7th ed.
  p. ; cm.
Includes bibliographical references and index.
ISBN 978-1-4160-5627-0 (pbk.: alk. paper)
1. Medicine—Terminology. 2. Human anatomy—Terminology. 3. English language—Glossaries, vocabularies, etc. 4. Spanish language—Conversation and phrase books (for medical personnel) I. Title.
[DNLM: 1. Terminology as Topic—Programmed Instruction. W 18.2 L5805b 2009]
R123.L46 2009
610.1'4—dc22

                                              2008025742

Publishing Director: Andrew Allen
Publisher: Jeanne Olson
Developmental Editors: Carolyn Kruse; Rebecca Swisher
Publishing Services Manager: Patricia Tannian
Senior Project Manager: Sarah Wunderly
Design Direction: Paula Catalano
Artist: Jeanne Robertson

Printed in Canada

Last digit is the print number: 9   8   7   6   5   4   3   2   1

Reviewers

Margaret Batson RN, MSN
Nursing Instructor
San Joaquin Delta College
Stockton, California

LaShunda Mechelle Blanding-Smith, MS-Management
Registered Health Information Administrator
Instructor
Alabama State University
Montgomery, Alabama

Gertrude Frangipani, RN, BS, MBA
Instructor
Learning Tree University
Chatsworth, California

Cindy L. Iavagnilio MSN, RN, CRNA
Assistant Professor of Nursing
Saint Mary's College
Notre Dame, Indiana

Patricia A. Ireland, CMT, FAAMT
Certified Medical Transcriptionist
Author, Instructor, Freelance Medical/Technical Editor
San Antonio, Texas

Jo Ann Kilsby, CMT, RHIT, FAAMT
Instructor
Austin Community College
Austin, Texas

Joseph L. Monaco, PA-C, MSJ
Interim Chair, Physician Assistant Program
Seton Hall University
South Orange, New Jersey

Melissa Ann Redding
Anatomy and Physiology Instructor
Science Department Chair
Washington Community High School
Washington, Illinois

Laura Shaffer, MS, LOTR
Instructor
Health Sciences Center
Louisiana State University
Shreveport, Louisiana

Carrie Stein, CMT
Medical Transcription Course Facilitator
Gatlin Education Services
Fort Worth, Texas

Tricia Tyhurst, CPC, CPC-H, BA-Ed
Instructor
University of Montana
Helena, Montana

Meredith Wallace PhD, APRN-BC
Associate Professor and Elizabeth DeCamp McInerney
    Chair of Health Sciences
Fairfield University School of Nursing
Fairfield, Connecticut

Charles Kent Williston, BA, MS
Instructor
Traviss Career Center
Lakeland, Florida

Acknowledgments

Several individuals have contributed to the refreshing approach of the seventh edition of *Building a Medical Vocabulary*. Suggestions from instructors and students have been incorporated, as well as in-depth analyses by an outstanding group of reviewers.

The new Pharmacology Section on the Companion CD was made possible by Erinn Kao, PharmD. Patricia Ireland, CMT, FAAMT, provided professional expertise in the preparation of the health care reports. I am also indebted to the companies who have allowed use of illustrations that vividly enhance the written word and bring life to explanations of medical terms.

The production of this book would not be possible without the producers, editors, proofreaders, and all others whose expertise has produced a book that I am sure will be valuable to students in their search for understanding of the medical language.

Words cannot adequately express my gratitude to Developmental Editor Carolyn Kruse who provides humor, steadfast encouragement, and herculean efforts during the preparation of many editions of this book, as well as *Quick and Easy Medical Terminology*.

Peggy Leonard, MT, MEd

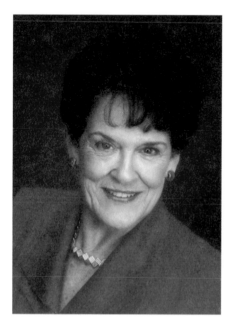

Peggy C. Leonard

DEDICATED TO

the instructors and students
whose enthusiasm and influence
have helped shaped this book

and to my family
who support me in so many ways

Preface

TO THE INSTRUCTOR

The seventh edition of *Building a Medical Vocabulary* is now even more interactive! Instructors and students have depended on this easy-to-use text for years. Although each profession and each specialty has its own particular terminology, much of the medical language is understood by all members of the health team and is the focus of this book. The book is useful in a medical terminology course or as self-paced material for anyone pursuing a career in the health professions.

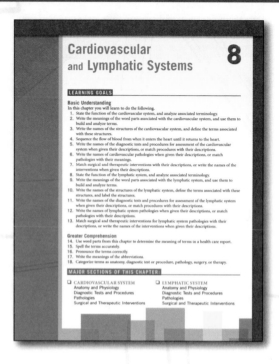

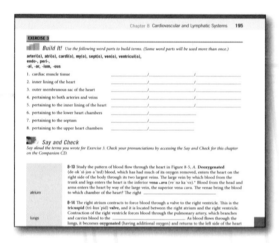

The Most Interactive Text on the Market!
After learning the meaning of word parts and how they are combined using a logical, step-by-step learning method, the student begins recognizing and writing new terms in the first chapter! Immediate involvement and feedback within the programmed method provide intrinsic motivation that is not found in other systems, and your students will have fun using this book. The new activities Build It, Word Analysis, and Say and Check help students to not only read and write terms, but also to analyze terms and understand the spoken language.

A Strong Foundation Section Precedes the Well-Organized Body Systems Section.
Chapters 1 through 7 provide a foundation for chapters about the body systems. *It is important that students study the foundation chapters in the sequence in which they are presented.* Students will learn many word parts, as well as concepts pertaining to body structure and body fluids in the foundation material. For instructors who have used previous editions, you will be delighted to find an even stronger foundation for the other chapters.

Body Systems (Chapters 8 through 17) Can Be Taught and Studied in Any Sequence.
Although terminology is given primary emphasis, the book can also be used as an introductory anatomy and physiology book. Because instructors can easily change the sequence of the body systems chapters, the book adapts well for use in conjunction with anatomy, physiology, or introductory medical science courses. A Function First section provides a quick overview of each system's purpose.

You will especially appreciate the organization of systems chapter material: anatomy and physiology, diagnostic tests and procedures, pathologies, and surgical and therapeutic interventions.

Learning Goals and End-of-Chapter Exercises Are Classified as Basic or Greater Comprehension.
Basic understanding requires labeling, recall of the meaning of word parts and medical terms, photo identification, word building, and analysis. Greater comprehension includes spelling, pronunciation, abbreviations, reading health care reports, categorizing terms (an application exercise), and a Challenge section. You determine and inform the students of your expectations. Instructors often have the students work all of the review, then exercise more specificity when choosing examination questions.

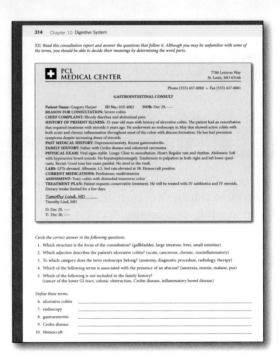

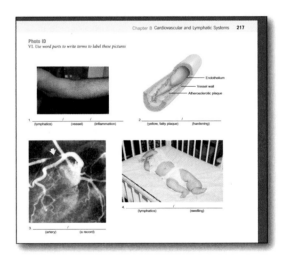

NEW! Word Building and Word Analysis Exercises.

New exercises that require students to use word parts to build terms or to break words into their component parts equip students to decipher unfamiliar terms when they are encountered in practice, thus improving the student's ability to communicate in the specialized language of health care.

NEW! More Labeling Exercises, Plus Numerous Exercises Within the Chapters.

Labeling exercises reinforce word building and visually reinforce terms. Section exercises reinforce learning by helping students recall the meaning of word parts and terms they learned in the section. The variety keeps the student interested, and includes pronouncing terms aloud, then checking them with the Companion CD.

NEW! Key Point Boxes.

Key points are shown highlighted in color to help students focus on the most important material.

NEW! Medical Process Highlighted.

The medical process of patient presentation, diagnostic testing, pathology determination, and therapeutics administration is reinforced in the introductory chapters, setting terminology within its medical context. In addition to teaching categories of terms, orientation to the medical process reinforces how those terms fit into patient presentation, diagnostics, and care, involving the student in the center of the "arena" of medicine by understanding its world of terms.

NEW! More Healthcare Reports Than Ever.

Students are inspired by health care documents that reflect patient diagnosis and treatment using terms and abbreviations they have learned. Records include history and physical, consultation, and pathology reports.

NEW! Expanded Art Program Has Even More Full-Color Illustrations and Photos.

Full-color art throughout the book enhances learning and makes difficult concepts easier to understand.

End-of-Chapter Reviews Help Students Measure How Much They Learn.

A variety of question types are included in *comprehensive* end-of-chapter reviews. Types of questions include labeling diagrams, fill-in-the-blanks, medical record exercises, writing terms, multiple-choice questions, and pronunciation practices that can be used in class when time permits. To facilitate learning beyond memorization, a new Challenge exercise introduces students to unfamiliar terms that they can analyze using word parts they know.

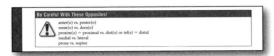

Caution Boxes alert the student to discriminate between similar terms.

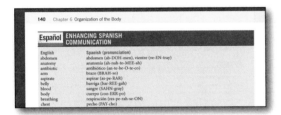

Spanish Translations are Presented.
Living in Venezuela several years ago, I learned the Spanish language. I am pleased to offer translation of many medical terms. This edition's instructor's curriculum resource also has matching exercises for the Spanish translations, if you wish to use them for extra-credit assignments.

Extra Learning Material in the Appendix.
Extra material is provided, along with an alphabetized listing of abbreviations, word parts, and Spanish translations.

NEW! Spanish Usage Appendix
A new appendix that includes common medical questions and phrases allows students to put Spanish medical terms to use with phrases such as "Are you in pain?" and "I am going to take your blood pressure."

NEW! Genetics Appendix
With the sequencing of the human genome, students will need to be exposed to terms about genetics. This new appendix gets them ready!

Comprehensive Review Chapter
Provides an all-chapter review in preparation for final examination or as a self-test for students to realize how much they've learned.

Comprehensive Glossary/Index
The students will love the glossary/index that provides the pronunciation, meaning, and page references for more than 2000 terms.

Software is Fun and Challenging
The software introduces a gaming aspect and provides another way for students to determine how much they have learned. The testing mode (in addition to the study mode) offers the option of having students print their results as proof of completion.

New Pharmacology Information.
Pharmacology for each chapter is available on the Companion CD if you wish to use it.

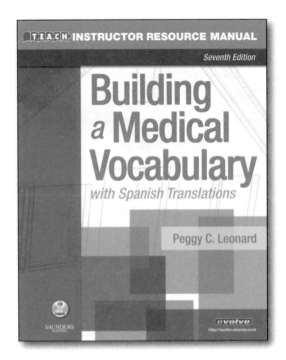

NEW! TEACH Manual—Including the Instructor's Curriculum Resource—with a CD.
A comprehensive curriculum resource is available to instructors by contacting Elsevier Health Sciences. It includes both printed material and software with access to over 2000 questions that can be used to produce your own tests. Several types of questions are included, along with classroom exercises, art from the text, transparency masters, and several summary tables designed especially for classroom use.

Evolve Course Management *evolve*
The Evolve website provides a course management platform for instructors who want to post course materials online. Elsevier Health Sciences provides hosting and technical support. The Student area includes study tips, updates, and links. The Instructor area includes the Instructor's Curriculum Resource, the Computerized Test Bank, and the Electronic Image Collection.

TO THE STUDENT

Here Is Your Blueprint for Learning Medical Terminology!

Imagine being able to read and write medical words the first day you begin studying. You will have this experience shortly as you begin studying *Building a Medical Vocabulary*. You will soon be breaking medical terms down into easier parts that will help you understand their meaning.

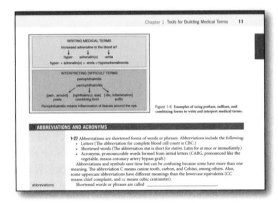

You'll Have Lots of Tools to Make Learning Easy.

Frames make learning easy! You will find the readability of a textbook, even though it is organized into frames. It is important to write your answers in the blanks, because writing increases retention of the material.

A Good Foundation Is Essential.

Be sure to study Chapters 1 through 7 in the order in which they are presented, because each chapter builds on the material learned in the previous chapter. Read all the material within a chapter, including the tables and illustration captions. Then study chapters 8 through 17 as directed by your instructor. Chapter 18 is a review of the whole text.

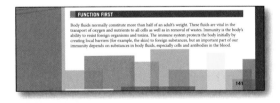

Function First Sections Explain WHY Each System Is Important.

Each of the body systems chapters (8 through 17) opens with a Function First section that gives you an overview of the function of each body system.

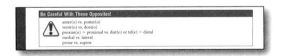

Caution! Students at Work!

Be careful of similar terms. The Caution Boxes help you distinguish between terms that look alike but have different meanings.

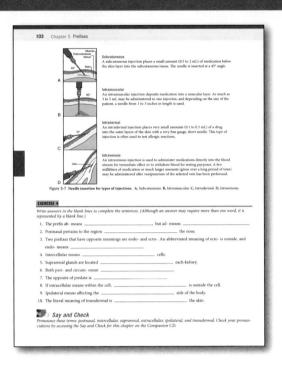

Know if You Understand a Section Before Moving Ahead.

Read a section. Then work the corresponding exercise to reinforce your learning. Working the exercises throughout the chapter lets you "chunk" the material into manageable pieces.

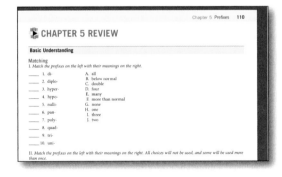

Measure How You Are Doing by Using the End-Of-Chapter Review Before the Test.

Complete the end-of-chapter review and check your answers in Appendix VI to ensure that you understand each chapter's material. Additional practice questions are provided on the Companion CD.

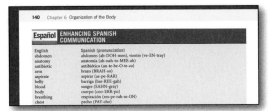

Real-Life Practice Opportunities!
Imagine yourself working in your chosen health care field. The case studies and health reports you read in this book are just like the ones you will be reading when you are a health care professional! You will be fully prepared to understand the day-to-day medical terminology you will encounter.

Index/Glossary

Preparing for a Mid-Term or Final Exam?
Use the Index/Glossary to review terms for the big exams. It has the definitions and the pages on which the terms were introduced, so you know where to find terms as you review. To prepare for the final, complete Chapter 18—it reviews the entire text!

You are about to embark on learning an entirely new language, but you have discovered a fun and easy way to do it! After the first chapter, medical terms that seem difficult now will be easy. Some terms will be easier to remember than others, but challenge yourself to understand every term in every chapter.

Spanish Translations Make Your Education More Valuable!
Spanish translations of selected medical terms are presented at the end of each chapter. Even if you do not speak Spanish, knowing some medical terminology in Spanish will help you put Spanish-speaking patients more at ease. The new Spanish usage appendix will help you place medical terms within conversational Spanish.

Have Fun with the Companion CD
Additional visuals and practice exercises on the Companion CD will help you measure how much you learned. You can work in study mode until you feel ready to try the test mode for each chapter. Your scores in the test mode are recorded and can also be printed.

The CD is also valuable in learning pronunciations. Say and Check allows you to practice pronunciation as you work certain exercises, and then use the CD to check yourself. In addition, the listing of medical terms at the end of each chapter is the same as the audio chapter glossary on the CD. Be sure that you LOOK at the terms as you practice pronouncing them. After listening to pronunciations, review the list and be sure that you know the meaning of each term.

Don't Be Intimidated by Long Drug Names!
Pharmacology material for each chapter is found on the Companion CD. You are not expected to remember the names of drugs, but you should recognize the meanings of the drug classes. Because new drugs are introduced and other drugs are removed each year, it is important to consult current drug reference materials. Sources such as *Mosby's Drug Consult, Mosby's Drug Guide for Health Professions,* the *Physician's Desk Reference (PDR),* the *Nurse's Drug Reference (NDR),* and *Drug Facts and Comparisons* (updated monthly) provide current information.

Contents

Pharmacology for each chapter is available on the Companion CD.

Tools for Building Medical Terms

1

Word Building, Word Parts, Forming Plurals, and Pronunciation

LEARNING GOALS

Basic Understanding
In this chapter you will learn to do the following.
1. Use the programmed learning format to learn medical terminology.
2. Identify the roles of word roots, prefixes, suffixes, and combining forms.
3. Identify examples of combining forms, prefixes, and suffixes.
4. Demonstrate correct usage of the combining vowel by correctly joining word parts to write medical terms.
5. Use the pronunciation rules inside the front cover of this book to pronounce words correctly.
6. Use the rules learned in this chapter to write the singular or plural forms of medical terms.
7. Demonstrate understanding of the use of the reference material.

MAJOR SECTIONS OF THIS CHAPTER:

- ❏ LEARNING BY THE PROGRAMMED METHOD
- ❏ FOUNDATIONS OF WORD BUILDING
- ❏ WORD ROOTS, COMBINING FORMS, PREFIXES, AND SUFFIXES
- ❏ COMBINING WORD PARTS
- ❏ EPONYMS
- ❏ ABBREVIATIONS AND ACRONYMS
- ❏ PRONUNCIATION OF MEDICAL TERMS
- ❏ PLURALS OF MEDICAL TERMS
- ❏ ENHANCING SPANISH COMMUNICATION
- ❏ PHARMACOLOGY

FUNCTION FIRST

The material in this chapter is important because it is the beginning foundation on which you will build a medical vocabulary. It explains word building and teaches you how to break down a word into its parts.

Each chapter introduces new terms and uses those you learned in previous chapters. You will gradually build a strong medical vocabulary foundation that will enable you to recognize and write thousands of medical words. It is important to study material in the order in which it is presented within a chapter. It is also important to study Chapters 1 through 7 in sequential order. These early chapters form the foundation for learning material about the body systems presented in Chapters 8 through 17.

LEARNING BY THE PROGRAMMED METHOD

1-1 It is important to study the first seven chapters in the sequence presented in this book, because these chapters are the foundation for learning terms presented in all other chapters.

Programmed learning consists of blocks of information, often containing blanks in which you will write answers. After writing an answer, you will check to see if it is correct by comparing your answer with that in the left column, called the answer column.

1-2 A frame is a block of information preceded by a number. Each frame is given a separate number, and most frames contain at least one blank in which you will write an answer. After writing your answer in a blank, you will check to see if it is correct.

> ➤ **KEY** POINT <u>Cover the answer column while you are filling in the blanks</u>. To do this, position the bookmark so that it covers only the answer column. After writing your answer in a blank, check it by sliding the bookmark down just enough to see the answer (Figure 1-1). When you are not using the bookmark to cover the answer column, use it to mark your place in the book.

1-3 You have just read two frames. Information contained in frames throughout this book will help you learn medical terms. A block of information with a number is called

frame

a _____.

Write the answer in the preceding blank and check it immediately. Some students prefer to write their answers on a separate sheet of paper so that they can rework the material later. It is important to write your answer because writing it will help you to remember it better than if you just think of the answer. Always check your answer immediately and say it aloud if possible. This is especially helpful when you are not familiar with the term. Saying an answer aloud helps you remember it. If you make an error, look back at previous frames to see where you went wrong. Otherwise, you may repeat the error without realizing why it is incorrect.

1-4 This text provides frequent exercises to reinforce what you are learning. Answers to the exercises and reviews are in Appendix VI, Solutions to Review Exercises. The end-of-the-chapter reviews help integrate what you have learned in a chapter.

EXERCISE 1

Write answers in the blanks.

1. In programmed learning, a block of information preceded by a number is called a _____.

2. Position the bookmark so that it covers only the _____ column.

3. It is important to _____ your answer because this will help you remember better than just thinking of the answer.

4. After writing the answer in the blank, always _____ it using the information in the answer column.

(Use Appendix VI to check your answers.)

FOUNDATIONS OF WORD BUILDING

1-5 Word building is a system of learning the meaning of various word parts to understand and write new words. Because it is impractical to memorize the medical dictionary, you will use a

building

system of word _____ to learn medical terms.

1-6 Pay close attention to spelling.

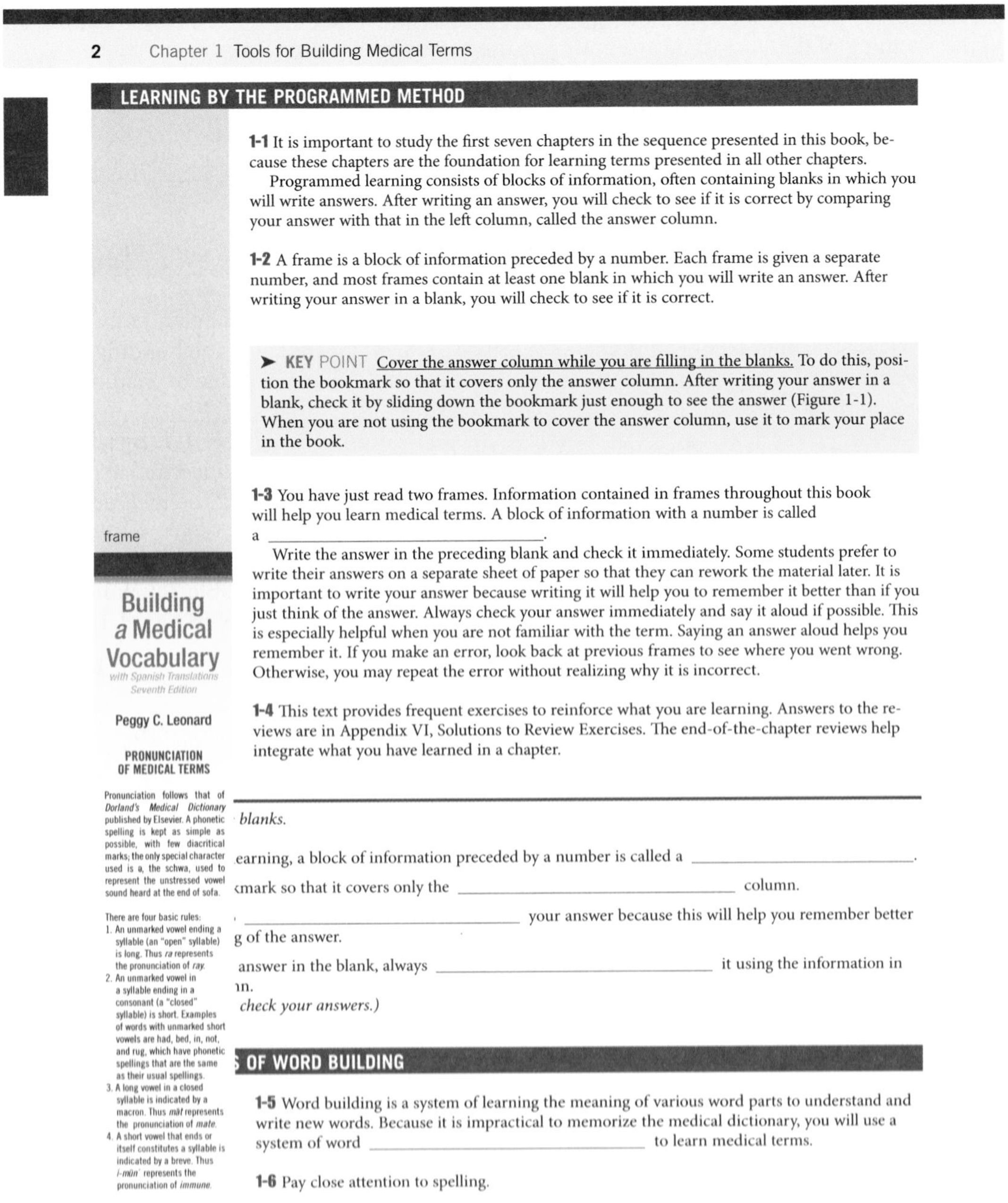

LEARNING BY THE PROGRAMMED METHOD

1-1 It is important to study the first seven chapters in the sequence presented in this book, because these chapters are the foundation for learning terms presented in all other chapters.

Programmed learning consists of blocks of information, often containing blanks in which you will write answers. After writing an answer, you will check to see if it is correct by comparing your answer with that in the left column, called the answer column.

1-2 A frame is a block of information preceded by a number. Each frame is given a separate number, and most frames contain at least one blank in which you will write an answer. After writing your answer in a blank, you will check to see if it is correct.

> ➤ **KEY** POINT <u>Cover the answer column while you are filling in the blanks.</u> To do this, position the bookmark so that it covers only the answer column. After writing your answer in a blank, check it by sliding down the bookmark just enough to see the answer (Figure 1-1). When you are not using the bookmark to cover the answer column, use it to mark your place in the book.

1-3 You have just read two frames. Information contained in frames throughout this book will help you learn medical terms. A block of information with a number is called

frame

a _____.

Write the answer in the preceding blank and check it immediately. Some students prefer to write their answers on a separate sheet of paper so that they can rework the material later. It is important to write your answer because writing it will help you to remember it better than if you just think of the answer. Always check your answer immediately and say it aloud if possible. This is especially helpful when you are not familiar with the term. Saying an answer aloud helps you remember it. If you make an error, look back at previous frames to see where you went wrong. Otherwise, you may repeat the error without realizing why it is incorrect.

1-4 This text provides frequent exercises to reinforce what you are learning. Answers to the reviews are in Appendix VI, Solutions to Review Exercises. The end-of-the-chapter reviews help integrate what you have learned in a chapter.

**Building
a Medical
Vocabulary**
with Spanish Translations
Seventh Edition

Peggy C. Leonard

**PRONUNCIATION
OF MEDICAL TERMS**

Pronunciation follows that of *Dorland's Medical Dictionary* published by Elsevier. A phonetic spelling is kept as simple as possible, with few diacritical marks; the only special character used is ə, the schwa, used to represent the unstressed vowel sound heard at the end of sofa.

There are four basic rules:
1. An unmarked vowel ending a syllable (an "open" syllable) is long. Thus *ra* represents the pronunciation of *ray*.
2. An unmarked vowel in a syllable ending in a consonant (a "closed" syllable) is short. Examples of words with unmarked short vowels are had, bed, in, not, and rug, which have phonetic spellings that are the same as their usual spellings.
3. A long vowel in a closed syllable is indicated by a macron. Thus *māt* represents the pronunciation of *mate*.
4. A short vowel that ends or itself constitutes a syllable is indicated by a breve. Thus *ĭ-mūn* represents the pronunciation of *immune*.

blanks.

earning, a block of information preceded by a number is called a _____.

kmark so that it covers only the _____ column.

_____ your answer because this will help you remember better g of the answer.

answer in the blank, always _____ it using the information in n.

check your answers.)

OF WORD BUILDING

1-5 Word building is a system of learning the meaning of various word parts to understand and write new words. Because it is impractical to memorize the medical dictionary, you will use a system of word _____ to learn medical terms.

1-6 Pay close attention to spelling.

Figure 1-1 Checking your answer. Position the bookmark so it covers only the answer column. Check your answers by sliding the bookmark down.

> ➤ **KEY** POINT <u>A change of only one letter can result in a different term.</u> Be careful when writing a term. Example: the ilium is a pelvic bone, and the ileum is part of the small intestine.

In addition to checking your answer each time, you will also check the

spelling

_____.

WORD ROOTS, COMBINING FORMS, PREFIXES, AND SUFFIXES

1-7 Most medical terms are composed of word parts that have their origins in Greek or Latin. Although familiarity with either of these two languages would facilitate learning medical terms, it is not necessary. We will be learning the English translation of many Greek or Latin word parts used in medical terminology.

➤ **KEY** POINT Word roots, combining forms, prefixes, and suffixes are word parts. Learning the meaning of these word parts eliminates the necessity of memorizing each new term you encounter. In this chapter, it is important to learn to recognize word roots, prefixes, and suffixes in terms and how to combine them to write medical terms.

parts

Word roots, combining forms, prefixes, and suffixes are called word _____.

WORD ROOTS

root

1-8 Most words, even ordinary words, have a word root. The word root is the main body of the word. It is usually accompanied by a prefix or suffix or both. Word roots are the building blocks for many terms related to anatomy, diagnosis, and medical procedures. You see by reading this information that most words have a word _____.

Look at the Greek and Latin words and their associated word roots in Table 1-1. By adding prefixes and suffixes, you will soon begin writing medical terms. (Don't be concerned about learning the meaning of the word parts for Chapter 1, because all of them will be included in subsequent chapters.)

1-9 You will sometimes learn two word roots that have the same meaning. Table 1-1 shows the Greek word root nephr for kidney, as well as the Latin word root ren for kidney.

➤ **KEY** POINT Remember this guideline for using Greek vs. Latin roots. As a general rule, Latin roots are used to write words naming and describing structures of the body, whereas Greek roots are used to write words naming and describing diseases, conditions, diagnosis, and treatment. As with most rules, there are exceptions.

Use this as a guideline only, because you will quickly learn exceptions. For example, both nephric and renal mean pertaining to the kidney. Likewise, both dermal and cutaneous mean pertaining to the skin (Figure 1-2).

When two medical terms have the same meaning but look very different, it is probably because the origins of the word roots are from two different languages, Greek and _____.

Latin

TABLE 1-1	Examples of Word Roots		
Greek Word	**Word Root**	**Latin Word**	**Word Root**
karkinos (crab, cancer)	carcin	*articulus* (joint)	articul
lithos (stone)	lith	*cauda* (tail)	caud
nephros (kidney)	nephr	*fungi* (fungus)	fung
stomatos (mouth)	stomat	*oris* (mouth)	or
		renes (kidney)	ren

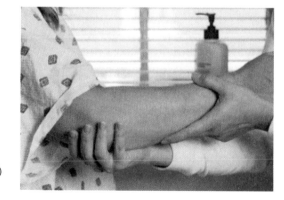

Figure 1-2 Examination of the skin. A patient's skin, the body's largest and most visible organ, can produce valuable information about his or her health. The scientific name of the skin is dermis, so named after the Greek term *derma. Cutis* (Latin) also means skin. Both dermal and cutaneous mean pertaining to the skin.

COMBINING FORMS

1-10 Many words would be difficult to pronounce if they were written without a vowel to join the word roots. A vowel (usually "o") is often inserted between word roots to make the word easier to pronounce. A word root with a vowel attached is called a combining form and looks like this: speed(o).

> ➤ **KEY** POINT A combining form ends in an enclosed vowel. Combining forms are recognized as word parts that end in an enclosed vowel. In speedometer, the combining form speed(o) is joined with another part of the word, meter. The parentheses are not included when the combining form joins other word parts.

form

Study Table 1-2 and observe that a combining vowel is added to a word root to write a combining _____.

cephal(o)

1-11 Some compound words are composed of two word roots or words. The term cephalometer is composed of two word roots, cephal and meter. Write the combining form for cephal: _____.

Collarbone and eyelid are examples of two words joined to form a new term.
You will learn the combining form for word roots because word roots are often combined with other word parts. Combining forms act as the foundation for most terms (Figure 1-3).

TABLE 1-2	Examples of Word Roots and Combining Forms	
Word Root	**Combining Form**	**Use in a Word**
blephar	blephar(o)	blepharospasm
cephal	cephal(o)	cephalometry
fung	fung(i)	fungicide
or	or(o)	oropharynx
path	path(o)	pathology

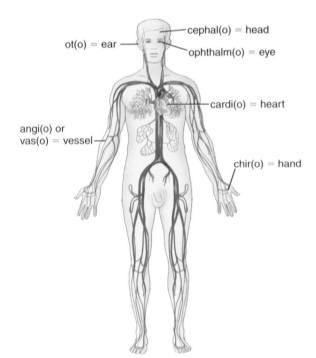

ot(o) = ear
cephal(o) = head
ophthalm(o) = eye
cardi(o) = heart
angi(o) or vas(o) = vessel
chir(o) = hand

Figure 1-3 Combining forms are the foundations of most terms. All body structures have corresponding combining forms.

EXERCISE 2

Write either CF *(for combining form) or* WR *(for word root) after each of the following word parts:*

1. aden(o) _____
2. bil(i) _____
3. cyan _____

4. derm(a) _____
5. duoden _____
6. electr _____

7. gloss(o) _____
8. hemat _____
9. ren _____

(Use Appendix VI to check your answers.)

PREFIXES

1-12 A prefix is a word part that is placed before a word root to modify its meaning.

> ➤ **KEY** POINT <u>A prefix written alone is usually followed by a hyphen</u>. An-, anti-, and peri- are examples of prefixes.

hyphen

When written alone, a prefix is usually followed by a _____.

1-13 In anhydrous, hydrous refers to water and the prefix an- means without. Combining the two meanings, anhydrous means without _____.

water

1-14 In subnormal, sub- means below. In subnormal, which part of the word is the prefix? _____

sub-

Normal is a familiar word that we use to mean agreeing with the regular and established type. Its meaning is changed when a prefix is added. Subnormal means _____ normal.

below

SUFFIXES

1-15 A suffix is attached to the end of a word or word part to modify its meaning. Suffixes are joined to combining forms to write nouns (names; the subject of the sentence), adjectives (descriptive words), and verbs (action words).

> ➤ **KEY** POINT <u>A suffix written alone is usually preceded by a hyphen</u>. The hyphen placed before a suffix indicates that another part precedes it. In the term tonsillitis, -itis means inflammation.

suffix

Blepharitis means inflammation of the eyelid. The word part blephar refers to the eyelid and is the word root. The word part -itis means inflammation and is being used as what part of the word? _____

dyspnea

1-16 Occasionally a word is composed of only a prefix and a suffix. Join dys- and -pnea to write a new word: _____. The prefix dys- means bad, painful, or difficult, and -pnea means breathing. Dyspnea means difficult breathing.

Visualize the relationship of prefixes, combining forms, and suffixes as you study Figure 1-4.

EXERCISE 3

Write CF (for combining form), P (for prefix), or S (for suffix) for each of the following word parts:

1. brady- _____
2. -cele _____
3. eu- _____

4. -graphy _____
5. hydr(o) _____
6. -iasis _____

7. mal- _____
8. phon(o) _____
9. -pathy _____

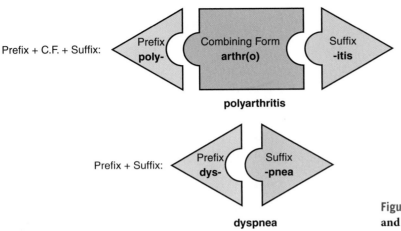

Prefix + C.F. + Suffix: Prefix **poly-**   Combining Form **arthr(o)**   Suffix **-itis**

polyarthritis

Prefix + Suffix: Prefix **dys-**   Suffix **-pnea**

dyspnea

Figure 1-4 The relationship of prefixes, combining forms, and suffixes.

EXERCISE 4

A prefix or suffix is underlined in each of the following terms. Write either P (for prefix) or S (for suffix) after each term:

1. <u>ad</u>hesion _____

2. adeno<u>pathy</u> _____

3. bili<u>ary</u> _____

4. derm<u>al</u> _____

5. <u>endo</u>cardial _____

6. hemato<u>logy</u> _____

7. <u>hypo</u>glossal _____

8. <u>micro</u>scope _____

9. <u>pre</u>natal _____

(Use Appendix VI to check your answers.)

COMBINING WORD PARTS

1-17 You have learned that medical terms are composed of word roots, combining forms, prefixes, and suffixes. You will now learn to combine these word parts to write medical terms.

➤ **KEY** POINT <u>In writing terms, you don't always use the combining vowel.</u> A rule that will help you when writing medical terms is this: Use the combining vowel before suffixes that begin with a consonant and before another word root.

Observe the use of the rule in building terms with these suffixes:

Combining Form	Suffixes	Term and Meaning
	+ -ic	= otic, pertaining to the ear
	+ -itis	= otitis, inflammation of the ear
ot(o) = ear	+ -logy	= otology, study of the ear
	+ -plasty	= otoplasty, plastic surgery of the ear
	+ -rrhea	= otorrhea, discharge from the ear
	+ -tomy	= ototomy, incision of the ear

(There are exceptions to the rule, and you will learn the exceptions as you progress through the material. For now, remember to drop the vowel before a suffix that begins with a vowel.) The rule for using the combining vowel shows us that the combining vowel is used in two cases. In one case, the combining vowel is used before a suffix that begins with a

consonant _____.

1-18 The combining vowel is also used to join two combining forms. When combining gastr(o), meaning stomach, and enter(o), meaning intestine, gastroentero results. (Of course, this is not a complete word because it needs a suffix.) Combine gastr(o) + enter(o) + -logy to write a term that means the study of the stomach, intestines, and related structures:

gastroenterology _____.

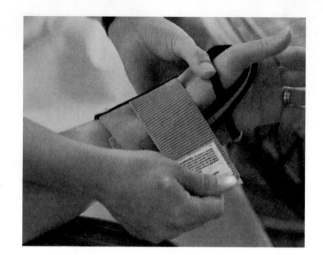

Figure 1-5 A carpal support. Maintaining the wrist in a resting position is important in preventing further irritation of the inflamed nerve in carpal tunnel syndrome, a painful disorder of the wrist and hand. It may develop spontaneously without a known cause or may result from disease or injury. A common cause is repetitive movements of the hands and wrists, such as in factory work or typing. Surgery may be required to relieve severe symptoms of long duration.

---

carpal

1-19 The wrist is also called the carpus. Write a word that means pertaining to the wrist by combining carp(o), meaning wrist, and -al, meaning pertaining to:

_____.

A carpal support holds the wrist in a given position (Figure 1-5).

1-20 The combining form aort(o) means aorta, and -itis means inflammation. Join the two word parts to write a term that means inflammation of the aorta:

aortitis

_____. (Check your spelling carefully.)

EXERCISE 5

Build It! *Combine the word parts to write medical terms.*

1. tonsill(o) + -itis   _____

2. ur(o) + -emia   _____

3. cardi(o) + aortitis   _____

4. ur(o) + genital   _____

5. enter(o) + -itis   _____

6. enter(o) + cyst   _____

(Use Appendix VI to check your answers.)

1-21 The word-building rules are summarized in Table 1-3.

> ➤ **KEY** POINT In general, most prefixes require no change before they are joined with other word parts. Notice that prefixes are not included in the rule concerning use of the combining vowel. That is because most prefixes require no change before they are joined with other word parts. (A few exceptions will be noted later.)

TABLE 1-3	Word-Building Rules

Joining Combining Forms

The combining vowel is usually retained between two combining forms.

Example: gastr(o) + enterology = gastroenterology

Joining Combining Forms and Suffixes

The combining vowel is usually retained when a combining form is joined with a suffix that begins with a consonant.

Example: enter(o) + -logy = enterology

The combining vowel is usually omitted when a combining form is joined with a suffix that begins with a vowel.

Example: enter(o) + -ic = enteric

Joining Other Word Parts and Prefixes

Most prefixes require no change when they are joined with other word parts.

Examples: peri- + appendicitis = periappendicitis; dys- + -pnea = dyspnea

---

EXERCISE 6

Build It! *Combine the word parts to write terms.*

1. peri- + appendicitis   _____

2. uni- + lateral   _____

3. anti- + septic   _____

4. an- + -emia   _____

(Use Appendix VI to check your answers.)

---

combining

1-22 If you correctly answered Exercises 5 and 6, you have learned the rules for using word parts to write medical terms. In this program, you will be using combining forms, prefixes, and suffixes to build many new words.

A combining form will be recognized as a word part that has a vowel enclosed in parentheses as its ending. For example, you may not know the meaning of thorac(o), but you recognize that thorac(o) is which type of word part? _____ form

anti-
tri-

1-23 Prefixes will be designated by placing a hyphen after the word part, such as pre-. The hyphen indicates that something follows this word part. Which of the following word parts are prefixes? metr(o), anti-, tri-, -scope _____ and

_____

Remember that the hyphen follows the prefix when the prefix is shown alone. If the hyphen comes before the word part, the word part is a suffix. This tells us that -scope is which type of

suffix

word part? _____

EXERCISE 7

Use CF (for combining form), P (for prefix), or S (for suffix) to designate each of the following word parts as a combining form, a prefix, or a suffix.

1. alkal(o) _____

2. bil(i) _____

3. -capnia _____

4. chol(e) _____

5. hypo- _____

6. neo- _____

7. -pepsia _____

8. post- _____

9. primi- _____

10. ven(o) _____

EXERCISE 8

Build It! *Combine the following word parts to write medical terms.*

1. acid(o) + -osis _____

2. acr(o) + -megaly _____

3. anti- + -emesis _____

4. bronch(o) + -scopy _____

5. dys- + -phagia _____

6. hypo- + thyroid(o) + -ism _____

7. leuk(o) + cyt(o) + -osis _____

8. mal- + absorption _____

9. my(o) + metr(o) + -ium _____

10. thromb(o) + phleb(o) + -itis _____

(Use Appendix VI to check your answers.)

1-24 You will also learn to recognize word parts as components of other words. To help you distinguish the component parts of medical terms, the words will often be divided by a diagonal line between the component parts.

For example, how many component parts are there in the word aden/oma?

two _____

How many component parts does peri/ophthalm/itis have?

three _____

> ➤ **KEY** POINT To interpret a new word, begin by looking at the suffix. Recognizing suffixes will help you identify the word as a noun, a verb, or an adjective. You will know the meaning of many suffixes after studying Chapters 3 and 4. After deciding the meaning of the suffix, go to the beginning of the word and read across from left to right, interpreting the remaining elements to develop the full sense of the term.

Using the suggested method, the interpretation of word parts in peri/ophthalm/itis is inflammation, around, eye. The full sense of the term is inflammation of tissues around the eye. See Figure 1-6 to summarize what you have learned about writing and interpreting medical terms.

1-25 Now that you have learned about word parts and how to analyze terms, you need to be aware that some terms do not follow the rules you have learned. In other cases, two spellings are accepted. Whenever you are in doubt, check a medical dictionary. Two spellings of the same term usually come about through popular use. (For example, both thoracentesis and thoracocentesis mean surgical puncture of the chest wall.) As we progress through the material, such exceptions are noted.

EPONYMS

1-26 Eponyms are names for diseases, organs, procedures, or body functions that are derived from the name of a person. A cesarean section, a surgical procedure in which the abdomen and uterus are incised to deliver an infant, is an eponym and is named after the manner in which Julius Caesar was supposedly born. Parkinson disease and Alzheimer disease are also eponyms.

Word building will not be as helpful when analyzing eponyms. Nevertheless, it is important to remember these terms also.

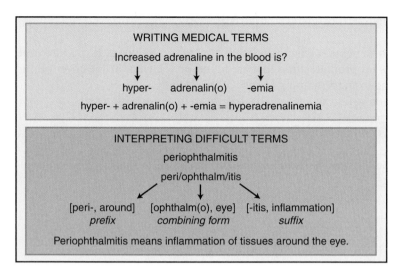

Figure 1-6 **Examples of using prefixes, suffixes, and combining forms to write and interpret medical terms.**

ABBREVIATIONS AND ACRONYMS

1-27 Abbreviations are shortened forms of words or phrases. Abbreviations include the following:
- Letters (The abbreviation for complete blood cell count is CBC.)
- Shortened words (The abbreviation stat is short for *statim,* Latin for at once or immediately.)
- Acronyms, pronounceable words formed from initial letters (CABG, pronounced like the vegetable, means coronary artery bypass graft.)

Abbreviations and symbols save time but can be confusing because some have more than one meaning. The abbreviation C means canine tooth, carbon, and Celsius, among others. Also, some uppercase abbreviations have different meanings than the lowercase equivalents (CC means chief complaint, and cc means cubic centimeter).

abbreviations   Shortened words or phrases are called _____.

> ➤ **KEY** POINT <u>Using abbreviations and symbols can be dangerous.</u> The Institute for Safe Medication Practices publishes lists of what are considered dangerous abbreviations and recommends that certain terms be written in full because they are easily mistaken for one with another meaning (for example, qn, meaning nightly or at bedtime, is misinterpreted as qh, which means every hour). Abbreviations are presented in this book because many are still commonly used, but particular caution must be taken in both using and reading abbreviations. If a common abbreviation is missing, you may wish to check to see if its use is discouraged by the Institute for Safe Medication Practices. The Institute's website address is www.ismp.org.

EXERCISE 9

Match the examples in the left column with the type of term in the right column.

_____ 1. CAD   A. abbreviation

_____ 2. D&C   B. eponym

_____ 3. Gram stain

_____ 4. Foley catheter

_____ 5. lig.

_____ 6. OSHA

_____ 7. Raynaud disease

_____ 8. stat.

PRONUNCIATION OF MEDICAL TERMS

dren

i

an

short

lo

short

1-28 A medical term is easier to remember when you know how to pronounce it. If you have not already done so, study the rules for pronunciation that are found on the front inside cover of this book. Do this before proceeding to the remaining frames of this chapter.

In the term adrenaline (ə-dren´ə-lin), which syllable has the primary accent?

_____

In adrenalitis (ə-dre″nəl-i´tis), which syllable has the primary accent?

_____

Which syllable receives secondary emphasis in angiectomy (an″je-ek´tə-me)?

_____

Is the "a" in angiectomy pronounced as a long or short "a"?

_____

1-29 In ankylosis (ang″kə-lo´sis), which is the primary accented syllable?

_____

Is the vowel in the sis syllable pronounced as a long or short "i"?

_____

1-30 Be aware that there are different ways to pronounce some medical terms. Pronunciation will be shown as new terms are introduced in later chapters. In addition, an alphabetical list of terms is presented in the Index/Glossary. The list includes the pronunciations and definitions for most medical terms presented in this book.

EXERCISE 10

Write answers in the blanks to review your understanding of the rules of pronunciation used in this book.

1. How many syllables does the term hypercalcemia (hi″pər-kal-se´me-ə) have?

_____

2. Using the pronunciation of hypercalcemia shown in number 1, which syllable receives the primary accent?

_____

3. Using the pronunciation of hypercalcemia shown in number 1, which syllable receives a secondary accent?

_____

4. Using the pronunciation of hypercalcemia shown in number 1, list all vowels that are pronounced as long vowels:

_____

(Use Appendix VI to check your answers.)

PLURALS OF MEDICAL TERMS

1-31 When you see a noun in its singular form, you will learn to write a plural for that term, but be aware that sometimes more than one plural is acceptable. Although plurals of many medical terms are formed using rules you may already know, it is important to learn rules that apply when terms have special endings.

Many plurals are formed by simply adding an "s" to the singular term. Write plurals by adding an "s" to these singular terms:

abrasions   abrasion _____

lacerations   laceration _____

TABLE 1-4 Forming Plurals of Nouns with Special Endings

If the Singular Ending Is	The Plural Ending Is	Examples (Singular)	Examples (Plural)
is (Some words ending in is form plurals by dropping the is and adding ides, as in epididymis and epididymides.)	es	diagnosis, prognosis, psychosis	diagnoses, prognoses, psychoses
um	a	atrium, ileum, septum, bacterium	atria, ilea, septa, bacteria
us (Some singular forms ending in us form plurals by dropping the us and adding either era or ora, for example viscus and viscera and corpus and corpora. Others form plurals by simply adding es, for example virus becomes viruses.)	i	alveolus, bacillus, bronchus	alveoli, bacilli, bronchi
a	ae	vertebra, patella, petechia	vertebrae, patellae, petechiae
ix (Through common use, appendixes and cervixes have become acceptable plural forms.)	ices	appendix, varix, cervix	appendices, varices, cervices
ex	ices	cortex	cortices
ax	aces	thorax	thoraces (thoraxes is also acceptable)
ma	s or mata	carcinoma, sarcoma	carcinomas or carcinomata, sarcomas or sarcomata
on (Some singular forms ending in on form plurals by adding s, for example, chorion becomes chorions.)	a	protozoon, spermatozoon	protozoa, spermatozoa
nx	nges	phalanx, larynx	phalanges, larynges

1-32 Many nouns that end in "s", "ch", or "sh" form their plurals by adding "es". The plural of abscess is abscesses. Write plurals by adding "es" to these terms:

branches   branch _____

brushes   brush _____

sinuses   sinus _____

1-33 Singular nouns that end in "y" preceded by a consonant form their plurals by changing the "y" to "i" and adding "es". For example, the plural of allergy is allergies. Change the "y" to "i" and add "es" to write plurals of these nouns:

capillaries   capillary _____

extremities   extremity _____

ovaries   ovary _____

1-34 Use Table 1-4 to learn the rules for forming other plurals of medical terms, but be aware that there are a few exceptions and that only major rules are included. Many dictionaries show the plural forms of nouns and can be used as references. Also notice that some terms have more than one acceptable plural.

EXERCISE 11

Write the plural form for each of the following singular nouns.

1. capsule _____

2. cataract _____

3. calculus _____

4. cortex _____

5. diagnosis _____

6. meninx _____

7. neurosis _____

8. protozoon _____

9. vertex _____

10. virus _____

Write the singular form of each plural noun.

11. appendices _____   15. sarcomata _____

12. fungi _____   16. spermatozoa _____

13. larynges _____   17. syndromes _____

14. prognoses _____   18. thrombi _____

(Use Appendix VI to check your answers.)

ENHANCING SPANISH COMMUNICATION

Spanish translation of selected terms is presented at the end of each chapter. Appendix II of *Building a Medical Vocabulary* has comprehensive lists of both English-Spanish and Spanish-English translations for easy reference.

Español | ENHANCING SPANISH COMMUNICATION

The sounds of Spanish vowels do not vary and must be fully and distinctly pronounced. This does not apply to double vowels. Use these rules to pronounce vowels:

Spanish vowel	Pronounce as	Spanish vowel	Pronounce as
a	a in mama	u	u in rule or the sound of oo in spool (The u is generally silent in these syllables: que, gue, and gui.)
e	a in day		
i	i in police		
o	o in so	y	e in see, but sounds like j if it follows n

Some consonants have similar sounds in English and Spanish. Some significant differences are noted here.

Spanish	Pronunciation	Spanish	Pronunciation
c	k or s, except ch pronounced like church	ñ	blending of n and y as in canyon
		q	k
d	sometimes as th		
		r	trilled r
g	similar to g in go, except pronounced as h before e or i	rr	strongly trilled r
h	not pronounced	z	s
j	h		
ll	blending of l and y, or simply y as in yet		

Phonetic pronunciation is presented with the stressed syllable in uppercase letters, as in the example BO-cah. In this term, the first syllable is stressed. Boca is the Spanish word for mouth.

PHARMACOLOGY

Pharmacology is the study of the preparation, properties, uses, and actions of drugs. Drugs are used in medicine to prevent, diagnose, and treat disease and to relieve pain. Another term for medicines is pharmaceuticals. Beginning with Chapter 2, additional information about medications is presented for each chapter on the Companion CD.

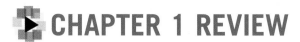 CHAPTER 1 REVIEW

Work the following review section. The review helps you know whether you have learned the material or not. After completing all sections of the review, check your answers with the solutions found in Appendix VI. (Don't be concerned about learning the meaning of the word parts for Chapter 1, because all of them will be included in subsequent chapters.)

Use the Companion CD for additional questions and a fun way to review. However, the CD does not replace the comprehensive written reviews at the end of each chapter.

Describing

I. Describe the role of each of the following word parts:

1. combining form _____

2. prefix _____

3. suffix _____

4. word root _____

Identifying Word Parts

II. Use CF (for combining form), P (for prefix), or S (for suffix) to designate each of the following word parts as a combining form, a prefix, or a suffix.

1. bil(i) _____		6. intra- _____	
2. crani(o) _____		7. multi- _____	
3. -ectomy _____		8. -oid _____	
4. gigant(o) _____		9. -plegia _____	
5. -iatrics _____		10. spher(o) _____	

Build It!

III. Using the rules you have learned in Chapter 1, combine the word parts to write medical terms.

1. hypo- + derm(o) + -ic _____

2. leuk(o) + -emia _____

3. melan(o) + -oid _____

4. my(o) + cardi(o) + -al _____

5. thromb(o) + -osis _____

Writing Plurals

IV. Write a singular or plural form for each term that is given.

1. atrium _____		6. ganglion _____	
2. bulla _____		7. indices _____	
3. bursae _____		8. microvillus _____	
4. cervices _____		9. septum _____	
5. enchondromata _____		10. syndrome _____	

Checking Spelling

V. *Use the Index/Glossary to check the spelling of these terms. Circle all misspelled terms and write their correct spellings:*

canser   cerebrotomy   colorrhaphy   neurolysis   ofthalmoplasty

Pronunciation

VI. *Use the Index/Glossary to check the pronunciations of the following terms. Complete the table by indicating the syllable that has the primary accent, all syllables containing a long vowel, and all syllables containing a short vowel. The first term is done as an example:*

	Syllable with primary accent	Syllable(s) with long vowel	Syllable(s) with short vowel
1. adipose	*ad*	*pos*	*ad, i*
2. aerosol			
3. cortisone			
4. lactose			
5. nephroscope			

Say and Check

VII. *Practice saying each of the following terms aloud. Check to see if you are correct by accessing the Say and Check for this chapter on the Companion CD that accompanies this text and listening to each term.*

1. adenopathy   (ad″ə-nop´ə-the)

2. cephalometer   (sef″ə-lom´ə-tər)

3. cutaneous   (ku-ta´ne-əs)

4. dermal   (dər´məl)

5. endocardial   (en″do-kahr´de-əl)

6. hematology   (he″mə-tol´ə-je)

7. hypoglossal   (hi″po-glos´əl)

8. otoplasty   (o´to-plas″te)

9. tonsillitis   (ton″sĭ-li´tis)

10. unilateral   (u″nĭ-lat´ər-əl)

(Check your answers with the solutions in Appendix VI. Pay particular attention to spelling. If most of your answers are correct, you are ready to move on to Chapter 2.)

Medicine
and Its Specialties

*Using Combining Forms to Build Terms
about Medical Specialties*

2

Basic Understanding

In this chapter you will learn to do the following.
1. Recognize prefixes, suffixes, combining forms, and word roots in medical words.
2. Write the meanings of the word parts and use them to build and analyze terms.
3. Match the terms for medical specialists with the areas in which they specialize, or write the medical specialties when given the area of expertise.
4. Identify the specialty associated with various medical conditions.
5. Match the terms for health professions presented in this chapter with their descriptions, or write the health professions when given their descriptions.
6. List five categories for classifying medical terms that are used in this book.

Greater Comprehension

7. Spell medical terms accurately.
8. Write the meanings of the abbreviations, including those in a health report presented in this chapter.
9. Pronounce medical terms correctly using the phonetic system that is presented in this book.

MAJOR SECTIONS OF THIS CHAPTER:

- ❏ MEDICINE AND ITS SPECIALTIES
- ❏ OTHER HEALTH PROFESSIONS
- ❏ MEDICAL RECORDS
- ❏ CATEGORIES OF MEDICAL TERMS

Terms printed in boldface type in Chapters 2 through 17 are included in the Pronunciation List located near the end of each chapter.

MEDICINE AND ITS SPECIALTIES

prefix

2-1 You have learned that prefixes, suffixes, and combining forms are word parts that are used to write medical terms. Which word part is placed before a word root to modify its meaning?
_____

You will learn many word parts as you study each chapter. Beginning now, you are expected to remember the meanings of word parts and terms that are introduced. Pronunciations will also be shown the first time a medical term is introduced.

combining

2-2 Some word parts end in an enclosed vowel—for example, psych(o). You recognize this type of word part as a _____ form.

This chapter introduces several combining forms associated with the medical specialties. You will also learn a few prefixes and suffixes that are used in naming both the specialties and the specialists.

suffix

2-3 Which word part is attached to the end of a word or word part to modify its meaning?
_____

Suffixes are added to other word parts (mainly combining forms) to write terms. Study the following suffixes and remember their meanings.

Suffixes Used in Writing Medical Specialists and Their Specialties

Suffix Terms about Specialists	Meaning	Suffix Terms about Specialties	Meaning
-er, -ist	one who	-ac, -al, -ic, -logic, -logical	pertaining to
-iatrician	practitioner	-iatrics, -iatry	medical profession or treatment
-logist	one who studies; specialist	-logy	study or science of

one

2-4 The suffixes -er and -ist mean _____ who. You know many terms that contain these suffixes—for example, practitioner, one who practices, and specialist, one who is devoted to a special field or occupation. In medicine, a specialist is a person who has advanced education and training in one area of practice, such as internal medicine, dermato/logy, or cardio/logy.

study

2-5 The suffix -logy means the _____ or science of, and the suffix -logist means one who studies or a specialist.

Also notice that several suffixes in the list, including -logic and -logical, mean pertaining to.

2-6 The suffixes that are mentioned in the last two frames are not used exclusively in writing medical terms. You will be able to think of many words that use these word parts. The suffixes -iatrics and -iatry are more specific for medicine and mean the medical _____ or a medical treatment.

profession

EXERCISE 1

Match the suffixes in the left column with their meaning in the right column. Some choices will be used more than once.

_____ 1. -ac   _____ 5. -ic   A. medical profession or treatment
_____ 2. -er   _____ 6. -ist   B. one who
                                              C. one who studies; specialist
_____ 3. -iatrician   _____ 7. -logist   D. practitioner
_____ 4. -iatry   _____ 8. -logy   E. pertaining to
(Use Appendix VI to check your answers.)   F. study or science of

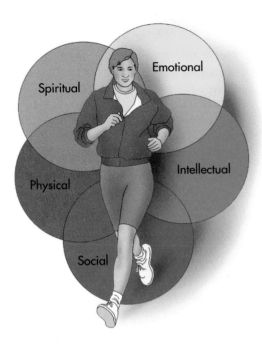

Figure 2-1 Holistic health. This viewpoint recognizes the integrated aspects of a person's physical, emotional, intellectual, social, and spiritual needs.

2-7 The term medicine has several meanings, including a drug or a remedy for illness. A second meaning of medicine is the art and science of diagnosis, treatment, and prevention of disease. Medicine recognizes that a person is a composite of physical, social, spiritual, emotional, and intellectual needs (Figure 2-1).

> ➤ **KEY** POINT <u>The holistic viewpoint considers the person as a functioning whole.</u> **Holistic**˙ (ho-lis´tik) health encompasses the perspective of the individual as an integrated system in which the separate parts interact and influence one another.

Recognizing that a person is a composite of physical, social, emotional, spiritual, and intellectual needs is a _____ viewpoint.

holistic

2-8 Family practice is a medical specialty that encompasses several branches of medicine and coordinates health care for all members of a family. A family practice physician often acts as the **primary health care provider,** referring complex disorders to other specialists. The family practice physician has largely replaced the concept of a general practitioner (GP).

2-9 Internal medicine is a clinical (nonsurgical) specialty of medicine that deals specifically with the diagnosis and treatment of diseases of the internal structures of the body. The specialist is called an **internist** (in-tur´nist).

> ➤ **KEY** POINT <u>Don't confuse an internist with the term intern.</u> An intern in many clinical programs is any immediate postgraduate trainee. A physician intern is in postgraduate training, learning medical practice under supervision before being licensed as a physician. An internist, however, is a licensed medical specialist.

internist

A physician who specializes in internal medicine is an _____.
Study the following combining forms associated with the medical specialties and remember the names of the medical specialties.

˙Holistic (Greek: *holos,* whole).

Combining Forms: Selected Medical Specialties

Combining Form(s)	Meaning	Medical Specialty	Medical Specialist
cardi(o)	heart	cardiology (kahr″de-ol′ə-je)	cardiologist (kahr″de-ol′ə-jist)
crin(o)	to secrete	endocrinology (en″do-krĭ-nol′ə-je)	endocrinologist (en″do-krĭ-nol′ə-jist)
dermat(o)	skin	dermatology (dur″mə-tol′ə-je)	dermatologist (dur″mə-tol′ə-jist)
esthesi(o)	feeling or sensation	anesthesiology (an″əs-the″ze-ol′ə-je)	anesthesiologist (an″əs-the″ze-ol′ə-jist)
gastr(o), enter(o)	stomach, intestines*	gastroenterology (gas″tro-en″tər-ol′ə-je)	gastroenterologist (gas″tro-en″tər-ol′ə-jist)
ger(a), ger(o), geront(o)	elderly or aged	geriatrics (jer″e-at′riks)	geriatrician (jer″e-ə-trish′ən)
gynec(o)	female	gynecology (gi″nə-, jin″ə-kol′ə-je)	gynecologist (gi″nə-, jin″ə-kol′ə-jist)
immun(o)	immune	immunology (im″u-nol′ə-je)	immunologist (im″u-nol′ə-jist)
ne(o), nat(o)	new, birth	neonatology (ne″o-na-tol′ə-je)	neonatologist (ne″o-na-tol′ə-jist)
neur(o)	nerve	neurology (noo-rol′ə-je)	neurologist (noo-rol′ə-jist)
obstetr(o)	midwife	obstetrics (ob-stet′riks)	obstetrician (ob″stə-trĭ′shən)
onc(o)	tumor	oncology (ong-kol′ə-je)	oncologist (ong-kol′ə-jist)
ophthalm(o)	eye	ophthalmology (of″thəl-mol′ə-je)	ophthalmologist (of″thəl-mol′ə-jist)
orth(o), ped(o)	orth(o) means straight ped(o) means child (sometimes, foot)	orthopedics (or″tho-pe′diks)	orthopedist (orthopedic surgeon) (or″tho-pe′dist)
ot(o), laryng(o)	ear, larynx	otolaryngology (o″to-lar″ing-gol′ə-je)	otolaryngologist (o″to-lar″ing-gol′ə-jist)
path(o)	disease	pathology (pə-thol′ə-je)	pathologist (pə-thol′ə-jist)
ped(o)	child (sometimes, foot)	pediatrics (pe″de-at′riks)	pediatrician (pe″de-ə-trĭ′shən)
psych(o)	mind	psychiatry (si-ki′ə-tre)	psychiatrist (si-ki′ə-trist)
radi(o)	radiant energy, radiation (sometimes, radius)	radiology (ra″de-ol′ə-je)	radiologist (ra″de-ol′ə-jist)
rheumat(o)	rheumatism	rheumatology (roo″mə-tol′ə-je)	rheumatologist (roo″mə-tol′ə-jist)
rhin(o)	nose	rhinology (ri-nol′ə-je)	rhinologist (ri-nol′ə-jist)
ur(o)	urinary tract (sometimes, urine)	urology (u-rol′ə-je)	urologist (u-rol′ə-jist)

*enter(o) sometimes refers specifically to the small intestine.

 Say and Check

Pronounce the terms for the medical specialties and specialists in the list you just read. Use the Companion CD to check your pronunciations. Refresh your memory of the rules of pronunciation by referring to the pronunciation guide inside the front cover if needed.

EXERCISE 2

Write meanings for these combining forms.

1. crin(o) _____
2. esthesi(o) _____
3. gastr(o) _____
4. geront(o) _____
5. gynec(o) _____

6. laryng(o) _____
7. nat(o) _____
8. ne(o) _____
9. orth(o) _____
10. rhin(o) _____

EXERCISE 3

Write the combining form you just learned for the following meanings.

1. child _____
2. ear _____
3. eye _____
4. foot _____
5. heart _____

6. immune _____
7. mind _____
8. nerve _____
9. skin _____
10. urinary tract _____

skin

2-10 You may already know some of the terms that are associated with the medical specialties. If you do not recognize the combining forms used in the following frames, look back at the listing that you just studied. For example, **dermato/logy** is the medical specialty concerned with the diagnosis and treatment of diseases of the _____.

A person with acne problems or skin allergies would be treated by a **dermatologist.**

2-11 Combine derm(o) and -al to write a term that means pertaining to the skin:

dermal (dur´məl)

_____.
Dermato/logic (dur″mə-to-loj´ik) and **dermato/logical** (dur″mə-to-loj´ĭ-kəl) also refer to the skin. Whether one chooses to say dermatologic or dermatological depends on one's preference. Remember that both -ic and -al mean pertaining to. The ending -ical makes use of both suffixes. Many adjectives accept either ending.

2-12 The study of the heart and its function is **cardio/logy.** A physician who specializes in cardiology is a **cardiologist.**
Combine cardi(o) and -ac to write a term that means pertaining to the heart:

cardiac
(kahr´de-ak)

_____.
In a cardi/ac arrest, the heart has stopped beating. In the term **cardiac,** cardi(o) means heart and -ac means pertaining to. If the heart stops beating, the patient has had a cardiac arrest.

2-13 Write the name of the specialist in ophthalmology by combining ophthalm(o) and

ophthalmologist

-logist: _____.
Ophthalmo/logy is the branch of medicine that specializes in the study, diagnosis, and treatment of disorders of the eye.
Ophthalmic (of-thal´mik), **ophthalmologic** (of″thəl-mə-loj´ik), and **ophthalmological**

eye

(of″thəl-mə-loj´ĭ-kəl) mean pertaining to the _____.

2-14 Pathology is the general study of the characteristics, causes, and effects of disease.

> ➤ **KEY** POINT Pathology has many specialties and subspecialties. A pathologist is certified in **clinical** or **anatomic pathology** or both. A **clinical pathologist** is a physician who is certified in the laboratory study of disease, and there are many subspecialties. An **anatomic pathologist** is certified in the study of the effects of disease on the structure of the body. Subspecialties include surgical pathologists and those who specialize in autopsies. When surgical specimens are obtained, a surgical pathologist studies the appearance of the tissue, a technician specially trained in this area prepares thin slices of the tissue, then the tissue is examined microscopically. During a surgery the surgical pathologist sometimes performs a frozen section method to determine how the operation should be modified or completed.

disease

The terms **patho/logic** (path″o-loj´ik) and **patho/logical** (path″o-loj´ĭ-kəl) mean morbid or pertaining to pathology or caused by _____.

2-15 The **endo/crine** (en´do-krīn, en´do-krin) glands secrete chemical messengers called hormones (hor´mōnz) into the bloodstream. These hormones play an important role in regulating the body's metabolism. The prefix endo- means inside. The suffix -crine, from the combining form crin(o), means to secrete.

> ➤ **KEY** POINT Glands that secrete hormones into the bloodstream are endocrine glands. One example of an endocrine gland is the adrenal (ə-dre´nəl) gland, which secretes adrenaline (epinephrine) into the bloodstream.

A **gland** is an organ with specialized cells that secrete material not related to their ordinary metabolism.

The science of the endocrine glands and the hormones they produce is **endocrinology.**

endocrinologist

A specialist in endocrinology is called an _____.

2-16 An/esthesio/logy is the branch of medicine concerned with the administration of anesthetics (an″əs-thet´iks) and with their effects. The physician who administers anesthetics during

anesthesiologist

surgery is an _____. An **anesthetic** is a drug or agent that is capable of producing a complete or total loss of feeling. The prefix an- means no, not, or without. The literal interpretation of anesthesiology is the study of no feeling, but you need to remember that it is the branch of medicine concerned with the administration of drugs that produce a loss of feeling.

An **an/esthetist** (ə-nes´thə-tist) is a nurse or other person trained in administering anesthetics.

2-17 Gastro/entero/logy is the study of diseases affecting the gastrointestinal tract, including the stomach and intestines. A physician who specializes in gastric disorders is a

gastroenterologist

_____.

Gastr/ic (gas´trik) means pertaining to the stomach.

2-18 Three combining forms—ger(a), ger(o), and geront(o)—mean old age or the aged. The scientific study of all aspects of the aging process and issues encountered by older persons is **geronto/logy** (jer″on-tol´ə-je). The branch of medicine that deals with the problems of aging and the diseases of older persons is **geriatrics.** A physician who specializes in gerontology is a

geriatrician

_____.

The selection of the correct combining form may be confusing. Common usage determines which term is proper. Practice will help you to remember.

2-19 Gyneco/logy is devoted to treating diseases of the female reproductive organs, including the breasts. A physician who specializes in the treatment of females is a

gynecologist

_____.

2-20 Many gynecologists also specialize in obstetrics. **Obstetrics** (OB) deals with pregnancy, labor, delivery, and immediate care after childbirth; however, obstetr(o) means midwife. Midwives assisted women during childbirth before obstetrics developed as a medical specialty.

Write the name of the physician who specializes in obstetrics:

obstetrician

_____.

Two adjectives that mean pertaining to obstetrics are **obstetric** and **obstetrical.**

> ➤ **KEY** POINT Nurse midwives manage normal pregnancies, labor, and childbirth. A **nurse midwife** is a registered nurse with advanced education and clinical experience in obstetrics and care of newborns. Nurse midwives work with women having normal pregnancies and uncomplicated deliveries.

2-21 Neo/nato/logy is the branch of medicine that specializes in the care of newborns, infants from birth to 28 days of age. A physician who specializes in neonatology is a

neonatologist

_____.

> ➤ **KEY** POINT Newborns are given a physical examination (PE) soon after birth. In general, weight triples and height increases by 50% in the first year of a healthy infant's life. Head circumference is also measured (Figure 2-2), and subsequent measurements are taken for the first few years. A rapidly rising head circumference suggests increased pressure inside the skull, and an unusually small head may indicate underdevelopment of the brain.

2-22 The word root for child is ped(o). **Pediatric** (pe″de-at′rik) means pertaining to children. **Ped/iatrics** is devoted to the study of children's diseases. Because diseases of children are often quite different from diseases encountered later in life, most parents prefer to take their children

pediatrics

to a physician who specializes in _____.

The suffix -iatrician, which means practitioner, is used to write the name of the physician who specializes in pediatrics. A **ped/iatrician** specializes in the development and care of infants and children and in the treatment of their diseases.

2-23 Onco/logy, a rapidly changing specialty, is concerned with the study of malignancy. The combining form onc(o) means tumor. Tumor as used here means an uncontrolled growth of tissue. Oncology is particularly concerned with malignant (mə-lig′nənt) tumors and their treatment. **Malignant*** means tending to become worse, spread, and cause death.

oncologist

A specialist who practices oncology is an _____.

*Malignant (Latin: *malignus,* bad disposition).

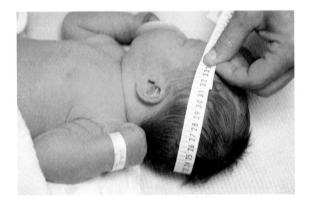

Figure 2-2 Cephalometry: measuring the head of a newborn. This is the appropriate placement of the measuring tape to obtain the head circumference of a newborn.

EXERCISE 4

Build It! *Build medical terms for the following definitions by using the word parts you have learned. The first question is done as an example.*

1. heart specialist   *cardio / logist*

2. endocrine gland specialist   _____ / _____ / _____

3. female specialty   _____ / _____

4. gastroenterology specialist   _____ / _____ / _____

5. heart specialty   _____ / _____

6. specialist in treating malignancies   _____ / _____

7. specialty of an anesthesiologist   _____ / _____ / _____

8. specialty of caring for newborns   _____ / _____ / _____

(Use Appendix VI to check your answers.)

2-24 Cancer refers to any of a large group of diseases that are characterized by the presence of a malignant tumor. These tumors are called **carcinomas** (kahr″sǐ-no′məz). Invasive carcinoma is a malignant tumor that infiltrates and destroys surrounding tissues and may continue spreading. **Remission** (re-mish′ən), whether spontaneous or the result of therapy, is the disappearance of the characteristics of a malignant tissue. Each cancer is distinguished by its site, nature, or clinical course. Everyone should know the seven warning signs of cancer (Table 2-1).

Tumors that do not invade surrounding tissue or spread to distant sites are referred to as **benign** (bə-nīn′) tumors. In other words, benign tumors are not _____.

malignant

Any new abnormal growth, either benign or malignant, is a neoplasm (ne′o-plaz-m).

2-25 An **oto/logist** (o-tol′ə-jist) specializes in **otology** (o-tol′ə-je), the study of the ear, including the diagnosis and treatment of its diseases and disorders. Physicians who specialize in ear, nose, and throat disorders are ear, nose, and throat (ENT) specialists, or otolaryngologists. The combining form ot(o) means ear and laryng(o) means **larynx** (lar′inks), or the voice box. **Oto/laryngo/logy** commonly refers to the branch of medicine dealing with diseases and disorders of the ears, nose, throat, and nearby structures. An **otolaryngologist** is a physician who practices otolaryngology. **O/tic** (o′tik) means pertaining to the ear.

Rhino/logy focuses on the diagnosis and treatment of disorders involving the nose. Write the

rhinologist

name of the physician who specializes in rhinology: _____.

2-26 **Psych/iatry** is a medical specialty that deals with the causes, treatment, and prevention of mental, emotional, and behavioral disorders. A physician who specializes in psychiatry is a **psychiatrist**.

TABLE 2-1   **Seven Warning Signs of Cancer**
Change in bowel or bladder habits
A sore that does not heal
Unusual bleeding or discharge from any body orifice
Thickening or a lump in the breast or elsewhere
Indigestion or difficulty in swallowing
Obvious change in a wart or mole
Nagging cough or hoarseness

Created by the American Cancer Society.

psychologist
(si-kol´ə-jist)

Clinical psycho/logy (si-kol´ə-je) is concerned with the diagnosis, treatment, and prevention of a wide range of personality and behavioral disorders. One who is trained in this area is a **clinical** _____. Clinical psychology is a branch of psychology rather than a branch of medicine.

2-27 Immuno/logy is one of the most rapidly expanding areas of science, and immun(o) is the combining form for immune. This branch of science involves assessment of the patient's immune defense mechanism against disease, hypersensitivity, and many diseases now thought to be associated with the immune mechanism. This mechanism involves the natural defenses that protect the body from pathogenic organisms and malignancies, but it is also involved in allergies, excessive reactions to common and often harmless substances in the environment.

immunologist

The specialist in immunology is an _____. Sometimes immunology is combined with the identification and treatment of allergies.

2-28 Almost all words that contain the combining form rheumat(o) pertain to rheumatism (roo´mə-tiz-əm). **Rheumatology** is the branch of medicine that deals with rheumatic disorders. One may think of **rheumatism** as just one disease, but it is any of a variety of disorders marked by inflammation, degeneration, or other problems of the connective tissues of the body, especially the joints and related structures.

rheumatologist

A specialist in rheumatology is a _____.

> ➤ **KEY** POINT Ancient Greeks thought humors became imbalanced. They believed that one's health was determined by the mixture of humors, certain fluids within the body. The word *rheum* meant a watery discharge; rheumatism was thought to be caused by a flowing of humors in the body and was thus named.

2-29 The combining form radi(o) means radiation or radiant energy. (Sometimes radi[o] is used to mean radius, a bone of the forearm, but usually it refers to radiant energy.) **Radio/logy** is the use of various forms of radiant energy (such as x-rays) in the diagnosis and treatment of disease. The physician who studies and interprets radiographs (x-ray examinations) is a

radiologist

_____. Two terms that mean pertaining to radiology are **radiologic** (ra˝de-o-loj´ik) and **radiological** (ra˝de-o-loj´ĭ-kəl).

> ➤ **KEY** POINT Sometimes radiology is called roentgenology. **Roentgenology** (rent˝gən-ol´ə-je), a branch of radiology dealing with the use of roentgen rays (x-rays), is named after its discoverer, Wilhelm Conrad Röntgen. Radiology includes the use of other forms of radiant energy for diagnostic and therapeutic purposes.

The combining form therapeut(o) means treatment, because **therapy** means treatment, and **therapeutic** means pertaining to treatment.

2-30 X-rays that pass through the patient expose the radiographic film or digital image receptor to create the image.

> ➤ **KEY** POINT X-radiation passes through different substances in the body in varying degrees. Where there is greater penetration, the image is black or darker; where the x-rays are absorbed by the subject, the image is white or light gray. Thus air appears black, fat appears dark gray, muscle tissue appears light gray, and bone appears very light or white. Heavy substances, such as lead or steel, appear white because they absorb the rays and prevent them from reaching the image receptor (see thumbtack in Figure 2-3).

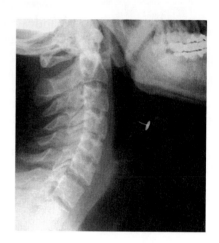

Figure 2-3 Radiograph of an aspirated thumbtack. The lodged tack appears white because it absorbs the x-rays and prevents them from reaching the film or image receptor. Also note the different appearances of air, soft tissue, bone, and teeth.

Substances that do not permit the passage of x-rays are described as **radiopaque** (ra″de-o-pāk′). When radi(o) is joined with the word opaque*, one "o" is omitted to facilitate pronunciation. The combining form radi(o) is also joined with lucent† to form the term **radiolucent** (ra″de-o-loo′sənt), which describes substances that readily permit the passage of x-rays.

Write the term that means not permitting the passage of x-rays or other radiant energy:

radiopaque

_____.

2-31 Radio/therapy (ra″de-o-ther′ə-pe) is the treatment using radiation to destroy cancer cells. The radiation may be applied by directing a beam of radiation toward the tumor with a machine that delivers radiation doses many times higher in intensity than those that are used for diagnosis. The radiation may be introduced through the bloodstream or surgically implanted. Radiation therapy is also called **radiation oncology.**

Radiotherapy can produce undesirable side effects because of incidental destruction of normal body tissues. Most of the side effects disappear with time and include nausea and vomiting, hair loss, ulceration or dryness of mucous membranes, and suppression of bone marrow activity.

2-32 The combining form ur(o) means urine or urinary tract. **Urology** is concerned with the urinary tract in both genders, as well as the male genital tract. A specialist in urology is a

urologist

_____.

Urologic (u″ro-loj′ik), **urological** (u″ro-loj′ĭ-kəl), and **urinary** (u′rĭ-nar″e) mean pertaining to the urine or the urinary system. A uro/logic examination is an examination of the urinary tract.

2-33 A **neuro/logist** is a physician who specializes in _____, the field of medicine that deals with the nervous system and its disorders.

neurology

The combining form neur(o) means nerve. A nerve cell is called a **neuron** (noor′on) (Figure 2-4). In many words, neur(o) refers to the nervous system, which is composed of the brain, spinal cord, and nerves.

2-34 Neurosurgery (noor′o-sur″jər-e) is surgery involving the brain, spinal cord, and/or peripheral nerves. Build a word combining neur(o) with surgeon that means a surgeon who specializes in surgery of the nervous system: _____.

neurosurgeon
(noor″o-sur′jən)

---

*Opaque (Latin: *opacus,* dark, obscure).
†Lucent (Latin: *lux,* light).

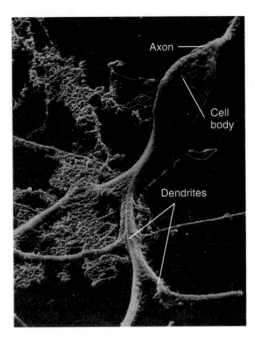

Figure 2-4 A neuron. A scanning electron micrograph of a typical nerve cell, a neuron.

The labels in the figure read: Axon, Cell body, Dendrites.

2-35 The term surgery is derived from a Greek word that means handwork. **Surgery** includes several branches of medicine that treat disease, injuries, and deformities by manual or operative procedures. The term surgery also refers to the work performed by a surgeon or the place where surgery is performed. Surgery that deals with operations of all kinds is called general

surgery

_____. There are many other surgical specialties, such as those dealing exclusively with the head and neck, hand, and urinary system. OR is the abbreviation for operating room, the place where surgeries are performed.

Small incisions through the skin and the use of scopes provide access to various body cavities, providing a faster, less painful recovery with fewer visible scars. In addition, more surgeries are being performed using the body's natural openings. For example, brain tumors can sometimes be removed through the nose. Accessing abdominal organs through the mouth, nose, vagina, or rectum avoids the need to cut through sensitive tissues and holds the promise of providing speedier recoveries.

2-36 Plastic surgery is the repair or reconstruction of tissue or organs by means of surgery. The combining form plast(o) means repair. Reconstructive surgery is an aspect of plastic surgery. It includes procedures such as resetting broken facial bones, restoring parts of the body destroyed by cancer, and correcting birth defects.

Aesthetic plastic surgery has greatly increased in the last few years, particularly that involving the face and breasts. Another notable trend is the increasing number of men who are having cosmetic surgery, with hair replacement leading the list. The medical specialist who performs

plastic

plastic surgery is called a _____ surgeon.

2-37 Ortho/pedics is a branch of surgery that deals with the preservation and restoration of the bones and associated structures. The specialist is called an **orthoped/ist** or an **orthopedic surgeon** (Figure 2-5).

The combining form orth(o) means straight, and ped(o) refers to child or foot (pes-,* pod[o], and -pod also refer to foot). The orthopedist originally straightened children's bones and corrected deformities. Today an orthopedist specializes in disorders of the bones and associated structures in people of all ages. The specialty that is concerned with diseases and disorders of the

orthopedics

bones and associated structures is _____.

---

*Latin: *pes,* foot.

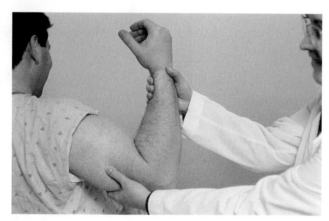

Figure 2-5 Orthopedist examining a patient. Orthopedics is a branch of medicine that specializes in the prevention and correction of disorders of the muscular and skeletal systems of the body.

EXERCISE 5

Build It! *Build medical terms for the following definitions by using the word parts you have learned.*

1. ear specialist   _____/_____

2. specialist in immune disorders   _____/_____

3. specialty for bones and associated structures _____/_____/_____

4. specialty practiced by psychiatrists   _____/_____

5. surgical specialty for the nervous system   _____/_____

6. urinary tract specialist   _____/_____

---

epidemiologist
(ep″ĭ-de″me-ol′ə-jist)

2-38 An **epidemic** attacks several people in a region at the same time. The field of medicine that studies the factors that determine the frequency and distribution of diseases is **epidemiology** (ep″ĭ-de″me-ol′ə-je). The specialist is an _____. A physician with this specialty may be assigned the responsibility of directing infection control programs within a hospital. An epidemiologist nurse also has special training and experience in the control of infections.

2-39 There are many other areas in which physicians specialize. **Preventive medicine** is concerned with preventing the occurrence of both mental and physical illness and disease. **Emergency medicine** deals with acutely ill or injured patients who require immediate medical treatment.

> ➤ **KEY** POINT Acute and chronic have opposite meanings. **Acute** (ə-kūt′) means having a short and relatively severe course. The opposite of acute is **chronic** (kron′ik), existing over a long period.

In the emergency room, patients are often prioritized according to their need for treatment. This method of sorting according to the patients' needs for care is called **triage** (tre-ahzh′, tre′ahzh). Write the term that means the sorting and prioritizing of patients for treatment:

triage

_____.

Emergency department (ED) more accurately describes the place in a hospital where emergencies are handled, than emergency room, and the terminology is evolving to reflect this fact.

2-40 Some physicians specialize in sports medicine, which is concerned with prevention, diagnosis, and treatment of sports injuries. A specialist in **forensic** (fə-ren′zik) **medicine** deals with the legal aspects of health care. Aerospace medicine is concerned with the effects of living and working in an artificial environment beyond Earth's atmosphere and forces of gravity. The effect of zero gravity on an astronaut's health would be an aspect of

aerospace

_____ medicine.

EXERCISE 6

Match the medical specialists with the areas in which they specialize.

_____ 1. anesthesiologist
_____ 2. dermatologist
_____ 3. geriatrician
_____ 4. gynecologist
_____ 5. neonatologist
_____ 6. neurologist
_____ 7. oncologist
_____ 8. otolaryngologist
_____ 9. pathologist
_____ 10. pediatrician

A. children
B. disease in general
C. ear, nose, and throat
D. feeling or sensation
E. females
F. nervous system
G. newborns
H. older persons
I. skin
J. tumors

EXERCISE 7

Write the specialty associated with the following conditions or situations:

1. heart attack _____

2. interpreting a radiograph _____

3. deficiency of the immune system _____

4. hormonal deficiency _____

5. nosebleed _____

6. miscarriage _____

7. irritable bowel disease _____

8. urinary infection _____

9. broken wrist _____

10. rheumatoid arthritis _____
(Use Appendix VI to check your answers.)

OTHER HEALTH PROFESSIONS

2-41 Sophisticated medical care would not be possible without a great variety of health professionals. Physicians rely on the competence of co-workers, those trained in medical specialties, as well as nurses and other allied health workers, who have completed a course of study in a field of health and whose specialized knowledge is vitally important in the diagnosis and treatment of disease.

A **physician assistant** (PA) is a person certified by the American Academy of Physician Assistants. Depending on their skill, their experience, and legal regulations, physician assistants can deliver primary patient care much like a licensed physician. Sometimes they work under the supervision of a

assistant

licensed physician. PA is an abbreviation for physician _____.

Study the meanings of the word parts in the following list.

Word Parts: Medicine and Allied Health Professions

Combining Forms	Meanings	Prefixes	Meanings
bi(o)	life or living	an-	no, not, or without
dent(i), dent(o), odont(o)	tooth	endo-	inside
opt(o), optic(o)	vision		
or(o)	mouth	**Suffix**	**Meaning**
pharmac(o)	drugs or medicine	-crine	secrete
therapeut(o)	treatment		

drugs

2-42 The combining form pharmac(o) refers to drugs or medicine. **Pharmaco/logy** (fahr″mə-kol′ə-je) is the study of _____, including their origin, nature, properties, and effects. A **pharmacy** is a place for the preparation and dispensing of drugs and medicinal supplies by **pharmacists** and their assistants. The science of formulating, dispensing, and providing information on drugs is also called pharmacy. (See the Companion CD for more information on pharmacology.)

RN

2-43 Nursing is one of the oldest and most familiar fields of medicine (Figure 2-6). The **registered nurse** (RN) is licensed to practice by a state board of nurse examiners or other state authority. The abbreviation for registered nurse is _____.

practical

A **licensed practical nurse** (LPN) is educated in basic nursing techniques and works under the supervision of a registered nurse. The LPN is a graduate of a school of practical nursing. LPN means a licensed _____ nurse. (LVN is **licensed vocational nurse.**)

As health care has become more complex, many nursing specialties, such as the nurse practitioner, nurse educator, nurse anesthetist, and nurse midwife, have developed.

laboratory

2-44 Medical laboratory personnel are skilled in the performance of clinical laboratory procedures used in diagnosis and the evaluation of patient progress. In descending order of responsibility and education, laboratory personnel include **medical technologists, medical technicians,** and laboratory assistants. The place in which these individuals work is a medical _____.

life

2-45 The combining form bi(o) means _____ or living. **Bio/hazards** (bi′o-haz″ərds) are objects or substances that are harmful or potentially harmful to humans, other organisms, or the environment. The biohazard symbol is recognized internationally and warns of harmful or potentially harmful agents (Figure 2-7).

radiologist

2-46 A **radio/logic technologist** operates diagnostic imaging equipment and assists radiologists. A radiologic technologist works under the supervision of a physician who specializes in radiology, a _____.

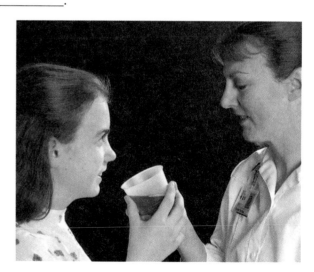

Figure 2-6 Nurse with young patient. Keeping patients calm and reassured is only one of the varied duties of the modern nurse.

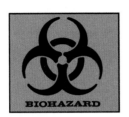

Figure 2-7 Biohazard label. Laboratories, doctors' offices, and other organizations that work with possible disease-causing organisms that require special conditions for containment must post signs bearing this special biohazard symbol.

therapist

2-47 A **physical therapist** is specially trained to provide physical therapy to patients (Figure 2-8). A professional who is skilled in physical therapy is called a physical

_____.

Rehabilitation medicine is concerned with restoring the ability to live and work as normally as possible after an injury or illness. **Physical therapy,** which is often part of rehabilitation, is the treatment of body ailments by nonmedicinal means. It uses natural agents such as water, heat, massage, and exercise in the treatment of disease.

Occupational therapists work to develop fine motor skills used for activities of daily living (ADLs) such as those required for eating, dressing, and maintaining hygiene. Other services include the assessment and preparation for returning to work after an injury or illness (Figure 2-9).

respiratory

2-48 Respiratory therapy is the treatment of disorders in which breathing may be impaired. Any disease in which breathing is affected would be a concern of those who work in _____ therapy. A **respiratory therapist** is a specialist who holds a degree in respiratory therapy.

Medical records, medical transcription, medical coding, tumor registry, dietetics, and research are only a few of the many fields that are associated with health care.

tooth

2-49 The combining forms dent(i), dent(o), and odont(o) mean _____. **Dent/istry** (den´tis-tre) is concerned with the teeth, the oral cavity, and associated structures, as well as the prevention, diagnosis, and treatment of disease and the restoration of defective or missing tissue. This includes the prevention of tooth and gum disease.

Or/al means pertaining to the mouth. The science of operative procedures on the mouth is oral surgery. If someone were having wisdom teeth pulled, it would probably be done by a specialist called an **oral** _____.

surgeon

2-50 The combining forms opt(o) and optic(o) mean vision. A person who deals with **optic/al** (op´tĭ-kəl) glasses and other devices used to correct vision is an **optic/ian** (op-tish´ən). An optician specializes in correcting vision.

vision

Opto/metry (op-tom´ə-tre) is the measurement of _____. In optometry, the irregularities of vision are diagnosed. Corrective lenses are often prescribed. An **opto/metr/ist** (op-tom´ə-trist) is a specialist concerned with vision. Do not confuse this term with the physician, ophthalmologist.

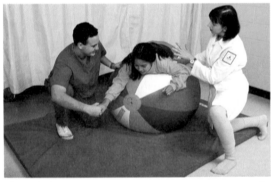

Figure 2-8 Physical therapists with young patient. The therapists are using exercise to help the patient strengthen and coordinate body movements.

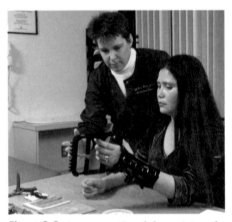

Figure 2-9 An occupational therapist working with a patient.

EXERCISE 8

Build It! Use the following word parts to complete these sentences.

endo-
bi(o), or(o), pharmac(o), radi(o), therapeut(o)
-al, -crine, -ic, -logic, -logy

1. The study of drugs and their effects is _____/_____.

2. Objects or substances that are harmful to humans or the environment are called _____ hazards.

3. A person who operates diagnostic imaging equipment is known as a _____/_____ technologist.

4. A term that means pertaining to the mouth is _____/_____.

5. Pertaining to treatment is _____/_____.

6. Glands that secrete hormones are _____/_____ glands.

MEDICAL RECORDS

2-51 Medical specialties and other health professions use health records as written forms of communication to document information that is relevant to the care of the patient (Pt). Medical reports communicate the patient's health status to other health professionals and to insurance companies and federal and state agencies. Inpatients (IPs) are persons who have been admitted to a hospital or other health care facility for at least an overnight stay. Outpatients (OP) are persons who are not admitted to a hospital and are being treated in an office, clinic, hospital, or other health care facility. Medical records must be maintained for outpatients as well as inpatients. The abbreviation IP means _____.

inpatient

2-52 There are many types of medical reports, including those for the history and physical (H&P) examination, operative (surgical) reports, consultation notes and letters, medication records, and laboratory and radiology reports. Medical reports often include statistical data (patient's legal name; date of birth [DOB]; file number, which may be the patient's social security number [SSN]; physician's name, etc.) and a signature line. DOB means _____ of birth.

date

   Representative samples are included in this book in Chapters 7-17 to give you experience understanding health care records. After you have learned several medical terms, you will be asked to read and explain various terms that are in medical reports and to apply terminology in practical situations. The following example, a history and physical examination summary, documents the patient's medical history along with findings from the physical examination (PE). Learn the common abbreviations that are shown on the report in Figure 2-10.

2-53 The Health Insurance Portability and Accountability Act (HIPAA) is a federal privacy act that went into effect in 2003. It gives the patient certain rights, including the rights to request restrictions of protected health information and to receive confidential communications concerning one's own medical condition and treatment. HIPAA is a federal _____ act concerning a patient's medical records.

privacy

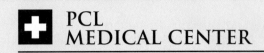

PCL MEDICAL CENTER

7700 Lexicon Way
St. Louis, MO 63146

Phone (555) 437-0000 • Fax (555) 437-0001

HISTORY AND PHYSICAL

H&P

Pt — **PATIENT NAME:** Margaret Ann Gordon   **ID #:** 009-3002   **DATE:** May 4, ----

Hx — <u>**HISTORY**</u>

CC — **CHIEF COMPLAINT:** Fever with mild dyspnea.

HPI — **HISTORY OF PRESENT ILLNESS:** The patient complains of malaise and loss of appetite. She has a productive cough.

PMH — **PAST MEDICAL HISTORY:** This 63-year-old female patient has a history of bronchitis, myocardial infarction (status post CABG one year ago), and deep venous thrombosis with pulmonary embolism.

FH — **FAMILY HISTORY:** Mother is living at age 85 with congestive heart failure. Father is deceased with a history of COLD and type 2 DM.

ROS — **REVIEW OF SYSTEMS:** Unremarkable except respiratory as noted.

PE — <u>**PHYSICAL EXAMINATION**</u>

GENERAL APPEARANCE: A well-developed, obese female who is coughing and appears feverish.

VS — **VITAL SIGNS:** Vital signs show T 100.8, P 98, R 28, BP 160/94. Exam limited to chest: Fine crackles at bilateral lung bases with some wheezes. Increased dyspnea on exertion.

DIAGNOSTIC DATA: O_2 saturation level 92% on 2 L oxygen. WBCs 24.5. Chest x-ray shows increased right lung density. No pneumothorax or pleural effusion. Increasing right lung infiltrate with masslike density, right hilum. Sputum collected for culture.

Dx — <u>**DIAGNOSIS:**</u> Community-acquired pneumonia

Tx — <u>**TREATMENT PLAN:**</u> IV antibiotics pending sputum culture results. Bronchodilator, such as Alupent. Expectorant, such as guaifenesin.

Ruth Wong, MD
Ruth Wong, MD
Pulmonologist

RW:pai
D: May 4, ----
T: May 5, ----

Figure 2-10 An example of a health care report. The H&P is one of the first documents prepared when a patient arrives for care.

EXERCISE 9

Write the meaning of these abbreviations.

1. CC _____

2. Dx _____

3. FH _____

4. H&P _____

5. HPI _____

6. Hx _____

7. OP _____

8. PE _____

9. PMH _____

10. ROS _____

11. Tx _____

12. VS _____

(Use Appendix VI to check your answers.)

EXERCISE 10

Write a word in each blank space to answer these questions.

1. What is the term for persons who have been admitted to a hospital or other health care facility for at least an overnight stay? _____

2. What is the term for patients who are not hospitalized and are being treated in an office, clinic, or other health care facility? _____

3. What is the abbreviation for the federal privacy act that gives the patient certain rights concerning his or her own health information? _____

(Use Appendix VI to check your answers.)

CATEGORIES OF MEDICAL TERMS

2-54 All medical specialties follow a process to study an illness and then treat it. The process includes knowledge of anatomy, uses diagnostic tests, determines the pathology, and treats the problem with surgical or other therapeutic means. As you study medical terminology, you will observe that terms are used in a variety of ways that correspond to this process. It will be helpful to keep the medical process in mind, as certain word parts indicate how a term is used.

> ➤ **KEY** POINT Here are the categories used in this book:
> • **Anatomy** (ə-nat´ə-me), the science of the structure of the body and the relation of its parts: the names of structures and related words, such as colon (large intestine) and colonic (pertaining to the colon). Anatomy is presented by body systems in Chapters 8-17.
> • **Diagnostic** (di˝əg-nos´tik) tests and procedures: terms used to describe disease (fever, headache) and the tests used to establish a **diagnosis** (di˝əg-no´sis), the determination of the cause of a disease. Diagnostic tests include clinical studies (measurement of blood pressure), laboratory tests (determination of blood gases), and radiologic studies (chest x-ray examination). You will learn many suffixes in Chapter 3 that form the basis of diagnostic terms.
> • **Pathology:** the names of diseases or disorders (influenza, leukemia). Several suffixes that form the basis of terms used to write pathologies are presented in Chapter 4.
> • **Surgery:** operative procedures (tonsillectomy, removal of the tonsils). You will learn many suffixes in Chapter 3 that form the basis of surgical terms.
> • **Therapy:** treatment of a disease or abnormal condition. Therapeutic terms include prescribed drugs (such as antibiotics) and physical treatments (such as electric stimulation to enhance the healing process).

anatomy

The femur is commonly called the thigh bone. Femur is the name of a structure. The appropriate category for femur is _____.

EXERCISE 11

Categorize the terms in the left column by selecting A, B, C, D, or E.

_____ 1. antibiotics

_____ 2. colon

_____ 3. blood gases

_____ 4. leukemia

_____ 5. removal of the tonsils

A. anatomy
B. diagnostic test or procedure
C. pathology
D. surgery
E. therapy

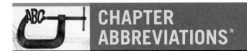

CHAPTER ABBREVIATIONS*

Abbreviations are shortened forms of written words or phrases that are used in place of the whole. For example, MD means doctor of medicine. However, MD has other meanings, including medical department and maximum dose.

Remember that certain abbreviations have been placed on a "do not use" list when an error in reading could jeopardize patient safety (Table 2-2). Some abbreviations have been included in this chapter because of their common use.

ADL	activity of daily living	**LVN**	licensed vocational nurse
CC	chief complaint	**MD**	doctor of medicine
DOB	date of birth	**OB**	obstetrics
Dx	diagnosis	**OP**	outpatient
ED	emergency department	**OR**	operating room
ENT	ear, nose, and throat	**PA**	physician assistant
FH	family history	**PE**	physical examination
GP	general practitioner	**PMH**	past medical history
H&P	history and physical	**Pt**	patient
HIPAA	Health Insurance Portability and Accountability Act	**RN**	registered nurse
		ROS	review of systems
HPI	history of present illness	**SSN**	social security number
Hx	history	**Tx**	treatment
IP	inpatient	**VS**	vital signs
LPN	licensed practical nurse		

*Many of these abbreviations share their meanings with other terms.

TABLE 2-2 The Joint Commission Official "Do Not Use" List,* 2007

Do Not Use	Potential Problem	Use Instead
U (unit)	Mistaken for "O" (zero), the number "4" (four) or "cc"	Write "unit"
IU (International Unit)	Mistaken for IV (intravenous) or the number 10 (ten)	Write "International Unit"
Q.D., QD, q.d., qd (daily)	Mistaken for each other	Write "daily"
Q.O.D., QOD, q.o.d, qod (every other day)	Period after the Q mistaken for "I" and the "O" mistaken for "I"	Write "every other day"
Trailing zero (X.0 mg)†	Decimal point is missed	Write "X mg"
Lack of leading zero (.X mg)	Decimal point is missed	Write "0.X mg"
MS	Can mean morphine sulfate or magnesium sulfate	Write "morphine sulfate"
MSO₄ and MgSO₄	Confused for each other	Write "magnesium sulfate"
Additional Abbreviations, Acronyms, and Symbols (for Possible Future Inclusion in the Official "Do Not Use" List)		
> (greater than)	Misinterpreted as the number "7" (seven) or the letter "L"	Write "greater than"
< (less than)	Confused for each other	Write "less than"
Abbreviations for drug names	Misinterpreted owing to similar abbreviations for multiple drugs	Write drug names in full
Apothecary units	Unfamiliar to many practitioners Confused with metric units	Use metric units
@	Mistaken for the number "2" (two)	Write "at"
cc	Mistaken for U (units) when poorly written	Write "mL" or "milliliters"
μg	Mistaken for mg (milligrams) resulting in 1000-fold overdose	Write "mcg" or "micrograms"

*Applies to all orders and all medication-related documentation that is handwritten (including free-text computer entry) or on preprinted forms.
†Exception: A "trailing zero" may be used only where required to demonstrate the level of precision of the value being reported, such as for laboratory results, imaging studies that report size of lesions, or catheter or tube sizes. It may not be used in medication orders or other medication-related documentation.

Medical care is changing and is influenced by increased knowledge of diseases, increased public awareness, and rapid advances in science and technology. Many new professions in the medical field have evolved in recent years, and no doubt more will continue to evolve as increasing emphasis is placed on promotion of wellness as well as the treatment of disease.

Congratulations! You are well on your way to learning medical terminology.

PREPARING FOR A TEST OF THIS CHAPTER
STUDY THE WORD LISTS

Review all lists of word parts and their meanings. If you have problems remembering certain word parts, use index cards to prepare flash cards with a word part on one side and its meaning on the reverse side. Review the cards several times before the test.

Be Careful With These!

-ist (one who) vs. -iatry (medical profession or treatment)
-logy (study of) vs. -logist (one who studies; specialist)
ne(o) (new) vs. neur(o) (nerve)
or(o) (mouth) vs. ur(o) (urinary tract or urine) vs. ot(o) (ear)
intern (one in postgraduate training) vs. internist (a physician)

WORK THE REVIEW SECTION

Work the following review section. The review helps you know if you have learned the material. The written exercises are divided into Basic Understanding (I through VIII) and Greater Comprehension (IX through XI). Your instructor will advise you concerning parts of the review you are to work. After completing all sections of the review, check your answers with the solutions found in Appendix VI.

 Say and Check

Review each term in the Pronunciation List at the end of the chapter. Look at the spelling of each term and be sure that you know its meaning. If you cannot recall its meaning, look up the term in the glossary and reread the frames that pertain to the term. Say each term aloud and click on the Chapter 2 pronunciations included on the Companion CD, listening as the terms are pronounced. Additional questions are included on the CD.

▶ CHAPTER 2 REVIEW

Basic Understanding

Identifying Word Parts

I. *Use slashes to divide the following terms into their component parts and identify the parts as* CF *(for combining form),* P *(for prefix), or* S *(for suffix). Example: neonatologist = neo/nato/logist; neo is CF; nato is CF; logist is S.*

1. cardiac   _____

2. gynecologist   _____

3. ophthalmological _____

4. pathology   _____

5. psychiatry   _____

Writing the Meanings

II. *Write the meanings of these word parts.*

1. bi(o)   _____

2. -crine   _____

3. dent(o)   _____

4. endo-   _____

5. optic(o)   _____

6. opt(o)   _____

7. or(o)   _____

8. pharmac(o)   _____

9. rhin(o)   _____

10. ur(o)   _____

Listing

III. *List five categories used in this book for classifying medical terms.*

1. _____

2. _____

3. _____

4. _____

5. _____

Matching

IV. Match the medical specialists with the areas in which they specialize.

_____ 1. anesthesiologist

_____ 2. dermatologist

_____ 3. endocrinologist

_____ 4. geriatrician

_____ 5. gynecologist

_____ 6. neurologist

_____ 7. oncologist

_____ 8. ophthalmologist

_____ 9. otolaryngologist

_____ 10. pediatrician

_____ 11. psychiatrist

_____ 12. rhinologist

A. children
B. drugs that produce loss of feeling or sensation
C. ear, nose, and throat
D. eyes
E. females
F. hormones and the glands that secrete them
G. mental, emotional, and behavioral disorders
H. nervous system
I. nose
J. older persons
K. skin
L. tumors

V. Match health professions in the left column with their descriptions in the right column.

_____ 1. pharmacists

_____ 2. physical therapists

_____ 3. radiologic technologists

_____ 4. rehabilitation therapists

_____ 5. respiratory therapists

A. dispense and provide information about drugs
B. operate diagnostic imaging equipment
C. restore one's ability to live and work as normally as possible after an injury
D. treat body ailments by nonmedicinal means
E. treat disorders in which breathing is impaired

Word Analysis

VI. Break the following terms into their word parts and define each word part. The first one is done as an example.

1. dental   _dent/al; dent(o) means tooth, -al means pertaining to_ _____

2. gastric   _____

3. neurology _____

4. oncology _____

5. otic   _____

Multiple Choice

VII. *Circle the correct answer to complete each of these sentences.*

1. A 65-year-old man has a history of heart problems. Which type of specialist should he see for care of his heart condition? (cardiologist, endocrinologist, laryngologist, orthopedist)

2. Cynthia is pregnant. Which type of specialist should she see to care for her during her pregnancy, labor, and delivery? (gerontologist, obstetrician, orthopedist, otologist)

3. Which term means a person who is not a physician but is trained in administering drugs that cause a loss of feeling? (anesthesiologist, anesthesist, anesthetics, anesthetist)

4. Which of the following physicians specializes in the diagnosis and treatment of newborns through the age of 28 days? (geriatrician, gynecologist, neonatologist, urologist)

5. John suffers from persistent digestive problems. His primary care physician refers him to which of the following specialists? (gastroenterologist, immunologist, rheumatologist, toxicologist)

6. Sally injures her arm while ice skating. The emergency room physician orders an x-ray film. Which type of physician is a specialist in interpreting x-ray films? (gynecologist, ophthalmologist, plastic surgeon, radiologist)

7. Sally's x-ray film reveals a fractured radius, one of the bones of her forearm. Dr. Bonelly, a bone specialist, puts a cast on Sally's arm. Which type of specialist is Dr. Bonelly? (dermatologist, orthopedist, otologist, rhinologist)

8. What does the word neuron mean?
(medical specialty that deals with the nervous system, nerve cell, neurosurgery, specialist in diseases of the nervous system)

9. Which physician specializes in diagnosis of disease using clinical laboratory results?
(clinical pathologist, gastroenterologist, internist, surgical pathologist)

10. Which term describes a substance that does not permit the passage of x-rays?
(radiopaque, roentgen, roentgenology, x-radiation)

Writing Terms

VIII. *Write a term for each of the following descriptions.*

1. a specialist in internal medicine _____

2. existing over a long period _____

3. having a severe and relatively short duration _____

4. method of prioritizing patients according to their need _____

5. permitting the passage of radiant energy _____

6. pertaining to the heart _____

7. study of the characteristics, causes, and effects of disease _____

8. surgery of the nervous system _____

9. tending to become worse, spread, and cause death _____

10. the secretions of endocrine glands _____

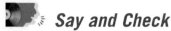 **Say and Check**

Say aloud the terms you wrote for Exercise VIII. Use the Companion CD to check your pronunciations.

Greater Comprehension

Spelling

IX. *Circle all misspelled terms and write their correct spellings:*

cardiak   dermatologic   obstetrics   optometry   sychiatry

Interpreting Abbreviations

X. *Write the meaning of each of these abbreviations:*

1. CC _____

2. GP _____

3. LVN _____

4. OB _____

5. OR _____

Pronunciation

XI. *The pronunciation syllables are shown for several medical words. Indicate which syllable has the primary accent by marking it with an ´.*

1. anesthesiology (an əs the ze ol ə je)

2. forensic (fə ren zik)

3. gastroenterology (gas tro en tər ol ə je)

4. orthopedics (or tho pe diks)

5. radiologic (ra de o loj ik)

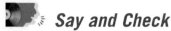 **Say and Check**

Say aloud the five terms in Exercise XI. Use the Companion CD to check your pronunciations. In addition, be prepared to pronounce aloud these terms in class:

anesthesiologist	gynecology	ophthalmic	psychiatry
anesthetic	larynx	orthopedist	radiopaque
benign	neonatologist	otic	rheumatologist
gastroenterologist	obstetrical	otolaryngology	rhinology
geriatrician	oncology	pediatrician	triage

(Use Appendix VI to check your answers.)

PRONUNCIATION LIST

This listing of terms from Chapter 2 matches the Chapter 2 Glossary on the Companion CD. Use the Companion CD to review the terms. Look closely at the spelling of each term as it is pronounced, pronounce it aloud, and be sure you know the meaning of each term.

acute
anatomic pathologist
anatomic pathology
anatomy
anesthesiologist
anesthesiology
anesthetic
anesthetist
benign
biohazard
carcinoma
cardiac
cardiologist
cardiology
chronic
clinical pathologist
clinical pathology
clinical psychologist
clinical psychology
dentistry
dermal
dermatologic
dermatological
dermatologist
dermatology
diagnosis
diagnostic
emergency medicine
endocrine
endocrinologist
endocrinology
epidemic
epidemiologist
epidemiology

family practice
forensic medicine
gastric
gastroenterologist
gastroenterology
geriatrician
geriatrics
gerontology
gland
gynecologist
gynecology
holistic
immunologist
immunology
internal medicine
internist
larynx
licensed practical nurse
licensed vocational nurse
malignant
medical technician
medical technologist
neonatologist
neonatology
neurologist
neurology
neuron
neurosurgeon
neurosurgery
nurse midwife
obstetric
obstetrical
obstetrician
obstetrics

occupational therapist
oncologist
oncology
ophthalmic
ophthalmologic
ophthalmological
ophthalmologist
ophthalmology
optical
optician
optometrist
optometry
oral
oral surgeon
orthopedic surgeon
orthopedics
orthopedist
otic
otolaryngologist
otolaryngology
otologist
otology
pathologic
pathological
pathology
pediatric
pediatrician
pediatrics
pharmacist
pharmacology
pharmacy
physical therapist
physical therapy
physician assistant

plastic surgery
preventive medicine
primary health care provider
psychiatrist
psychiatry
radiation oncology
radiologic
radiologic technologist
radiological
radiologist
radiology
radiolucent
radiopaque
radiotherapy
registered nurse
rehabilitation medicine
remission
respiratory therapist
respiratory therapy
rheumatism
rheumatologist
rheumatology
rhinologist
rhinology
roentgenology
surgery
therapeutic
therapy
triage
urinary
urologic
urological
urologist
urology

Español ENHANCING SPANISH COMMUNICATION

English	Spanish (pronunciation)
acute	agudo (ah-GOO-do)
aged	envejecido (en-vay-hay-SEE-do)
anesthetic	anestésico (ah-nes-TAY-se-co)
benign	benigno (bay-NEEG-no)
cancer	cáncer (KAHN-ser)
child	niña (NEE-nya), niño (NEE-nyo)
chronic	crónico (CRO-ne-co)
diagnostic	diagnóstico (de-ag-NOS-te-co)
disease	enfermedad (en-fer-may-DAHD)
ear	oreja (o-RAY-hah)
eye	ojo (O-ho)
gland	glándula (GLAN-doo-lah)
gynecology	ginecología (he-nay-co-lo-HEE-ah)
heart	corazón (co-rah-SON)
hormone	hormona (or-MOH-nah)
intestine	intestino (in-tes-TEE-no)
life	vida (VEE-dah)
malignant	maligno (mah-LEEG-no)
mind	mente (MEN-te)
muscle	músculo (MOOS-coo-lo)
nerve	nervio (NERR-ve-o)
neurology	neurología (nay-oo-ro-lo-HEE-ah)
nose	nariz (nah-REES)
optician	óptico (OP-te-co)
pathology	patología (pah-to-lo-HEE-ah)
pregnancy	embarazo (em-bah-RAH-so)
psychiatry	psiquiatría (se-ke-ah-TREE-ah)
psychology	psicología (se-co-lo-HEE-ah)
radiation	radiación (rah-de-ah-se-ON)
stomach	estómago (es-TOH-mah-go)
surgeon	cirujano(a) (se-roo-HAH-no) (na)
surgery	cirugía (se-roo-HEE-ah)
therapy	tratamiento (trah-tah-me-EN-to)
throat	garganta (gar-GAHN-tah)
urinary system	sistema urinario (sis-TAY-mah oo-re-NAH-re-o)
urine	orina (o-REE-nah)
urology	urología (oo-ro-lo-HEE-ah)
x-ray	radiografía (rah-de-o-grah-FEE-ah)

Diagnostic, Therapeutic, and Surgical Terms

3

Using Suffixes to Build Medical Terms

LEARNING GOALS

Basic Understanding

In this chapter you will learn to do the following:

1. Write the meanings of the word parts and use them to build and analyze terms.
2. Match suffixes pertaining to diagnosis with their meanings or write their meanings.
3. Identify the procedures a physician uses during a physical examination.
4. Recognize several types of diagnostic imaging procedures.
5. Recognize several combining forms associated with therapy, and write the meanings of therapeutic terms or match them with their meanings.
6. Match suffixes pertaining to surgical procedures with their meanings or write their meanings.
7. Recognize combining forms for selected body structures in medical terms and write their meanings or match them with their meanings.

Greater Comprehension

8. Spell medical terms accurately.
9. Write the meaning of the abbreviations.
10. Pronounce medical terms correctly.

MAJOR SECTIONS OF THIS CHAPTER:

❑ SUFFIXES PERTAINING TO DIAGNOSIS
❑ BASIC EXAMINATION PROCEDURES
❑ DIAGNOSTIC RADIOLOGY

❑ THERAPEUTIC INTERVENTIONS
❑ SUFFIXES PERTAINING TO SURGICAL PROCEDURES
❑ COMBINING FORMS FOR SELECTED BODY STRUCTURES

FUNCTION FIRST

You will learn a number of suffixes in this chapter and use them to write new terms. Certain terms and their related suffixes have the same meaning. For example, both -scope and a scope mean an instrument for viewing. Most suffixes are not words in themselves and are attached to the end of a word or word part. To make the suffixes easier to remember, they are presented in groups.

The suffix that is added to a word part (mainly a combining form) generally determines its category. Some students find it helpful to know what types of words are formed by the use of various suffixes. For these students information about parts of speech is provided. It is logical that a suffix coincides with how its meaning is used in speech. For example, an instrument is a noun, so thermometer, an instrument for measuring temperature, is a noun.

SUFFIXES PERTAINING TO DIAGNOSIS

3-1 Diagnosis (di″əg-no′sis) is the identification of a disease or condition by a scientific evaluation of physical signs, symptoms, history, tests, and procedures. Compare diagnosis with **prognosis** (prog-no′sis), which means the predicted outcome of a disease.

> ➤ **KEY** POINT <u>Signs are objective; symptoms are subjective.</u> **Signs** are definitive evidence of an illness or disordered function. **Symptoms** are subjective evidence as perceived by the patient, such as pain.

sign
symptom

Indisputable evidence, such as a rash, is which—a sign or a symptom? _____

Is itching of the skin a sign or a symptom? _____
Itching and rash are both diagnostic terms.

3-2 Diagnostic (di″əg-nos′tik) terms are used to describe the signs and symptoms of disease (such as rash and itching), as well as the tests used to establish a diagnosis. The tests include basic examination procedures, clinical studies (measuring blood pressure), laboratory tests (determination of blood gases), and radio/logic (ra″de-o-loj′ik) studies, which relate to the use of radiant energy (such as a chest x-ray study).

Laboratory (lab) tests, ranging from simple to sophisticated studies, identify and quantify substances to evaluate organ functions or establish a diagnosis. Within normal limits (WNL) is a phrase sometimes used by physicians to describe the results of a laboratory test.

Both laboratory and radiologic tests that are used to establish a diagnosis are

diagnostic

_____ terms.

3-3 Suffixes that pertain to diagnosis are used to describe signs and symptoms, as well as tests and procedures that are used to diagnose disease. Some diseases are named for the diagnostic term. An abnormal condition of the respiratory system, bronchiectasis, is named for the dilation of the bronchial walls. Dilation, also called **dilatation** (dil″ə-ta′shən), is the condition of being stretched or dilated beyond the normal dimensions, or the process of being dilated. Write the

dilatation

term that is a synonym for dilation: _____.

All the suffixes in the list below form nouns unless otherwise noted. Read each suffix and its meaning. It is necessary to take time to study each suffix and its meaning. It is also helpful to think of words you may know that can help you to remember the meaning. Throughout this chapter, make flash cards for word parts and their meanings. Review with the flash cards several times before the test.

Suffixes: Diagnosis

Signs and Symptoms

-algia, -dynia	pain	-rrhea	flow or discharge
-ectasia, -ectasis	dilatation (dilation, enlargement) or stretching of a structure or part	-rrhexis	rupture
		-spasm	twitching, cramp
-edema	swelling	-stasis	stopping, controlling
-emesis	to vomit, vomiting		
-malacia	soft, softening	**Procedures**	
-megaly	enlargement	-gram	a record
-oid (forms adjectives and nouns)	resembling	-graph	instrument used to record
		-graphy	process of recording
		-meter	instrument used to measure
-penia	deficiency	-scope	instrument used for viewing
-rrhage, -rrhagia	excessive bleeding or hemorrhage	-scopy	visual examination

ear

3-4 Both **oto/dynia** (o″to-din′e-ə) and **ot/algia** (o-tal′je-ə) mean a pain in the

_____ or earache.

eye

ophthalmalgia
(of´thəl-mal´jə)

deficiency

enlargement

discharge

-rrhexis
hemorrhage

swelling

ophthalmomalacia
(of-thal´mo-mə-la´shə)

controlling

twitching

bone

3-5 Ophthalmo/dynia (of-thal″mo-din´e-ə) means pain in the _____.
Use -algia to write another term that means pain in the eye:
_____.

3-6 The suffix -penia means _____. **Calci/penia**
(kal″sĭ-pe´ne-ə) means a deficiency of calcium.

3-7 You may be more familiar with the prefix mega-, but -megaly also means enlarged or enlargement. **Cardio/megaly** (kahr″de-o-meg´ə-le) means _____ of the heart.

3-8 Several suffixes in the list begin with rr. **Oto/rrhea** (o″to-re´ə) means a _____ from the ear.

3-9 Write a suffix that means rupture: _____.
Both -rrhage and -rrhagia mean excessive bleeding or _____.

3-10 Several suffixes are also terms that can stand alone. **Emesis** (em´ə-sis) means the material expelled in vomiting, and **edema** (ə-de´mə) is the presence of abnormally large amounts of fluid in the tissues, resulting in swelling. The suffix -edema means swelling.
Blephar(o) is a combining form that means eyelid. **Blephar/edema** (blef″ə-rĭ-de´mə) is _____ of the eyelid.
An outstanding example of edema is seen in the late stages of **elephantiasis** (el″ə-fən-ti´ə-sis), a parasitic disease generally seen in the tropics (Figure 3-1). The excessive swelling is caused by obstruction of the lymphatic vessels by the parasites.

3-11 Malacia (mə-la´shə) means softening. Use a combining form before -malacia to write a word that means abnormal softening of the eye: _____.

3-12 Stasis (sta´sis), the term, means the same as the suffix -stasis, which means stopping or _____.

3-13 Spasm means cramp or twitching. **Blepharo/spasm** (blef´ə-ro-spaz″əm) means _____ of the eyelid.

3-14 The combining form oste(o) means bone. If something is described as **oste/oid** (os´te-oid), it resembles _____.

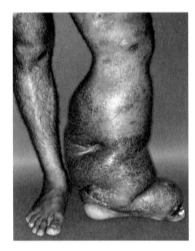

Figure 3-1 Lymphedema. Extensive swelling, caused by chronic obstruction of the lymphatic vessels, occurs in the late stages of elephantiasis.

recording

record

electrocardiograph
(e-lek″tro-kahr′de-o-graf″)

otoscope (o′to-skōp)

ophthalmoscopy
(of″thəl-mos′kə-pe)

3-15 Electro/cardio/graphy (e-lek″tro-kahr″de-og′rə-fe), the process of recording the electrical impulses of the heart, is one example of a diagnostic procedure. The suffix -graphy means the process of _____. An **electro/cardio/gram** (e-lek″tro-kahr′de-o-gram″) is a record or tracing of the electrical impulses of the heart, because -gram means the _____ that is produced in this procedure. This is abbreviated as either ECG or EKG. The combining form electr(o) means electricity, and the suffix -graph means an instrument used for recording. Use electr(o) + cardi(o) + -graph to write the name of the instrument used in electrocardiography: _____(Figure 3-2).

3-16 Oto/scopy (o-tos′kə-pe) means an examination of the outer ear, including the eardrum (Figure 3-3). Write a word that means the lighted instrument used in otoscopy: _____.

3-17 Using otoscopy as a model, write a term that means examination of the interior of the eye with an **ophthalmoscope** (of-thal′mə-skōp): _____ (Figure 3-4).

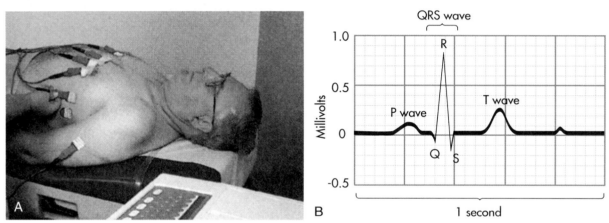

Figure 3-2 Electrocardiography. A, A patient undergoing electrocardiography, the making of graphic records produced by electrical activity of the heart muscle. The instrument, an electrocardiograph, is shown. The electrical impulses that are given off by the heart are picked up by electrodes (sensors) and conducted into the electrocardiograph through wires. **B,** An enlarged section of an ECG, a tracing that represents the heart's electrical impulses, which are picked up and conducted to the electrocardiograph by electrodes or leads connected to the body. The pattern of the graphic recording indicates the heart's rhythm and other actions. The normal ECG is composed of the labeled parts shown in the drawing. Each labeled segment represents a different part of the heartbeat. Electrocardiography is a valuable diagnostic tool.

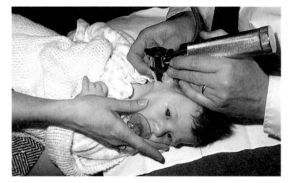

Figure 3-3 Otoscopy. An otoscope is being used to visually examine the ear, including the eardrum.

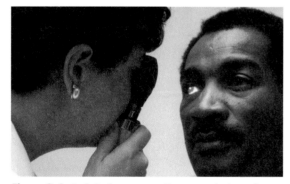

Figure 3-4 Ophthalmoscopy. Proper technique for ophthalmoscopic visualization of the interior of the eye.

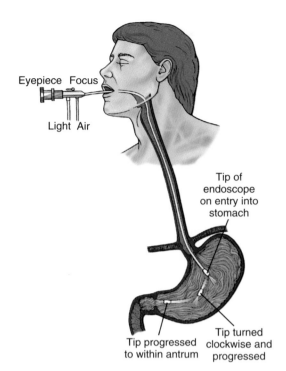

Eyepiece Focus

Light Air

Tip of
endoscope
on entry into
stomach

Tip progressed   Tip turned
to within antrum clockwise and
progressed

Figure 3-5 An example of a flexible endoscope. This endoscope is being used to examine the interior of the stomach via the esophagus. Depending on the structure to be examined, the physician chooses either a flexible or a rigid endoscope. Most of the stomach interior can be examined.

3-18 An **endo/scope** (en´do-skōp) is an illuminated optic instrument for the visualization of the interior of a body cavity or organ. Although the endoscope is generally introduced through a natural opening (for example, introduction of an endoscope into the mouth and through the esophagus to examine the interior of the stomach; Figure 3-5), it may also be inserted through an incision (for example, insertion of an endoscope into the chest cavity through an incision in the chest wall).

Endoscopy (en-dos´kə-pe) is visual inspection of a cavity of the body by means of an endoscope. Write the term that means a diagnostic procedure that uses an endoscope:

endoscopy   _____.

3-19 A **catheter** ` (kath´ə-tər) is a hollow flexible tube that can be inserted into a cavity of the body to withdraw or to instill fluids, perform tests, or visualize a vessel or cavity (for example, to view inside blood vessels). The introduction of a catheter is **catheterization** (kath˝ə-tur-ĭ-za´shən). To introduce a catheter within the body is to **catheterize** (kath´ə-ter-īz). Write the name of the device used in catheterization: _____.

catheter

A Latin term **cannula** (kan´u-lə) is also used to mean a hollow flexible tube that is inserted into vessels, ducts, or cavities.

_____

`Catheter (Greek: *katheter,* something lowered).

EXERCISE 1

Match the suffixes in the left column with their meanings in the right column.

_____ 1. -algia	A. controlling	
_____ 2. -ectasis	B. dilatation	
	C. enlargement	
_____ 3. -edema	D. excessive bleeding	
_____ 4. -emesis	E. pain	
	F. softening	
_____ 5. -malacia	G. swelling	
_____ 6. -megaly	H. vomiting	
_____ 7. -rrhagia		
_____ 8. -stasis		

EXERCISE 2

Write the suffix that means the following:

1. deficiency   _____

2. flow or discharge   _____

3. resembling   _____

4. rupture   _____

5. twitching or cramp _____

EXERCISE 3

Build It! *Use the following word parts to build terms. (Some word parts will be used more than once.)*

blephar(o), calc(i), cardi(o), ophthalm(o), oste(o), ot(o), -dynia, -malacia, -megaly, -oid, -penia, -rrhea, -scopy, -spasm

1. abnormal softening of the eye   _____/_____

2. calcium deficiency   _____/_____

3. discharge from the ear   _____/_____

4. earache   _____/_____

5. enlargement of the heart   _____/_____

6. examination of the eye   _____/_____

7. resembling bone   _____/_____

8. twitching of the eyelid   _____/_____

Say and Check

Pronounce the terms you wrote in Exercise 3. Use the Companion CD to check your pronunciations.

BASIC EXAMINATION PROCEDURES

3-20 Basic examinations are performed to assess the patient's condition. Vital signs are measured and recorded for most patients. Vital signs actually include only the measurements of pulse rate, respiration rate, and body temperature; however, they can vary and sometimes include other measurements. Although not strictly a vital sign, blood pressure is customarily included. The measurements of pulse rate, respiration rate, and body temperature are included when one

vital   checks the _____ signs of a patient.

3-21 The **pulse** is the rhythmic expansion of an artery that occurs as the heart beats; it may be felt with a finger (Figure 3-6). The pulse rate is the number of pulse beats per minute. A normal pulse rate in a resting state is 60 to 100 beats per minute. The rhythmic expansion of an artery

pulse   that occurs as the heart beats is called the _____.

3-22 The **respiration rate** is the number of breaths per minute. The rise and fall of the patient's chest is observed while counting the number of breaths and noting the ease with which breathing is accomplished. The number of breaths per minute is the

respiration   _____ rate.

3-23 The measurement of body temperature is also a vital sign. Therm(o), the combining form for heat, is used to write thermo/meter, an instrument for measuring temperature. Body temperature is the level of heat produced and sustained by the body processes. Variation and changes in

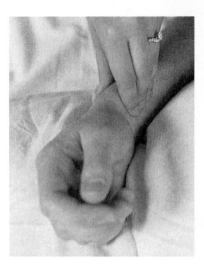

Figure 3-6 Assessment of the radial pulse. The pulse is easily detected over an artery that is close to the surface of the body and lies over a bone. Radi(o) sometimes means radiant energy, but in this case it is used to mean radius, a bone of the forearm, for which the artery is named.

body temperature may indicate disease. Normal adult body temperature as measured orally is 98.6° F or 37° C (F and C are abbreviations for Fahrenheit and Celsius). A thermo/meter is a(n) _____ for measuring temperature.

instrument

Temperature measurement can be accomplished by several means: most commonly oral, rectal, under the arm, or in the ear (Figure 3-7). Electronic measurement has decreased the time required for accurate measurement. One piece of equipment that contains a probe covered by a disposable sheath can be used to measure temperature under the tongue, in the rectum, or under the arm. For tympanic membrane (eardrum) temperature measurement, a specially designed probe similar to an otoscope is required.

mouth

3-24 An **oral** (or´əl) **thermometer** is placed in the _____. A **rectal** (rek´təl) **thermometer** is inserted in the **rectum** (rek´təm). Rectal temperatures are generally slightly higher than oral temperatures. Measurements of temperature under the arm and **tympanic thermometers** vary somewhat from those obtained by oral or rectal means. Special under-the-arm **axillary** (axill(o) means armpit) thermometers for newborns are available.

3-25 Blood pressure is the pressure exerted by the circulating volume of blood on the walls of the arteries and veins and on the chambers of the heart. Blood pressure is discussed in detail in Chapter 8. One combining form for chest is steth(o). The **stetho/scope** (steth´o-skōp) is placed on the chest to listen to heart sounds, particularly closing of the heart valves. The

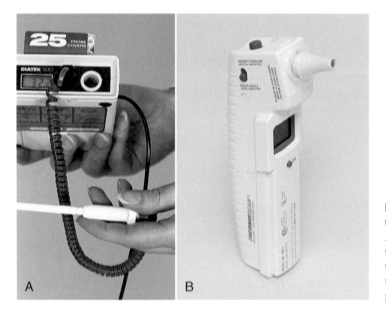

Figure 3-7 Devices for electronic temperature measurement.
A, Thermometer for measuring temperature orally, rectally, or under the arm. **B,** Tympanic membrane thermometer that uses a probe placed in the ear.

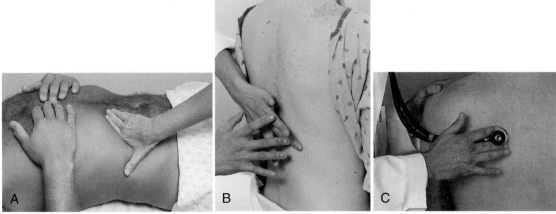

Figure 3-8 Three aspects of the physical examination. These techniques help in assessing the internal organs. **A,** Palpation. **B,** Percussion. **C,** Auscultation with a stethoscope.

stethoscope is also used to hear sounds of breathing and intestinal action and to take blood pressure. Write the name of the instrument placed on the chest to hear heart sounds:

stethoscope

_____ . A stethoscope is being used to listen to the patient's breathing in Figure 3-8, C.

3-26 A physical examination (PE) is an investigation of the body to determine its state of health, using any of several techniques, which include the following:

- inspection The examiner uses the eyes to observe the patient.
- **palpation** (pal-pa´shən): The examiner feels the texture, size, consistency, and location of certain body parts with the hands; (Figure 3-8, A.)
- **percussion** (pər-kŭ´shən): The examiner taps the body with the fingertips or fist to evaluate the size, borders, and consistency of internal organs and to determine the amount of fluid in a body cavity; (Figure 3-8, B.)
- **auscultation** (aws″kəl-ta´shən): The examiner listens for sounds within the body to evaluate the heart, blood vessels, lungs, intestines, or other organs or to detect the fetal heart sound in pregnant women. Auscultation is performed most commonly with a stethoscope (Figure 3-8, C.)

palpation
percussion
auscultation

Using the hands to feel the location or size of the liver is an example of _____. Tapping the chest with the fingertips is an example of _____. Listening to the heart with a stethoscope is an example of _____.

walk

3-27 Ambulation (am″bu-la´shən) means the act of walking. **Ambulant** (am´bu-lənt) describes a person who is able to _____. It is also accurate to say that a walking person is **ambulatory** (am´bu-lə-tor″e). A person's ability to ambulate is one observation an examiner would make by inspection.

EXERCISE 4

Write a word to complete each sentence.

1. The rhythmic expansion of an artery that occurs as the heart beats is called the _____.

2. Counting the number of breaths per minute measures the _____ rate.

3. The name of the procedure in which the physician listens with a stethoscope for sounds within the body is

   _____.

4. The name of the procedure in which the physician taps the patient's body with the fingertips to evaluate an internal

   organ is _____.

5. The name of the procedure in which the physician feels the texture, size, consistency, and location of body parts with

   the hands is _____.

6. The term for the act of walking is _____.

Say and Check

Say aloud the terms you wrote for Exercise 4. Use the Companion CD to check your pronunciations.

DIAGNOSTIC RADIOLOGY

3-28 Radiology is the branch of medicine concerned with x-rays and **radioactive** substances and with the diagnosis and treatment of disease using any of the various sources of radiant energy. Diagnostic radiology is used to establish or confirm a diagnosis. Learn the word parts below and their meanings.

Word Parts: Radiology

Combining Form	Meaning	Prefix	Meaning
ech(o), son(o)	sound	ultra-	excessive
electr(o)	electricity		
fluor(o)	emitting or reflecting light		
radi(o)*	radiant energy		
tom(o)	to cut		

*radi(o) sometimes means radius, a bone of the forearm.

3-29 Radio/graphy was the predominant means of diagnostic imaging for many years, with x-rays providing film images of internal structures. Almost everyone is familiar with a chest x-ray examination (see Figure 9-7).

This is a common type of diagnostic radiology. An x-ray image is a **radio/graph**; however, you have learned that -graph refers to an instrument used for recording. We see the same common usage in the word photograph, which refers to the picture obtained in photography. We

radiograph   commonly refer to a **radiographic** film as a _____, rather than a radiogram.

3-30 X-rays that pass through the patient expose the radiographic film or digital image receptor to create the image. X-radiation passes through different substances in the body to varying degrees, causing the image to appear dark, varying shades of gray, and white (see Figure 2-3). You learned in the previous chapter that substances that do not permit the passage of x-rays are

radiopaque   described as _____.

3-31 Additional diagnostic imaging modalities include the following:

- Contrast imaging
- Computed tomography (CT), formerly known as **computed axial tomography** (CAT)
- Nuclear scans (placing radioactive materials into body organs for the purpose of imaging)
- Magnetic resonance imaging (MRI)
- Sono/graphy (also called ultra/sono/graphy, **echo/graphy,** or ultra/sound)

3-32 Contrast imaging is the use of radiopaque materials to make internal organs visible on x-ray images. A contrast medium may be injected into a vessel, swallowed, or introduced into a body cavity, resulting in greater visibility of internal organs or cavities outlined by the contrast

contrast

material. This type of imaging is called _____ imaging. One example is a barium enema, the introduction of barium sulfate, a radiopaque contrast medium, into the rectum. A barium enema increases visibility of the inner contours of the lower intestinal tract (Figure 3-9).

3-33 Fluoro/scopy (floo-ros´kə-pe) is a method of viewing x-ray images in real time so that motion can be seen, and radiography provides a permanent record of the image at a particular point in time. Fluoroscopy and radiography are both used to follow the movement of the barium sulfate through the upper and lower portions of the gastro/intestinal (GI) tract. The studies are called upper GI series (or barium swallow) and lower GI series (barium enema), respectively.

fluoroscope
(floor´o-skōp)

Write the name of the instrument used in fluoroscopy: _____. This device projects an x-ray image on a monitor. Barium enemas and barium swallows are done for diagnosis of certain types of obstruction, ulcers, tumors, or other abnormalities.

tomography
(to-mog´rə-fe)

3-34 CT is the abbreviation for **computed** _____. This technique produces an image of a detailed cross section of tissue similar to what one would see if the body or body part were actually cut into sections. The tom(o) in tomo/graphy means to cut. The procedure, however, is painless and non/invasive, meaning it does not require the skin to be broken or a cavity or organ of the body to be entered. A CT scanner and a **tomogram** (to´mo-gram), the record produced, are shown in Figure 3-10.

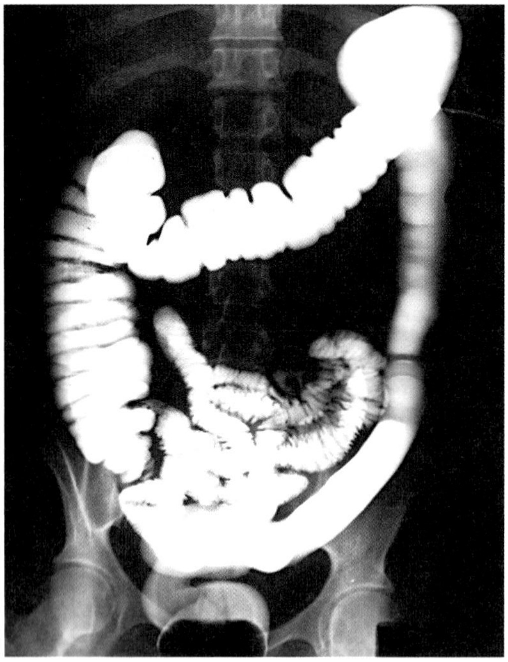

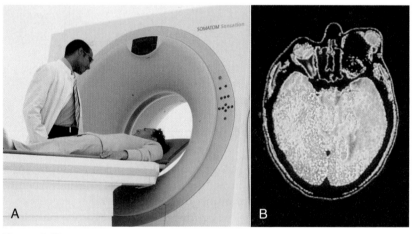

Figure 3-10 **Computed tomography of the brain. A,** Positioning of patient for computed tomography. **B,** Computed tomographic scan of the brain.

Figure 3-9 Contrast imaging. In this example of a barium enema, radiopaque barium sulfate is used to make the large intestine clearly visible.

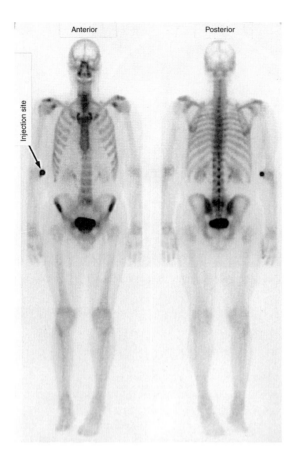

Anterior   Posterior

Injection site

Figure 3-11 Nuclear medicine. Administering a radiopharmaceutical that accumulates in a specific organ or structure provides information about its function, and to some degree its structure.

3-35 Nuclear medicine involves administering **radio/pharmaceuticals** (ra″de-o-fahr″mə-soo′tĭ-kəlz) to a patient orally, into the vein, or by having the patient breathe the material in vapor form. Computerized scanners called gamma cameras detect the radioactivity emitted by the patient and map its location to form an image of the organ or system (Figure 3-11). You remember that oral administration is by _____. Pharmaceuticals (fahr″mə-soo′tĭ-kəlz) are medicinal drugs, and radiopharmaceuticals are those that are radioactive.

mouth

> ➤ **KEY** POINT <u>An integrated system often presents a more complete picture</u>. **Positron emission tomography** (PET) is a type of computerized radiographic technique using radioactive substances to examine the metabolic activity of various body structures, such as the brain. A hybrid of both computed tomography and PET or emission scanning presents a more complete picture than attempting to correlate the two studies separately.

magnetic

3-36 MRI is the abbreviation for _____ **resonance** (rez′o-nəns) **imaging.** It is a noninvasive technique for visualizing internal structures and creates images based on the magnetic properties of chemical elements within the body, rather than using ionizing radiation such as x-rays. In addition, it produces superior soft-tissue resolution (Figure 3-12). Soft-tissue resolution distinguishes adjacent structures. Patients must remain motionless for a time and may experience anxiety because of being somewhat enclosed inside the scanner. The newer, open MRI scanners have eliminated much of the anxiety and can accommodate larger patients.

3-37 **Sono/graphy** (sə-nog′rə-fe) is known by different names, including **ultrasonography** (ul″trə-sə-nog′rə-fe) and diagnostic **ultrasound** (ul′trə-sound). The prefix ultra- means _____. Most of these names use the combining form son(o), which means sound. Sonography is the process of imaging deep structures of the body by sending and receiving high-frequency sound waves that are reflected back as echoes from tissue

excessive

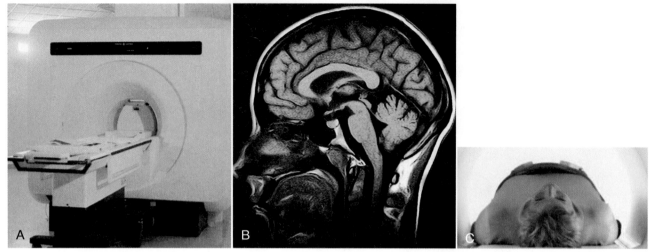

Figure 3-12 Magnetic resonance imaging (MRI). A, Clinical setting for magnetic resonance imaging. **B,** Image of the head. **C,** An open MRI.

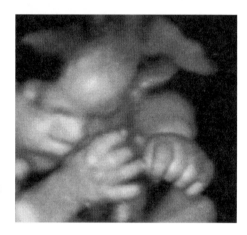

Figure 3-13 Ultrasound of third-trimester fetus. Utilizing sound waves at high frequency, ultrasound imaging provides two- and three-dimensional images of internal organs, including images of a developing fetus.

interfaces. Conventional sonography provides two-dimensional images, but the more recent scanners are capable of showing a three-dimensional perspective. Sonography is very safe because it is not invasive and does not use ionizing radiation. It has many medical applications, including imaging of the fetus (Figure 3-13).

EXERCISE 5

Write a word in each blank to complete these sentences.

1. The use of radiopaque materials to make internal organs visible on x-ray examination is called

   _____ imaging.

2. CT means computed _____.

3. Nuclear medicine involves placing _____ materials into body organs for the purpose of imaging.

4. Creating images based on the magnetic properties of chemical elements within the body is MRI, which means magnetic _____ imaging.

5. Ultrasonography provides imaging of internal structures by measuring and recording _____ waves.

THERAPEUTIC INTERVENTIONS

treatment	**3-38** **Therapeutic** (ther″ə-pu′tik) means pertaining to therapy or _____. Therapy is a term as well as a suffix, -therapy. Learn the following word parts and their meanings.

Word Parts: Treatment

Combining Form	Meaning	Combining Form	Meaning
algesi(o)	sensitivity to pain	therapeut(o)	treatment
chem(o)	chemical	therm(o)	heat
cry(o)	cold		
esthesi(o)	feeling or sensation	**Suffix**	**Meaning**
narc(o)	stupor	-therapy	treatment
pharmac(o), pharmaceut(i)	drugs or medicine		

treat	**3-39** Therapeutic radiology uses radiation to _____ cancer. Radiation therapy, also called radiation onco/logy, is the treatment of cancer using ionizing radiation, such as x-rays (Figure 3-14). The literal translation of onco/logy is the study of
tumors	_____, but radiation oncology is treatment of tumors using ionizing radiation.
	The source of radiation can be either external or internally implanted radioactive substances. The goal of this type of therapy is to deliver a maximum dose of radiation to the cancerous tissue and a minimal dose to the surrounding healthy tissue. A natural consequence of this type of therapy, unfortunately, is at least some damage to normal cells. Radiation oncology is used to
cancer	treat _____.
	3-40 In addition to radiation, several approaches are used to treat cancer, including surgery to remove the cancer and **chemo/therapy** (ke″mo-ther′ə-pe), which is treatment of disease by chemical agents. The combining form chem(o) means chemical.
neoplasms	**Anti/neo/plastics** (an″te-, an″ti-ne″o-plas′tiks) are medications that are used to treat malignant _____. Many malignant tumors are curable if detected and treated in the early stage.
cryotherapy (kri″o-ther′ə-pe)	**3-41** Both heat and cold are used in treatment. Treating with heat is called **thermotherapy** (thur″mo-ther′ə-pe). Use cry(o) to write a term that means treating with cold temperatures: _____.

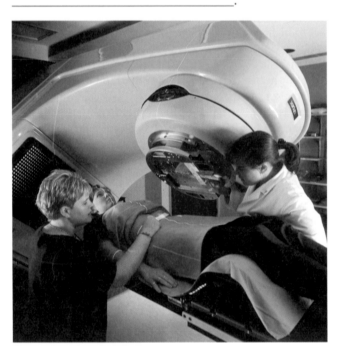

Figure 3-14 **Radiation therapy.**

medicine (drugs)

3-42 **Pharmaco/therapy** (fahr″mə-ko-ther′ə-pe) is the treatment of diseases with _____. A medication is a drug or medicine. Over-the-counter (OTC) medications can be obtained without a prescription, but a prescription drug (R$_x$) can be dispensed to the public only with an order by a properly authorized person. Some abbreviations that are commonly used by physicians when writing prescriptions follow.

Common Abbreviations Used in Writing Prescriptions

Abbreviation	Meaning	Abbreviation	Meaning
a.c.	before meals (ante cibum)	p.r.n.	as the occasion arises, as needed (pro re nata)
ad lib.	freely as needed, at pleasure (ad libitum)		
aq.	water (aqua)	q.i.d.	four times a day (quater in die)
b.i.d.	twice a day (bis in die)	stat.	immediately (statim)
NPO	nothing by mouth (nil per os)	t.i.d.	three times a day (ter in die)

without

3-43 You have heard of the word esthetic, also spelled aesthetic, which pertains to the sense of beauty or to sensation (feeling). The prefix an- means not or without; esthesi(o) refers to feeling (nervous sensation). **An/esthetic** (an″əs-thet′ik) means characterized by or producing anesthesia, and the same term is applied to a drug that brings about this numbing effect. Literal translation of an/esthesia (an″es-the′zhə) is _____ feeling but **anesthesia** means loss of sensation or loss of the ability to feel pain. The term anesthesia is formed by combining an- + esthesi(o) + -ia. (An "i" is dropped to avoid double "i" and to facilitate pronunciation.)

3-44 Anesthesia can occur with or without loss of consciousness. Anesthesia may be local, regional, or general. Local anesthesia is confined to one area of the body. Brief surgical or dental procedures can be performed when anesthesia is administered to a localized area; therefore it is called local anesthesia. When an anesthetic blocks a group of nerve fibers, regional anesthesia occurs. In this case, loss of feeling occurs in a certain region of the body. For this reason, it is called regional anesthesia.

general

General anesthesia produces a state of unconsciousness with absence of sensation over the entire body. The drugs producing this state are called _____ anesthetics.

3-45 Certain drugs called neuromuscular (noor″o-mus′ku-lər) blocking agents may be used to stop muscle contraction during surgery. **Neuro/muscul/ar** means pertaining to the _____ and muscles. Later you will study how the nerves and muscles interact to bring about movement.

nerves

3-46 An **an/alges/ic** (an″əl-je′zik) is a drug that relieves pain. The term results from combining an- + algesi(o) + -ic, but notice that one "i" is omitted to facilitate pronunciation. The combining form algesi(o) means sensitivity to _____.

pain

An analgesic such as aspirin is a type of **pharmaceutical** (fahr″mə-soo′tĭ-kəl). The term pharmaceutical means pertaining to pharmacy or drugs, but it also means a medicinal drug.

3-47 A **narcotic** (nahr-kot′ik) is a substance that produces insensibility or _____. The term also means a narcotic drug. Narcotic analgesics alter perception of pain, induce a feeling of euphoria, and may induce sleep. Repeated use of narcotics may result in physical and psychological dependence. In large amounts (for example, in an overdose [OD]), narcotics can depress respiration.

stupor

EXERCISE 6

Write a word in each blank to complete these sentences.

1. A drug that relieves pain is a/an _____.

2. Partial or complete loss of sensation is _____.

3. Drugs that are used to stop muscle contraction are _____ blocking agents.

4. A word that means pertaining to treatment is _____.

5. A/An _____ is a substance that produces insensibility or stupor.

6. Treatment of cancer using ionizing radiation is called _____ oncology.

7. Treatment with heat is called _____.

8. Treatment with cold temperatures is _____.

SUFFIXES PERTAINING TO SURGICAL PROCEDURES

operative

3-48 You learned earlier that surgery is a medical specialty concerned with operative procedures; therefore suffixes that pertain to surgical procedures are used to write words about _____ means of treating injury or disease.

All the suffixes in the following list are used to name various surgical procedures, and all form nouns when combined with other word parts.

Suffixes: Surgical Procedures

Suffix	Meaning
-centesis	surgical puncture to aspirate or remove fluid
-ectomy	excision (surgical removal or cutting out)
-lysis	process of loosening, freeing, or destroying
-pexy	surgical fixation (fastening in a fixed position)
-plasty	surgical repair
-rrhaphy	suture (uniting a wound by stitches)
-scope	instrument used for viewing (also used in diagnostic procedures)
-scopy	visual examination with a lighted instrument (not always a surgical procedure)
-stomy	formation of an opening
-tome	an instrument used for cutting
-tomy	incision (cutting into tissue)
-tripsy	surgical crushing

puncture

3-49 The suffix -centesis means surgical puncture. **Amnio/centesis** (am″ne-o-sen-te´sis) is surgical _____ of the **amnion** (am´ne-on), the thin membrane that surrounds the fetus during pregnancy. A small amount of **amniotic** (am″ne-ot´ik) fluid is removed for analysis to aid in the diagnosis of fetal abnormalities.

nerve

3-50 You learned in the last chapter that neur(o) means _____. **Neur/ectomy** (noo-rek´tə-me) is partial or total excision of a nerve. (Note that partial or total is implied. Literal translation does not always indicate the full meaning.)

3-51 Neuro/lysis (noo-rol´ĭ-sis) means destruction of nerve tissue or loosening of adhesions (ad-he´zhənz) surrounding a nerve. Fibrous structures called **adhesions** form when two structures abnormally attach to each other.

neurotripsy
(noo″ro-trip´se)

Change the suffix of neurolysis to form a word that specifically means surgical crushing of a nerve: _____.

-pexy

3-52 The suffix that means surgical fixation or fastening in a fixed position is _____.

ophthalmoplasty
(of-thal´mo-plas˝te)
incision

3-53 You learned earlier that ophthalm(o) means eye. Combine ophthalm(o) and -plasty to write a new term: _____. The term you just wrote means surgical repair of the eye.
    Ophthalmo/tomy (of˝thəl-mot´ə-me) is _____ of the eye (in this case, the eyeball).

-tome

3-54 Write the suffix that means an instrument used for cutting: _____.

> ➤ KEY POINT Be sure you can distinguish between the words incision and excision. **Incision** is cutting into. **Excision** is cutting out or removal.

-scopy

3-55 The suffix that means a visual examination with a lighted instrument is _____, and the instrument used is a scope, which can also be a suffix.

ear

3-56 **Oto/plasty** (o´to-plas˝te) is surgical repair of the _____.
    Rhinoplasty (ri´no-plas˝te) is surgical repair of the nose. This is a plastic surgery on the nose, either reconstructive or cosmetic (Figure 3-15).

3-57 Wounds are physical injuries to body tissue, whether caused by an accident or surgery. Where cutting or tearing has occurred, sutures or other materials (staples or wire) hold tissues together while wound healing takes place. To **suture** is to stitch together cut or torn edges of tissue with silk, catgut, wire, or synthetic material. Write the suffix that means suture:

-rrhaphy

_____.

    Superficial wounds often heal on their own or by the use of an adhesive spray or skin closure tapes. Deep wounds or those located where movement opens the cut edges generally require stronger materials such as sutures or staples (Figure 3-16).

> ➤ KEY POINT Absorbable vs. nonabsorbable suture material. Absorbable suture is digested over time by body enzymes. Catgut, prepared from the intestines of mammals (originally cats), is one of the best examples of absorbable suture material. Nonabsorbable suture either is left in the body, where it becomes embedded in scar tissue, or is removed when healing is complete. Silk, cotton, wire, and certain synthetic materials are not absorbed by the body and are examples of nonabsorbable sutures.

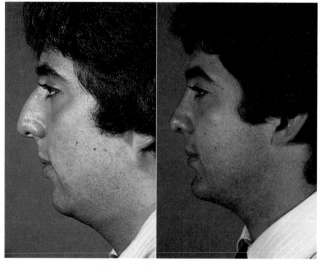

Figure 3-15 **Rhinoplasty.**

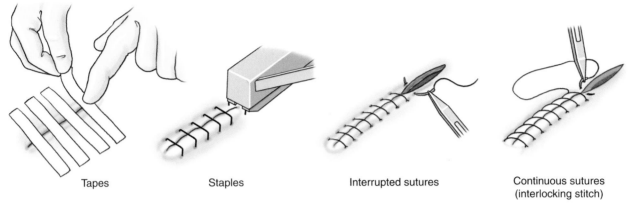

| Tapes | Staples | Interrupted sutures | Continuous sutures (interlocking stitch) |

Figure 3-16 Common skin closures.

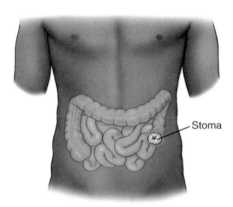

Stoma

Figure 3-17 Stoma. This is an example of surgical creation of a stoma, in this case an artificial anus, on the abdominal wall after removal of much of the large intestine.

3-58 Approximate (ə-prok´sĭ-māt″) means to bring close together by suture or other means. The act of bringing closer together is approximation. Tissue approximation can be accomplished with materials other than suture, such as tape, clips, and staples. In some instances, special adhesives that bond almost instantly can be sprayed on a wound to

approximate

_____ the skin, thus eliminating the need for stitches.

3-59 Perhaps you have heard of a **stoma,** which is a small opening, either natural or artificially created (Figure 3-17). The suffix that means formation of an opening is

-stomy

_____ and is derived from the same root as stoma.

EXERCISE 7

Match the suffixes in the left column with their meanings in the right column.

_____ 1. -centesis   _____ 6. -scopy

_____ 2. -ectomy   _____ 7. -stomy

_____ 3. -pexy   _____ 8. -tome

_____ 4. -plasty   _____ 9. -tomy

_____ 5. -rrhaphy   _____ 10. -tripsy

A. excision
B. formation of an opening
C. incision
D. instrument used for cutting
E. surgical crushing
F. surgical fixation
G. surgical puncture
H. surgical repair
I. suture
J. visual examination

EXERCISE 8

Use the following word parts to build terms. (Some word parts will be used more than once.)

amni(o), neur(o), ophthalm(o), ot(o), -centesis, -ectomy, -lysis, -plasty, -tripsy

1. excision of a nerve   _____/_____

2. surgical destruction of a nerve   _____/_____

3. surgical puncture of the amnion   _____/_____

4. surgical repair of the ear   _____/_____

5. surgical repair of the eye   _____/_____

6. surgical crushing of a nerve   _____/_____

Say and Check

Say aloud the terms you wrote for Exercise 8. Use the Companion CD to check your pronunciations.

COMBINING FORMS FOR SELECTED BODY STRUCTURES

3-60 Some combining forms for body structures are presented in this section. This list is not intended to be complete. You learned some combining forms in the previous chapter, and many more will be presented in later chapters. Adding various suffixes to the combining forms will determine how the resulting term is used in a sentence. Practice learning the combining forms in the same manner that you learned the list of suffixes pertaining to surgical procedures.

Combining Forms: Selected Body Structures

Combining Form(s)	Meaning	Combining Form(s)	Meaning
aden(o)	gland	mamm(o), mast(o)	breast
angi(o)	vessel	nephr(o), ren(o)	kidney
append(o), appendic(o)	appendix	oste(o)	bone
blephar(o)	eyelid	steth(o)	thorax (chest)
cerebr(o), encephal(o)	brain; cerebr(o) sometimes means cerebrum, the main portion of the brain	trache(o)	trachea (windpipe)
		tonsill(o)	tonsil
		vas(o)	vessel; ductus deferens (also called vas deferens, excretory duct of the testicle)
chir(o)	hand		
col(o), colon(o)	colon or large intestine		
cutane(o), derm(a), dermat(o)	skin		

colonoscope
(ko-lon′o-skōp)

3-61 Both **colono/scopy** (ko″lən-os′kə-pe) and **colo/scopy** (ko-los′ko-pe) mean an examination of the lining of the colon with a special instrument. The instrument is a _____, also called a **coloscope** (kol′o-skōp).

suture

3-62 **Colectomy** (ko-lek′tə-me) is excision of the colon (or a portion of it). **Colo/pexy** (ko′lo-pek″se) is surgical fixation of the colon, and **colo/rrhaphy** (ko-lor′ə-fe) is _____ of the colon.

blepharoplasty
(blef′ə-ro-plas″te)

3-63 Write a term that means surgical repair of the eyelid: _____.

hand

3-64 **Chiro/plasty** (ki′ro-plas″te) is plastic surgery on the _____.

3-65 Angio/plasty (an´je-o-plas˝te) means plastic surgery on vessels (in this case, blood vessels). **Angio/rrhaphy** (an˝je-or´ə-fe) means repair of a vessel by _____.

> ➤ **KEY** POINT <u>Be careful not to misspell terms that contain rrh</u>. Note that angiorrhaphy is spelled with two r's.

3-66 Osteo/tomy (os˝te-ot´ə-me) is cutting of a bone. Write a word that means the instrument used in osteotomy: _____.

suture

osteotome
(os´te-o-tōm´)
incision

3-67 Tracheo/tomy (tra˝ke-ot´ə-me) is an _____ made into the trachea (tra´ke-ə) through the neck. This procedure may be performed as an emergency measure to gain access to the airway below a blockage. Use -stomy to build a word that means the opening into the **trachea** through which a tube may be inserted: _____.

3-68 Combine aden(o) and -ectomy: _____. This new term means surgical removal of a gland.

tracheostomy
(tra´ke-os´tə-me)
adenectomy
(ad˝ə-nek´tə-me)

3-69 Use append(o) to write a word that means surgical removal of the appendix: _____.

3-70 Use mast(o) to write a term that means excision of a breast: _____.
   Mammo/plasty (mam´o-plas˝te) is surgical repair of the breast.

appendectomy
(ap˝en-dek´tə-me)

mastectomy
(mas-tek´tə-me)

> ➤ **KEY** POINT <u>Mammoplasty can enlarge or reduce the breasts</u>. Plastic surgery is performed to enlarge small breasts, to reduce or lift large or sagging breasts, or to reconstruct a breast after removal of a tumor. Enlarging the breasts is called augmentation mammoplasty (Figure 3-18).

3-71 Encephalo/tomy (en-sef˝ə-lot´ə-me) and **cerebro/tomy** (ser˝ə-brot´ə-me) mean _____ of the brain. Not all word parts that have the same meaning are interchangeable. You will learn which to use as you study them.
   Write a word that means the instrument used in encephalotomy: _____.

incision

encephalotome
(en-sef´ə-lə-tōm)

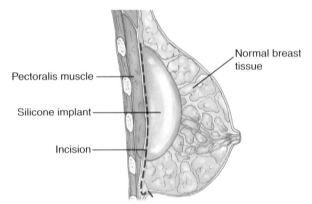

Pectoralis muscle

Normal breast tissue

Silicone implant

Incision

Figure 3-18 Augmentation mammoplasty. This type of augmentation is achieved by inserting envelopes filled with silicone gel (*shown here*) or saline beneath normal breast tissue or beneath the muscle of the chest. An incision below the breast causes the least obvious scarring.

EXERCISE 9

Write the meaning of the underlined part in each of the following words.

1. neuro<u>lysis</u> _____
2. <u>ophthalmo</u>plasty _____
3. color<u>rhaphy</u> _____
4. <u>oto</u>plasty _____
5. <u>encephalo</u>tomy _____
6. mammo<u>plasty</u> _____
7. <u>angio</u>rrhaphy _____
8. <u>adenectomy</u> _____
9. cerebro<u>tomy</u> _____
10. <u>blepharo</u>plasty _____

EXERCISE 10

Build It! *Use the following word parts to build terms. (Some word parts will be used more than once.)*

angi(o), append(o), blephar(o), chir(o), colon(o), encephal(o), mamm(o), oste(o)
-ectomy, -plasty, -rrhaphy, -scopy, -tome, -tomy

1. examination using a colonoscope _____/_____
2. excision of the appendix _____/_____
3. incision of the brain _____/_____
4. instrument for cutting bone _____/_____
5. surgical repair of the breast _____/_____
6. surgical repair of the eyelid _____/_____
7. surgical repair of the hand _____/_____
8. suture of a vessel _____/_____

Say and Check

Say aloud the terms you wrote for Exercise 10. Use the Companion CD to check your pronunciations.

CHAPTER ABBREVIATIONS*

a.c.	before meals *(ante cibum)*	**OD**	overdose; right eye *(oculus dexter)*
ad lib.	freely as needed, at pleasure *(ad libitum)*	**OTC**	over the counter (drug that can be obtained without a prescription)
aq.	water *(aqua)*	**PE**	physical examination
b.i.d.	twice a day *(bis in die)*	**PET**	positron emission tomography
C	Celsius	**p.r.n.**	as the occasion arises, as needed *(pro re nata)*
CT, CAT	computed tomography, computed axial tomography	**q.i.d.**	four times a day *(quater in die)*
ECG, EKG	electrocardiogram	**Rx**	prescription
F	Fahrenheit	**stat.**	immediately *(statim)*
MRI	magnetic resonance imaging	**t.i.d.**	three times a day *(ter in die)*
NPO	nothing by mouth *(nil per os)*	**WNL**	within normal limits

*Many of these abbreviations share their meanings with other terms.

Be Careful with These!

-gram (a record) vs. -graph (an instrument) vs. -graphy (a process)
-rrhage (excessive bleeding) vs. -rrhea (discharge) vs. -rrhexis (rupture)
-tome (cutting instrument) vs. -tomy (cutting into)
-tomy (cutting into) vs. -stomy (formation of an opening)
incision (cutting into) vs. excision (cutting out, removal)
diagnosis (identification of disease) vs. prognosis (predicted outcome)
sign (objective) vs. symptom (subjective)

▶ CHAPTER 3 REVIEW

Basic Understanding

Matching

I. *Match the following surgical suffixes with their meanings.*

_____ 1. -centesis	A. excision
_____ 2. -ectomy	B. formation of an opening
	C. surgical crushing
_____ 3. -pexy	D. surgical fixation
_____ 4. -plasty	E. surgical puncture
	F. surgical repair
_____ 5. -rrhaphy	G. suture
_____ 6. -scopy	H. visual examination
_____ 7. -stomy	
_____ 8. -tripsy	

Matching

II. *Match the following diagnostic suffixes with their meanings.*

_____ 1. -algia	A. dilatation
_____ 2. -ectasia	B. enlargement
	C. excessive bleeding
_____ 3. -edema	D. flow or discharge
_____ 4. -emesis	E. pain
	F. resembling
_____ 5. -malacia	G. rupture
_____ 6. -megaly	H. softening
	I. swelling
_____ 7. -oid	J. vomiting
_____ 8. -rrhagia	
_____ 9. -rrhea	
_____ 10. -rrhexis	

Word Analysis

III. *Break the following terms into their component parts and state the meaning of each word part. The first one is done as an example.*

1. amniocentesis   *amnio/centesis; amni/o, amnion; -centesis, surgical puncture*

2. blepharoplasty   _____

3. coloscopy   _____

4. echography   _____

5. electrocardiograph   _____

6. fluoroscope   _____

7. osteoid   _____

8. tomogram   _____

IV. *Write the meaning of these types of therapeutic terms:*

1. antineoplastics _____

2. chemotherapy _____

3. pharmacotherapy _____

4. thermotherapy _____

V. *Label these three aspects of the physical examination.*

1. _____   2. _____   3. _____

Multiple Choice

VI. *Circle one answer for each of the following questions.*

1. Susie tells the doctor that she has a sore throat. Which term describes the sore throat?
   (diagnosis, prognosis, sign, symptom)

2. Mr. Jones has plastic surgery on his hand. What is the name of this procedure?
   (carpectomy, chiroplasty, ophthalmoplasty, otoplasty)

3. Which word means stopping or controlling? (phobia, ptosis, spasm, stasis)

4. A 70-year-old man is told he has an enlarged heart. Which term describes his condition?
   (cardiomegaly, carditis, coronary artery disease, megalomania)

5. Which term means a record of the electrical impulses of the heart?
   (echography, electrocardiogram, electrocardiograph, electrocardiography)

6. Which term specifically means an opening into the trachea?
   (tracheoplasty, tracheostomy, tracheotome, tracheotomy)

7. Which term means removal of a gland? (adenectomy, adenotomy, appendotomy, appendectomy)

8. Which term means abnormal softening of the eye?
   (ophthalmalgia, ophthalmomalacia, ophthalmoscopy, ophthalmotomy)

9. Which term means an earache? (otodynia, otology, otoscope, otoscopy)

10. Which diagnostic procedure produces an image of a detailed cross-section of tissue similar to what one would see
    if the organ were actually cut into sections?
    (computed tomography, contrast imaging, electrocardiography, nuclear medicine imaging)

Writing Terms

VII. *Write a term for each clue that is given.*

1. excessive bleeding _____

2. excision of the colon _____

3. incision of the eye _____

4. instrument used in encephalotomy _____

5. plastic surgery of the ear _____

6. surgical crushing of a nerve _____

7. surgical fixation of the colon _____

8. suture of a vessel _____

9. swelling of the eyelid _____

10. visual examination of the ear _____

Say and Check

Say aloud the terms you wrote for Exercise VII. Use the Companion CD to check your pronunciations.

GREATER COMPREHENSION

Spelling
VIII. *Circle all misspelled terms and write their correct spellings.*

cerebrotomy   colorrhaphy   nurotripsy   ofthalmoplasty   simptom

Interpreting Abbreviations
IX. *Write the meaning of each of these abbreviations.*

1. CT _____

2. CAT _____

3. ECG _____

4. EKG _____

5. MRI _____

Pronunciation
X. *Indicate the primary-accented syllable in each of the following terms by marking it with an ´.*

1. appendectomy (ap en dek tə me)

2. calcipenia (kal sĭ pe ne ə)

3. encephalotomy (en sef ə lot ə me)

4. neurolysis (nŏŏ rol ĭ sis)

5. sonography (sə nog rə fe)

Say and Check

Say aloud the five terms in Exercise X. Use the Companion CD to check your pronunciations. In addition, be prepared to pronounce aloud these terms in class:

adhesions	dilatation	malacia	otoscopy
angiorrhaphy	electrocardiogram	neurectomy	stasis
blepharedema	electrocardiography	ophthalmalgia	suture
chiroplasty	encephalotomy	osteoid	tracheostomy
colonoscope	fluoroscopy	otorrhea	ultrasonography

Challenge

XI. Break these words into their component parts and write their meanings. Even if you have not seen these terms before, you may be able to break them apart and determine their meanings. The first is done as an example.

1. appendicitis   *appendic/itis: inflammation of the appendix*

2. chirospasm   _____

3. encephalitis   _____

4. rhinoplasty   _____

5. tracheoscopy   _____

(Use Appendix VI to check your answers.)

 PRONUNCIATION LIST

Use the Companion CD to review the terms that have been presented. Look closely at the spelling of each term as it is pronounced and be sure you know the meaning of each term.

adenectomy	colectomy	malacia	positron emission
adhesions	colonoscope	mammoplasty	tomography
ambulant	colonoscopy	mastectomy	prognosis
ambulation	colopexy	narcotic	pulse
ambulatory	colorrhaphy	neurectomy	radioactive
amniocentesis	coloscope	neurolysis	radiograph
amnion	coloscopy	neuromuscular	radiographic
amniotic	computed axial	neurotripsy	radiopharmaceuticals
analgesic	tomography	ophthalmalgia	rectal thermometer
anesthesia	computed tomography	ophthalmodynia	rectum
anesthetic	cryotherapy	ophthalmomalacia	respiration rate
angioplasty	diagnosis	ophthalmoplasty	rhinoplasty
angiorrhaphy	dilatation	ophthalmoscope	signs
antineoplastic	echography	ophthalmoscopy	sonography
appendectomy	edema	ophthalmotomy	spasm
approximate	electrocardiogram	oral thermometer	stasis
auscultation	electrocardiograph	osteoid	stethoscope
axillary	electrocardiography	osteotome	stoma
blepharedema	elephantiasis	osteotomy	suture
blepharoplasty	emesis	otalgia	symptoms
blepharospasm	encephalotome	otodynia	therapeutic
calcipenia	encephalotomy	otoplasty	thermotherapy
cannula	endoscope	otorrhea	tomogram
cardiomegaly	endoscopy	otoscope	trachea
catheter	excision	otoscopy	tracheostomy
catheterization	fluoroscope	palpation	tracheotomy
catheterize	fluoroscopy	percussion	tympanic thermometer
cerebrotomy	incision	pharmaceutical	ultrasonography
chemotherapy	magnetic resonance	pharmacotherapy	ultrasound
chiroplasty	imaging		

Español ENHANCING SPANISH COMMUNICATION

English	Spanish (pronunciation)
anesthesia	anestesia (ah-nes-TAY-se-ah)
appendix	apéndice (ah-PEN-de-say)
bone	hueso (oo-AY-so)
brain	cerebro (say-RAY-bro)
breast	seno (SAY-no)
diagnosis	diagnóstico (de-ag-NOS-te-co)
dilatation	dilatación (de-lah-tah-se-ON)
edema	hidropesía (e-dro-pay-SEE-ah)
electricity	electricidad (ay-lec-tre-se-DAHD)
enlargement	aumento (ah-oo-MEN-to)
eyelid	párpado (PAR-pah-do)
hand	mano (MAH-no)
heat	calor (cah-LOR)
hemorrhage	hemorragia (ay-mor-RAH-he-ah)
instrument	instrumento (ins-troo-MEN-to)
narcotic	narcótico (nar-CO-te-co)
pain	dolor (do-LOR)
physical examination	examen físico (ek-SAH-men FEE-se-co)
rupture	ruptura (roop-TOO-rah)
sound	sonido (so-NE-do)
spasm	espasmo (es-PAHS-mo)
suture	sutura (soo-TOO-rah)
swelling	hinchar (in-CHAR)
symptom	síntoma (SEEN-to-mah)
temperature	temperatura (tem-pay-rah-TOO-rah)
trachea	tráquea (TRAH-kay-ah)
vessel	vaso (VAH-so)
vomiting	vómito (VO-me-to)
wound	lesión (lay-se-ON)

Diseases and Disorders

4

*Using Suffixes to Build Terms
about Diseases and Disorders*

LEARNING GOALS

Basic Understanding
In this chapter you will learn to do the following:
1. Write the meanings of the word parts and use them to build and analyze terms.
2. Match suffixes pertaining to pathologies with their meanings or write their meanings.
3. Match miscellaneous suffixes for medical terms with their meanings or write their meanings.
4. Recognize combining forms for diseases and disorders and write their meanings or match them with their meanings.
5. Match the combining forms that describe color with their meanings or write their meanings.
6. Recognize several terms associated with diseases and disorders and write their meanings.
7. List four general types of microorganisms and the four classifications of bacteria.
8. Recognize several terms associated with bioterrorism.
9. Name the major causes of cancer deaths in men and women in the United States.
10. Recognize ways in which cancer cells metastasize.

Greater Comprehension
11. Spell medical terms accurately.
12. Write the meanings of the abbreviations.
13. Pronounce medical terms correctly.

MAJOR SECTIONS OF THIS CHAPTER:

- ❏ WORD PARTS PERTAINING TO PATHOLOGIES
- ❏ MISCELLANEOUS SUFFIXES
- ❏ COMBINING FORMS AND RELATED SUFFIXES
- ❏ ADDITIONAL COMBINING FORMS

- ❏ CLASSIFICATION OF DISEASE
- ❏ MICROORGANISMS AND INFECTIOUS DISEASES
- ❏ BIOTERRORISM
- ❏ DEATH AND CANCER STATISTICS

WORD PARTS PERTAINING TO PATHOLOGIES

diseases

4-1 Suffixes joined to combining forms are used to write the names of many diseases or disorders. Patho/logies are terms that represent the names of _____ or disorders. All the suffixes in the following list are used to write nouns.

Word Parts: Pathologies

Combining Form	Meaning	Suffix	Meaning
cancer(o), carcin(o)	cancer	-itis	inflammation
lith(o)	stone or calculus	-lith	stone or calculus
onc(o)	tumor	-mania	excessive preoccupation
path(o)	disease	-maniac	a person who shows excessive preoccupation
Suffix	**Meaning**	-oma	tumor
-cele	hernia (protrusion of all or part of an organ through the wall of the cavity that contains it)	-osis	condition (often an abnormal condition; sometimes an increase)
		-pathy	disease
-emia	condition of the blood	-phobia	abnormal fear
-ia-, -iasis	condition	-ptosis	prolapse (sagging)

tumor

onc(o)

4-2 Carcin/oma (kahr″sĭ-no´mə) is cancer or a cancer/ous tumor, because carcin(o) means cancer and -oma means _____.

You also know a combining form that means tumor, which is _____.

4-3 Many tumors are benign. For example, an **angi/oma** (an″je-o´mə) is a benign tumor made up of blood vessels or lymph vessels (Figure 4-1).

4-4 The suffix that means inflammation is -itis. **Ophthalm/itis** (of″thəl-mi´tis) is inflammation of the _____.

eye

appendix

otitis (o-ti´tis)

breast

nerve

Appendic/itis (ə-pen″dĭ-si´tis) is inflammation of the _____.

Write a term that means inflammation of the ear: _____.

Tonsillitis (ton″sĭ-li´tis) means inflammation of the tonsils, and **mast/itis** (mas-ti´tis) is inflammation of the _____.

Oste/itis (os″te-i´tis) is inflammation of a bone, and **neuritis** (noo-ri´tis) is inflammation of a _____.

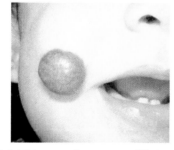

Figure 4-1 This type of angioma is filled with blood vessels. It is often called a birthmark because it is commonly found during infancy. It grows at first but may spontaneously disappear in early childhood. It can be surgically removed if bleeding or injury is a problem, or later for cosmetic reasons.

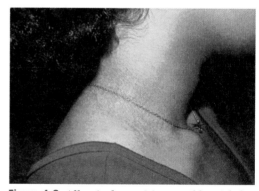

Figure 4-2 Allergic dermatitis caused by nickel in the necklace. Allergic dermatitis usually results from contact with jewelry, metal clasps, or coins. Other types of allergic dermatitis may be caused by contact with poison ivy, other metals, or chemicals, including latex, dyes, and perfumes.

adenitis (ad″ə-ni′tis)	Write a term that means inflammation of a gland: _____.
skin	**Dermat/itis** (dur″mə-ti′tis) is inflammation of the _____.

One type of dermatitis is caused by an allergic reaction (Figure 4-2).

4-5 The list of suffixes that pertain to pathologies contains a word that means protrusion of all or part of an organ through an abnormal opening. That word is

hernia (hur′ne-ə)
herniation

_____. This is also called **herniation** (hur″ne-a′shən).

An **encephalo/cele** (en-sef′ə-lo-sēl″) is _____ of part of the brain through an opening in the skull, also called **cerebral** (sə-re′brəl, ser′ə-brəl) hernia (Figure 4-3).

4-6 Phobia (fo′be-ə) means any persistent and irrational fear of something. The suffix -phobia

fear

means abnormal _____.

sagging

4-7 As a suffix, -ptosis (to′sis) means prolapse or _____. As a term, **ptosis** has two meanings. It can mean the same as the suffix. It is also sometimes used to mean prolapse of one or both eyelids (Figure 4-4).

-mania

4-8 A suffix that means excessive preoccupation is _____. **Mania** is a term that also means an emotional disorder (see Chapter 15). In **klepto/mania** (klep″to-ma′ne-ə), there is an excessive preoccupation that leads to an uncontrollable and recurrent urge to steal.

4-9 Pyro/mania (pi″ro-ma′ne-ə) is a disorder characterized by excessive preoccupation with

pyromaniac
(pi″ro-ma′ne-ak)

seeing or setting fires. A person having characteristics of pyromania is a _____.

4-10 Several suffixes mean condition. **Hyster/ia** is a condition so named because ancient Greeks believed that hysterical women suffered from a disturbed condition of the uterus (hyster(o)

condition

means uterus). **Neur/osis** (noo-ro′sis) is a nervous _____ or disorder that is not caused by a demonstrable structural change. The suffix -iasis also means condition.

disease

4-11 Both path(o) and the corresponding suffix -pathy mean _____. Literal interpretation of **adeno/pathy** (ad″ə-nop′ə-the) is any disease of a gland; however, it means enlargement of a gland, especially a gland of the lymphatic (lim-fat′ik) system (Figure 4-5).

4-12 Ophthalmopathy (of″thəl-mop′ə-the) means any disease of the eye.
Write a word that means any disease of the ear: _____.

otopathy
(o-top′ə-the)
blood

4-13 The suffix -emia means a condition of the _____.
Bacter/emia (bak″tər-e′me-ə) is the presence of bacteria in the blood.

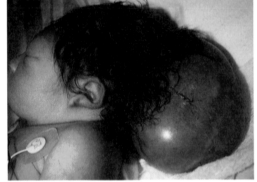

Figure 4-3 **An encephalocele.** Herniation of part of the brain and its covering through a defect in the skull.

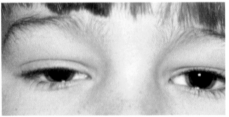

Figure 4-4 **Blepharoptosis.** Note the drooping of the right upper eyelid.

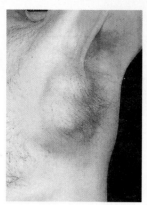

Figure 4-5 Enlarged lymph node. This particular type of adenopathy is enlargement of the axillary node, a gland of the lymphatic system located under the arm.

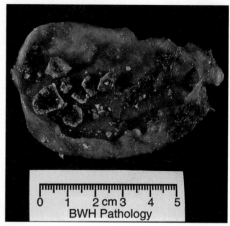

Figure 4-6 Gallstones in the gallbladder after removal. These stones may cause inflammation, jaundice, and pain and can lead to obstruction of the gallbladder.

-lith

4-14 A calculus is a stone. **Calculi** are abnormal stones formed in body tissues and are usually associated with the urinary tract (kidney stones) or the gallbladder or its ducts (Figure 4-6). Write a suffix that means a calculus: _____.

EXERCISE 1

Circle the correct answer to complete each sentence.

1. The suffix -iasis means (condition, dilatation, disease, excessive).
2. The suffix -itis means (deficiency, inflammation, sagging, soft).
3. The suffix -phobia means abnormal (bleeding, deficiency, fear, preoccupation).
4. The suffix -ptosis means (decreased, disease, fear, prolapse).
5. The suffix that means excessive preoccupation is (-mania, -maniac, -phobia, -ptosis).
6. The suffix that means tumor is (-oid, -oma, -osis, -rrhagia).
7. The suffix that means disease is (-pathy, -penia, -phobia, -ptosis).
8. The suffix that means hernia is (-cele, -megaly, -rrhea, -stasis).
9. The suffix that means blood is (-algia, -dynia, -emia, -emesis).
10. The suffix that means a stone or calculus is (-cele, -lith, -malacia, -megaly).

EXERCISE 2

Word Analysis. *Break these words into their component parts. Then write the meaning of each term.*

1. adenopathy _____
2. carcinoma _____
3. neurosis _____
4. otitis _____

 Say and Check

Say aloud the terms in Exercise 2. Use the Companion CD to check your pronunciations.

EXERCISE 3

Build It! *Use the following word parts to complete these sentences.*

angi(o), bacter(i), dermat(o), encephal(o), -cele, -emia, -itis, -oma

1. Inflammation of the skin is _____/_____.

2. A benign tumor made up of vessels is _____/_____.

3. Herniation of part of the brain through an opening in the skull is _____/_____.

4. The presence of bacteria in the blood is _____/_____.

Say and Check

Say aloud the terms you wrote for Exercise 3. Use the Companion CD to check your pronunciations.

MISCELLANEOUS SUFFIXES

4-15 Read through this list of suffixes and their meanings. Thinking of familiar words that contain these suffixes and using them on flashcards will help you remember their meanings.

Several suffixes mean pertaining to. You may be wondering how you know which suffix to use, and practice with flashcards will help you remember. **Neur/al** (noor´əl) means pertaining to a _____ or the nerves.

nerve

Miscellaneous Suffixes

Suffix	Meaning	Suffix	Meaning
-able, -ible	capable of, able to	-iac	one who suffers
-al, -ary, -eal, -ive, -tic	pertaining to	-opia	vision
-ase	enzyme	-ose	sugar
-eum, -ium	membrane	-ous	pertaining to or characterized by
-ia, -ism	condition or theory	-y	state or condition

breast

4-16 Mamm/ary (mam´ər-e) means pertaining to the _____.

cerebral

4-17 Combine cerebr(o) and -al to write a word that means pertaining to the brain: _____.

blepharal (blef´ə-ral)

4-18 Use -al to write a word that means pertaining to the eyelid: _____. The suffix -al is more commonly used than -eal; however, remember that -eal also means pertaining to.

pertaining

4-19 Divis/ive means _____ to something that causes division or dissension.

You have already learned that -ic means pertaining to, but -tic also means pertaining to. You will study the meaning of cyanosis later in this chapter; cyano/tic means pertaining to cyanosis.

4-20 You learned that pyro/mania is a disorder characterized by excessive preoccupation with seeing or setting fires. Mania could be broken down further to mean mani-, meaning mental aberration or madness, + -ia, condition; however, we recognize -mania as excessive preoccupation. A pyro/maniac is _____ affected with a compulsion to set fires.

one

vision	**4-21** Learning in Chapter 2 that opt(o) means vision should make it easier to remember that the suffix -opia also means _____.
capable	**4-22** Preventable means capable of being prevented. Both -able and -ible are used to mean _____ of.
membrane (mem´brān)	**4-23** The suffixes -eum and -ium mean _____. Perhaps you have heard of the **peritoneum** (per″ĭ-to-ne´əm), a membrane that lines the abdominal and pelvic cavities.

4-24 Two suffixes that may look similar but are very different are -ase and -ose. Words ending in -ase usually refer to enzymes (en´zīms), and those that end in -ose are usually sugars.

> ➤ **KEY** POINT Enzymes are often named by changing -ose to -ase. **Enzymes** cause chemical changes in other substances, such as sugars, and are usually named by adding -ase to the combining form of the substance on which they act.

The enzyme **lact/ase** (lak´tās) acts on the sugar **lact/ose** (lak´tōs). The combining form lact(o) means milk, and lactose is the main sugar found in milk. Lactose intolerance is a sensitivity disorder in which one cannot digest milk because of an inadequate production of the enzyme

lactase	_____.
characterized	**4-25** The suffix -ous means pertaining to or _____ by. According to one definition, the term suspicious means characterized by or indicative of suspicion.
condition	**4-26** The suffix -y means _____ and is often used to write other common suffixes, such as -pathy.

EXERCISE 4

Match suffixes in the left column with their meanings in the right column.

_____ 1. -able
_____ 2. -ase
_____ 3. -eum
_____ 4. -iac
_____ 5. -ism
_____ 6. -opia
_____ 7. -ose
_____ 8. -ous
_____ 9. -tic
_____ 10. -y

A. capable of
B. condition or theory
C. enzyme
D. membrane
E. one who suffers
F. pertaining to
G. pertaining to or characterized by
H. state or condition
I. sugar
J. vision

EXERCISE 5

Word Analysis. *Break these words into their component parts. Then write the meaning of each term.*

1. blepharal _____

2. cerebral _____

3. lactase _____

4. mammary _____

5. neural _____

(Use Appendix VI to check your answers.)

 Say and Check

Say aloud the terms in Exercise 5. Use the Companion CD to check your pronunciations.

COMBINING FORMS AND RELATED SUFFIXES

specialist

4-27 A few combining forms and suffixes are so often combined that they remain fixed and easily recognized. For example, log(o) means knowledge or words. The suffix -logist, meaning one who studies or a specialist, results when log(o) is combined with -ist. You have already learned that the suffix -logist means one who studies or a _____.

4-28 Study the following list of word parts and their meanings. All the suffixes are used to form nouns, with the exception of those ending in -ic and -tic. The suffixes -genic, -lytic, -phagic, and -trophic are used to form adjectives, words that modify or describe nouns. The suffix -ic can also be used to form words with several of the combining forms presented.

Selected Combining Forms and Related Suffixes

Combining Forms and Meanings	Suffixes and Meanings (if Different from the Combining Form)
cyt(o) means cell	-cyte
gen(o) means beginning, origin	-gen, that which generates; -genic (produced by or in); -genesis (producing or forming)
kinesi(o) means movement	-kinesia, -kinesis (movement, motion)
leps(o) means seizure	-lepsy
log(o) means knowledge or words	-logy (study or science of); -logist (one who studies)
lys(o) means destruction, dissolving	-lysin (that which destroys); -lysis (process of destroying); -lytic (capable of destroying; note the change in spelling)
megal(o) means large, enlarged	-megaly (enlargement)
metr(o) means measure; uterine tissue	-meter (instrument used to measure); -metry (process of measuring)
path(o) means disease	-pathy
phag(o) means eat, ingest	-phagia, -phagic, -phagy (eating, swallowing)
phas(o) means speech	-phasia
plas(o) means formation, development	-plasia (formation or development); -plasma (substance of cells)
plast(o) means repair	-plasty (surgical repair)
pleg(o) means paralysis	-plegia
schis(o), schiz(o), schist(o) mean split, cleft	-schisis
scler(o) means hard*	-sclerosis (hardening)
scop(o) means to examine, to view	-scope (instrument used for viewing); -scopy (process of visually examining)
troph(o) means nutrition	-trophic, -trophy

*Scler(o) sometimes means the sclera, the tough white outer coat of the eyeball.

4-29 A **micro/scope** (mi´kro-skōp) is an instrument for viewing objects that must be magnified so they can be studied. The process of viewing things with a microscope is

_____.

microscopy
(mi-kros´kə-pe)

4-30 **Hemo/lysis** (he-mol´ə-sis) is the destruction of red blood cells that results in the liberation of hemoglobin (he´mo-glo˝bin), a red pigment. A substance that causes hemolysis is a _____. This is also called a **hemolytic** (he˝mo-lit´ik) substance or agent. **Hemolyze** (he´mo-līz) is a verb that means to destroy red blood cells and cause them to release hemoglobin.

hemolysin
(he-mol´ə-sin)

4-31 The combining form megal(o) means large or enlarged. The suffix that means enlargement is _____ .

-megaly

4-32 A **patho/gen** (path´o-jən) is any agent or microorganism (mi˝kro-or´gən-iz-əm) that produces disease. **Patho/genic** (path-o-jen´ik) means capable of causing _____.

disease

4-33 A **carcino/gen** (kahr-sin´ə-jen) is a carcinogenic substance, one that produces cancer. The production or origin of cancer is called _____. Some commonly known carcinogens are listed in Table 4-1.

carcinogenesis
(kahr˝sĭ-no-jen´ə-sis)

4-34 **Cephalo/metry** (sef˝ə-lom´ə-tre) (cephal(o) means head) is measurement of the dimensions of the head. A device or instrument for measuring the head is a _____.

cephalometer
(sef˝ə-lom´ə-tər)

4-35 A **phago/cyte** (fa´go-sīt) is a cell that can ingest and destroy particulate substances such as bacteria. **Ingest** means to _____.

eat

4-36 **Epi/lepsy** (ep´ĭ-lep˝se) refers to a group of **neurologic** (noor˝o-loj´ik) disorders characterized by seizures. Literal translation of this term does not give the full meaning. Write this term that refers to a group of neurologic disorders characterized by seizures: _____.

epilepsy

4-37 **Dys/trophic** (dis-tro´fik) muscle deteriorates because of defective nutrition or metabolism. Any disorder caused by defective nutrition or metabolism is called a _____.

dystrophy (dis´trə-fe)

4-38 Kinesis is used both as a word and as the suffix -kinesis to mean _____.

movement

4-39 It will be easier to remember the meaning of -megaly if you associate it with mega-. Write a word of your choice that begins with mega-: _____. It is likely that the word large is part of the word's meaning.

4-40 Many words that contain the suffix -phag have something to do with _____ or swallowing.

eating

4-41 The suffix -phasia means _____.

speech

4-42 Because plas(o) means formation or development, the corresponding suffix is

_____.

-plasia

TABLE 4-1   Selected Commonly Known Carcinogens

Alcoholic beverage consumption	Coal tar	Smokeless tobacco
Arsenic	Coke oven emissions	Solar radiation and exposure to sunlamps and sunbeds
Asbestos	Environmental tobacco smoke	Soots
Benzene	Mustard gas	Tobacco smoking
Benzidine	Quartz	Vinyl chloride
Cadmium	Silica	

From Phipps WJ, Monahan FD, Sands JK et al: *Medical-surgical nursing: health and illness perspectives*, ed 7, St Louis, 2003, Mosby.

-plegia	**4-43** Pleg(o) means paralysis, and its corresponding suffix is _____.
-schisis	**4-44** Schis(o), schiz(o), and schist(o) mean split or cleft, and the corresponding suffix is _____.
-sclerosis	**4-45** Combine scler(o) and -osis to write a suffix that means hardening: _____. **Sclerosis** (sklə-ro´sis) is also a term that means hardening.

EXERCISE 6

Match the following suffixes in the left column with their meanings in the right column.

_____ 1. -cyte

_____ 2. -genic

_____ 3. -kinesia

_____ 4. -lepsy

_____ 5. -lysin

_____ 6. -lysis

_____ 7. -lytic

_____ 8. -plasty

_____ 9. -scope

_____ 10. -scopy

A. capable of destroying
B. cell
C. instrument used for viewing
D. movement
E. process of destroying
F. process of examining visually
G. produced by or in
H. surgical repair
I. seizure
J. that which destroys

EXERCISE 7

Match the following suffixes in the left column with their meanings in the right column.

_____ 1. -megaly

_____ 2. -meter

_____ 3. -metry

_____ 4. -pathy

_____ 5. -phagia

_____ 6. -phasia

_____ 7. -plegia

_____ 8. -schisis

_____ 9. -sclerosis

_____ 10. -trophy

A. disease
B. eating or swallowing
C. enlargement
D. hardening
E. instrument used to measure
F. nutrition
G. paralysis
H. process of measuring
I. speech
J. split or cleft

EXERCISE 8

Change the suffix in each underlined term to write a new word to complete these sentences. (No. 1 is done as an example.)

1. The instrument used in <u>microscopy</u> is a _____*microscope*_____.

2. The term for a substance that causes <u>hemolysis</u> is _____.

3. An adjective that means pertaining to <u>hemolysis</u> is _____.

4. <u>Ophthalmitis</u> is one type of a larger category that means any disease of the eye; this category is

   _____.

5. A <u>carcinogenic</u> substance is called a _____.

6. Measurement of the head using a <u>cephalometer</u> is called _____.

7. A <u>phagocytic</u> cell is called a _____.

8. A neurologic disorder in which <u>epileptic</u> seizures occur is called _____.

Say and Check

Say aloud the terms you wrote for Exercise 8. Use the Companion CD to check your pronunciations.

ADDITIONAL COMBINING FORMS

4-46 Most medical terms have one or more combining forms as their foundation. You will learn many new combining forms as you study later chapters pertaining to the body systems or the body in general. Some common combining forms will be introduced in this section. It is sometimes easier to learn them in groups, such as combining forms that describe color and commonly used combining forms.

   Study these combining forms for colors with their meanings. Again, try to think of words that you know that will help you remember the combining forms. For example, it will be easy to remember that chlor(o) means green if you think of chlorophyll, the pigment that makes plants green.

Combining Forms: Color

Combining Form	Meaning	Combining Form	Meaning
alb(o), albin(o), leuk(o), occasionally leuc(o)	white	erythr(o)	red
		melan(o)	black
chlor(o)	green	xanth(o)	yellow
cyan(o)	blue		

white

black

cyan(o)

4-47 An **albino** (al-bi´no) is an individual with congenital (kən-jen´ĭ-təl) absence of pigment in the skin, hair, and eyes. The skin and hair appear _____ because of the lack of pigment. An albino has a hereditary condition known as **albinism** (al´bĭ-niz-əm). Congenital conditions are those that exist at, or before, birth.

   Albinism is characterized by partial or total lack of the pigment called melanin (mel´ə-nin). **Melan/in** is a _____ or dark brown pigment that naturally occurs in the hair, skin, and eyes but is partially or totally lacking in albinos (Figure 4-7).

4-48 **Cyan/osis** (si˝ə-no´sis) is a bluish discoloration of the skin and mucous (mu´kəs) membranes caused by a deficiency of oxygen in the blood (Figure 4-8). The part of the term cyanosis that means blue is _____.

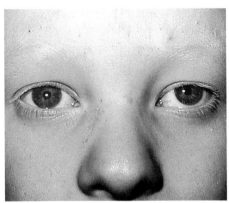

Figure 4-7 The white hair and pale skin of albinism. This condition is characterized by partial or total lack of melanin pigment in the body.

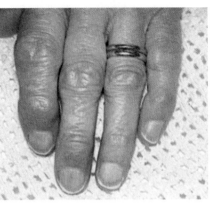

Figure 4-8 Cyanosis. The bluish discoloration is generally not as obvious as the extremely cyanotic skin of this patient.

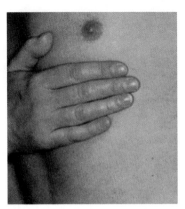

Figure 4-9 Jaundice. Note the contrast in the examiner's hand and the yellow discoloration of the skin of a patient with an acute liver disorder.

➤ **KEY** POINT <u>Mucous membranes secrete mucus.</u> Because they secrete mucus (mu´kəs), they are named mucous membranes. Membranes are sheets of tissue that cover or line various cavities or parts of the body that open to the outside, such as the lining of the mouth. (Note the different spelling of the body fluid mucus vs. the adjective mucous.)

red

4-49 Erythro/cytes (ə-rith´ro-sītz) are _____ blood cells. (Erythrocytes are not actually red but are so named because they contain a red-pigmented protein.)

yellow

4-50 Xantho/derma (zan″tho-der´mə) is a _____ coloration of the skin, as in jaundice (jawn´dis). **Jaundice** is characterized by the yellow discoloration of the skin, mucous membranes, and **sclerae** (sklēr´e) (white outer part of the eyeballs) and is caused by an increased amount of bilirubin in the blood (Figure 4-9).

EXERCISE 9

Write the color associated with each of the following combining forms.

1. alb(o)   _____
2. chlor(o)   _____
3. cyan(o)   _____
4. erythr(o) _____

5. leuk(o)   _____
6. melan(o)   _____
7. xanth(o)   _____

EXERCISE 10

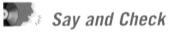 ***Build It!*** *Use the following word parts to complete these sentences.*

albin(o), cyan(o), erythr(o), xanth(o), -cyte, -derma, -ism, -osis

1. The literal translation of _____/_____ is yellow skin.
2. A bluish discoloration of the skin and mucous membranes is _____/_____.
3. A red blood cell, translated literally as red cell, is _____/_____.
4. An albino has a condition known as _____/_____.

Say and Check

Say aloud the terms you wrote for Exercise 10. Use the Companion CD to check your pronunciations.

4-51 Study the following list of commonly used combining forms. Again, try to think of words that you know that will help you remember the combining forms and put them on flash cards.

Commonly Used Combining Forms

Combining Form	Meaning	Combining Form	Meaning
bi(o)	life or living	nas(o), rhin(o)	nose
cephal(o)	head	pod(o)	foot
hist(o)	tissue	pyr(o)	fire
lact(o)	milk	tox(o), toxic(o)	poison
muscul(o), my(o)	muscle		

study

living

4-52 Bio/logy (bi-ol´ə-je) is the _____ of life and living things.
    Bi/opsy (bi´op-se) is the examination of tissue from the _____ body. A biopsy is either removal of a small piece of living tissue or the tissue excised or aspirated. **Aspiration** (as″pĭ-ra´shən) is drawing in or out by suction, usually aided by the use of a syringe or a suction device. The term also means the drawing of a foreign substance, such as the gastric contents, into the respiratory tract while taking a breath.

> ➤ KEY POINT Know the difference between a biopsy and an autopsy. In a **biopsy**, tissue is removed from a living body, sectioned, and viewed through a microscope to establish a precise diagnosis. In an **autopsy** (aw´top-se), organs and tissues of a dead body are studied to determine the cause of death or pathologic conditions. An autopsy is the same as a **postmortem** examination.

4-53 Histo/logy (his-tol´ə-je) is the study of the structure, composition, and function of tissues. A microscope is used to study the minute cells that make up tissue. Stated simply, histo/logy means the study of tissue. One who specializes in histology is a _____.

histologist
(his-tol´ə-jist)

4-54 Toxic (tok´sik) is another word for poisonous. The use of tox(o) and toxic(o) originates with a Greek word that means archery or the archer's bow. Ancient Greeks smeared poison on arrowheads that were used in hunting. In a regular dictionary, you will find the word toxophilite, one fond of archery. But in medical words, tox(o) almost always means _____. A **tox/in** (tok´sin) is a poison. If a substance is poisonous, it is said to be a toxic substance.

poison

4-55 Cyt(o) is the combining form for cell, so **cyto/toxic** (si´to-tok″sik) agents are those used to kill or poison _____, such as in cancer treatment. Cells are discussed in Chapter 6.

cells

4-56 Combine toxic(o) and -logy to write a word that means the science or study of poisons: _____.

    A specialist in toxicology is a _____.

toxicology
(tok″sĭ-kol´ə-je)
toxicologist
(tok″sĭ-kol´ə-jist)

4-57 Cephal/ic (sə-fal´ik) means pertaining to the _____.

head

4-58 You have learned that rhin(o) means nose. Another combining form that means nose is nas(o). Combine nas(o) and -al to write a word that means pertaining to the nose: _____.

nasal (na´zəl)

4-59 You learned that chir(o) means hand. Write the combining form from the list that means foot: _____.

pod(o)

my(o)	**4-60 Muscul/ar** (mus´ku-lər) means pertaining to muscle. Write the second combining form that means muscle: _____. Now write a term that means muscular pain by combining my(o) and -algia:
myalgia (mi-al´jə)	_____.

EXERCISE 11

Match each combining form in the left column with its meaning in the right column.

_____ 1. bi(o)

_____ 2. cephal(o)

_____ 3. electr(o)

_____ 4. hist(o)

_____ 5. my(o)

_____ 6. pod(o)

_____ 7. therm(o)

A. foot
B. electric
C. head
D. heat
E. living
F. muscle
G. tissue

EXERCISE 12

Build It! *Use these word parts to complete the following terms.*

bi(o), cephal(o), hist(o), my(o), nas(o), pod(o), pyr(o), toxic(o)

1. Pertaining to the head is _____ic.

2. The study of tissue is _____logy.

3. The examination of tissue from the living body to establish a diagnosis is called _____opsy.

4. Muscular pain is _____algia.

5. The study of poisons is _____logy.

6. Pain in the foot is called _____algia.

7. Pertaining to the nose is _____al.

8. An uncontrollable urge to see or set fires is _____mania.

CLASSIFICATION OF DISEASE

4-61 All parts of the body can be affected by disease.

> ➤ KEY POINT The term disease has two meanings. **Disease** (dĭ-zēz´) is a condition of abnormal structure or function of the body, or the term can refer to a specific illness or disorder characterized by a recognizable set of signs and symptoms.

Disorder (dis-or´dər) generally refers to a disruption or interference with normal functions, as a mental or nutritional disorder. Although the two terms seem similar, the general term

disease

that you will use for a condition of abnormal structure or function is _____.

4-62 There are several ways to classify diseases. A classification based on structure or function would be as follows:

- organic diseases, which are associated with a demonstrable physical change in an organ or tissues; for example, a tumor
- functional disorders, which are marked by signs or symptoms but no physical changes; for example, most psychologic disorders

physical

It is important to remember that organic diseases, unlike functional disorders, are associated with a demonstrable _____ change.

Classification of diseases according to cause includes infectious (caused by pathogenic organisms; for example, bacterial infections), hereditary, degenerative (deterioration of structure or function), traumatic, **auto/immune** (aw″to-ĭ-mūn′) (altered function of the immune system resulting in the production of antibodies against one's own cells), and related to nutritional deficiencies. The body's defense system is discussed in Chapter 7. The combining form aut(o) means self.

EXERCISE 13

Match the types of diseases and disorders in the left column with their descriptions in the right column.

_____ 1. functional disorder

_____ 2. infectious disease

_____ 3. organic disease

A. caused by pathogenic organisms
B. demonstrable physical change
C. signs or symptoms without physical change

idiopathic

iatrogenic
nosocomial

4-63 Other terms that are applied to various circumstances when disease occurs are idio/pathic (idi[o] means individual) diseases, iatro/genic (iatr[o] means physician or treatment) disorders, and nosocomial* (nos[o] means disease) infections. An **idiopathic disease** (id″e-o-path′ik) develops without an apparent or known cause (for example, high blood pressure for which there is no known cause). An **iatrogenic disorder** (i-at″ro-jen′ik) is an unfavorable response to medical treatment (for example, a transfusion reaction). **Nosocomial infections** (nos″o-ko′me-əl in-fek′shəns) are hospital-acquired infections (for example, infection of a surgical wound). More specifically, this type of infection was not present or incubating before the patient's admission to the hospital and is acquired 72 hours or longer after admission.

A disease that develops without an apparent or known cause is an _____ disease.

An unfavorable response to medical treatment is an _____ disorder, and a hospital-acquired infection is a _____ infection.

MICROORGANISMS AND INFECTIOUS DISEASES

4-64 Infectious diseases are caused by pathogenic organisms. **Contagious** (kən-ta′jəs) means capable of being transmitted from one individual to another. When contagious diseases are passed from one person to another, there is transmission of the disease.

> ➤ KEY POINT A **communicable disease** (kə-mu′nĭ-kə-bəl dĭ-zēz′), also called a contagious disease, is transmitted from one person or animal to another by one of these means:
> • directly by contact with discharges or airborne droplets from an infected person
> • indirectly via substances (for example, bloodborne transmission through contact with blood or body fluids that are contaminated with blood) or inanimate objects (such as a contaminated spoon)
> • via carriers called vectors (for example, mosquitoes, which transmit malaria)

communicable

A contagious disease is also called a _____ disease.

*Nosocomial (Greek: *nosokomeian,* hospital).

TABLE 4-2 Transmission of Infectious Diseases and Selected Examples*

Direct Contact
Common cold (9)
Genital warts (13)
Infectious mononucleosis (9)
Ringworm (16; also indirect contact)

Indirect Contact
Infected needles (acquired immunodeficiency syndrome; also direct contact, 13)
Infected secretions or droplets (influenza, 9)
Infected food (salmonellosis, hepatitis A, 10)
Airborne (tuberculosis, 9)
Infected blood (hepatitis B; also direct contact, 13)
Insect bite (malaria, 5)
Maternal-fetal infection (congenital syphilis, 13)

*The number within the parentheses indicates the chapter in which the condition is discussed.

A number of infectious diseases will be studied in this book (Table 4-2). Study the word parts that pertain to disease in the following list.

Word Parts: Disease

Word Part	Meaning	Combining Forms for Microorganisms	
iatr(o)	physician or treatment	bacter(i), bacteri(o)	bacteria
idi(o)	individual	fung(i), myc(o)	fungus
nos(o), path(o)	disease	staphyl(o)	grapelike cluster; uvula
seps(o)	infection	strept(o)	twisted
sept(i), sept(o)*	infection	vir(o), virus(o)	virus

*Also means septum.

EXERCISE 14

Match word parts with their meanings.

_____ 1. iatr(o)
_____ 2. idi(o)
_____ 3. nos(o)
_____ 4. seps(o)
_____ 5. staphyl(o)
_____ 6. strept(o)

A. disease
B. grapelike cluster
C. individual
D. infection
E. physician or treatment
F. twisted

4-65 Pathogenic microorganisms generally include various types of bacteria, fungi, viruses, and protozoa. **Micro/bio/logy** (mi″kro-bi-ol′ə-je) is a special branch of biology. Micro/bio/logists study bacteria, fungi, viruses, and other small organisms. Very small or microscopic organisms are called _____. **Virulence** (vir′u-ləns) means the degree of disease-causing capability of a microorganism.

microorganisms

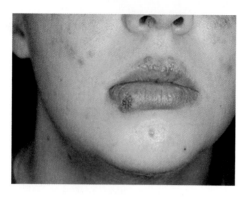

Figure 4-10 Fever blisters. This infection is caused by a virus that has an affinity for mucous membranes, particularly around the mouth and nose.

VIRUSES

4-66 A **virus** (vi′rəs) is a minute microorganism that replicates only within a cell of a living plant or animal, because viruses have no independent metabolic activity. Pathogenic viruses are responsible for human diseases such as influenza, hepatitis, and fever blisters (Figure 4-10). Microorganisms that can only replicate inside cells of another living organism are called

viruses   _____.

> ➤ **KEY** POINT <u>Viruses are much smaller than bacteria, fungi, and protozoa.</u> Because of their small size, viruses generally require the use of an electron microscope, which uses a beam of electrons rather than visible light. In contrast, a microbiologist uses a light microscope to view most bacteria, fungi, or protozoa.

BACTERIA

4-67 **Bacteria** (bak-tēr′e-ə) are unicellular micro/organisms that are classified according to their shape as spheric (cocci), rod-shaped (bacilli), spiral (spirochetes and spirilla), and comma-shaped (vibrios).

> ➤ **KEY** POINT <u>Most bacteria are helpful rather than harmful.</u> They are responsible for decay and are used extensively in food production, as in vinegar, sour cream, and cheese. Bacteria are also beneficial in the intestinal tract, where they are responsible for production of vitamin K. Normal bacterial flora of the skin help prevent the establishment of pathogenic bacteria. Only a few of the total number of species of bacteria are pathogenic.

Gram stain is a special staining technique that serves as a primary means of identifying and classifying bacteria. Gram-positive bacteria appear violet (purple) by this method, and gram-negative bacteria appear pinkish. Examine the **cocci** (kok′si) and **bacilli** (bə-sil′i) in Figure 4-11, and then write answers in these blanks.

spheric   The bacteria in Figure 4-11, *A,* are gram-positive cocci. This is determined by noting their
violet or purple   shape, which is _____, and their color, which is
elongated (rod-   _____. The bacteria in Figure 4-11, *B,* are gram-negative
shaped); pinkish   bacilli. This is determined by noting their shape, which is _____, and their color, which is _____.

4-68 Summarizing information in the previous frame, spheric bacteria are called

cocci   _____.
bacilli   Rod-shaped bacteria are called _____.
Bacteria that stain pink or red after undergoing Gram staining are called gram-
negative   _____, whereas bacteria that stain violet or purple are
positive   gram-_____.

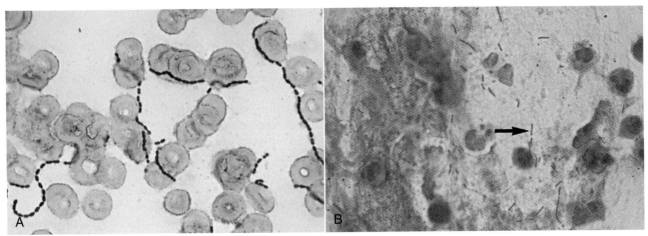

Figure 4-11 Gram stains of direct smears. Body fluids were collected, stained, and examined for the presence of leukocytes, bacteria, or other significant findings. **A,** Gram-positive cocci. The cocci are arranged in chains. Cells are also present on the smear. **B,** Gram-negative bacilli *(arrow)* are shown in the presence of numerous leukocytes.

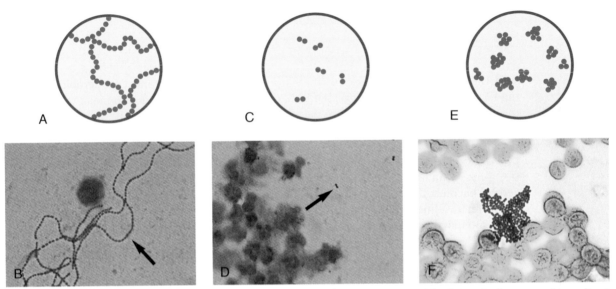

Figure 4-12 Three coccal arrangements. A, Schematic drawing of streptococci, cocci in chains. **B,** Streptococci in a direct smear. **C,** Schematic drawing of diplococci, cocci in pairs. **D,** Diplococci in a direct smear. **E,** Schematic drawing of staphylococci, cocci arranged in grapelike clusters. **F,** Staphylococci in a direct smear.

4-69 Cocci are often seen in particular arrangements when viewed with the microscope. For this reason, cocci are further classified according to their arrangement. Although there are others, three commonly seen arrangements are shown in Figure 4-12.

twisted

Learning these arrangements will give more meaning when you hear words such as streptococcal (often shortened to strep) and staphylococcal (staf″ə-lo-kok´əl) (often shortened to staph) infections. Although the combining form strept(o) means _____, **strepto/cocci** (strep″to-kok´si) appear to grow in a chain that does not necessarily appear twisted.

4-70 Strep throat is a common way of saying **strepto/coccal pharyng/itis** (strep″to-kok´əl far″in-ji´tis). Coccal means pertaining to cocci. The combining form pharyng(o) means pharynx or throat. In strep throat, inflammation of the throat is caused by what type of bacteria?

streptococci

_____ There are many types of streptococci, and not all streptococci cause pharyngitis.

staphylococci
(staf´ə-lo-kok´si)

4-71 The combining form staphyl(o) means a grapelike cluster. Cocci that are arranged like a cluster of grapes are called _____. You may have heard of someone having a staph infection. Staph is an abbreviation for staphylococci. The number of MRSA (methicillin-resistant *Staphylococcus aureus*) infections has risen, but this potentially deadly infection is usually preventable by practicing good hygiene. MRSA bacteria are resistant to many of the most powerful antibiotics.

The combining form staphyl(o) is also used to mean uvula (u´vu-lə), a structure that hangs like a bunch of grapes from the soft palate in the back of the mouth. When staphyl(o) is joined to cocci, it refers to a type of bacteria. When it is not joined to cocci, you will have to decide which meaning is intended.

diplococci

4-72 When cocci occur in pairs, they are called **diplococci** (dip˝lo-kok´si). The reason they remain in pairs is incomplete separation after cell division. Cocci in pairs (double cocci) are called _____. One well-known diplococcus is the bacteria that causes gonorrhea.

EXERCISE 15

List four general types of microorganisms.

1. _____   3. _____

2. _____   4. _____

anaerobic
(an´ə-ro´bik)

4-73 The need for oxygen varies with each species of bacteria, but most are aerobic. The combining form aer(o) means air or gas, but sometimes the usage is extended to mean oxygen. Two meanings of **aerobic** (ār-o´bik) are requiring oxygen (air) to maintain life and growing or occurring in the presence of oxygen. Use the prefix an- to write a term that means the opposite of aerobic: _____. Anaerobic bacteria (for example, the bacteria that cause tetanus) grow in the complete or almost complete absence of oxygen. **Tetanus** (tet´ə-nəs) is an acute, potentially fatal infection of the central nervous system caused by an anaerobic bacillus, *Clostridium tetani*. The bacteria can infect wounds and produce a lethal neurotoxin. Tetanus injections or booster shots (see Chapter 7) are generally recommended for persons who have a wound and have not been immunized within the past 5 years.

bacteria

4-74 An **anti/septic** (an˝tĭ-sep´tik) is a substance that inhibits the growth of microorganisms without necessarily killing them. **Bacterio/static** (bak-tēr˝e-o-stat´ik) means inhibiting the growth of bacteria. However, **bacteri/cidal** (bak-tēr˝ĭ-si´dəl) means killing _____. Both these terms can be written using either bacter(i) or bacteri(o), but note the more commonly used terms.

botulism

4-75 Bacterial food poisoning results from eating food that is contaminated by certain types of bacteria. One type is caused by various species of *Salmonella* and is characterized by fever and digestive signs and symptoms that include nausea, vomiting, and diarrhea beginning 8 to 48 hours after eating contaminated food. Similar symptoms caused by another type of bacteria, *Staphylococcus*, usually appear much sooner and usually last only a few hours. **Botulism** (boch´ə-liz-əm), an often fatal form of food poisoning, is caused by a toxin produced by the anaerobic bacterium *Clostridium botulinum*. Most botulism occurs after eating improperly canned or improperly cooked foods. Of the types of bacterial food poisoning described, the one that is caused by a toxin and can be fatal is called _____.

spiral

4-76 **Spirochetes** (spi´ro-kētz) are _____-shaped bacteria. Note the spiral shape of the spirochete in Figure 4-13. The special technique called dark-field preparation is used to search for spirochetes that cause **syphilis** (sif´ĭ-lis). The slide is examined using a microscope in which the spirochetes appear many times larger (400 times or more) than their actual size. The organism can often be observed in material from a chancre, the painless skin lesion that begins at the infection site in the early stages of syphilis. Syphilis is a sexually

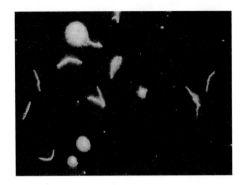

Figure 4-13 Dark-field preparation demonstrating the spirochete of syphilis. The organism, *Treponema pallidum,* can be observed in material from a chancre in the early stages of syphilis using a special dark-field preparation. The organisms are long, tightly coiled spirals that are motile.

transmitted disease (STD), formerly called venereal disease. STDs are usually acquired by sexual intercourse or genital contact.

Vibrios (vib´re-os) are comma-shaped bacteria. **Cholera** (kol´ar-ə) and several other epidemic forms of gastro/enter/itis (gas″tro-en″tər-i´tis), inflammation of the stomach and intestines, are caused by various types of pathogenic vibrios.

FUNGI

4-77 Fungi (fun´ji) are microorganisms that feed by absorbing organic molecules from their surroundings. They may be parasitic and may invade living organic substances. Yeasts and molds are included in this group.

> ➤ **KEY** POINT <u>Only a few of the known fungi are pathogenic to humans</u>. *Candida albicans,* a microscopic fungus, is normally present in the mouth, intestinal tract, and vagina of healthy individuals. Infections may occur under certain circumstances, particularly when immunity is deficient (Figure 4-14). Athlete's foot and ringworm are other diseases caused by fungi.

Ringworm is so named because of the shape of the lesion on the skin. Ringworm is not caused by a worm but by a _____.

fungus

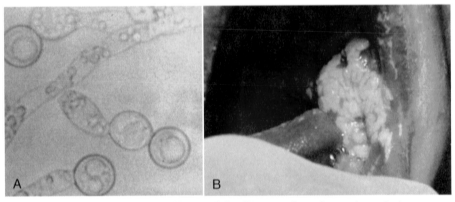

A   B

Figure 4-14 Oral infection caused by *Candida albicans,* a fungal organism. A, Appearance of the microscopic fungi, showing the way in which the fungi multiply by budding. **B,** Thrush, an oral infection of the mouth, caused by *C. albicans.*

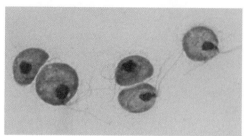

Figure 4-15 *Trichomonas* in a stained smear. *Trichomonas* is a sexually-transmitted protozoon that is pathogenic to humans. Five protozoa are shown. The flagella, the hairlike projections that the protozoa use for movement, are visible.

PROTOZOA

4-78 Protozoa (pro″tə-zo′ə) are the simplest organisms of the animal kingdom.

> ➤ **KEY** POINT <u>Only a few species of protozoa are pathogenic to humans.</u> **Malaria** (mə-lar′e-ə), an infectious illness caused by one or more of several species of pathogenic protozoa, is transmitted by the bite of an insect vector, the female *Anopheles* mosquito. In its acute form, the disease is characterized by anemia, enlarged spleen, chills, and fever. **Trichomoniasis** (trik″o-mo-ni′ə-sis), another human protozoal infection, is a sexually transmitted disease. A stained preparation of these protozoa is shown in Figure 4-15.

4-79 Typical laboratory microscopes provide low power and high power magnifications of 100× and 400×, meaning 100 times and 400 times the actual sizes of the objects viewed. Each microscopically-viewed area is called a field of vision. As an estimation of quantity, microscopy laboratory reports often cite the number of organisms per high-power field (HPF), not just in reporting bacteria but also in other areas such as the study of urine or in hematology. Sometimes the number of organisms or cells per low-power field (LPF) is reported. HPF and LPF are abbreviations for microscopic high- and _____-power field, respectively.

low

EXERCISE 16

Match the types of bacteria in the left column with clues in the right column.

_____ 1. bacilli

_____ 2. diplococci

_____ 3. spirochetes

_____ 4. staphylococci

_____ 5. streptococci

_____ 6. vibrios

A. comma-shaped bacteria
B. rod-shaped bacteria
C. spheric bacteria in grapelike clusters
D. spheric bacteria in pairs
E. spheric bacteria in twisted chains
F. spiral bacteria

BIOTERRORISM

4-80 Weapons of mass destruction (WMD) have been a concern for many years but have come to the forefront as acts of terrorism have increased. The Federal Emergency Management Agency (FEMA) and the Centers for Disease Control and Prevention (CDC) use the following categories to define weapons of mass destruction:

B   Biologic
N   Nuclear
I   Incendiary (incendiaries, flammable substances used to ignite fires, or explosives)
C   Chemical
E   Explosive (A bomb constructed and deployed in a manner other than conventional military action is an improvised explosive device [IED]. These types of bombs may be partially composed of conventional military explosives attached to a detonating mechanism.)

living

Health care providers must be trained to recognize and deal with these emergencies. Biologic weapons of mass destruction use _____ organisms that are pathogenic to humans.

4-81 Bio/terrorism (bi″o-ter′ər-izm) is the use of pathogenic biologic agents to cause terror in a population.

> ➤ **KEY** POINT <u>High priority agents of bioterrorism pose a risk to national security</u>. Biologic agents are placed on this list largely for the following reasons:
> - They can be easily disseminated (distributed over a general area) or transmitted from person to person.
> - They cause high mortality and have a major public health impact.
> - They can cause public panic and social disruption.
> - They require special action for public health preparedness.

bioterrorism

The use of pathogenic biologic agents to cause terror in a population is known as _____. The CDC lists the highest priority agents as those that cause the following diseases: anthrax, botulism, plague, smallpox, tularemia, and viral hemorrhagic fevers. Botulism, a type of bacterial food poisoning, was described in the previous section. It is suggested that you use a medical dictionary to learn additional facts about these diseases. The CDC defines other categories of biologic agents that could be used or engineered for mass dissemination. Many hospitals are implementing emergency preparedness plans to deal with threats or acts of bioterrorism.

EXERCISE 17

Write words in the blanks to complete these sentences.

1. WMD is the abbreviation for _____ of mass destruction.

2. CDC is the abbreviation for Centers for _____ Control and Prevention.

3. The use of pathogenic biologic agents to cause terror in a population is called _____.

4. A term that means scattered or distributed over a general area is _____.

DEATH AND CANCER STATISTICS

cancer

4-82 You have already learned that neoplasms are also called tumors, and malignant neoplasm is the same as _____.

> ➤ **KEY** POINT <u>The term cancer is used in two ways</u>. **Cancer** (kan′sər) is a neoplasm characterized by uncontrolled and unregulated growth of cells that tend to invade surrounding tissue and to spread (metastasize). The term cancer also refers to a group of more than 200 diseases characterized by the presence of malignant cells.

4-83 Cancer can occur in persons of all ages, can occur anywhere in the body, and is the second most common cause of death in the United States. Many potential causes of cancer are recognized, but the majority of cancers are attributed to cigarette smoking, exposure to carcinogenic chemicals, radiation, and ultraviolet rays. Carcino/genic refers to the ability to

cause

_____ cancer.

development

4-84 Carcino/genesis is the _____ of cancer. In **metastasis** (mə-tas′tə-sis), cells move from their primary location. Common sites to which cells metastasize are lymph nodes, bone, lung, brain, and liver. There are four ways in which cancer cells **metastasize** (mə-tas′tə-sīz), or form new cancers in other places (Table 4-3).

TABLE 4-3	Modes of Metastasis of Cancer Cells from Malignant Tumors

1. Direct invasion of surrounding tissue
2. Invasion of the bloodstream, where the cancer cells may be carried to distant sites
3. Invasion of lymphatic vessels, where the cancer cells may be transported to implant in the lymph nodes or other distant sites
4. Spread of cancer cells throughout a body cavity

4-85 The National Center for Health Statistics lists heart disease as the number one cause of adult deaths in the United States, and cancer is listed as number two. Currently, one of four deaths in the United States is caused by cancer. In spite of the growing optimism with improvements in prevention, early detection, and treatment of many forms of cancer, the total number of recorded cancer deaths in the United States continues to increase slightly because of the aging and expanding population.

heart

The main cause of adult deaths in the United States is _____ disease, and the second leading cause of death is cancer.

Although cancer is sometimes regarded as a disease of older individuals, it is also the second leading cause of death among children ages 1 to 14 years in the United States, with accidents being the most common cause of death.

4-86 Each year the American Cancer Society (ACS) estimates the number of new cancer cases and deaths expected in the United States. Most skin cancers and most in situ cancers are not included in cancer predictions and statistics about cancer deaths. *In situ* is Latin and means localized and not invading the surrounding tissue. A word that means *in situ* is

localized

_____. The incidence of cancer and cancer death varies by type in men and women. Look at estimated incidences and deaths for men and women in Table 4-4. Look first at the estimated new cases in American men. The site of the greatest number of

prostate

estimated new cancer cases in men is the _____.

In women, what is the site of the greatest number of estimated new cancer cases?

breast
lung

_____

Notice that cancer of the _____ and bronchus ranks number one in estimated deaths from cancer for all adults.

4-87 Lung cancer remains a highly lethal disease, although significant improvements in treatment have occurred. The most important cause of lung cancer is tobacco smoking. Besides cigarettes, exposure to airborne asbestos, uranium, radon, and high doses of ionizing radiation have been linked to increased incidence of lung cancer, according to the American Cancer Society.

cigarettes
(or smoking)

However, the greatest cause of lung cancer is _____.

Cigarette smoking increases the risk of lung cancer more than the risk of cancer at any other site, but cigarette smoking—as well as pipe smoking—also multiplies the risk of cancers of the lip, mouth, tongue, and throat.

TABLE 4-4	Estimated New Cases and Cancer Deaths for Adults by Gender, United States, 2007

Men	Women
Estimated New Cases for the Three Major Causes	
Prostate (29%)	Breast (26%)
Lung and bronchus (15%)	Lung and bronchus (15%)
Colon and rectum (10%)	Colon and rectum (11%)
Estimated Deaths for the Three Major Causes	
Lung and bronchus (31%)	Lung and bronchus (26%)
Prostate (9%)	Breast (15%)
Colon and rectum (9%)	Colon and rectum (10%)

Data from Cancer Statistics, 2007, CA, *Cancer for Clin* 57:1, 2007.
Excludes basal and squamous cell skin cancers and in situ carcinomas.

cervix

4-88 Table 4-4 gives only the major causes of estimated new cancer cases and deaths in the United States, and cervical cancer is not listed. But worldwide, cervical cancer is the third most common type of cancer in women. Cervical cancer starts in the cervix, the lower part of the uterus (womb) that opens at the top of the vagina. Almost all cervical cancers are caused by HPV (human papillomavirus), for which a vaccine was developed in 2006. Cervical cancer is cancer of the _____.

cancer

4-89 The development of cervical cancer is very slow, and the pre/cancerous condition can be detected by a test called a Pap smear. Pre/cancerous means likely to become _____.
 The unique aspect of cervical cancer is that a vaccine, the first approved vaccine targeted to prevent a specific type of cancer, is available; it prevents precancerous lesions for most types of cervical cancer. Read more about the risk factors and prevention of cervical cancer in Chapter 13.

EXERCISE 18

Describe four ways in which cancer metastasizes:

1. _____

2. _____

3. _____

4. _____

EXERCISE 19

Write a word in each blank to complete these sentences.

1. The number one cause of death in the United States is _____ disease.

2. The number two cause of death in the United States is _____.

3. A vaccine that prevents most types of _____ cancer is available.

CHAPTER ABBREVIATIONS*

ACS	American Cancer Society	LPF	low-power field
CDC	Centers for Disease Control and Prevention	MRSA	methicillin-resistant *Staphylococcus aureus*
FEMA	Federal Emergency Management Agency	staph	staphylococci
HPF	high-power field	STD	sexually transmitted disease
HPV	human papillomavirus	strep	streptococci
IED	improvised explosive device	WMD	weapons of mass destruction

*Many of these abbreviations share their meanings with other terms.

Be Careful with These!

-ase (enzyme) vs. -ose (sugar)
-ia (condition) vs. -iac (one who suffers)
iatrogenic (unfavorable response to medical treatment) vs. idiopathic (disease without an apparent or known cause)
-lysin (that which destroys) vs. -lytic (capable of destroying)
-phagia (eating, swallowing) vs. -phasia (speech)
-plasia (formation, development) vs. -plasty (surgical repair)

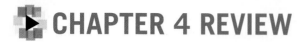 **CHAPTER 4 REVIEW**

Basic Understanding

Matching

I. Match suffixes in the left column with their meanings in the right column.

_____ 1. -cele
_____ 2. -emia
_____ 3. -iasis
_____ 4. -lith
_____ 5. -mania
_____ 6. -oma
_____ 7. -phobia
_____ 8. -ptosis

A. abnormal fear
B. calculus
C. condition
D. condition of the blood
E. excessive preoccupation
F. hernia
G. prolapse
H. tumor

II. Match combining forms for colors and their meanings.

_____ 1. alb(o)
_____ 2. chlor(o)
_____ 3. cyan(o)
_____ 4. erythr(o)
_____ 5. melan(o)
_____ 6. xanth(o)

A. black
B. blue
C. green
D. red
E. white
F. yellow

Multiple Choice

III. Circle the correct answer to complete each sentence.

1. Julie experiences redness of the skin around her recently acquired earrings. What is Julie's condition called? (dermatitis, malacia, mastitis, ptosis)

2. When James and Cynthia's baby is born, it has a yellow discoloration of the skin and mucous membranes. Which condition is most likely? (albinism, cyanosis, jaundice, myalgia)

3. Johnny, a college student, sees the physician and is told that his appendix is inflamed. What is the name of his condition? (appendectomy, appendicitis, appendorrhexis, appendotomy)

4. Karen sustains a severe head injury in which there is herniation of the brain through an opening in the skull. What is the name of this pathology? (cerebritis, cerebrotomy, encephalocele, encephaloplasty)

5. Ken suffers an abnormal fear of heights. What type of pathology does he have? (dilatation, mania, phobia, ptosis)

6. What is the term for examination of tissue from a living body? (autopsy, biopsy, postmortem, ptosis)

7. Which term means any disease of the ear? (adenopathy, ophthalmopathy, osteitis, otopathy)

8. Histology means the study of which of the following? (disease, function, structure, tissue)

9. Which of the following means a cell that can ingest and destroy particulate substances? (carcinogen, erythrocyte, leukocytosis, phagocyte)

10. Which of the following is a verb that means to destroy red blood cells and cause them to release hemoglobin? (hemolysin, hemolysis, hemolytic, hemolyze)

11. Which of the following is a general term for a disease associated with a demonstrable physical change? (autoimmune disease, communicable disease, functional disorder, organic disease)

12. Which of the following terms applies to a hospital-acquired infection? (iatrogenic, idiopathic, nosocomial, therapeutic)

13. Which of the following causes the most deaths in the United States? (automobile accidents, cancer, heart disease, homicides)

14. Which type of cancer causes the greatest number of deaths in males in the United States? (prostate, lung, colon, rectum)

15. Which of the following is the most common type of cancer in women in the United States? (breast, lungs, cervical, colon)

16. What is a common name for streptococcal pharyngitis? (infectious mononucleosis, ringworm, salmonellosis, strep throat)

Listing

IV. *Name four general types of microorganisms and describe at least one outstanding feature.*

1. _____

2. _____

3. _____

4. _____

V. *List four general types of bacteria.*

1. _____   3. _____

2. _____   4. _____

VI. *Describe four ways in which cancer cells metastasize.*

1. _____

2. _____

3. _____

4. _____

Photo ID

VII. *Use word parts to write terms to label pictures 1 through 4.*

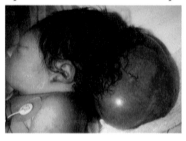

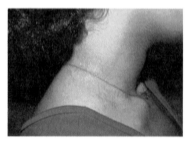

1. _____/_____   2. _____/_____
    (brain)   (hernia)   (skin)   (inflammation)

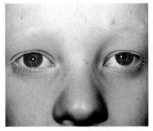

3. _____/_____
   (white)   (condition)

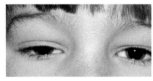

4. _____/_____
   (eyelid)   (prolapse)

Writing Terms

VIII. *Write a term for each clue that is given.*

1. a red (blood) cell _____

2. a substance that causes hemolysis _____

3. a substance that produces cancer _____

4. any disease of the eye _____

5. excessive preoccupation with fires _____

6. inflammation of a bone _____

7. muscular pain _____

8. pertaining to the nose _____

9. stones _____

10. viewing things with a microscope _____

 ## Say and Check

Say aloud the terms you wrote for Exercise VIII. Use the Companion CD to check your pronunciations.

Greater Comprehension

Spelling

IX. *Circle all misspelled terms and write their correct spellings.*

angioma   blepharal   cefalic   epilepsy   serebral

Interpreting Abbreviations

X. *Write the meanings of these abbreviations.*

1. ACS _____

2. FEMA _____

3. HPF _____

4. IED _____

5. WMD _____

Pronunciation

XI. Indicate the primary-accented syllable in each term by marking it with an ´.

1. adenopathy (ad ə nop ə the)

4. hemolytic (he mo lit ik)

2. autopsy (aw top se)

5. lactose (lak tōs)

3. cephalometry (sef ə lom ə tre)

 Say and Check

Say aloud the five terms in Exercise XI. Use the Companion CD to check your pronunciations. In addition, be prepared to pronounce aloud these terms in class:

albinism	carcinogenesis	hemolyze	otopathy
anaerobic	cerebral	jaundice	phagocyte
angioma	dystrophic	microscopy	ptosis
biopsy	encephalocele	neurologic	staphylococci
blepharal	hemolysin	ophthalmopathy	xanthoderma

Challenge

XII. Break these words into their component parts and write their meanings. Perhaps you haven't seen the terms before, but you may be able to break them apart and determine their meanings.

1. blepharitis _____

2. leukocyte _____

3. myocele _____

4. neurogenic _____

5. xanthous _____

(Check your answers with the solutions in Appendix VI.)

 PRONUNCIATION LIST

Use the Companion CD to review the terms that have been presented. Look closely at the spelling of each term as it is pronounced and be sure you know the meaning of each term.

adenitis	bioterrorism	disease	idiopathic disease
adenopathy	blepharal	disorder	ingest
aerobic	botulism	dystrophic	jaundice
albinism	calculi	dystrophy	kleptomania
albino	cancer	encephalocele	lactase
anaerobic	carcinogen	enzyme	lactose
angioma	carcinogenesis	epilepsy	malaria
antiseptic	cephalic	erythrocyte	mammary
appendicitis	cephalometer	fungi	mania
aspiration	cephalometry	hemolysin	mastitis
autoimmune	cerebral	hemolysis	melanin
autopsy	cholera	hemolytic	metastasis
bacilli	cocci	hemolyze	metastasize
bacteremia	communicable disease	hernia	microbiology
bacteria	contagious	herniation	microorganisms
bactericidal	cyanosis	histologist	microscope
bacteriostatic	cytotoxic	histology	microscopy
biology	dermatitis	hysteria	muscular
biopsy	diplococci	iatrogenic disorder	myalgia

nasal
neural
neuritis
neurologic
neurosis
nosocomial infections
ophthalmitis
ophthalmopathy
osteitis
otitis

otopathy
pathogen
pathogenic
peritoneum
phagocyte
phobia
postmortem
protozoa
ptosis
pyromania

pyromaniac
sclera
sclerosis
spirochetes
staphylococci
streptococcal pharyngitis
streptococci
syphilis
tetanus
tonsillitis

toxic
toxicologist
toxicology
toxin
trichomoniasis
vibrios
virulence
virus
xanthoderma

Español ENHANCING SPANISH COMMUNICATION

English	Spanish (pronunciation)
bacilli	bacilos (bah-SE-los)
biopsy	biopsia (be-OP-see-ah)
calculus	cálculo (CAHL-coo-lo)
enzyme	enzima (en-SEE-mah)
fear	miedo (me-AY-do)
fever	fiebre (fe-AY-bray)
fire	fuego (foo-AY-go)
foot (pl., feet)	pie (PE-ay), pies (PE-ays)
head	cabeza (cah-BAY-sah)
hernia	hernia (AYR-ne-ah), quebradura (kay-brah-DOO-rah)
inflammation	inflamación (in-flah-mah-se-ON)
influenza	gripe (GREE-pay)
membrane	membrana (mem-BRAH-nah)
movement	movimiento (mo-ve-me-EN-to)
nutrition	nutrición (noo-tre-se-ON)
paralysis	parálisis (pah-RAH-le-sis)
parasite	parásito (pah-RAH-se-to)
prolapse	prolapso (pro-LAHP-so)
seizure	ataque (ah-TAH-kay)
speech	habla (AH-blah), lenguaje (len-goo-AH-hay)
stone	cálculo (CAHL-coo-lo)
sugar	azúcar (ah-SOO-car)

Colors	Los Colores
black	negro (NAY-gro)
blue	azul (ah-SOOL)
green	verde (VERR-day)
red	rojo (ROH-ho)
white	blanco (BLAHN-co)
yellow	amarillo (ah-mah-REEL-lyo)

Prefixes

Using Prefixes, Suffixes, and Combining Forms to Build Medical Terms

LEARNING GOALS

Basic Understanding

In this chapter you will learn to do the following:
1. Use prefixes to build and analyze terms.
2. Match prefixes pertaining to numbers or quantities with their meanings or write their meanings.
3. Recognize prefixes pertaining to position or direction in medical terms and write their meanings.
4. Use a- or an- correctly to write terms of negation.
5. Match other prefixes used in medical terms with their meanings or write their meanings.

Greater Comprehension
6. Spell medical terms accurately.
7. Write the meanings of the abbreviations.
8. Pronounce medical terms correctly.

MAJOR SECTIONS OF THIS CHAPTER:

❏ **PREFIXES THAT PERTAIN TO NUMBERS OR QUANTITY**
❏ **PREFIXES THAT PERTAIN TO POSITION OR DIRECTION**
❏ **PREFIXES RELATED TO NEGATION**

❏ **USING OTHER PREFIXES TO BUILD TERMS**
❏ **COMMON ABBREVIATIONS IN MEDICAL RECORDS**

FUNCTION FIRST

You have learned that prefixes, suffixes, and combining forms are word parts that are used to write medical terms. Prefixes are placed before words to modify their meanings.

Most prefixes, including those ending with a vowel, can be added to the remainder of the word without change. You will encounter some exceptions, however. Prefixes in this chapter will be grouped as those pertaining to numbers or quantity, to position or direction, and to negation, plus some miscellaneous prefixes.

PREFIXES THAT PERTAIN TO NUMBERS OR QUANTITY

5-1 Study the following prefixes that pertain to numbers or quantity. Many of the prefixes in the list are used in everyday language, so think of words you may know that can help you remember their meanings.

Prefixes: Numbers or Quantity

Prefix Specific Numbers	Meaning	Prefix Quantities	Meaning
mono-, uni-	one	ana-	excessive
bi-, di-	two	diplo-	double
tri-	three	hemi-, semi-	half, partly
quad-, quadri-, tetra-	four	hyper-	excessive, more than normal
centi-	one hundred or one hundredth (1/100)	hypo-	beneath or below normal
		multi-, poly-	many
milli-	one thousandth (1/1000)	nulli-	none
		pan-	all
		primi-	first
		super-, ultra-	excessive

one

5-2 A mono/logue is a speech performed by _____ actor.

one

5-3 The terms monorail and unicorn contain prefixes that mean one. Both a mono/rail and a uni/corn have _____ rail and horn, respectively.

two

5-4 Carbon di/oxide (CO_2) contains _____ atoms of oxygen.

> ➤ **KEY** POINT <u>Prefixes identify the type of cycle</u>. Uni/cycles, bi/cycles, and tri/cycles are named according to the number of wheels (Figure 5-1).

three

5-5 In tri/angle, tri/fecta, and tri/mester, the tri- refers to _____.

four

5-6 **Quad/ruplets** (kwod-rōōp´letz) are four offspring born at one birth, and a quadr/angle is an enclosure that has _____ sides.

four

5-7 Carbon tetra/chloride (CCl_4) has _____ chloride atoms.

centi-

5-8 When trying to remember the meaning of **centi/grade** (sen´tĭ-grād), it is helpful to remember that centigrade is a temperature scale in which 0° is the freezing point and 100° is the boiling point of water at sea level (Figure 5-2). Centigrade is the same as **Celsius** (sel´se-əs), named after the Swedish scientist, Anders Celsius. Write the prefix used to write the term centigrade, which means 100: _____.

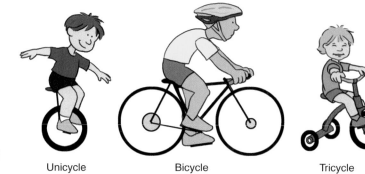

Figure 5-1 Using the prefixes uni-, bi-, and tri-. The terms unicycle, bicycle, and tricycle describe the number of wheels each cycle has.

Unicycle   Bicycle   Tricycle

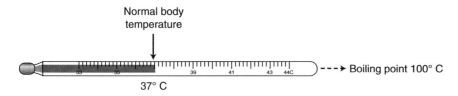

Normal body
temperature

37° C

- - - ▶ Boiling point 100° C

Figure 5-2 Degrees Centigrade. Centigrade, or degrees Celsius, is so named because 0° is the freezing point and 100° is the boiling point of water at sea level using this temperature scale. The normal adult body temperature, as measured orally, is 37° Centigrade.

centimeter
(sen´tĭ-me˝tər)

milligram
(mil´ĭ-gram)

two

half

semipermeable
(sem˝e-pur´me-ə-bəl)

super-

excessive

below

5-9 Add a prefix to meter to write a term for a unit of length equal to one hundredth of a meter _____.

5-10 A **milli/meter** (mil´ĭ-me˝tər) is one thousandth of a meter. Write a term that means one thousandth of a gram: _____.

5-11 Dipl/opia (dĭ-plo´pe-ə) means double vision. How many images of a single object are seen in diplopia? _____ (Note that one "o" is dropped when diplo- is joined with -opia to facilitate pronunciation.)

5-12 In both hemi/sphere and semi/circle, the prefixes mean _____.

5-13 Semi- sometimes means partial, as in semi/dry, moderately dry. Add a prefix to permeable to write a term that means partially but not wholly permeable: _____.
   A semipermeable membrane is one that allows the passage of some substances but prevents the passage of others based on differences in the size, charge, or solubility (Figure 5-3).

5-14 Hyper/active (hi˝pər-ak´tiv) means excessively active. Hyper/sensitive means excessively sensitive. In addition to hyper-, two more prefixes mean excessive: ultra- and _____.

5-15 Ultrasonic (ul˝trə-son´ik) is descriptive of sound frequencies so high they cannot be perceived by the human ear. In ultra/sonography, images of deep structures of the body are obtained by measuring and recording the reflection of high-frequency sound waves.
   Ultra/violet (ul˝trə-vi´ə-lət) describes light beyond the visible spectrum at its violet end. These rays have powerful properties, including sunburn and tanning of the skin, as well as uses in medicine in the diagnosis and treatment of disease (Figure 5-4).
   In both ultrasonic and ultraviolet, you need to remember that ultra- means _____.

5-16 A prefix that means the opposite of hyper- is hypo-. In the word hypo/derm/ic (hi˝po-dur´mik), hypo- means _____.

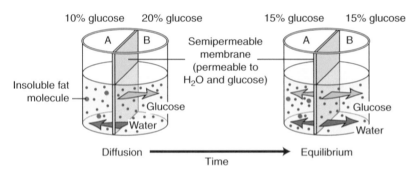

Figure 5-3 Semipermeable membrane. Some particles in a fluid move from an area of higher concentration to an area of lower concentration, but other particles cannot move across the membrane because of size, charge, or solubility.

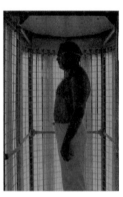

Figure 5-4 A patient with a skin disorder receives ultraviolet treatment.

many	**5-17** In the terms multi/tude and poly/unsaturated, the prefixes mean _____. In multimedia, multinational, and polyester the prefixes are used to mean, or at least imply, many.
nulli-	**5-18** Null is a word that means having no value, nothing, or equal to zero. Write the prefix that means none: _____.
pan-	**5-19 Pan/demic** (pan-dem´ik) means occurring throughout (in other words, affecting all) the population of a country, a people, or the world. Write the prefix that means all: _____.
first	**5-20** Primitive humans were some of the first people on earth. Primary means what position in rank or importance? _____

EXERCISE 1

Match the prefixes in the left column with their meanings in the right column. The choices on the right may be used more than once.

_____ 1. bi-

_____ 2. di-

_____ 3. mono-

_____ 4. quad-

_____ 5. tri-

_____ 6. uni-

A. one
B. two
C. three
D. four

EXERCISE 2

Write the meaning of these prefixes.

1. hemi-   _____

2. multi-   _____

3. nulli-   _____

4. poly-   _____

5. primi-   _____

EXERCISE 3

Identify and state the meaning of the prefixes in these terms.

1. centigrade   _____

2. diplopia   _____

3. hyperactive   _____

4. hypodermic   _____

5. millimeter   _____

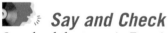 ## Say and Check

Say aloud the terms in Exercise 3. Use the Companion CD to check your pronunciations.

PREFIXES THAT PERTAIN TO POSITION OR DIRECTION

5-21 Several important prefixes pertain to position or direction. Study the following list. Again, think of familiar words to help you remember their meanings, and practice with flashcards.

Prefixes: Position or Direction

Prefix	Meaning	Prefix	Meaning
ab-	away from	intra-	within
ad-	toward	ipsi-	same
ante-, pre-	before in time or in place	meso-, mid-, medio-	middle
circum-, peri-	around	para-	near, beside, or abnormal
dia-	through	per-	through or by
ecto-, ex-, exo-, extra-	out, without, away from	post-	after, behind
en-, end-, endo-	inside	retro-	behind, backward
epi-	above, on	super-, supra-	above, beyond
hypo-, infra-, sub-	beneath, under	sym-, syn-	joined, together
inter-	between	trans-	across

ab-

5-22 Ab/duct (ab-dukt´) means to carry away by force or draw away from a given position. The prefix that means away from is _____. The prefix ad- is the opposite of ab-. In chemical **addiction** (ə-dik´shən) a person has a compulsive need for a certain drug or, in other words, is drawn toward a habit-forming drug.

before

5-23 Both ante- and pre- mean _____ in time or place. A preview is shown before a show or performance. After is the opposite of before, and the corresponding prefix for after is post-. To postdate a check is to write a date after the date that the check is written. The prefix post- in many medical terms also means behind. **Post/nasal** (pōst-na´zəl) means lying or occurring behind the nose. Another prefix, retro-, means behind or backward, as in the term retroactive, which means extending back to a prior time or condition.

around

5-24 The perimeter is the outer boundary or the line that is drawn around the outside of an area. Both peri- and circum- mean _____.

dia-

5-25 The diameter passes through the center of a circle. The prefix in diameter that means through is _____. Another prefix, per-, means through or by. To **perspire**˙ (pur-spīr´) is to excrete fluid through the pores of the skin.

across

A **trans/dermal** (trans-dur´məl) drug is one that can be absorbed through unbroken skin (Figure 5-5). An example is the patch to prevent motion sickness. The literal translation of trans/dermal is _____ the skin.

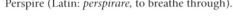

˙Perspire (Latin: *perspirare*, to breathe through).

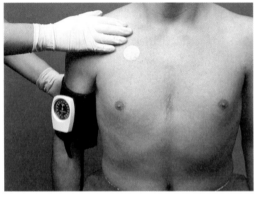

Figure 5-5 Transdermal drug delivery. Application of a nitroglycerin patch.

inside	**5-26** Several prefixes, ecto-, ex-, exo-, and extra-, mean out, without, or away from. For instance, exit means to go out. Practice will help you know which prefix to use when writing terms. Enclose means to close up inside something. Both en- and endo- mean _____.
inter-	**5-27** An interval is a space of time between events. Write the prefix that means between: _____.
intra-	**5-28** Intracollegiate activities occur within a college or are engaged in by members of a college. The prefix that means within is _____.

> ➤ **KEY** POINT <u>Know the difference among intracellular, intercellular, and extracellular.</u> **Intracellular** means within the cell, and **extracellular** means situated outside a cell or the cells of the body. **Intercellular** means located between cells. For example, the space between cells is called the intercellular space (Figure 5-6).

epi-	**5-29** Write the prefix from the list that means above or on: _____. The prefixes super- and supra- can also mean above and sometimes mean beyond. Supernormal is beyond normal human powers. **Supra/renal** (soo″prə-re′nəl) pertains to a location above a
above	kidney, so suprarenal glands are located _____ the kidneys.
under	**5-30** The prefixes hypo-, infra-, and sub- mean beneath or _____. **Hypo/dermic** (hi″po-dur′mik) means beneath the skin. A hypodermic needle is used to inject a drug or medication under the skin or into blood vessels and for withdrawing a fluid, such as blood. Following are four important types of injections:

* **sub/cutaneous** (sub″ku-ta′ne-əs), beneath the skin
* **intra/muscular** (in″trə-mus′ku-lər), within a muscle
* **intra/dermal** (in″trə-dur′məl), within the dermis (dur′mis), the layer of skin that contains the blood vessels
* **intra/venous** (in″trə-ve′nəs), within a vein, because venous means pertaining to a vein

under	The literal translation of subcutaneous is _____ the skin.

In a subcutaneous injection, the needle is placed into the subcutaneous tissue beneath the skin. Study the four types of injections in Figure 5-7 and be able to describe each type.

5-31 The prefix ipsi- means same. **Ipsi/lateral** (ip″sĭ-lat′ər-əl) means affecting the same side of the body. The opposite of this, **contra/lateral** (kon″trə-lat′ər-əl), means affecting the opposite side of the body. The prefix contra- means against, but here it is used to mean opposite or opposed to a particular side of the body.

middle	**5-32** The prefix mid- means _____. Two other prefixes that mean middle are meso- and medio-.
beside	**5-33** Parallel lines run beside each other. Para- means _____.
together	**5-34** Both sym- and syn- mean joined or _____. A **syn/drome** (sin′drōm) is a set of symptoms that occur together and collectively characterize a particular disease or condition.

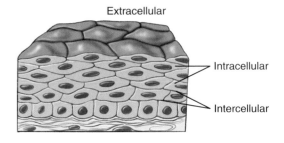

Figure 5-6 Locations relative to cells. Extracellular is outside the cell, intracellular is within the cell, and intercellular is between cells.

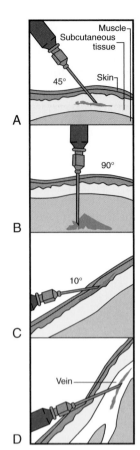

Subcutaneous
A subcutaneous injection places a small amount (0.5 to 2 mL) of medication below the skin layer into the subcutaneous tissue. The needle is inserted at a 45° angle.

Intramuscular
An intramuscular injection deposits medication into a muscular layer. As much as 3 to 5 mL may be administered in one injection, and depending on the size of the patient, a needle from 1 to 3 inches in length is used.

Intradermal
An intradermal injection places very small amounts (0.1 to 0.3 mL) of a drug into the outer layers of the skin with a very fine gauge, short needle. This type of injection is often used to test allergic reactions.

Intravenous
An intravenous injection is used to administer medications directly into the bloodstream for immediate effect or to withdraw blood for testing purposes. A few milliliters of medication or much larger amounts (given over a long period of time) may be administered after venipuncture of the selected vein has been performed.

Figure 5-7 Needle insertion for types of injections. A, Subcutaneous. **B,** Intramuscular. **C,** Intradermal. **D,** Intravenous.

EXERCISE 4

Write answers in the blank lines to complete the sentences. (Although an answer may require more than one word, it is represented by a blank line.)

1. The prefix ab- means _____, but ad- means _____.

2. Postnasal pertains to the region _____ the nose.

3. Two prefixes that have opposite meanings are endo- and ecto-. An abbreviated meaning of ecto- is outside, and endo- means _____.

4. Intercellular means _____ cells.

5. Suprarenal glands are located _____ each kidney.

6. Both peri- and circum- mean _____.

7. The opposite of predate is _____.

8. If intracellular means within the cell, _____ is outside the cell.

9. Ipsilateral means affecting the _____ side of the body.

10. The literal meaning of transdermal is _____ the skin.

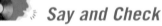 *Say and Check*

Pronounce these terms: postnasal, intercellular, suprarenal, extracellular, ipsilateral, and transdermal. Use the Companion CD to check your pronunciations.

PREFIXES RELATED TO NEGATION

5-35 When a prefix of negation is placed before a term, it forms a new word with the opposite meaning. For example, **symptomatic** (simp″to-mat′ik) means having symptoms, and **asymptomatic** (a″simp-to-mat′ik) means without (not having) symptoms.

Prefixes: Negation

Prefix	Meaning
a-, an-	no, not, without
in-	not or inside (in)

5-36 **Hydrous** (hi′drəs) means containing water. **Anhydrous** (an-hi′drəs) means absence of water.

> ➤ **KEY** POINT Learn these rules for using a- or an-:
> • Use a- before a consonant.
> • Use an- before a vowel or the letter h.

5-37 **Trauma** (traw′mə, trou′mə) means a wound or injury, whether physical or emotional. **Traumatic** (trə-mat′ik) means pertaining to or occurring as the result of trauma (injury).
  Write a word that means not inflicting or causing damage or injury: _____.

atraumatic
(a″traw-mat′ik)
in-

5-38 Another prefix that means not, as in the term inconsistent, is _____. Sometimes in- means inside, as in the terms include and **inhale** (in-hāl′), to breathe in.

EXERCISE 5

Use either a- or an- to write words that have the opposite meanings of these terms.

1. The opposite of esthesia is _____.
2. The opposite of hydrous is _____.
3. The opposite of plastic is _____.
4. The opposite of traumatic is _____.
5. The opposite of symptomatic is _____.

EXERCISE 6

Use in- to write words that have the opposite meaning.

1. The opposite of consistent is _____.
2. The opposite of animate is _____.
3. The opposite of attentive is _____.
4. The opposite of capable is _____.
5. The opposite of visible is _____.

USING OTHER PREFIXES TO BUILD TERMS

5-39 There are additional prefixes that you need to know to write medical terms. Their meanings should be easy to remember, because many of them are used in everyday language. Note that some prefixes have more than one meaning and may pertain to two classifications, such as position and time. An example is post-, which means after to describe time or behind to describe position. Study the list of miscellaneous prefixes, using word association to help you remember their meanings.

Miscellaneous Prefixes

Prefix Related to Size	Meaning	Prefix Related to Description	Meaning
macro-, mega-, megalo-	large or great	ana-	upward or again
micro-	small	anti-, contra-	against
		brady-	slow
Related to Time		dys-	bad, difficult
ante-, pre-, pro-	before	eu-	good, normal
post-	after or behind	mal-	bad
		pro-	favoring, supporting
		tachy-	fast

before

5-40 The prefixes ante-, pre-, and pro- mean before in time. **Pre/cancerous** (pre-kan´sər-əs) is a term that is used to describe an abnormal growth that is likely to become cancerous. Preadmission certification is a system whereby physicians are required to obtain advance approval for nonemergency admission for many patients. With pre/admission, the approval is obtained _____ the person is admitted to the hospital.

post-

5-41 The prefix that means after in time is _____.
Post/anesthetic (pōst″an-əs-thet´ik) describes the time after anesthetic is administered, and **post/infectious** describes the time after an infection.

large

5-42 The prefixes mega- and megalo- mean large, and you see them in common terms such as megalith and megalopolis, a very _____ stone and city, respectively.

5-43 When referring to size, **macro/scopic** (mak″ro-skop´ik) structures are large enough to be seen by the naked eye. If the structures are so small that they can be seen only with a microscope, they are called _____ structures.

microscopic
(mi″kro-skop´ik)

small

5-44 **Micr/ot/ia** (mi-kro´shə) is an unusually small size of the external ear (one "o" is omitted to facilitate pronunciation). Literal translation of microtia is _____ ear (Figure 5-8).

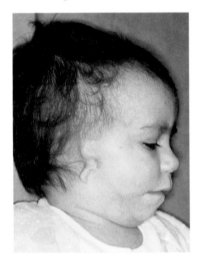

Figure 5-8 Microtia. This example shows the unusual size that results from underdevelopment of the external ear. Otoplasty, reconstructive surgery of the ear, is generally performed before the child reaches school age.

against

5-45 Both anti- and contra- mean _____, as in the terms **anti/perspirant** (an″te-, an″ti-pur′spər-ant″) and **contra/ceptive** (kon″trə-sep′tiv). An antiperspirant inhibits or prevents perspiration (sweating). A contraceptive prevents conception or diminishes the likelihood of conception.

The prefix that means the opposite of against is pro-, which means favoring or supporting (in other words, for). "Weighing the pros and cons" is commonly understood.

fast

slow

5-46 The prefixes brady- and tachy- have opposite meanings, slow and _____, respectively. You learned that -phasia means speech. **Brady/phasia** (brad″ĭ-fa′zhə) means an abnormally _____ manner of speech, often associated with mental illness. The opposite of bradyphasia is **tachy/phasia** (tak″e-fa′zhə), rapid speech, as may be present in the manic phase of bipolar disorder.

bad

5-47 Both dys- and mal- mean _____, but dys- can also mean difficult, as in the term **dys/lexia** (dis-lek′se-ə), which means difficulty in reading, often reversing letters or having difficulty distinguishing letter sequences. **Malaise** (mă-lāz′) is a vague feeling of bodily discomfort and fatigue.

5-48 **Fatigue** (fə-tēg′) is a state of exhaustion or a loss of strength or endurance. A second definition of fatigue is loss of the ability to respond to stimuli that normally evoke muscular contraction or other activity. **Lethargy** (leth′ər-je), more severe than fatigue, is a state of dullness, sluggishness, or prolonged sleepiness or drowsiness. A person suffering

lethargy

_____ is said to be **lethargic** (lə-thar′jik).

normal

5-49 The prefix eu- means good or _____. **Eu/phoria** (u-for′e-ə) is a feeling or state of well-being, and **dys/phoria** (dis-for′e-ə) is characterized by depression and anguish.

EXERCISE 7

Match the prefixes in the left column with their meaning(s) in the right column. The choices on the right may be used more than once.

_____ 1. anti-	A. against	
_____ 2. brady-	B. bad	
_____ 3. contra-	C. fast	
_____ 4. dys-	D. good or normal	
_____ 5. eu-	E. large	
_____ 6. mal-	F. slow	
_____ 7. micro-	G. small	
_____ 8. macro-		
_____ 9. megalo-		
_____ 10. tachy-		

EXERCISE 8

 Build It! *Use the following prefixes to complete these sentences.*

brady-, contra-, dys-, eu-, macro-, mal-, micro-, post-, pre-, tachy-

1. An abnormally fast manner of speech is _____phasia.

2. A vague feeling of bodily discomfort and fatigue is _____aise.

3. An abnormal growth that is likely to become cancerous is described as _____cancerous.

4. Objects that are large enough to be seen by the naked eye are described as _____scopic structures.

5. A feeling of well-being is _____phoria.

6. The description of the time after anesthetic is administered is _____anesthetic.

7. An unusually small size of the external ear is _____otia.

8. Difficulty in reading is _____lexia.

9. The term for a device or technique that prevents conception is _____ceptive.

10. Abnormally slow speech is _____phasia

 Say and Check

Say aloud the terms that resulted when you added prefixes in Exercise 8. Use the Companion CD to check your pronunciations.

COMMON ABBREVIATIONS IN MEDICAL RECORDS

Study the following abbreviations.

CHAPTER ABBREVIATIONS*

Units of Measure

cm	centimeter
dL	deciliter
g	gram
kg	kilogram
L	liter
mcg	microgram
mg	milligram
mL	milliliter

Medication Administration

b.i.d.	twice a day (*bis in die*)
h	hour (*hora*)
IV	intravenous
min	minutes
p.o.	orally (*per os*)
p.r.n.	as needed (*pro re nata*)
q.	every
t.i.d.	three times per day (*ter in die*)

History and Examinations

A&O	alert and oriented
BP	blood pressure
CC	chief complaint
DOB	date of birth
Dx	diagnosis
HEENT	head, eye, ear, nose, and throat
HPI	history of the present illness
Hx	history
L&W	living and well
P	pulse
PE	physical examination
R	respirations
ROM	range of motion
ROS	review of systems
T	temperature
TFT	thyroid function test
WD, WN	well developed, well nourished
WNL	within normal limits

*Many of these abbreviations share their meanings with other terms.

5-50 You will encounter dozens of abbreviations in medical records. Many are concerned with medication administration, units of measure, or information obtained from the history or examinations. Study the following list as a first step to understanding abbreviations in medical records. Practice using flashcards of the abbreviations and their meanings or use the electronic flashcards available on the Evolve site.

5-51 Timing of medication as well as the units of measure for medicines are extremely important in medical therapy! If a patient were to receive 2 g of a medication b.i.d., you would know that he or she was getting two grams of medication _____ per day. How a medication is administered is often abbreviated as well. IV indicates the medication is given within the veins, or intravenously. What route does p.o. indicate? _____

twice

orally or by mouth

5-52 If a patient visited a physician complaining of indigestion, the physician would write that indigestion was the patient's CC, or _____ complaint.

chief

5-53 The physician's next step would be to take a history of the present illness, abbreviated _____, by asking questions about it. Another part of the history (Hx) would include questions about the various body systems, and information from those questions would be documented in a section called review of systems, abbreviated _____.

HPI

ROS

physical

5-54 Then the physician may perform a PE, or _____ examination, and perhaps order some diagnostic tests.

diagnosis

5-55 Once the physician has arrived at a Dx, or _____, therapy is prescribed to address the problem or control the symptoms of the problem, or both.

EXERCISE 9

Write the meanings of the abbreviations for questions 1-20.

1. cm _____
2. dL _____
3. g _____
4. kg _____
5. L _____
6. mcg _____
7. mg _____
8. mL _____
9. A&O _____
10. BP _____
11. CC _____
12. DOB _____
13. Dx _____
14. Hx _____
15. P _____
16. PE _____
17. R _____
18. ROM _____
19. ROS _____
20. T _____

EXERCISE 10

Write the abbreviation for each of the following:

1. twice per day _____
2. hour _____
3. intravenously _____
4. minutes _____
5. orally _____
6. as needed _____
7. every _____
8. three times per day _____
9. living and well _____
10. well developed _____
11. within normal limits _____
12. history of the present illness _____

Be Careful with These!

in- (not) vs. in- (inside)
infra- (under) vs. intra- (within)

Opposites:
ab- (away from) vs. ad- (toward)
ante-, pre- (before) vs. post- (after)
en-, end-, endo- (inside) vs. ecto-, exo-, extra- (outside)
hyper- (more than normal) vs. hypo- (less than normal)
macro- (large) vs. micro- (small)
nulli- (none) vs. pan- (all)
super-, supra- (above) vs. hypo-, infra-, sub- (below)

CHAPTER 5 REVIEW

Basic Understanding

Matching

I. *Match the prefixes on the left with their meanings on the right.*

_____ 1. di-

_____ 2. diplo-

_____ 3. hyper-

_____ 4. hypo-

_____ 5. nulli-

_____ 6. pan-

_____ 7. poly-

_____ 8. quad-

_____ 9. tri-

_____ 10. uni-

A. all
B. below normal
C. double
D. four
E. many
F. more than normal
G. none
H. one
I. three
J. two

II. *Match the prefixes on the left with their meanings on the right. All choices will not be used, and some will be used more than once.*

_____ 1. ab-

_____ 2. di-

_____ 3. hemi-

_____ 4. milli-

_____ 5. mono-

_____ 6. multi-

_____ 7. poly-

_____ 8. semi-

_____ 9. super-

_____ 10. supra-

_____ 11. tetra-

A. away from
B. excessive
C. half, partly
D. many
E. one
F. one hundred or one hundredth
G. one thousand or one thousandth
H. toward
I. two
J. three
K. four

Multiple Choice

III. *Circle the correct answer in each of the following questions.*

1. What does primi- mean? (above, beneath, excessive, first)

2. What does tachy- mean? (bad, good, fast, slow)

3. What does dys- mean? (difficult, good, normal, slow)

4. What does hypo- mean? (above, after, before, beneath)

5. Which term describes a structure that can be seen with the naked eye? (macroscopic, microscopic, ophthalmoscopic, ophthalmoscopy)

6. What does the prefix in antibiotic mean? (against, before, effective, supporting)

7. What does the prefix in hemisphere mean? (all, double, favoring, half)

8. What is the meaning of the prefix in bilateral? (one, two, three, four)

9. Which type of injection places a small amount of drug into the outer layers of the skin? (intradermal, intramuscular, intravenous, subcutaneous)

10. Which term means a set of symptoms that occur together and characterize a particular disease or condition? (dysphoria, symptomatic, syndrome, tachyphasia)

Labeling

IV. *Use word parts to write terms to label 1 to 3.*

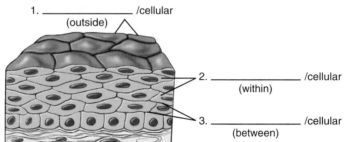

1. _____ /cellular
   (outside)

2. _____ /cellular
   (within)

3. _____ /cellular
   (between)

Word Analysis

V. *Pronounce each term aloud, then divide it into its component word parts, stating the meaning of the word parts.*

1. macroscopic _____

2. microtia _____

3. postnasal _____

4. tachyphasia _____

5. transdermal _____

Writing Terms

VI. *Use a- or an- to write terms that have the opposite meanings of these words.*

1. esthesia vs. _____

2. hydrous vs. _____

3. plastic vs. _____

4. symptomatic vs. _____

5. traumatic vs. _____

VII. *Write a term for each of the following:*

1. abnormally slow speech _____

2. behind the nose _____

3. decreased size of the external ear _____

4. double vision _____

5. occurring on the opposite side _____

6. descriptive of extremely high sound frequencies _____

7. descriptive of light beyond the visible spectrum _____

8. located between cells _____

9. permeable to selective substances _____

10. state of exhaustion _____

Say and Check

Say aloud the terms you wrote for Exercise VII. Use the Companion CD to check your pronunciations.

Greater Comprehension

Spelling
VIII. *Circle all misspelled terms and write their correct spellings.*

adiction   antiperspirant   ipselateral   postanethetic   suprarenal

Interpreting Abbreviations
IX. *Write the meaning of these abbreviations*

1. A&O _____

2. DOB _____

3. IV _____

4. p.r.n. _____

5. ROS _____

Pronunciation
X. *Indicate the primary accented syllable by marking it with an ´.*

1. abduct (ab dukt)

2. contraceptive (kon trə sep tiv)

3. hypodermic (hi po dur mik)

4. syndrome (sin drōm)

5. transdermal (trans dur məl)

Say and Check

Say aloud the five terms in Exercise X. Use the Companion CD to check your pronunciations. In addition, be prepared to pronounce aloud these terms in class:

anhydrous	euphoria	macroscopic	semipermeable
atraumatic	fatigue	malaise	subcutaneous
bradyphasia	intradermal	microtia	suprarenal
diplopia	ipsilateral	pandemic	symptomatic
dyslexia	lethargic	precancerous	ultrasonic

Challenge
XI. *Break these words into their component parts and write their meanings. Even if you have not seen these terms before, you may be able to break them apart and determine their meanings.*

1. adduct _____

2. exoskeleton _____

3. periappendicitis _____

4. prenatal _____

5. symbiosis _____

PRONUNCIATION LIST

Use the companion CD to review the terms that have been presented. Look closely at the spelling of each term as it is pronounced, and be sure you know the meaning of each term.

abduct	dysphoria	lethargic	quadruplets
addiction	euphoria	lethargy	semipermeable
anhydrous	extracellular	macroscopic	subcutaneous
antiperspirant	fatigue	malaise	suprarenal
asymptomatic	hydrous	microscopic	symptomatic
atraumatic	hyperactive	microtia	syndrome
bradyphasia	hypodermic	milligram	tachyphasia
Celsius	inhale	millimeter	transdermal
centigrade	intercellular	pandemic	trauma
centimeter	intracellular	perspire	traumatic
contraceptive	intradermal	postanesthetic	ultrasonic
contralateral	intramuscular	postinfectious	ultraviolet
diplopia	intravenous	postnasal	
dyslexia	ipsilateral	precancerous	

Español ENHANCING SPANISH COMMUNICATION

English	Spanish (pronunciation)
fatigue	fatiga (fah-TEE-gah)
hypodermic	hipodérmico (e-po-DER-me-co)
microscope	microscopio (me-cros-CO-pe-o)
perspire	sudar (soo-DAR)
trauma	daño (DAH-nyo), herida (ay-REE-dah)

Organization of the Body

6

Organizational Scheme, Anatomic and Directional Terms, Body Regions and Cavities

Basic Understanding
In this chapter you will learn to do the following:
1. Recognize the relationship of cells, tissues, and organs.
2. Name four main types of tissue.
3. Write the meanings of combining forms for position and direction, and name the related anatomic terms or match the terms with their meanings.
4. Label the directional terms and planes of the body.
5. Write the combining forms for body regions and body cavities when given their meanings, or match the combining forms with their meanings.
6. Identify the four abdominal quadrants.
7. Identify the nine abdominopelvic divisions used by anatomists.
8. Write terms that relate to the body as a whole when given their meanings, or match the terms with their meanings.

Greater Comprehension
9. Spell medical terms accurately.
10. Write the meanings of the abbreviations.
11. Pronounce medical terms correctly.

MAJOR SECTIONS OF THIS CHAPTER

- ❑ **THE BODY'S ORGANIZATIONAL SCHEME**
- ❑ **ANATOMIC POSITION AND DIRECTIONAL TERMS**
- ❑ **BODY REGIONS AND BODY CAVITIES**
- ❑ **TERMS RELATED TO THE BODY AS A WHOLE**

FUNCTION FIRST

Order and organization are outstanding features of the human body. All its parts, from tiny atoms to visible structures, work together as a functioning whole.

THE BODY'S ORGANIZATIONAL SCHEME

6-1 The body's organizational structure has several levels. These are illustrated in Figure 6-1. From simplest to complex, the levels are as follows:

- atoms or ions (for example, carbon, oxygen, hydrogen, nitrogen)
- molecules (for example, proteins, sugars, water)
- organelles (specialized structures within cells—for example, the nucleus)
- cells (fundamental units of life)
- tissues (similar cells acting together to perform a function)
- organs (tissue types working together to perform one or more functions, such as the lungs)
- body systems (several organs working together to accomplish a set of functions)
- total organism (a human capable of carrying on life functions)

chemical

The simplest level is the _____ level.

6-2 The human body consists of trillions of cells.

> ➤ **KEY** POINT <u>The cell is the fundamental unit of all living matter</u>. The typical cell found in humans consists of a nucleus and cytoplasm, surrounded by a cell membrane. Chromosomes, the determinants of inherited characteristics, are located in the nucleus (Figure 6-2).

There are numerous types of body cells (blood cells, bone cells, liver cells, and many others), but all share certain characteristics such as metabolism, building up of substances, and breaking down of substances for the body's use. Chromosomes, threadlike structures within the nucleus of a cell, contain deoxyribonucleic acid (DNA), which functions in the transmission of genetic information. Write the abbreviation for the material in cells that contains genetic infor-

DNA

mation: _____ .

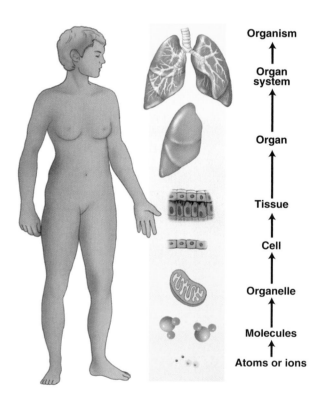

Figure 6-1 Organizational scheme of the body. The formation of the human organism progresses from different levels of complexity. All its parts, from tiny atoms to visible structures, work together to make a functioning whole.

EXERCISE 1

Four levels of human organization are organelles, cells, organs, and tissues. List these levels in order from simple to more complex levels:

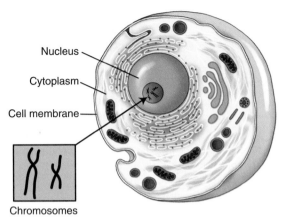

Figure 6-2 **Basic cell structure, diagrammatic repre- senta-tion.** Chromosomes are threadlike structures in the nucleus of a cell that function in the transmission of genetic information. Each chromosome consists of a double strand of deoxyribonucleic acid (DNA).

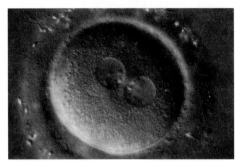

Figure 6-3 **Fertilized human egg.** Joining of the male and female nuclei determines the gender as well as the characteristics of the individual who will develop.

EXERCISE 2

Name the three major parts of a cell.

1. _____   2. _____   3. _____

6-3 Every individual begins life as a single cell, a fertilized egg (Figure 6-3). This single cell divides into two cells, then four, eight, and so on, until maturity. During development, cells become specialized. Cells that have the ability to divide without limit and give rise to specialized cells are called stem cells. They are abundant in a fetus and in cord blood of a newborn. Stem cells are used in bone marrow transplants and can be used in research for organ or tissue regeneration. These undifferentiated cells that can give rise to other types of cells are called

stem

_____ cells.

6-4 In humans, each somatic cell has 23 pairs of chromosomes. The combining forms somat(o) and som(a) mean body. Somatic (so-mat´ik) cells are all the cells of the body except the sex cells,

body

sperm and ova (singular: ovum). Somat/ic means pertaining to the _____.

> ➤ KEY POINT Each chromosome has a double strand of DNA. Genes, the biologic units of inheritance, are arranged in a linear pattern along the length of each strand of DNA. A **genetic disorder** (also called an inherited disorder) is a disease or condition that is determined by one's genes or a change in the number or structure of the chromosomes. Some genetic disorders are listed in Table 6-1. See also Appendix III for genetic terminology.

An abnormality in the chromosomes themselves, or too many chromosomes, usually results in defects. **Down syndrome** (sin´drŏm), the most common chromosomal abnormality of a gen-

---

TABLE 6-1 **Selected Genetic Disorders**	
albinism (4)*	hemophilia (7)
cystic fibrosis (9)	Huntington disease (15)
diabetes mellitus (10, 17)	muscular dystrophy (15)
Down syndrome (6, 13)	rheumatoid arthritis (15)
gout (14)	sickle cell anemia (7)

*The number in parentheses indicates the chapter in which the disorder is explained.

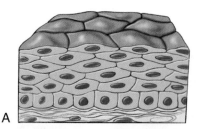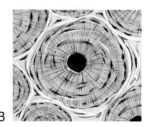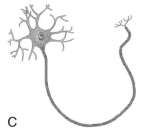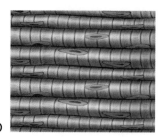

A   B   C   D

Figure 6-4 Types of tissue. There are four basic types of tissue composed of different types of microscopic cells. **A,** Epithelial tissue appears as sheetlike arrangements of epithelial cells. **B,** Connective tissue. The example is bone cells, which form the densest type of connective tissue. **C,** Nerve tissue. A single neuron is shown. Neurons tend to bind with other neurons or communicate with one another by electrical impulses. **D,** Muscle tissue is composed of cells that have the ability to contract when stimulated by a nerve.

Down

eralized syndrome, is a congenital (kən-jen´ĭ-təl) condition characterized by varying degrees of mental retardation and multiple defects (see Figure 13-11). The incidence is generally associated with advanced age of the mother. **Congenital** (Latin: *congenitus,* born together) means existing at, and usually before, birth. This example of a congenital defect, usually caused by an extra chromosome 21, is _____ syndrome.

6-5 A tissue is a group of cells that have similar structure and function as a unit. Using the following information, learn the four types of tissues in Figure 6-4.

Figure 6-4, *A* **Epithelial** (ep˝ĭ-the´le-əl) tissue forms the covering of body surfaces, both inside and on the surface of the body; an example is the outer layer of the skin.

Figure 6-4, *B* Connective tissue supports and binds other body tissues and parts; examples are bone and cartilage.

Figure 6-4, *C* Nervous tissue coordinates and controls many body activities; it is found in the brain, spinal cord, and nerves.

Figure 6-4, *D* Muscle tissue produces movement; an example is skeletal muscle that makes bending of the arm possible.

tissue

A group of cells that have similar structure and function as a unit is called a _____.

6-6 Organs are made up of two or more tissue types that work together to perform one or more functions and form a more complex structure. You are familiar with many organs, such as the liver, the lungs, and the reproductive organs.

A body system consists of several organs that work together to accomplish a set of functions. See Table 6-2 for a listing of the major body systems and their functions. Body systems will be covered in Chapters 8 through 17 of this book. Some systems will be combined in the same chapter; for example, the cardiovascular and lymphatic systems are presented in Chapter 8. You

heart

have already learned that cardi(o) means the _____.

TABLE 6-2	**Major Body Systems**
Body System	**Major Functions**
Cardiovascular system	Delivers oxygen, nutrients, and vital substances throughout the body; transports cellular waste products to the lungs and kidneys for excretion
Lymphatic system	Helps maintain the internal fluid environment; produces some types of blood cells; regulates immunity
Respiratory system	Brings oxygen into the body and removes carbon dioxide and some water waste
Digestive system	Provides the body with water, nutrients, and minerals; removes solid wastes
Urinary system	Filters blood to remove wastes of cellular metabolism; maintains the electrolyte and fluid balance
Reproductive system	Produces offspring
Muscular system	Makes movement possible
Skeletal system	Provides protection, form, and shape for the body; stores minerals and forms some blood cells
Nervous system	Coordinates the reception of stimuli; transmits messages to stimulate movement
Integumentary system	Provides external covering for protection; regulates the body temperature and water content
Endocrine system	Secretes hormones and helps regulate body activities

EXERCISE 3

Write a word in each of the blanks to complete these sentences.

1. Every individual begins life as a single _____.

2. Similar cells acting together to perform a function are called _____.

3. Tissue types working together to perform a function are called a/an _____.

4. The type of tissue that supports and binds other body tissues and parts is called _____ tissue.

5. The tissue type that forms the covering of body surfaces is _____ tissue.

6. The type of tissue that produces movement is _____ tissue.

7. The tissue type that coordinates and controls many body activities is _____ tissue.

8. All cells of the body except the sex cells are called _____ cells.

9. Undifferentiated cells that give rise to specialized cells are called _____ cells.

10. The term that means existing at or before birth is _____.

EXERCISE 4

Descriptions are given below the pictures of four types of body tissue. Label each picture with one of the following: connective, epithelial, muscle, or nervous.

1. _____
tissue is composed of neurons.

2. _____
tissue forms the covering of body surfaces.

3. _____
tissue supports and binds other body tissues.

4. _____
tissue is composed of cells that can contract.

ANATOMIC POSITION AND DIRECTIONAL TERMS

6-7 Anatomy (ə-nat´ə-me) is the study, description, and classification of structures and organs of the body. Anatomists use directional terms and planes to describe the position and direction of the body. Locations and positions are always described relative to the body in the **anatomic** (an″ə-tom´ik) **position**—that is, the position that a person has while standing erect with the arms at the sides and the palms forward, as shown in Figure 6-5.

In the anatomic position, the palms are forward. The palm* is the hollow of the hand. **Palm/ar** (pahl´mər) pertains to the _____.

palm

Plantar† (plan´tər) pertains to the sole. Write the word that means pertaining to the sole: _____.

plantar

6-8 In the anatomic position, the chest faces forward. The combining form thorac(o) means chest. The scientific name of the chest is the **thorax** (thor´aks). **Thoraco/tomy** (thor″ə-kot´ə-me) is incision into the _____. Thoracotomy refers to any incision of the chest wall.

chest (thorax)

The thorac/ic (thə-ras´ik) region is the area of the chest. **Thoracic** means pertaining to the chest.

*Palm (Latin: *palma*).
†Plantar (Latin: *planta*, sole).

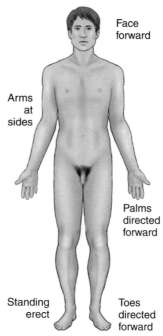

Figure labels: Face forward, Arms at sides, Palms directed forward, Standing erect, Toes directed forward

Figure 6-5 Anatomic position. The person is standing erect with the arms at the sides and the palms forward.

chest

thoracodynia

suprathoracic
(soo″ prə-thə-ras′ik)
across

frontal (frun′təl)

transverse
(trans-vərs′)

midsagittal
(mid-saj′ĭ-təl)

anterior (an-tēr′e-ər)

posterior
(pos-tēr′e-ər)
lateral (lat′ər-əl)

6-9 Thoraco/dynia (thor″ə-ko-din′e-ə) is a type of pain in the _____.
(It differs from **angina pectoris** [an-ji′nə, an′jə-nə pek′to-ris], a heart disease in which the chest pain results from interference with the supply of oxygen to the heart muscle.) A term for pain in the chest is _____.

Two directional terms that pertain to the chest are written by combining the prefixes supra- and trans- with thoracic. Write a term that means pertaining to a location above the chest: _____.

Trans/thorac/ic (trans″thə-ras′ik) means through the chest cavity or _____ the chest wall.

6-10 Body or **anatomic planes,** imaginary flat surfaces, are used to identify the position of the body (Figure 6-6). Locations and positions are described relative to the body in the anatomic position. Complete these sentences while studying Figure 6-6:
The _____ **plane** divides the body into front and back portions. This plane is also called the coronal (kor′ə-nəl) plane.
A _____ **plane** divides the body into upper and lower portions.

A **sagittal** (saj′ĭ-təl) **plane** divides the body into right and left sides. A _____ **plane** divides the body into equal right and left halves.

6-11 Aspects refer to the surface of the figure when seen from various perspectives. The aspects shown in Figure 6-6 are used to describe locations of various structures or parts. The front is called the _____ aspect.

The back of the figure is the _____ aspect.

The side of the figure is the _____ aspect.

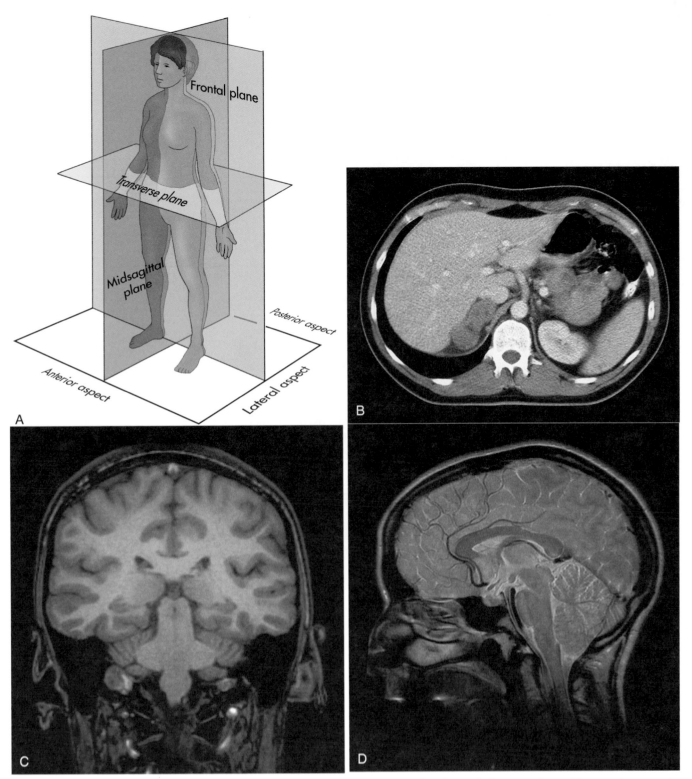

Figure 6-6 Anatomic reference planes and aspects. A, The frontal, transverse, and midsagittal planes are shown. The anterior, posterior, and lateral aspects are used to describe locations of various structures or parts. **B,** Computed tomography (CT) of the abdomen, transverse image. **C,** Magnetic resonance imaging (MRI) of a frontal or coronal scan through the head, showing the brain. Note the ears on the sides of the head. **D,** MRI of a sagittal scan through the head.

EXERCISE 5

Label the body planes and aspects that are indicated on the illustration.

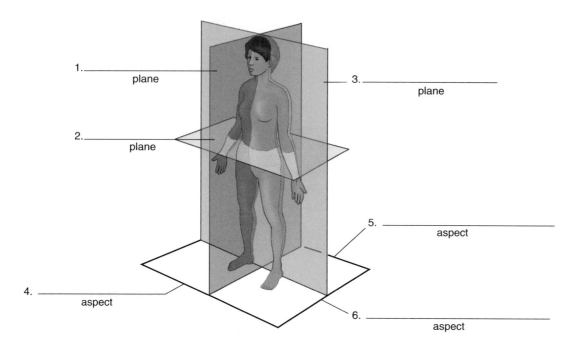

1. _____ plane
2. _____ plane
3. _____ plane
4. _____ aspect
5. _____ aspect
6. _____ aspect

Study the following combining forms used in directional terms. Associate the combining forms with words you already know. For example, it may be easier to remember that tel(e) means far or distant if you think of a telephone, which allows you to talk with someone distant from you.

Combining Forms: Directional Terms

Combining Form	Term	Meaning
anter(o)	anterior	nearer to or toward the front
poster(o)	posterior	nearer to or toward the back
ventr(o)	ventral	belly side
dors(o)	dorsal	directed toward or situated on the back side
medi(o)	medial, median	middle or nearer the middle
later(o)	lateral	farther from the midline of the body or from a structure
super(o)	superior	uppermost or above
infer(o)	inferior	lowermost or below
proxim(o)	proximal	nearer the origin or point of attachment
dist(o), tel(e)	distal	far or distant from the origin or point of attachment
caud(o)	caudad or caudal	in an inferior position
cephal(o)	cephalad	toward the head

front

6-12 Anterior means nearer to or toward the front. **Antero/medial** (an″tər-o-me′de-əl) indicates the aspect that is toward the _____ and toward the middle.

6-13 In humans, the anterior or front side is also the ventral (ven′trəl) surface. **Ventral** refers to the belly side. **Ventro/median** (ven″tro-me′de-ən) is another way of saying anteromedial, but the latter is more common.

ventral

In humans, the anterior or front side is the same as the _____ surface. In dogs, for example, the ventral surface is not the front side.

6-14 The opposite of anterior is posterior (pos-tēr´e-ər). **Posterior** means directed toward or situated at the back. **Postero/external** (pos″tər-o-ek-stur´nəl) indicates that something is situated on the outside of a posterior part. Thus posteroexternal is situated _____ and outside. **Postero/internal** (pos″tər-o-in-tər´nəl) is situated behind and _____.

behind

within (inside)

front

    Antero/posterior (an″tər-o-pos-tēr´e-ər) (AP) pertains to both the _____ and the back sides, or from the front to the back of the body.

6-15 In radiology, directional terms are used to specify the direction of the x-ray beam from its source to its exit surface before striking the film. In an anteroposterior projection, the x-ray beam strikes the anterior aspect of the body first. In other words, the beam passes from _____ to back. **Postero/anterior** (pos″tər-o-an-tēr´e-ər), abbreviated PA, means from the posterior to the anterior surface, or, in other words, from _____ to front.

front

back

Positions for some common radiographic projections of the chest are shown in Figure 6-7.

6-16 Both **dorsal** (dor´səl) and posterior mean directed toward or situated on the back side. **Dorso/ventral** (dor″so-ven´trəl) pertains to the back and _____ surfaces. (Note the order in which the two word parts are presented. The importance of the order becomes obvious when one is describing the path of a bullet, for example. Dorsoventral sometimes means passing from the back to the belly surface.)

belly (front)

    Lateral means side, so **dorso/lateral** (dor″so-lat´ər-əl) means behind and to one side of the body. Use another word part that you learned that means behind to write a different term that means behind and to one side: _____.

posterolateral
(pos″tər-o-lat´ər-əl)

side

    Medial (me´de-əl) and **median** (me´de-ən) mean pertaining to the middle or midline of a body or structure.
    Medio/lateral (me″de-o-lat´ər-əl) means from the middle to one _____. This term also denotes the direction of a line, as in the path of a bullet or an x-ray beam.

6-17 Lateral means side and denotes a position away from the midline of the body. Write the combining form for anterior: _____. Write a new word using lateral that means situated in front and to one side: _____.

anter(o)

anterolateral
(an″tər-o-lat´ər-əl)

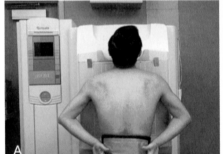
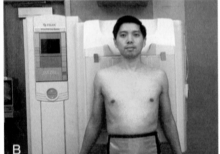
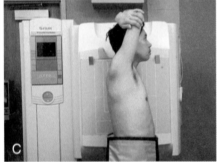

Figure 6-7 Patient positioning for a chest x-ray examination. A, In a posteroanterior (PA) projection, the anterior aspect of the chest is closest to the image receptor. **B,** In an anteroposterior (AP) projection, the posterior aspect of the chest is closest to the image receptor. **C,** In a left lateral chest projection, the left side of the patient is placed against the image receptor.

side	**6-18 Uni/lateral** (u″nĭ-lat′ər-əl) means affecting only one _____.
sides	**Bi/lateral** (bi-lat′ər-əl) pertains to two _____. In other words, bilateral refers to both sides of the body.
back	**Postero/medial** (post″tər-o-me′de-əl) means situated in the middle of the _____ side of an organism.
front	**6-19** Anatomists use the term **superior** (soo-pēr′e-ər) to indicate uppermost or situated above. **Antero/superior** (an″tər-o-soo-pēr′e-ər) indicates a position in _____ and above.
posterosuperior (pos″tər-o-soo-pēr′e-ər)	Using the combining form for posterior, build a word that means behind and above: _____.
above	**Super/ficial** (soo″pər-fish′əl) means situated on or near the surface. Superficial radiation therapy is sometimes used for surface lesions such as skin tumors. Superficial comes from a similar-appearing Latin word that contains super(o), the combining form that means uppermost or situated _____.
below	**6-20** Inferior (in-fēr′e-ər) is the opposite of superior. There may be certain products that you consider inferior to your favorite brand. When you consider something inferior, you believe that product is lower in value than something else. **Inferior** means lower or below. In anatomy, inferior means situated _____. It is often used in reference to the lower surface of a structure or the lower of two or more similar structures.
middle	**Infero/median** (in″fər-o-me′de-ən) means situated in the _____ of the underside. Only a few medical words use the combining form infer(o). The prefix sub- is more often used in medicine to indicate under or below.
tail	**6-21** The combining form caud(o) means toward the tail or the end of the body away from the head. **Caudad** (kaw′dad) or **caudal** (kaw′dəl) pertains to a _____ or tail-like structure. In human anatomy, it also means inferior.
caudal	Another word in human anatomy that means the same as inferior is _____, which also refers to the tail.
	6-22 The combining form proxim(o) means near. **Proxim/al** (prok′sĭ-məl) refers to something that is near. Proximal describes the position of structures that are nearest their origin or point of attachment. The end of the thigh bone that joins with the hip bone is the
proximal	_____ end.
distal	**6-23 Distal** (dis′təl) is the opposite of proximal. If the upper end of the thigh bone is proximal, the lower end of the thigh bone is _____ to the hip bone.
proximal	Which is nearer its origin, a structure that is proximal or one that is distal? _____
distant	Another combining form, tel(e), also means distant. A tele/cardio/gram (tel″ə-kahr′de-o-gram) registers the heart impulses of patients in _____ places. With a **telecardiogram,** the cardiologist and the patient may be in different cities, and the heart tracing is sent by phone.
	6-24 The combining form cephal(o) means head, and the suffix -ad means toward. **Cephalad** (sef′ə-lad) means toward the head. **Dorso/cephalad** (dor″so-sef′ə-lad) means situated toward the back of the head. Write another word using -ic that means pertaining to the head:
cephalic (sə-fal′ik)	_____.

EXERCISE 6

Complete the table by writing the meaning of each word part that is listed. Also write the corresponding anatomic term for 1 through 12. (Numbers 2 and 8 have two anatomic terms each.) The first one is done as an example.

Combining Form	Meaning	Anatomic Term
1. anter(o)	*front*	*anterior*
2. caud(o)		
3. cephal(o)		
4. dist(o)		
5. dors(o)		
6. infer(o)		
7. later(o)		
8. medi(o)		
9. poster(o)		
10. proxim(o)		
11. super(o)		
12. ventr(o)		

Say and Check

Say aloud the anatomic terms you wrote for Exercise 6. Use the Companion CD to check your pronunciations.

down

up

side

6-25 Locations and directions are generally described relative to the body in the anatomic position. Physicians rely on additional positions for examination or surgery. **Prone*** (prōn) and **supine**† (soo-pīn´, soo´pīn) are terms used to describe the position of persons who are lying face downward and lying on the back, respectively (Figure 6-8, *A* and *B*). If a person is prone, is the face turned up or down? _____

Pronation (pro-na˝shən) and **supination** (soo˝pĭ-na´shən) are generally used to indicate positioning of the hands and feet, but their complete meanings include the act of lying prone or face downward and assumption of a supine position. Pronation of the arm is the rotation of the forearm so that the palm faces downward.

Supination is the rotation of a joint that allows the hand or foot to turn upward. Supination of the wrist allows the palm to turn _____. Compare pronation and supination of the wrist in Figure 6-8, *C*.

Recumbent (re-kum´bənt) means lying down. The lateral recumbent position is assumed by the patient lying on the side, because lateral means pertaining to the _____.

*Prone (Latin: *pronus,* inclined forward). †Supine (Latin: *supinus,* lying on the back, face upward).

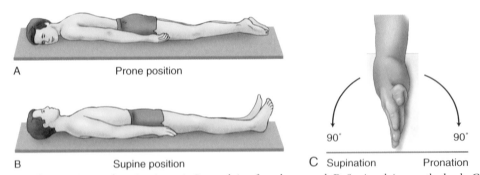

A   Prone position

B   Supine position

C Supination   Pronation

90°   90°

Figure 6-8 Comparison of pronation and supination. **A,** Prone, lying face downward. **B,** Supine, lying on the back. **C,** Supination and pronation of the elbow and wrist joints which permit the palm of the hand to turn up or downward.

EXERCISE 7

Label the body positions with one of these two terms: prone or supine.

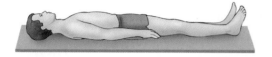
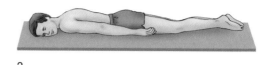

1. _____   2. _____

BODY REGIONS AND BODY CAVITIES

trunk

6-26 The body is made up of two major regions:
- head, neck, and trunk (chest, abdomen, and pelvis)
- extremities (arms and legs)
  The chest, abdomen (ab´də-mən, ab-do´mən), and pelvis make up the body's
  _____. The trunk has two major cavities that contain internal organs.
  Learn the following combining forms that are used to describe the body.

Selected Combining Forms: Body

Combining Form	Meaning	Combining Form	Meaning
abdomin(o)	abdomen	pelv(i)	pelvis
acr(o)	extremities (arms and legs)	peritone(o)	peritoneum
axill(o)	armpit	pod(o)	foot
cephal(o)	head	som(a), somat(o)	body
crani(o)	cranium (skull)	spin(o)	spine
dactyl(o)	finger or toe	thorac(o), steth(o)	thorax (chest)
encephal(o)	brain	viscer(o)	viscera (large abdominal organs)
herni(o)	hernia		
omphal(o), umbilic(o)	umbilicus (navel)		

abdominothoracic
(ab-dom˝ĭ-no-thə-ras´ik)

6-27 The **abdomen** is that part of the body lying between the thorax and the pelvis. Write a word that means pertaining to the abdomen and thorax by combining abdomin(o) + thorac(o) + -ic:
_____.

6-28 Because of its large area and numerous internal organs, the abdomen is frequently subdivided using imaginary lines to indicate points of reference. There are two methods of using imaginary lines to divide the abdomen into regions. Dividing the abdomen into four quadrants (kwod´rəntz) is a convenient way to designate areas in the abdominal (ab-dom´ĭ-nəl) cavity (Figure 6-9, *A*). Refer to the diagram to answer the following:

upper
lower

Quadrant is a term that means any one of four corresponding parts. RUQ and LUQ refer to the right and left _____ quadrants, respectively. RLQ and LLQ refer to the right and left _____ quadrants.

quadrant

Abdominal quadrants are used to describe the location of pain or of body structures. The system of naming four abdominal areas that are determined by drawing two imaginary lines through the umbilicus is the four-_____ system. Principal organs contained in the four abdominal quadrants are shown in Table 6-3.

6-29 Anatomists describe the abdomen as having nine regions, shown in Figure 6-9, *B*. The nine-region system is also used in clinical and surgical settings. Some of the terms may be unfamiliar, but try to remember the divisions. When the terms are studied in more detail in later chapters, they will acquire more meaning. Look at Figure 6-9, *B*, while working this frame.

hypochondriac
(hi˝ po-kon´dre-ak)

The upper lateral regions beneath the ribs are the right and left _____ **regions.**

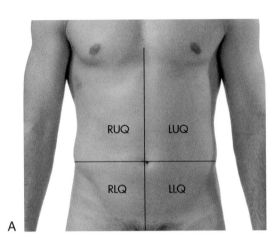

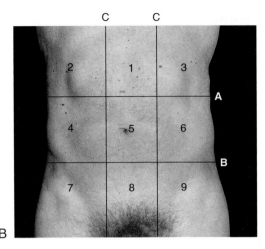

Figure 6-9 Two systems of using imaginary lines to divide the abdomen into regions. A, Quadrants of the abdomen, four divisions of the abdomen determined by drawing a vertical line and a horizontal line through the umbilicus. *RUQ, LUQ, RLQ,* and *LLQ* are abbreviations for right upper quadrant, left upper quadrant, right lower quadrant, and left lower quadrant respectively. **B,** The nine anatomical regions of the abdomen, determined by four imaginary lines *A, B, C,* and *C.* The regions are: *1,* epigastric; *2,* right hypochondriac; *3,* left hypochondriac; *4,* right lumbar; *5,* umbilical; *6,* left lumbar; *7,* right inguinal (or iliac); *8,* hypogastric; *9,* left inguinal (or iliac).

TABLE 6-3 Abdominal Quadrants and Their Contents	
Right upper quadrant (RUQ)	Contains the right lobe of the liver, gallbladder, right kidney, and parts of the large and small intestines
Left upper quadrant (LUQ)	Contains the left lobe of the liver, stomach, pancreas, left kidney, spleen, and parts of the large and small intestines
Right lower quadrant (RLQ)	Contains the right ureter, right ovary and uterine tube, appendix, and parts of the large and small intestines
Left lower quadrant (LLQ)	Contains the left ureter, left ovary and uterine tube, and parts of the large and small intestines

epigastric
(ep″ĭ-gas′trik)
umbilical
(əm-bil′ĭ-kəl)
lumbar (lum′bahr,
lum′bər)
hypogastric
(hi″po-gas′trik)
iliac (il′e-ak)
inguinal
(ing′gwĭ-nəl)

Between the hypochondriac regions lies the _____ **region.** The stomach is in this region.

The _____ region lies just below the epigastric region. The **umbilical region** is that of the navel, or umbilicus.

The right and left _____ **regions** lie on each side of the umbilical region.

The lower middle region is called the _____ **region.**

Finally, the two lower lateral regions are the right and left _____ or _____ **regions.**

6-30 The first region that you named in the preceding frame was the hypochondriac region. (You have probably also heard the term **hypochondriac** applied to a person who has a false belief of suffering from some disease. Ancient Greeks believed that organs in the hypochondriac region of the abdomen were the cause of melancholy and imaginary diseases, hence the term hypochondriac.) **Abdomin/al** means pertaining to the _____.

abdomen

EXERCISE 8

Label the abdominal quadrants that are indicated on the diagram with these abbreviations; LLQ, LUQ, RLQ, RUQ.

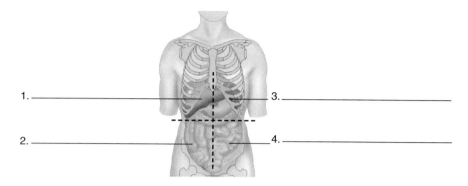

1. _____   3. _____

2. _____   4. _____

back (posterior)
front (belly)

6-31 The body has two major cavities, spaces that contain internal organs. The two principal body cavities are the dorsal cavity and the ventral cavity. We learned previously that dorsal means situated toward the _____ surface of the body. Ventral means situated toward the _____ surface.

cranial, spinal

6-32 The dorsal and ventral cavities are subdivided as shown in Figure 6-10. The **dorsal cavity** is divided into the _____ cavity and the _____ cavity.
   The **cranial** (kra´ne-əl) **cavity** contains the brain, and the spinal (spi´nəl) cavity contains the spinal cord and the beginnings of the spinal nerves. The cranial and spinal cavities are divisions of the _____ body cavity.

dorsal

6-33 The **ventral cavity** is the anterior body cavity. It is subdivided into the thoracic, abdominal, and pelvic (pel´vik) cavities. You have learned that thoracic means pertaining to the _____. (The combining form steth(o) is used in the term stethoscope, but thorac(o) is used in referring to the thoracic or chest cavity.) The thoracic cavity contains several divisions, which you will learn in a later chapter. The abdominal and pelvic cavities are not separated by a muscular partition, and together they are often called the **abdomino/pelvic** (ab-dom˝ĭ-no-pel´vik) **cavity.** The muscular **diaphragm** (di´ə-fram) separates the thoracic cavity from the abdominopelvic cavity.

thorax (chest)

pelvic

6-34 The **pelvis** is the lower portion of the trunk of the body. You learned that pelv(i) is the combining form for pelvis. The cavity formed by the pelvis is the _____ cavity.
   The pelvic cavity contains the urinary bladder, the lower portion of the large intestine, the rectum, and the male or female reproductive organs. However, organs such as the stomach, spleen, and liver are contained in the _____ cavity.

abdominal

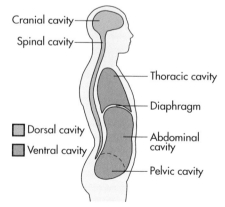

Figure 6-10 The body has two principal body cavities, the dorsal and ventral cavities, each further subdivided. The dorsal cavity is divided into the cranial cavity and the spinal cavity. The ventral cavity is divided into the thoracic cavity and the abdominopelvic cavity, which is subdivided into the abdominal cavity and the pelvic cavity.

EXERCISE 9

Build It! *Label the body cavities by building terms using these word parts. (The suffixes may be used more than once.)*

abdomin(o), crani(o), pelv(i), spin(o), thorac(o), -al, -ic

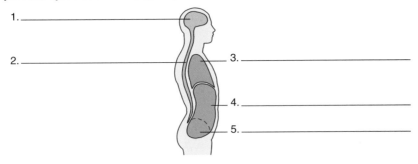

1. _____

2. _____

3. _____

4. _____

5. _____

6-35 The abdominopelvic cavity is lined with a membrane called the **peritoneum** (per″ĭ-to-ne′əm). This membrane also covers the internal organs (Figure 6-11). Write the name of the membrane that lines the abdominopelvic cavity and covers the internal organs:

peritoneum

_____.

There are two types of peritoneum:
- The **parietal** (pə-ri′ə-təl) **peritoneum** lines the abdominal and pelvic walls.
- The **visceral** (vis′ər-əl) **peritoneum** contains large folds that weave in between the organs, binding them to one another and to the walls of the cavity.

parietal

The peritoneum that lines the abdominopelvic cavity is _____ peritoneum.

Organs within the ventral body cavity, especially the abdominal organs, are called **viscera**

visceral

(vis′ər-ə). Peritoneum that invests the viscera is called _____ peritoneum.

6-36 Build a word that means pertaining to the peritoneum using the suffix -eal:

peritoneal
(per″ĭ-to-ne′əl)

_____.

Serous membranes such as the peritoneum secrete a lubricating fluid that allows the organs to slide against one another or against the cavity wall. The peritoneal cavity is the space between the parietal peritoneum and the visceral peritoneum.

6-37 Write a word using -plasty that means surgical repair of the abdomen:

abdominoplasty
(ab-dom′-ĭ-no-plas″te)

_____. (This type of plastic surgery, when done for aesthetic reasons to tighten the abdominal muscles, is commonly called a tummy tuck.)

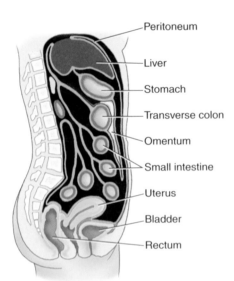

Peritoneum

Liver

Stomach

Transverse colon

Omentum

Small intestine

Uterus

Bladder

Rectum

Figure 6-11 The peritoneum (tan) in a median sagittal section of a female. This extensive membrane lines the entire abdominal wall and is reflected over the viscera. The free surface of the peritoneum is smooth and lubricated by a fluid that permits the viscera to glide easily against the abdominal wall and against one another.

6-38 **Ascites** (ə-si´tēz) is abnormal accumulation of serous fluid in the peritoneal cavity, sometimes resulting in considerable **distension** (enlargement, stretching) of the abdomen (Figure 6-12).

abdomen

Abdomino/centesis (ab-dom″ĭ-no-sen-te´sis) is surgical puncture of the _____. **Abdominal paracentesis** (par″ə-sen-te´sis) is another name for abdominocentesis. This procedure is performed to remove fluids or to inject a therapeutic agent. It is most often done to remove excess fluid, ascites, from the peritoneal cavity (Figure 6-13). The removal of the excess fluid in the peritoneal cavity is called abdominal

paracentesis

_____.

6-39 The body's **extremities** are the four limbs. Each arm, elbow, forearm, wrist, hand, and associated fingers make up one of the body's upper extremities. Each thigh, knee, leg, ankle, foot, and associated toes make up one of the lower extremities. Fingers and toes are digits. When referring to the bones of the digits, phalanges is the proper term. When referring to a digit in its entirety (multiple phalanges plus surrounding soft tissues), digit, finger, or toe should be used. Many medical terms use combining forms for the body extremities—hands, feet, and phalanges (bones

acr(o)
extremities
acrocyanosis
(ak″ro-si″ə-no´sis)
extremities

of the fingers and toes). The combining form for extremities is _____. In **acro/paralysis** (ak″ro-pə-ral´ĭ-sis), movement of the _____ is impaired.

Build a word by combining acr(o), cyan(o), and -osis: _____.

Literal translation of this new word is a blue condition of the _____. This is an intermittent cyanosis of the extremities, caused by exposure to cold or emotional stimuli. **Acrocyanosis** is also called **Raynaud** (ra-nō´) sign or **phenomenon** (Figure 6-14).

extremities

6-40 **Acro/megaly** (ak″ro-meg´ə-le) is a disorder in which there is enlargement of the _____. In acromegaly there is enlargement of many parts of the skeleton, particularly the distal portions such as the nose, ears, jaws, fingers, and toes (see Figure 17-14). It is caused by increased secretion of growth hormone by the pituitary (pĭ-too´ĭ-tar″e) gland.

6-41 The suffix -osis means condition but sometimes implies a disease or abnormal increase. It usually indicates an abnormal noninflammatory condition. **Inflammation** is tissue reaction to injury and is recognized by pain, heat, redness, and swelling.

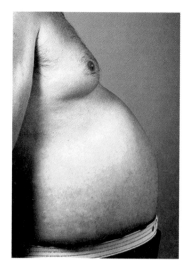

Figure 6-12 Ascites. This abnormal accumulation of a fluid in the peritoneal cavity is treated with dietary therapy and drugs. Abdominal paracentesis may be performed to relieve the pressure of the accumulated fluid.

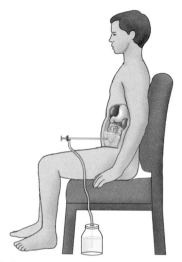

Figure 6-13 Paracentesis. This procedure in which fluid is withdrawn from a body cavity is performed to remove excess fluid from the abdomen.

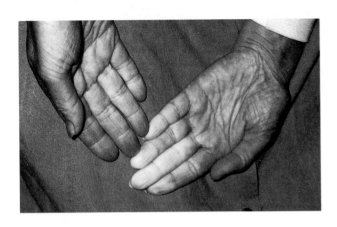

Figure 6-14 Raynaud phenomenon occurs in Raynaud disease. This intermittent lack of circulation of the fingers, toes, and sometimes ears and nose, with severe paleness, often accompanied by pain, is usually brought on by cold or emotional stimuli.

skin

     Literal translation of **dermat/osis** (dur″mə-to′sis) is a _____ condition. Its true meaning is any disease of the skin in which inflammation is not present. In-flammation of the skin is called **dermatitis. Acro/dermat/itis** (ak″ro-dur″mə-ti′tis) is inflamma-tion of the skin of the _____, especially the hands and feet.

extremities

     Write another word that, translated literally, means surgical repair of the skin: _____. In this surgery, skin grafts are used to cover destroyed or lost skin.

dermatoplasty
(dur′mə-to-plas″te)

6-42 The combining form dactyl(o) usually refers to a finger but sometimes to a toe. Fingers and toes are also called **digits** (dij′its). Whenever you see dactyl(o) or digit, immediately think of a finger or toe. A **dactylo/gram** (dak-til′o-gram) is a mark or record of a fingerprint. The part of the word that refers to the finger is dactyl(o). The process of taking fingerprints is

dactylography
(dak″tə-log′ra-fe)

_____.
    Dactyl/itis (dak″tə-li′tis) is inflammation of a finger or toe.
    Dactylo/spasm (dak′tə-lo-spaz″əm) is a cramping or twitching of a digit. Write this word that means cramping of a finger or toe: _____.

dactylospasm

6-43 The combining form for hand is chir(o). Use chir(o) and -spasm to form a new word: _____. Writer's cramp is a form of **chirospasm.**

chirospasm
(ki′ro-spaz″əm)
hand
hands

    Chiro/plasty (ki′ro-plas″te) is surgical repair of the _____.
    Chiro/pod/y (ki-rop′ə-de) literally refers to the _____ and feet and was once a term for podiatry (po-di′ə-tre). A **pod/iatrist** (po-di′ə-trist) specializes in the care of _____. The specialized field dealing with the foot, including its anatomy, pathology, and medical and surgical treatment, is

feet

podiatry

_____..

6-44 A **podo/gram** (pod′o-gram) is a print or record of the foot. The term footprint is more commonly used than _____.

podogram

EXERCISE 10

Write combining forms for the following terms:

1. chest   _____

2. extremities   _____

3. finger or toe   _____

4. pelvis   _____

5. spine   _____

6. skull   _____

Break the following terms into their component parts and state the meaning of each word part.

1. abdominocentesis _____

2. acromegaly _____

3. chiroplasty _____

4. dactylography _____

5. dermatoplasty _____

6. peritoneum _____

7. podiatrist _____

8. visceral _____

Say and Check

Say aloud the terms in Exercise 11. Use the Companion CD to check your pronunciations.

TERMS RELATED TO THE BODY AS A WHOLE

6-45 A disease or a disorder in one structure can affect the functioning of the body as a whole. In Chapter 4, you learned how an infectious disease such as influenza can spread from one person to someone else. Infections occur when the body is invaded by pathogenic microorganisms. Infection is just one of several causes of an abnormal elevation of the body temperature, which is called fever or **pyr/exia** (pi-rek´se-ə). The latter term is written using a combining form pyr(o), which means fire; however, pyrexia means a _____ or a febrile condition.

fever

    Febrile (feb´ril) pertains to fever. **A/febrile** (a-feb´ril) means _____ fever.

without

    An **anti/pyretic** (an″te-, an″ti-pi-ret´ik) is an agent that is effective against _____. **Anti/febrile** (an″te-, an″ti-feb´ril) and antipyretic both mean effective against fever. Aspirin is a well-known antipyretic.

fever

6-46 A **pyro/gen** (pi´ro-jən) is a substance or agent that produces fever, such as some bacterial toxins. **Hyper/pyrexia** (hi″pər-pi-rek´se-ə) denotes a highly elevated body temperature, because hyper- means excessive or more than normal. This can be produced by physical agents such as hot baths or hot air, or by reaction to infection. A body temperature that is much greater than normal is called _____. An abnormally high temperature is considered to be **hyperpyrexial** (hi″pər-pi-rek´se-əl).

hyperpyrexia

6-47 **Anti/infective** (an″te-in-fek´tiv) means capable of killing infectious micro/organisms or of preventing them from spreading. An agent that is capable of this action is also called an antiinfective. The literal translation of antiinfective is acting _____ infection. **Anti/microb/ial** (an″te-, an″ti-mi-kro´be-əl) agents act against **microbes** (mi´krōbz), another name for microorganisms. Antimicrobial means the same as antiinfective.

against

    There are many types of antiinfectives. Because the term anti/bio/tic (an″te-, an″ti-bi-ot´ik) contains the combining form bi(o), we know that **antibiotics** act against _____ microscopic organisms. Antibiotics are derived from microorganisms or they are produced semisynthetically and are used to treat infections, largely bacterial infections. Read more about other types of antiinfectives in the Chapter Pharmacology section on the Companion CD.

living

6-48 Inflammation is the body's protective response to irritation or injury. You are familiar with some of the signs of inflammation, such as heat and redness. **Antiinflammatory** (an″te-in-flam´ə-tor″e) means acting _____ inflammation. In other words, it means counteracting or reducing inflammation.

against

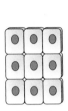
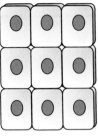
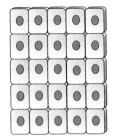

Original tissue   Increase in tissue size by hypertrophy   Increase in tissue size by hyperplasia

Figure 6-15 **A representation of tissue enlargement by hypertrophy and hyperplasia.**

6-49 Earlier in this chapter, you studied how tissue is a collection of similar cells acting together to perform a particular function. The suffix -plasia means formation. Several terms that contain -plasia are used to describe abnormal tissue formation. **Dys/plasia** (dis-plaʹzhə) is the abnormal development of tissues or organs. **A/plasia** (ə-plaʹzhə) is the lack of development of an organ or tissue. Translated literally, aplasia means _____ development.

without

An/otia (an-oʹshə), congenital absence of one or both ears, is an example of aplasia.

    Hypo/plasia (hiʺpo-plaʹzhə) is less severe than aplasia; it is the underdevelopment of an organ or tissue and usually results from fewer than the normal number of cells.

hyperplasia (hiʺpər-plaʹzhə)

6-50 Write a new term by combining hyper- and -plasia: _____. Literal translation of the word parts yields "increased development," but you will need to remember that **hyper/plasia** means an abnormal increase in the number of normal cells in tissue. Hyperplasia contrasts with another term, **hyper/trophy** (hyper-, increased; -trophy, nutrition), which means an increase in the size of an organ caused by an increase in the size of the cells rather than the number of cells. Figure 6-15 will help you understand the difference between hyperplasia and hypertrophy. It may be helpful to note that, despite the technical difference between hyperplasia and hypertrophy, these terms are sometimes used interchangeably to indicate increased size of a body part.

    Cells of the heart are particularly prone to hypertrophy (hi-purʹtrə-fe). In other words, the heart increases in size by enlarging individual cells. An enlargement of the adult heart may be caused by an increased workload. This differs from hyperplasia, in which the number of cells increases. The new cells may be either benign or malignant, so hyperplasia does not necessarily mean that the new cells are cancerous.

6-51 However, a change in the structure and orientation of cells, characterized by a loss of differentiation and reversal to a more primitive form, is characteristic of malignancy. This change in cell structure is called **ana/plasia** (anʺə-plaʹzhə). The prefix ana- means upward, excessive, or again. The important thing to remember about anaplasia is that it is especially characteristic of

malignancy

_____.

    Normal somatic cells divide to produce two identical daughter cells in a predictable manner. Cell growth or function is changed in aplasia, anaplasia, dysplasia, hypoplasia, or hyperplasia, but an important difference is that anaplastic cells are characteristic of carcinoma. Study Table 6-4 to understand the difference in these terms.

TABLE 6-4	Comparison of Abnormal Tissue Formation		
Term	**Cell Division**	**Significance**	**Metastasis**
aplasia	Essentially absent	Organ or tissue does not develop	No
hypoplasia	Reduced	Underdevelopment of organ or tissue	No
hyperplasia	Increased	More tissue development; enlargement of organ	No
dysplasia	Continuous or inappropriate	Cellular deviation from the normal, which may progress to anaplasia in certain organs (example: uterus)	No
anaplasia	Rapid and abnormal cells	Characteristic of malignancy	Possible

Build It! *Use these word parts to write terms to complete these sentences. (Some will be used more than once.)*

pyr(o), a-, ana-, dys-, hyper-, hypo-, -gen, -plasia

1. An agent that causes fever is a/an   _____/_____.

2. Abnormal development of tissue or organs is called   _____/_____.

3. Lack of development of an organ or tissue is   _____/_____.

4. Underdevelopment of an organ or tissue is   _____/_____.

5. Abnormal increase in the number of normal cells in tissue is _____/_____.

6. A change in the structure and orientation of cells that is
   characteristic of malignancy is   _____/_____.

Say and Check

Say aloud the terms you wrote for Exercise 12. Use the Companion CD to check your pronunciations.

6-52 You have learned that both som(a) and somat(o) refer to the body in general. The death of a person, **somatic** (so-mat´ik) **death,** is usually defined as absence of electrical activity of the brain for a specified period under rigidly defined circumstances. Practice will help you learn which word part to use in writing terms about the body.

body
somat(o)

Somato/genic (so″mə-to-jen´ik) means originating in the _____. The part of somatogenic that means body is _____.

6-53 You have already learned that cephal(o) refers to the head and that cephal/ad means toward the _____.

head

The combining form encephal(o) means the brain and is so called because the brain is located inside the head. **Electro/encephalo/graphy** (e-lek″tro-ən-sef´ə-log´rə-fe) is the process of recording electrical activity of the brain and can be used to determine somatic death.

6-54 An **electro/encephalo/gram** (e-lek″tro-en-sef´ə-lo-gram″) is a record produced by the electrical impulses of the _____. (You see why the abbreviation EEG is commonly used!) The instrument used to record electrical impulses of the brain is an **electroencephalograph** (e-lek″tro-ən-sef´ə-lo-graf″).

brain

Encephal/itis (en-sef´ə-li´tis) is _____ of the brain. There are many types of encephalitis, but a large percentage of cases are caused by viruses. The symptoms include mild to severe convulsions, coma, and even death in some cases.

inflammation

Encephalo/pathy (en-sef″ə-lop´ə-the) is any _____ of the brain.

disease

body

6-55 Som/esthetic (so″mes-thet´ik) pertains to _____ feeling. The "a" is dropped from som(a) to facilitate pronunciation. A particular part of the brain, the somesthetic area, is responsible for receiving and pinpointing where and what sensations occur in the body. A lesion in this part of the brain could affect one's ability to read, write, or speak and also one's ability to recognize objects by touch. A lesion is a wound or other pathologic change in body tissue.

mind

6-56 Somato/psych/ic (so″mə-to-si´kik) pertains to both body and _____. Somatopsychic disorders are physical disorders that influence mental activity. A brain lesion (physical disorder) often produces significant intellectual difficulties and memory loss (mental activities).

Physiology is the study of the function of the body. **Psycho/physio/logic** (si″ko-fiz″e-o-loj´ik), also called **psycho/somatic** (si″ko-so-mat´ik), disorders are the opposite of somatopsychic. Extreme or prolonged emotional states that influence the physical body's functioning are psychophysiologic disorders. Emotional factors may precipitate conditions such as high blood pressure.

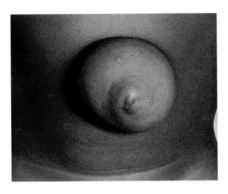

Figure 6-16 Omphalocele. An umbilical hernia is a skin-covered protrusion of intestine through a weakness in the abdominal wall around the umbilicus. The hernia often closes spontaneously within 2 years, but large hernias may require surgical closure.

You learned that physi(o) means nature. In psychophysiologic disorders, the natural functioning of the body is influenced by emotional factors.

mind

6-57 Psychosomatic is also the commonly used term that refers to the interaction of the mind, or psyche, and the body. You have learned that psych(o) means _____.
Psych/ic (si′kik) has two meanings: **Psychic** means pertaining to the mind, or the term refers to a person with the ability to read the minds of others.

umbilicus
umbilicus

6-58 Omphalus (om′fə-ləs) is another name for the **umbilicus** (əm-bil′ĭ-kəs) or navel.
Omphal/ic (om-fal′ik) means pertaining to the _____.
    An **omphalo/cele** (om′fə-lo-sēl″) is a congenital hernia of the _____.
Babies are sometimes born with an omphalocele, protrusion of part of the intestine through a defect in the abdominal wall at the umbilicus (Figure 6-16). Write the formal name for an um-

omphalocele

bilical (əm-bil′ĭ-kəl) hernia: _____.

6-59 A hernia can occur through any weakness or defect in the peritoneum that lines the abdominal or pelvic cavities. In addition to the umbilicus, frequent sites of such weaknesses are old surgical scars and the inguinal (ing′gwĭ-nəl) (groin) and **femoral** (fem′or-əl) (thigh) canals (Figure 6-17). Read the information that accompanies the illustration and write answers in the blanks. A hernia that occurs through an inadequately healed surgical site is an

incisional

_____ hernia.
    The type of hernia that occurs if a loop of intestine descends through the femoral canal into

femoral
inguinal

the groin is a _____ hernia.
    A direct or indirect hernia that occurs in the groin is an _____ hernia.
    Hernio/plasty (hur′ne-o-plas″te), surgical repair of a hernia, is sometimes used specifically to denote repair using a mesh patch or plug to reinforce the area of the defect.

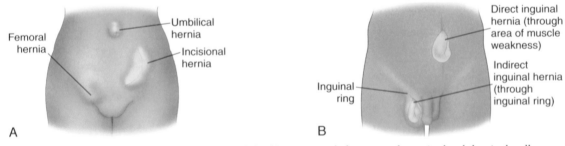

Femoral hernia

Umbilical hernia

Incisional hernia

Direct inguinal hernia (through area of muscle weakness)

Inguinal ring

Indirect inguinal hernia (through inguinal ring)

A

B

Figure 6-17 Common types of abdominal hernias. A, Umbilical hernias result from a weakness in the abdominal wall around the umbilicus. An incisional hernia is herniation through inadequately healed surgery. In a femoral hernia, a loop of intestine descends through the femoral canal into the groin. **B,** Inguinal hernias are of two types. A direct hernia occurs through an area of weakness in the abdominal wall. In an indirect hernia a loop of intestine descends through the inguinal canal, an opening in the abdominal wall for passage of the spermatic cord in males and a ligament of the uterus in females.

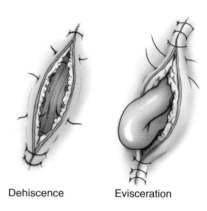

Figure 6-18 Dehiscence and evisceration. Both are complications of wound healing and involve a splitting open of the wound, but evisceration is the total separation of all wound layers and protrusion of internal organs (for example, part of the intestine) through the open wound.

Dehiscence   Evisceration

6-60 Wounds are physical injury to body tissue, whether caused by accident or surgery.

> ➤ **KEY** POINT <u>Several factors slow the process of healing</u>. Infection slows the healing process. Other factors are:

presence of foreign material
decaying tissue
movement (lack of immobilization) of the
    wound

poor blood circulation
decreased number of white blood cells
deficiency of antibodies
malnutrition in the individual

6-61 Deep wounds or those in an area of movement, such as near a joint, may require sutures or another means of holding the tissue together while healing occurs. Movement retards healing and can lead to **dehiscence** (de-his´əns), a splitting open or rupture of a wound after it has closed. It also means the separation of a surgical incision, typically an abdominal incision. Write

dehiscence

this term that means a splitting open: _____.

evisceration

Evisceration (e-vis″ər-a´shən) is the protrusion of internal organs through an open wound. If an internal organ protrudes through a dehiscence, this is called _____. Compare dehiscence and evisceration (Figure 6-18).

umbilicus
inflammation

6-62 Omphal/oma (om″fə-lo´mə) is a tumor of the _____.
   Omphal/itis (om″fə-li´tis) is _____ of the umbilicus.
   Write a term that means hemorrhage from the umbilicus by combining omphal(o) and

omphalorrhagia
(om″fə-lo-ra´jə)
rupture

-rrhagia: _____.

   Omphalorrhexis (om″fə-lo-rek´sis) means _____ of the umbilicus.

EXERCISE 13

Write a word in each blank to complete the sentences.

1. Omphalus is another name for the navel, also called the _____.

2. The death of a person is called _____ death.

3. Electroencephalography is the process of recording electrical activity of the _____.

4. Congenital herniation of the navel is called _____.

5. A term that means pertaining to the body and the mind is psychosomatic or _____.

6. A splitting open of a wound is called _____.

7. The protrusion of internal organs through an open wound is _____.

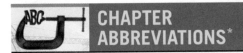

CHAPTER ABBREVIATIONS*

AP	anteroposterior (also others)	**LUQ**	left upper quadrant
DNA	deoxyribonucleic acid	**PA**	posteroanterior (also others)
EEG	electroencephalogram	**RLQ**	right lower quadrant
LLQ	left lower quadrant	**RUQ**	right upper quadrant

*Many of these abbreviations share their meanings with other terms.

Be Careful With These Opposites!

anter(o) vs. poster(o)
ventr(o) vs. dors(o)
proxim(o) = proximal vs. dist(o) or tel(e) = distal
medial vs. lateral
prone vs. supine

▶ CHAPTER 6 REVIEW

Basic Understanding

📊 *Build It!*

I. *Build terms using these word parts to identify these illustrations. (Prefix may be used more than once.)*

hyper-, -plasia, -trophy

Original tissue

1. Increase tissue size by
_____/_____

2. Increase tissue size by
_____/_____

Matching

II. *Using the diagram, identify the following abdominal regions with the correct letter (A-I). The first region is done as an example.*

1. epigastric   _B_   4. left iliac   _____   7. right iliac   _____

2. hypogastric   _____   5. left lumbar   _____   8. right lumbar   _____

3. left hypochondriac _____   6. right hypochondriac _____   9. umbilical   _____

III. *Match each directional term with its meaning, A through H. (Selections may be used more than once.)*

_____ 1. anterior

_____ 2. distal

_____ 3. dorsal

_____ 4. inferior

_____ 5. lateral

_____ 6. medial

_____ 7. posterior

_____ 8. proximal

_____ 9. superior

_____ 10. ventral

A. above
B. back
C. below
D. far
E. front
F. middle
G. near
H. side

Sequencing

IV. *Four levels of human organization are body systems, cells, organs, and tissues. List these in order from simple levels to more complex levels.*

1. _____

2. _____

3. _____

4. _____

Multiple Choice

V. *Circle the correct answer for each of the following.*

1. Similar cells acting together to perform a function defines a/an (body system, organ, organism, tissue).

2. Pete is trying to explain the two methods of drawing imaginary lines to designate abdominal areas. He explains that dividing the abdomen into (bilateral areas, eight regions, six regions, four quadrants) is a convenient way to describe the location of pain or of body structures.

3. A term that means from the middle to one side is (anteromedian, anterolateral, mediolateral, posteromedial).

4. Dr. Ray explains in a radiology report that a fracture has occurred in the distal portion of the thigh bone. Distal means (farther from the origin, in the middle of the bone, nearer the origin, on the side of the bone).

5. Which plane divides the body into anterior and posterior portions? (frontal, midsagittal, sagittal, transverse)

6. Which term means inflammation of the brain? (cephaloitis, craniitis, encephalitis, sephalitis)

7. What is the term that means lying face downward? (ambulatory, prone, proximation, supine)

8. Shelley has a noninflammatory skin condition. What is the skin condition called?
(dermatitis, dermatosis, pyosis, pyrexia)

9. What is another name for the navel? (angina, ascites, omphalocele, umbilicus)

10. Which of these terms means a muscular partition that separates the thoracic and abdominopelvic cavities? (diaphragm, paracentesis, peritoneum, pyrogen)

Writing Terms

VI. *Write words for the following:*

1. pertaining to above the chest   _____

2. affecting only one side   _____

3. lying flat on the back   _____

4. pertaining to the peritoneum   _____

5. pertaining to the sole   _____

6. inflammation of the skin   _____

7. pertaining to the abdomen and pelvis   _____

8. cramping of the hand   _____

9. abnormal development of tissue   _____

10. a record of electrical impulses of the brain _____

Say and Check

Say aloud the terms you wrote for Exercise VI. Use the Companion CD to check your pronunciations.

Greater Comprehension

Spelling
VII. *Circle all misspelled terms and write their correct spelling:*

abdomin   acrosyanosis   hyperpyrexia   palmar   superficial

Interpreting Abbreviations
VIII. *Write the meaning of each of these abbreviations:*

1. AP _____

2. DNA _____

3. LLQ _____

4. RLQ _____

5. RUQ _____

Pronunciation
IX. *The pronunciation is shown for several medical words. Indicate the primary accented syllable in each term with an ´.*

1. bilateral (bi lat ər əl)

2. cephalic (sə fal ik)

3. omphalic (om fal ik)

4. posterosuperior (pos tər o soo pēr e ər)

5. visceral (vis ər əl)

Say and Check
Say aloud the five terms in Exercise IX. Use the Companion CD to check your pronunciations. In addition, be prepared to pronounce aloud these terms in class:

abdominothoracic	antiinfective	dorsoventral	midsagittal
acromegaly	ascites	electroencephalography	omphalocele
anaplasia	caudad	hyperplasia	psychosomatic
anotia	chiropody	hyperpyrexia	supination
anteromedial	diaphragm	hypertrophy	transthoracic

Challenge
X. *Break these words into their components parts, and write their meanings. Even if you have not seen these terms before, you may be able to break them apart and determine their meanings.*

1. cephalocentesis_____

2. dactyledema _____

3. dorsodynia _____

4. extraperitoneal _____

5. thoracostomy _____

(Check your answers with the solutions in Appendix VI.)

PRONUNCIATION LIST

Use the Companion CD to review the terms that have been presented. Look closely at the spelling of each term as it is pronounced and be sure you know the meaning of each term.

abdomen
abdominal
abdominal paracentesis
abdominocentesis
abdominopelvic cavity
abdominoplasty
abdominothoracic
acrocyanosis
acrodermatitis
acromegaly
acroparalysis
afebrile
anaplasia
anatomic plane
anatomic position
anatomy
angina pectoris
anotia
anterior
anterolateral
anteromedial
anteroposterior
anterosuperior
antibiotics
antifebrile
antiinfective
antiinflammatory
antimicrobial
antipyretic
aplasia
ascites
bilateral
caudad
caudal
cephalad
cephalic
chiroplasty
chiropody
chirospasm

congenital
cranial cavity
dactylitis
dactylogram
dactylography
dactylospasm
dehiscence
dermatitis
dermatoplasty
dermatosis
diaphragm
digits
distal
distension
dorsal
dorsal cavity
dorsocephalad
dorsolateral
dorsoventral
Down syndrome
dysplasia
electroencephalogram
electroencephalograph
electroencephalography
encephalitis
encephalopathy
epigastric region
epithelial
evisceration
extremities
febrile
femoral
frontal plane
genetic disorder
hernioplasty
hyperplasia
hyperpyrexia
hyperpyrexial
hypertrophy

hypochondriac
hypochondriac region
hypogastric region
hypoplasia
iliac
inferior
inferomedian
inflammation
inguinal regions
lateral
lumbar regions
medial
median
mediolateral
microbes
midsagittal plane
omphalic
omphalitis
omphalocele
omphaloma
omphalorrhagia
omphalorrhexis
omphalus
palmar
parietal peritoneum
pelvis
peritoneal
peritoneum
plantar
podiatrist
podiatry
podogram
posterior
posteroanterior
posteroexternal
posterointernal
posterolateral
posteromedial
posterosuperior

pronation
prone
proximal
psychic
psychophysiologic
psychosomatic
pyrexia
pyrogen
quadrant
Raynaud phenomenon
recumbent
sagittal plane
somatic death
somatogenic
somatopsychic
somesthetic
superficial
superior
supination
supine
suprathoracic
telecardiogram
thoracic
thoracodynia
thoracotomy
thorax
transthoracic
transverse plane
umbilical region
umbilicus
unilateral
ventral
ventral cavity
ventromedian
viscera
visceral peritoneum

Español ENHANCING SPANISH COMMUNICATION

English	Spanish (pronunciation)
abdomen	abdomen (ab-DOH-men), vientre (ve-EN-tray)
anatomy	anatomía (ah-nah-to-MEE-ah)
antibiotic	antibiótico (an-te-be-O-te-co)
arm	brazo (BRAH-so)
aspirate	aspirar (as-pe-RAR)
belly	barriga (bar-REE-gah)
blood	sangre (SAHN-gray)
body	cuerpo (coo-ERR-po)
breathing	respiración (res-pe-rah-se-ON)
chest	pecho (PAY-cho)
face	cara (CAH-rah)
fever	fiebre (fe-AY-bray)
finger	dedo (DAY-do)
fingerprint	impresión digital (im-pray-se-ON de-he-TAHL)
hip	cadera (cah-DAY-rah)
kidney	riñon (ree-NYOHN)
leg	pierna (pe-ERR-nah)
liver	hígado (EE-ga-do)
navel	ombligo (om-BLEE-go)
palm	palma (PAHL-mah)
rib	costilla (cos-TEEL-lyah)
skull	cráneo (CRAH-nay-o)
sole	planta (PLAHN-tah)
thigh	muslo (MOOS-lo)
toe	dedo del pie (DAY-do del PE-ay)
urinary bladder	vejiga (vah-HEE-gah)
uterus	útero (OO-tay-ro)
wrist	muñeca (moo-NYAY-cah)

Body Fluids and Immunity

7

Cellular Needs, Blood and Its Terminology, and the Immune System

LEARNING GOALS

Basic Understanding
In this chapter you will learn to do the following:
1. Recognize general facts about body fluids, and analyze associated terms.
2. Write the meaning of word parts pertaining to body fluids and immunity, and use them to build and analyze terms.
3. Recognize the types of body fluid and the kinds of imbalances that affect metabolism.
4. Name the functions of and the principal conditions that affect the formed elements of the blood, or match the terms with their meanings.
5. Write the name of blood pathologies when given the description of the condition, or match the terms with the description.
6. Write terms that describe coagulation, or match the terms with their descriptions.
7. List several body defense mechanisms.
8. Define active versus passive immunity and natural versus artificial immunity.
9. Name several nonspecific body defense mechanisms, and describe the two aspects of specific immune response.

Greater Comprehension
10. Define terms that are presented in health care reports.
11. Recognize the meaning of several signs and symptoms of anemia.
12. Spell medical terms accurately.
13. Pronounce medical terms correctly.
14. Write the meanings of the abbreviations.
15. Categorize terms as anatomy, diagnostic test or procedure, pathology, surgery, or therapy.

MAJOR SECTIONS OF THIS CHAPTER:

- ❏ CELLULAR NEEDS AND BODY FLUIDS
- ❏ COMPOSITION OF BLOOD
- ❏ BLOOD DISORDERS
- ❏ ANEMIAS AND ABNORMAL HEMOGLOBINS
- ❏ BLOOD COAGULATION, TRANSFUSIONS, AND BONE MARROW TRANSPLANTS
- ❏ IMMUNITY

FUNCTION FIRST

Body fluids normally constitute more than half of an adult's weight. These fluids are vital in the transport of oxygen and nutrients to all cells as well as in removal of wastes. Immunity is the body's ability to resist foreign organisms and toxins. The immune system protects the body initially by creating local barriers (for example, the skin) to foreign substances, but an important part of our immunity depends on substances in body fluids, especially cells and antibodies in the blood.

CELLULAR NEEDS AND BODY FLUIDS

between
within

7-1 Body fluids are the plasma (liquid part) of the circulating blood, the intercellular fluid, and the intracellular fluid. You have learned the meaning of intercellular and intracellular, so inter/cellular fluid is that fluid _____ cells, and intra/cellular fluid is that fluid _____ cells.

> ➤ **KEY** POINT <u>Body fluids serve many functions.</u> Although body fluids are vital in transporting oxygen and nutrients throughout the body, they are also involved in eliminating wastes and transporting other essentials, including immune substances, enzymes, and hormones.

water

7-2 Water is the most important component of body fluids. Body fluids are not distributed evenly throughout the body, and they move back and forth between compartments that are separated by cell membranes. The most important component of body fluids is

_____.

Chemical and microscopic studies are performed on various body fluids to determine the body's internal status. Laboratory tests are commonly used to detect, identify, and quantify substances; evaluate organ functions; help establish or confirm a diagnosis; and aid in the management of disease.

intracellular

7-3 An adult body's weight is made up of approximately 60% fluid and 40% solids (Figure 7-1). Looking at the illustration, you see that most of the fluid is _____ fluid, meaning that it is located within the cells. **Cellul/ar** (sel´u-lər) means pertaining to (or consisting of) cells, because cellul(o) means little cell or compartment. You know that intracellular and extracellular are terms that describe location relative to cells.

extracellular

7-4 Fluid that is not contained within the cells, the _____ fluid, is either plasma or interstitial (in″tər-stish´əl) fluid. Only about one fourth of the extracellular fluid is **plasma** (plaz´mə), the liquid part of the blood. The **interstitial**˙ (in″tər-stish´əl) **fluid** fills the spaces between most of the cells of the body and is transported away from the tissues by the lymphatic system. If anything interferes with that transportation, the fluid accumulates in the interstitial spaces, resulting in a condition called edema, which you studied in an earlier chapter.

˙Interstitial (Latin: *interstitium,* space or gap in a tissue or structure).

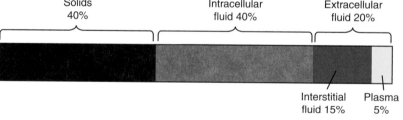

Figure 7-1 The body's fluid compartments. Fluid makes up 60% of the adult's body weight, and most of that is intracellular fluid. Two types of extracellular fluid are interstitial fluid and plasma.

EXERCISE 1

Build It! *Use these prefixes to build terms to complete these sentences.*

extra-, inter-, intra-

1. More than half of all body fluid is contained within cells and is called _____cellular fluid.

2. Fluid outside cells is called _____cellular fluid.

3. The fluid that fills the spaces between most of the body cells is _____stitial fluid.

FLUID BALANCE

7-5 The regulation of the amount of water in the body is called fluid balance.

> ➤ **KEY** POINT <u>Fluid balance is maintained through intake and output of water.</u> Water is obtained by drinking fluids and eating foods. Water leaves the body via urine, feces, sweat, tears, and other fluid discharges. This balance depends on the proper intake of water and the elimination (output) of body wastes, including excess water (Figure 7-2). Note that most of the fluid gained by the body is through drinking water, and most of the fluid is excreted in the urine.

The fluid balance depends on proper functioning of several body systems, particularly the urinary system. **Dehydration** (de″hi-dra′shən) (excessive loss of water from body tissue) or generalized edema (swelling caused by excessive accumulation of fluid in the body tissues) can occur if the body cannot maintain fluid balance. This regulation of the amount of water in the body is called _____ balance.

fluid

7-6 Several combining forms will be used in this chapter to describe body fluids. You already know that cyt(o) and -cyte mean _____.

cell

7-7 Fluid balance is one aspect of **homeo/stasis** (ho″me-o-sta′sis) (home[o], constant + -stasis, controlling), a relative constancy in the internal environment of the body. When the body is healthy, the tissue fluid that bathes and maintains the cells remains fairly constant within very limited normal ranges. Homeostasis is naturally maintained by sensing and control mechanisms that promote healthy survival. The combining form home(o) means _____ or sameness, and -stasis, in this case, means controlling.

constant

Learn the meanings of the word parts in the following list.

Word Parts: Body Fluids

Word Part	Meaning	Word Part	Meaning
Combining Forms for Selected Compartments		**Combining Forms for Selected Electrolytes**	
angi(o), vascul(o)	vessel	calc(i)	calcium
cellul(o)	little cell or compartment	kal(i)	potassium
		natr(o)	sodium
Miscellaneous Combining Forms			
home(o)	sameness; constant		
hydr(o)	water		

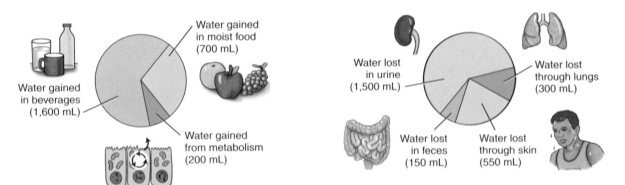

Water gained in beverages (1,600 mL)

Water gained in moist food (700 mL)

Water gained from metabolism (200 mL)

Water lost in urine (1,500 mL)

Water lost through lungs (300 mL)

Water lost in feces (150 mL)

Water lost through skin (550 mL)

Figure 7-2 Avenues of fluid intake and output. The kidneys are the main regulators of fluid loss. Generally, fluid intake equals fluid output so that the total amount of fluid in the body remains constant. Water is the most important constituent of the body and is essential to every body process. Depriving the body of needed water eventually leads to dehydration.

Match each word part in the left column with its meaning in the right column. (Choices A through G may be used more than once.)

_____ 1. angi(o)

_____ 2. calc(i)

_____ 3. cellul(o)

_____ 4. home(o)

_____ 5. hydr(o)

_____ 6. kal(i)

_____ 7. natr(o)

_____ 8. vascul(o)

A. calcium
B. little cell or compartment
C. potassium
D. sameness or constant
E. sodium
F. vessel
G. water

electricity

7-8 The nervous system and endocrine system work together to bring about homeostasis by affecting various functions, including the heartbeat, respiration, blood pressure, body temperature, and the concentration of electrolytes (e-lek´tro-līts) in the body fluids. **Electrolytes** are molecules that conduct an electrical charge. Some examples of electrolytes in body fluids are calcium, potassium, and sodium. To remember that electrolytes conduct an electric charge, it may be helpful to recall that electr(o) means _____.

calcium
potassium

hyponatremia
(hi″po-nə-tre´me-ə)

7-9 Certain diseases, conditions, and medications may lead to an imbalance of the electrolytes. **Hypo/calc/emia** (hi″po-kal-se´me-ə) is a deficiency of _____ in the blood. **Hypo/kal/emia** (hi″po-kə-le´me-ə) is a deficiency of _____ in the blood. Write a word that means a deficiency of sodium in the blood: _____. **Hyper/calcemia, hyper/kalemia,** and **hyper/natremia** are greater than normal blood levels of calcium, potassium, and sodium, respectively. Proper quantities of electrolytes are critical to normal metabolism and function.

water
head

7-10 In chemistry, hydr(o) refers to hydrogen, but more commonly hydr(o) means water. **Hydro/cephaly** (hi″dro-sef´ə-le) appears to mean _____ in the _____. In medical terms, some interpretation is needed in dividing words into their components. Hydrocephaly is more commonly called **hydrocephalus** (hi″dro-sef´ə-ləs). Hydrocephalus means a condition characterized by abnormal accumulation of cerebrospinal (ser″ə-bro-spi´nəl) fluid (see Chapter 15) within the skull, causing enlargement of the head, mental retardation, and convulsions (Figure 7-3).

Treatment of hydrocephalus generally consists of surgical intervention to correct the cause or to shunt the excess fluid away from the skull. **Shunt** (shunt), as a verb, means to redirect the flow of a body fluid from one cavity or vessel to another. The device that is implanted in the body to redirect the fluid is also called a shunt (noun). Write this new term for what is often used in treating hydrocephalus: _____. Remember, the word can be used as a verb or a noun.

shunt

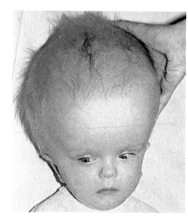

Figure 7-3 Four-month-old child with hydrocephalus. Hydrocephalus is usually caused by obstruction of the flow of cerebrospinal fluid. If hydrocephalus occurs in an infant, the soft bones of the skull push apart as the head increases progressively in size.

EXERCISE 3

Divide these terms into their component parts, and state the meanings of the terms.

1. homeostasis _____

2. hydrocephalus _____

3. hyperkalemia _____

4. hypernatremia _____

5. hypocalcemia _____

Say and Check

Say aloud the terms in Exercise 3. Use the Companion CD to check your pronunciations.

EXERCISE 4

In your own words, describe the following terms:

1. dehydration _____

2. edema _____

3. electrolytes _____

4. fluid balance _____

5. shunt _____

Say and Check

Say aloud the terms in Exercise 4. Use the Companion CD to check your pronunciations.

TYPES OF BODY FLUIDS

7-11 Although one may first think of blood when speaking of body fluids, there are many others including **lymph** (limf), saliva, urine, mucus, spinal fluid, tears, gastric juices, perspiration, and pus. The proper functioning of all body systems is dependent on body fluids.

➤ **KEY** POINT Several body fluids are associated with specific body systems. For example, cerebrospinal fluid bathes the brain and spinal cord and is associated with the nervous system. Urine is formed and excreted by the urinary system.

fluids

Blood, lymph, saliva, and urine are all examples of body _____.

7-12 Blood and lymph are the fluids that we generally associate with the **cardio/vascul/ar** (kahr″de-o-vas′ku-lər) (cardi[o], heart; vascul[o], vessel; -ar, pertaining to) and lymphatic (lim-fat′ik) systems. These fluids circulate throughout the body, providing nutrients for cells and transporting wastes for removal.

➤ **KEY** POINT Lymph is the fluid that circulates through the lymphatic vessels. As blood circulates, needed substances move across the vessel walls into the fluid that surrounds the body cells and fluid accumulates in the tissue spaces. This excess fluid is normally transported away from the tissues by the **lymphatic system**. The fluid is called lymph.

blood
lymph

The fluid _____ is carried by the cardiovascular system, and the fluid _____ is carried by the lymphatic system.

7-13 As blood circulates, it remains inside blood vessels in humans, so it is an **intra/vascular** fluid. Write this term that means within a vessel by combining intra-, vascul(o), and -ar: _____.

intravascular

Study the word parts and their meanings in the following list.

Word Parts: Selected Body Fluids

Word Part	Meaning	Word Part	Meaning
hem(a), hem(o), hemat(o), -emia	blood	muc(o)	mucus
		py(o)	pus
hidr(o)	sweat, perspiration	sial(o)	saliva; salivary glands
hydr(o)	water	ur(o)	urine; urinary tract

EXERCISE 5

Match each combining form in the left column with the correct body fluid in the right column. (Choices A through G may be used more than once.)

_____ 1. hem(o)

_____ 2. hemat(o)

_____ 3. hidr(o)

_____ 4. hydr(o)

_____ 5. muc(o)

_____ 6. py(o)

_____ 7. sial(o)

_____ 8. ur(o)

A. blood
B. mucus
C. perspiration
D. pus
E. saliva
F. urine
G. water

perspiration
hidr(o)

7-14 More than a million tiny structures called sweat glands are found in the skin. Sweat, or **perspiration** (per″spĭ-ra′shən), contains water, salts, and other waste products. These substances are excreted through pores in the skin when one perspires, and this serves as a means of ridding the body of wastes and regulating the body temperature. Another name for sweat is _____.

The combining form for sweat is _____. Do not confuse this combining form with hydr(o), which has the same pronunciation.

7-15 It is easy to confuse the terms excrete and secrete. **Secretion** (se-kre′shən) is the process of discharging a substance into a cavity. For example, saliva (sə-li′və) is secreted into the mouth to keep the mouth moist, along with other functions. **Excretion** (eks-kre′shən) is the body's way of eliminating waste substances. Perspiration is excreted through pores in the skin. Substances that are secreted or excreted are called secretions or excretions, respectively.

Saliva is the clear fluid secreted by the salivary (sal′ĭ-var-e) glands in the mouth. It serves to moisten the oral cavity, to aid in chewing and swallowing, and contains an enzyme that initiates digestion of starch. The combining form that means saliva is

sial(o)

_____. This combining form also means the salivary glands.

mucus

7-16 **Mucus** (mu′kəs) is the slippery secretion of glands within mucous membranes. **Muc/ous** (mu′kəs) means composed of or secreting _____. Mucous membranes line cavities or canals of the body that open to the outside, such as the digestive tract. Note the difference in spelling and meaning of the terms mucus (noun) and mucous (adjective).

7-17 Pus (pus) is the liquid product of infection. The combining form that means pus is

_____.

py(o)

> ▶ **KEY** POINT <u>Bacterial infection is the most common cause of pus production.</u> Pus is a thick fluid that is made up of the remains of liquefied necrotic tissue that has become infected, usually by bacteria. Pus is composed of protein substances, fluid, bacteria, and white blood cells (or their remains). It is generally yellow; if it is red, this suggests blood from the rupture of small vessels.

7-18 Discharges from infected tissue are described as **purulent** (pu´roo-lənt) or **suppurative** (sup´u-ra″tiv). Both terms mean pertaining to, consisting of, or producing pus. **Sanguinous** (sang´gwi-nəs) means containing blood.

Write the term that begins with a "p" that is used to describe infected tissue:

purulent

_____.

Write the term that begins with an "s" that is used to describe infected tissue:

suppurative

blood

_____.

Sanguinous means containing _____.

7-19 A localized collection of pus in a cavity surrounded by inflamed tissue is called an **abscess** (ab´ses) (Figure 7-4). The inflamed tissue may disintegrate and become necrotic (nə-krot´ik), increasing the difficulty of delivering medication to the site of infection and slowing the healing process. The combining form necr(o) means death. In **necrosis** (nə-kro´sis), there is localized tissue death in response to either injury or disease, and the tissue is described as **necrotic.** Abscesses may need to be excised or surgically drained for healing to occur.

abscess

A localized collection of pus in a cavity is an _____.

7-20 A **hemat/oma** (he″mə-to´mə) is a localized collection of blood, usually clotted, in an organ, space, or tissue, resulting from a break in the wall of a blood vessel. The term hematoma (hemat[o], blood + -oma, tumor) is derived from the old meaning of tumor, a swelling, because there is a raised area wherever a hematoma exists. Hematomas can occur almost anywhere in the body. They are especially dangerous when they occur inside the skull, but most hematomas are not serious. Bruises are familiar forms of hematomas.

You will use the suffix -oma to write words for tumors of many kinds, but you'll also need to remember that a localized collection of blood in an organ, tissue, or space is called a

hematoma

_____.

blood

7-21 Translated literally, hyper/emia (hi″pər-e´me-ə) means excessive _____. You need to know that **hyperemia** is an excess of blood in part of the body caused by increased blood flow, as one often sees in inflammation. In hyperemia, the overlying skin usually becomes reddened and warm.

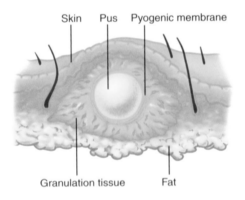

Skin   Pus   Pyogenic membrane

Granulation tissue   Fat

Figure 7-4 An abscess. The pus is contained within a thin pyogenic membrane that is surrounded by harder granulation tissue, the tissue's response to the infection.

EXERCISE 6

Match the terms in the left column with the descriptions in the right column.

_____ 1. excretion

_____ 2. hematoma

_____ 3. hyperemia

_____ 4. pus

_____ 5. sanguinous

_____ 6. secretion

_____ 7. suppurative

A. containing blood
B. excess of blood in some part that is caused by increased blood flow
C. localized collection of blood in an organ, space, or tissue
D. pertaining to or consisting of pus
E. process of discharging a substance into a cavity
F. process of eliminating waste substances
G. the liquid product of infection

COMPOSITION OF BLOOD

7-22 Blood, the most studied of all body fluids, is composed of a liquid portion, plasma, and several formed elements (cells or cell fragments).

> ➤ **KEY** POINT   Hematology (he″mə-tol´ə-je) is the study of blood and blood-forming tissues. The combining form hemat(o) means blood, but in the word hematology, the definition includes the blood-forming tissues, in other words, the bone marrow and lymphoid tissue (spleen, thymus, tonsils, and lymph nodes).

blood

hematologist

(he″mə-tol´ə-jist)

Hemato/logic (he″mə-to-loj´ik) means pertaining to hematology or the study of the _____. Change the ending of hematology to create a word that means one who studies blood: _____.
    Learn these word parts.

Word Parts: Aspects of the Blood

Word Part	Meaning	Word Part	Meaning
Combining Forms for Blood Cells		**Miscellaneous Combining Forms**	
chrom(o)	color	aer(o)	air or gas
cyt(o), -cyte	cell	is(o)	equal
hemoglobin(o)	hemoglobin	necr(o)	death
kary(o), nucle(o)	nucleus		
morph(o)	shape; form	**Miscellaneous Suffixes**	
norm(o)	normal	-ant	that which causes
phil(o)	attraction	-ate	to cause an action or the
poikil(o)	irregular		result of an action
spher(o)	round	-cidal	killing
		-poiesis	production
Combining Forms for Blood Clotting		-poietin	that which causes production
coagul(o)	coagulation		
fibrin(o)	fibrin		
thromb(o)	thrombus; clot		

EXERCISE 7

Match each word part in the left column with its meaning in the right column.

_____ 1. aer(o)

_____ 2. chrom(o)

_____ 3. cyt(o)

_____ 4. is(o)

_____ 5. kary(o)

_____ 6. morph(o)

_____ 7. necr(o)

_____ 8. phil(o)

_____ 9. poikil(o)

_____ 10. spher(o)

A. air
B. attraction
C. cell
D. color
E. death
F. equal
G. irregular
H. nucleus
I. round
J. shape or form

7-23 Hemato/poiesis (he″mə-to-, hem″ə-to-poi-e′sis) is the production of blood, specifically the formation and development of its cells. Write this new word by joining hemat(o) and -poiesis:

hematopoeisis

_____.

Hematopoiesis occurs in the bone marrow (specifically the red bone marrow), the soft, spongelike material in the cavity of bones. When you hear the term bone marrow failure, it is failure of the hematopoietic function of the bone marrow. In other words, in bone marrow failure, the red bone marrow does not produce _____ cells.

blood

EXERCISE 8

These three terms look similar. Divide them into their component parts and explain the differences in their meanings.

1. hematologic   _____

2. hematopoiesis _____

3. hematopoietic _____

Say and Check

Say aloud the terms in Exercise 8. Use the Companion CD to check your pronunciations.

7-24 Blood clots when it is removed from the body. **Coagulation** (ko-ag″u-la′shən) is the formation of a clot (Figure 7-5). Blood coagulation is a series of chemical reactions in which special fibers (fibrin) entrap blood cells, resulting in a blood clot.

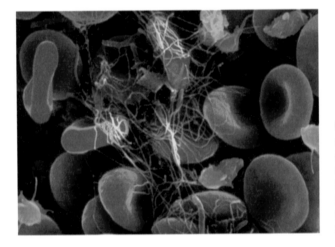

Figure 7-5 Blood coagulation. This scanning electron micrograph has been colored to emphasize the different structures. Red blood cells *(red)* are entangled with the fibrin *(yellow)*. Note the thin center and the thick edges that give red blood cells a concave appearance. The platelets *(blue)*, which initiate clotting, are also visible.

against
coagulation

Blood transfusions and many hematologic studies require blood that has not coagulated. An **anti/coagulant** (an″te-, an″ti-ko-ag´u-lənt) is used to prevent blood from clotting. You have learned that anti- is a prefix that means against. An anti/coagulant acts _____ coagulation. In other words, it prevents blood from clotting. Another word for blood clotting is _____.

anticoagulant

A **coagul/ant** (ko-ag´u-lənt) promotes or accelerates coagulation, because -ant means that which causes. A substance that prevents coagulation is called an _____.

Another suffix, -ate, means to cause an action or the result of an action. Thus **coagulate** (ko-ag´u-lāt) has two meanings, either to cause to clot or to become clotted. When you read that blood coagulates when removed from the body, it means that the blood clots.

coagulopathy
(ko-ag″u-lop´ə-the)

7-25 Write a word that means any disease (disorder) of coagulation: _____.

Exposure to air is not the reason that blood coagulates when removed from the body. A circulating anticoagulant normally prevents blood from clotting within the body. An anticoagulant can also be placed in blood as soon as it is removed from the body to prevent

coagulation

_____.

in vitro

7-26 In vitro[*] (in ve´tro) means occurring in a laboratory test tube (or glass) or occurring in an artificial environment. Because the anticoagulant is placed in the blood in an artificial environment (outside the body), this is in vitro use of an anticoagulant. A Latin term meaning in an artificial environment or outside the body is _____.

clotting
(coagulation)

Some patients tend to form clots within blood vessels, a serious condition that can result in death. For these patients, a physician prescribes in vivo (in ve´vo) anticoagulants to prevent _____. **In vivo**[†] is a Latin term that means occurring in a living organism.

[*]In vitro (Latin: *in,* within; *vitreus,* glassware).
[†]In vivo (Latin: *in,* within; *vivo,* alive).

EXERCISE 9

The following terms look similar. Divide them into their component parts, and explain the differences in their meanings.

1. anticoagulant _____

2. coagulant _____

3. coagulate _____

4. coagulopathy _____

🔊 Say and Check

Say aloud the terms in Exercise 9. Use the Companion CD to check your pronunciations.

7-27 Laboratory tests often require treating blood with an anticoagulant to prevent clotting. The blood in the tube in Figure 7-6 has been treated with an anticoagulant. The formed elements are erythrocytes (ə-rith´ro-sīts), leukocytes (loo´ko-sīts), and thrombocytes. Thrombo/cyte (throm´bo-sīt) is another name for a blood **platelet** (plat´lət). The layer that is made up of leukocytes and platelets is sometimes called the buffy coat.

> ➤ **KEY** POINT <u>An **erythro/cyte** is a red blood cell (RBC), often simply called red cell or red corpuscle (kor´pəs-əl).</u> A **corpuscle** is defined as any small mass or cell. Many structures, including red blood cells, are corpuscles. Normally, erythrocytes are biconcave disks that have no nucleus when seen in circulating blood. Their major function is transportation of oxygen and carbon dioxide. Look again at the shape of the red blood cells in Figure 7-5.

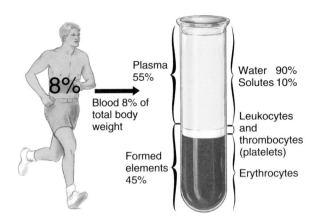

8%

Plasma 55%

Blood 8% of total body weight

Formed elements 45%

Water 90%
Solutes 10%

Leukocytes and thrombocytes (platelets)

Erythrocytes

Figure 7-6 Blood components. The blood in this test tube has been treated with anticoagulant to prevent clotting and has been centrifuged to separate its components. Red blood cells, the heaviest of the three components, make up the bottom layer. The middle layer of white blood cells and platelets is often called the buffy coat. The liquid part of treated blood (plasma) constitutes the upper layer. Any of these blood components can be given in a transfusion.

hemat(o)

The **hemato/crit** (he-mat´ə-krit) measures the percentage of red blood cells in a volume of blood. The part of hematocrit that means blood is _____. (Hematocrit is often abbreviated Hct.) The hematocrit is not a difficult concept. It simply tells us what percentage of the blood is made up of red blood cells. Normal values are based on packed red cell volume, which is determined by centrifuging the blood. Exact normal values vary among children, men, and women, but they usually range between 37% and 54%. (The hematocrit can also be calculated based on the size and number of red cells in a minute sample of blood.)

platelet

7-28 The suffix in the term thrombocyte implies that it is a cell; however, thrombocytes are not typical cells but simply cell fragments without a nucleus (see Figure 7-5). **Thrombocyte** is another name for a blood _____.

erythrocytes

7-29 Erythro/cyt/ic (ə-rith″ro-sit´ik) means pertaining to erythrocytes. **Erythro/poiesis** (ə-rith″ro-poi-e´sis) is the production of _____.
    Erythro/poietin (ə-rith″ro-poi´ə-tin), a hormone that is produced in the kidneys, stimulates erythropoiesis. (Note the slight change in the suffix -poiesis. The suffix -poietin means a substance that causes production.) Erythropoietin acts on stem cells of the red bone marrow to produce erythrocytes.

7-30 The white blood cell (WBC) is another important type of blood cell.

➤ **KEY** POINT White blood cells are referred to as **leukocytes**. The primary function of leukocytes is to protect the body against pathogenic organisms. Leukocytes are also called white cells or white corpuscles.

disease

You remember from Chapter 4 that patho/genic means capable of causing _____.

7-31 The blood of healthy persons has normal numbers of erythrocytes and leukocytes. This number is determined by blood counts. A leukocyte count is a determination of the number

white
red

of _____ blood cells. An erythrocyte count is the evaluation of the number of _____ blood cells.

7-32 Erythrocytes, **leukocytes,** and thrombocytes (more commonly called blood platelets) are the formed elements of the blood.
    A thrombo/cyte is not a cell that has clotted. It is a cell fragment that initiates the formation of a clot. You need to remember that another name for a blood platelet is a

thrombocyte

_____.

➤ **KEY** POINT Learn the difference between internal vs. external blood clots. The combining form thromb(o) means **thrombus** (throm´bəs), a blood clot that is attached to a vessel wall and tends to obstruct a blood vessel or a cavity of the heart. Be aware that some specialists differentiate between a blood clot (occurring in a test tube) and a thrombus (occurring internally).

EXERCISE 10

Write the medical term, as well as the common name of the formed elements of the blood.

Medical Term	Common Name
1. _____	_____
2. _____	_____
3. _____	_____

 Say and Check

Say aloud the terms you wrote for Exercise 10. Use the Companion CD to check your pronunciations.

7-33 A stained blood smear, as shown in Figure 7-7, *A*, allows examination of the erythrocytes, leukocytes, and blood platelets. The cells and platelets are stained for microscopic examination. A normal red cell in circulating blood has matured and lost its nucleus; however, a white blood cell still has a nucleus. There are five major types of leukocytes that can be classified by the presence or absence of granules (granulo/cytes or a/granulo/cytes) in the cytoplasm and their staining characteristics.

Types of White Blood Cells

Granulocytes	Combining Form
neutrophil (noo´tro-fil), sometimes abbreviated neut	neutrophil(o), neutr(o)
eosinophil (e˝o-sin´o-fil), abbreviated eos	eosinophil(o), eosin(o)
basophil (ba´so-fil), abbreviated baso	basophil(o)

Agranulocytes	
lymphocyte (lim´fo-sīt), abbreviated lymph	lymphocyt(o), sometimes lymph(o)
monocyte (mon´o-sīt), abbreviated mono	monocyt(o), sometimes mon(o)

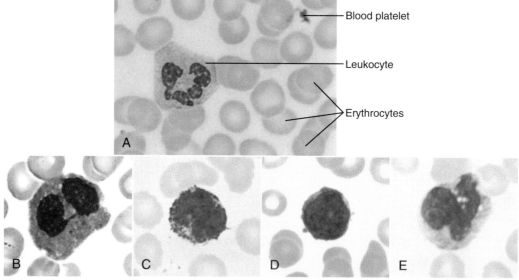

Figure 7-7 Human blood, stained. A, A leukocyte, a blood platelet, and erythrocytes are labeled. The leukocyte is a segmented neutrophil. **B,** An eosinophil. **C,** A basophil. **D,** A lymphocyte. **E,** A monocyte.

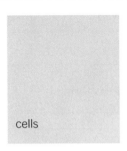

cells

The leukocyte in Figure 7-7, *A,* is a neutrophil. Neutrophils, eosinophils, and basophils have granules and are called **granulo/cytes** (gran´u-lo-sītz˝). The combining form phil(o) in these terms means attraction. Neutro/phils are so named because they are easily stained with (attracted to) neutral dyes. The granules of eosino/phils appear orange because they stain with eosin, an acid dye (Figure 7-7, *B*). On the other hand, the granules of baso/phils are stained dark by basic dyes (Figure 7-7, *C*). Lymphocytes and monocytes are **a/granulo/cytes** (a-gran´u-lo-sītz), meaning _____ that lack granules (Figure 7-7, *D* and *E*).

EXERCISE 11

List the five major types of WBCs.

1. _____   4. _____

2. _____   5. _____

3. _____

Say and Check

Say aloud the terms you wrote for Exercise 11. Use the Companion CD to check your pronunciations.

A differential white cell count is an examination and enumeration of the distribution of leukocytes in a stained blood smear. This laboratory test provides information related to infections and various diseases and is included in a complete blood cell count (cbc).

7-34 Poly/morpho/nuclear (pol˝e-mor˝fo-noo´kle-ər), a word often encountered when one is reading about leukocytes, is often shortened to **polymorph** (pol´e-morf) and is abbreviated PMN. **Polymorphonuclear** means having a nucleus that is divided in such a way that the cell may appear to have several nuclei, such as in the neutrophil in Figure 7-7, *A*. The combining form morph(o) means form or shape. In the term polymorphonuclear, poly- means

many

_____, morph(o) means shape, and nuclear pertains to a nucleus. A leukocyte with a nucleus that is divided in such a way that it appears multiple is polymorphonuclear.

nucleus

7-35 The word part for nucleus is nucle(o) or kary(o). A **nucleo/protein** (noo˝kle-o-pro´tēn) is a protein found in the _____. **Karyomegaly** (kar˝e-o-meg´ə-le) is abnormal enlargement of a cell nucleus.

nucleus

Nucle/oid (noo´kle-oid) means resembling a _____.

EXERCISE 12

Word Analysis. *Divide these terms into their component parts, and explain the meanings of the terms.*

1. karyomegaly   _____

2. polymorphonuclear   _____

3. nucleoid   _____

4. nucleoprotein   _____

Say and Check

Say aloud the terms in Exercise 12. Use the Companion CD to check your pronunciations.

BLOOD DISORDERS

clot

7-36 Thrombo/genesis (throm″bo-jen′ə-sis) is the formation of a blood _____ or a thromb/us (plural: **thrombi** [throm′bi]).

thrombus
thrombus

   Thrombo/lysis (throm-bol′ĭ-sis) is dissolution or destruction of a clot that has formed in a blood vessel. In other words, thrombolysis is destruction of a _____.
   Thromb/osis (throm-bo′sis) is the presence of a _____.
If a thrombus does not dissolve spontaneously, or if a thrombolytic agent cannot be used, the clot may need to be surgically removed, a procedure known as a **thromb/ectomy** (throm-bek′tə-me). **Thrombo/lytic** (throm″bo-lit′ik) means capable of dissolving a thrombus.
   A piece of a thrombus, a bit of tissue or tumor, or a bubble of gas or air that circulates in the blood stream until it becomes lodged in a vessel is an **embolus** (em′bo-ləs). **Embolism** (em′bə-liz-əm) is the presence of an embolus.

thrombocytes

7-37 Thrombo/cyto/penia (throm″bo-si″to-pe′ne-ə) is a decrease in the number of _____. This is also called **thrombopenia** (throm″bo-pe′ne-ə). Because thrombo/cytes are important in the process of blood coagulation, thrombocytopenia, if severe, results in a bleeding disorder.
   Thrombo/cyt/osis (throm″bo-si-to′sis) means an increase in the number of thrombocytes in the circulating blood. You learned that -osis means condition, but sometimes it implies an increased condition.

blood

7-38 Literal translation of hemo/lysis (he-mol′ə-sis) is destruction of _____.
Hemolysis is destruction of the red blood cell membrane, resulting in the release of **hemoglobin** (he′mo-glo″bin), the red pigment of blood (Figure 7-8). Because you have learned three combining forms that mean blood, you may be wondering how one knows which form to use. Common usage determines the proper form. Even though hemato/lysis is a good word, hemolysis is much better known.

destruction
(hemolysis)

   A **hemo/lysin** (he-mol′ə-sin) is a substance that causes _____ of red blood cells. When blood is placed in water or another substance that hemolyzes it, the destruction refers to the dissolving of the erythrocytes, which burst and release their red pigment.

7-39 Infectious mononucleosis (mon″o-noo″kle-o′sis) is an acute infection caused by the Epstein-Barr virus. It is characterized by fever, sore throat, swollen lymph glands, leukocytosis with atypical lymphocytes, abnormal liver function, and enlargement of the spleen. **Leukocytosis**

increase
white

(loo″ko-si-to′sis) means an _____ in the number of _____ blood cells.
   Young people are most often affected. Treatment is primarily symptomatic, with analgesics to control pain and enforced bed rest to prevent serious complications of the liver or spleen.

7-40 Staphylo/cocc/emia (staf″ə-lo-kok-se′me-ə) is staphylococci in the blood. The blood is normally free of microorganisms. **Bacter/emia** (bak″tər-e′me-ə) is the presence of

bacteria
streptococci

_____ in the blood. **Streptococc/emia** (strep″to-kok-se′me-ə), a type of bacter/emia, is the presence of _____ in the blood. A blood culture is helpful in detecting and identifying many types of bacteria that cause bacteremia. A sensitivity test provides information about which antibiotic is likely to be most effective for treatment.

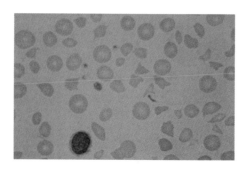

Figure 7-8 Hemolysis. This preparation of stained blood shows one WBC and several RBCs and blood platelets. Several of the RBCs have irregular shapes and a variety of sizes with significant space between some of the cells, suggesting hemolysis in which some of the red cells were destroyed.

> ➤ **KEY** POINT <u>Systemic (sis-tem´ik) means pertaining to the whole body rather than to a</u> <u>specific area of the body.</u> **Septic/emia** (sept[i], infection + -emia, blood) (sep″tĭ-se´me-ə) is a systemic infection in which pathogens have spread from some part of the body and are not only present in the circulating blood but are multiplying and causing blood infection. This is also called sepsis, and the patient is described as septic.

The presence of microbial toxins in the blood is **tox/emia** (tok-se´me-ə), a serious condition. A unique type of toxemia is seen in toxic shock syndrome (TSS). The severity of the disease is caused by toxins of a pathogenic strain of *Staphylococcus* and can become life-threatening unless it is recognized and treated. It is most common in menstruating females using high-absorbency tampons but has been seen in other persons. Although toxemia is generally reserved to describe the presence of toxins in the blood, it is sometimes used to mean severe and progressive (for example, toxemia of pregnancy).

blood

7-41 Literal translation of leuk/emia (loo-ke´me-ə) is white _____, and it is so called because of the large number of white cells in the blood of patients with this disease. **Leukemia** is a progressive, malignant disease of the **hemato/poietic** (he″mə-to-, hem″ə-to-poi-et´ik) (blood-forming) organs, characterized by a sharp increase in the number of leukocytes, as well as the presence of immature forms of leukocytes in the blood and bone marrow. A malignancy in which there is a sharp increase in the number of leukocytes is

leukemia

leukocytopenia
(loo″ko-si″to-pe´ne-ə)

_____.

Write a word using leuk(o), cyt(o), and -penia: _____. This is often shortened to **leukopenia** (loo″ko-pe´ne-ə). Either word means a decrease or deficiency in the number of leukocytes.

blood

7-42 An/emia (ə-ne´me-ə) literally means without _____. Because no one can live without blood, the name anemia is an exaggeration of the condition.

deficiency

Erythro/cyto/penia (ə-rith″ro-si″to-pe´ne-ə) is a _____ of erythrocytes. Erythrocytopenia can be shortened to **erythropenia** (ə-rith″ro-pe´ne-ə). Either word means a deficiency in the number of red blood cells.

7-43 Anemia, however, is a deficiency in the number of red blood cells or a deficiency in hemoglobin, or sometimes a reduction in both red cells and hemoglobin.

> ➤ **KEY** POINT <u>Anemia is not a disease but a sign of various diseases.</u> The severity of signs and symptoms depends on the severity of the anemia. Severe anemia may be accompanied by signs and symptoms that stem from diminished oxygen-carrying capacity of the blood.

Table 7-1 lists classic signs and symptoms of anemia. Several new terms are included in the table. **Tachycardia** (tak″ĭ-kahr´de-ə) means an increased pulse rate; it will be studied in the next chapter. Analyzing its word parts, tachy- means _____,

fast

cardi(o) means heart, and -ia means condition. One "i" is omitted to facilitate pronunciation.

TABLE 7-1   Classic Signs and Symptoms of Anemia

- Pallor (color of nail beds, palms, and mucous membranes of the mouth and conjunctivae are more reliable than skin color for assessing paleness)
- Tachycardia (increased pulse rate)
- Heart murmur
- Angina (chest pain)
- Decreased number of erythrocytes, hemoglobin, or both
- Congestive heart failure
- Dyspnea (difficult breathing)
- Shortness of breath
- Fatigue on exertion
- Headache
- Dizziness
- Syncope (fainting)
- Tinnitus (ringing in the ears)
- Gastrointestinal symptoms (anorexia, nausea, sore tongue and mouth)
- Constipation or diarrhea

Dys/pnea (disp´ne-ə) means difficult breathing because the suffix, -pnea, means breathing. You will learn more about dyspnea in Chapter 9. Note that **pallor** (pal´ər), named after the Latin term, refers to an unnatural paleness or absence of color. The table defines **syncope**[*]

fainting

ringing

(sing´kə-pe) as _____ and **tinnitus**[†] (tin´ĭ-təs, tĭ-ni´təs) as _____ in the ears.

7-44 Iron deficiency anemia results when there is a greater demand for iron than the body can supply. It can be caused by blood loss or insufficient intake or absorption of iron from the intestinal tract. Iron deficiency anemia is often treated successfully with iron tablets and a well-balanced diet.

Ancient Greeks drank water in which iron swords had been allowed to rust, thinking that they derived strength from the sword. The French steeped iron filings in wine and then drank it! Like the French wine with added iron, some modern products contain iron and vitamins with substantial alcohol. It is said that long ago, Ozark mountain people stuck nails in apples and let the nails rust. They removed the nails and fed the apples to their children. If the children's anemia improved after eating the apples, it is possible that they had

iron

_____ deficiency anemia.

7-45 Because coagulation involves several factors, a bleeding disorder can result from any number of deficiencies, including a deficiency of vitamin K. Classic **hemo/philia** (he″mo-fil´e-ə) is a hereditary bleeding disorder in which there is deficiency of one coagulation factor called anti/hemophilic (an″te-, an″ti-he″mo-fil´ik) factor (AHF) VIII. Other types of hemophilia may result from the deficiencies of other coagulation or clotting factors. In hemophilia there is spontaneous bleeding or prolonged bleeding after a minor injury. Perhaps the naming of hemophilia came about because of excessive and prolonged bleeding that occurs in the disorder, leading to an inaccurate conclusion that affected individuals had an affinity or attraction to blood.

Prolonged bleeding leads to a deficiency of both red blood cells and hemoglobin. This

anemia

condition is called _____.

leukocytosis

7-46 An increase in the number of leukocytes is _____. You learned earlier that leukemia is characterized by leukocytosis. But there is a major difference between leukemia and most conditions that cause leukocytosis. In leukemia, the production of leukocytes is uncontrolled, and many of the leukocytes produced are immature and nonfunctional.

Leukocytosis may be transitory and often accompanies a bacterial, but not usually a viral, infection. Because the main function of leukocytes is protection against harmful invading microorganisms such as bacteria, this should help you remember which type of cell is likely to increase

leukocytes

during a bacterial infection: _____.

7-47 Infection is sometimes confused with inflammation. Inflammation is a protective response of body tissues to irritation or injury, often resulting in elimination of offending agents and establishment of conditions necessary for repair. Infection (the presence of living microorganisms within the tissue) is but one cause of inflammation. Which of these two words is part of the

inflammation

body's natural defense? _____

> ➤ **KEY** POINT The cardinal signs of acute inflammation are redness, heat, swelling, and pain, sometimes accompanied by loss of function (Figure 7-9). Pain is actually a symptom rather than a sign but is included as one of the four cardinal signs.

Inflammation may be acute or chronic, lasting for months or even years. In chronic inflammation, the injurious agent persists or repeatedly injures tissue and can be debilitating to the individual.

---

[*]Syncope (Greek: *synkoptein,* to cut short).
[†]Tinnitus (Latin: *tinnire,* to tinkle).

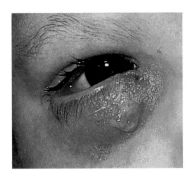

Figure 7-9 Sty. This infection of a gland of the eyelid shows two of the cardinal signs of inflammation: redness and swelling. It is not difficult to imagine that the sty has the other two signs of inflammation, pain and warmth, in the area around the sty.

7-48 Anemia and polycythemia represent abnormalities in the number of erythrocytes. Leukemia, leukocytosis, and leukopenia are abnormalities in the number of leukocytes. An increase or a decrease in blood platelets is also abnormal.

erythrocytes

Erythro/cyt/osis (ə-rith″ro-si-to′sis) means an increase in the number of _____. There is an increase in the number of erythrocytes in **polycythemia.** There are two forms of this condition, primary polycythemia (also called **polycythemia vera** [pol″e-si-the′me-ə ve′rə]) and secondary polycythemia. In both there is an increase

erythrocytes

in the number of _____.

Primary polycythemia is a serious disorder in which the bone marrow overproduces many types of cells and is associated with a chromosomal defect. Secondary polycythemia occurs as a physiologic response to prolonged exposure to high altitude or to lung or heart disease. In the described situations, insufficient oxygen in the tissue brings about the response. Sometimes the cause of secondary polycythemia is not known.

There is also an increase in the number of leukocytes in this disease, as well as the more marked erythrocytosis. This increased cell mass results in a sluggish flow of blood through the blood vessels. The increased red cell mass leads to several secondary alterations, such as elevated blood pressure, increased viscosity, and thrombotic tendencies. Viscosity is the ability or inability of a fluid to flow well. A solution with high viscosity is thick and flows more slowly than one of lower viscosity. Thrombotic tendencies favor formation of

thrombi

_____.

7-49 Principal conditions that are associated with abnormalities in the blood cells and platelets are listed in Table 7-2. The table lists a few terms that you have not yet studied.

granulocyte

A/granulo/cyt/osis means absence of what type of blood cell? _____

Disseminated (dĭ-sem′ĭ-nāt″əd), meaning scattered or distributed over a considerable area, intra/vascul/ar coagulation (DIC) is a grave coagulopathy (ko-ag″u-lop′ə-the) in which there is generalized intravascular clotting. A coagulo/pathy is any disorder of

coagulation

_____.

TABLE 7-2	Principal Conditions Affecting Blood Cells and Platelets	
Conditions Involving Erythrocytes	**Conditions Involving Leukocytes**	**Conditions Involving Blood Platelets**
Anemia	Leukocytosis	Disseminated intravascular coagulation
Bone marrow failure	Leukopenia	Thrombocytopenia
Hemolysis	Agranulocytosis	Thrombocytosis
Polycythemia	Leukemia (acute or chronic)	

EXERCISE 13

Write a word in each blank to complete these sentences.

1. Another name for a blood platelet is _____.

2. A clot in a vessel or the heart is _____.

3. Thrombogenesis is the formation of a blood _____.

4. Destruction of a thrombus is _____.

5. Destruction of red blood cells, resulting in the release of hemoglobin, is called _____.

6. A progressive, malignant disease of the hematopoietic organs, characterized by a sharp increase in the number of leukocytes, is called _____.

7. Leukopenia means a deficiency of _____.

8. An increase in the number of thrombocytes is called _____.

9. A term for a deficiency in the number of red blood cells, a deficiency in hemoglobin, or sometimes a reduction in both red cells and hemoglobin is _____.

10. The meaning of syncope is _____.

ANEMIAS AND ABNORMAL HEMOGLOBINS

7-50 Hemoglobin (Hb, Hgb), the iron-containing pigment of erythrocytes, carries oxygen from the lungs to tissues throughout the body. Microscopic variations in the erythrocytes are often observed in anemias and can be seen on a stained blood smear. A microscope is used to view cells and other objects too small to be seen with the naked eye. A micro/cyte (mi´kro-sīt) is a

small   _____ cell. **Microcytes** are undersized red blood cells sometimes seen in anemia. A condition in which there is an increase in the number of undersized red blood cells can be named by combining micr(o) + cyt(o) + -osis:

microcytosis   _____.
(mi˝kro-si-to´sis)

7-51 Macro/cyte (mak´ro-sīt) usually refers to a large erythrocyte. Macrocytes are seen in certain types of anemia. An increase in the number of larger-than-normal erythrocytes is called

macrocytosis   _____. **Macrocyte** and **megalo/cyte** (meg´ə-lo-sīt) both
(mak´ro-si-to´sis)   mean large cell (usually erythrocytes).

    With use of a microscope, erythro/cytes can be studied to determine whether they appear normal. If erythrocytes appear to be of normal size, we refer to them as **normocytes** (nor´mo-sīts) or we describe them as **normocytic** (nor˝mo-sit´ik).

7-52 Combine an- + is(o) + cyt(o) + -osis to write a word that means that cells are not of equal
anisocytosis   size: _____. Anisocytosis is common in the blood of people
(an-i˝so-si-to´sis)   who are anemic.
equal   **Iso/tonic** (i˝so-ton´ik) means _____ tension. Isotonic also denotes a solution in which body cells can be bathed without damage to the cells through diffusion of water into or out of the cells, because the concentration of electrolytes in the solution is equal to that in the cell. A solution in which cells can be placed without damage to the
isotonic   cells or change in their general appearance is an _____ solution.

round   **7-53** A sphere is round. A **sphero/cyte** (sfēr´o-sīt) is a _____ cell. A normal red blood cell is biconcave, resembling a disk indented on opposite sides. A sphero/cyte
round   is a red blood cell that is less concave than normal and appears _____.
       Using spherocyte and -osis, write a term that means the presence of spherocytes in the
spherocytosis   blood: _____.
(sfēr´o-si-to´sis)

7-54 **Poikilo/cytes** (poi´kĭ-lo-sītz″) are red blood cells that have an abnormal shape. The combining form poikil(o) means irregular. If a red blood cell has an irregular shape, we call it a

poikilocyte
poikilocytosis
(poi″kĭ-lo-si-to´sis)

_____. The presence of poikilocytes in the blood is

_____.

Poikilocytes are seen in several disorders, including sickle (sik´əl) cell anemia. People with **sickle cell anemia,** a hereditary anemia that mainly afflicts blacks, inherit an abnormal type of hemoglobin. Their red blood cells appear elongated and sickled and are highly fragile. In vivo hemolysis occurs, resulting in hemolytic anemia. Sickle cells are irregularly shaped erythrocytes, so they are also poikilocytes.

7-55 **Hypo/chrom/ia** (hi″po-kro´me-ə) is a condition in which the red blood cells have a

below

_____ normal amount of color. They are described as **hypochromic** (hi″po-kro´mik) cells. Cells that have more than the normal amount of color—in

hyperchromic
(hi″pər-kro´mik)

other words, excessive pigmentation—are described as _____ cells.

Hemo/globin is the red pigment found inside erythrocytes that gives blood its red color. **Globins** (glo´binz) or **globulins** (glob´u-linz) are types of proteins; therefore hemo/globin is a

blood

type of protein found in _____. Hemoglobin is often abbreviated Hb or Hgb.

7-56 Observe several abnormal types of erythrocytes (Figure 7-10). You can see that

smaller
larger
size
shape

microcytes are _____ than normal, macrocytes are _____ than normal, anisocytes are erythrocytes that vary in _____, and poikilocytes are erythrocytes that have an unusual _____. In anemia, erythrocytes usually do not have

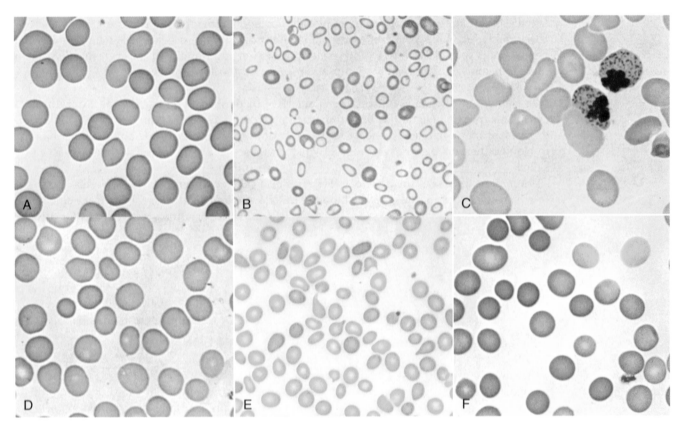

Figure 7-10 Morphologic variations of red blood cells in a stained blood smear. A, Normal erythrocytes. **B,** Hypochromic microcytes. A few cells are normal, but most have central paleness and small diameter. **C,** Macrocytes in pernicious anemia. In addition to erythrocytes of a larger size than normal, two immature ones still have a nucleus. These cells also show anisocytosis and/or poikilocytosis. **D,** Anisocytosis. Note the varying sizes of erythrocytes. **E,** Poikilocytes. Several erythrocytes have abnormal shapes. **F,** Spherocytes. About half of the cells show dense staining and a round shape.

TABLE 7-3	Two Classifications of Anemia

Morphologic Classification (Based on the Appearance of Red Cells in Stained Smear)
1. Normocytic normochromic (from sudden blood loss, hemolytic anemias, kidney disorders, and certain chronic diseases)
2. Macrocytic normochromic (deficiency of vitamin B_{12} or folic acid is a leading cause of certain chronic diseases)
3. Microcytic hypochromic (insufficient iron or hemoglobin production, chronic blood loss)

Etiologic Classification (Based on Cause)
1. Increased loss or destruction of red cells (bleeding or hemolysis caused by heredity or change in the red cell environment)
2. Decreased or defective production of red cells (deficiencies in diet; defective absorption; bone marrow interference, such as malignancies, toxic drugs, or irradiation)

a normal appearance. Table 7-3 shows two ways in which anemias are classified, one on the basis of appearance of red cells and the other on the basis of cause.

7-57 Some anemias are hereditary and are caused by abnormal hemoglobins. Use hemoglobin(o) to write a word that literally means any disease of the hemoglobins:

hemoglobinopathy
(he″mo-glo″bin-op′ə-the)
_____.
The hemoglobinopathies are a group of diseases caused by or associated with the presence of abnormal hemoglobin in the blood.

7-58 Because hemoglobins are proteins, they move at various speeds across paper or starch gel, based on their electrical charge, their size, and their mobility. **Hemoglobin electrophoresis** (e-lek″tro-fə-re′sis) is used to identify abnormal hemoglobin.
Hemoglobins are generally identified by letters or sometimes by their place of occurrence and discovery. Normal adult hemoglobin is designated hemoglobin A. There are many abnormal types. One type of abnormal hemoglobin, S, is found in sickle cell anemia. Abnormal hemoglobins such as Hb S generally result in distortion and fragility of the erythrocytes, causing

dissolve
them to hemolyze more readily. Hemo/lyze means that the erythrocytes _____.

7-59 Hemo/lytic anemia is a disorder characterized by premature destruction of the erythrocytes. This type of anemia may be an inherited disorder; may be associated with some infectious diseases; or may occur as a response to drugs, various toxic agents, or certain incompatibilities in blood or tissue types. The disorder in which erythrocytes are destroyed prematurely is

hemolytic
called _____ anemia.
Hemolytic disease of the newborn (HDN) is also called **erythro/blast/osis fetalis** (ə-rith″ro-blas-to′sis fe-tal′əs). The blood of infants who are born with this type of hemolytic anemia contains **erythro/blasts** (ə-rith′ro-blasts) (immature erythrocytes), and it is for this reason the condition was named erythroblastosis fetalis.

> ► KEY POINT <u>The cause of erythroblastosis fetalis may be an Rh factor incompatibility of the mother and the fetus.</u> The disease results from an incompatibility of the blood groups of the mother and fetus, such as the Rh (Rhesus) factor, ABO blood groups, or other blood incompatibilities. Diagnosis is confirmed during pregnancy by amniocentesis and analysis of the amniotic fluid.

Treatment may consist of an **intrauterine** (in″trə-u′tər-in) (within the uterus) transfusion or immediate exchange transfusions after birth. In Rh factor incompatibility, sensitization to the Rh factor can be prevented by injection of the mother with a preparation such as RhoGAM. Hemolytic reactions involving the ABO blood groups are generally less severe than those involving the Rh factor.

7-60 Write a word that means the opposite of plastic by using either a- or an-:

aplastic (a-plas′tik)
_____. You previously learned that plast(o) means repair.

Aplastic means having no tendency to develop new tissue. In aplastic anemia, the bone marrow is diseased and produces few cells.

Irregularities in the blood often indicate abnormal conditions of various body systems; however, certain diseases or disorders are associated mainly with the blood or bone marrow and are called **dyscrasias** (dis-kra´zhəz).* Some examples of the latter, such as leukemia and aplastic anemia, have already been discussed.

---

*Dyscrasia (Greek: *dys,* bad; *krasis,* mingling).

EXERCISE 14

Write words for the following meanings.

1. an undersized erythrocyte   _____

2. an increase in the number of oversized erythrocytes   _____

3. presence of cells of unequal size   _____

4. a red blood cell that appears round   _____

5. an irregularly shaped erythrocyte   _____

6. excessive pigmentation of erythrocytes   _____

7. decreased pigmentation of erythrocytes   _____

8. a disease associated with abnormal hemoglobin   _____

9. having no tendency to develop new tissue   _____

10. red pigment found in erythrocytes   _____

 ## Say and Check

Say aloud the terms you wrote for Exercise 14. Use the Companion CD to check your pronunciations.

BLOOD COAGULATION, TRANSFUSIONS, AND BONE MARROW TRANSPLANTS

fibrin

fibrinolysin
(fi˝brĭ-nol´ə-sin)
thrombus

platelets

7-61 Coagulation of the blood is a series of chemical reactions that result in a blood clot. **Fibrin** (fi´brin) is formed when blood clots. Fibrino/gen (fi-brin´o-jən) is a precursor of _____. **Fibrinogen** is a protein that is changed into fibrin in the process of coagulation.

Fibrino/lysis (fi˝brĭ-nol´ə-sis) is the destruction of fibrin. Write a word that means a substance that can dissolve fibrin: _____.

A fibrinolysin can dissolve a blood clot, which is another name for a _____. Heparin and warfarin (Coumadin) are in vivo anticoagulants that are used to prevent blood clots. The blood of persons taking anticoagulants is tested regularly using laboratory tests such as PT and PTT (abbreviations for prothrombin [pro-throm´bin] time and partial thromboplastin [throm˝bo-plas´tin] time). **Prothrombin** and **thromboplastin** are factors involved in different parts of the coagulation process, and the tests provide information about various stages of the coagulation process. The importance of accurate and reliable prothrombin time measurements has resulted in a standardized reporting system for prothrombin times called the International Normalized Ratio (INR).

7-62 Blood coagulation saves lives when it occurs in response to injury. It can result in death, however, if it occurs in the circulating blood. An internal blood clot, a thrombus, usually starts with tissue damage and is particularly life-threatening if the clot occurs in the heart or if it breaks off and is taken by the bloodstream to the brain or heart. Thrombocyt/osis, an increase in the number of blood _____, can also cause thrombosis. Blood coagulation brings about hemo/stasis (he˝mo-sta´sis, he˝mos´tə-sis). Stasis means stoppage of flow. **Hemo/stasis** can mean arrest of bleeding or interruption of blood flow through a vessel or to any part of the body.

> ➤ **KEY** POINT <u>Bleeding disorders can be as serious a problem of blood coagulation as thrombosis.</u> The most common cause of bleeding disorders is thrombocyto/penia, an insufficiency of blood platelets, resulting from either decreased production or survival or increased destruction. In addition, malfunction or absence of any of the coagulation factors causes at least some degree of bleeding tendency. Hemostasis may be delayed in these cases, resulting in the loss of large amounts of blood. A transfusion may be necessary to replace the lost blood.

7-63 The prefix trans- means through or across. The introduction of whole blood or blood components into the bloodstream of a person is called a **blood transfusion** (trans-fu´zhən). In the earliest transfusions, blood was passed directly _____ from one person to another. When blood is used for transfusion, grouping or typing of the blood is necessary. Blood typing determines the blood group of a person. There are four main ABO blood groups (A, B, O, and AB). Rh (Rhesus) factors are also always considered. There are also several other genetically determined factors on the red blood cells. Blood typing tests determine a person's blood type by mixing blood with commercially prepared sera (and blood cells, for reverse type) and observing for agglutination (ə-gloo″tĭ-na´shən). In this type of **agglutination,** aggregates or small clumps of erythrocytes form, which may be visible macro/scopically or perhaps only micro/scopically (Figure 7-11).

Write the term that is another name for blood clumping: _____.

across

agglutination

7-64 A transfusion reaction is an adverse reaction to the blood a person receives in a transfusion. Among the most common reactions are those that result from blood group incompatibilities. In other words, something in the donor's blood is not compatible with the blood of the recipient. Symptoms of transfusion reactions vary in degree from mild to severe. Some are manifested immediately, whereas others may not occur for several days. Blood group incompatibilities often result in agglutination or hemolysis of the erythrocytes. Hemo/lysis is _____ of the erythrocytes.

destruction

> ➤ **KEY** POINT <u>Certain diseases can be transmitted to the recipient through blood transfusion.</u> Various screening tests are performed to avoid using infected blood. Screening generally includes testing for several types of **hepatitis** (hep″ə-ti´tis)—hepatitis A, B, C, and D; human **immunodeficiency** (im″u-no-də-fish´ən-se) virus (the agent that causes acquired immunodeficiency syndrome [AIDS]); cytomegalovirus (CMV); and syphilis (rapid plasma reagin test [RPR] is commonly used). Certain areas of the United States are beginning to also test for the West Nile virus, which causes West Nile encephalitis.

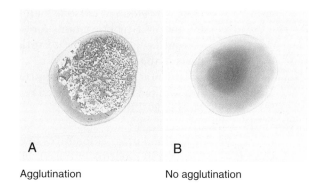

A Agglutination

B No agglutination

Figure 7-11 **Observing macroscopic agglutination in the laboratory. A,** Agglutination. This test on a glass slide using blood and commercially prepared serum results in visible small clumps, agglutination. **B,** No macroscopic agglutination. No visible clumping but microscopic examination is required to verify that agglutination has not occurred.

7-65 Autologous* (aw-tol′ə-gəs) and homologous† (ho-mol′ə-gəs) are terms that are often associated with blood transfusions or skin grafts. In an **autologous transfusion,** blood is removed from a donor and stored for a variable period before it is returned to the donor's circulation. In

autologous

an _____ **graft,** tissue is transferred from one site to another on the same body.

In contrast, a **homologous graft** is a tissue removed from a donor for transplantation to a recipient of the same species. This is also called an **allograft** (al′o-graft). A transplant from one's identical twin is an **iso/graft** (i′so-graft), but a transplantation from all other individuals of one's species is an allo/graft. Best results occur with an isograft or when the donor is closely related to the recipient. Transplantation of certain organs, such as kidneys, has a high degree of success.

7-66 Bone marrow transplants are used in treating patients with leukemia or aplastic anemia. **Allo/gene/ic** (al″o-jə-ne′ik), also called **allo/genic** (al″o-jen′ik), bone marrow transplants have a lower success rate than many organ transplants, such as transplant of the kidneys. For this reason, autologous transplants are preferred, using marrow previously obtained from the patient and stored, then reinfused when needed.

In allogeneic bone marrow transplants, a donor with a close human leukocyte antigen type is selected. The recipient is given chemotherapy or irradiation to destroy the diseased cells and much of the normal bone marrow. Bone marrow cells are aspirated from the donor's hip, repeating many times to obtain sufficient marrow. The cells are treated with anticoagulant and prepared for intravenous transfusion into the patient. Subsequent problems may include infection and graft versus host disease (immune response caused by incompatibility of the donor cells and recipient tissues).

*Autologous (Greek: *autos,* self).
†Homologous (Greek: *homos,* same).

EXERCISE 15

Use the following word parts to build terms to complete these sentences. (Some word parts will be used more than once.)

coagul(o), fibrin(o), hem(o), -ation, -gen, -lysin, lysis, -stasis

1. Destruction of fibrin is _____.

2. A series of chemical reactions that result in a blood clot is _____.

3. Interruption of blood flow through a vessel is _____.

4. The term for a substance that can dissolve a blood clot is _____.

5. A term for a protein that is changed into fibrin when coagulation takes place is _____.

Say and Check

Say aloud the terms you wrote for Exercise 15. Use the Companion CD to check your pronunciations.

EXERCISE 16

Write words in the blanks to complete these sentences.

1. A term for aggregation of cells into clumps or masses is _____.

2. A/An _____ reaction is an adverse reaction to the blood a person receives.

3. The term for the transfusion of a person's own blood after it has been collected in advance and stored is a/an _____ transfusion.

4. A/An _____ graft is tissue removed from a donor for transplantation to a recipient of the same species.

5. In vivo anticoagulants are given to persons to prevent blood _____.

IMMUNITY

7-67 Our bodies have many defenses, including immunity, which usually protects us from pathogenic organisms and other foreign substances. **Immunity** (ĭ-mu´nĭ-te) is the protection against infectious disease conferred by immunization, previous infection, or other factors. The immune reaction that can occur in a blood transfusion is part of the same system that provides protection against disease-causing organisms. We are continually exposed to pathogens and other harmful substances. Patho/gens are microorganisms that are capable of causing

disease

_____.

Study the word parts for immunity.

Word Parts: Immunity

Word Part	Meaning	Word Part	Meaning
aut(o)	self	-phylaxis	protection
immun(o)	immune	ana-	upward, excessive, or again

> ➤ **KEY** POINT Any substance that is capable, under appropriate conditions, of inducing a specific immune response is an **antigen** (an´tĭ-jən). Antigens may be bacteria, tissue cells, toxins, or foreign proteins. The body's natural ability to counteract microorganisms or toxins is called **resistance** (re-zis´təns). **Susceptibility** (sə-sep″tĭ-bil´ĭ-te) is a lack of resistance. For example, when we are exposed to the influenza virus, we do not become ill if our body has sufficient resistance.

susceptibility

The term for lacking resistance (or being susceptible) is _____.

7-68 Two types of body defenses are nonspecific resistance and specific resistance. Nonspecific defensive mechanisms are directed against all pathogens and include unbroken skin, phagocytes, inflammation, and proteins such as **complement** (kom´plə-mənt) and interferon (in″tər-fēr´on) (Figure 7-12). **Interferon** is of particular importance because it is formed when cells are exposed to a virus. Additional nonspecific defenses include mucus of mucous membranes, which traps foreign particles; hairlike projections (cilia) that form the lining of the respiratory tract and transport dust and microorganisms out of the body; beneficial normal flora that prevent the overgrowth of undesirable organisms; the composition and outward flow of urine; chemicals in human tears; and acids of the stomach, vagina, and skin, which help destroy invading microorganisms.

Phago/cyt/osis (fa″go-si-to´sis) is the ingestion and destruction of microorganisms and cellular debris by certain cells. The combining form phag(o) means to eat. Certain tissue cells called **macrophages** (mak´ro-fāj-ez) and leukocytes are the primary phagocytic cells. **Phago/cyt/ic** means pertaining to phagocytes or phagocytosis. Phagocytes (fa´go-sīts) are cells

ingest (or eat)

that _____ microorganisms and cellular debris.

7-69 The second type of defense, specific defense mechanisms, is selective (specific) for particular pathogens. This specific resistance is called immunity, and it protects us from a particular disease or condition. Both specific and nonspecific defenses occur simultaneously and work together to overcome pathogens. Resistance to a particular disease is called

immunity

_____.

Specific defense incorporates cell-mediated immunity and antibody-mediated immunity. White blood cells called T lymphocytes (also called T cells) are responsible for cell-mediated immunity. B lymphocytes (also called B cells) are responsible for antibody-mediated immunity.

against

7-70 Anti/bodies (an´tĭ-bod″ēz) are formed _____ antigens. People do not generally form antibodies against their own body cells; however, this happens in **autoimmune** (aw″to-ĭ-mūn´) **diseases,** a group of diseases characterized by altered function of the immune system that results in the production of antibodies against one's own cells. The condition

autoimmune

in which one forms antibodies against one's own cells is an _____ disease.

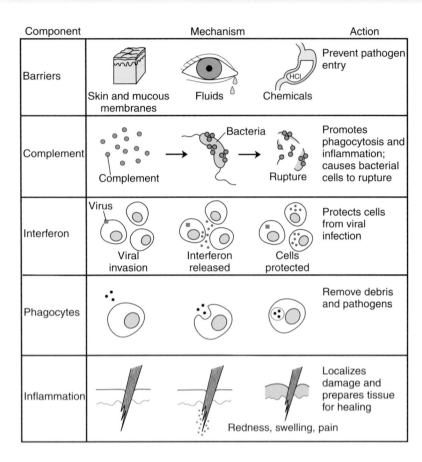

Component	Mechanism	Action
Barriers	Skin and mucous membranes	Fluids	Chemicals	Prevent pathogen entry
Complement	Complement → Bacteria → Rupture	Promotes phagocytosis and inflammation; causes bacterial cells to rupture
Interferon	Virus — Viral invasion	Interferon released	Cells protected	Protects cells from viral infection
Phagocytes		Remove debris and pathogens
Inflammation	Redness, swelling, pain	Localizes damage and prepares tissue for healing

Figure 7-12 Nonspecific defense mechanisms.
This is the body's initial defense against pathogens and foreign substances. Unlike cell-mediated immunity or antibody-mediated immunity, these defense mechanisms are nonspecific and directed against all types of invaders.

7-71 Antibodies are immunoglobulins (im″u-no-glob′u-linz) and are classified as IgA, IgD, IgE, IgG, or IgM. The combining form immun(o) means immune. An antibody interacts with the antigen that induced its synthesis. **Immuno/globulins,** or antibodies, are found in the blood plasma and act _____ harmful invading microorganisms.

against

Specific antibodies provide us with immunity against disease-causing organisms. We generally acquire antibodies either by having a disease or by receiving a vaccination (vak″sĭ-na′shən). A vaccination causes our bodies to produce _____.

antibodies

7-72 Polio vaccine contains polio antigen, which causes the formation of polio _____. After receiving the polio vaccine, one is immunized against poliomyelitis (po″le-o-mi″ə-li′tis) for a specific length of time.

antibodies

Occasionally the interaction of our defense mechanisms with an antigen results in injury. This excessive reaction to an antigen is called **hyper/sensitivity** (hi″pər-sen″sĭ-tiv′ĭ-te). Write this word that means a heightened reaction to an antigen: _____.

hypersensitivity

Anaphylaxis (an″ə-fə-lak′sis) or **anaphylactic** (an″ə-fə-lak′tik) **reactions** are exaggerated, life-threatening hypersensitivity reactions to a previously encountered antigen. The suffix -phylaxis means protection, and ana- means upward, excessive, or again. With a wide range in the severity of symptoms, the reactions may include generalized itching, difficult breathing, airway obstruction, and shock. Insect stings and penicillin are two common causes of anaphylactic shock, a severe and sometimes fatal systemic hypersensitivity reaction.

7-73 **Allergies** (al′ər-jēz) are conditions in which the body reacts with an exaggerated immune response to common, harmless substances, most of which are found in the environment.

➤ **KEY** POINT An **allergen** (al′ər-jen) is a substance that can produce an allergic reaction but is not otherwise harmful. Some common allergens are certain foods, pollen, animal dander, feathers, and house dust.

allergens

against

active
passive

Essentially harmless substances that cause allergies are called _____.
Allergy testing is used to identify the specific allergens. The most common is skin testing, which
exposes the patient to small quantities of the suspected allergens.

In an allergic reaction, injured cells release a substance called **histamine** (his´tə-mēn), which
causes dilation of the capillaries (the smallest blood vessels), an increase in gastric secretion,
and contraction of smooth muscle of several internal organs. Histamine is responsible for
the symptoms of hay fever: teary eyes, sneezing, and swollen membranes of the upper
respiratory tract. An **anti/histamine** (an″te-, an″ti-his´tə-mēn), a preparation that acts
_____ histamine, usually relieves the symptoms.

7-74 Immunization (im″u-nĭ-za´shən) is the process by which resistance to an infectious disease
is induced or augmented.

> ➤ **KEY** POINT Remember the difference between active and passive immunity. Active immu-
> nity occurs when the individual's own body produces an immune response to a harmful antigen.
> Passive immunity results when the immune agents develop in another person or animal and then
> are transferred to an individual who was not previously immune. This second type of immunity
> is borrowed immunity that provides immediate protection but is effective for only a short time.

Immunity that an individual develops in response to a harmful antigen is
_____ immunity. Borrowed immunity that is effective for
only a short time is _____ immunity.

7-75 In both active and passive immunity, the recognition of specific antigens is called specific
immunity. The terms natural and artificial refer to how the immunity is obtained (Figure 7-13).

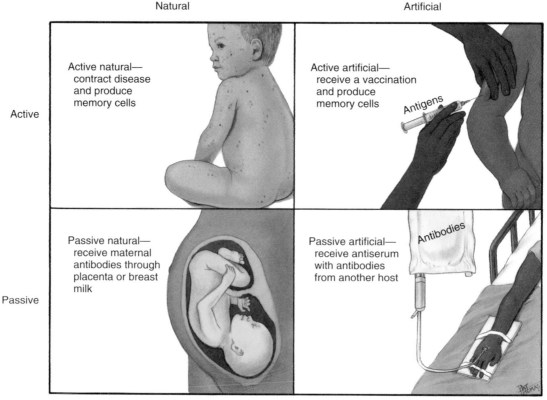

Natural   Artificial

Active

Active natural—
contract disease
and produce
memory cells

Active artificial—
receive a vaccination
and produce
memory cells   Antigens

Passive

Passive natural—
receive maternal
antibodies through
placenta or breast
milk

Passive artificial—
receive antiserum
with antibodies
from another host   Antibodies

Figure 7-13 Four types of specific immunity. Active natural and passive natural immunities, as the names imply,
occur through the normal activities of either an individual contracting a disease or a fetus being exposed to maternal antibodies. Both active artificial and passive artificial immunities require deliberate actions of receiving
vaccinations or antibodies.

A **vaccination** is any injection or ingestion of inactivated or killed microbes or their products that is administered to induce immunity. Vaccinations are available to immunize against many diseases such as typhoid, diphtheria, polio, measles, and mumps. Depending on its type, vaccine is administered orally or by injection. Vaccination is a form of **prophylaxis*** (pro″fə-lak′sis), prevention of or protection against disease.

antibodies

toxin (or poison)

7-76 Toxoids (tok′soidz) contain toxins, which are antigens. Toxoids cause our bodies to produce _____, thus providing us with immunity. Tox/oid, when broken down into its components, means resembling a _____. Actually, a **toxoid** is simply a toxin that has been treated to eliminate its harmful properties without destroying its ability to stimulate antibody production.

A toxoid is a helpful form of toxin. However, words containing tox(o) usually refer to substances that have an adverse effect. For example, a **cyto/toxin** (si′to-tok″sin) has harmful effects

cells

on _____. **Cyto/tox/icity** (si″to-tok-sis′ĭ-te) is the degree to which an agent possesses a specific destructive action on cells. This term is used in referring to the lysis of cells by immune phenomena, and it is also used to describe the activity of antineoplastic drugs that selectively kill cells. Anti/neo/plastic means inhibiting or preventing the development of neoplasms, malignant tumors.

Tox/icity (tok-sis′ĭ-te) is the degree to which something is poisonous or a condition that results from exposure to a toxin or to toxic amounts of a substance that does not cause adverse effects in smaller amounts.

7-77 **Immuno/compromised** (im″u-no-kom′prə-mīzd) pertains to an immune response that has been weakened by a disease or an **immuno/suppressive** (im″u-no-sə-pres′iv) agent. Radiation and certain drugs are **immuno/suppressants** (im″u-no-sə-pres′ənts), meaning that they

immune

suppress the _____ response.

To **transplant** (trans-plant′) is to transfer tissue. The tissue that is transplanted is called a transplant (trans′plant). Note that the pronunciation of the term depends on its usage as a verb or a noun. When tissue is transplanted from one person to another, rejection (re-jek′shən) is often a problem. **Rejection** is an immune reaction to the donor's tissue cells, with ultimate destruction of the transplanted tissue. Medications are used to suppress immune reactions, but the drugs have side effects. Rejection is still the most common problem encountered in transplantation of tissue from one person to another.

7-78 Immunodeficiency diseases are a group of health conditions caused by a defect in the immune system and are generally characterized by susceptibility to infections and chronic diseases. One of the most publicized immunodeficiency diseases is AIDS, a viral disease involving a defect in cell-mediated immunity that is manifested by various opportunistic infections. Infections caused by normally nonpathogenic organisms in a host whose resistance has been decreased are called opportunistic infections. There is no known cure for AIDS, and the prognosis is poor. Some persons with AIDS are susceptible to malignant neoplasms, especially Kaposi sarcoma (see Figure 13-17).

AIDS is caused by either of two varieties of the human immunodeficiency virus, designated HIV-1 and HIV-2. AIDS is transmitted by sexual intercourse or exposure to contaminated body fluid of an infected person. It was originally found in homosexual men and intravenous drug users but now occurs increasingly in heterosexual men and women, and in babies born of

immunodeficiency

infected mothers. AIDS means acquired _____ syndrome.

---

*Prophylaxis (Greek: *prophylax*, advance guard).

EXERCISE 17

Write words in the blanks to complete these sentences.

1. A foreign substance that induces production of antibodies is called a/an _____.

2. Lacking resistance is being _____ to a disease.

3. Phagocytosis of pathogens is part of the body's _____ defense mechanism.

4. Antibody-mediated immunity is part of the body's _____ defense mechanism.

5. _____ immunity occurs when an individual's body produces an immune response to a harmful antigen.

6. AIDS is an abbreviation for acquired _____ syndrome.

CHAPTER ABBREVIATIONS*

AHF	antihemophilic factor	**INR**	International Normalized Ratio
AIDS	acquired immunodeficiency syndrome	**lymph**	lymphocyte
baso	basophil	**mono**	monocyte
CBC, cbc	complete blood cell count	**neut**	neutrophil
CMV	cytomegalovirus	**PMN**	polymorphonuclear
DIC	disseminated intravascular coagulation	**PT**	prothrombin time (also physical therapy)
eos	eosinophil	**PTT**	partial thromboplastin time
Hb, Hgb	hemoglobin	**RBC**	red blood cell, red blood cell count
HCT, Hct	hematocrit	**Rh**	rhesus (a blood group)
HDN	hemolytic disease of the newborn	**RPR**	rapid plasma reagin
HIV	human immunodeficiency virus	**WBC**	white blood cell, white blood cell count

*Many of these abbreviations share their meanings with other terms.

Be Careful with These!

hidr(o) vs. hydr(o)
autologous vs. homologous
excretion vs. secretion
mucus vs. mucous

 # CHAPTER 7 REVIEW

Basic Understanding

Matching

I. *Match descriptions in the left column with A, B, or C.*

_____ 1. body defense

_____ 2. blood platelet

_____ 3. contains hemoglobin

_____ 4. initiates coagulation

_____ 5. transports oxygen

A. leukocyte
B. erythrocyte
C. thrombocyte

II. *Match each type of immunity with its description in the right column.*

_____ 1. active natural

_____ 2. active artificial

_____ 3. passive artificial

_____ 4. passive natural

A. contracting a disease
B. exposure of the fetus to maternal antibodies
C. receiving a vaccination
D. receiving an injection of antibodies

True or False

III. *Mark each statement T for true or F for false.*

_____ 1. Body fluids move back and forth between compartments that are separated by cell membranes.

_____ 2. Blood is an intravascular fluid.

_____ 3. Respiration is the main way that water is lost from the body.

_____ 4. Most extracellular fluid is plasma.

_____ 5. Lymph is the fluid that circulates through the lymphatic vessels.

Build It!

IV. *Use word parts to build terms to label the illustration.*

1. _____ / _____
   (clot)   (cell)

2. _____ / _____
   (white)   (cell)

3. _____ / _____
   (red)   (cell)

Word Analysis

V. *Divide these terms into their component parts, and define the terms.*

1. cellular   _____

2. coagulant   _____

3. hematopoiesis _____

4. hypocalcemia _____

5. necrotic   _____

Say and Check

Say aloud the terms in Exercise V. Use the Companion CD to check your pronunciations.

Listing

VI. *Name five nonspecific body defenses.*

1. _____

2. _____

3. _____

4. _____

5. _____

VII. *Name two types of specific body defenses.*

1. _____

2. _____

Fill in the Blanks

VIII. *Write a word in each blank to complete these sentences.*

1. Mr. Perkins' physician tells him that he has hypokalemia, probably resulting from the use of diuretics. Hypokalemia means that Mr. Perkins has an inadequate amount of _____ in the blood.

2. Blood _____ is a series of chemical reactions that result in a blood clot.

3. Fluid that is located between cells and in tissue spaces is called _____ fluid.

4. Mrs. Klott forms a blood clot, called a/an _____, after surgery.

5. Mrs. Klott's physician prescribes an in vivo _____ after she develops a blood clot.

6. A vital function of body fluids is to transport nutrients and remove body _____.

7. A relative constancy in the internal environment of the body is called _____.

8. An examination and enumeration of the distribution of leukocytes in a stained blood smear is called a/an _____ white cell count.

9. Destruction of the red blood cell membrane resulting in the release of hemoglobin is called _____.

10. A term given to a group of malignant diseases characterized by abnormal numbers and forms of immature white blood cells in the blood is _____.

Multiple Choice

IX. *Circle the correct answer in these sentences.*

1. The name of the substance from which fibrin originates is (fibrinogen, fibrinolysis, thrombogen, thrombolysis).

2. The degree of disease-causing capability of an organism is called (resistance, sensitivity, susceptibility, virulence).

3. Transportation of oxygen to body cells is a major function of (blood platelets, erythrocytes, leukocytes, thrombocytes).

4. A term that means having no tendency to repair itself or develop into new tissue is (analytic, anisocytosis, aplastic, hemolytic).

5. The surgical procedure whereby living organs are transferred from one part of the body to another or from one individual to another is (rejection, transmission, transplant, transreaction).

6. Intracellular fluid is found (around, between, inside, outside) cells.

7. One of the specific body defense mechanisms is (cell-mediated immunity, intact skin, interferon, phagocytosis).

8. A normal defensive response of the body to a pathogen is (erythropia, infection, inflammation, xanthoderma).

9. The most abundant body fluid is (extracellular, interstitial, intracellular, plasma).

10. A decrease in the number of blood platelets is called (hemophilia, leukemia, leukocytosis, thrombopenia).

Writing Terms

X. *Write a term for each of the following meanings.*

1. any erythrocyte of irregular shape   _____

2. below normal sodium in the blood   _____

3. body's ability to resist infectious disease _____

4. blood clotting   _____

5. dissolving of a thrombus   _____

6. a homologous graft   _____

7. localized collection of pus in a cavity _____

8. neutral-staining granulocyte   _____

9. production of blood   _____

10. within cells   _____

 Say and Check

Say aloud the terms you wrote for Exercise X. Use the Companion CD to check your pronunciations.

Greater Comprehension

Health Care Reports

XI. *Read the following consultation report and define the terms or abbreviations that follow the report. Although you may be unfamiliar with some of the terms, you should be able to determine their meanings by considering their word parts.*

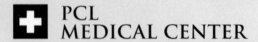 **PCL MEDICAL CENTER**

7700 Lexicon Way
St. Louis, MO 63146

Phone (555) 437-0000 • Fax (555) 437-0001

CONSULTATION

Patient Name: Thomas Byerly   **ID No.:** 007-0001   **Date:** Feb 11, ----
Date of Birth: Nov 6, ----   **Sex:** Male   **PCP:** Jay Miller, MD
REASON FOR CONSULTATION: Neutropenia, thrombocytopenia
HISTORY OF PRESENT ILLNESS: This 70-year-old white man with history of coronary artery disease and melanoma underwent a 4-vessel coronary artery bypass grafting on Jan 10/----. He was readmitted to the hospital on Jan 22/---- with wound dehiscence and wound infection. He was treated with vancomycin but had supratherapeutic vancomycin levels and was switched to Timentin. He has had decreasing white cell counts and has been mildly neutropenic since being switched. His WBC count today is 3.4 with an absolute neutrophil count of 1.53.
PAST MEDICAL HISTORY:

1. Coronary artery disease
2. Remote history of melanoma
3. Deep vein thrombosis
4. Hypertension
5. Anemia

ALLERGIES: Coumadin and tape
MEDICATIONS: Aspirin 325 mg daily; Lopressor 25 mg b.i.d.; Timentin 3.2 mg IV every 6 hours, lisinopril 20 mg daily
LABORATORY VALUES: WBCs 3.4, Hgb 9.3, platelets 210, with absolute neutrophil count of 1.53. CRP 2.3. Culture of wound grew *Staphylococcus.*
ASSESSMENT:

1. Neutropenia, most likely due to medications. The patient's white count was normal on admission to the hospital. In the case of medication-related thrombocytopenia, Timentin and/or vancomycin could be the cause of this hematologic abnormality. The fact that the patient may have immune deficiency with his history of melanoma and anemia should be investigated.
2. *Staphylococcus* wound infection, healed.

Define:

1. neutropenia _____

2. thrombocytopenia _____

3. melanoma _____

4. dehiscence _____

5. supratherapeutic _____

6. thrombosis _____

7. anemia _____

8. b.i.d. _____

9. hematologic _____

10. immune deficiency _____

XII. *Read the following physical examination report and define the terms or abbreviations that follow the report. Although you may be unfamiliar with some terms, you should be able to determine their meanings by considering their word parts.*

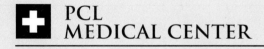

PCL MEDICAL CENTER

7700 Lexicon Way
St. Louis, MO 63146

Phone (555) 437-0000 • Fax (555) 437-0001

PHYSICAL EXAMINATION

Patient Name: George Thompson   **ID No.:** 007-0002   **Date:** Apr 23, ----
Date of Birth: Dec 26, ----   **Age:** 45   **Sex:** Male
GENERAL APPEARANCE: Dyspneic with pallor. Complains of malaise.
PHYSICAL EXAMINATION:
   VITAL SIGNS: Vital signs are WNL.
   HEENT: Normocephalic, atraumatic.
   NECK: No JVD, bruits, or lymphadenopathy.
   LUNGS: Decreased breath sounds bilaterally.
   HEART: Regular rate and rhythm.
   ABDOMEN: Soft, nontender, nondistended. No hepatosplenomegaly.
   EXTREMITIES: No edema, clots, clubbing, or cyanosis.
   NEUROLOGIC: Alert, oriented ×3, gait WNL.
LABORATORY DATA: WBCs 5.6, Hgb 8.8, Hct 26.5, Na 127
IMPRESSION:
1. Iron deficiency anemia secondary to chronic blood loss
2. Worsening hyponatremia
3. Exacerbation of COPD
DISPOSITION:
1. Anemia: Has required parenteral iron in the past secondary to inability to tolerate iron by mouth. Have his blood typed and cross-matched for a 2-unit transfusion. Set up consult with Gastroenterology for upper and lower GI eval.
2. Hyponatremia: Some improvement after infusion of normal saline today. Recommend fluid restriction.
3. COPD: Set up consult with Pulmonology for treatment recommendations.

Define:

1. dyspneic _____
2. pallor _____
3. malaise _____
4. bilaterally _____
5. edema _____
6. Hgb _____
7. Hct _____
8. hyponatremia _____
9. WNL _____
10. normocephalic _____

XIII. *Read the following bone marrow transplant report and define the terms or abbreviations that follow the report. Although you may be unfamiliar with some terms, you should be able to determine their meanings by considering their word parts.*

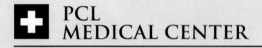

PCL MEDICAL CENTER

7700 Lexicon Way
St. Louis, MO 63146

Phone (555) 437-0000 • Fax (555) 437-0001

BONE MARROW TRANSPLANT CLINIC OUTPATIENT NOTE

Patient Name: Amber L. Wells   **ID No.:** 007-0004   **Date:** Dec 13, ----

CC: Patient is a 25-year-old woman who is 53 days status post allogeneic hematopoietic stem cell transplant for the second time for an overlap MPD/MDS who is seen today in routine follow-up.

HPI: The patient complains of some intermittent upper abdominal and bilateral flank pain. It is mild in nature. It is not associated with any nausea, vomiting, or diarrhea. She has some occasional hot flashes but no documented fevers. Overall she is doing well.

ROS: No nausea, vomiting, diarrhea, skin rash, fever, shortness of breath, chest pain, extremity edema, problems with her PIC line, or bleeding complications.

MEDICATIONS

1. Cyclosporin 100 mg p.o. b.i.d.
2. Prednisone 20 mg p.o. daily
3. Septra DS, 1 p.o. on Mondays, Wednesdays, and Fridays
4. Acyclovir 800 mg p.o. b.i.d.
5. Zantac 150 mg p.o. b.i.d.
6. Maalox p.r.n.
7. Synthroid 0.05 mg p.o. daily
8. Coumadin 5 mg p.o. daily
9. Compazine p.r.n.
10. Restoril p.r.n.
11. Natural Tears p.r.n.
12. Homeopathic medicines p.r.n.
13. Sudafed p.r.n.
14. Potassium 20 mEq p.o. daily

PE: Vital signs show blood pressure 108/73, temperature 98.4, heart rate 90, respirations 18, oxygen saturation 98% on room air; weight is stable at 61.2 kg. In general she is in no acute distress, alert and oriented ×4. Mouth and throat are clear. Lungs are clear. Cardiovascular exam reveals no murmurs or gallops. Extremity exam reveals trace bilateral lower extremity edema. Skin exam is within normal limits with no evidence of GVHD.

LABORATORY DATA: Chemistries are all within normal limits, including a potassium of 3.7 and a magnesium of 1.6. Liver function tests are within normal limits. CBC shows a white count of 12.4, hemoglobin 12, platelet count 323,000. INR is 2.46.

IMPRESSION: Amber Wells is a 25-year-old woman who is 53 days status post allogeneic transplant. She has no evidence of ongoing graft-versus-host disease (GVHD) and is on a fairly rapid steroid taper. She has engrafted well. There are no acute problems today.

PLAN: Followup with me on Jan 3, ---- or sooner p.r.n.

Josette L. Sims, MD
Josette L. Sims, M.D.
Hematologist

JS:pai
D: Dec 13, ----
T: Dec 14, ----

Define:

1. CC _____

2. HPI _____

3. ROS _____

4. PE _____

5. allogeneic   _____

6. hematopoietic stem cell   _____

7. oriented ×4   _____

8. intermittent   _____

9. p.r.n.   _____

10. GVHD   _____

Matching

XIV. *Match the signs and symptoms of severe anemia in the left column with the correct meaning in the right column:*

_____ 1. dyspnea

_____ 2. pallor

_____ 3. syncope

_____ 4. tinnitus

A. difficult breathing
B. fainting
C. loss of appetite
D. nausea
E. paleness
F. ringing in the ears

Spelling

XV. *Circle all misspelled terms and write their correct spelling:*

bacteremia   cellular   fibrinolisis   polymorfonuclear   toxisity

Interpreting Abbreviations

XVI. *Write the meaning of these abbreviations:*

1. AHF   _____

2. CBC   _____

3. Hgb   _____

4. HIV   _____

5. PT   _____

Pronunciation

XVII. *The pronunciation is shown for several medical words. Indicate the primary accented syllable in each term with an ´.*

1. coagulopathy (ko ag u lop ǝ the)

2. erythropoietin (ǝ rith ro poi ǝ tin)

3. allogenic (al o jen ik)

4. necrotic (nǝ krot ik)

5. prophylaxis (pro fǝ lak sis)

Say and Check

Say aloud the five terms in Exercise XVII. Use the Companion CD to check your pronunciations. In addition, be prepared to pronounce aloud these terms in class:

agglutination	disseminated	homologous	perspiration
agranulocytosis	eosinophil	hydrocephalus	phagocytic
autologous	erythroblastosis fetalis	immunocompromised	suppurative
coagulation	globulins	immunosuppressant	syncope
cytotoxicity	hemoglobin	monocyte	tinnitus

Categorizing Terms

XVIII. *Categorize the terms in the left column by selecting A, B, C, D, or E.*

_____ 1. hematocrit

_____ 2. in vivo anticoagulant

_____ 3. leukocyte

_____ 4. septicemia

_____ 5. thrombectomy

A. anatomy
B. diagnostic test or procedure
C. pathology
D. surgery
E. therapy

Challenge

XIX. *Break these words into their components parts, and write their meanings. Even if you have not seen these terms before, you may be able to break them apart and determine their meanings.*

1. eosinophilia _____

2. erythroid _____

3. hemoglobinometer _____

4. leukopoiesis _____

5. thromboid _____

(Use Appendix VI to check your answers.)

 PRONUNCIATION LIST

Use the practice CD to review the terms that have been presented. Look closely at the spelling of each term as it is pronounced and be sure you know the meaning of each term.

abscess	coagulate	fibrinolysin	hyperemia
agglutination	coagulation	fibrinolysis	hyperkalemia
agranulocytes	coagulopathy	globins	hypernatremia
agranulocytosis	complement	globulins	hypersensitivity
allergen	corpuscle	granulocytes	hypocalcemia
allergies	cytotoxicity	hematocrit	hypochromia
allogeneic	cytotoxin	hematologic	hypochromic
allogenic	dehydration	hematologist	hypokalemia
allograft	disseminated	hematology	hyponatremia
anaphylactic reactions	dyscrasias	hematoma	immunity
anaphylaxis	dyspnea	hematopoiesis	immunization
anemia	electrolytes	hematopoietic	immunocompromised
anisocytosis	embolism	hemoglobin	immunodeficiency
antibodies	embolus	hemoglobin electrophoresis	immunoglobulins
anticoagulant	eosinophil	hemoglobinopathy	immunosuppressant
antigen	erythroblastosis fetalis	hemolysin	immunosuppressives
antihistamine	erythroblasts	hemolysis	in vitro
aplastic	erythrocyte	hemophilia	in vivo
autoimmune diseases	erythrocytic	hemostasis	infectious mononucleosis
autologous graft	erythrocytopenia	hepatitis	interferon
autologous transfusion	erythrocytosis	histamine	interstitial fluid
bacteremia	erythropenia	homeostasis	intrauterine
basophil	erythropoiesis	homologous graft	intravascular
blood transfusion	erythropoietin	hydrocephalus	isograft
cardiovascular	excretion	hydrocephaly	isotonic
cellular	fibrin	hypercalcemia	karyomegaly
coagulant	fibrinogen	hyperchromic	leukemia

leukocyte
leukocytopenia
leukocytosis
leukopenia
lymph
lymphatic system
lymphocyte
macrocyte
macrocytosis
macrophages
megalocyte
microcytes
microcytosis
monocyte
mucous
mucus
necrosis
necrotic
neutrophil

normocytes
normocytic
nucleoid
nucleoprotein
pallor
perspiration
phagocytic
phagocytosis
plasma
platelet
poikilocyte
poikilocytosis
polycythemia
polycythemia vera
polymorph
polymorphonuclear
prophylaxis
prothrombin
purulent

pus
rejection
resistance
saliva
sanguinous
secretion
septicemia
shunt
sickle cell anemia
spherocyte
spherocytosis
staphylococcemia
streptococcemia
suppurative
susceptibility
syncope
systemic
tachycardia

thrombectomy
thrombi
thrombocyte
thrombocytopenia
thrombocytosis
thrombogenesis
thrombolysis
thrombolytic
thrombopenia
thromboplastin
thrombosis
thrombus
tinnitus
toxemia
toxicity
toxoid
transplant
vaccination

Español ENHANCING SPANISH COMMUNICATION

English	Spanish (pronunciation)
allergy	alergia (ah-LEHR-he-ah)
anemia	anemia (ah-NAY-me-ah)
blood sample	muestra de sangre (moo-AYS-trah day SAHN-gray)
clot	coágulo (co-AH-goo-lo)
constipation	estreñimiento (es-tray-nye-me-EN-to)
destruction	destrucción (des-trooc-se-ON)
diarrhea	diarrea (de-ar-RAY-ah)
dizziness	vértigo (VERR-te-go)
excretion	excreción (ex-cray-se-ON)
fainting	languidez (lan-gee-DES), desmayo (des-MAH-yo)
fiber	fibra (FEE-brah)
fluid	fluido (floo-EE-do)
headache	dolor de cabeza (do-LOR day cah-BAY-sa)
injury	daño (DAH-nyo)
leukemia	leucemia (lay-oo-SAY-me-ah)
lymph	linfa (LEEN-fa)
lymphatic	linfático (lin-FAH-te-co)
mucus	moco (MO-co)
oxygen	oxígeno (ok-SEE-hay-no)
protection	proteccion (pro-tec-se-ON)
perspiration	sudor (soo-DOR)
redness	rojo (RO-ho)
ringing	zumbido (zoom-BEE-do)
saliva	saliva (sah-LEE-vah)
sweat	sudor (soo-DOR)
swelling	prominencia (pro-me-NEN-se-ah)
tears	lágrimas (LAH-gre-mahs)
tests	pruebas (proo-AY-bahs)
transfusion	transfusión (trans-foo-se-ON)
water	agua (AH-goo-ah)
wound	lesión (lay-se-ON)

Cardiovascular
and Lymphatic Systems

LEARNING GOALS

Basic Understanding
In this chapter you will learn to do the following:

1. State the function of the cardiovascular system, and analyze associated terminology.
2. Write the meanings of the word parts associated with the cardiovascular system, and use them to build and analyze terms.
3. Write the names of the structures of the cardiovascular system, and define the terms associated with these structures.
4. Sequence the flow of blood from when it enters the heart until it returns to the heart.
5. Write the names of the diagnostic tests and procedures for assessment of the cardiovascular system when given their descriptions, or match procedures with their descriptions.
6. Write the names of cardiovascular pathologies when given their descriptions, or match pathologies with their meanings.
7. Match surgical and therapeutic interventions with their descriptions, or write the names of the interventions when given their descriptions.
8. State the function of the lymphatic system, and analyze associated terminology.
9. Write the meanings of the word parts associated with the lymphatic system, and use them to build and analyze terms.
10. Write the names of the structures of the lymphatic system, define the terms associated with these structures, and label the structures.
11. Write the names of the diagnostic tests and procedures for assessment of the lymphatic system when given their descriptions, or match procedures with their descriptions.
12. Write the names of lymphatic system pathologies when given their descriptions, or match pathologies with their descriptions.
13. Match surgical and therapeutic interventions for lymphatic system pathologies with their descriptions, or write the names of the interventions when given their descriptions.

Greater Comprehension
14. Use word parts from this chapter to determine the meaning of terms in a health care report.
15. Spell the terms accurately.
16. Pronounce the terms correctly.
17. Write the meanings of the abbreviations.
18. Categorize terms as anatomy, diagnostic test or procedure, pathology, surgery, or therapy.

MAJOR SECTIONS OF THIS CHAPTER:

❑ **CARDIOVASCULAR SYSTEM**
  Anatomy and Physiology
  Diagnostic Tests and Procedures
  Pathologies
  Surgical and Therapeutic Interventions

❑ **LYMPHATIC SYSTEM**
  Anatomy and Physiology
  Diagnostic Tests and Procedures
  Pathologies
  Surgical and Therapeutic Interventions

FUNCTION FIRST

The cardiovascular system circulates blood throughout the body, delivering nutrients and other essential materials to the fluids surrounding the cells, removing waste products, and conveying the wastes to organs where they can be excreted. As blood circulates, interstitial fluid accumulates in the tissue spaces. This excess fluid is normally transported away from the tissues by another vascular network that helps maintain the internal fluid environment—the lymphatic system. The lymphatic system helps maintain the internal fluid environment of the body by returning proteins and tissue fluids to the blood, aids in the absorption of fats into the bloodstream, and helps to defend the body against microorganisms and disease.

CARDIOVASCULAR SYSTEM

ANATOMY AND PHYSIOLOGY

8-1 The heart and blood vessels make up the **cardio/vascul/ar** (cardi[o], heart + vascul[o], vessel + -ar, pertaining to) (kahr″de-o-vas′ku-lər) system.

> ➤ **KEY** POINT The vast network of blood vessels delivers oxygen, nutrients, and vital substances to the interstitial fluids surrounding all the body's cells. Blood vessels include arteries (ahr′tə-rēz), arterioles (ahr′tēr′e-ōlz), capillaries (kap′ĭ-lar″ēz), venules (ven′ūlz), and veins (vānz) (Figure 8-1).

vessel

　　Vascul/ar (vas′ku-lər) means pertaining to a _____, specifically a blood vessel. Learn these word parts that are used to describe the anatomy and physiology of the cardiovascular system.

Word Parts: Cardiovascular Anatomy and Physiology

Combining Form	Meaning	Combining Form	Meaning
Main Components of the Cardiovascular System		**Other Word Parts**	
angi(o), vas(o), vascul(o)	vessel	atri(o)	atrium
aort(o)	aorta	coron(o)	crown
arter(o), arteri(o)	artery	mediastin(o)	mediastinum
arteriol(o)	arteriole	ox(i)	oxygen
cardi(o)	heart	pulmon(o)	lung
phleb(o), ven(i), ven(o)	vein	sept(o)*	septum; partition
venul(o)	venule	sin(o)	sinus
		steth(o), thorac(o)	chest
Tissues of the Heart		valv(o), valvul(o)	valve
endocardi(o)	endocardium	ventricul(o)	ventricle
myocardi(o)	myocardium	**Suffix**	**Meaning**
pericardi(o)	pericardium	-ole	small

*Sept(o) sometimes means infection.

8-2 The arteries are shown in red and the veins are shown in blue in Figure 8-1. This oversimplifies blood circulation, but it will help you remember that, in general, **arteries** carry oxygen-rich blood to body tissues and **veins** carry oxygen-poor blood back to the heart.

　　You already know that cardi(o) means heart. You also need to remember that arter(o) and arteri(o) mean artery. **Arteri/al** (ahr-tēr′e-əl) means pertaining to one or more

arteries

_____.

8-3 **Arteri/ole** means little artery when translated literally, because -ole means little. The combining form for arteriole is _____. **Capillaries** are microscopic blood vessels that receive blood from the arterioles. Capillaries are so small that erythrocytes must pass through them in single file. Blood and tissue fluids exchange various substances across the capillary walls.

arteriol(o)

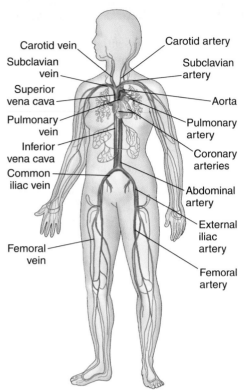

Figure 8-1 The cardiovascular system, the heart, and blood vessels. Two major components of the vascular network are shown, the arteries *(red)* and the veins *(blue)*. Only the larger or more common blood vessels are labeled.

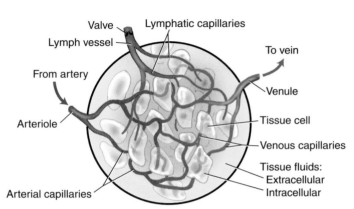

Figure 8-2 A capillary bed showing the relationship of blood vessels. Blood that is rich in oxygen is carried by the arteries, which branch many times to become arterioles. Arterioles branch to become capillaries, the site of oxygen and carbon dioxide exchange. Oxygen-poor blood is returned to the heart through the venules, which flow into the veins. The veins carry the blood to the two largest veins, the superior and inferior venae cavae, which empty into the heart. Venae cavae is plural for vena cava.

8-4 The capillaries join arterioles and venules (Figure 8-2). You will be using three combining forms that mean vein: phleb(o), ven(i), and ven(o). Phleb(o) is used more often to write medical terms, but you will need to remember that **veni/puncture** (ven´ĭ-punk˝chər) means puncture of a _____. Both venipuncture and **phlebo/tomy** (flə-bot´ə-me) mean opening of a vein to draw blood for laboratory analysis. Translated literally, phlebotomy means _____ of a vein. **Phlebotomists** (flə-bot´ə-mists) are persons with special training in the practice of drawing blood. **Ven/ous** (ve´nəs) means pertaining to the veins.

    Venules join the capillaries and veins. The combining form venul(o) means venule.* **Venul/ar** (ven´u-lər) means pertaining to, composed of, or affecting venules.

    Arterio/ven/ous (ahr-tēr˝e-o-ve´nəs) means pertaining to both _____ and veins.

8-5 Blood circulation is the circuit of blood through the body, from the heart through the arteries, arterioles, capillaries, venules, and veins and back to the heart. Circulation means movement in a regular or circular fashion. If you study blood circulation more closely, you learn that it consists of many events that occur simultaneously.

> ➤ **KEY** POINT <u>Two important types of circulation occur each time the heart beats:</u>
> - **Systemic circulation** (sis-tem´ik sur˝ku-la´shən): the general circulation that carries oxygenated blood from the heart to the tissues of the body and returns the blood with much of its oxygen exchanged for carbon dioxide back to the heart.
> - **Pulmonary circulation** (pool´mo-nar˝e sur˝ku-la´shən): the circuit that the blood makes from the heart to the lungs for the purpose of ridding the body of carbon dioxide and picking up oxygen.

*Venule (Latin: *venula,* small vein).

Margin answers:
vein

incision

arteries

systemic

The general circulation that transports oxygen to all tissues of the body is
_____ circulation.

The combining form pulmon(o) means lung, and the suffix -ary means pertaining to.
Pulmon/ary (pool´mo-nar˝e) means pertaining to the lungs. The heart has four chambers: right
atrium (a´tre-əm) (RA), right **ventricle** (ven´trĭ-kəl) (RV), left atrium (LA), and left ventricle
(LV). Study and label Figure 8-3 as you read about pulmonary and systemic circulation.

arteries

8-6 All tissues of the body, including heart tissue and lung tissue, receive oxygen via the systemic
circulation. However, you will need to remember that pulmonary circulation provides the means
for the blood to take on oxygen from air that we take into our lungs. Oxygen-deficient blood
leaves the heart via the pulmonary _____. After oxygenation,
which takes place in the lungs, the blood is returned to the heart via the pulmonary

veins

_____..

> ➤ **KEY** POINT The naming of pulmonary arteries and veins is different from that of other
arteries and veins in the body. You have learned that, in general, arteries transport blood rich
in oxygen and veins transport blood that has had much of its oxygen removed. Pulmonary arteries transport deoxygenated blood to the lungs. After the blood absorbs oxygen in the lungs,
the pulmonary veins transport the blood back to the heart before it is pumped throughout the
body.

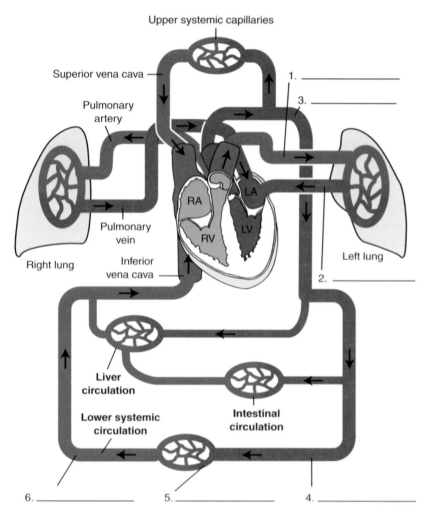

Upper systemic capillaries

Superior vena cava

1. _____

3. _____

Pulmonary
artery

RA

LA

Pulmonary
vein

LV

RV

Right lung

Inferior
vena cava

Left lung

2. _____

Liver
circulation

**Lower systemic
circulation**

**Intestinal
circulation**

6. _____   5. _____   4. _____

**Figure 8-3 Schematic drawing of blood circulation
and the relationship of blood vessels.** *Arrows* indicate the direction of blood flow through the heart to
the lungs and the major vessels of the cardiovascular
system. *RA, RV, LA,* and *LV* are abbreviations for the
four chambers of the heart. Blood circulation consists
of two types of circulation: pulmonary circulation and
systemic circulation. Label the diagram as indicated.
Pulmonary circulation: Pulmonary arteries carry
oxygen-deficient blood *(blue)* to the lungs, where it is
oxygenated. Label the left pulmonary artery, *(1).* Oxygenated blood is returned to the heart via pulmonary
veins. Label the left pulmonary vein, *(2).* **Systemic circulation:** Oxygen-rich blood *(red)* is pumped from
the heart into the aorta *(3)* and is routed to arteries
that branch to become arterioles, which branch to become capillaries. Label the artery *(4)* and capillary *(5).*
In the capillaries, blood is provided to the tissues of
the body and the blood, with much of its oxygen exchanged for carbon dioxide, passes into the venules,
then the veins. Label the vein indicated by number *6.*
Blood then returns to the heart via veins called the superior and inferior venae cavae.

EXERCISE 1

Beginning with artery, list the six components of the cardiovascular system (2 through 5) to indicate the flow of blood as it circulates back toward the heart. Numbers 1 and 6 are done as an example.

1. *artery* _____

2. _____

3. _____

4. _____

5. _____

6. *superior and inferior venae cavae*

EXERCISE 2

Match the combining forms in the left column with the structures in the right column. (Selections A to E may be used more than once.)

_____ 1. arter(o)

_____ 2. arteri(o)

_____ 3. arteriol(o)

_____ 4. phleb(o)

_____ 5. pulmon(o)

_____ 6. ven(i)

_____ 7. ven(o)

_____ 8. venul(o)

A. arteriole
B. artery
C. lung
D. vein
E. venule

---

chest

8-7 The muscular heart is the center of the cardiovascular system. It beats normally about 70 times per minute, or more than 100,000 times per day. In the adult, it weighs 230 grams to 340 grams (about ½ pound) and is the size of a clenched fist. The heart lies in the thorac/ic cavity. You learned earlier that the thoracic cavity is the _____ cavity.

The heart lies just left of the midline of the body, between the lungs, in a space called the **mediastinum** (me″de-əs-ti′nəm). The media/stinum is an area in the chest cavity between the lungs. The mediastinum contains the heart and its large vessels, the trachea, the esophagus, and nearby structures such as the lymph nodes. Write this new word, which refers to the area between the lungs: _____.

mediastinum

8-8 Special arteries supply blood to the heart itself. The combining form coron(o) means crown. **Coronary** (kor′ə-nar″e) means encircling in the manner of a crown. Blood vessels that supply oxygen to the heart encircle it in a crownlike fashion (Figure 8-4). Arteries that supply blood to the heart are _____ **arteries.**

coronary

The wall of the heart consists primarily of cardiac muscle tissue, **myocardium** (mi″o-kahr′de-əm). You probably remember that my(o) means muscle. The term myocardium is the product of combining my(o) with cardi(o) and -ium, which means membrane. (One "i" is dropped to facilitate pronunciation.) My(o) and cardi(o) are often used together, so it is easier to remember that myocardi(o) means myocardium.

The important thing to remember about myocardium is that it comprises most of the heart and is what type of tissue? _____ The myocardium is made up of muscle fibers that contract, resulting in a wringing type of movement that squeezes blood from the heart with each beat. **Myocardial** (mi″o-kahr′de-əl) means pertaining to the myocardium.

muscle

8-9 A membranous sac, the **pericardium** (per″ĭ-kahr′de-əm), encloses the heart, as shown in Figure 8-4. The pericardium, which is attached to the heart, is composed of an inner layer (**visceral pericardium** or **epicardium**) and an outer, tougher layer (**parietal** [pə-ri′ə-təl] **pericardium**). Epi/cardium (ep″ĭ-kahr′de-um) is so named because it lies on the surface of the heart. The pericardium, a tough fibrous tissue that constitutes the outermost sac, fits loosely around the heart and protects it.

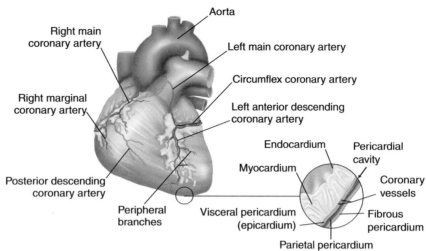

Figure 8-4 Coronary arteries and heart tissues. The two main coronary arteries are the left coronary artery (LCA) and right coronary artery (RCA). The three layers of the heart, beginning with the innermost layer, are endocardium, myocardium, and epicardium (also called the visceral pericardium).

around

The prefix peri- means around. Peri/card/ium is a membrane _____ the heart. (Again, when cardi[o] is combined with -ium, one "i" is dropped.) **Peri/cardial** (per″e-kahr´de-əl) means pertaining to the pericardium. The space between the two pericardial layers is the **pericardial cavity.** Because peri- and cardi(o) are often combined, it is easier to learn that pericardi(o) means the pericardium. Write a term that means pertaining to the pericardium using the suffix -al: _____.

pericardial
inside

Translated literally, **endo/card/ium** (en″do-kahr´de-um) is the membrane _____ the heart. The endocardium is the membrane that forms the lining inside the heart. The combining form endocardi(o) means endocardium. **Endocardial** (en″do-kahr´de-əl) means pertaining to the endocardium.

8-10 The four-chambered heart is separated into right and left chambers by a partition called the **septum** (sep´təm).

> ➤ **KEY** POINT The combining form sept(o) has two meanings. Sept(o) means either septum or infection; however, the term septum always means a dividing wall or partition. Septum may be used in describing structures other than the heart, but the word always means a dividing wall or partition.

septal (sep´təl)

Using the suffix -al, write a term that means pertaining to the septum: _____.

8-11 In addition to being divided longitudinally into right and left chambers by a septum, each side of the heart is further divided into an atrium (plural: atria) and a ventricle. This can be seen in the simple drawing of blood circulation in Figure 8-3, but also locate these four chambers in Figure 8-5.

The two upper chambers of the heart are the right and left atria. The two lower chambers of the heart are the right and left ventricles. The combining form atri(o) means atrium or atria. Using septal as a model, write a term that means pertaining to the atrium:

atrial

_____.

8-12 The heart has both a left ventricle and a right ventricle. **Ventricular** (ven-trik´u-lər) means pertaining to a ventricle. Combine atri(o), ventricul(o), and -ar to write a term that is abbreviated AV or A-V and means pertaining to an atrium and a ventricle of the heart:

atrioventricular
(a″tre-o-ven-trik´u-lər)

_____

The term ventricle is also applied to a chamber of the brain. Therefore ventricul(o) refers to a ventricle of either the heart or the brain. By analyzing other parts of the term or the sentence, one can often determine which organ is affected, the brain or the heart.

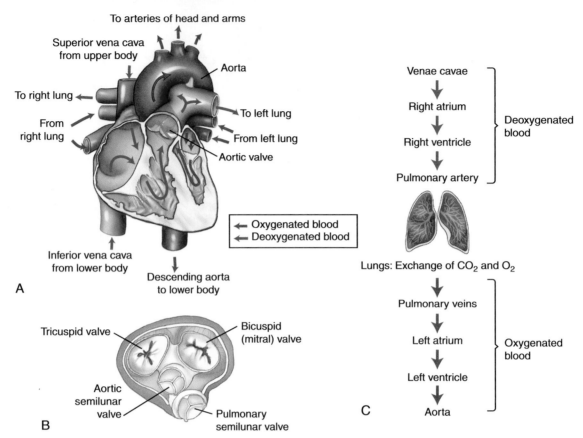

Figure 8-5 Circulation of blood through the heart. A, Anterior cross-section showing the heart chambers. Arrows indicate the direction of blood flow through the heart. **B,** Heart valves (viewed from above), the structures that prevent backflow of blood by opening and closing with each heartbeat. **C,** Schematic representation of deoxygenated or oxygenated status of the blood as it flows through the heart.

EXERCISE 3

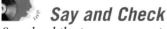 **Build It!** *Use the following word parts to build terms. (Some word parts will be used more than once.)*

endo-, peri-, arteri(o), atri(o), cardi(o), my(o), sept(o), ven(o), ventricul(o), -al, -ar, -ium, -ous

1. cardiac muscle tissue   _____/_____/_____

2. inner lining of the heart   _____/_____/_____

3. outer membranous sac of the heart   _____/_____/_____

4. pertaining to both arteries and veins   _____/_____/_____

5. pertaining to the inner lining of the heart _____/_____/_____

6. pertaining to the lower heart chambers _____/_____

7. pertaining to the septum   _____/_____

8. pertaining to the upper heart chambers _____/_____

Say and Check

Say aloud the terms you wrote for Exercise 3. Use the Companion CD to check your pronunciations.

8-13 Study the pattern of blood flow through the heart in Figure 8-5, *A*. **Deoxygenated** (de-ok´sĭ-jən-a˝ted) blood, which has had much of its oxygen removed, enters the heart on the right side of the body through its two largest veins. The large vein by which blood from the trunk and legs enters the heart is the inferior **vena cava** (ve´nə ka´və).* Blood from the head and arms enters the heart by way of the large vein, the superior vena cava. The venae cavae bring the blood to which chamber of the heart? The right _____

atrium

8-14 The right atrium contracts to force blood through a valve to the right ventricle. This is the **tricuspid** (tri-kus´pid) **valve,** and it is located between the right atrium and the right ventricle. Contraction of the right ventricle forces blood through the pulmonary artery, which branches and carries blood to the _____. As blood flows through the lungs, it becomes **oxygenated** (having additional oxygen) and returns to the left side of the heart by way of the pulmonary veins. The pulmonary veins bring the blood to the left atrium.

lungs

The left atrium contracts and forces blood into the left ventricle. The flow of blood from the left atrium to the left ventricle is controlled by the **mitral** (mi´trəl) _____, also called the **bicuspid valve.** This richly oxygenated blood is then pumped into the aorta (a-or´tə) from the left ventricle. The **aorta** is the largest artery of the body. It branches into smaller arteries to carry blood all over the body.

valve

8-15 In normal heart function, valves close and prevent backflow of blood when the heart contracts.

> ➤ **KEY** POINT Valves between the atria and ventricles are **atrioventricular valves**. The tricuspid valve is the name of the valve between the right atrium and the right ventricle, and the bicuspid, or mitral, valve is the valve between the left atrium and left ventricle (see Figure 8-5, *B*). Cuspid refers to the little flaps of tissue that make up the valve. The left atrioventricular valve is generally called the mitral valve in medicine, so named because the two valve flaps are shaped somewhat like the mitered corner joints of a picture frame.

Remembering that bi- means two, the bi/cuspid valve has _____ flaps. The tricuspid valve has three flaps of tissue.

two

8-16 Once again, look at Figure 8-5 and locate the pulmonary valve. It regulates the flow of blood from the right ventricle to the pulmonary trunk, which divides into _____ arteries that lead to the lungs. Pulmonary means pertaining to the lungs, and vessels that carry blood from the heart to the lungs are **pulmonary arteries.** Note that vessels that carry blood from the lungs back to the heart are **pulmonary** _____.

pulmonary

After flowing from the left atrium to the left ventricle, blood leaves the heart by way of the _____ **valve,** which regulates the flow of blood into the aorta. The pulmonary and aortic valves are also called **semilunar** (sem˝e-loo´nər) **valves** (because of the half-moon appearance of the valve cusps).

veins

aortic (a-or´tik)

8-17 Only a few words use the combining form valv(o), but all pertain to a valve. **Valv/al** (val´vəl) and **valv/ar** (val´vər) both pertain to a _____. **Valv/ate** (val´vāt) means pertaining to or having valves.

valve

Valvula means a valve, especially a small valve. The combining form valvul(o) is also used in words to mean valve. **Valvul/ar** (val´vu-lər), having valves, is a synonym for valvate.

---

*Vena cava (Latin: *vena,* veins; *cava,* cavity).

EXERCISE 4

Match the term with its meaning. Each term is used only once.

_____ 1. large vein by which blood enters the heart

_____ 2. structure that closes and prevents backflow of blood

_____ 3. type of valves located between the atria and the ventricles

_____ 4. valve leading to the aorta from the left ventricle

_____ 5. valves with a half-moon appearance of the cusps

A. aortic
B. atrioventricular
C. semilunar
D. valve
E. vena cava

8-18 It is important to remember that both atria contract simultaneously, followed by simultaneous contraction of both ventricles. The cardiac conduction system, composed of highly specialized tissue that is capable of producing and conveying electrical impulses, is responsible for the coordinated contraction (Figure 8-6).

Find the **sino/atrial** (si″no-a′tre-əl) (SA) **node,** located at the junction of the right atrium and the superior vena cava. Electrical impulses arise spontaneously in the SA node and stimulate contraction. The SA node is the natural pacemaker of the heart. The SA node is also called the sinus node. The combining form sin(o) means sinus. A sinus is a cavity or channel. Perhaps you are more familiar with the sinuses near the nose (air cavities that sometimes drain or become inflamed in sinus/itis). The term sinusitis does not use the combining form.

Use sin(o) + atrial to write the name of the natural pacemaker of the heart, the

sinoatrial _____ node.

8-19 The electrical impulse generated by the SA node travels through both atria to the **atrio/ventricul/ar** (AV) **node,** which in turn conducts the impulse to the atrioventricular bundle (AV bundle, called also the bundle of His) and then to the **Purkinje** (pər-kin′je) **fibers** and walls of the ventricles. This highly specialized system results in simultaneous contraction of the atria, followed by contraction of the ventricles.

atrioventricular   AV node means the _____ node. This special type of cardiac tissue is located near the septal wall between the left and right atria. The atria contract while the electrical impulse is briefly delayed in the AV node.

Another name for the atrioventricular bundle or AV bundle is the bundle of His, named after the Swiss physician Wilhelm His, Jr. Purkinje fibers are the termination of the bundle branches. These fibers, spread throughout the right and left ventricles, are specialized to carry the impulse at a high velocity and cause the ventricles to contract.

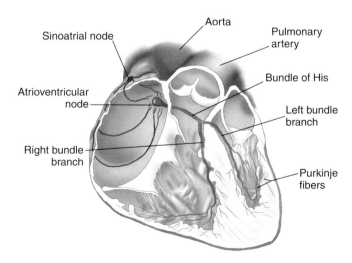

Figure 8-6 Conduction system of the heart. The electrical impulse originates in the heart, and contraction of the heart's chambers is coordinated by specialized heart tissues.

8-20 The heart and blood vessels work together to provide a continuous supply of oxygen and nutrients to cells throughout the body. Observe the difference in thickness of blood vessels in Figure 8-7.

> ➤ **KEY** POINT <u>Arteries, veins, and capillaries are lined with endothelium, a layer of epithelial cells, which secretes substances that prevent blood clotting and regulate the tone of the vessels.</u> Arteries and veins have three additional layers: an inner layer, a muscular layer, and a white fibrous outer layer. Arteries are thicker than veins, and their outer layer is elastic, allowing them to expand as the heartbeat forces blood into them.

arteries

Arteries carry blood away from the heart. For this reason, blood pressure is much higher in _____ than in veins. Veins also contain valves at various intervals to control the direction of the blood flow back to the heart.

8-21 The aorta is the main trunk of the systemic arterial system (Figure 8-8). Arteries branch out either directly or indirectly from the aorta, which arises from the left ventricle of the heart. Each artery is responsible for conveying oxygen and nutrients to specific organs and tissues, as indicated in Figure 8-9.

To identify and discuss location, anatomists divide the aorta into three major portions: the ascending aorta, the aortic arch, and the descending aorta. The descending aorta is further divided into the thoracic and the abdominal aorta.

ascending

8-22 As the aorta emerges from the left ventricle, it stretches upward. At this point it is called the _____ aorta. It gives off two branches, the right and left coronary arteries, that transport blood to the heart. The ascending aorta then turns to the left, forming an arch that is called the arch of the aorta, or the aortic arch.

thoracic
abdominal
aorta

The descending aorta is a continuation of the aortic arch. The portion of the descending aorta in the thorax is called the _____ aorta. The portion of the descending aorta in the abdomen is called the _____ aorta.

Aort/ic (a-or´tik) means pertaining to the _____.
Intra/aortic (in″trə-a-or´tik) means within the aorta.

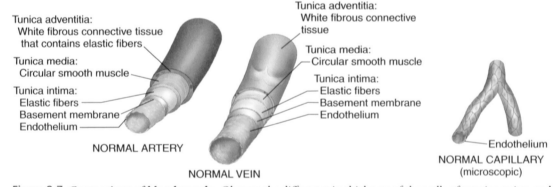

Figure 8-7 **Comparison of blood vessels.** Observe the difference in thickness of the walls of arteries, veins, and capillaries. A capillary wall consists of a single layer of endothelial cells. Arteries are thicker than veins, and their outer walls contain elastic fibers. The thickness of the outer wall varies with the location of the artery.

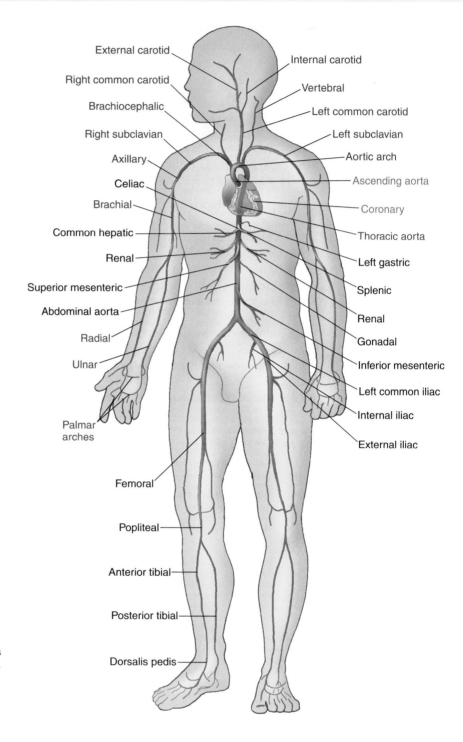

Figure 8-8 Anterior view of the aorta and its principal arterial branches. Labels for the ascending, arch, thoracic, and abdominal aorta and their corresponding arteries are shown in *red, green, purple,* and *black,* respectively.

EXERCISE 5

Write the meanings of the combining forms listed below.

Combining Form   Meaning

1. aort(o) _____

2. endocardi(o) _____

3. mediastin(o) _____

4. myocardi(o) _____

5. pericardi(o) _____

6. valvul(o) _____

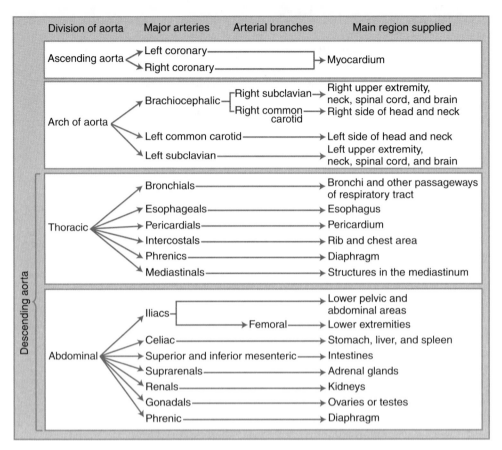

Figure 8-9 **The aorta and its branches.** Schematic presentation of the divisions of the aorta and the corresponding regions of the body to which blood is supplied.

EXERCISE 6

Write a word in each blank to complete these sentences that describe circulation.

Oxygen-poor blood is delivered to the right side of the heart via the two largest veins, the superior and inferior

(1) _____   _____. The blood from these two largest

veins is emptied into the chamber of the heart called the right (2) _____. When

the heart contracts, blood is forced through the tricuspid valve to the lower chamber, called the

(3) _____   _____. Another contraction of the

heart forces the blood into the pulmonary artery, which branches and carries blood to the

(4) _____, where it picks up oxygen. The pulmonary veins take blood back to the

heart chamber called the (5) _____   _____. The

flow of blood from the left atrium to the left ventricle is controlled by the (6) _____

valve. Blood is then pumped into the largest artery in the body, the (7) _____. This

vessel branches many times to become arteries, which again branch many times to become the smallest arteries, called

(8) _____, which in turn branch to become the smallest vessels, where oxygen is de-

livered to body tissues. These vessels, called (9) _____, are composed of only a single

layer of cells and are continuous with venules, which in turn are continuous with larger vessels called

(10) _____. These vessels are directly or indirectly connected with the venae cavae.

DIAGNOSTIC TESTS AND PROCEDURES

arteries

hypotension
(hi″po-ten′shən)

diastolic
(di″ə-stol′ik)

8-23 The heart rate and blood pressure (BP) give a preliminary indication of how the heart is functioning. Arteries are popularly used to measure blood pressure, and the reading is a reflection of cardiac output and arterial resistance. In other words, blood pressure measures the amount of pressure on the walls of the arteries. The blood pressure reading is a reflection of the quantity of blood flow from the heart and resistance in the walls of the _____.

8-24 **Hyper/tension** (hi″pər-ten′shən), abbreviated HTN, is increased blood pressure. Decreased blood pressure is _____.

Recall that blood pressure is measured using an apparatus called a sphygmomanometer* (sfig″mo-mə-nom′ə-ter) (Figure 8-10). A direct measurement can be obtained only by measuring pressure within a vessel or the heart itself, as in heart catheterization, which is described later in this section.

Blood pressure is at its highest point when the ventricles contract. This is known as **systole** (sis′to-le). Relaxation of the ventricles is **diastole** (di-as′to-le).[†] See the blood flow in the atria and ventricles during contraction and relaxation of the heart (Figure 8-11). The blood pressure measured when the ventricles contract is the **systolic** (sis-tol′ik) **pressure.** The blood pressure measured when the ventricles relax is called the _____ **pressure**. Four factors that increase blood pressure are increased cardiac output, increased blood volume, increased blood viscosity, and loss of elasticity of the arterial walls.

8-25 Recall also that the rhythmic expansion of an artery lying near the surface of the skin can be felt with the finger. This is known as the **pulse** (puls). All arteries have a pulse, but the one most often used is the radial artery on the anterolateral aspect of the wrist.

A normal pulse rate in a resting state is 60 to 100 beats per minute. An increased pulse rate (greater than 100 beats per minute) is **tachy/cardia** (tak″ĭ-kahr′de-ə). Using brady-, write a

---

*Sphygmomanometer (Greek: *sphygmos,* pulse + *manos,* thin + *metron,* measure).
[†]Diastole (Greek: *diastole,* expansion).

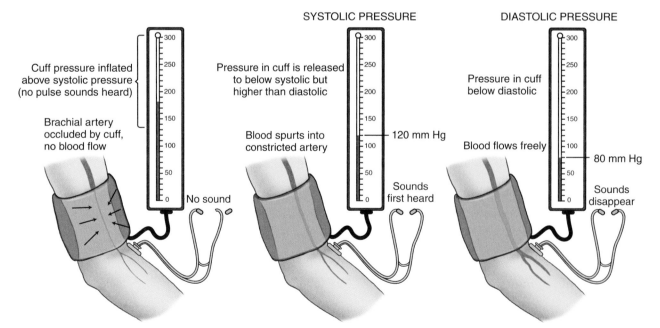

Figure 8-10 Measurement of blood pressure. Systolic pressure is due to ventricular contraction. Diastolic pressure occurs when the ventricles relax. The sounds heard through the stethoscope result from blood flow in the artery. The first sound heard represents the systolic pressure. As the pressure declines, the last sound heard represents the diastolic pressure. This example represents a normal blood pressure reading of 120/80 mm Hg (the height of mercury in a graduated column on the blood pressure apparatus). In arteriosclerosis the arteries lose their elasticity and cannot expand when blood is pumped into them.

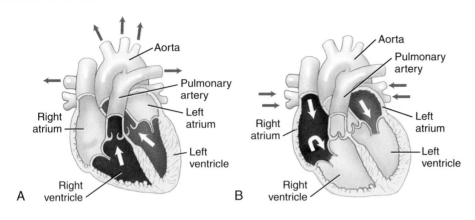

Figure 8-11 Blood flow during systole and diastole. A, Systole, contraction of the ventricles. **B,** Diastole, relaxation of the ventricles.

bradycardia
(brad″e-kahr″de-ə)

word that means a decreased pulse rate (less than 60 beats per minute):

_____.

8-26 The electrical impulses arising in the SA node and carried by the cardiac conduction system produce electrical currents that can be measured in **electro/cardio/graphy** (e-lek″tro-kahr″de-og´rə-fe), the process of recording the electrical currents of the heart. Each segment of the ECG shows the electrical cycle of the heart (Figure 8-12). Recall that the record produced in electrocardiography is an _____, and the name of the instrument is an **electrocardiograph** (e-lek″tro-kahr´de-o-graf″). Normal heart rhythm is called sinus rhythm.

electrocardiogram
(e-lek″tro-kahr´de-o-gram″)

A **Holter** (hōl´tər) **monitor** is a portable electrocardiograph that a person can wear while conducting normal daily activities. This device records heart activity over time and during various activities to aid in the diagnosis of cardiac problems that occur intermittently.

8-27 Laboratory tests for cardiovascular disorders include testing for fats and cardiac enzymes in the blood. **Lipids** (lip´idz) are fatty substances in the body and include **cholesterol** (kə-les´tər-ol″) and **triglycerides** (tri-glis´ər-īdz). High levels of these two lipids are associated with greater risk of **arteriosclerosis** (ahr-tēr″e-o-sklə-ro´sis), hardening of the arteries. Two lipids associated with a greater risk of cardiovascular disease are triglycerides and

cholesterol

_____.

Lipo/proteins (lip″o, li″po-pro´tēnz) are special proteins that transport lipids in the blood. The elevation of **low-density lipoproteins** (LDLs) is associated with an increased risk of cardiovascular disease. High levels of **high-density lipoproteins** (HDLs) are associated with decreased cardiac risk profiles.

8-28 Certain enzymes are released into the bloodstream by damaged heart muscle. Levels of these enzymes can be measured in blood tests called the **lactate dehydrogenase** (lak´tāt de-hi´dro-jən″ās) **test** (LDH) and **creatine kinase** (kre´ə-tin ki´nās) **test** (CK), also called cre-

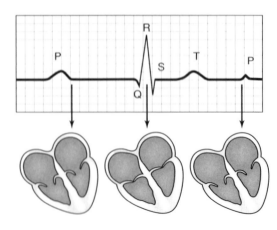

Figure 8-12 Electrocardiogram showing the location of the major waves. The P wave begins the cycle and represents the contraction of the atria when forcing the blood into the ventricles. The QRS complex represents the contraction of the ventricles when forcing the blood into both the pulmonary and systemic circulation. Relaxation of the heart occurs at the T wave. The cycle begins again with the new P wave.

heart

atine phosphokinase (fos″fo-ki′nās) (CPK). Levels of these enzymes usually rise within a few hours after a heart attack. LDH and CPK are blood tests to assess _____ damage.

8-29 Several diagnostic procedures are used to help assess heart disease, many of which are noninvasive. Examination of a chest x-ray gives information about the size and position of the heart.

   Stress tests measure the heart's response during controlled physiologic stress, usually exercise. In the treadmill exercise test (or **treadmill stress test**), an ECG and other measurements are taken while the patient walks on an inclined treadmill at varying speeds and inclines. Measuring the heart's response while exercising in this manner is called a treadmill _____ test.

stress

The **thallium stress test** and other nuclear medicine procedures also measure cardiovascular function, particularly in coronary artery disease.

8-30 Diagnostic procedures are often able to detect abnormalities before the heart is damaged. Because each procedure has special benefits, several may be performed. **Echo/cardio/graphy** (ek″o-kahr″de-og′rə-fe) is the use of ultrasonography (ul″trə-sə-nog′rə-fe) in diagnosing heart disease. A record of the heart obtained by directing ultrasonic waves through the chest wall is an

echocardiogram
(ek″o-kahr′de-o-gram″)

_____. Figure 8-13 is an echocardiogram that shows the chambers of the heart and a large thrombus.

   Doppler echocardiography gives information about the direction and pattern of blood flow within the heart. Doppler scanning and additional specialized radiographic procedures provide additional information about heart functions.

8-31 Cardiac MRI, magnetic resonance imaging, may be done, as well as computed tomography. The latter produces cross-sectional images of an organ similar to what one would see if the organ were actually cut into sections. The record produced by tomography is a _____.

tomogram
(to′mo-gram)

   Positron emission tomography is used in other areas also but is especially helpful in examining blood flow in the heart and blood vessels. In this procedure the patient is injected with a radioactive element, which becomes concentrated in the heart, and color-coded images are produced.

8-32 **Arterio/graphy** (ahr″tēr-e-og′rə-fe) is radiography of arteries after injection of radiopaque material into the bloodstream. Literally, this word means recording of the arteries. Build a word that means the film produced in arteriography: _____ (Figure 8-14). Through common usage, **arteriograph** (ahr-tēr′e-o-graf) is used interchangeably with arteriogram, just as photo/graph is used to mean the record (picture) produced in photography.

arteriogram
(ahr-tēr′e-o-gram)

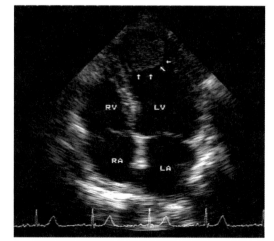

Figure 8-13 Echocardiogram. The heart is viewed from the top, and the four chambers (*RV* [right ventricle], *RA* [right atrium], *LV* [left ventricle], *LA* [left atrium]) are visible, as well as a large thrombus, indicated by the *arrows*.

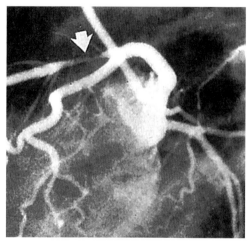

Figure 8-14 Arteriogram. Radiographic image after injection of a radiopaque contrast medium reveals blockage of an artery (*arrow*).

The combining form phot(o) means light. **Coronary arteriography** is a radiographic procedure used to study coronary arteries.

Digital subtraction angiography (DSA) provides computer-enhanced radiographic images of blood vessels filled with contrast material.

8-33 **Aorto/graphy** (a″or-tog′rə-fe) is radiography of the aorta after introduction of a contrast medium. The film produced by aortography is an _____. Different areas of the aorta are generally studied, rather than visualizing all of its divisions. Thoracic, abdominal, and renal aortography are examples of areas of the aorta that are studied. Radiology of the aorta in the abdominal area is called abdominal _____.

8-34 There are also several invasive tests available to diagnose cardiovascular disease. **Cardiac catheterization** (kath″ə-tur-ĭ-za′shən) is a diagnostic procedure in which a catheter (kath′ə-tər) is introduced through an incision into a large blood vessel of the arm, leg, or neck and threaded through the circulatory system to the heart. Pressures and patterns of blood flow can be determined in catheterization (Figure 8-15).

The catheter enables the use of contrast media that enhance x-ray images of the heart and its vessels. A radiographic procedure that produces an **angiogram** (an′je-o-gram″) is called **angiography** (an″je-og′rə-fe). Radiography of the coronary arteries is coronary _____. Cardiac angiography, also called **angiocardiography** (an″je-o-kahr″de-og′rə-fe), is radiography of the heart and its vessels.

Electrophysiologic studies use electrode catheters to pace the heart and can identify disturbances in the rhythm of the heart that would otherwise be inapparent.

aortogram
(a-or′to-gram)

aortography

angiography

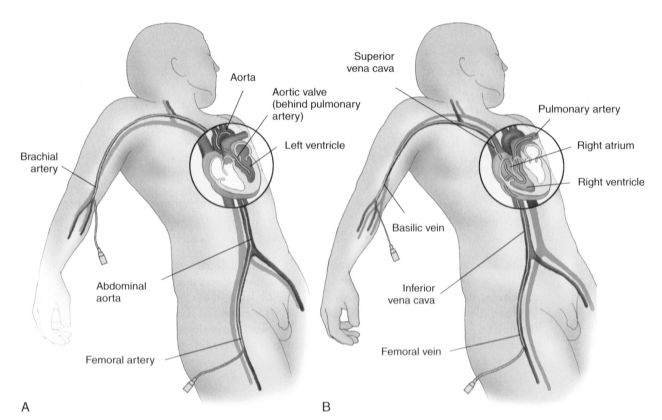

A   B

Figure 8-15 Heart catheterization. A, Left-sided. **B,** Right-sided. Progress of the catheter is monitored by fluoroscopy as it is threaded through blood vessels to reach the heart. Fluoroscopy gives the physician immediate images of the location of the catheter throughout the procedure. The right side of the heart may be the only side examined, because left-sided heart catheterization is riskier than that of the right.

EXERCISE 7

Build It! *Use the following word parts to build terms. (Some word parts will be used more than once, some not at all.)*

brady-, tachy-, aort(o), arteri(o), cardi(o), electr(o), steth(o), -ia, -gram, -graph, -graphy, -scope

1. instrument used to record electrical currents of the heart   _____/_____/_____

2. increased pulse rate   _____/_____/_____

3. radiography of the aorta   _____/_____

4. film produced in radiography of the arteries   _____/_____

5. instrument used to listen to heart sounds   _____/_____

Say and Check

Say aloud the terms you wrote for Exercise 7. Use the Companion CD to check your pronunciations.

EXERCISE 8

Write a word in each blank to complete these sentences.

1. Increased blood pressure is _____.

2. Decreased pulse is _____.

3. Relaxation of the ventricles is called _____.

4. Blood pressure that is measured when the ventricles contract is the _____ pressure.

5. A portable electrocardiograph that a person can wear is a _____ monitor.

6. Cholesterol and triglycerides are fatty substances called _____.

7. LDL and HDL are special proteins called _____.

8. Cardiac ultrasonography is called _____.

Say and Check

Say aloud the terms you wrote for Exercise 8. Use the Companion CD to check your pronunciations.

PATHOLOGIES

HEART PATHOLOGIES

8-35 Cardiovascular disease is any abnormal condition characterized by dysfunction of the heart and blood vessels. Diagnosis and treatment of cardiovascular disorders have improved, but cardiovascular disease remains the major cause of death in the United States.

Heart disease can be classified in many ways. One method is based on whether the cause of the heart dysfunction developed away from the heart (as in diseases of the arteries), or if the heart itself was the primary site of the dysfunction. The leading cause of death in the United States is _____ disease.

cardiovascular

Learn the meaning of these word parts that are used to describe heart abnormalities.

Additional Word Parts: Heart Pathologies

Word Part	Meaning	Word Part	Meaning
rhythm(o), rrhythm(o)	rhythm	scler(o), -sclerosis	hard, hardening
de-	down, from, or reversing	-stenosis	narrowing, stricture

8-36 Primary cardiac diseases include those caused by structural cardiac defects, as well as inflammation and infection that originate within the heart. Defects are sometimes present in one of the four chambers of the heart, in one of the heart valves, or in the septum that divides the two sides of the heart. If heart disease is present at birth, it is a **congenital heart disease.**

atrium

Atrio/megaly (a″tre-o-meg′ə-le) is abnormal enlargement of an _____ of the heart.

8-37 A **ventricular septal defect** is an abnormal opening in the septum dividing the right and the left ventricles. Look at Figure 8-11 and be sure that you can locate where a ventricular septal defect would occur. This defect is a type of congenital heart disease. An **atrial septal defect** is also a congenital heart disease. An atrial septal defect is an abnormal opening in the part of the

atria

septum that separates the right and the left _____.

8-38 There are other congenital heart diseases, but atrial septal defects and ventricular septal defects account for 30% to 40% of heart diseases that are present at birth. Almost all congenital heart defects (those present at birth) interrupt the normal flow of blood through the heart and vessels. **Heart murmurs**—abnormal heart sounds—are often heard. Cyanosis may also be

blue (or bluish)

present. Cyan/osis is a _____ discoloration of the skin and mucous membranes that results from insufficient oxygen to the tissues.

Three other congenital heart diseases are **patent ductus arteriosus** (duk′təs ahr-tēr″e-o′səs) (PDA), **coarctation of the aorta**, and **tetralogy of Fallot** (tĕ-tral′ə-je ov fə-lo′). Patent ductus arteriosus is an abnormal opening between the pulmonary artery and the aorta. There is narrowing of a part of the aorta in coarctation of the aorta. There are four congenital heart defects in tetralogy of Fallot, named for the French physician. It may be difficult to remember the types of defects, but it is important to remember that these three diseases are congenital heart diseases and surgery may be indicated.

8-39 Normally the intervals between pulses are of equal length. Remembering that a- means no

without

or without, **a/rrhythmia** (ə-rith′me-ə) is _____ rhythm. The combining forms rrhythm(o) and rhythm(o) mean rhythm. Arrhythmia is the same as arhythmia and is the more common spelling.

A variation in the normal rhythm of the heartbeat is an arrhythmia. Although this term is more commonly used, **dys/rhythm/ia** (dis-rith′me-ə) would be more technically correct. Dysrhythmia is a disturbance of rhythm. Common usage generally determines whether one uses one "r" or two in medical terms that pertain to rhythm. Write the new term that means an abnormal,

dysrhythmia

disordered, or disturbed rhythm: _____.

Heart flutters are rapid contractions of either the atria or the ventricles and can be seen on the electrocardiogram. Heart **palpitations**˙ (pal″pĭ-ta′shənz), however, are subjective sensations of a pounding or racing heart. It can be associated with heart disease, but some persons experience palpitations and yet have no evidence of heart disease. In these cases, the palpitations are believed to be emotional responses to stress.

8-40 **Ventricular fibrillation** (fĭ-brĭ-la′shən) is a severe cardiac arrhythmia in which ventricular contractions are too rapid and uncoordinated for effective blood circulation. A cardiac arrhyth-

fibrillation

mia marked by rapid, uncoordinated contractions is called _____.

Sometimes a defibrillator is used to alleviate fibrillation. (The prefix de- is used to mean down, from, or reversing. It is in the latter sense that it is used here.) A **defibrillator** (de-fib″rĭ-la′tər) is an electronic apparatus that has defibrillator paddles that are used to make contact with the patient and deliver a preset voltage of electricity to shock the heart (Figure

fibrillation

8-16). **Defibrillation** (de-fib″rĭ-la′shən) stops _____. Ventricular fibrillation is often a cause of cardiac arrest. Another name for cardiac arrest is **a/systole** (a-sis′to-le), which means absence of heartbeat or contraction.

8-41 You learned earlier that the heart has a special structure, the sinoatrial node, where electrical impulses arise and stimulate contraction. Impairment in the conduction of the impulse from the SA node to other parts of the heart is known as a **heart block.** When the electrical impulse is not conducted throughout the heart, normal heart contraction does not occur. This condition is

---

˙Palpitations (Latin: *palpitare*, to move frequently and rapidly).

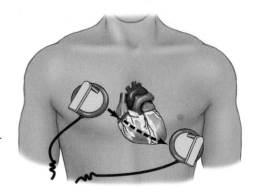

Figure 8-16 **Flow of current when defibrillator paddles are applied.** The paddles, usually applied over special defibrillator pads on the patient's chest, deliver an electrical shock at a preset voltage to the myocardium. *Arrows* indicate the flow of the electrical current as it passes through the heart.

block

known as a heart _____. The condition may be asymptomatic and require no intervention, but implantation of an artificial pacemaker (described later in the surgical intervention section) may be necessary in complete heart block.

8-42 Atrial fibrillation, a cardiac arrhythmia characterized by disorganized electrical activity in the atria, results in reduced stroke volume (the amount of blood ejected by a ventricle during contraction) but is not as life-threatening as ventricular fibrillation. Other arrhythmias that can be detected by electrocardiography include bradycardia, tachycardia, premature ventricular contractions (PVC), and atrio/ventricular block (AVB).

In **paroxysmal** (par″ok-siz′məl) **atrial tachycardia** (PAT), the patient may detect palpitations and a racing heartbeat (150 to 250 beats per minute) that occur and stop suddenly. Paroxysmal means occurring in sudden, repeated episodes.

Atrio/ventricular block is a disorder of impulse transmission between the atria and the

ventricles

_____.

8-43 In many types of heart disease, the heart attempts to compensate for its deficit by working harder. Cardio/megaly (kahr″de-o-meg′ə-le) may result. **Cardio/megaly** is

enlargement

_____ of the heart.

smallness

Micro/cardia (mi-kro-kahr′de-ə), the opposite of cardiomegaly, is abnormal _____ of the heart.

8-44 Insufficient blood flow to an area is termed **ischemia** (is-ke′me-ə). If the myocardial demand for oxygen exceeds the capability of diseased coronary arteries, myocardial

ischemia

_____ results. The patient may experience chest pain, often called **angina pectoris**[*] (an-ji′nə, an′jə-nə pek′to-ris), or simply angina. The pain usually radiates along the neck, jaw, and shoulder and down the left arm. The pain may be relieved by rest or medication.

8-45 Myocardial infarction (in-fahrk′shən), MI, is necrosis of a portion of cardiac muscle caused by an obstruction or a blood clot in a coronary artery. Cells die when deprived of oxygen. The death of cells in an area of the myocardium because of oxygen deprivation is myocardial infarction (Figure 8-17). A myocardial infarction is a heart attack. **An/ox/ia** means an abnormal

oxygen

condition characterized by absence of _____. A localized area of damaged tissue resulting from anoxia is called an **infarct**[†] (in′fahrkt).

MI is the most common cause of death in the United States. Whether death occurs after MI largely depends on the resulting damage to the myocardium. Those who survive often suffer complications of heart function. When areas of the myocardium die because of lack of oxygen,

infarction

this is called myocardial _____.

Rest is an important part of recovery after a heart attack. The patient is usually left with some heart damage, often resulting in failure of the heart to function normally. This deficiency of the heart is called **cardiac insufficiency.** If the damage is too severe, surgical intervention may be necessary.

---

[*]Angina pectoris (Latin: *angor,* strangling; *pectus,* breast or chest).
[†]Infarct (Latin: *infarcire,* to stuff).

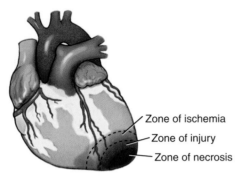

Zone of ischemia
Zone of injury
Zone of necrosis

Figure 8-17 Myocardial infarction. Also called a heart attack, myocardial infarction is necrosis of a portion of cardiac muscle. It is usually caused by an obstruction in a coronary artery.

EXERCISE 9

Build It! *Use the following word parts to build terms. (Some word parts will be used more than once.)*

an-, dys-, micro-, atri(o), cardi(o), cyan(o), ox(i), rrhythm(o), -ia, -megaly, -osis

1. Enlargement of an atrium of the heart　　　　　　　＿＿＿＿＿＿＿＿/＿＿＿＿＿＿＿＿＿

2. Bluish discoloration of the skin and mucous membranes　＿＿＿＿＿＿＿＿/＿＿＿＿＿＿＿＿＿

3. A variation in the normal rhythm of the heartbeat　＿＿＿＿＿/＿＿＿＿＿＿＿/＿＿＿＿＿＿＿

4. Abnormal smallness of the heart　　　　　　　＿＿＿＿＿＿/＿＿＿＿＿＿＿/＿＿＿＿＿＿＿

5. Abnormal condition of absence of oxygen　　　＿＿＿＿＿＿/＿＿＿＿＿＿＿/＿＿＿＿＿＿＿

Say and Check

Say aloud the terms you wrote for Exercise 9. Use the Companion CD to check your pronunciations.

congestive

8-46 MI and other disorders in which there is insufficient oxygen to the heart may lead to **congestive heart failure** (CHF), also called congestive heart disease. CHF is an abnormal condition that reflects impaired cardiac function. The patient experiences weakness, breathlessness, and edema. Edema is an abnormal accumulation of fluid in the interstitial spaces of tissue. This condition is called ＿＿＿＿＿＿＿＿＿＿＿＿＿＿＿＿ heart failure.

narrowing

8-47 Heart valves can also be defective, resulting in the valves not opening fully, as in **valvul/ar stenosis. Stenosis** (stə-no´sis) means narrowing. When a valve is stenos/ed, it becomes constricted or narrower. Valvular stenosis is ＿＿＿＿＿＿＿＿＿＿＿＿＿＿＿＿ of the opening created by the valve. Stenosis of any of the heart's valves can decrease blood circulation.

　　Valves may also become infected and inflamed. **Valvul/itis** (val″vu-li´tis) is inflammation of a valve, especially a heart valve. Build a new word that specifically means inflammation of the valves of the heart by using a combining form that means heart + valvulitis:

cardiovalvulitis
(kahr″de-o-val″vu-li´tis)

＿＿＿＿＿＿＿＿＿＿＿＿＿＿＿＿＿＿＿＿.
　　Weakening of one or both mitral cusps when the heart contracts is called **mitral valve prolapse** (MVP). Prolapse means sagging. When a valve prolapses, such as in MVP, the valve sags rather than opening fully. Symptoms vary from absent to severe, and the condition may be associated with sounds heard through a stethoscope, including a clicking sound or heart murmur.

rheumatic

8-48 Rheumatic (roo-mat´ik) fever, usually occurring in childhood, may develop as a delayed reaction to an inadequately treated infection of the upper respiratory tract by certain pathogenic streptococci (group A beta-hemolytic). The disease may affect the brain, heart, joints, or skin. **Rheumatic heart disease** is damage to heart muscle and heart valves caused by episodes of rheumatic fever. Permanent damage to the heart or the valves may occur. This type of damage is called ＿＿＿＿＿＿＿＿＿＿＿＿＿＿＿＿ heart disease.

8-49 Cardio/myo/pathy (kahr″de-o-mi-op´ə-the) is a general diagnostic term that designates primary myocardial disease. In other words, the disease originated in the myocardium. A disease of the myocardium that is not attributable to outside causes that results in insufficient oxygen,

cardiomyopathy	damaged valves, or high blood pressure is called a _____. **Myocarditis** (mi″o-kahr-di′tis) is an example of a cardiomyopathy.
inflammation	Myocard/itis means _____ of the myocardium. This may be caused by an infection, rheumatic fever, a chemical agent, or a complication of another disease.
endocarditis (en″do-kahr-di′tis)	**8-50** Inflammation of the inner lining of the heart is _____. Endocarditis is caused by infectious microorganisms that invade the lining of the heart, quite often the valves.
pericarditis (per″ĭ-kahr-di′tis)	Using -itis, build a word that means inflammation of the pericardium: _____. In pericarditis, the pericardium becomes inflamed owing to an infectious microorganism, a cancerous growth, or a variety of other causes.
hemopericardium	**8-51 Hemo/pericardium** (he″mo-per″ĭ-kahr′de-əm) is an effusion (ə-fu′zhen)* of blood into the pericardial space. **Effusion** means the escape of fluid into a part, such as a cavity. Blood in the pericardial space is called _____. An accumulation of fluid in the pericardial space can lead to compression of the heart, which is called **cardiac tamponade** (tam″pon-ād′).
low	**8-52 Shock** is a life-threatening condition in which there is inadequate blood flow to the body's tissues. It is usually associated with inadequate cardiac output, hypotension, and tissue damage. Causes of shock include hemorrhage or dehydration resulting in hypo/vol/emia. The term **hypovolemia** (hi″po-vo-le′me-ə) means an abnormally _____ circulating blood volume.

*Effusion (Latin: *effusion,* pour out).

EXERCISE 10

Write the names of the cardiac pathologies represented by the following definitions. The first letter of each term is given as a clue.

1. enlarged heart c_____

2. rapid and uncoordinated ventricular contractions f_____

3. absence of heart contractions a_____

4. a localized area of damaged tissue resulting from insufficient oxygen i_____

5. insufficient blood flow to an area i_____

6. inflammation of the valves of the heart c_____

7. inflammation of the pericardium p_____

8. a word that means narrowing s_____

9. inflammation of the lining of the heart e_____

10. a life-threatening condition in which blood flow is inadequate s_____

Say and Check

Say aloud the terms you wrote for Exercise 10. Use the Companion CD to check your pronunciations.

BLOOD VESSEL PATHOLOGIES

8-53 Arteries, arterioles, capillaries, venules, and veins make up the network of blood vessels that carry blood. The dilation and constriction of blood vessels influence blood pressure and the distribution of blood to various parts of the body. The vaso/motor (va″zo-, vas″o-mo′tər) center located in the brain regulates vasoconstriction (va″zo-, vas″o-kən-strik′shən) and vasodilation (va″zo-, vas″o-di-la′shən), thus influencing the diameter of the blood vessels.

vasodilation	**Vaso/dilation** is stretching or dilation of a vessel. In the word vasodilation, dilation means expansion or stretching. An increase in the diameter of a blood vessel is _____. The opposite of vasodilation is **vaso/constriction.** When blood vessels constrict, they become narrow. A decrease in the diameter of blood vessels is vasoconstriction. Learn the meaning of these word parts used to describe disorders of the blood vessels.

Additional Word Parts: Blood Vessel Pathologies

Word Part	Meaning
aneurysm(o)	aneurysm
ather(o)	yellowish, fatty plaque
embol(o)	embolus

	8-54 The coronary arteries supply blood to the heart tissue. A heart attack may be preceded by **coronary artery disease** (CAD), an abnormal condition of the coronary arteries that causes a reduced flow of oxygen and nutrients to the myocardium. Arterio/sclerosis (ahr-tēr″e-o-sklə-ro′sis) is a thickening and loss of elasticity of the walls of the arteries. Literal interpretation of
hardening	arterio/scler/osis is _____ of the arteries. **Arterio/sclero/tic** (ahr-tēr″e-o-sklə-rot′ik) **heart disease** (ASHD) is hardening and thickening of the walls of the coronary arteries. This reduces the oxygen supply to the myocardium and may lead to a heart attack.
	8-55 Athero/sclerosis (ath″ər-o-sklə-ro′sis), a form of arteriosclerosis, is characterized by the formation of fatty deposits on the walls of arteries (Figure 8-18). Only a few words use the combining form ather(o), which means yellow, fatty plaque. Write the term that means a form of arteriosclerosis characterized by the formation of fatty deposits on the walls of arteries:
atherosclerosis	_____. The yellowish plaques in atherosclerosis are cholesterol, other lipids, and cellular debris that accumulate in the inner walls of arteries. As atherosclerosis progresses, the vessel walls become fibrotic and calcified and the **lumen** (cavity) narrows, resulting in reduced blood flow. The plaque creates a risk for **occlusion** (o-kloo′zhən) (blockage) or thrombosis and is one of the major causes of coronary heart disease, angina pectoris, myocardial infarction, and other cardiac disorders. An occlusion is an obstruction or closure.
coronary	**8-56** Formation of a blood clot in a coronary artery is **coronary thrombosis** (throm-bo′sis). **Coronary occlusion** is a closing off of a _____ artery. The occlusion may result from a thrombus, but it is more likely to be caused by a narrowing of the lumen of the blood vessel. Myocardial infarction occurs if an occlusion is complete and no blood is being supplied to an area of the myocardium. A blood clot in a vessel in the brain is one cause of a **cerebro/vascular accident** (CVA). This abnormal condition is characterized by occlusion of a vessel of the brain by an embolus, throm-

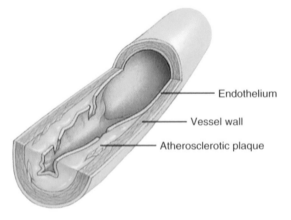

Endothelium

Vessel wall

Atherosclerotic plaque

Figure 8-18 Partial blockage of an artery by plaque in atherosclerosis. The endothelium is a layer of epithelial cells that lines blood and lymph vessels as well as the heart and many closed cavities of the body. As lipids, calcium, fibrin, and other cellular substances are deposited within the lining of the arteries, an inflammatory response results from the efforts to heal the endothelium.

Figure 8-19 Types of stroke. A, Hemorrhagic stroke. Blood vessel bursts and allows blood to seep into brain tissue until clotting stops the seepage. **B,** Thrombotic stroke. Plaque can cause a clot that blocks blood flow to form. **C,** Embolic stroke. A blood clot or other embolus reaches an artery in the brain, lodges there, and blocks the flow of blood.

  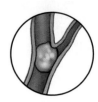

A Hemorrhagic stroke   B Thrombotic stroke   C Embolic (embolitic) stroke

---

cerebrovascular

bus, or cerebrovascular hemorrhage or spasm and results in ischemia of the brain tissues (Figure 8-19). CVA, also called stroke, is an abbreviation for _____ accident.

8-57 Scler/osis is a condition characterized by abnormal hardening of tissue. Build a word that means hardening of the aorta: _____.

aortosclerosis
(a-or″to-sklə-ro´sis)

Stenosis (stə-no´sis) means constriction or narrowing of a passage or orifice. **Stricture** (strik´chər) is also used in this sense. Two terms often have the same meaning because words are derived from both the Latin and the Greek languages. In **aortic stenosis,** narrowing of the aorta, blood cannot flow efficiently from the left ventricle into the aorta, and the condition may lead to congestive heart failure. **Aortic insufficiency** (AI), also called **aortic regurgitation,** is somewhat less severe, but blood flows back into the left ventricle during diastole because the aortic valve does not close completely. The heart will work harder in an attempt to deliver needed oxygen and nutrients to all the body's cells.

Build a word that means inflammation of the aorta by using the combining form for aorta plus the suffix for inflammation: _____. **Angio/card/itis** (an″je-o-kahr-di´tis) is inflammation of the heart and large blood vessels.

aortitis (a″or-ti´tis)

narrowing

8-58 Angio/stenosis (an″je-o-stə-no´sis) is _____ of the diameter of a vessel. Any disease of the arteries is an **arterio/pathy** (ahr-tēr″e-op´ə-the). Use arter(o) to write a word that means inflammation of an artery: _____.

arteritis
(ahr″tə-ri´tis)

Peripheral vascular disease is blockage or narrowing of arteries that results in interference of adequate blood flow to the extremities, especially those conditions affecting the lower extremities. Atherosclerosis is one cause of this condition.

8-59 An **aneurysm** (an´u-riz″əm) is a localized dilation or ballooning out of the wall of a blood vessel. Aneurysms can occur in many blood vessels, but most aneurysms are arterial. This is because pressure is higher in the arteries, particularly the aorta. Use the combining form aneurysm(o) to write words about aneurysms. **Aneurysm/al** (an″u-riz´məl) means pertaining to an _____.

aneurysm

An aneurysm may rupture, causing hemorrhage, or thrombi may form in the dilated vessel and give rise to emboli (em´bə-li) that may obstruct smaller vessels.

8-60 Aneurysms tend to occur at specific sites, most commonly in the abdominal aorta (Figure 8-20). Most patients are asymptomatic until the aneurysm ruptures. Aneurysms may be first discovered by routine examination or during radiographic study performed for another reason. Computed tomography and ultrasound are usually helpful in establishing a diagnosis. Aortography, also called aortic arteriography, is performed for all patients who are to undergo surgical repair of a thoracic aneurysm. The radiographic process in which the aorta and its branches are injected with contrast media for visualization is called _____.

aortography

8-61 An **angi/oma** (an″je-o´mə) is a benign tumor of either blood or lymph vessels. Angiomas are not malignant and sometimes disappear spontaneously. An angioma is either a **hem/angi/oma** (he-man″je-o´mə) or a **lymph/angi/oma** (lim-fan″je-o´mə). A hemangioma is a tumor of _____ vessels. (Note that the vowel is dropped from hem[a] and lymph[o] when they are joined with combining forms that begin with a vowel.) A lymph/angi/oma is a tumor composed of lymph vessels.

blood

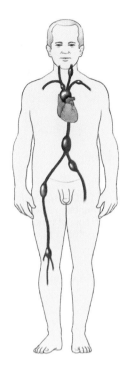

Figure 8-20 **Common anatomic sites of arterial aneurysms.**

EXERCISE 11

Build It! *Use the following word parts to build terms. (Some word parts will be used more than once.)*

aneurysm(o), angi(o), arteri(o), cardi(o), lymph(o), -al, -itis, -oma, -sclerosis, -stenosis

1. narrowing of the diameter of a vessel   _____/_____

2. pertaining to a localized dilation of the wall of a blood vessel   _____/_____

3. a tumor composed of lymph vessels   _____/_____/_____

4. thickening and loss of elasticity of the arteries   _____/_____/_____

5. inflammation of the heart and large blood vessels   _____/_____/_____

Say and Check

Say aloud the terms you wrote for Exercise 11. Use the Companion CD to check your pronunciations.

	8-62 Varicose (var´ĭ-kōs) **veins** are swollen and knotted and occur most often in the legs. They result from sluggish blood flow in combination with weakened walls and incompetent valves in the veins. Unlike arteries, which have substantially more muscle and elastic tissue, veins have flaplike valves that prevent blood from flowing backward. Defective valves allow the blood to collect in the veins, which become swollen and knotted (Figure 8-21). This condition is called
varicose	_____ veins.
phlebitis (flə-bi´tis)	**8-63** Using phleb(o), build a word that means inflammation of a vein: _____.

Thrombo/phleb/itis (throm″bo-flə-bi´tis) is inflammation of a vein associated with a blood clot. **Venous thrombosis,** formation of a thrombus within a vein, may be a complication of phleb/itis. It may also result from an injury to the leg or prolonged bed confinement.

Hemorrhoids (hem´ə-roidz) are a type of varicose veins in the lower rectum or anus (see Figure 10-22, *B*).

8-64 Phlebo/stasis (flə-bos´tə-sis) may be a spontaneous slowing down of blood flow in a vein or the result of a deliberate act in which one compresses the vein to control the flow of blood temporarily. In many words, -stasis will be used for either of these two meanings.

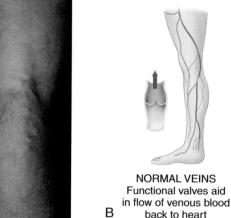

Figure 8-21 Varicose veins. A, The appearance of superficial varicose veins. **B,** Comparison of normal veins and varicose veins. Sluggish blood flow, weakened walls, and incompetent valves contribute to varicose veins in the legs, a common location for these enlarged and twisted veins near the surface of the skin.

NORMAL VEINS
Functional valves aid in flow of venous blood back to heart

VARICOSE VEINS
Failure of valves and pooling of blood in superficial veins

vein	You will need to remember that phlebostasis means either a spontaneous venous stasis or stopping the flow of blood in a _____ by application of a tourniquet (toor´nĭ-kət) on an extremity. A **tourniquet** is a device applied around an extremity to control the circulation and prevent the flow of blood to or from the distal area.

EXERCISE 12

Write a word in each blank to complete these sentences.

1. A term for a localized dilation or ballooning out of the wall of a blood vessel is _____.

2. CAD is an abbreviation that means _____ artery disease.

3. A closing off of a coronary artery is called coronary _____.

4. Formation of a blood clot in a coronary artery is coronary _____.

5. Formation of fatty deposits on the walls of arteries is a form of arteriosclerosis, called _____.

6. Hardening of the aorta is _____.

7. The term for inflammation of a vein associated with a blood clot is _____.

8. Narrowing of the diameter of the aorta is called aortic _____.

Say and Check

Say aloud the terms you wrote for Exercise 12. Use the Companion CD to check your pronunciations.

SURGICAL AND THERAPEUTIC INTERVENTIONS

8-65 Cardio/pulmonary resuscitation (re-sus″ĭ-ta´shən) (CPR) is a basic emergency procedure for life support, consisting of manual external cardiac massage and artificial respiration. Pulmonary refers to the lungs, so cardio/pulmonary pertains to the heart and lungs. The artificial respiration can be mouth-to-mouth breathing or a mechanical form of ventilation.

CPR is used in cases of cardiac arrest to establish effective circulation and ventilation in order to prevent irreversible cerebral damage resulting from anoxia. CPR is an abbreviation for

cardiopulmonary

_____ resuscitation.

8-66 You learned earlier that the SA node is called the pacemaker of the heart. A second meaning of pacemaker is an artificial **cardiac pacemaker,** a small battery-powered device that is generally used to increase the heart rate by electrically stimulating the heart muscle. Depending on the patient's need, a cardiac pacemaker may be permanent or temporary and may fire only on demand or at a constant rate (Figure 8-22). Severe bradycardia may indicate the need for an arti-

pacemaker

ficial cardiac _____.

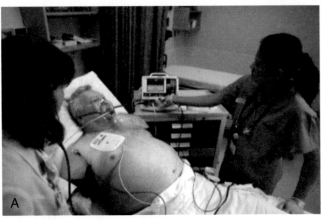
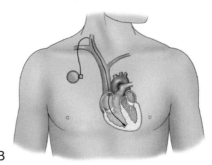

Figure 8-22 **An external pacemaker vs. an internal cardiac pacemaker.** **A,** An external pacemaker is used temporarily in a hospital setting by delivering electrical current through the skin. This procedure, initiated by the nurse, may be used until a more definitive therapy is available. **B,** An internal or artificial cardiac pacemaker provides an electrical current that travels from the battery through a conducting wire to the myocardium and stimulates the heart to beat.

cardioverter	**8-67 Cardio/version** (kahr´de-o-vur˝zhən) uses electrical shock to restore the normal rhythm of the heart with a device that delivers a direct-current shock. An automatic implantable **cardioverter** (kahr´de-o-vər˝tər) is a device that detects sustained ventricular tachycardia or fibrillation and terminates it by a shock that restores the normal rhythm (Figure 8-23). This implanted device is called an automatic implantable _____.
pericardium	**8-68 Peri/cardio/centesis** (per˝e-kahr˝de-o-sen-te´sis) is surgical puncture of the _____. This procedure is performed to draw off fluid that has accumulated in the pericardial space.
cardioplegic (kahr˝de-o-plej´ik)	**8-69** If surgery is to be performed on the heart, **cardio/plegia** (kahr˝de-o-ple´jə) may be necessary to stop myocardial contractions. Solutions used to stop the heart's action so that surgery may be performed on the heart are called _____ **solutions.** Surgeries involving the heart and major vessels generally require **cardiopulmonary** (kahr˝de-o-pool´mə-nar-e) **bypass,** a procedure in which the heart is bypassed by providing an
extracorporeal	**extra/corporeal**˙ (eks˝trə-kor-por´e-əl) (outside the body) device to pump blood. The term that means outside the body is _____. The blood is diverted from the heart and lungs to a pump oxygenator (ok´sĭ-jə-na˝tər), then returned directly to the aorta and pumped to the rest of the body (Figure 8-24).
atria	**8-70** Atrial or ventricular septal defects usually require surgical closure of the abnormal opening. **Atrio/septo/plasty** (a˝tre-o-sep´to-plas˝te) is surgical repair of the septum in the area between the right and left _____.
bypass	**8-71** The term **bypass** (bi´pas) is also used to mean bypass surgery. A **coronary artery bypass** is an open heart surgery in which a prosthesis or a section of a blood vessel is grafted onto one of the coronary arteries, bypassing a blocked or narrowed coronary artery in coronary artery disease. If a vessel from elsewhere in the patient's body is used to provide an alternate route for the blood to circumvent the obstructed coronary artery, the surgery is called a **coronary artery bypass graft** (CABG), pronounced "cabbage" (Figure 8-25). The vessels that are generally used are a segment of the saphenous (sə-fe´nəs) vein from the patient's leg or the mammary artery. A bypass is also called a **shunt**. One that circumvents a vessel that supplies blood to the heart is called a coronary artery _____.

˙Extracorporeal (Latin: _corpus,_ body).

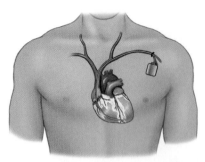

Figure 8-23 Implantable cardioverter-defibrillator. This surgically implanted electric device automatically terminates arrhythmias by delivering low-energy shocks to the heart, restoring proper rhythm when the heart begins beating too fast or erratically. It is generally attached to the chest wall and has a wire lead embedded in the heart.

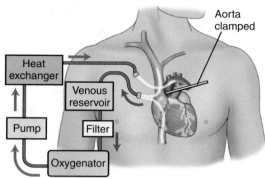

Figure 8-24 Components of a cardiopulmonary bypass system used during heart surgery.

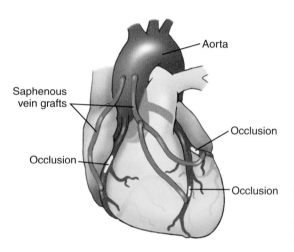

Figure 8-25 Coronary artery bypass graft using saphenous vein grafts. Sections of the patient's own saphenous veins located in the legs are grafted onto the coronary arteries to bypass the blocked coronary arteries.

➤ **KEY** POINT <u>Depending on the patient, there may be less-invasive surgeries for CAD that do not require cardiopulmonary bypass.</u> Options for the traditional CABG include minimally invasive direct coronary artery bypass (MIDCAB), off-pump coronary artery bypass (OP-CAB), and port-access and video-assisted CABGs.

Developments in cardiac surgery are heart transplantation and use of an artificial heart. Research continues to bring improvements in these two types of surgeries.

8-72 A variety of procedures, some not requiring extensive surgery, are available for treating vascular insufficiencies. Per/cutane/ous (per-, through + cutane[o], skin + -ous, pertaining to) means performed through the skin. Percutaneous procedures to improve blood flow in a particular vessel involve the use of a catheter, monitored by fluoroscopy, that is introduced through a blood vessel. The management of coronary artery occlusions by any of the catheter-based techniques is called **percutaneous coronary intervention** (PCI). These procedures include the compression or removal of plaque that may be preventing adequate blood flow. PCI is

percutaneous _____ coronary intervention and applies to a coronary artery.

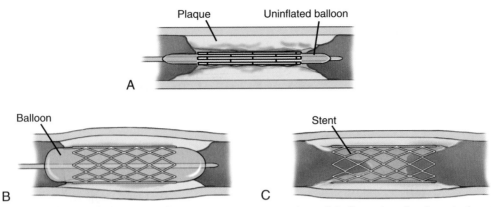

Figure 8-26 Balloon angioplasty and placement of a coronary artery stent. A small, balloon-tipped catheter is threaded into a coronary artery and inflated to compress the plaque. A stent, an expandable meshlike structure, is placed over the angioplasty site to keep the coronary artery open. **A,** The stent and uninflated balloon catheter is positioned in the artery. **B,** The stent expands as the balloon is inflated. **C,** The balloon is then deflated and removed, leaving the implanted stent.

> ➤ **KEY** POINT <u>PCI is invasive but nonsurgical management of coronary arteries.</u> PCI involves the use of catheters inserted into occluded or stenosed arteries. Plaque is compressed, destroyed, or cut away and removed. Procedures include laser-assisted angioplasty, percutaneous transluminal coronary angioplasty, implantation of coronary stents to keep the vessel open, and atherectomy.

repair

   As a term written alone, angio/plasty means surgical _____ of a blood vessel that has become damaged by disease or injury.

8-73 Laser-assisted angioplasty applies to arteries in general and is the opening of an occluded artery with laser energy delivered to the site through a fiberoptic probe. One type of PCI, **excimer laser coronary angioplasty,** is used to remove blockage in a coronary

artery

_____.

8-74 In **percutaneous transluminal coronary angioplasty** (PTCA) a catheter equipped with an inflatable balloon tip is inserted into a partially occluded coronary artery. After the catheter is passed through and just past the appropriate area, the balloon at the tip of the catheter is inflated, and the atherosclerotic plaque is compressed **(balloon angioplasty).** PTCA means percu-

angioplasty

taneous transluminal coronary _____.
   An **intracoronary stent** is sometimes inserted during PTCA to treat abrupt or threatened closure of a coronary artery. **Stents** (stents), sometimes containing drugs to discourage blood clots, are expandable meshlike structures that are placed over the angioplasty site to keep the vessel open by compressing the arterial walls (Figure 8-26). Intra/coronary (in″trə-kor′ə-nar″e) per-

artery

tains to the interior of a coronary _____.

8-75 Atherectomy (ath″ər-ek′tə-me) uses a specially designed catheter for cutting away plaque from the lining of an artery. Some atherectomies use a rotational blade to shave off the plaque, which is simultaneously extracted by suction (Figure 8-27). Cutting away plaque from the

atherectomy

interior of an artery with a rotational blade is a type of _____.

8-76 If less invasive procedures are either unsuccessful or not recommended (for example, total occlusion of a blood vessel), it may be possible to surgically remove plaque that has accumulated in an artery. In the case of coronary arteries, you read earlier that CABG or one of its options is often performed.
   End/arter/ectomy (end-ahr″tər-ek′tə-me) is surgical excision of arteriosclerotic plaque from

artery

the inner wall of an obstructed _____. Endarterectomy does

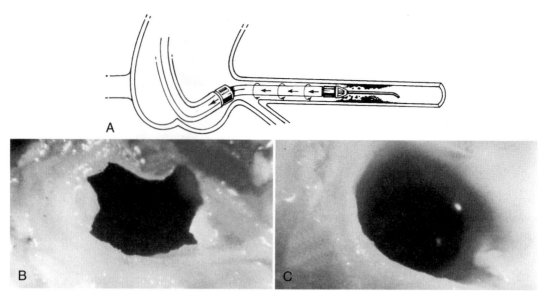

Figure 8-27 Extraction atherectomy for removing fatty or lipid material from the lumen of blood vessels. The catheter is positioned and monitored via fluoroscopy. **A,** The atherectomy catheter has cutting edges for excising the plaque and openings through which the plaque fragments are extracted. **B,** The coronary artery before atherectomy. **C,** The same coronary artery after atherectomy.

endarterectomy	not designate a particular artery. There are several sites in the body where plaque commonly forms. One of these is the carotid artery, and this occlusion causes restricted blood flow to the brain. Removal of arteriosclerotic plaque from an obstructed carotid artery, usually done to prevent stroke, is called **carotid** _____.
	8-77 The formation of a blood clot is often prevented by administration of an oral anticoagulant. Once a thrombus (blood clot) in an artery is formed, it is sometimes treated with a thrombo/lytic agent to dissolve the clot. This procedure may be recommended for a blood clot in a coronary artery in a patient with acute myocardial infarction. In this procedure, called **intra/vascular thrombo/lysis,** the thrombolytic agent is delivered through a catheter and infused into the clot, which often dissolves over a period of time. The use of a catheter to deliver a
thrombolysis	thrombolytic agent to dissolve a blood clot is called intravascular _____.
opening	**8-78 Angio/stomy** (an″je-os′tə-me) is formation of a new _____ into a blood vessel.
angiectomy (an″je-ek′tə-me)	Incision of a vessel is **angiotomy** (an″je-ot′ə-me). Use angi(o) to write a word that means the removal (excision) of a vessel: _____.
	8-79 Discomfort from varicose veins varies widely. Superficial varicose veins may primarily present a cosmetic problem. In such situations **sclero/therapy** (sklēr″o-ther′ə-pe), direct injection of a sclerosing agent, can be performed in an office setting and causes minimal discomfort. It successfully eliminates unsightly superficial varicose veins (see Figure 8-21) but does not prevent development of further varicosities.
	Conservative treatment of varicose veins includes elevation of the limb, compression stockings, and exercise. Surgical intervention for varicose veins involves tying off of the entire vein and removal of its incompetent tributaries. In selected patients the use of laser therapy delivered through a catheter may be an option in the treatment of varicosities.
vein	**Phleb/ectomy** (flə-bek′tə-me) is surgical removal of a _____. This procedure may involve removing only a segment of the vein. Phlebectomy may be necessary for treatment of varicose veins.
vein	**Phlebo/plasty** (fleb′o-plas″te) is plastic surgery of a _____.

EXERCISE 13

Build It! *Use the following word parts to build terms. (Some word parts will be used more than once.)*

end-, peri-, angi(o), arter(o), cardi(o), phleb(o), pulmon(o), -centesis, -ectomy, -plasty, -plegia, -stomy

1. surgical puncture of the pericardium   _____/_____/_____

2. formation of a new opening into a blood vessel   _____/_____/_____

3. stopping the heart's action   _____/_____/_____

4. plastic surgery on a vein   _____/_____/_____

5. surgical excision of plaque from the inner wall of an artery _____/_____/_____

Say and Check

Say aloud the terms you wrote for Exercise 13. Use the Companion CD to check your pronunciations.

clot	**8-80 Heparin** is prescribed in the treatment and prophylaxis (for example, to prevent a blood clot after surgery) of a variety of thromboembolic (throm″bo-em-bol′ik) disorders. **Thrombo/embol/ic** pertains to an embolus resulting from a blood _____. **Embol/ectomy** (em″bə-lek′tə-me), excision of the embolus, may be indicated, especially if the aorta or the common iliac artery is obstructed. In other cases, heparin is given and followed by frequent monitoring of the coagulation status of the patient's blood.

dilation	**8-81 Vaso/dilators** (va″zo-, vas″o-di′la-tərz) are medications that cause _____ of blood vessels. The pain of angina pectoris is often relieved by rest and vasodilation of the coronary arteries using **nitroglycerin,** a coronary vasodilator.
	
	    Calcium channel blockers are drugs that help diminish muscle spasms and are used primarily in treatment of spasms of the coronary artery.
	
	    Drugs called **beta blockers** are often given after a myocardial infarction to allow the heart to work less.

rhythm	**8-82 Digoxin** is a well-known drug that is prescribed in the treatment of congestive heart failure and certain arrhythmias. **Anti/arrhythmic** (an″te-ə-rith′mik) **drugs** prevent, alleviate, or correct an abnormal heart _____.
against	**8-83 Anti/hyper/tensive** (an″te-, an″ti-hi″pər-ten′siv) means acting _____ hypertension, or counteracting high blood pressure. The term also applies to agents that reduce high blood pressure. **Diuretics** (di″u-ret′ikz) are also used in the treatment of hypertension and act to reduce the blood volume through greater excretion of water by the kidneys.
antilipidemic	**8-84 Anti/lipid/emic** (an″te-, an″ti-lip″ĭ-de′mik) drugs are prescribed to reduce the risk of atherosclerotic cardiovascular disease. Combined with exercise and a low-fat diet, antilipidemic drugs lower cholesterol levels in the blood. Lower incidence of coronary heart disease and lower cholesterol levels are found in populations consuming a low-fat diet. Medications that lower cholesterol in the blood are called _____ drugs.

Read the surgical schedule and match the diagnoses in the left column with the surgical interventions in the right column. (All selections are used.)

SURGICAL SCHEDULE:

_____ 1. arrhythmia

_____ 2. atrial septal defect

_____ 3. blocked coronary artery

_____ 4. plaque in a peripheral artery

_____ 5. severe bradycardia

_____ 6. varicose veins

A. atherectomy
B. atrioseptoplasty
C. cardiac pacemaker
D. internal cardioverter
E. phlebectomy
F. PTCA

Match the drugs in the left column with their use in the right column. (All selections are used.)

_____ 1. antiarrhythmics

_____ 2. antihypertensives

_____ 3. antilipidemics

_____ 4. vasodilators

A. alleviate abnormal heart rhythm
B. dilate blood vessels
C. lower blood cholesterol levels
D. reduce blood pressure

LYMPHATIC SYSTEM

ANATOMY AND PHYSIOLOGY

8-85 The **lymphatic** (lim-fat´ik) **system,** also called the **lymphatics,** is composed of lymphatic vessels, a fluid called **lymph** (limf), **lymph nodes,** and three organs: the spleen, thymus, and tonsils. The system helps protect and maintain the internal fluid environment of the body by producing, filtering, and conveying lymph; absorbing and transporting fats to the blood system; and serving as an important part of the immune system. Lymph nodes filter lymph and trap substances, helping prevent the spread of infection or cancer cells. In addition, lymph nodes contain macro/phages that can phagocytize foreign substances. Lymphocytes undergo maturation in lymphatic tissue to become B lymphocytes (B cells) or T lymphocytes (T cells). B cells and T cells are involved in antibody- and cell-mediated immunity, respectively.

lymph

The fluid transported by the lymphatic vessels is _____.
Learn the meaning of the following word parts.

Word Parts: Lymphatic System

Combining Form	Meaning	Combining Form	Meaning
aden(o)	gland	lymphat(o)	lymphatics
adenoid(o)	adenoids	splen(o)	spleen
lymph(o)	lymph, lymphatics	thym(o)	thymus
lymphaden(o)	lymph node	tonsill(o)	tonsil
lymphangi(o)	lymph vessel		

Write the combining form for these structures of the lymphatic system.

1. adenoid _____

2. lymph node _____

3. lymph vessel _____

4. thymus _____

5. tonsil _____

8-86 Lympho/genous (lim-foj´ə-nəs) means both forming lymph or derived from lymph or the lymphatics. Write the word that means originating in the lymphatics: _____.

lymphogenous

8-87 Study the major parts of the lymphatic system (Figure 8-28). Only the major lymph vessels and nodes are shown. The smallest vessels of this system are lymph capillaries, which are found in almost all regions of the body. Look at the detailed drawing of the proximity of the lymphatic capillaries to the cardiovascular capillaries, venules, and arterioles. The lymphatic capillaries pick up _____ fluid that has collected from the normal course of blood circulation.

interstitial

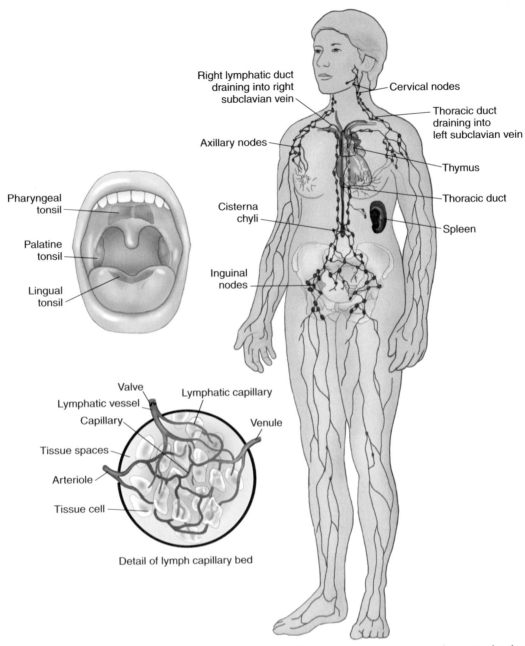

Figure 8-28 **Lymphatic system.** The close relationship to the cardiovascular system is shown in the detailed drawing. Lymph capillaries merge to form lymphatic vessels that join other vessels to become trunks that drain large regions of the body. The right lymphatic duct receives fluid from the upper right quadrant of the body and empties into the right subclavian vein. The thoracic duct, which begins with the cisterna chyli, collects fluid from the rest of the body and empties it into the left subclavian vein. The lymph nodes are small, bean-shaped structures distributed along the vessels. Also shown are the lymphatic organs: tonsils, thymus, and spleen.

Fluid enters but does not leave the lymph vessels because of valves that carry the fluid away from the tissue. The system depends on muscular contraction because there is no pump, and transport of fluid is slow. Lymph ducts eventually empty the lymph into the subclavian (səb-kla′ve-ən) veins, thus returning the fluid to the systemic circulation (Figure 8-29).

8-88 Note the bean-shaped lymph nodes along the course of the lymph vessels shown in Figure 8-28. The **cisterna chyli** (sis-tur′nə ki′li) and the ducts are structures that are formed by the merging of many lymph vessels and their trunks.

chest

As its name indicates, the thorac/ic duct is located in the _____.

8-89 Three types of lymph nodes are shown in the drawing. The combining form that you will use to write terms about lymph nodes is _____.

lymphaden(o)
neck

The **cervic/al** (sur′vĭ-kəl) **lymph nodes** are located in the area of the _____. In other chapters, you will study the combining forms cervic(o), axill(o), and inguin(o), which mean neck, armpit, and groin, respectively, as used here. For now, remember the locations of the cervical, **axillary** (ak′sĭ-lar″e), and **inguinal** (ing′gwĭ-nəl) lymph **nodes.**

8-90 Lymph is the fluid transported by the lymphatic vessels. Sometimes lymph(o) is used to mean lymphatics, but it is also a combining form for lymph. The combining form that you will use to write terms about lymph vessels is _____.

lymphangi(o)

8-91 Cells from malignant tumors may escape and be transported by the lymphatic circulation or the bloodstream to implant in lymph nodes and other organs far from the primary tumor. Cancer cells that wander into a lymph vessel may be trapped by the lymph nodes and begin growing there, or the cells may be carried to sites far from their origin. Lymph nodes are often examined to determine if cancer has spread to the lymphatics.

8-92 The **spleen** (splēn), the **tonsils** (ton′silz), and the **thymus** (thi′məs) contain lymphatic tissue and are specialized lymphatic organs. The spleen is a large organ situated in the upper left part of the abdominal cavity. **Splen/ic** (splen′ik) refers to the _____.

spleen

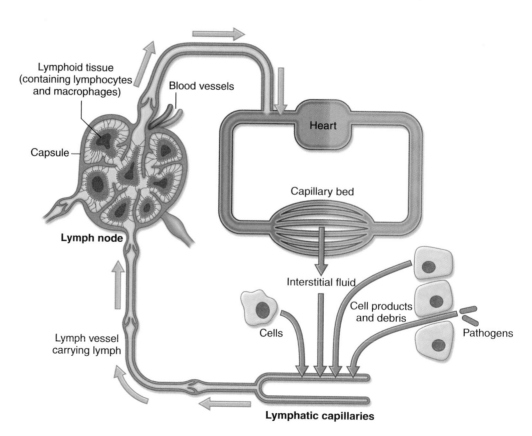

Figure 8-29 Circulation of lymph in the lymphatic system.

Although one can live without the spleen, it performs important tasks such as defense, production of lymphocytes and plasma cells, blood storage, and destruction and recycling of red blood cells and platelets.

Spleno/lymphatic (sple″no-lim-fat´ik) pertains to the spleen and the lymph nodes.

8-93 The thymus is also called the thymus gland because it is a glandlike body. It is located in the anterior mediastinal cavity and is important in the maturation of T cells, which are involved in cell-mediated immunity. The thymus usually obtains its greatest absolute size at puberty and then becomes smaller. **Thym/ic** (thi´mik) means pertaining to the _____.

thymus

8-94 When we see the word tonsil, we think of the pair of small, almond-shaped masses located at the back of the throat. These are the **palatine** (pal´ə-tīn) **tonsils** (the palate is the roof of the mouth) and are usually what one is referring to when the term tonsil is used. But one should be aware that the tonsils are small masses of lymphatic tissue of several types, including the palatine and **sub/lingual** (sub-, beneath + lingu[o], tongue + -al, pertaining to) **tonsils,** as well as the **adenoids. Tonsill/ar** (ton´sĭ-lər) means pertaining to a _____. The combining form adenoid(o) means adenoids.

tonsil

EXERCISE 17

Write a word in each blank to complete this paragraph.

As blood circulates, interstitial fluid accumulates in the tissue spaces. This excess fluid is normally transported away

from the tissues by a vascular network called the (1) _____ system. The system is

composed of vessels, nodes, the spleen, thymus, tonsils, and a fluid called (2) _____.

The fluid flows in one direction only, away from the tissue, and is eventually emptied into the subclavian

(3) _____, thus returning the fluid to the (4) _____

circulation. The spleen, the tonsils, and the thymus are specialized lymphatic organs. A term that means pertaining to

the spleen is (5) _____. Pertaining to the thymus is (6) _____.

Pertaining to the palatine tonsils is (7) _____.

DIAGNOSTIC TESTS AND PROCEDURES

8-95 The lymphatic channels and lymph nodes can be x-rayed after injection of radiopaque material into a lymphatic vessel. This procedure is called **lympho/graphy** (lim-fog´rə-fe). Write a word that means the picture produced in lymphography: _____.

lymphogram
(lim´fo-gram)

8-96 The lymphatic vessels are the focus of study in **lymph/angio/graphy** (lim-fan″je-og´rə-fe), radiology of the lymphatic vessels after the injection of a contrast medium. In lymphadeno/graphy, the lymph _____ are the focus of study.

nodes

Imaging of lymphoid organs can also be accomplished using computed tomography, magnetic resonance imaging, and nuclear magnetic imaging.

8-97 Biopsies of the lymph nodes are important tools for diagnosis of the spread of cancer and are routine after many surgeries in which cancerous organs are removed. Examination of the lymph nodes is important because cancer cells are often carried to the lymph nodes via

lymph

_____.

Blood tests provide additional information about the lymphatic system, especially tests related to immunity and specialized studies of both B and T lymphocytes.

EXERCISE 18

Write a word in each blank to complete these sentences.

1. Radiography of the lymphatic vessels and nodes after injection of radiopaque material is _____.

2. The lymphatic vessels are the focus of study in lymphangiography, whereas the lymph nodes are the focus in

   _____.

3. Removal of tissue from the lymph nodes to determine if cancer has spread from a nearby organ is called

   _____ of the lymph nodes.

 Say and Check

Say aloud the terms you wrote for Exercise 18. Use the Companion CD to check your pronunciations.

PATHOLOGIES

lymphatics

lymph

node

8-98 **Lymph/edema** (lim″fə-de′mə) means swelling of the subcutaneous tissue of an extremity as a result of obstruction of the lymphatics. The meaning of lymphedema is implied. You will need to remember that lymphedema means swelling of an extremity owing to obstruction of the _____. Primary lymphedema is hypoplasia and maldevelopment of the lymphatic system resulting in swelling and sometimes grotesque distortion of the extremities (Figure 8-30).

Acquired lymphedema results from trauma to the lymphatic ducts, such as surgical removal of lymph channels in mastectomy, obstruction of lymph drainage by malignant tumors, or the infestation of lymph vessels with parasites (see Figure 3-1). **Lympho/stasis** (lim-fos′tə-sis) is stoppage of _____ flow.

8-99 **Lymph/aden/itis** (lim-fad″ə-ni′tis) is inflammation of a lymph _____. This inflammatory condition can result from a bacterial infection or other inflammatory condition, and the location of the affected node is indicative of the site of the infection. For example, inflammation of a cervical lymph node indicates infection of a tooth; of the mouth, throat, or ear; or somewhere in the head (Figure 8-31). Antibiotics are generally indicated when bacterial infection is present.

Swelling of several lymph glands is characteristic of infectious mononucleosis, an acute viral infection that was discussed in the previous chapter.

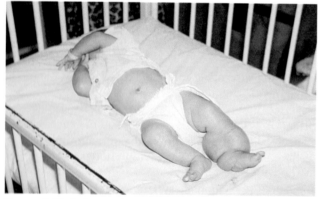

Figure 8-30 Primary lymphedema. Congenital lymphedema, as shown in the illustration, is usually apparent at birth and most often involves the legs.

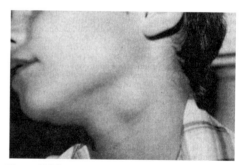

Figure 8-31 Lymphadenitis. The cervical lymph node is enlarged, firm, painless, and freely movable. The node may resolve without treatment or may eventually rupture and drain.

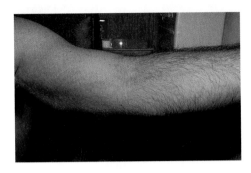

Figure 8-32 Streptococcal lymphangitis. This type of inflammatory condition of the lymph nodes is caused by streptococcal bacteria. Examination of the area distal to the affected node usually reveals the source of the infection.

8-100 Lymph/adeno/pathy (lim-fad″ə-nop′ə-the) is any disorder characterized by a localized or generalized enlargement of the lymph nodes or lymph vessels. As stated earlier, a lymphangioma, composed of a mass of dilated lymph vessels, is benign.

lymphatic

Literal interpretation of lymph/oma (lim-fo′mə) is a _____ tumor. A **lymphoma** is a type of neoplasm (tumor) of lymphoid tissue that originates in the system itself and is usually malignant. Two main types of lymphomas are Hodgkin disease and non-Hodgkin lymphoma.

Not all malignancies of the lymphatic system originate in the system itself. Cancer cells may be brought to the lymphatics via lymph and result in **lymphatic carcinoma.**

lymphatic

8-101 Lymph/ang/itis (lim″fan-ji′tis) is inflammation of a _____ vessel. (Note the spelling of lymphangitis, which uses the combining forms for lymph, vessel, and inflammation. Some of the vowels are omitted in the spelling of lymphangitis to facilitate pronunciation.) Lymphangitis is often the result of an acute streptococcal infection of one of the extremities (Figure 8-32).

8-102 Thrombo/lymphang/itis (thromb″bo-lim″fan-ji′tis) is inflammation of a lymph

vessel

_____ resulting from a blood clot.

splenopathy (sple-nop′ə-the)

Any disease of the spleen is called a _____.

enlargement

spleen

8-103 Spleno/megaly (sple″no-meg′ə-le) is _____ of the spleen. **Spleno/rrhagia** (sple″no-ra′jə) is hemorrhage from the _____. Because of its anatomic location, the spleen is often injured in abdominal trauma. Rupture of the spleen can occur from blunt trauma, such as a blow from a car accident.

splenoptosis (sple″nop-to′sis)

Combine splen(o) and -ptosis to write a term that means a downward displacement (sagging) of the spleen: _____.

thymopathy (thi-mop′ə-the)

8-104 A **thym/oma** (thi-mo′mə) is a tumor, usually benign, of the thymus. Any disease of the thymus is a _____.

adenoiditis (ad″ə-noid-i′tis)

8-105 Tonsill/itis (ton″sĭ-li′tis) is inflammation of the palatine tonsils. Inflammation of the adenoids is _____. When the adenoids are enlarged as a result of frequent infection, they can obstruct the passageway, and removal may be indicated.

EXERCISE 19

Match pathologies in the left column with the correct terms in the right column.

_____ 1. enlarged spleen

_____ 2. inflammation of a lymph vessel

_____ 3. inflammation of a lymph node

_____ 4. inflammation of the palatine tonsils

_____ 5. tumor originating in the lymphatics

A. lymphadenitis
B. lymphangitis
C. lymphoma
D. splenomegaly
E. tonsillitis

SURGICAL AND THERAPEUTIC INTERVENTIONS

excision

8-106 Penicillin and hot soaks are usually prescribed for lymphangitis. Infected lymph nodes often respond to antibiotic therapy or resolve on their own. **Lymphaden/ectomy** (lim-fad"ə-nek´tə-me) is _____ of a lymph node. This term is often accompanied by an adjective referring to the location of the node that is removed, such as cervical (referring to the neck) lymphadenectomy.

radiation

8-107 Treatment of lymphoma is determined by the type of lymphoma but can include intensive radiotherapy, chemotherapy, and biological therapies, including interferon. Radio/therapy is treatment of tumors using _____ to kill malignant cells and deter their proliferation.

splenectomy
(sple-nek´tə-me)

8-108 Splenoptosis, prolapse of the spleen, can be corrected by surgical fixation of the spleen. This surgery is called **spleno/pexy** (sple´no-pek"se).
　　A ruptured spleen often requires surgical intervention. **Spleno/rrhaphy** (sple-nor´ə-fe) is suture of the spleen. Surgical removal of the spleen is _____.

tonsillectomy
(ton"sĭ-lek´tə-me)

8-109 **Thymectomy** (thi-mek´tə-me) means removal of the thymus.
　　Excision of the tonsils is a _____. A tonsillectomy is performed to treat a chronic infection of the tonsils. An **adenoidectomy** (ad"ə-noid-ek´tə-me) is performed because the adenoids are enlarged, chronically infected, or causing obstruction. They are sometimes removed at the same time as a tonsillectomy as a prophylactic measure. A procedure in which tonsillectomy and adenoidectomy are performed at the same time is called a **tonsilloadenoidectomy** (ton"sĭ-lo-ad"ə-noid-ek´tə-me).

EXERCISE 20

Match interventions in the left column with the correct terms in the right column.

___ 1. diseased adenoids

___ 2. excision of the adenoids

___ 3. excision of the lymph nodes

___ 4. removal of the thymus

___ 5. suture of the spleen

___ 6. tumor of the thymus

A. adenoidectomy
B. adenoidopathy
C. lymphadenectomy
D. lymphangiectomy
E. splenectomy
F. splenorrhaphy
G. thymectomy
H. thymoma

EXERCISE 21

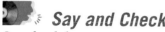 ***Build It!*** *Use the following word parts to build terms. (Some word parts will be used more than once.)*

lymph(o), splen(o), thym(o), tonsill(o), lymphaden(o), -ectomy, -edema, -ic, -pathy, -rrhagia

1. Pertaining to the thymus　　　　　　　　　　　　　 _____ / _____

2. Swelling from obstruction of the lymphatics　　　 _____ / _____

3. Hemorrhage from the spleen　　　　　　　　　　 _____ / _____

4. Surgical removal of the tonsils　　　　　　　　　 _____ / _____

5. Any disorder characterized by enlargement of the lymph nodes _____ / _____

Say and Check

Say aloud the terms you wrote for Exercise 21. Use the Companion CD to check your pronunciations.

CHAPTER ABBREVIATIONS*

AI	aortic insufficiency (and several others)
ASHD	arteriosclerotic heart disease
AV, A-V	atrioventricular
AVB	atrioventricular block
BP	blood pressure
CABG	coronary artery bypass graft
CAD	coronary artery disease
CHF	congestive heart failure
CK (CPK)	creatine kinase (formerly called creatine phosphokinase)
CPR	cardiopulmonary resuscitation
CVA	cerebrovascular accident (also costovertebral angle)
DSA	digital subtraction angiography
HDL	high-density lipoprotein
HTN	hypertension
LA	left atrium
LDH	lactate dehydrogenase (enzyme elevated after MI)

LDL	low-density lipoprotein
LV	left ventricle
MI	myocardial infarction
MIDCAB	minimally invasive direct coronary artery bypass
mm Hg	millimeters of mercury
MVP	mitral valve prolapse
OPCAB	off-pump coronary artery bypass
PAT	paroxysmal atrial tachycardia
PCI	percutaneous coronary intervention
PDA	patent ductus arteriosus (also posterior descending [coronary] artery)
PTCA	percutaneous transluminal coronary angioplasty
PVC	premature ventricular contraction
RA	right atrium
RV	right ventricle
SA	sinoatrial

*Many of these abbreviations share their meanings with other terms.

► CHAPTER 8 REVIEW

Basic Understanding

Labeling
I. *Using this illustration of a capillary bed, write combining forms for the structures that are indicated. (Line 1 is done as an example.) Write two combining forms for line 2 (artery) and three combining forms for line 4 (vein), as indicated on the drawing.*

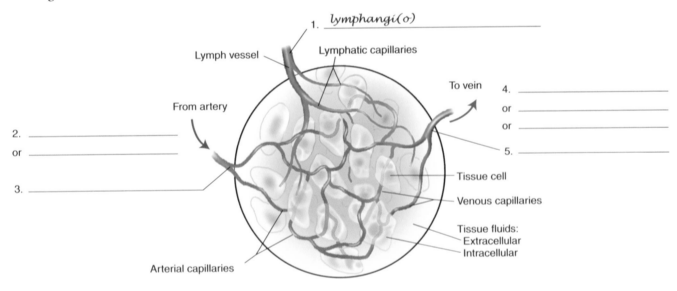

1. lymphangi(o)

Lymph vessel Lymphatic capillaries

To vein 4. ____

or ____

or ____

From artery

2. ____

or ____

3. ____

5. ____

Tissue cell

Venous capillaries

Tissue fluids:
Extracellular
Intracellular

Arterial capillaries

II. *Write combining forms for the structures of the lymphatic system that are indicated on the diagram.*

1. _____

2. _____

3. _____

4. _____

5. _____

Matching

III. *Use all selections to match terms in the left column with their descriptions in the right column.*

_____ 1. arterioles

_____ 2. aorta

_____ 3. atria

_____ 4. capillaries

_____ 5. pulmonary arteries

_____ 6. pulmonary veins

_____ 7. veins

_____ 8. venae cavae

_____ 9. venules

_____ 10. ventricles

A. lower chambers of the heart
B. the largest artery
C. two large veins that communicate with the right atrium
D. upper chambers of the heart
E. vessels that carry blood from the heart to the lungs
F. vessels that carry blood from the lungs to the heart
G. vessels that convey blood from the venules toward the heart
H. vessels that join arteries and capillaries
I. vessels that join arterioles and venules
J. vessels that join capillaries and veins

IV. *Match terms in the left column with their descriptions in the right column.*

_____ 1. cardiac septum

_____ 2. endocardium

_____ 3. mediastinum

_____ 4. myocardium

_____ 5. pericardium

A. area in the chest cavity that contains the heart
B. cardiac muscle tissue
C. inner lining of the heart
D. sac which encloses the heart
E. wall between the left and right sides of the heart

Listing

V. *Name three functions of the lymphatic system.*

1. _____

2. _____

3. _____

Photo ID

VI. *Use word parts to write terms to label these pictures*

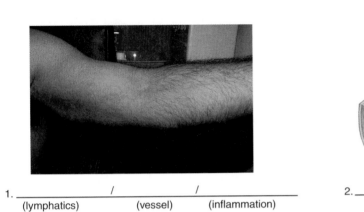

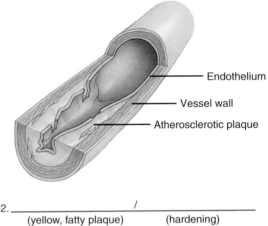

1. _____ / _____ / _____
   (lymphatics)   (vessel)   (inflammation)

2. _____ / _____
   (yellow, fatty plaque)   (hardening)

Endothelium

Vessel wall

Atherosclerotic plaque

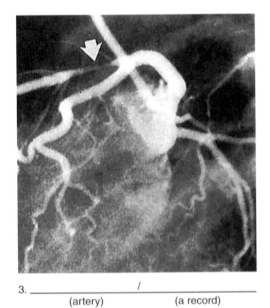

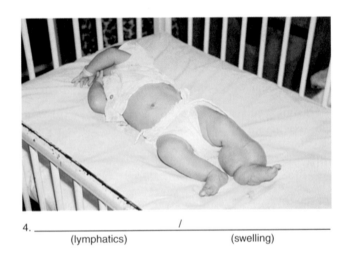

3. _____ / _____
   (artery)   (a record)

4. _____ / _____
   (lymphatics)   (swelling)

Word Analysis

VII. *Divide these terms into their component parts, and state the meaning of each term.*

1. adenoidectomy _____

2. angiography _____

3. anoxia _____

4. atriomegaly _____

5. cardiovascular _____

6. echocardiography _____

7. endarterectomy _____

8. hemopericardium _____

9. phlebectomy _____

10. thrombophlebitis _____

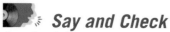 **Say and Check**

Say aloud the terms in Exercise VII. Use the Companion CD to check your pronunciations.

VIII. *Circle the correct answer for each of the following questions.*

1. Charlie, a 60-year-old man, has just been diagnosed as having a coronary occlusion. He is most at risk for which of the following? (atrioventricular block, congenital heart disease, myocardial infarction, rheumatic fever)

2. Charlie is told that he has a form of arteriosclerosis in which yellowish plaque has accumulated on the walls of the arteries. What is the name of this form of arteriosclerosis?
(aortostenosis, atherosclerosis, cardiomyopathy, coarctation)

3. Charlie's physician advises surgery. Which surgery is generally prescribed for coronary occlusion?
(automatic implantable cardiopulmonary bypass, cardioverter, coronary artery bypass, pericardiocentesis)

4. Kristen, a 28-year-old woman, is told she has inflammation of the lining of the heart. What is the medical term for this heart pathology? (coronary heart disease, endocarditis, myocarditis, pericarditis)

5. Jayne suffered ventricular fibrillation during coronary angiography. What procedure did the physician use to stop fibrillation? (atherectomy, endarterectomy, cardiopulmonary resuscitation, defibrillation)

6. Jim developed a blood clot in a coronary artery. What is Jim's condition called?
(myocardial infarction, coronary artery bypass, coronary thrombosis, fibrillation)

7. Baby Seth is born with cyanosis and a heart murmur. Which congenital heart disease does the neonatologist think is more likely? (atrial septal defect, atrioventricular block, megalocardia, pericarditis)

8. Ten-year-old Zack had a sore throat for several days before he developed painful joints and a fever. Which disease does the physician suspect that can cause damage to the heart valves?
(aortic valve sclerosis, aortic valve stenosis, mitral valve prolapse, rheumatic fever)

9. Ed experiences pain in his legs that is caused by blockage of arteries in the lower extremities. What is the name of his condition? (angiocarditis, lymphangioma, peripheral artery disease, varicose veins)

10. Carol has an angiogram that shows a ballooning out of the wall of a cerebrovascular artery. Which condition does Carol have? (aneurysm, angioma, arteriosclerosis, coronary thrombosis)

Writing Terms

IX. *Write one word for each of the following clues.*

1. a tumor of the thymus _____

2. abnormal hardening of the aorta _____

3. absence of a heartbeat _____

4. agent that causes dilation of blood vessels _____

5. increased blood pressure _____

6. increased pulse _____

7. inflammation of a lymphatic vessel _____

8. narrowing of the diameter of a vessel _____

9. removal of the tonsils _____

10. suture of the spleen _____

Say and Check

Say aloud the terms you wrote for Exercise IX. Use the Companion CD to check your pronunciations.

Greater Comprehension

Health Care Reports

X. *Read the following Cardiac Consult and answer the questions that follow the report. Although you may be unfamiliar with some of the terms, you should be able to answer the questions by determining the meanings of word parts.*

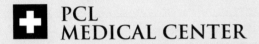
PCL
MEDICAL CENTER

7700 Lexicon Way
St. Louis, MO 63146

Phone (555) 437-0000 • Fax (555) 437-0001

CARDIAC CONSULT

Patient Name: Dwight Moore   **Hospital No.:** 008:1200   **Date:** Oct 8, ----

CHIEF COMPLAINT: Increased tiredness

HISTORY OF PRESENT ILLNESS: 68-year-old man with history of multiple CVAs with increased lethargy and swallowing dysfunction. CT scan revealed a new cerebellopontine ischemic CVA. Cardiac workup revealed no atrial fibrillation or other significant arrhythmia on telemetry. INR 2.8 to 3.0. Hypercoagulable workup was unremarkable.

PMH: HTN, CHF, MI, CAD, ASHD, multiple CVAs, and hypercholesterolemia

PAST SURGICAL HISTORY: Right and left carotid endarterectomies

SOCIAL HISTORY: Married with supportive family. Is a retired engineer.

REVIEW OF SYSTEMS:

 HEENT: No jugular vein distention. Throat congested. Tympanic membranes intact.

 CARDIOPULMONARY: Lungs with bibasilar crackles. Regular rate and rhythm.

 GASTROINTESTINAL: Abdomen soft, nontender; positive bowel sounds, no hepatosplenomegaly.

 MUSCULOSKELETAL: No clubbing, clots, cyanosis, or edema.

 NEUROMUSCULAR: Left hemiparesis, left facial droop.

John L. Wilson, MD

John L. Wilson, MD

JLW:pai

D: Oct 8, ----

T: Oct 9, ----

---

1. Describe the meaning of Mr. Moore's ischemic CVA: _____

_____

2. Describe the diagnostic test that was used to diagnose the present illness: _____

_____

3. Is the patient experiencing atrial fibrillation? _____

Define atrial fibrillation: _____

_____

4. Is the patient experiencing arrhythmia? _____

Define arrhythmia: _____

_____

5. Define telemetry: _____

_____

6. Define right and left carotid endarterectomies: _____

_____

Write out the meanings of these abbreviations:

7. HTN _____

8. CHF _____

9. MI _____

10. CAD _____

11. ASHD _____

XI. *Read the case study (SOAP Note) and define the underlined words or abbreviations.*

PCL MEDICAL CENTER

7700 Lexicon Way
St. Louis, MO 63146

Phone (555) 437-0000 • Fax (555) 437-0001

CASE STUDY (SOAP NOTE)

Patient Name: Henry I. Wilson   **ID No.:** 008-1201   **Date:** Mar 7, ----

SUBJECTIVE: 58-year-old man came to Clinic with midsternal chest pain radiating to both shoulders. Patient has an unremarkable history, denies smoking, drinks socially, no illicit drug abuse. Family history shows that his father died of a <u>myocardial infarction</u> at age 68. His mother, 78, is living with <u>hypertension</u> and <u>hypercholesterolemia</u> that developed in midlife.

OBJECTIVE: BP 160/94, apical heart rate 100 and regular, respirations 24, weight 208 pounds, height 6'1". HEENT: Head normocephalic, atraumatic. TMs intact. Neck: No carotid bruits or JVD. Lungs clear to <u>auscultation</u> bilaterally. Extremities: No clubbing, clots, cyanosis, or edema. <u>ECG</u> is WNL. Cardiac enzymes are WNL. Cholesterol 250. Thallium stress test showed chest pain with exertion and demonstrated a need for <u>cardiac catheterization</u>. Cardiac Cath: <u>Coronary angiography</u> showed blockage in three main coronary arteries.

ASSESSMENT: 1. Hypercholesterolemia; 2. coronary artery disease; 3. <u>angina pectoris</u>

PLAN: <u>CABG</u> in the AM. Need stat lipids, CBC, chemistries, and chest x-ray.

Define:

1. myocardial infarction _____

2. hypertension _____

3. hypercholesterolemia _____

4. auscultation _____

5. ECG _____

6. cardiac catheterization _____

7. coronary angiography _____

8. angina pectoris _____

9. CABG _____

XII. Write out and define the underlined terms/abbreviations in this partial Emergency Department Treatment Record.

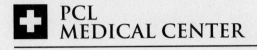 **PCL**
MEDICAL CENTER

7700 Lexicon Way
St. Louis, MO 63146

Phone 555.437.0000 • Fax 555.437.0001

EMERGENCY DEPARTMENT TREATMENT RECORD

Patient Name: Gus Abell   **ID No:** 008-1202   **Date:** Apr 3, ----
Mode of Arrival: EMS   **DOB:** Oct 13, ----   **Sex:** Male

PREHOSPITAL COURSE: This 65-year-old man was brought from the nursing home in full cardiac arrest at 1455 hours. The <u>EMS</u> had given 3 rounds of epinephrine, 2 rounds of atropine, and shock ×1 in the field. Patient was in <u>asystole</u> when he arrived.

PRIMARY INTERVENTIONS: <u>CPR</u> was begun at 1500 hours. Patient was in a bag mask by ventilation at 100% O_2, and the patient had an IO in the left tibia. A triple lumen was inserted into the left femoral and right femoral veins. One liter of normal saline was bolused. Epinephrine was given and repeated in 3 minutes; 1 amp of bicarb was given. There was spontaneous return of pulse at 1508 hours, and CPR was stopped.

Dopamine drip was started at 5 mcg/min and was titrated up to 20 mcg/min. The patient was <u>tachycardic</u> at that point, up to 120 to 130 beats per minute, and his blood pressure remained tenuous at 70 to 80 <u>systolic</u>. The patient was then started on Levophed drip at 0.5 mcg/min, and this was titrated up to 20 mcg/min. The dopamine was decreased to a level of 5 mcg/min. The patient's blood pressure improved to 120 systolic on the Levophed drip. The patient also received a radial <u>arterial</u> line for blood pressure monitoring.

Define:

1. EMS _____

2. asystole _____

3. CPR _____

4. tachycardic _____

5. systolic _____

6. arterial _____

Spelling

XIII. Circle all misspelled terms and write their correct spelling:

adenoidectomy   athrosclerosis   diastole   iskemia   mediastinum

Interpreting Abbreviations

XIV. Write the meanings of these abbreviations:

1. AV _____

2. CABG _____

3. CHF _____

4. CPR _____

5. MI _____

Pronunciation

XV. *The pronunciation is shown for several medical words. Indicate the primary accented syllable with an ´.*

1. cardiomyopathy (kahr de o mi op ə the)

2. lymphadenopathy (lim fad ə nop ə the)

3. lymphography (lim fog rə fe)

4. pericardial (per ĭ kahr de əl)

5. vasodilation (va zo, vas o di la shən)

 Say and Check

Say aloud the five terms in Exercise XV. Use the Companion CD to check your pronunciations. In addition, be prepared to pronounce aloud these terms in class:

aneurysmal	bypass	mitral	phlebostasis
angiocarditis	cardioverter	myocardium	splenoptosis
aortography	dysrhythmia	nitroglycerin	tonsilloadenoidectomy
arteriosclerotic	endarterectomy	palpitations	vasodilator
bradycardia	lymphedema	pericardium	ventricular

Categorizing Terms

XVI. *Classify the terms in the left column (1-10) by selecting A, B, C, D, or E.*

_____ 1. angiography

_____ 2. angiostenosis

_____ 3. atrioseptoplasty

_____ 4. aortosclerosis

_____ 5. lymphoma

_____ 6. lymphangitis

_____ 7. lymphography

_____ 8. phlebectomy

_____ 9. vasodilators

_____ 10. venule

A. anatomy
B. diagnostic test or procedure
C. pathology
D. surgery
E. therapy

Challenge

XVII. *Break these words into their component parts, and write their meanings. Even if you have not seen these terms before,* you may be able to break them apart and determine their meanings.

1. aneurysmectomy _____

2. epicardial _____

3. lymphangiectasia _____

4. pericardiostomy _____

5. vasculitis _____

(Use Appendix VI to check your answers.)

PRONUNCIATION LIST

Use the Companion CD to review the terms that have been presented. Look closely at the spelling of each term as it is pronounced and be sure you know the meaning of each term.

adenoidectomy
adenoiditis
adenoids
aneurysm
aneurysmal
angiectomy
angina pectoris
angiocardiography
angiocarditis
angiogram
angiography
angioma
angiostenosis
angiostomy
angiotomy
anoxia
antiarrhythmic drugs
antihypertensive
antilipidemic
aorta
aortic
aortic insufficiency
aortic regurgitation
aortic stenosis
aortic valve
aortitis
aortogram
aortography
aortosclerosis
arrhythmia
arterial
arteries
arteriogram
arteriograph
arteriography
arteriole
arteriopathy
arteriosclerosis
arteriosclerotic heart
    disease
arteriovenous
arteritis
asystole
atherectomy
atherosclerosis
atrial
atrial fibrillation
atrial septal defect
atriomegaly
atrioseptoplasty

atrioventricular
atrioventricular block
atrioventricular node
atrioventricular valves
atrium
axillary nodes
balloon angioplasty
beta blockers
bicuspid valve
bradycardia
bypass
calcium channel blockers
capillaries
cardiac catheterization
cardiac insufficiency
cardiac pacemaker
cardiac tamponade
cardiomegaly
cardiomyopathy
cardioplegia
cardioplegic solutions
cardiopulmonary bypass
cardiopulmonary
    resuscitation
cardiovalvulitis
cardiovascular
cardioversion
cardioverter
carotid endarterectomy
cerebrovascular accident
cervical lymph nodes
cholesterol
cisterna chyli
coarctation of the aorta
congenital heart disease
congestive heart failure
coronary
coronary arteries
coronary arteriography
coronary artery bypass
coronary artery bypass
    graft
coronary artery disease
coronary occlusion
coronary thrombosis
creatine kinase test
defibrillation
defibrillator
deoxygenated
diastole

diastolic pressure
digital subtraction
    angiography
digoxin
diuretics
Doppler echocardiography
dysrhythmia
echocardiogram
echocardiography
effusion
electrocardiogram
electrocardiograph
electrocardiography
electrophysiologic studies
embolectomy
endarterectomy
endocardial
endocarditis
endocardium
epicardium
excimer laser coronary
    angioplasty
extracorporeal
fibrillation
heart block
heart flutters
heart murmur
hemangioma
hemopericardium
heparin
high-density lipoproteins
Holter monitor
hypertension
hypotension
hypovolemia
infarct
inguinal nodes
intraaortic
intracoronary stent
intravascular thrombolysis
ischemia
lactate dehydrogenase test
laser-assisted angioplasty
lipids
lipoproteins
low-density lipoproteins
lumen
lymph
lymph nodes
lymphadenectomy

lymphadenitis
lymphadenopathy
lymphangiography
lymphangioma
lymphangitis
lymphatic carcinoma
lymphatic system
lymphatics
lymphedema
lymphogenous
lymphogram
lymphography
lymphoma
lymphostasis
mediastinum
microcardia
mitral valve
mitral valve prolapse
myocardial
myocardial infarction
myocarditis
myocardium
nitroglycerin
occlusion
oxygenated
palatine tonsils
palpitations
parietal pericardium
paroxysmal atrial
    tachycardia
patent ductus arteriosus
percutaneous coronary
    intervention
percutaneous transluminal
    coronary angioplasty
pericardial
pericardial cavity
pericardiocentesis
pericarditis
pericardium
peripheral vascular disease
phlebectomy
phlebitis
phleboplasty
phlebostasis
phlebotomists
phlebotomy
positron emission
    tomography
pulmonary

Continued

pulmonary arteries
pulmonary circulation
pulmonary veins
pulse
Purkinje fibers
rheumatic heart disease
sclerosis
sclerotherapy
semilunar valve
septal
septum
shock
shunt
sinoatrial node
spleen
splenectomy
splenic
splenolymphatic
splenomegaly

splenopathy
splenopexy
splenoptosis
splenorrhagia
splenorrhaphy
stenosis
stents
stricture
sublingual tonsils
systemic circulation
systole
systolic pressure
tachycardia
tetralogy of Fallot
thallium stress test
thromboembolic
thrombolymphangitis
thrombophlebitis
thymectomy

thymic
thymoma
thymopathy
thymus
tonsillar
tonsillectomy
tonsillitis
tonsilloadenoidectomy
tonsils
tourniquet
treadmill stress test
tricuspid valve
triglycerides
valval
valvar
valvate
valvula
valvular
valvular stenosis

valvulitis
varicose veins
vascular
vasoconstriction
vasodilation
vasodilator
veins
vena cava
venipuncture
venous
venous thrombosis
ventricle
ventricular
ventricular fibrillation
ventricular septal defect
venular
venules
visceral pericardium

Español ENHANCING SPANISH COMMUNICATION

English	Spanish (pronunciation)
artery	arteria (ar-TAY-re-ah)
blood pressure	presión sanguínea (pray-se-ON san-GEE-nay-ah)
capillary	capilar (cah-pe-LAR)
catheter	catéter (cah-TAY-ter)
cholesterol	colesterol (co-les-tay-ROL)
high blood pressure	hipertensión, presión alta (e-per-ten-se-ON, pray-se-ON AHL-tah)
murmur	murmullo (moor-MOOL-lyo)
narrow	estrecho (es-TRAY-cho)
obstruction	obstrucción (obs-trooc-se-ON)
pulse	pulso (POOL-so)
rhythm	ritmo (REET-mo)
spleen	bazo (BAH-so)
tonsil	tonsila (ton-SEE-lah), amígdala (ah-MEEG-dah-lah)
varicose veins	venas varicosas (VAH-nahs vah-re-CO-sas)
vein	vena (VAY-nah)
weakness	debilidad (day-be-le-DAHD)

Respiratory System

9

LEARNING GOALS

Basic Understanding

In this chapter you will learn to do the following:

1. State the function of the respiratory system, and analyze associated terminology.
2. Write the meaning of the word parts associated with the respiratory system, and use the word parts to build and analyze terms.
3. Write the names of the structures of the respiratory system when given their descriptions, define the terms associated with these structures, and label the structures.
4. Distinguish between structures of the upper respiratory tract and those of the lower respiratory tract.
5. Write or recognize the sequence of the flow of air from the atmosphere through the respiratory structures.
6. Match structures of the respiratory system with the instruments and procedures that are used to study them, or write the names of the procedures when given their descriptions.
7. Match terms for respiratory system pathologies with their meanings, or write the names of the pathologies when given their descriptions.
8. Match terms for surgical and therapeutic interventions for respiratory system pathologies with descriptions of the interventions, or write the names of the interventions when given their descriptions.

Greater Comprehension

9. Use word parts from this chapter to define terms in a health care report.
10. Spell the terms accurately.
11. Pronounce the terms correctly.
12. Write the meanings of the abbreviations.
13. Categorize terms as anatomy, diagnostic test or procedure, pathology, surgery, or therapy.

MAJOR SECTIONS OF THIS CHAPTER:

❑ ANATOMY AND PHYSIOLOGY
   Upper Respiratory Passageways
   Lower Respiratory Passageways
❑ DIAGNOSTIC TESTS AND
   PROCEDURES

❑ PATHOLOGIES
   Disordered Breathing
   Upper Respiratory Abnormalities
   Lower Respiratory Abnormalities
❑ SURGICAL AND THERAPEUTIC
   INTERVENTIONS

FUNCTION FIRST

The primary function of the respiratory system is to provide oxygen for the body and to remove carbon dioxide. Secondary functions are maintaining the acid-base balance, producing speech, facilitating smell, and maintaining the body's heat and water balances.

ANATOMY AND PHYSIOLOGY

oxygen

9-1 The **respiratory** (res′pĭ-rə-tor″e) **system** cooperates with the circulatory system to provide _____ for body cells and to expel waste carbon dioxide through breathing. The exchange of these gases is involved in both internal and external respiration. This chapter focuses on external respiration.

> ➤ **KEY** POINT <u>External respiration gets oxygen into the blood; internal respiration moves oxygen from the blood to the tissues.</u> External respiration is the process involved in breathing, the ventilation of the lungs, and the exchange of oxygen (O_2) and carbon dioxide (CO_2) between the air in the lungs and the blood. The delivery of oxygen by the blood to body cells with the removal of carbon dioxide is internal respiration.

inspiration

9-2 Breathing is alternate inspiration (in″spĭ-ra′shən) and expiration (ek″spĭ-ra′shən) of air into and out of the lungs. **Inspiration** (in, into + spir[o], to breathe + -ation, process) is the process of breathing in. The drawing of air into the lungs is _____. It is also called **in/halation** (in″hə-la′shən).

Expelling air from the lungs, the act of breathing out or letting out one's breath, is **expiration.** This is the same as **exhalation.**

lungs

9-3 In studying the respiratory system, you will often see breathing referred to as pulmonary (pool′mo-nar″e) ventilation,* or simply, **ventilation.** You learned earlier that **pulmon/ary** pertains to the _____.

The respiratory tract is the complex of organs and structures that perform pulmonary ventilation and the exchange of oxygen and carbon dioxide between the air and the blood as it circulates through the lungs. See the names and locations of the structures in Figure 9-1.

---

*Ventilation (Latin: *ventilare*, to fan).

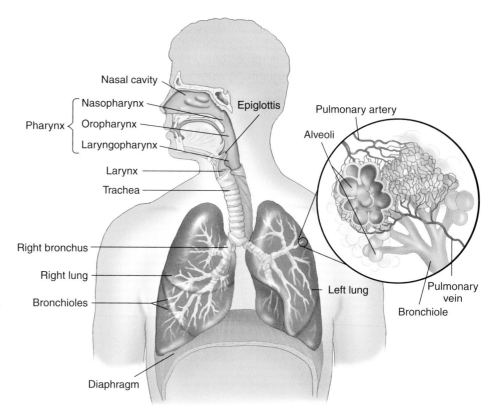

Figure 9-1 Structures of the respiratory system. The nose, nasal cavity, paranasal sinuses (shown in Figure 9-2), pharynx, and larynx comprise the upper respiratory tract. The trachea, bronchi, bronchioles, alveoli, and lungs comprise the lower respiratory tract.

9-4 The conducting passages of this system are known as the upper respiratory tract and the lower respiratory tract. The nose, nasal cavity, paranasal (par″ə-na′zel) sinuses, pharynx (far′inks), and larynx (lar′inks) comprise the upper respiratory tract. The trachea (tra′ke-ə), bronchi (brong′ki), bronchioles (brong′ke-ōlz), alveoli (al-ve′o-li), and lungs belong to the

lower

_____ respiratory tract (Figure 9-2).

> ➤ **KEY** POINT Be careful with the pronunciation of pharynx and larynx. These two terms are often mispronounced. Say the two pronunciations aloud: pharynx (far′inks) and larynx (lar′inks).

Study the following word parts and be sure you know their meanings.

Word Parts: Respiratory Anatomy and Physiology

Combining Form	Meaning	Combining Form	Meaning
Upper Respiratory Tract		thorac(o)	chest
epiglott(o)	epiglottis	trache(o)	trachea
laryng(o)	larynx		
nas(o), rhin(o)	nose	**Word Parts Used to Describe Function**	
palat(o)	palate	acid(o)	acid
pharyng(o)	pharynx	alkal(o)	alkaline; basic
sin(o), sinus(o)	sinus	ox(i)	oxygen
		phas(o)	speech
		phon(o)	voice
Lower Respiratory Tract		spir(o)	to breathe
alveol(o)	alveoli		
bronch(o), bronchi(o)	bronchi	**Suffixes**	
bronchiol(o)	bronchioles	-ation	process
lob(o)	lobe	-capnia	carbon dioxide
phren(o)	diaphragm or mind	-pnea	breathing
pleur(o)	pleura	-ptysis	spitting
pneum(o)	lungs or air		
pneumon(o), pulm(o), pulmon(o)	lungs		

UPPER RESPIRATORY PASSAGEWAYS

9-5 Looking at Figure 9-2, follow the passage of air through the respiratory system by writing the names of respiratory structures in the blanks: Air first enters the body through the

nose

_____, where it is warmed, moistened, and filtered. Regardless of whether air is taken in by the nose or the mouth, it passes to the pharynx, a muscular tube about 13 cm (5 inches) long in an adult. The pharynx also functions as part of the digestive system in the swallowing of food. Air then passes over the vocal cords in the larynx before reaching the **trachea,** also known as the windpipe. The trachea divides into two primary

bronchioles

bronchi, which divide further into many _____. Oxygen and carbon dioxide are exchanged within the alveoli.

EXERCISE 1

Arrows in this diagram represent the pathway of air from the nose to the lung capillaries. Write the names of the structures represented by the blanks.

Nose → Nasal cavity → Nasopharynx → 1. _____ → Laryngopharynx →

2. _____ → Trachea → 3. _____ → Bronchioles →

4. _____ → Lung capillaries

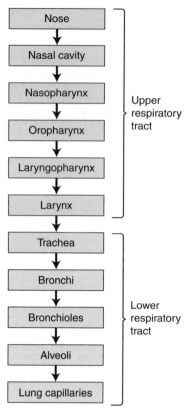

Figure 9-2 **Pathway of air from the nose to the capillaries of the lungs.**

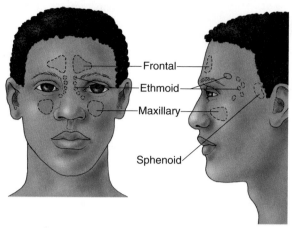

Figure 9-3 Paranasal sinuses. These air-filled, paired cavities in various bones around the nose are lined with mucous membranes. Their openings into the nasal cavity are easily obstructed.

9-6 The respiratory tract is lined with mucous membranes. Organs of the upper respiratory tract filter, moisten, and warm the air as it is inhaled. The combining forms nas(o) and rhin(o) mean _____. Already knowing that laryng(o) means larynx should help you remember that pharyng(o) means _____.
Common names for the **larynx** and pharynx are voicebox and throat, respectively.

The external part of the nose contains two openings, the nostrils, also called the **nares** (na′rēz), singular **naris.** The hollow interior of the nose is separated into right and left cavities by the **nasal septum.** Literal interpretation of para/nasal sinuses means the air cavities _____ the nose. The **paranasal sinuses** (par″ə-na′zəl si′nəs-əs) are pairs of air-filled cavities in various bones that surround the nasal cavity and open into it. The types of paranasal sinuses are shown in Figure 9-3.

9-7 Both cartilage and bone give structure to the nose. The nasal septum is composed of cartilage. Build a word using endo- that means inside (within) the nose: _____.
Retro/nasal (ret″ro-na′zəl) and **supra/nasal** (soo″prə-na′səl) mean behind the nose and above the nose, respectively.

The anterior portion of the **palate** (pal′ət), or roof of the mouth, separates the nasal cavity and the oral cavity. **Or/al** means pertaining to the mouth, and **nas/al** (na′zəl) means pertaining to the _____. The palate consists of bone and the membrane that covers it. Because the anterior portion contains bone, it is called the hard palate. The soft palate is the fleshy posterior portion of the palate. The pendant, fleshy tissue that hangs from the soft palate is the palatine **uvula** (u′vu-lə). The combining form palat(o) means palate. **Palatine** (pal′ə-tīn) refers to the _____.

9-8 The naso/lacrimal (na″zo-lak′rĭ-məl) duct opens into the nasal cavity. The **nasolacrimal duct** is a tubular passage that carries fluid (tears) from the eye to the _____ cavity. Now you can understand why the nose fills with fluid when a person cries. **Lacrimal** pertains to tears.

Answer column:
nose
pharynx

near

endonasal
(en″do-na′zəl)

nose

palate

nasal

The nose has nerve endings that detect many odors. **Olfactory**[*] (ol-fak´tə-re) pertains to the sense of smell. **Olfaction** (ol-fak´shən), the sense of smell, is a function of the nose.

9-9 The **pharynx** serves as a passageway for both the respiratory and digestive tracts. In referring to parts of the pharynx, three divisions are recognized (see Figure 9-1): the nasopharynx (na″zo-far´inks), the oropharynx (or″o-far´inks), and the laryngopharynx (lə-ring″go-far´inks). The **naso/pharynx** is that part of the pharynx that lies behind the nose. The **oro/pharynx** lies behind

mouth

the _____. The **laryngopharynx** is that part of the pharynx that lies near the larynx.

9-10 The nasopharynx is the upper part of the pharynx and is continuous with the nasal passages. The **auditory tube,** formerly called the **eustachian** (u-sta´ke-ən) **tube,** is a narrow channel connecting the middle ear and the nasopharynx. The opening to the auditory tube is in the nasopharynx. The adenoids are also located in the nasopharynx.

nasopharynx

    Naso/pharyng/eal (na″zo-fə-rin´je-əl) pertains to the _____.

pharynx

    Pharyng/eal (fə-rin´je-əl) means pertaining to the pharynx. **Oro/pharyngeal** (or″o-fə-rin´je-əl) means pertaining to the mouth and _____. This term also pertains to the oropharynx. The oropharynx contains the palatine tonsils, which are visible when the mouth is open wide. The lowest part of the pharynx is called the laryngopharynx. It is here that the pharynx divides into the larynx and the esophagus. Air passes through the larynx, and food passes through the esophagus.

larynx; pharynx

9-11 Laryngeal means pertaining to the larynx. **Laryngo/pharyng/eal** (lə-ring″go-fə-rin´je-əl) refers to the _____ and the _____.

    The **glottis** (glot´is) is the vocal apparatus of the larynx. It consists of the vocal cords and the opening between them. The **vocal cords,** also called vocal folds, are a pair of strong bands of elastic tissue with a mouthlike opening through which air passes, creating sound.

glottis

These vocal folds are part of the vocal apparatus of the larynx called the _____.

    Muscles open and close the glottis during inspiration and expiration, and they regulate the vocal cords during the production of sound. Muscles also close off a lidlike structure that covers the glottis during swallowing. The lidlike structure, the **epiglottis** (ep″ĭ-glot´is), is composed of cartilage and covers the larynx during the swallowing of food.

9-12 Foreign bodies may be aspirated into the nose, throat, or lungs on inspiration. If a person inspires while attempting to swallow, food may be accidentally aspirated into the larynx. Spontaneous coughing is the body's effort to clear the obstructed airway. Respiration stops if complete obstruction of the airway occurs.

    In usual situations, food does not enter the larynx but passes on to the esophagus. Food does

epiglottis

not enter the larynx because a lidlike structure, the _____, is closed. **Epiglottides** (ep″ĭ-glot´ĭ-dēs) is the plural of epiglottis, hence the term epiglottiditis (ep″ĭ-glot″ĭ-di´tis).

---

[*]Olfactory (Latin: *olfacere,* to smell).

EXERCISE 2

Word Analysis. *Divide the following words into their component parts, and write the meaning of each term.*

1. inspiration _____

2. paranasal _____

3. pharyngeal _____

4. pulmonary _____

5. retronasal _____

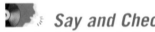

Say and Check

Say aloud the terms in Exercise 2. Use the Companion CD to check your pronunciations.

EXERCISE 3

Write the names of respiratory structures to complete these sentences.

1. The structure that is commonly called the throat is the _____.

2. The hollow interior of the nose is separated into two cavities by the nasal _____.

3. The glottis is the vocal apparatus of the _____.

4. The upper respiratory tract consists of the nose, nasal cavity, paranasal _____, pharynx, and larynx.

5. The lidlike structure called the _____ covers the larynx during the swallowing of food.

LOWER RESPIRATORY PASSAGEWAYS

9-13 Infections of the upper respiratory tract are common and often spread to the lower respiratory tract. The lower respiratory tract, a continuation of the upper respiratory tract, begins with the trachea. Trache/al (tra´ke-əl) means pertaining to the trachea. Endo/tracheal (en˝do-tra´ke-əl) means within the trachea.

In addition to the trachea, the lower respiratory tract includes two primary bronchi and several secondary bronchi, bronchioles, alveolar ducts, and alveoli. The two lungs are composed of millions of alveoli and their related ducts, bronchioles, and bronchi.

bronchi   The trachea branches into the right and left primary _____. Bronchi are lined with cilia, hairlike projections that propel mucus up and away from the lower airway. Bronchi branch to become **bronchioles,** structures that lead to alveolar ducts. At the ends of the ducts are the **alveoli,** small pockets where carbon dioxide and oxygen are exchanged between the inspired air and capillary blood.

9-14 Most of the lower respiratory passageways are located in the chest cavity.

> ➤ KEY POINT The **mediastinum** is the middle portion of the thoracic cavity between the two lungs. In the mediastinum, the trachea (windpipe) divides into the right and left primary bronchi; bronch(o) and bronchi(o) mean bronchi. Bronchial tubes is another term for bronchi (singular is bronchus).

bronchi   **Bronchi/al** means pertaining to the _____.
Bronchioles are small airways that extend from the bronchi into the lungs. Translated literally, bronchi/ole means little bronchus.

Alveolar means pertaining to the alveoli. **Broncho/alveolar** (brong˝ko-al-ve´ə-lər) means pertaining to a bronchus and alveoli. Write a word that means between alveoli:

interalveolar   _____.
(in˝tər-al-ve´ə-lər)

9-15 Both lungs are composed of millions of alveoli and their related ducts, bronchioles, and bronchi.

> ➤ KEY POINT The two lungs have similar characteristics, but have a different number of lobes. Each lung is conical and has an apex (uppermost portion) and a base (lower portion). Note in Figure 9-1 that the left lung has two lobes and the right lung has three lobes.

apex   **Apical** (ap´ĭ-kəl) refers to the _____, or the uppermost portion of the lung. The depression where blood vessels enter and leave the lung is called the **hilum** (hi´ləm).

9-16 Each lung is surrounded by a membrane called the **pleura** (ploor´ə) (plural is pleurae). One layer of the membrane, the **visceral pleura,** covers the lung's surface. The other layer, the **parietal** (pə-ri´ə-təl) **pleura,** lines the walls of the thoracic cavity. **Visceral·** means pertaining to the viscera, the large internal organs enclosed within a body cavity, especially the abdominal cavity. Parietal† pertains to the outer wall of a cavity or organ.

Two types of pleurae are the visceral pleura and the parietal pleura. The visceral pleura

lungs

surrounds the _____; the parietal pleura lines the walls of the thoracic cavity. Between the two pleurae is a space called the **pleural cavity,** which contains a thin film of pleural fluid that acts as a lubricant as the lungs expand and contract during respiration.

9-17 The combining form pleur(o) means pleura. **Pleur/al** (ploor´əl) pertains to the

pleura
outside

_____.

Extrapleural (eks″trə-ploor´əl) means _____ the pleural cavity.

lungs

9-18 Both pulmonary and **pulmonic** mean pertaining to the _____ or the respiratory system, but pulmonary is more commonly used.

Extrapulmonary (eks″trə-pool´mo-nar″e) means outside, or not connected with, the lungs.

below

Sub/pulmonary (səb-pool´mo-nar″e) means _____ the lung.

9-19 Normal lungs are highly elastic and fill the chest cavity during inspiration, pressing down on the diaphragm. The **diaphragm** (di´ə-fram), the muscular partition that separates the thoracic and abdominal cavities, contracts and increases the size of the thoracic cavity during inspiration. It aids respiration by moving up and down as we exhale and inhale (Figure 9-4).

The formal anatomic name for the diaphragm is **diaphragma** (di″ə-frag´mə). **Diaphragma/tic**

diaphragm

(di″ə-frag-mat´ik) means pertaining to the _____. The diaphragm is pierced by several openings through which pass the aorta, the vena cava, and the esophagus.

> ➤ **KEY** POINT <u>The combining form phren(o) means both diaphragm and mind.</u> Ancient Greeks believed that the midriff was the seat of emotions; the Greek word *phren* was applied to this area as a structure, as well as the center of emotions. For this reason diaphragm and mind have the same combining form, phren(o).

Phren/ic (fren´ik) has two meanings, either pertaining to the diaphragm or pertaining to the mind. **Sub/phrenic** (səb-fren´ik) means located beneath the diaphragm. When studying respira-

diaphragm

tion, phren(o) probably refers to the muscular partition that separates the chest and abdominal cavities, the _____.

·Visceral (Latin: *viscus,* internal organ). †Parietal (Latin: *paries,* wall).

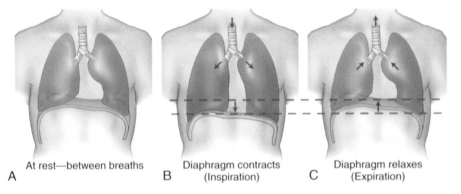

A   At rest—between breaths
B   Diaphragm contracts (Inspiration)
C   Diaphragm relaxes (Expiration)

Figure 9-4 Changes in the lungs and diaphragm during respiration. A, Diaphragm relaxed, just before inspiration. **B,** Inspiration. The diaphragm contracts, moving downward and increasing the size of the thoracic cavity. Inspiration is also aided by contraction of the intercostal muscles, which are between the ribs. Air moves into the lungs until pressure inside the lungs equals atmospheric pressure. **C,** Expiration. Respiratory muscles relax, and the chest cavity decreases in size as air moves from the lungs out into the atmosphere.

EXERCISE 4

Build It! *Use the following word parts to build terms. (Some word parts will be used more than once.)*

endo-, extra-, sub-, alveol(o), bronch(o), phren(o), pleur(o), pulmon(o), trache(o), -al, -ar, -ary, -ic

1. pertaining to the diaphragm _____/_____

2. pertaining to a bronchus and alveoli _____/_____/_____

3. pertaining to within the trachea _____/_____/_____

4. pertaining to outside the pleural cavity _____/_____/_____

5. pertaining to beneath the lungs _____/_____/_____

Say and Check

Say aloud the terms you wrote for Exercise 4. Use the Companion CD to check your pronunciations.

EXERCISE 5

1. The lower respiratory tract begins with a structure called the _____.

2. Bronchi branch to become _____.

3. Tiny structures of the respiratory system where carbon dioxide and oxygen are exchanged between the inspired air and capillary blood are _____.

4. The uppermost part of the lung is called the _____.

5. Each lung is surrounded by a membrane called the _____.

DIAGNOSTIC TESTS AND PROCEDURES

nasal

9-20 Physical assessment of the respiratory structures often begins with examination of the nose and throat, often using a nasal speculum for examination of the interior of the nose. A **naso/scope** (na´zo-skōp) is a speculum that is used for inspecting the _____ cavity.

The color of the mucous membranes and the presence of swelling, bleeding, or discharge are noted. One finding is septal deviation, a structural defect of the nasal septum in which it is shifted toward one side of the nose or the other (Figure 9-5).

polyp

pharynx

9-21 It may also be possible to see a **nasal polyp** with the help of a nasoscope. A polyp (pol´ip) is a growth or mass protruding from a mucous membrane. Polyps are usually (but not always) benign. They can grow on almost any mucous membrane. If such a growth occurs in the nasal cavity or in the sinuses, it is called a nasal _____.

A **pharyngo/scope** (fə-ring´go-skōp) is an instrument for examining the lining of the structure that is commonly called the throat, the _____.

instrument

9-22 Laryngo/scopy (lar″ing-gos´kə-pe), examination of the larynx with an endoscope, is generally performed by a specialist. A **laryngoscope** (lə-ring´gə-skōp) is the _____ used in laryngoscopy.

If further study is needed, a physician may order a radiographic examination of the larynx, **laryngography** (lar″ing-gog´rə-fe). This procedure usually includes the pharynx, as well as the larynx.

tracheoscopic

bronchoscope
(brong´ko-skōp)

9-23 Viewing the interior of the trachea is a **tracheoscopy** (tra″ke-os´kə-pe). This is also called a _____ examination.

Add a suffix to bronch(o) to form a word that means an instrument for viewing the bronchi: _____.

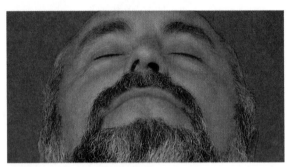

Figure 9-5 Deviated septum. This shifted partition of the nasal cavity may obstruct the nasal passages. Severe septal deviation may be corrected by rhinoplasty or septoplasty.

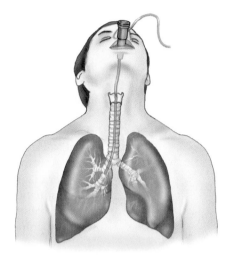

Figure 9-6 Bronchoscopy. Visual examination of the tracheobronchial tree using a bronchoscope. Other uses for this procedure include suctioning, obtaining a biopsy specimen or fluid, and removing foreign bodies.

bronchogram
(brong′ko-gram)

Broncho/scopy (brong-kos′kə-pe) or **broncho/scopic** (brong″ko-skop′ik) **examination** is direct viewing of the bronchi (Figure 9-6). **Broncho/graphy** (brong-kog′rə-fe) involves the use of x-rays after instillation of an opaque solution. The film obtained by broncho/graphy is a _____. This procedure is seldom used, having been replaced by computed tomography.

mediastinoscope
(me″de-ə-sti′no-skōp)

9-24 Mediastino/scopy (me″de-as″tĭ-nos′kə-pe) is examination of the mediastinum by means of an endoscope inserted through an incision of the chest. This procedure allows direct inspection of the mediastinum and biopsy of tissue, using an instrument called a _____.

9-25 Radiography of the chest, commonly called a chest x-ray, is a valuable tool in studying the lungs as well as nearby structures. Examine the chest x-ray in Figure 9-7, and study the relationship of the lungs with other structures in the chest cavity. The air in the lungs appears black. Note also the white appearance of bone (collarbone, breastbone, and ribs). The breasts and other soft tissues appear gray. In looking at the respiratory structures, it is understandable why the trachea and bronchial branches are referred to as the tracheobronchial tree.

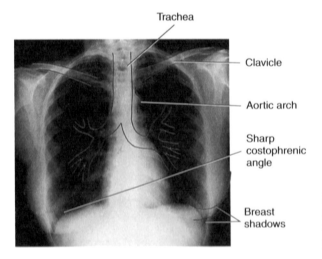

Trachea

Clavicle

Aortic arch

Sharp costophrenic angle

Breast shadows

Figure 9-7 A normal radiograph of the chest. Do not be concerned about the meanings of all the terms in the chest x-ray film. The clavicle is the collarbone, and the costophrenic angle is the angle between the diaphragm and the chest wall at the bottom of the lung.

The muscular structure that contracts and relaxes during inspiration and expiration is the

diaphragm

_____.

vessels

9-26 Pulmonary angio/graphy (an″je-og′rə-fe) is radiology of the _____ of the lungs after injection of a contrast medium. Pulmonary angiography is primarily performed on patients with suspected thromboembolic (throm″bo-em-bol′ik) disease. A thrombus is an internal blood clot. If part of it breaks off, the clot fragment can travel in the bloodstream to another site. Any foreign object that circulates in the bloodstream and becomes lodged in a vessel is called an embolus. **Thrombo/embol/ic** pertains to obstruction of a blood vessel with material from a blood clot that is carried by the bloodstream from its site of origin.

Other diagnostic radiologic studies of respiratory organs include computed tomography, magnetic resonance imaging, and lung scans. A lung scan uses radioactive material to test blood flow or air distribution in the lungs. Information about the flow of blood in the lungs is helpful in diagnosing pulmonary embo/lism, the presence of an embolus in the lungs.

9-27 The lung volume in normal quiet breathing is approximately 500 mL; however, forced maximum inspiration raises this level considerably. **Spiro/metry** (spi-rom′ə-tre) is a measurement of the amount of air taken into and expelled from the lungs (Figure 9-8). The combining form spir(o) as used here means breath or breathing. The instrument used is a

spirometer
(spi-rom′ə-tər)

_____.

The largest volume of air that can be exhaled after maximal inspiration is the vital capacity (VC). A reduction in vital capacity often indicates a loss of functioning lung tissue.

Spirometry measures ventilation (the ability of the lungs to move air) and is one type of pulmonary function test (PFT) that helps determine the capacity of the lungs to exchange oxygen and carbon dioxide effectively.

9-28 A **pulse oxi/meter** (ok-sim′ə-tər) is a photo/electric device for determining the oxygen saturation of the blood in a pulsating capillary bed (Figure 9-9). The finger probe is most commonly used for monitoring the patient's oxygenation status in a hospital, during pulmonary rehabilitation programs, or during stress testing; however, an ear oximeter is sometimes used. The name of the procedure that determines the oxygen saturation of the blood in a pulsating

oximetry

capillary bed is **pulse** _____.

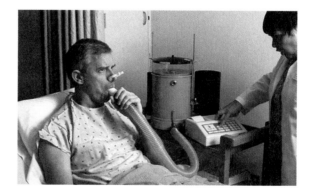

Figure 9-8 Spirometry. Evaluation of the air capacity of the lungs uses a spirometer, such as the one shown. The spirometer is used to assess pulmonary function by measuring and recording the volume of inhaled and exhaled air.

Figure 9-9 Oximetry, noninvasive monitoring of oxygen saturation. A, The oximeter shows an oxygen saturation of 95%. **B,** The earlobe is a common site for measurement during exercise. **C,** The finger probe is most frequently used for stationary measurements.

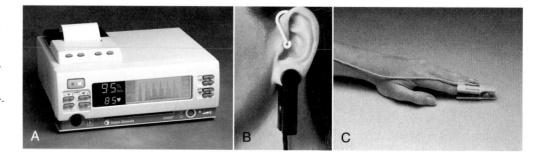

9-29 The use of percussion, described in Chapter 3, is helpful in assessing the lungs (see Figure 3-8, *B*). Chest auscultation (see Figure 3-8, *C*), listening to breath sounds, provides information about the flow of air through the tracheo/bronchial tree. Abnormal sounds that are heard during inspiration include rhonchi (rong´ki), wheezes, crackles (also called **rales** [rahlz]), and friction rub (Figure 9-10).

Abnormal sounds can be heard when a stethoscope is used to evaluate the sound of air moving in and out of the lungs. This procedure is called _____.

auscultation

9-30 A **rhonchus*** (rong´kəs) is an abnormal sound consisting of a continuous rumbling sound that clears on coughing. A **wheeze** is a musical noise that sounds like a squeak. **Crackles** are discontinuous bubbling noises during inspiration that are not cleared by coughing. A **friction rub** is a dry, grating sound. If the friction rub is heard over the pleural area, it may be a sign of lung disease, although it may be normal if heard over another area such as the liver.

Practice enables development of the ability to distinguish these abnormal sounds. Another sound, **stridor**† (stri´dər) is an abnormal high-pitched musical sound caused by an obstruction in the trachea or larynx, most often heard during inspiration. Write the term that is an abnormal high-pitched sound associated with an obstruction in the trachea or larynx:

_____.

stridor

9-31 Arterial blood gas (ABG) analysis is a blood test that measures the amount of oxygen, carbon dioxide, and pH in a blood sample collected from an artery. ABG is the abbreviation for _____ blood gas.

arterial

Other laboratory tests include cultures for bacteria or fungi in sputum or material collected from throat swabs. **Phlegm** (flem) is abnormally thick mucus secreted by the membranes of the respiratory passages. **Sputum** (spu´təm) is phlegm or other material that is coughed up from the lungs.

---

*Rhonchus (Greek: *rhonchos,* snore).
†Stridor (Latin: *stridor,* harsh sound).

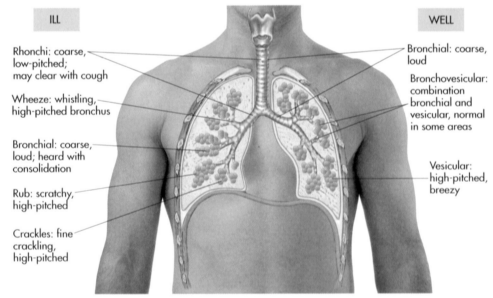

Figure 9-10 Breath sounds in the ill and well patient. Common terms used to describe sounds heard in the ill patient are rhonchi, wheeze, friction rub, and crackles, as well as coarse, loud bronchial sounds heard with consolidation. Consolidation means the process of becoming solid, as when the lungs become firm and inelastic in pneumonia.

EXERCISE 6

Match these structures with the instrument or procedure that is used to study them.

_____ 1. blood vessels of the lung   _____ 4. voice box

_____ 2. nose   _____ 5. windpipe

_____ 3. throat

A. laryngoscope
B. nasoscope
C. pharyngoscope
D. pulmonary angiography
E. tracheoscope

EXERCISE 7

Build It! *Use the following word parts to build terms. (Some word parts will be used more than once.)*

bronch(o), laryng(o), ox(i), pharyng(o), spir(o), -graphy, -meter, -metry, -scope, -scopy

1. a device that determines oxygen saturation   _____/_____

2. measurement of the amount of air taken into and expelled from the lungs   _____/_____

3. process of visualizing the bronchi with x-rays   _____/_____

4. examination of the larynx with an endoscope   _____/_____

5. instrument for examining the pharynx   _____/_____

Say and Check

Say aloud the terms you wrote for Exercise 7. Use the Companion CD to check your pronunciations.

PATHOLOGIES
DISORDERED BREATHING

apnea (ap′ne-ə)

9-32 Disorders of the respiratory system are a major cause of illness and death. Acute or chronic respiratory problems can progress rapidly and become life-threatening emergencies. Chronic lung disease often causes heart disease because of the lungs' functional role in circulation. Pulmonary hypertension is a condition of abnormally high blood pressure in the pulmonary circulation, caused by resistance of blood flow in the vessels of the lung. This brings about an increased workload for the heart and eventually leads to heart failure.

You learned earlier that -pnea is a suffix that means breathing. Choose either a- or an- to write a word that means absence of spontaneous breathing: _____.

9-33 Sleep apnea is a sleep disorder characterized by transient periods of cessation of breathing. The two primary types are central sleep apnea (from failure of stimulation by the nervous system) and obstructive sleep apnea (from collapse or obstruction of the airway).

Cheyne-Stokes (chān stōks) **respiration** (CSR) is an abnormal pattern of respiration that is characterized by alternating periods of apnea and deep, rapid breathing, occurring more frequently during sleep.

breathing

9-34 Many pathologies can cause shortness of breath (SOB). Remembering that dys- means bad or difficult, **dys/pnea** (disp-ne′ə) is labored or difficult _____.
Dys/pne/ic (disp-ne′ik) is an adjective that means pertaining to or caused by dyspnea.

> ➤ KEY POINT Anoxia is more severe than hypoxia. **An/ox/ia** (ə -nok′se-ə) means an absence or deficiency of oxygen in body tissues below the level needed for proper functioning. **Hypoxia** (hi-pok′se-ə) is a reduction of oxygen in body tissues to levels below those required for normal metabolic functioning. Note the spelling of hyp/ox/ia (the o of hypo- has been dropped). Anoxia is more severe than hypoxia, but both mean oxygen deficiency.

Asphyxia* (as-fik´se-ə) or **asphyxiation** (as-fik˝se-a´shən) is a condition caused by insufficient intake of oxygen. Extrinsic† causes, those originating outside the body, include drowning, crushing injuries of the chest, and inhalation of carbon monoxide. Intrinsic‡ causes include hemorrhage into the lungs or pleural cavity, foreign bodies in the throat, and diseases of the air passages. Asphyxia is caused by lack of _____.

oxygen

9-35 Cyanosis, dyspnea, and tachycardia accompanied by mental disturbances are seen in asphyxia. In extreme cases, convulsions, unconsciousness, and death may occur. **Tachy/cardia** (tachy-, fast + -cardi(o), heart + -ia, condition) means an increased heart rate.

Write the term that means a condition caused by insufficient intake of oxygen (be careful with the spelling): _____.

asphyxia or asphyxiation

9-36 Hyper/pnea (hi˝pər-, hi˝pərp-ne´ə) is an exaggerated deep or rapid respiration. It occurs normally with exercise and abnormally in several conditions, including pain, fever, hysteria, or inadequate oxygen. The latter can occur in cardiac or respiratory disease. A literal translation of hyper/pnea is excessive _____.

breathing

Hyper/pnea may lead to **hyper/ventilation** (hi˝pər-ven˝tĭ-la´shən)—excessive aeration of the lungs—which commonly reduces carbon dioxide levels in the body. Carbon dioxide contributes to the acidity of body fluids, and if too much carbon dioxide is lost, alkalosis results. **Alkal/osis** (al˝-kə-lo´sis) is a pathologic condition resulting from the accumulation of basic substances or from the loss of acid by the body. Transient alkalosis can be caused by hyperventilation. Transient§ means not lasting or of brief duration.

9-37 The abbreviation pH means potential hydrogen and is the symbol for hydrogen ion concentration, a calculated scale that represents the relative acidity or alkalinity of a solution; a value of 7.0 is neutral, below 7.0 is acidic, and above 7.0 is alkaline. The normal pH of body fluids (plasma and intracellular and interstitial fluids) is 7.35 to 7.45. Is normal plasma slightly acid or alkaline? _____

alkaline

> ➤ KEY POINT The state of equilibrium of the blood pH is called the acid-base balance. Cellular metabolism produces substances such as excess carbon dioxide that would upset the pH balance were it not for buffer systems of the blood, along with respiratory and urinary functions that help keep the pH constant. The expelling of carbon dioxide during exhalation is part of the regulatory mechanism that maintains the constancy of the pH—that is, the acid-base balance.

9-38 The combining form alkal(o) means alkaline or basic. Alkal/osis is an alkaline condition. **Alkal/emia** (al˝kə-le´me-ə) is increased alkalinity of the blood. Alkal/emia is an aspect of alkalosis, the general term for accumulation of basic substances in the body fluids. The opposite of alkalosis is **acid/osis** (as˝ĭ-do´sis). The combining form acid(o) means acid. A pathologic condition that results from accumulation of acid or depletion of alkaline substances is called

_____.

acidosis

9-39 The suffix -capnia refers to carbon dioxide. **Hyper/capnia** (hi˝pər-kap´ne-ə) means greater than normal amounts of carbon dioxide in the blood. **Hypo/ventilation** (hi˝po-ven˝tĭ-la´shən), a reduced amount of air entering the pulmonary alveoli, results in hypercapnia. Carbon dioxide contributes to the acidity of blood. Does hypercapnia result in lowering or increasing blood pH? _____

lowering

Within minutes, the lungs begin to compensate for any acid-base imbalance by increasing the excretion of carbon dioxide through faster or deeper breathing.

---

*Asphyxia (*a-*, no + Greek: *phyxis*, pulse).
†Extrinsic (Latin: *extrinsecus*, situated on the outside).
‡Intrinsic (Latin: *intrinsecus*, situated on the inside).
§Transient (Latin: *trans*, to go by).

TABLE 9-1	Potential Causes of Acid-Base Imbalances
Acidemia	**Alkalemia**
Ingestion of highly acidic drugs	Ingestion of alkaline drugs
Severe diarrhea	Intense hyperventilation
Severe diabetes	Vomiting of gastric acid
Asphyxia	Metabolic problems
Vomiting of lower intestinal contents	
Disease, particularly respiratory or kidney failure	

absence

hypocapnia

acidemia

9-40 **Hypo/capnia** (hi″po-kap′ne-ə) is the opposite of hypercapnia and means an abnormally low level of carbon dioxide in the blood. **A/capnia** (ă-kap′ne-ə) is a synonym for hypocapnia, although in its strictest sense a/capnia means _____ of carbon dioxide.

Would hyperventilation lead to hypercapnia or hypocapnia? _____

9-41 **Acid/emia** (as″ĭ-de′me-ə) is an arterial blood pH below 7.35, whereas alkal/emia is recognized as a blood pH above 7.45. Either of these conditions can be considered an acid-base imbalance. Look at some conditions listed in Table 9-1 that can lead to an acid-base imbalance.

Asphyxia leads to which condition, alkalemia or acidemia? _____

EXERCISE 8

Build It! *Use the following word parts to build terms. (Some word parts will be used more than once.)*

a-, an-, dys-, hypo-, alkal(o), ox(i), phren(o), -capnia, -dynia, -emia, -ia, -osis, -pnea

1. absence or deficiency of oxygen _____/_____/_____

2. abnormally low level of carbon dioxide _____/_____

3. labored or difficult breathing _____/_____

4. cessation of breathing _____/_____

5. condition of accumulation of basic substances in the body _____/_____

Say and Check

Say aloud the terms you wrote for Exercise 8. Use the Companion CD to check your pronunciations.

EXERCISE 9

Write a word in each blank to complete these sentences.

1. Asphyxia is a condition caused by insufficient intake of _____.

2. Exaggerated deep or rapid breathing is _____.

3. Increased aeration of the lungs is _____.

4. A greater than normal amount of carbon dioxide is _____.

5. A term for an arterial blood pH below 7.35 is _____.

9-42 Acute respiratory failure is a sudden inability of the lungs to maintain normal respiratory function. It may be caused by an obstruction in the airways or failure of the lungs. Respiratory failure leads to hyp/ox/ia. Acute (or adult) respiratory distress syndrome (ARDS) is severe pulmonary congestion characterized by respiratory insufficiency and hypoxemia and can result in acute respiratory failure.

Hyp/ox/emia (hi″pok-se′me-ə) is decreased oxygen in the _____. Once again, notice the spelling. You learned earlier that asphyxia is caused by insufficient intake of oxygen. This leads to hypoxemia, hypercapnia, loss of consciousness, and death if not corrected.

9-43 In **ortho/pnea** (or″thop-ne′ə), breathing is difficult except in an upright position. Analyze ortho/pnea (orth[o], straight + -pnea, breathing). In orthopnea, the person experiences chronic airflow limitation (CAL) and must sit or stand to breathe deeply or comfortably. Write the term that means a condition in which breathing is difficult except in an upright position: _____. Two comfortable positions that help orthopneic patients breathe more comfortably are shown in Figure 9-11.

9-44 Adults normally have a respiration rate of about 12 to 20 breaths per minute. **Eu/pnea** (ūp-ne′ə) means normal breathing. If a person were breathing at a rate of 25 breaths per minute at rest, this would be **tachypnea.** The word tachy/pnea (tak″ip-ne′ə, tak″e-ne′ə) means _____ breathing.

The opposite of this is slow breathing, or _____. A graphic representation of various patterns of breathing is shown in Figure 9-12.

In another condition, **hypo/pnea** (hi-pop′ne-ə), the breathing is shallow, in addition to being slow. This may be appropriate in a well-conditioned athlete but can occur either if it is painful to breathe or if there is damage to the brain stem.

9-45 Abnormalities in the diaphragm will affect breathing, because the diaphragm normally moves downward as the lungs expand during inspiration. **Phreno/dynia** (fren″o-din′e-ə) is pain in the diaphragm. Paralysis of the diaphragm is **phreno/plegia** (fren″o-ple′jə). **Phreno/ptosis** (fren″op-to′sis, fren″o-to′sis) is a prolapsed or downward displacement of the diaphragm. Use phren(o) to write a word that means inflammation of the diaphragm: _____.

blood

orthopnea

fast
bradypnea
(brad″e-ne′ə,
brad-ip′ne-ə)

phrenitis (frə-ni′tis)

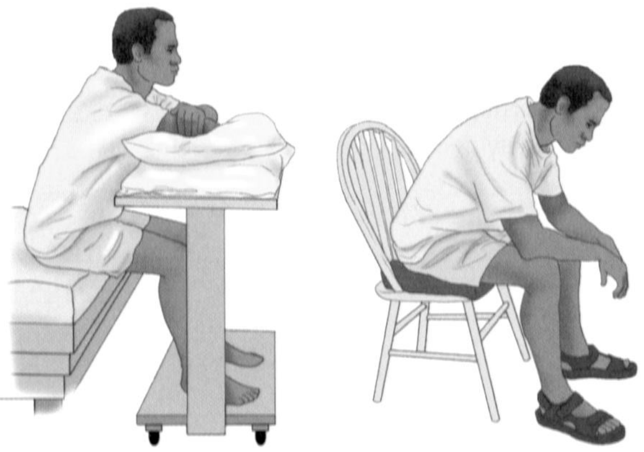

Figure 9-11 **Two positions for the orthopneic patient.** These positions ease the work of breathing for persons with chronic airflow limitation (CAL).

Normal (Eupnea) — Regular at a rate of 12-20 breaths per minute

Bradypnea — Slower than 12 breaths per minute

Tachypnea — Faster than 20 breaths per minute

Hyperpnea — Deep breathing, faster than 20 breaths per minute

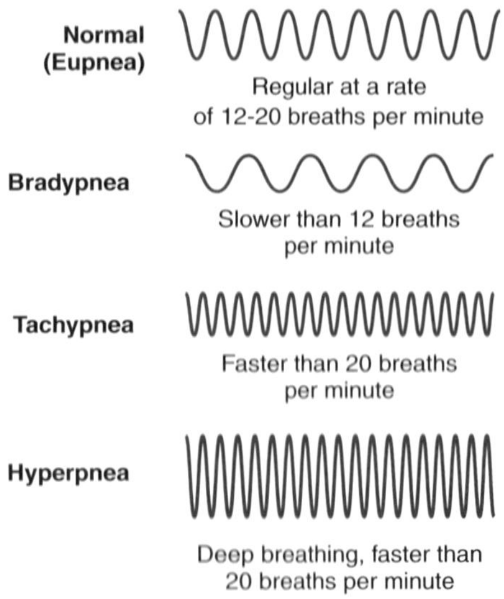

Figure 9-12 **Selected patterns of respiration.** An example of normal respiration is compared with those seen in bradypnea, tachypnea, and hyperpnea.

EXERCISE 10

Word Analysis. *Break the following terms into their component parts. Then write the meaning of each term.*

1. bradypnea _____

2. eupnea _____

3. hypoxemia _____

4. orthopnea _____

5. phrenoplegia _____

6. tachypnea _____

Say and Check

Say aloud the terms in Exercise 10. Use the Companion CD to check your pronunciations.

UPPER RESPIRATORY ABNORMALITIES

respiration (or breathing)

9-46 An upper airway obstruction is any significant interruption in the airflow through the nose, mouth, pharynx, or larynx. Laryngoscopy may be helpful in locating and removing the cause of the obstruction. If the cause is not removed, respiratory arrest occurs. Respiratory arrest is cessation of _____.

inflammation

9-47 During infections and allergies, swelling may block the passages and cause fluid to accumulate in the sinuses. A sinus headache can result from the pressure within the sinuses. **Sinus/itis** (si″nəs-i′tis) is _____ of one or more paranasal sinuses. A structural defect of the nose can also result in sinusitis.

rhinitis (ri-ni′tis)

9-48 Build a word using rhin(o) that means inflammation of the mucous membranes of the nose: _____. Acute rhinitis is also called **coryza**[*] (ko-ri′zə), meaning a profuse discharge of the mucous membranes of the nose. This is usually what is meant when speaking of an upper respiratory infection (URI).

nose

　　Rhino/rrhea (ri″no-re′ə) is discharge from the _____. This is commonly called a runny nose.

hemorrhage

9-49 Nosebleeds have many causes, including irritation of the nasal membranes, fragility of these membranes, violent sneezing, trauma, high blood pressure, vitamin K deficiency, or (particularly in children) picking the nose. **Rhinorrhagia** (ri″no-ra′jə) means profuse bleeding from the nose. Literal translation of rhino/rrhagia is _____ from the nose. Another medical term for nosebleed is **epistaxis** (ep″ĭ-stak′sis).

nose

nasal

9-50 A **rhino/lith** (ri′no-lith) is a calculus or stone in the _____. A calculus consists of inorganic substances, such as calcium and phosphate, that crystallize to form a hard mass resembling a pebble. A rhino/lith is a _____ calculus. The presence of nasal stones is **rhino/lith/iasis** (ri″no-lĭ-thi′ə-sis).

　　A rhinolith can interfere with breathing through the nose, making it more comfortable to breathe through the mouth.

9-51 Canker sores are ulcerations, especially inside the mouth. **Palat/itis** (pal″ə-ti′tis) is inflammation of the hard palate, the bony portion of the roof of the mouth.

　　Pharyng/itis (far″in-ji′tis) is inflammation or infection of the pharynx, usually causing symptoms of a sore throat. Sore throat (pharyngeal pain) is **pharyngo/dynia** (fə-ring″go-din′e-ə) or **pharyng/algia** (far″in-gal′jə).

[*]Coryza (Greek: *koryza*, catarrh).

Tonsill/itis (ton″sĭ-li′tis) is one reason for a sore throat. The tonsils are located in the oropharynx. Enlarged tonsils can fill the space behind the nares and may completely block the passage of air from the nose into the throat.

9-52 Other causes of a sore throat include strepto/coccal infections, **herpes simplex virus** (HSV), and infectious mono/nucleosis. It is important to receive an antibiotic for strep infections, because untreated strep infections sometimes lead to rheumatic fever (see Chapter 8). Herpes simplex, caused by the herpes simplex virus, usually produces small, transient, irritating, and sometimes fluid-filled blisters on the skin and mucous membranes. Infections tend to occur particularly around the nose and mouth.

nasopharyngitis
(na″zo-far″in-ji′tis)

Inflammation of the nasopharynx is _____. Various infectious organisms cause pharyngitis or nasopharyngitis.

pharynx
pharyngopathy
(far″ing-gop′ə-the)
laryngitis
(lar″in-ji′tis)

9-53 Pharyngo/myc/osis (fə-ring″go-mi-ko′sis) is a fungal condition of the _____.
Write a word that means any disease of the pharynx: _____.

9-54 Build a word that means inflammation of the larynx: _____. This condition would probably result in temporary loss of voice. Inflammation of the larynx may be caused not only by infectious microorganisms but also by overuse of the voice, allergies, or irritants.

larynx

A person with laryngitis often suffers only minor discomfort. If the larynx becomes painful, the person has **laryng/algia** (lar″in-gal′jə), which is pain of the _____.
You may be wondering if you could combine laryng(o) with -dynia, which also means pain. Although some people would know what you mean, this term is not generally used.

9-55 A/phonia (a-fo′ne-ə) is a condition characterized by the inability to produce normal speech sounds that results from overuse of the vocal cords, organic disease, or emotional problems, such as anxiety. The combining form phon(o) means voice. Laryngitis may result in absence of voice, which is called _____.

aphonia
difficult (weak)

Dys/phonia (dis-fo′ne-ə) means _____ voice. Dysphonia is not related to the ability to pronounce words. It is the same as hoarseness and may precede aphonia.

speech

9-56 The combining form phas(o) means speech. Literal translation of dys/phas/ia is difficult _____. **Dysphasia** (dis-fa′zhə) is impairment of speech, characterized by a lack of coordination and an inability to arrange words in their proper order, a problem resulting from a brain lesion. Difficulty in speech caused by a brain lesion is called

dysphasia

_____.

absence

9-57 A/phasia (ə-fa′zhə) is the _____ of speech. Aphasia is an inability to communicate through speech or writing, as a result of dysfunction of the brain. A person who has aphasia is said to be aphasic (ə-fa′zik).

EXERCISE 11

Build It! *Use the following word parts to build terms. (Some word parts will be used more than once.)*

a-, dys-, pharyng(o), phas(o), phon(o), rhin(o), sinus(o), -dynia, -ia, -itis, -rrhea

1. discharge from the nose _____/_____

2. impairment of speech _____/_____/_____

3. inflammation of one or more paranasal sinuses _____/_____

4. throat pain _____/_____

5. inability to communicate _____/_____/_____

Say and Check

Say aloud the terms you wrote for Exercise 11. Use the Companion CD to check your pronunciations.

polyp

9-58 You learned earlier that a polyp is a tumor-like growth, usually benign, that projects from a mucous membrane. A growth of this type on the vocal cords is called a laryngeal _____ (Figure 9-13).

Although painless, laryngeal polyps cause hoarseness. They are generally caused by smoking, allergies, or abuse of the voice, and eliminating the cause often relieves the hoarseness. Surgery can be performed using direct laryngoscopy if rest does not correct the problem.

larynx

9-59 Laryngo/plegia (lə-ring″go-ple′jə) is paralysis of the muscles of the _____. Spasmodic closure of the larynx (spasm of the larynx) is **laryngospasm** (lə-ring′go-spaz″əm). Any disease of the larynx is a **laryngopathy** (lar-ing-gop′ə-the).

inflammation

The epiglottis prevents food from entering the larynx and the trachea during swallowing. **Epiglott/itis** (ep″ĭ-glŏ-ti′tis) or **epiglottid/itis** is _____ of the epiglottis.

9-60 The common cold is a contagious viral infection of the upper respiratory tract. Some of its major characteristics are rhinitis, rhinorrhea, tearing and eye discomfort, and sometimes low-grade fever. **Rhin/itis** is inflammation of the nasal membranes. **Rhino/rrhea** is

discharge

_____ from the nasal membranes.

The barking cough of **croup** (kro͞op) is often accompanied by difficulty in breathing and stridor. Croup is an acute viral infection of the upper and lower respiratory tract that occurs primarily in infants and young children.

9-61 Diphtheria (dif-thĕr′e-ə) and **pertussis** (pər-tus′is) are two acute contagious respiratory diseases. They are both caused by specific pathogenic bacteria and are both preventable by vaccination. Immunization for diphtheria and pertussis is usually begun in conjunction with tetanus immunization early in infancy. The exotoxin of the tetanus bacillus affects the nervous system, resulting in paralysis. For this reason, the common name of tetanus is lockjaw. It is easy to

diphtheria

misspell the term diphtheria. Write the term here: _____.

Pertussis is commonly called whooping cough, named for the coughing that ends in a loud whooping inspiration. It occurs primarily in infants and young children but can occur in anyone who has not been immunized.

9-62 A **corona/virus** (kə-ro′nə-vi″rus), named for its appearance under an electron microscope, has been identified as the organism responsible for severe acute respiratory syndrome (SARS). It is spread by close contact with an infected person. Illness generally begins with a fever and body aches, and some people experience mild respiratory symptoms. After 3 to 7 days, a lower respiratory phase begins and patients may develop a dry cough and have trouble breathing.

Severity of the disease ranges from causing mild illness to death. The Centers for Disease Control and Prevention reports a fatality rate of approximately 3%. SARS is the abbreviation

severe

for _____ acute respiratory syndrome.

9-63 Influenza is a highly contagious respiratory infection that is caused by various strains of influenza virus. Three main types (type A, type B, and type C) have been identified, but new strains emerge at regular intervals (for example, Asian flu virus and bird flu). Influenza is charac-

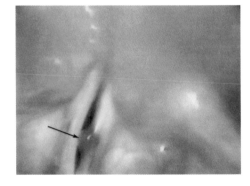

Figure 9-13 A laryngeal polyp. This hemorrhagic polyp *(arrow)* on the vocal cord occurs most commonly in adults who smoke, have many allergies, live in dry climates, or abuse the voice.

terized by fever, sore throat, cough, muscle ache, and weakness. Yearly vaccination is recommended for health care personnel, the elderly, and debilitated persons.

This highly contagious disease that is characterized by fever, respiratory symptoms, muscle aches, and weakness is _____.

influenza

EXERCISE 12

Match terms in the left columns with the clues in the right column.

_____ 1. coryza   _____ 4. pharyngitis

_____ 2. laryngitis   _____ 5. rhinolithiasis

_____ 3. pertussis

A. sore throat usually accompanies this condition
B. acute rhinitis
C. sometimes called whooping cough
D. sometimes results in temporary loss of voice
E. the presence of nasal calculi

 Say and Check

Say aloud the terms in Exercise 12. Use the Companion CD to check your pronunciations.

LOWER RESPIRATORY ABNORMALITIES

9-64 The lower respiratory tract is a common site of infections, obstructive conditions, and malignancies. As you learned in Chapter 4, although cancer of the lung and bronchi are not the most common types of cancer, they cause the greatest number of adult cancer deaths. Fatigue is common in chronic respiratory conditions. Clubbing is a sign that is often associated with advanced chronic pulmonary disease. An abnormal enlargement of the distal fingers and toes, clubbing is most easily seen in the distal fingers (Figure 9-14).

Several unnatural surface features of the chest can be seen during a physical examination. Both pigeon chest and funnel chest are skeletal abnormalities of the chest. The breastbone has a prominent anterior projection in pigeon chest, and it is depressed in funnel chest (Figure 9-15). Breathing is generally not affected in either of these structural defects. A prominent anterior projection of the breastbone is characteristic of which skeletal abnormality, pigeon chest or funnel chest? _____ chest

pigeon

9-65 Flail chest occurs when multiple rib fractures cause instability of the chest wall. The lung underlying the injury contracts and bulges with each inspiration and expiration. This condition must be surgically corrected to prevent hypoxia.

Barrel chest—a large, rounded thorax—may be normal in some individuals but may also be a sign of pulmonary emphysema. The common name for a large, rounded thorax is _____ chest.

barrel

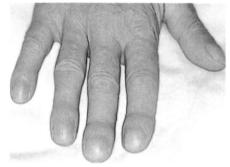

Figure 9-14 Clubbing. Abnormal enlargement of the distal phalanges is seen in advanced chronic pulmonary disease, but may be associated with other disorders, such as cyanotic heart disease and chronic kidney disease.

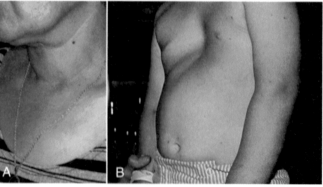

Figure 9-15 Comparison of two structural problems of the chest, pigeon chest and funnel chest. A, Pigeon chest, a congenital structural defect characterized by prominent sternal protrusion. **B,** Funnel chest, indentation of the lower sternum.

EXERCISE 13

Match the following unnatural chest features with their outstanding characteristics.

_____ 1. barrel chest   _____ 3. funnel chest

_____ 2. flail chest   _____ 4. pigeon chest

A. contracting and bulging of the lung during inspiration and expiration
B. depression of the breastbone
C. prominent anterior projection of the breastbone
D. rounded chest

---

aplasia

9-66 The suffix -plasia means formation or development. **A/plasia** (ə-pla´zhə) means absence of formation or development. Incomplete formation or development of the lung is the same as _____ of the lung.

infant

9-67 Respiratory distress syndrome (RDS) is an acute lung disease of the newborn that occurs most often in premature babies. In most cases, the infant dies only a few days after birth or recovers with no after effects. Sudden infant death syndrome (SIDS) is the unexpected and sudden death of an apparently normal and healthy infant that occurs during sleep and may be linked with respiration. SIDS means sudden _____ death syndrome.
    Learn the meanings of the word parts in the following list.

Word Parts: Respiratory Pathologies

Combining Form	Meaning	Prefix	Meaning
anthrac(o)	coal	meta-	change; next, as in a series
atel(o)	imperfect or incomplete	**Suffix**	**Meaning**
coni(o)	dust	-ation	process
embol(o)	embolus	-pnea	breathing
fibr(o)	fiber or fibrous	-ptosis	prolapse
thromb(o)	thrombus	-ptysis	spitting
		-stenosis	narrowing

inflammation

9-68 Laryngo/trache/al (lə-ring″go-tra´ke-əl) means pertaining to the larynx and the trachea. **Laryngotracheitis** (lə-ring″go-tra″ke-i´tis) means _____ of the larynx and trachea. If the larynx, trachea, and bronchi are inflamed, it is called **laryngo/tracheo/bronch/itis** (lə-ring″go-tra″ke-o-brong-ki´tis).
    Tracheo/malacia (tra″ke-o-mə-la´shə) is softening of the trachea, and **tracheo/stenosis** (tra″ke-o-stə-no´sis; trache[o] + -stenosis, narrowing) is narrowing of the lumen of the trachea.

painful

Trache/algia (tra″ke-al´jə) means a _____ trachea.

bronchitis
(brong-ki´tis)
bronchopathy
(brong-kop´ə-the)
bronchi

9-69 Broncho/pulmonary (brong″ko-pool´mə-nar″e) pertains to the bronchi and lungs. Build a word that means inflammation of the bronchi by combining bronch(o) and -itis: _____.
    Bronchogenic (brong-ko-jen´ik) means originating in a bronchus. Use bronch(o) to write a word that means any disease of the bronchi: _____.
    Broncho/lith/iasis (brong″ko-lĭ-thi´ə-sis) is a condition in which stones are present in the _____.

dilation

9-70 Literal translation of bronchi/ectasis (brong″ke-ek´tə-sis) is _____ of the bronchi; however, **bronchiectasis** is an abnormal condition of the bronchial tree that is characterized by irreversible dilation and destruction of the bronchial walls. Signs and symptoms include chronic sinusitis, a constant cough producing a great deal of sputum, hemoptysis (hem[o], blood + -ptysis, spitting), and persistent crackles.

9-71 Broncho/spasm (brong´ko-spaz″əm) means bronchial spasm. Bronchospasm brings about **broncho/constriction** (bron″ko-kən-strik´shən), resulting in an acute narrowing and obstruction of the respiratory airway. There is usually a cough with generalized wheezing, a chief characteristic of asthma and bronchitis.

Asthma is characterized by recurring episodes of paroxysmal (par″ok-siz′məl) wheezing and dyspnea, constriction of the bronchi, coughing, and viscous bronchial secretions. It is also called bronchial asthma. **Paroxysmal** refers to a sudden recurrence or intensity of symptoms.

bronchioles

9-72 **Bronchiol/ectasis** (brong″ke-o-lek′tə-sis) is dilation of the _____.
Bronchiolitis (brong″ke-o-li′tis) means inflammation of the bronchioles.

EXERCISE 14

Build It! *Use the following word parts to build terms. (Some word parts will be used more than once.)*

a-, bronch(i), bronchiol(o), laryng(o), pulmon(o), trache(o), -ary, -ectasis, -itis, -plasia

1. absence of formation or development _____/_____

2. inflammation of the larynx and trachea _____/_____/_____

3. inflammation of the bronchioles _____/_____

4. irreversible dilation and destruction
    of the bronchial walls _____/_____

5. pertaining to the bronchi and lungs _____/_____/_____

Say and Check

Say aloud the terms you wrote for Exercise 14. Use the Companion CD to check your pronunciations.

lungs

9-73 The two highly elastic lungs are the main components of the respiratory system. **Pneumon/ia** (noo-mo′ne-ə), or **pneumonitis** (noo″mo-ni′tis), means inflammation of the _____. Several microorganisms including bacteria, viruses, and fungi have been identified as causes of pneumonia, but the disease is often caused by pneumo/cocci, a type of pathogenic coccal bacteria. This type of pneumonia is called **pneumo/coccal pneumonia.** A vaccine is available for pneumococcal pneumonia and is recommended for persons over 65 years of age and/or those with immunodeficiencies.

Lobar pneumonia involves one or more of the five major lobes of the lungs. **Broncho/pneumon/ia** (brong″ko-noo-mo′ne-ə) involves both the bronchi and the lungs and is usually a result of the spread of infection from the upper to the lower respiratory tract.

abscess

9-74 A **pulmonary abscess** (lung abscess) is a complication of an infection of the lung. A localized cavity containing pus and surrounded by inflamed lung tissue is a lung _____.

pleural

9-75 **Pleural effusion** (ə-fu′zhən) is a collection of nonpurulent fluid in the _____ cavity (Figure 9-16). Non/purulent means not containing pus. If pleural effusion contains pus, it is called **pyo/thorax** or **empyema** (em″pi-e′mə). This condition is an extension of infection from

pleural

nearby structures. Empyema is when the _____ effusion contains pus.

Untreated empyema can lead to **pulmonary fibrosis,** also called fibrosis of the lungs. The combining form fibr(o) means fiber or fibrous (tough, threadlike). Pulmonary fibrosis is a

fibrous

_____ condition of the connective tissue of the lungs, resulting from the formation of scar tissue.

chest

9-76 **Hydrothorax** (hi″dro-thor′aks) is a noninflammatory accumulation of fluid in one or both pleural cavities. Literal interpretation of hydro/thorax is watery _____.

An accumulation of blood and fluid in the pleural cavity is called **hemo/thorax** (he″mo-thor′aks). Trauma, such as a knife wound, is the most common cause of hemothorax, but it can occur as a result of inflammation or tumors. Write this new term that means blood

hemothorax

and fluid in the pleural cavity: _____.

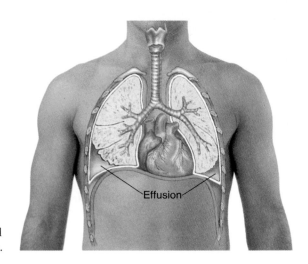

Figure 9-16 Pleural effusion. Abnormal accumulation of fluid in the pleural space is characterized by fever, chest pain, dyspnea, and nonproductive cough.

blood

pleura

pleuritis

lungs

pleura

9-77 Pneumo/thorax (noo″mo-thor′aks) is air or gas in the pleural cavity; it leads to collapse of the lung. This may be the result of an open chest wound that permits the entrance of air, rupture of a vesicle on the surface of the lung, or a severe bout of coughing; it may even occur spontaneously without apparent cause. (Both pneumothorax and hemothorax are illustrated in Figure 9-17.)
   Pneumo/hemo/thorax (noo″mo-he″mo-thor′aks) is an accumulation of air and _____ in the pleural cavity.

9-78 Pleur/itis (ploŏ-ri′tis) is inflammation of the _____.
Pleurisy (ploor′ĭ-se) is another name for pleuritis. Pleurisy may be caused by an infection, injury, or tumor, or it may be a complication of certain lung diseases. A sharp pain on inspiration is characteristic of pleurisy. A pleural friction rub may be heard on auscultation.
   Pleurisy is another name for _____.

9-79 Pleuro/pneumon/ia (ploor″o-noŏ-mo′ne-ə) is a combination of pleurisy and pneumonia. You will need to remember that pleuropneumonia is inflammation of both the pleura and the _____.

9-80 Pleuro/dynia (ploor″o-din′e-ə) is pain of the pleura. This can be caused by inflammation of the pleura or by **pleural adhesions,** in which the pleural membranes stick together or to the wall of the chest and produce pain on movement or breathing. Adhesion means a sticking together of two surfaces that are normally separated. Pleural adhesion may be associated with pleur/itis, which is inflammation of the _____.

Figure 9-17 Two abnormal conditions of the chest cavity. A, Pneumothorax is air or gas in the chest cavity. The *arrows* indicate the two situations that result in pneumothorax. *Arrow 1* represents an open chest wound that permits the entrance of air into the pleural space. *Arrow 2* represents a tear within the lung that allows air to enter the pleural space. **B,** Hemothorax, blood in the pleural cavity, below the left lung. The massive hemothorax shown has caused much of the left lung to collapse.

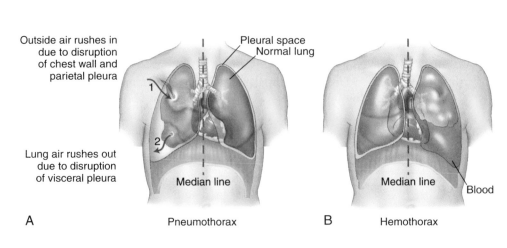

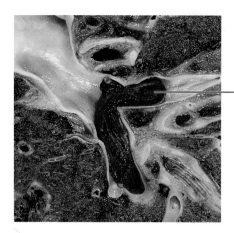

— Embolus

Figure 9-18 Embolus. This particular internal blood clot broke loose and traveled from a lower extremity and is now located in a pulmonary artery branch.

lung

9-81 Pulmonary edema is an accumulation of extravascular fluid in _____ tissue. Pulmonary edema also involves the alveoli and progresses to fluid entering the bronchioles and bronchi. Dyspnea on exertion is one of the earliest symptoms of pulmonary edema. As the condition becomes more advanced, the patient may become orthopneic. Acute pulmonary edema is an emergency situation. Congestive heart failure is the most common cause of pulmonary edema.

In **congestive heart failure,** the work demanded of the heart is greater than its ability to perform. Decreased output of blood by the left ventricle produces congestion and engorgement of the pulmonary vessels with escape of fluid into pulmonary tissues. Congestive heart failure

pulmonary

can result in the lung disorder, _____ edema.

pulmonary

9-82 A **pulmon/ary embolus** (em´bo-ləs) is an obstruction of the _____ artery or one of its branches (Figure 9-18). Obstruction of a large pulmonary vessel can cause sudden death.

EXERCISE 15

Match these pathologies with their descriptions.

_____ 1. accumulation of extravascular fluid in lung tissue

_____ 2. air or gas in the pleural cavity

_____ 3. blood and fluid in the pleural cavity

_____ 4. inflammation of the lungs

_____ 5. localized pus-containing cavity surrounded by inflamed lung tissue

_____ 6. noninflammatory accumulation of fluid in one or both pleural cavities

_____ 7. nonpurulent fluid in the pleural cavity

_____ 8. obstruction of a pulmonary artery or one of its branches

A. hemothorax
B. hydrothorax
C. pleural effusion
D. pneumonia
E. pneumothorax
F. pulmonary abscess
G. pulmonary edema
H. pulmonary embolus

dust

9-83 The lungs of a newborn are pink. The adult lung darkens as a result of dust, soot, or other environmental pollutants. **Pneumo/coni/osis** (noo˝mo-ko˝ne-o´sis) is any disease of the lung caused by chronic inhalation of dust, usually mineral dust of either occupational or environmental origin.

The combining form coni(o) means dust. Pneumoconiosis is a condition (disease) of the lungs caused by inhalation of _____.

coal

9-84 Anthracosis (an-thrə-ko´sis), asbestosis (as˝bes-to´sis), and silicosis (sil˝ĭ-ko´sis) are three kinds of pneumoconiosis. The combining form anthrac(o) means coal. **Anthrac/osis** is a chronic lung disease characterized by the deposit of _____ dust in the lungs. It occurs in coal miners and is aggravated by cigarette smoking.

asbestos

Asbest/osis is a chronic lung disease that results from prolonged exposure to
_____. It may occur in asbestos miners and workers or those exposed to asbestos building materials. **Mesothelioma** (me″zo-the″le-o′mə), a rare malignant tumor, sometimes develops and is almost always fatal. The mesothelium is a layer of epithelial cells that covers the pleura and the peritoneum.

pneumoconiosis

Silic/osis is a lung disorder caused by long-term inhalation of silica dust, which is found in sands, quartzes, and many other stones. This lung disorder is a type of
_____.

9-85 Chronic obstructive pulmonary disease (COPD), also called chronic obstructive lung disease (COLD), is a nonspecific designation that includes a group of progressive and irreversible respiratory problems in which dyspnea and chronic cough are prominent features. The mechanism of air trapping is explained in Figure 9-19. Airflow obstruction ultimately occurs. Emphysema, chronic bronchitis, asthmatic bronchitis, bronchiectasis, and cystic fibrosis are often included in this group. COPD is aggravated by cigarette smoking and air pollution.

Emphysema[*] (em″fə-se′mə), characterized by overinflation and destructive changes in alveolar walls, is probably the most severe COPD. Permanent hyperinflation of the lungs occurs as alveoli are destroyed, and alveolar air is trapped, thus interfering with exchange of carbon dioxide and oxygen.

Overinflation and destruction of the alveolar walls are major characteristics of

emphysema

_____.

9-86 **Cystic fibrosis** is an inherited disorder of the exocrine glands that involves the lungs, pancreas, and sweat glands. Heavy secretion of thick mucus clogs the bronchi and leads to a chronic cough and persistent upper respiratory infections. Excessive salt loss (three to six times the normal concentrations) in the perspiration of persons who have cystic fibrosis forms the basis of the sweat test, a laboratory test to determine the amount of sodium and chloride excretion from the sweat glands. The disease is usually diagnosed in infancy or early childhood. The

fibrosis

sweat test is performed to diagnose cystic _____.

9-87 **Atel/ectasis** (atel[o], imperfect + -ectasis, stretching) (at″ə-lek′tə-sis) is an abnormal condition characterized by the collapse of all or part of a lung. Failure of the lungs to expand fully at birth is called primary atelectasis. Other causes of atelectasis include obstructions of the airways, compression of the lung as a result of fluid or air, and pressure from a tumor.

atelectasis

Write the name of this abnormal condition in which there is incomplete expansion of a lung at birth or airlessness of a lung that once functioned: _____.

---

[*]Emphysema (Greek: *en*, inside; *physema*, a blowing).

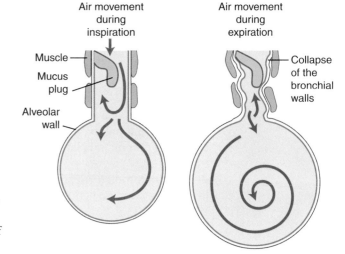

Figure 9-19 Mechanisms of air trapping in chronic obstructive pulmonary disease. Air trapping is the result of an inefficient expiratory effort. As the rate of respiration increases, breathing becomes shallower and the amount of trapped air increases.

9-88 Tuberculosis (too-ber″ku-lo´sis) (TB) is an infectious disease that often is chronic and commonly affects the lungs, although it may occur in other parts of the body. Pulmonary tuberculosis affects the _____.

lungs

Resistance to tuberculosis depends a great deal on a person's general health. Early symptoms of tuberculosis (loss of energy, appetite, and weight) may go unnoticed. Fever, night sweats, and spitting up of bloody or purulent sputum may not occur until a year or more after the initial exposure to the disease. The disease is named after **tubercles** (too´bər-kəlz), which are small, round nodules produced in the lungs by the infective bacteria.

9-89 Liquefaction of the tubercles not only results in tubercular cavities in the lungs but can also cause the production of a large quantity of highly infectious sputum that is raised when the infected person coughs.

out

To **ex/pectorate** (ek-spek´tə-rāt) is to cough up and spit _____ material from the lungs and air passages. (The material coughed up from the lungs is sputum.) Blood-stained sputum is often produced in tuberculosis. **Hemo/ptysis** (he-mop´tĭ-sis) is the spitting of blood or blood-stained sputum.

EXERCISE 16

Write terms for the following meanings.

1. a lung disease characterized by the deposit of coal dust in the lungs _____

2. any disease of the lung characterized by chronic inhalation of dust _____

3. collapse of all or part of a lung _____

4. spitting of blood or blood-stained sputum _____

EXERCISE 17

Multiple Choice
Circle the correct answer.

1. Overinflation and destructive changes in alveolar walls are characteristics of which of the following? (congenital atelectasis, emphysema, mesothelioma, pleuropneumonia).

2. Which of the following represents a group of progressive and irreversible respiratory problems in which dyspnea is a prominent feature? (COPD, cystic fibrosis, embolism, pulmonary edema).

3. Which of the following is *not* a type of pneumoconiosis? (anthracosis, asbestosis, emphysema, silicosis)

4. Which of the following is an inherited disorder of the exocrine glands that involves the lungs, pancreas, and sweat glands? (congestive heart failure, cystic fibrosis, pneumohemothorax, pulmonary edema)

 Say and Check

Say the terms in the last two exercises aloud. Use the Companion CD to check your pronunciations.

SURGICAL AND THERAPEUTIC INTERVENTIONS

9-90 Asphyxiation, the inability to breathe, requires immediate corrective measures to prevent damage or death. Removal of a foreign body in the airway may be needed before oxygen and artificial respiration are administered. One method of dislodging food or other obstruction from the windpipe is the **Heimlich** (hīm´lik) **maneuver** (Figure 9-20).

Artificial respiration may be manual, as in the lifesaving procedure **cardiopulmonary resuscitation** (CPR), or provided by a mechanical ventilator, a device used to provide assisted respiration and usually temporary life support. CPR consists of artificial respiration and external cardiac massage.

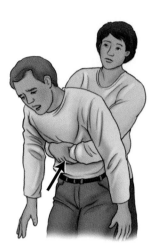

Figure 9-20 Heimlich maneuver. The rescuer grasps the choking person from behind, placing the thumb side of the fist against the victim's abdomen, in the midline, slightly above the navel and well below the breastbone. Abruptly pulling the fist firmly upward will often force the obstruction up the windpipe.

opening

A **tracheo/stomy** (tra″ke-os′tə-me), surgical creation of an _____ in the trachea, may be necessary in upper airway obstruction. A tracheostomy requires a **tracheo/tomy** (tra″ke-ot′ə-me), an incision into the trachea through the neck below the larynx.

9-91 A tracheostomy is not always an emergency procedure and can be temporary or permanent. A tracheostomy is performed after a **laryngectomy** (lar″in-jek′tə-me) or when prolonged mechanical ventilation is needed. A tube is inserted through an incision in the neck into the trachea. There are many types of tracheostomy tubes; some permit speech.

Sometimes a person has a stoma at the base of the neck. Surgical creation of this type of opening into the trachea is called a tracheostomy. A general term for a mouthlike opening is a

stoma

_____.

9-92 In COPD or other problems in hypoxic patients, oxygen therapy may be prescribed by the physician. Oxygen is sometimes administered after general surgery.

In patients who can breathe but are hypoxic, oxygen is delivered through tubing via a simple face mask, nasal prongs, a **Venturi mask,** or **trans/tracheal** (trans-tra′ke-əl) oxygen (TTO) delivery. A Venturi mask and a transtracheal oxygen system deliver a more consistent and accurate oxygen concentration. Compare the four types of airway management shown in Figure 9-21. The term **nasal cannula** (kan′u-lə) refers to either of the two small tubes that are inserted into the nares. Other types of cannulas (cannulae) may be inserted into a duct or cavity to either deliver medication or drain fluid. The nasal cannula shown in Figure 9-21, *B*, delivers oxygen. TTO delivers oxygen to the lungs through a flexible catheter that is inserted directly into the trachea.

9-93 Oxygen is administered in hypoxic patients to increase the amount of oxygen in circulating blood. It is also administered during anesthesia, because oxygen functions as a carrier gas for the delivery of anesthetic agents to the tissues of the body. An overdose of oxygen can have toxic effects, which include respiratory depression and damage to the lungs. Using hyp/ox/emia as a model, write a word that means increased oxygen content of the blood:

hyperoxemia
(hi″pər-ok-se′me-ə)

_____.

9-94 Endo/tracheal intubation is the management of the patient with an airway catheter inserted through the mouth or nose into the trachea. An endotracheal tube may be used to maintain a patent (open and unblocked) airway or to maintain a closed system with a ventilator.

Naso/tracheal (na″zo-tra′ke-əl) **intubation** is insertion of a tube through the nose into the trachea. **Orotracheal** (or″o-tra′ke-əl) **intubation** is insertion of a tube through the mouth into

trachea

the _____. Compare these two types of intubation with a **tracheostomy tube** that is used for prolonged airway management (Figure 9-22).

9-95 Mechanical ventilation is the use of an artificial device to assist in breathing. It is a means of supporting patients until either they recover sufficiently to breathe independently or the decision is made to withdraw respiratory support.

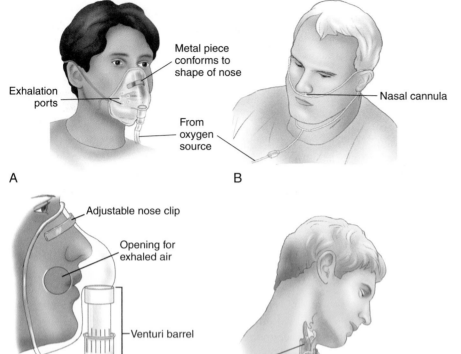

Figure 9-21 **Four means of administering oxygen. A,** A simple oxygen mask delivers high concentrations of oxygen and is used for short-term oxygen therapy or in an emergency. **B,** The nasal cannula, a device that delivers oxygen by way of two small tubes that are inserted into the nostrils. **C,** The Venturi mask, a face mask designed to allow inspired air to mix with oxygen. **D,** Transtracheal oxygen is a long-term method of delivering oxygen directly into the lungs.

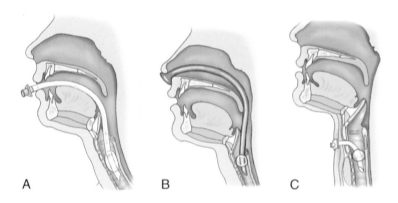

Figure 9-22 **Comparison of endotracheal intubation and a tracheostomy tube. A,** Orotracheal intubation for short-term airway management. **B,** Nasotracheal intubation for short-term airway management. **C,** Tracheostomy tube for longer maintenance of the airway.

> ➤ KEY POINT The two major types of mechanical ventilation are negative pressure and positive pressure ventilation. In negative pressure ventilation, the chest is pulled outward by chambers that encase the chest or body and air rushes into the lungs. Portable ventilators of this type are sometimes used in the home (Figure 9-23, *A*). More acutely ill patients require positive pressure ventilators, which push air into the lungs (Figure 9-23, *B*).

Using an artificial device to assist a patient to breathe is called mechanical

ventilation   _____.

9-96 Oxygenation means the act or process of adding oxygen. Extra/corpor/eal means outside the body. **Extracorporeal membrane oxygenator** (ECMO) is a device used in a hospital to provide respiratory support by circulating the blood through an artificial lung, then returning the blood to the patient's circulatory system. It is used in newborns and occasionally in adults with acute respiratory distress syndrome.

oxygenator   ECMO is the abbreviation for extracorporeal membrane _____.

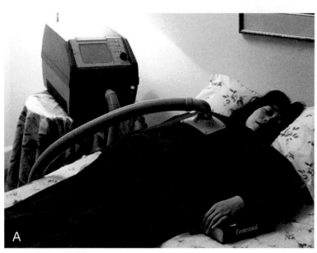
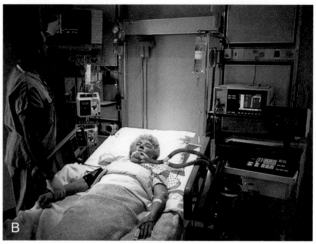

Figure 9-23 Negative pressure and positive pressure mechanical ventilation. A, Negative pressure ventilation. **B,** Positive pressure ventilation in a hospital setting.

9-97 The term thoracentesis (thor″ə-sen-te′sis) is a shortened form of the term **thoracocentesis** (thor″ə-ko-sen-te′sis). **Thora/centesis** is surgical puncture of the chest wall and pleural space with a needle to aspirate fluid or to obtain a specimen for biopsy. It has both therapeutic and diagnostic uses.

puncture

Thora/centesis is surgical _____ of the chest wall and can be used in the treatment of pleural effusion (Figure 9-24).

Thoracentesis is sometimes called pleurocentesis (ploor″o-sen-te′sis).

If fluid has accumulated in the lung itself, the procedure of puncturing the lung to drain the fluid contents is **pneumo/centesis** (noo″mo-sen-te′sis).

9-98 A **pneumonectomy** (noo″mo-nek′tə-me), either partial or complete, is usually required for treating lung cancer. Removal of a lung requires an open surgery that will provide full access to structures in the chest cavity. A total pneumon/ectomy is removal of an entire lung. If only part of the lung is removed, the surgery is called a partial pneumonectomy. **Pneum/ectomy** (noo-mek′tə-me) has the same meaning as pneumonectomy. Write a term that means a surgical

thoracotomy

incision into the chest: _____.

Either radiation or chemo/therapy or both may be used to destroy remaining tumor cells or in certain types of localized malignancies.

9-99 A **lob/ectomy** is an excision of a single lobe. Because other organs, such as the liver and brain, also have lobes, one has to specify pulmonary lobectomy, unless it is clear that the

lung

lobectomy refers to the _____.

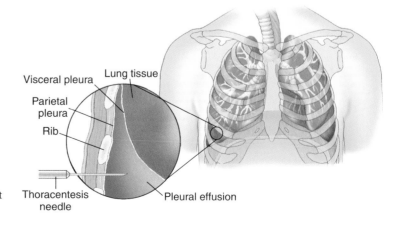

Figure 9-24 Insertion of the needle in thoracentesis. The actual site for insertion depends on the location of the effusion and the material that has escaped into the pleural space. Thoracocentesis means the same as thoracentesis, but the latter term is used more often.

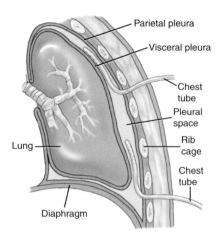

- Parietal pleura
- Visceral pleura
- Chest tube
- Pleural space
- Rib cage
- Chest tube
- Lung
- Diaphragm

Figure 9-25 Placement of chest tubes. A chest tube is a catheter that is inserted through the thorax into the pleural space and is attached to a water-seal chest drainage device. The chest tube is used to remove fluid or air after chest surgery and lung collapse.

A **thoraco/stomy** is an incision made into the chest wall to provide an opening for a chest tube. A chest tube is inserted into the pleural space to remove air and/or fluid and is commonly used after chest surgery (Figure 9-25).

9-100 Trauma of the head and face may result in the need for plastic surgery of various respiratory organs. However, rhino/plasty (ri′no-plas″te) is usually done for cosmetic reasons. **Rhino/plasty** is plastic surgery of the _____.

nose

Palato/plasty (pal′ə-to-plas″te) is surgical repair (reconstruction) of the palate. Palatoplasty, along with additional plastic surgery, is used to correct cleft palate, a congenital defect characterized by a fissure in the midline of the palate. Write the term that means plastic surgery of the palate: _____.

palatoplasty

9-101 Tracheoplasty (tra′ke-o-plas″te) is plastic surgery to repair the trachea. Write a term using sept(o), rhin(o), and -plasty: _____. This new term means plastic surgery of the nasal septum and the external nose. Surgical reconstruction of the nasal septum is **septoplasty** (sep′to-plas″te).

septorhinoplasty
(sep″to-ri′no-plas″te)

Thoraco/plasty (thor′ə-ko-plas″te) is a surgical procedure that involves removing ribs and allowing the chest wall to collapse a lung. The procedure, a therapeutic measure, is sometimes done to gain access during thoracic surgery. The procedure done to collapse a lung is called a _____.

thoracoplasty

EXERCISE 18

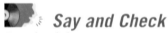 **Build It!** *Use the following word parts to build terms. (Some word parts will be used more than once.)*

laryng(o), pneumon(o), thorac(o), trache(o), -centesis, -ectomy, -plasty, -tomy

1. surgical removal of the voice box   _____/_____

2. surgical puncture of the chest wall and pleural space to aspirate fluid   _____/_____

3. plastic surgery to repair the trachea   _____/_____

4. incision into the trachea   _____/_____

5. partial or complete surgical removal of a lung   _____/_____

Say and Check

Say aloud the terms you wrote for Exercise 18. Use the Companion CD to check your pronunciations.

adenoids

9-102 For mild sleep apnea, weight loss or a change in sleeping position may reduce or correct the problem. A common nonsurgical method to prevent airway collapse is the use of continuous positive airway pressure (CPAP ventilation). A small electric compressor delivers positive pressure through a face mask during sleep (Figure 9-26).

Surgical intervention for sleep apnea may involve an **adenoid/ectomy** (ad″ə-noid-ek′tə-me), excision of the _____, **uvul/ectomy** (u″vu-lek′tə-me), excision of the uvula, the pendant tissue in the back of the pharynx, or surgical repair of the posterior oropharynx. Both conventional and laser surgeries are used for this purpose.

neoplasms

9-103 An anti/neoplas/tic is a treatment that acts against _____. These treatments are designed to kill or prevent the spread of cancer cells.

> ➤ **KEY** POINT <u>Many malignant lesions may be curable if detected in the early stage</u>. Treatment selection depends on the site, stage of the cancer, and unique characteristics of the individual. Some anti/cancer treatments include surgery, irradiation, and chemotherapy with anti-neoplastic agents. Irradiation uses radiant energy such as x-rays and radioactive substances to treat cancer.

9-104 A method of encouraging voluntary deep breathing after surgery or with patients who have chronic air obstruction involves use of an incentive spirometer, a small apparatus that provides visual feedback about the inspired volume of air (Figure 9-27). While in the hospital, a registered pulmonary function therapist (RPFT) is involved in respiratory treatments and evaluating progress. Patients may also be seen by a **pulmono/logist** (pool″mə-nol′ə-jist), a physician specializing in evaluating and treating lung disorders.

Nebulizers (neb′u-li″zərz) and inhalers are used to administer medications that are inhaled. **Bronchodilators** (brong″ko-di′la-tərz) are medications used in asthma and other respiratory conditions that constrict air passages. A broncho/dilator expands the bronchi (bronchodilation) and other air passages. An agent that dilates the bronchi is a

bronchodilator

_____. **Anti/asthmatics** (an″te-az-mat′iks) are medications that prevent or treat the symptoms of asthma.

9-105 Respiratory infections are generally treated with antibiotics, along with other medications that individual patients need. For example, **decongestants*** cause vasoconstriction of the nasal membranes, thereby eliminating or reducing swelling or congestion.

---

*Decongestant (*de-*, away or remove; Latin: *congerere*, to pile up).

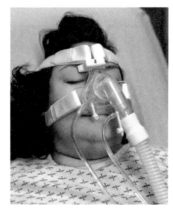

Figure 9-26 Noninvasive use of CPAP to alleviate mild sleep apnea. This machine may be used in the home setting to maintain adequate blood oxygen levels while sleeping.

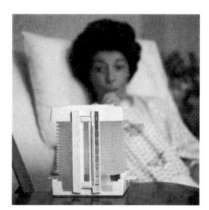

Figure 9-27 Incentive spirometry. A therapeutic means of encouraging deep breathing using a specially designed spirometer that provides visual feedback.

against	**Anti/histamines** (an″te-, an″ti-his′tə-mēnz) are also used to treat colds and allergies. Antihistamines act _____ histamine to reduce its effects. Histamine brings about many of the symptoms that occur with the common cold.
against	**9-106 Anti/tussive** (an″te-, an″ti-tus′iv) means _____ coughing. In other words, antitussive* means preventing or relieving coughing, or an agent that does so.
mucolytic (mu″ko-lit′ik)	Use muc(o) plus a suffix to write a word that means destroying or dissolving mucus: _____. **Muco/lytic** is a term that also means an agent that destroys or dissolves mucus. An abundance of mucus is produced in certain respiratory disorders, such as emphysema. Mucolytics and bronchodilators are often used in treating these patients to open their breathing passages.

*Antitussive (*anti-*, against; Latin: *tussis,* cough).

EXERCISE 19

Write words in the blanks to complete these sentences. The first letters of the answers are given as clues.

1. The inability to breathe is a_____.

2. Artificial respiration and external cardiac massage are administered in cardiopulmonary r_____.

3. In a hospital setting, artificial respiration is supplied by a mechanical v_____.

4. Surgical creation of an opening into the trachea is called a t_____.

5. COPD means chronic o_____ pulmonary disease.

6. TTO is the abbreviation for t_____ oxygen, which is a means of delivering oxygen to the lungs.

7. Insertion of a tube through the mouth into the trachea is called o_____ intubation.

8. Pneumocentesis is surgical puncture of a l_____ to drain fluid contents.

9. A t_____ is an incision made into the chest wall to provide an opening for a chest tube.

10. An agent that prevents coughing is called an a_____.

CHAPTER ABBREVIATIONS*

ABG	arterial blood gas	PFT	pulmonary function test
ARDS	acute or adult respiratory distress syndrome	pH	potential hydrogen; symbol for hydrogen ion concentration
CAL	chronic airflow limitation		
CO_2	carbon dioxide	RDS	respiratory distress syndrome
COLD	chronic obstructive lung disease	RPFT	registered pulmonary function therapist
COPD	chronic obstructive pulmonary disease	SARS	severe acute respiratory syndrome
CPAP	continuous positive airway pressure (for sleep apnea)	SIDS	sudden infant death syndrome
		SOB	shortness of breath
CPR	cardiopulmonary resuscitation	TB	tuberculosis
CSR	Cheyne-Stokes respiration	TTO	transtracheal oxygen
ECMO	extracorporeal membrane oxygenation	URI	upper respiratory infection
HSV	herpes simplex virus	VC	vital capacity
O_2	oxygen		

*Many of these abbreviations share their meanings with other terms. CO_2 and O_2 are chemical symbols.

▶ CHAPTER 9 REVIEW

Basic Understanding

Matching

I. *Match structures in the left column (1-7) with their characteristics or functions in the right column (A-G).*

_____ 1. alveolus
_____ 2. bronchus
_____ 3. diaphragm
_____ 4. larynx
_____ 5. nose
_____ 6. pharynx
_____ 7. trachea

A. a branch of the trachea
B. a muscular partition that facilitates breathing
C. commonly called the windpipe
D. connected with the paranasal sinuses
E. contains the palatine tonsils
F. contains the vocal cords
G. where oxygen and carbon dioxide exchange occurs

II. *Match diseases or disorders in the left column (1-7) with their characteristics in the right column (A-G).*

_____ 1. anthracosis
_____ 2. asthma
_____ 3. atelectasis
_____ 4. COPD
_____ 5. cystic fibrosis
_____ 6. emphysema
_____ 7. pertussis

A. accumulation of coal dust in the lungs
B. can result from disorders such as chronic bronchitis and chronic asthma
C. chronic respiratory infection and disorders of the pancreas and sweat glands
D. congenital, incomplete expansion of a lung or a portion of a lung
E. destruction of the alveolar walls that leads to hindered gas exchange
F. paroxysmal cough, ending in a whooping inspiration
G. paroxysmal dyspnea accompanied by wheezing

Labeling

III. *Label structures in the diagram with the corresponding combining form. The first one is done as an example. Note that number 2 and number 6 have two answers.*

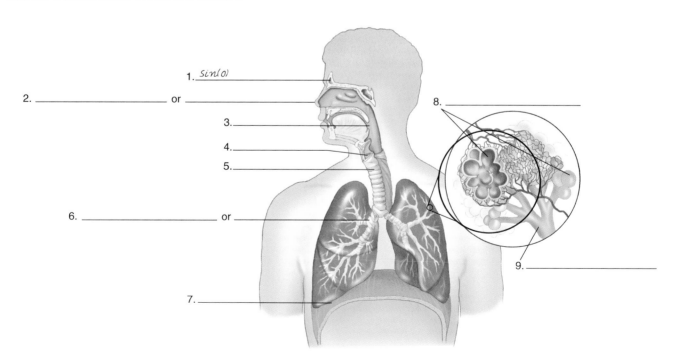

1. _Sin(0)_
2. _____ or _____
3. _____
4. _____
5. _____
6. _____ or _____
7. _____
8. _____
9. _____

Sequencing

IV. *Number the following structures to show the sequence of passage of air from the nose to the lungs. The first one is done as an example.*

nasal cavity ___1___   bronchi _____   larynx _____   pharynx _____

trachea _____   alveoli _____   bronchioles _____

Listing

V. *List five functions of the respiratory system.*

1. _____

2. _____

3. _____

4. _____

5. _____

Matching

VI. *Select A (upper respiratory tract) or B (lower respiratory tract) to identify the locations of these structures.*

1. alveolus _____   5. nose _____   A. upper respiratory tract
                                                          B. lower respiratory tract
2. bronchiole _____   6. pharynx _____

3. bronchus _____   7. trachea _____

4. larynx _____

Photo ID

VII. *Use word parts to write terms to label these pictures.*

Pleural space
Normal lung

Median line

1. _____/_____
      (air)   (chest)

Median line
Blood

2. _____/_____
      (blood)   (chest)

3. _____/_____
      (bronchi)   (visual examination)

Lung tissue
Visceral pleura
Parietal pleura
Rib
Thoracentesis needle
Pleural effusion

4. _____/_____
      (chest)   (surgical puncture)

VIII. *Label these patterns of respiration.*

Regular at a rate
of 12-20 breaths per minute

Slower than 12 breaths
per minute

Faster than 20 breaths
per minute

Deep breathing, faster than
20 breaths per minute

1. _____/_____
   (good)   (breathing)

2. _____/_____
   (slow)   (breathing)

3. _____/_____
   (fast)   (breathing)

4. _____/_____
   (greater than normal)   (breathing)

Multiple Choice

IX. *Circle one answer for each of the following multiple choice questions.*

1. Mrs. Smith's doctor tells her that she has pneumonia. What is another name for her diagnosis?
   (congestive heart disease, pneumonitis, pulmonary edema, pulmonary insufficiency)

2. Which term means coughing up and spitting out sputum? (expectoration, expiration, exhalation, extrapleural)

3. John R. is told that he suffers periodic absence of breathing. What is the name of his condition?
   (apnea, dyspnea, hyperpnea, hypopnea)

4. Which of the following activities is the respiratory system's greatest contribution to the acid-base balance?
   (exchange of CO_2 for O_2, maintaining body temperature, regulating water loss, taking in water)

5. What is the serous membrane that lines the walls of the thoracic cavity?
   (parietal pleura, rhinorrhea, silicosis, visceral pleura)

6. Which term refers to a sudden recurrence or intensity of symptoms?
   (atelectasis, extracorporeal, hypoventilation, paroxysmal)

7. Mrs. Sema has difficulty breathing except when sitting in an upright position. What is the term for her condition?
   (anoxia, hypocapnia, inspiration, orthopnea)

8. What is the term for reduced acidity of the body fluids, such as may occur in hyperventilation?
   (acid-base balance, acid-base compensation, acidosis, alkalosis)

9. The pulmonary specialist orders a test to measure the amount of air taken into and expelled from the lungs. What
   is the name of the test? (laryngoscopy, mediastinoscopy, spirometry, thoracometry)

10. What is effusion of fluid into the air spaces and tissue spaces of the lungs called? (pleuropneumonia, pneumonitis,
    pulmonary edema, pulmonary insufficiency)

Writing Terms

X. *Write a term for each of the following.*

1. an internal blood clot _____

2. difficult or weak voice _____

3. direct visualization
   of the bronchi _____

4. drawing in or out
   as by suction _____

5. inflammation of
   the throat _____

6. presence of
   nasal calculi _____

7. pertaining to the air
   sacs of the lung _____

8. radiographic examination
   of the larynx _____

9. profuse nosebleed _____

10. within the nose _____

Say and Check

Say aloud the terms you wrote for Exercise X. Use the Companion CD to check your pronunciations.

Greater Comprehension

Health Care Reports

XI. *Define the underlined terms or abbreviations in the following Pulmonary Function Clinic Note.*

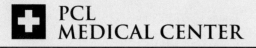

PCL MEDICAL CENTER

7700 Lexicon Way
St. Louis, MO 63146

Phone (555) 437-0000 • Fax (555) 437-0001

PULMONARY FUNCTION CLINIC NOTE

Patient Name: Fay Schmidt   **ID No.:** 009-3001   **Date:** Mar 6, ----
REFERRING PHYSICIAN: Ruth Wong, MD, Pulmonologist
THERAPY ORDERED: This 63-year-old female patient with <u>COPD</u> is seen at the request of Dr. Wong, who ordered <u>nebulizer</u> treatments with 1 mL albuterol and 0.5 mg Atrovent q. 4 h.
GOAL OF THERAPY: Treat <u>hypoventilation</u> and <u>hypoxemia</u>. Relieve <u>bronchospasm</u>, <u>bronchodilation</u>. Clearance of mucus. Also patient education.
ASSESSMENT: Bilateral lobes with decreased breath sounds before treatment. Patient had <u>paroxysmal</u> coughing spell during treatment with some <u>dyspnea</u> noted. Treatment stopped at patient request. Oxygen saturation level 95% on 1.5 L O_2 per <u>nasal cannula</u> after treatment.
DIAGNOSIS: Chronic obstructive pulmonary disease

Zoe Blum, RPFT, MS
Zoe Blum, RPFT, MS
Chief of Service

---

1. COPD _____

2. nebulizer _____

3. hypoventilation _____

4. hypoxemia _____

5. bronchospasm _____

6. bronchodilation _____

7. paroxysmal _____

8. dyspnea _____

9. nasal cannula _____

10. RPFT _____

XII. *Read the following History and Physical and answer the questions that follow it.*

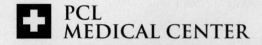

PCL MEDICAL CENTER

7700 Lexicon Way
St. Louis, MO 63146

Phone (555) 437-0000 • Fax (555) 437-0001

BRIEF HISTORY AND PHYSICAL EXAMINATION

Patient: Margaret Ann Gordon   **ID No.:** 009-3002   **Date:** May 4, ----

CHIEF COMPLAINT: Fever with mild dyspnea. Productive cough. Malaise and loss of appetite.

PAST HISTORY: This 63-year-old female patient, well known to me, has a history of bronchitis, myocardial infarction (status post CABG one year ago), and deep venous thrombosis with pulmonary embolism.

FAMILY HISTORY: Mother is living at age 85 with congestive heart failure. Father deceased with a history of COLD and type 2 DM.

PHYSICAL EXAM: Vital signs show T 100.8, P 98, R 28, BP 160/94. O_2 saturation level 92% on 2 L oxygen. Exam limited to chest: Fine crackles at bilateral lung bases with some wheezes. Increased dyspnea on exertion.

DIAGNOSTIC DATA: WBCs 24.6. Chest x-ray with increased right lung density. No pneumothorax or pleural effusion. Increasing right lung infiltrate with masslike density, right hilum. Sputum collected for culture.

DIAGNOSIS: Community-acquired pneumonia.

TREATMENT PLAN: IV antibiotics pending sputum culture results. Bronchodilator, such as Alupent. Expectorant, such as guaifenesin.

Ruth Wong, MD
Ruth Wong, MD
Pulmonologist

Write the answer from the report that corresponds to each of these descriptions.

1. a vague feeling of discomfort and fatigue   _____

2. abnormal accumulation of fluid in the pleural space   _____

3. abnormal musical respiratory sounds   _____

4. abnormal respiratory sounds that consist of discontinuous
   bubbling noises   _____

5. the presence of air or gas in the pleural space   _____

6. inflammation of the bronchi   _____

7. chronic obstructive lung disease   _____

8. the blockage of a pulmonary artery by a substance brought
   by the circulating blood   _____

9. therapeutic agent that relaxes the bronchioles   _____

10. therapeutic agent that assists in the coughing up of sputum _____

XIII. *Read the following partial report of a History and Physical Examination. Then define the underlined terms.*

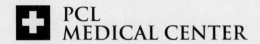

PCL
MEDICAL CENTER

7700 Lexicon Way
St. Louis, MO 63146

Phone (555) 437-0000 • Fax (555) 437-0001

PULMONARY CLINIC HISTORY AND PHYSICAL EXAM

Patient Name: Tonya Wells   **ID No.:** 009-3003   **Date:** 21 June ——
HISTORY: Patient is a 52-year-old woman, a former 23-pack-year smoker, with history of severe <u>idiopathic</u> <u>pulmonary hypertension</u> and class III dyspnea on exertion treated with bosentan 125 mg b.i.d. Recently started on <u>inhaled</u> Ventavis 6× to 9× per day per Pulmonary Clinic. Patient here in follow-up. She reports significant improvement in dyspnea on exertion since initiation of inhaled Ventavis. She began that medication on 5 May and has been using as prescribed every 2 to 3 hours. She describes some brief headaches associated with each dose, but these are tolerable. Previously she was able to walk only about half a block before becoming <u>dyspneic</u>. Now she is able to walk at least 2 blocks since starting on Ventavis. She continues to report a very mild intermittent dry cough. Denies <u>hemoptysis</u>, chest pain, and syncope. She has been using nocturnal <u>CPAP</u> at 9 cm of water pressure every night as prescribed. Has also been using 1 L oxygen bleed-in with CPAP; however, she is asking if she needs to continue this. She is tolerating bosentan and has had normal LFTs every month. She has been therapeutic on Coumadin, which is managed by the Coumadin Clinic.
ALLERGIES: Sulfa drugs, also some environmental allergies
MEDICATIONS

1. bosentan 125 mg p.o. b.i.d.
2. Ventavis 6 to 9 inhalations per day
3. Coumadin daily
4. lithium b.i.d.

1. idiopathic _____

2. pulmonary hypertension _____

3. inhaled _____

4. dyspneic _____

5. hemoptysis _____

6. CPAP _____

Spelling
XIV. *Circle all misspelled terms and write their correct spellings:*

acapnia   auscultation   bronchiectasis   laryngografy   pnumonitis

Pronunciation
XV. *The pronunciation is shown for several medical words. Indicate which syllable has the primary accent by marking it with an ´.*

1. laryngopathy (lar ing gop ə the)

2. parietal (pə ri ə təl)

3. pharyngeal (fə rin je əl)

4. spirometer (spi rom ə tər)

5. tracheostomy (tra ke os tə me)

Say and Check

Say aloud the five terms in Exercise XV. Use the Companion CD to check your pronunciations. In addition, be prepared to pronounce aloud these terms in class:

alveoli	bronchopulmonary	hyperpnea	spirometry
anthracosis	bronchoscopy	hypoxemia	subphrenic
antiasthmatic	coryza	pneumocentesis	tachypnea
antitussive	empyema	pyothorax	thoracostomy
asphyxia	hemoptysis	rhinolithiasis	uvulectomy
atelectasis			

Interpreting Abbreviations

XVI. *Write the meaning of these abbreviations.*

1. ABG _____

2. ECMO _____

3. HSV _____

4. SARS _____

5. URI _____

Categorizing Terms

XVII. *Classify the terms in the left columns (1-10) by selecting category A, B, C, D, or E.*

_____ 1. anthracosis   _____ 6. naris

_____ 2. antitussives   _____ 7. oximeter

_____ 3. bronchography   _____ 8. palatoplasty

_____ 4. coryza   _____ 9. percussion

_____ 5. epiglottis   _____ 10. rhonchus

A. anatomy
B. diagnostic test or procedure
C. pathology
D. surgery
E. therapy

Challenge

XVIII. *Break these words into their component parts, and write their meanings. Even if you have not seen these terms before, you may be able to break them apart and determine their meanings.*

1. bronchospirometry _____

2. laryngostomy _____

3. pharyngoplegia _____

4. pneumomycosis _____

5. sinoscopy _____

(Use Appendix VI to check your answers.)

PRONUNCIATION LIST

Use the Companion CD to review the terms that have been presented. Look closely at the spelling of each term as it is pronounced and be sure you know the meaning of each term.

acapnia	alkalemia	anoxia	antitussive
acidemia	alkalosis	anthracosis	aphasia
acidosis	alveolar	antiasthmatics	aphonia
adenoidectomy	alveoli	antihistamines	apical

aplasia
apnea
asbestosis
asphyxia
asphyxiation
asthma
atelectasis
auditory tube
bradypnea
bronchi
bronchial
bronchiectasis
bronchiolectasis
bronchioles
bronchiolitis
bronchitis
bronchoalveolar
bronchoconstriction
bronchodilators
bronchogenic
bronchogram
bronchography
broncholithiasis
bronchopathy
bronchopneumonia
bronchopulmonary
bronchoscope
bronchoscopic examination
bronchoscopy
bronchospasm
cardiopulmonary
    resuscitation
Cheyne-Stokes respiration
congestive heart failure
coronavirus
coryza
crackles
croup
cystic fibrosis
decongestants
diaphragm
diaphragma
diaphragmatic
diphtheria
dysphasia
dysphonia
dyspnea
dyspneic
emphysema
empyema
endotracheal intubation
epiglottides
epiglottiditis
epiglottis
epiglottitis
epistaxis
eupnea
eustachian tube

exhalation
expectorate
expiration
extracorporeal membrane
    oxygenator
extrapleural
extrapulmonary
friction rub
glottis
Heimlich maneuver
hemoptysis
hemothorax
herpes simplex virus
hilum
hydrothorax
hypercapnia
hyperoxemia
hyperpnea
hyperventilation
hypocapnia
hypopnea
hypoventilation
hypoxemia
hypoxia
influenza
inhalation
inspiration
interalveolar
lacrimal
laryngalgia
laryngeal
laryngectomy
laryngitis
laryngography
laryngopathy
laryngopharyngeal
laryngopharynx
laryngoplegia
laryngoscope
laryngoscopy
laryngospasm
laryngotracheal
laryngotracheitis
laryngotracheobronchitis
larynx
lobectomy
mediastinoscope
mediastinoscopy
mediastinum
mesothelioma
mucolytic
nares
naris
nasal
nasal cannula
nasal polyp
nasal septum
nasolacrimal duct

nasopharyngeal
nasopharyngitis
nasopharynx
nasoscope
nasotracheal intubation
nebulizers
olfaction
olfactory
oral
oropharyngeal
oropharynx
orotracheal intubation
orthopnea
oxygenation
palate
palatine
palatitis
palatoplasty
paranasal sinus
parietal pleura
paroxysmal
pertussis
pharyngalgia
pharyngeal
pharyngitis
pharyngodynia
pharyngomycosis
pharyngopathy
pharyngoscope
pharynx
phlegm
phrenic
phrenitis
phrenodynia
phrenoplegia
phrenoptosis
pleura
pleural
pleural adhesions
pleural cavity
pleural effusion
pleurisy
pleuritis
pleurodynia
pleuropneumonia
pneumectomy
pneumocentesis
pneumococcal pneumonia
pneumoconiosis
pneumohemothorax
pneumonectomy
pneumonia
pneumonitis
pneumothorax
pulmonary
pulmonary abscess
pulmonary angiography
pulmonary edema

pulmonary embolus
pulmonary fibrosis
pulmonic
pulmonologist
pulse oximeter
pulse oximetry
pyothorax
rales
respiratory system
retronasal
rhinitis
rhinolith
rhinolithiasis
rhinoplasty
rhinorrhagia
rhinorrhea
rhonchus
septoplasty
septorhinoplasty
silicosis
sinusitis
spirometer
spirometry
sputum
stridor
subphrenic
subpulmonary
supranasal
tachycardia
tachypnea
thoracentesis
thoracocentesis
thoracoplasty
thoracostomy
thromboembolic
tonsillitis
trachea
trachealgia
tracheomalacia
tracheoplasty
tracheoscopy
tracheostenosis
tracheostomy
tracheostomy tube
tracheotomy
transtracheal
tubercles
tuberculosis
uvula
uvulectomy
ventilation
Venturi mask
visceral
visceral pleura
vocal cords
wheeze

Español ENHANCING SPANISH COMMUNICATION

English	Spanish (pronunciation)
acidity	acidez (ah-se-DES)
asphyxia	asfixia (as-FEEC-se-ah)
asthma	asma (AHS-mah)
breathe	alentar (ah-len-TAR), respirar (res-pe-RAR)
breathing	respiración (res-pe-rah-se-ON)
cough	tos (tos)
diaphragm	diafragma (de-ah-FRAHG-mah)
erect, straight	derecho (day-RAY-cho)
imperfect	imperfecto (im-per-FEC-to)
influenza	gripe (GREE-pay)
lobe	lóbulo (LO-boo-lo)
lung	pulmón (pool-MON)
nose	nariz (nah-REES)
nostril	orificio de la nariz (or-e-FEE-se-o day lah nah-REES)
obstruction	obstrucción (obs-trooc-se-ON)
pneumonia	neumonía (nay-oo-mo-NEE-ah), pulmonía (pool-mo-NEE-ah)
respiration	respiración (res-pe-rah-se-ON)
throat	garganta (gar-GAHN-tah)
tonsil	tonsila (ton-SEE-lah), amígdala (ah-MEEG-dah-lah)
trachea	tráquea (TRAH-kay-ah)
voice	voz (vos)

Digestive System

10

LEARNING GOALS

Basic Understanding
In this chapter you will learn to do the following:
1. State the four major functions of the digestive system, and analyze associated terms.
2. Write the meanings of the word parts associated with the upper and lower digestive tract, and use them to build and analyze terms.
3. Write the names of the major structures of the digestive system, define the terms associated with these structures, and label the structures.
4. List the three classes of nutrients and their functions.
5. State the function of the accessory organs of digestion, and analyze associated terms.
6. Write the names of the diagnostic tests and procedures for assessment of the digestive system when given their descriptions, and match them with the digestive structures.
7. Match terms for digestive system pathologies with their meanings, or write the names of the pathologies when given their descriptions.
8. Match the pathologies of accessory organs of digestion with their meanings, or write the names of the pathologies when given their descriptions.
9. Match terms for surgical and therapeutic interventions for digestive tract and accessory organ pathologies with descriptions of the interventions, or write the names of the interventions when given their descriptions.

Greater Comprehension
10. Use word parts from this chapter to determine the meanings or answer questions about the terms in a health care report.
11. Spell the terms accurately.
12. Pronounce the terms correctly.
13. Write the meanings of the abbreviations.
14. Categorize terms as anatomy, diagnostic test or procedure, pathology, surgery, or therapy.

MAJOR SECTIONS OF THIS CHAPTER:

- ❑ **ANATOMY AND PHYSIOLOGY**
  Digestion and Nutrition
  Major Structures of the Digestive System
  Upper Digestive Tract
  Lower Digestive Tract
  Accessory Organs of Digestion
- ❑ **DIAGNOSTIC TESTS AND PROCEDURES**
- ❑ **PATHOLOGIES**
  Upper Digestive Tract
  Lower Digestive Tract
  Accessory Organs of Digestion
- ❑ **SURGICAL AND THERAPEUTIC INTERVENTIONS**
  Upper and Lower Digestive Tracts
  Accessory Organs of Digestion

FUNCTION FIRST

Four major functions of the digestive system are ingestion of food, digestion of food, absorption of nutrients, and elimination of wastes. Accessory organs of digestion have additional functions, including the production or storage of secretions that aid in the chemical breakdown of food, filtration of the blood and breakdown of toxic compounds, storage of iron and certain vitamins, synthesis of plasma proteins, and regulation of blood glucose levels.

ANATOMY AND PHYSIOLOGY

intestines

10-1 The digestive system is known by many names, including the digestive tract, the **alimentary** (al″ə-men′tər-e) **tract,** and the gastrointestinal (gas″tro-in-tes′tĭ-nəl) or GI system. **Gastro/intestin/al** refers to the stomach and the _____.

> ➤ KEY POINT The digestive tract is a long, muscular tube, lined with mucous membrane, that extends from the mouth to the anus. The upper GI (UGI) tract consists of the mouth, **pharynx** (far′inks) (called the throat in nonmedical language), esophagus, and stomach. The lower GI tract is made up of the small and large intestines. The accessory organs (salivary glands, liver, gallbladder, and pancreas) secrete fluids that aid in digestion and absorption of nutrients.

DIGESTION AND NUTRITION

10-2 Nutrition is the sum of the processes involved in the taking in, digestion, absorption, and use of food substances by the body. The digestive system provides the body with water, nutrients, and minerals and eliminates undigested food particles.

> ➤ KEY POINT Digestion can be divided into four stages. The stages from beginning to end can be divided into four separate functions: ingestion, digestion, absorption, and elimination.

mouth

The first function of the digestive system is ingestion, the way in which the body takes in nutrients. In humans, **ingestion** (in-jes′chən) is orally taking substances into the body. Ingestion means swallowing the substances; in other words, the substance is taken into the body through the _____.

10-3 Digestion (di-jes′chən), the second function of the digestive system, is the conversion of food into substances that can be absorbed in the GI tract.

> ➤ KEY POINT Digestion consists of mechanical and chemical processes. Mechanical digestion begins in the mouth with chewing and continues with churning actions in the stomach. Carbohydrates, proteins, and fats are transformed into smaller molecules through chemical digestion. The accessory organs contribute digestive fluids to aid this process.

digestion

The second activity of nutrition, called _____, consists of both mechanical and chemical processes that break down the food.

10-4 After swallowing, the digestive system moves the food particles along the digestive tract and mixes them with enzymes and other fluids. These movements are brought about by the contractions of smooth muscles of the digestive system. Be aware that some texts list movement of the food particles along the digestive tract as an additional function.

around

The movement of food particles through the digestive tract is called **peristalsis** (per″ĭ-stawl′sis). You learned earlier that peri- means _____.

The suffix -stalsis means contraction. The presence of food in the digestive tube stimulates a co-ordinated, rhythmic muscular contraction called peristalsis.

10-5 Absorption (ab-sorp´shən), the third function, is the process in which the digested food molecules pass through the lining of the small intestine into the blood or lymph capillaries. This passage of the simple molecules from the lining of the small intestine into the blood or lymph is

absorption   called _____. Assimilation is the process of incorporating nutritive material into living tissue and occurs either after or simultaneously with absorption.

10-6 The fourth function, **elimination** (e-lim˝ĭ-na´shən), is removal of undigested food particles (waste). Wastes are excreted (eliminated) through the anus in the form of feces. The anus is the opening of the large intestine to the outside. This last function of the digestive system is called

elimination   _____.
　　The elimination of undigested food particles is only one type of elimination of body wastes. Other body wastes include carbon dioxide excreted by the lungs and excess water and other substances excreted in the urine and through perspiration.

10-7 Alimentation (al˝ə-men-ta´shən) is the process of providing nourishment, or nutrition,* for the body. Good nutrition is essential for **metabolism** (mə-tab´ə-liz˝əm), the sum of all the physical and chemical processes that take place in living organisms and result in growth, generation of energy, elimination of wastes, and other body functions as they relate to the distribution of nutrients in the blood after digestion.

nutrition   　　Alimentation means providing _____ for the body.

10-8 A balanced diet is one that is adequate in energy-providing substances (carbohydrates and fats), tissue-building compounds (proteins), inorganic chemicals (water and mineral salts), vitamins, and certain other substances, such as bulk for promoting movement of the contents of the digestive tract. The recommended dietary allowances (RDAs) are the levels of daily intake of essential nutrients that are considered adequate to meet nutritional needs. RDA means

dietary   recommended _____ allowance.
　　Homeo/stasis is the state of dynamic equilibrium of the internal environment of the body. Homeostasis is maintained even though the amounts of various food substances and water that we take in vary. Learn the meanings of the following word parts that are used in discussing digestion and nutrition.

Word Parts: Digestion and Nutrition

Combining Forms Substances	Meaning	Suffixes Functions	Meaning
amyl(o)	starch	-dipsia	thirst
bil(i), chol(e)	bile or gall	-orexia	appetite
glyc(o)	sugar	-pepsia	digestion
lact(o)	milk	-stalsis	contraction
lip(o)	fats		
prote(o)	protein		

10-9 Carbohydrates, fats, and proteins are the three major classes of nutrients. Carbohydrates, the basic source of energy for human cells, include starches and sugars.
　　The combining form glyc(o) means sugar. **Glyco/lysis** (gli-kol´ə-sis) is the breaking down of

sugar   _____.

10-10 Glucose (gloo´kōs), a simple sugar, is the major source of energy for the body's cells. It is found in certain foods, especially fruits, and is also formed when more complex sugars and starches are broken down by the digestive system. The concentration of glucose in the blood in healthy individuals is maintained at a fairly constant level.

glucose   　　The type of sugar that is the main source of energy for the body is _____.

*Nutrition (Latin: *nutriens*, food that nourishes).

10-11 Starches, a second type of carbohydrate, break down easily and are eventually reduced to glucose before being absorbed into the blood. The combining form amyl(o) means starch. The digestive process whereby starch is converted into sugars is called **amylolysis** (am″ə-lol′ə-sis). The literal translation of amylo/lysis is _____ of starch.

destruction

10-12 Proteins are nitrogenous compounds that provide amino acids and building material for development, growth, and maintenance of the body. The combining form prote(o) means protein. **Proteo/lysis** (pro″te-ol′ĭ-sis) is breaking down (destruction, digestion) of _____. Proteolysis is necessary for digestion, because proteins must be chemically broken down before they can be absorbed.

protein

10-13 Fats, also called lipids (lip′ids), serve as an energy reserve. When stored in fat cells, they form lipoid tissue that helps to cushion and insulate vital organs. The combining form lip(o) means fats. Although **lipids** also include steroids, waxes, and fatty acids, lip(o) usually refers to fats. **Lip/oid** (lip′oid) means resembling _____.

fats

    Calories are units that are used to denote the energy value of food or the heat expenditure of an organism. Proteins, carbohydrates, and fats contain calories. Having about twice as many calories per gram as carbohydrates and proteins, fats are well suited for storage of unused calories.

10-14 Bile is a digestive chemical that breaks fats into smaller particles, preparing them for further action by lipases and absorption. Two combining forms meaning bile are chol(e) and _____.

bil(i)

10-15 Digestive enzymes act on food substances, causing them to break down into simpler compounds. Enzymes are usually named by adding -ase (meaning enzyme) to the combining form of the substance on which they act. For example, **lip/ase** (lip′ās, li′pās) breaks down lipids.

    The combining form lact(o) means milk. Remembering that -ose means sugar, write a new word that means the main sugar in milk (milk sugar): _____.

lactose

The enzyme lact/ase breaks down lactose. Lactose intolerance is a disorder caused by inadequate production of, or defect in, the enzyme lactase.

    Amylase (am′ə-lās) is an enzyme that breaks down starch. **Proteinase** (pro′tēn-ās) or **protease** (pro′te-ās) is an enzyme that breaks down protein.

10-16 Thirst is the desire for fluid, especially for water. Not only does water serve to transport food in the digestive tract, but it is also the principal medium in which chemical reactions occur. The suffix that means thirst is _____.

-dipsia

10-17 The normal desire for food is called the appetite. The suffix that you will use to write words about the appetite is _____.

-orexia

    The suffix that means digestion is _____. Normal digestion is **eu/pepsia** (u-pep′se-ə).

-pepsia

EXERCISE 1

Write the meanings of these word parts.

1. amyl(o) _____

2. chol(e) _____

3. glyc(o) _____

4. lact(o) _____

5. lip(o) _____

6. prote(o) _____

7. -dipsia _____

8. -orexia _____

9. -pepsia _____

10. -stalsis _____

EXERCISE 2

Match the terms in the left column with their descriptions in the right column.

_____ 1. absorption

_____ 2. alimentation

_____ 3. calories

_____ 4. carbohydrate

_____ 5. digestion

_____ 6. elimination

_____ 7. gastrointestinal

_____ 8. ingestion

_____ 9. lipids

_____ 10. proteolysis

A. breaking down of protein
B. conversion of food into substances that can be absorbed
C. fats
D. how the body takes in nutrients
E. pertaining to the stomach and intestines
F. removal of undigested food particles
G. the basic source of energy for human cells; includes glucose and starches
H. the process in which digested food molecules pass through the small intestine lining into the blood or lymph capillaries
I. the process of providing nourishment or nutrition for the body
J. units that denote the energy value of food

MAJOR STRUCTURES OF THE DIGESTIVE SYSTEM

lower

10-18 The structures that you are about to label make up the muscular tube portion of the digestion tract, which consists of the upper GI tract and the _____ GI tract.
The salivary glands, liver, gallbladder, and pancreas (the accessory organs) are already labeled. Note their locations in relation to the other structures. Learn the meanings of the following word parts.

Word Parts: Major Structures of the Digestive System

Structures	Combining Forms	Structures	Combining Forms
Upper GI Tract		**Lower GI Tract**	
mouth	or(o), stomat(o)	small intestine	enter(o)[†]
esophagus	esophag(o)	duodenum	duoden(o)
stomach	gastr(o)	jejunum	jejun(o)
		ileum	ile(o)
Accessory Organs of Digestion		large intestine	col(o), colon(o)[‡]
gallbladder	cholecyst(o)	rectum	rect(o)
common bile duct	choledoch(o)	anus	an(o)
liver	hepat(o)		
pancreas	pancreat(o)		
salivary glands	sialaden(o)[*]		

[*]Sometimes sial(o).
[†]Enter(o) sometimes means the intestines in general.
[‡]Col(o) and colon(o) sometimes refer specifically to the colon, the larger portion of the large intestine.

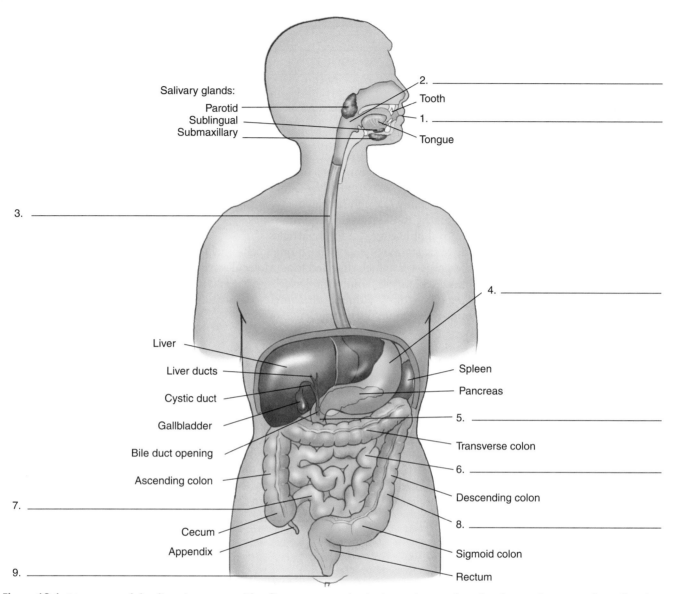

Figure 10-1 Structures of the digestive system. The alimentary tract, beginning at the mouth and ending at the anus, is basically a long, muscular tube. Several accessory organs (salivary glands, liver, gallbladder, and pancreas) are also shown.

10-19 Label the structures in Figure 10-1 as you read the following information.

Digestion begins in the mouth *(1)*. The teeth grind and chew the food before it is swallowed. The mass of chewed food is called a **bolus** (bo´ləs).

The pharynx *(2)* passes the bolus to the esophagus *(3)*, which leads to the stomach *(4)*, where food is churned and broken down chemically and mechanically.

The liquid mass, called **chyme** (kīm), is passed to the small intestine, where digestion continues and absorption of nutrients occurs. The three parts of the small intestine are shown: duodenum *(5)*, jejunum *(6)*, and ileum *(7)*.

Undigested food passes to the large intestine *(8)*, where much of the water is absorbed. It is stored in the rectum until it is eliminated through the anus *(9)*.

10-20 You already know the combining forms for several structures that you labeled. **Or/al** means pertaining to the _____.

A second combining form that means mouth is stomat(o). In general, or(o) is used in terms that describe the mouth as a structure and stomat(o) is used to write other terms, such as diagnostic and surgical terms. **Pharyng/eal** (fə-rin´je-əl) means pertaining to the _____.

mouth

pharynx

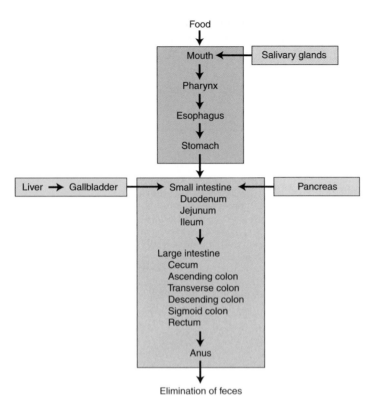

Figure 10-2 Pathway of food through the digestive system.

Oro/pharyng/eal (or″o-fə-rin′je-əl) means pertaining to the mouth and pharynx or pertaining to the oropharynx, the part of the pharynx posterior to the mouth—the throat.

10-21 The **esophagus** is a long, muscular canal that extends from the pharynx to the stomach. **Gast/ric** (gas′trik) means pertaining to the _____.

stomach

10-22 Both **intestin/al** (in-tes′tĭ-nəl) and **enter/ic** (en-ter′ik) mean pertaining to the _____. Most medical words concerning the intestines are formed using enter(o), but a few terms use enter(o) to specifically mean the small intestine (for example, **enter/itis** (en″tər-i′tis).

intestine

10-23 Enter/al (en′tər-əl) means within, by way of, or pertaining to the small intestine. Although enter(o) is used to write terms about the small intestine, you need to remember that enter(o) means either the small intestine or the _____ in general. Enteral tube feeding introduces food directly into the gastrointestinal tract.

intestines

10-24 The combining form col(o) means the large intestine. This combining form can also mean the **colon,** the structure that comprises most of the large intestine and where much of the water is absorbed as the wastes are moved along to the rectum. An adjective that means pertaining to the colon uses colon(o). Join colon(o) and -ic to write this term:

colonic (ko-lon′ik)

_____.

   Colic (kol′ik) means pertaining to the large intestine, but it also means spasm in any hollow or tubular soft organ accompanied by pain. You may be most familiar with infantile colic, which is colic occurring during the first few months of life.

10-25 The **rectum** (rek′təm) is the lower part of the large intestine. The **anus** (a′nəs) is the outlet of the rectum, and it lies in the fold between the buttocks. The anal canal is about 4 cm long. Solid wastes are eliminated via the anus. **Rectal** and **anal** (a′nəl) mean pertaining to the rectum and anus, respectively. The pathway of food through the digestive tract is summarized in Figure 10-2.

The digestive tract is lined with a mucous membrane, which secretes mucus for lubrication. Mucus is the slippery material produced by mucous membranes. The adjective used to describe a membrane that secretes mucus is **mucous** (mu′kəs). **Mucosa** (mu-ko′sə) is the same as a mucous membrane.

resembling

Muc/oid means _____ mucus.

EXERCISE 3

Write the meaning of these combining forms.

1. an(o) _____
2. cholecyst(o) _____
3. choledoch(o) _____
4. col(o) _____
5. duoden(o) _____
6. enter(o) _____
7. gastr(o) _____
8. hepat(o) _____
9. ile(o) _____
10. jejun(o) _____
11. or(o) _____
12. pancreat(o) _____
13. rect(o) _____
14. sialaden(o) _____
15. stomat(o) _____

EXERCISE 4

Build It! *Use the following word parts to build terms. (Some word parts will be used more than once.)*

colon(o), enter(o), gastr(o), muc(o), or(o), pharyng(o), -eal, -ic, -itis, -oid

1. inflammation of the small intestines _____/_____
2. pertaining to the stomach _____/_____
3. pertaining to the mouth and throat _____/_____/_____
4. pertaining to the large intestines _____/_____
5. resembling mucus _____/_____

Say and Check

Say aloud the terms you wrote for Exercise 4. Use the Companion CD to check your pronunciations.

UPPER DIGESTIVE TRACT

stomach

10-26 The oral cavity is the beginning of the digestive tract and, along with the esophagus and _____, comprises the upper digestive tract. The mouth contains many structures that hold the food in place and facilitate chewing (Figure 10-3).

Learn the following word parts that pertain to structures of the upper digestive tract.

Word Parts: Structures of the Upper Digestive Tract

Combining Forms	Meaning	Combining Forms	Meaning
or(o), stomat(o)	mouth	palat(o)	palate
Structures of the Mouth		pharyng(o)	pharynx
bucc(o)	cheek	sial(o)	saliva, salivary glands
cheil(o)	lip	sialaden(o)	salivary gland
dent(i), dent(o), odont(o)	teeth	**Other Structures**	
gingiv(o)	gums	esophag(o)	esophagus
gloss(o), lingu(o)	tongue	gastr(o)	stomach
mandibul(o)	mandible	pylor(o)	pylorus
maxill(o)	maxilla	vag(o)	vagus nerve

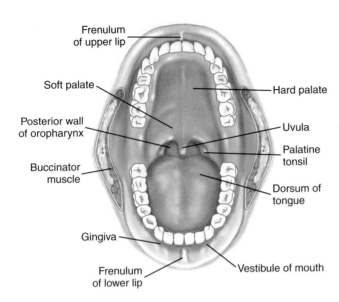

Frenulum
of upper lip

Soft palate

Posterior wall
of oropharynx

Buccinator
muscle

Gingiva

Frenulum
of lower lip

Hard palate

Uvula

Palatine
tonsil

Dorsum of
tongue

Vestibule of mouth

Figure 10-3 Mouth structures. The mouth is bounded anteriorly by the lips and contains the tongue and teeth. The roof of the mouth is the hard palate. Other aspects of the mouth include the gums, the uvula (the fleshy appendage in the back of the throat), the oropharynx, and the buccinator muscle (the main muscle of the cheek that is involved in chewing).

10-27 The **mandible** (man´dĭ-bəl) is the lower jaw, and the **maxilla** (mak-sil´ə) is the upper jaw. **Mandibul/ar** (man-dib´u-lər) means pertaining to the mandible, the _____ jaw.
    Maxill/ary (mak´sĭ-lar″e) means pertaining to the maxilla, or _____ jaw.

lower
upper

10-28 The roof of the mouth is formed by the bony arch of the hard palate and the fibrous soft palate. **Palat/ine** (pal´ə-tīn) pertains to the _____.
    The combining form bucc(o) means cheek, and the **bucc/al** (buk´əl) **cavity** pertains to the area between the teeth and the cheeks.
    The combining form cheil(o) means the _____.

palate

lip

10-29 The mucous membrane that provides support for the teeth is the gum. Another name for the gum is **gingiva. Gingiv/al** (jin´jĭ-vəl) pertains to the _____.

gums

10-30 Both gloss(o) and lingu(o) mean the tongue; therefore, **gloss/al** (glos´əl) and **lingu/al** (ling´gwəl) mean pertaining to the tongue. Most words involving the tongue use the combining form gloss(o). However, both **hypo/glossal** (hi″po-glos´əl) and **sub/lingual** (səb-ling´gwəl) mean _____ the tongue. Some medications are designed to be placed under the tongue, where they dissolve.

under

10-31 Glosso/pharyng/eal (glos″o-fə-rin´je-əl) refers to the _____ and the throat (or pharynx).

tongue

10-32 Three combining forms mean the teeth: dent(i), dent(o), and odont(o). **Dent/al** pertains to the teeth. **Inter/dental** (in″tər-den´təl) means between the _____.
    The dent- in denture refers to teeth. A **dent/ure** (den´chər) refers to a set of teeth, either natural or artificial, but is ordinarily used to designate artificial ones.
    Denti/lingual (den″tĭ-ling´wəl) pertains to the _____ and the tongue.

teeth

teeth

10-33 The primary or deciduous teeth, often called "baby teeth," begin to fall out and to be replaced with permanent teeth when a child is about 6 years of age. The wisdom teeth are the last teeth to erupt, generally between 17 and 25 years of age.
    There are 32 permanent teeth in a full set. The mouth has an upper and a lower dental arch, the curving shape formed by the arrangement of a normal set of teeth in the jaw. A complete set has 16 teeth in each dental arch. Observe the dental arch in Figure 10-4, *A.* Note that the illustration shows the teeth of the lower jaw, or _____ arch. The eight teeth on each side of the dental arch make up a quadrant. Label the teeth in a quadrant as you read the information that follows.

mandibular

There are two **incisors** (in-si´zərs) *(1)*, one **cuspid** (kus´pid) *(2)*, two **bicuspids** *(3)*, and three **molars** *(4)*. Anterior teeth generally fall out and are replaced sooner than posterior ones. The last molar, which is posterior to all other teeth, is known as the wisdom tooth.

10-34 The structure of a molar is shown in Figure 10-4, *B*. All teeth consist of two basic parts: the crown and the root or roots (embedded in the bony socket). A socket is a hollow or depression into which another part fits—in this case, the tooth. The part that projects above the gum is the _____.

The exposed part of the crown is covered by enamel, the hardest substance in the body. The soft tissue inside the tooth is the dental pulp, also called the **endodontium** (en˝do-don´she-əm). When the word endodontium is broken down into its component parts, its parts mean a membrane _____ the tooth, but you need to remember that it means dental pulp.

10-35 The tissue investing and supporting the teeth is **periodontium** (per˝e-o-don´she-əm). You learned that peri- means around, so peri/odont/ium is the tissue _____ the teeth. **Peri/odont/al** (per˝e-o-don´təl) means around a tooth, or pertaining to the periodontium.

10-36 Dentistry is the art and science of diagnosing, preventing, and treating diseases and disorders of the _____ and surrounding structures of the oral cavity. There are several dental specialties, each requiring additional training after graduation from dental school.

10-37 Orth/odont/ics is concerned with irregularities of alignment of _____ and associated facial problems. One who specializes in orthodontics, often using braces to straighten the teeth, is an **orthodontist**. One "o" is dropped when orth(o) is combined with odont(o) to facilitate pronunciation. You will see that one "o" is generally dropped when odont(o) is joined with prefixes or other combining forms that also end in "o."

A **peri/odont/ist** (per˝e-o-don´tist) specializes in the study and treatment of the periodontium. This specialty concerns the gingival tissue, as well as the other tissue that supports the teeth. What is the specialty of a periodontist? _____

An **end/odont/ist** is a dentist who specializes in the prevention and treatment of conditions that affect the dental pulp, tooth root, and surrounding tissue and the associated practice of root canal therapy. The specialty is **endodontics** (en˝do-don´tiks).

Left margin answers:
crown

inside

around

teeth

teeth

periodontics
(per˝e-o-don´tiks)

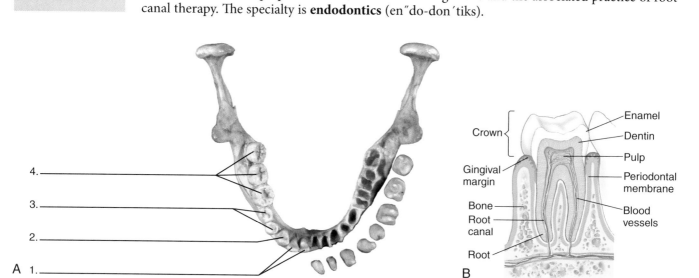

Figure 10-4 Designations of permanent teeth. A, Teeth of the lower jaw (mandibular arch). Half of the teeth are removed to demonstrate the sockets. **B,** Section of a molar tooth. All teeth follow a basic plan, consisting of two basic parts: the crown and the root or roots (embedded in the bony socket). The central cavity contains the root canal and tooth pulp, which are richly supplied with blood and lymph vessels, as well as nerves. The chief substance of the tooth, dentin, is similar to bone but harder and more compact. Dentin is covered by enamel on the crown. Enamel is the hardest substance in the body and is composed mainly of calcium phosphate. The cementum is a bonelike connective tissue that provides support to the tooth.

children	**10-38** A dentist who specializes in **ped/odont/ics** (pe-do-don´tiks) treats _____. Pedodontics is a branch of dentistry that deals with tooth and mouth conditions of children. A specialist in pedodontics is a **pedodontist.**
dental	**10-39** **Ger/odont/ics** (jer″o-don´tiks) is a branch of dentistry that deals with the dental problems of older persons. Note that the vowel is dropped from ger(o) when it is combined with odont(o). A **ger/odont/ist** is a dentist specializing in the _____ problems of older persons.

EXERCISE 5

Build It! *Use the following word parts to build terms. (Some word parts will be used more than once.)*

inter-, peri-, dent(o), lingu(o), mandibul(o), odont(o), palat(o), -al, -ar, -ine, -ist

1. pertaining to the tongue   _____/_____

2. pertaining to the lower jaw   _____/_____

3. practitioner who specializes in the gums and other tissues that support the teeth   _____/_____/_____

4. pertaining to the roof of the mouth   _____/_____/_____

5. pertaining to between the teeth   _____/_____/_____

Say and Check

Say aloud the terms you wrote for Exercise 5. Use the Companion CD to check your pronunciations.

starch	**10-40** Salivary glands, which are accessory organs of digestion, secrete saliva into the oral cavity. The mouth tastes what we consume and performs other functions of digestion by mixing the food with saliva, chewing, and voluntarily swallowing it. In addition, saliva contains amylase, which begins digestion of _____ in the mouth. The salivary glands are three paired glands (Figure 10-5).

> ➤ **KEY** POINT The names of the salivary glands indicate their location. The **par/otid** (pə-rot´id) **glands,** the largest salivary glands, are near the ears. The suffix -id means either having the shape of or a structure. The **sub/lingual glands** are located under the tongue. The **sub/mandibular** (sub″man-dib´u-lər) **glands** are located in the tissue of the mandible, rather than beneath it as the prefix sub- in the name implies.

10-41 Food that is swallowed passes from the mouth to the pharynx and the esophagus. Both the pharynx and the esophagus are muscular structures that move food along on its way to the stomach.

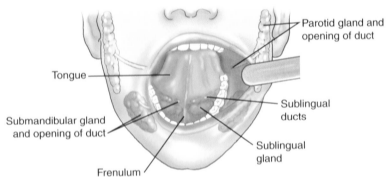

Figure labels: Tongue · Submandibular gland and opening of duct · Frenulum · Parotid gland and opening of duct · Sublingual ducts · Sublingual gland

Figure 10-5 Salivary glands. Three pairs of salivary glands (parotid, sublingual, and submandibular glands) consist of numerous lobes connected by vessels and ducts.

> ➤ **KEY** POINT <u>The esophagus is a muscular canal extending from the pharynx to the</u> <u>stomach.</u> The esophagus, about 24 cm (about 9½ inches) long, secretes mucus to facilitate the movement of food into the stomach, which is lined with mucous membrane. Upper and lower esophag/eal sphincters control the movement of food into and out of the esophagus. A **sphincter**[*] (sfingk´tər) consists of circular muscle that constricts a passage or closes a natural opening in the body.

esophagus

Esophag/eal (ə-sof″ə-je´al) means pertaining to the _____.

sphincter

10-42 The circular esophageal muscle that controls movement of food from the pharynx into the esophagus is called the upper esophageal sphincter. The lower esophageal _____ controls the movement of food into the stomach. This sphincter is also called the cardiac sphincter because the name of the portion of the stomach near the upper opening is the cardiac region. The region was so named because of its proximity to the heart.

behind

     Post/esophag/eal (pōst-ə-sof″ə-je´əl) means situated _____ the esophagus.

10-43 Examine Figure 10-6, *A*, to learn more about the structure of the stomach. Regions of the stomach are the **cardiac region,** the **fundus** (fun´dəs), the body, and the **pyloric** (pi-lor´ik) **region,** or **pylorus.**

[*]Sphincter (Greek: *sphincter*, that which binds tight).

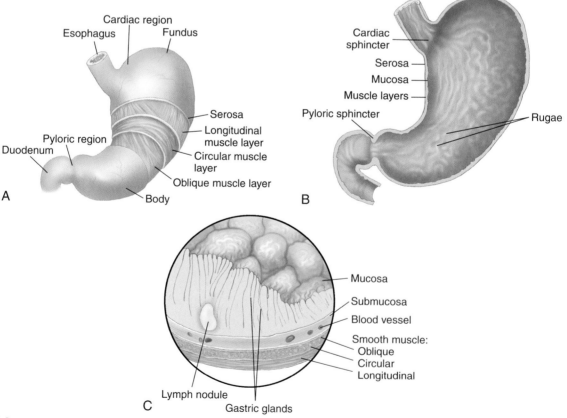

Figure 10-6 Features of the stomach. A, External view: The stomach is composed of the cardiac region, a fundus or round part, a body or middle portion, and a pyloric portion, which is the small distal end. The stomach has a serous coat (serosa) and three muscular layers. **B,** Internal view: The cardiac sphincter guards the opening of the esophagus into the stomach and prevents backflow of material into the esophagus. The stomach ends with the pyloric sphincter, which regulates outflow. The lining of the stomach, the mucosa, is arranged in temporary folds called rugae (visible in the empty stomach), which allow expansion as the stomach fills. **C,** Structure of the stomach wall: Longitudinal, circular, and oblique smooth muscle lie just beneath the serosa. All stomach layers are richly supplied with blood vessels and nerves. Gastric glands secrete gastric juice through gastric pits, tiny holes in the mucosa.

pyloric

The cardiac region lies near the upper opening from the esophagus. The round and most superior region of the stomach is the fundus. The main portion of the stomach is called the body. As the body of the stomach approaches the lower opening, it narrows and is called the _____ region.

The stomach ends with the pyloric sphincter, which regulates the outflow of stomach contents into the **duodenum,** the first part of the small intestine.

10-44 Look at Figure 10-6, B. The mucosa that lines the stomach is arranged in temporary folds called **rugae** (roo´je). Ruga (singular of rugae) means ridge, wrinkle, or fold. The rugae, most apparent when the stomach is empty, allow the stomach to expand as it fills.

serosa
(sēr-o´sə, sēr-o´zə)

The outer layer of the stomach is the _____. This type of visceral peritoneum holds the stomach in position by folding back on and over the structure.

Three muscle layers are present in the stomach, rather than two, which are found in other structures of the digestive tract (see Figure 10-6, C).

10-45 Place a prefix before gastric to write a word that means pertaining to the inside (interior) of the stomach: _____.

endogastric
(en´do-gas´trik)

The stomach is a temporary reservoir for food and is the first major site of digestion. After digestion, the stomach gradually feeds liquefied food (chyme) into the small intestine.

EXERCISE 6

Write a word in each blank to complete the following sentences. The first letter of each answer is given as a clue.

1. Another name for the mouth is the o_____ cavity.

2. The lower jaw is the m_____.

3. The upper jaw is the m_____.

4. The roof of the mouth is the p_____.

5. The buccal cavity pertains to the area between the teeth and the c_____.

6. Another name for the gum is g_____.

7. Glossal means pertaining to the t_____.

8. Sublingual means beneath the t_____.

9. Another name for the throat is the p_____.

10. Dental pulp is called e_____.

11. The tissue that invests and supports the teeth is p_____.

12. The dental specialty that is concerned with irregularities of the alignment of teeth and associated facial problems is

    o_____.

13. The branch of dentistry that deals with the tooth and mouth conditions of children is p_____.

14. The branch of dentistry that specializes in dental problems of older persons is g_____.

15. The three paired glands that secrete saliva into the oral cavity are the s_____ glands.

16. The muscular canal that extends from the mouth to the stomach is the e_____.

17. A circular muscle that constricts a passage or closes a natural opening in the body is called a s_____.

18. The lower region of the stomach is called the p_____ region.

LOWER DIGESTIVE TRACT

10-46 The intestines make up the lower digestive tract. The intestines are sometimes called the bowels. Extending from the pyloric opening to the anus, the intestinal tract is about 7.5 to 8.5 meters (about 24½ to 28 feet) long.

> ➤ **KEY** POINT The intestines include the small intestine and the large intestine. The adult small intestine, comprising more than three fourths of the length of the intestines, is 6 to 7 meters (about 20 to 23 feet) long. The large intestine is so named because it is larger in diameter than the small intestine, but it is less than one fourth as long.

small

Which is longer, the small intestine or the large intestine? _____ intestine

10-47 The small intestine finishes the process of digestion, absorbs the nutrients, and passes the residue on to the large intestine. In other words, the small intestine is responsible for two successive processes, digestion and _____, before passing the residue to the large intestine.

absorption

10-48 The small intestine consists of three parts: the duodenum (doo″o-de′nəm, doo-od′ə-nəm), the jejunum (jə-joo′nəm), and the ileum (il′e-əm). The structure of the small intestine is shown in Figure 10-7. Read the information that accompanies the drawing, and label the three parts of the small intestine.

Study the layers of the wall of the small intestine to write answers in these blanks. The innermost membrane is called the mucosa. Both the mucosa and submucosa have many folds and fingerlike projections called _____. Both these features increase the surface area of the mucosa. In addition, the **villi** function to absorb nutrients.

villi (vil′i)*

serosa

There are two layers of muscle and an outer membrane called the _____.

10-49 The duodenum is about 25 cm long, less than a foot long. **Duoden/al** (doo″o-de′nəl; doo-od′ə-nəl) means pertaining to the _____.

duodenum

10-50 The part of the small intestine below the duodenum is the **jejunum.** It is about 2.4 meters (about 8 feet) long and joins the ileum, which is the twisted end of the small intestine. **Jejun/al** means pertaining to the _____.

jejunum

*Villus, pl. villi (Latin: tuft of hair)

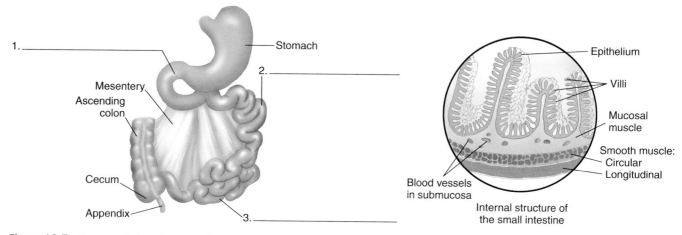

Figure 10-7 Characteristics of the small intestine. Label the three parts of the small intestine (1 to 3) as you read. The first portion, the duodenum *(1),* begins at the pyloric sphincter and is the shorter section. The second portion is the jejunum *(2),* which is continuous with the third portion, the ileum *(3).* The ileum is the longest of the three parts of the small intestine. Note that the small intestine decreases in diameter from its beginning at the duodenum to its ending, at the ileum. The internal structure is similar throughout its length. The wall *(inset)* has an inner lining of mucosa, two layers of muscle, and an outer layer of serosa.

| ileum | The **ileum** is the distal portion of the small intestine. Both **ile/ac** and **ile/al** mean pertaining to the _____. |

10-51 The large intestine is only about 1.5 meters (about 5 feet) long. The combining forms col(o) and colon(o) mean the colon (ko´lən) or the _____

large

intestine. The colon is only that portion of the large intestine extending from the cecum to the rectum, but colon is sometimes used to mean the large intestine in general.

The large intestine is anatomically divided into the cecum, colon, rectum, and anal canal. Learn the combining forms for the following structures.

Word Parts: Large Intestine

Combining Forms Structures	Meaning	Combining Forms Pathology	Meaning
append(o), appendic(o)	appendix	diverticul(o)	diverticula
cec(o)	cecum		
col(o), colon(o)	large intestine or colon		
proct(o)	anus, rectum		
sigmoid(o)	sigmoid colon		

10-52 Study the location of the parts of the large intestine in Figure 10-8.

The **cecum** (se´kəm) forms the first portion of the large intestine and is located just distal to the ileum. The combining form cec(o) means cecum. The **ileo/cecal** (il″e-o-se´kəl) **valve** is

cecum

located between the ileum and the _____. **Retro/cecal** (ret″ro-se´kəl) means behind the cecum.

10-53 The **vermiform appendix** is a wormlike structure that opens into the cecum. An appendix simply means an appendage, but its most common usage is in referring to the vermiform appendix just described. **Appendicular** means either pertaining to an appendage or pertaining to the

appendix

vermiform _____.

10-54 The colon makes up most of the 1.5 meters (5 feet) of large intestine. Different parts of the colon are designated as the ascending, transverse, descending, and **sigmoid** (sig´moid) **colon.**

sigmoid

The last part of the colon is the _____ colon.

Retro/col/ic (ret″ro-kol´ik) means behind the colon. Remembering that peri- means around,

around

the literal translation of peri/col/ic (per″e-kol´ik) is _____ the colon. **Pericolic** means pertaining to the tissue around the colon. In this term, "the tissue around the structure" is implied.

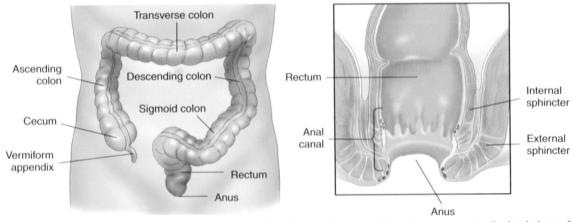

Figure 10-8 Features of the large intestine: the cecum, appendix, colon, and rectum. The colon is anatomically divided into four parts. The first part rises upward and is called the ascending colon. The transverse colon is the part that crosses the abdomen. The colon then descends on the left side of the abdomen and thus is called the descending colon. The last part is S-shaped and is called the sigmoid colon. The internal structure of a portion of the rectum and the anus are *shown on the right.*

rectum

10-55 The lower part of the large intestine is the rectum, which terminates in a narrow anal canal. This canal in turn opens to the exterior at the anus. **Feces** is body waste that is discharged from the bowels by way of the anus. Feces is also called stool or fecal material. **Defecation** (def″ə-ka′shən) is the elimination of feces from the rectum.

    Colo/rectal (ko″lo-rek′təl) means pertaining to or affecting the colon and the

_____.

rect(o)

10-56 The combining form proct(o) refers to the anus (a′nəs) or rectum. You have now learned two combining forms for rectum: proct(o) and _____. A **procto/logist** (prok-tol′ə-jist) specializes in treating disorders of the colon, rectum, and anus.

    Most medical terms that refer to the anus use proct(o), but you need to remember that an(o)

anus

also means anus. An/al refers to the _____, as in the phrases anal opening and anal canal.

10-57 The combining form enter(o) means intestines, sometimes referring to the small intestine only, but the term **gastro/entero/logy** is the study of the stomach and

intestines

_____ and associated diseases.

10-58 Structural features of both the small intestine and large intestine are well suited for their roles in the digestive system. As you studied earlier, the small intestine is responsible for further digestion of the chyme and absorption of nutrients.

> ➤ **KEY** POINT The large intestine has several important functions:
> - While moving wastes along its length, the large intestine absorbs water, sodium, and chloride. The large intestine is capable of absorbing 90% of the water and sodium it receives.
> - The large intestine secretes mucus, which binds fecal particles into a formed mass and lubricates the mucosa.
> - Bacteria in the large intestine are responsible for the production of several vitamins.
> - Feces is formed and expelled from the body.

EXERCISE 7

Match the structures in the left columns with either A, small intestine, or B, large intestine.

_____ 1. anal canal   _____ 5. ileum   A. small intestine

_____ 2. cecum   _____ 6. jejunum   B. large intestine

_____ 3. colon   _____ 7. rectum

_____ 4. duodenum

EXERCISE 8

Build It! *Use the following word parts to build terms. (Some word parts will be used more than once.)*

peri-, retro-, cec(o), col(o), duoden(o), ile(o), proct(o), -al, -ic, -logist

1. pertaining to the first part of the small intestine   _____/_____

2. specialist in treating disorders of the colon, rectum, and anus   _____/_____/_____

3. pertaining to behind the first portion of the large intestine   _____/_____/_____

4. pertaining to the third part of the small intestine   _____/_____

5. pertaining to the tissue around the colon   _____/_____/_____

Say and Check

Say aloud the terms you wrote for Exercise 8. Use the Companion CD to check your pronunciations.

ACCESSORY ORGANS OF DIGESTION

accessory

10-59 The liver, gallbladder, pancreas, and salivary glands produce substances that are needed for proper digestion and absorption of nutrients and are considered to be _____ organs to the digestive system.

> ➤ **KEY** POINT Accessory organs of digestion are digestive glands. These organs lie outside the digestive tract, yet they produce or store secretions that are conveyed to the digestive tract by ducts. The secretions aid in the breakdown of food.

10-60 The liver, gallbladder, and pancreas are located near the other digestive structures within the abdominal cavity. See these structures in Figure 10-9.

liver

The liver is the largest gland of the body and is essential for the maintenance of life. **Hepat/ic** (hə-pat′ik) means pertaining to the _____.

10-61 Production of bile is a major function of the liver. The bile is then transported to the gallbladder for storage.

> ➤ **KEY** POINT The liver has several important functions. In addition to production of bile, liver functions include the following:
> - breakdown of toxic compounds
> - involvement in the regulation of blood glucose
> - lipid metabolism
> - synthesis of plasma proteins
> - storage of iron and certain vitamins
> - filtering of the blood
> - excretion of bile pigments from the breakdown of hemoglobin
> - excretion of hormones and cholesterol

bile

A major function of the liver is the production of _____, which is transported to the gallbladder for storage. Bile aids in the digestion of fats.

liver

10-62 Hepato/lytic (hep″ə-to-lit′ik) means destructive of the _____. (The term hepatolytic is less common than **hepatotoxic** [hep′ə-to-tok″sik], which means essentially the same thing.)

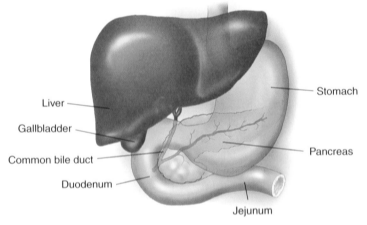

Liver
Gallbladder
Common bile duct
Duodenum
Jejunum
Stomach
Pancreas

Figure 10-9 Accessory organs of digestion. The liver, gallbladder, and pancreas are accessory digestive organs. The liver and pancreas have additional functions as well. More than 500 functions of the liver have been identified. The formation and excretion of bile for digestion of fats is one of its most commonly known activities. Bile is stored in the gallbladder and released when fats are ingested. The pancreas secretes many substances, including digestive enzymes and insulin.

liver

Extra/hepatic (eks″trə-hə-pat′ik) means situated or occurring outside the _____.
Supra/hepatic (soo″prə-hə-pat′ik) means above the liver.

bile

10-63 The combining forms chol(e) and bil(i) refer to bile or gall. **Biliary** (bil′e-ar-e) means pertaining to _____, but chol(e) is used more often to write terms. The organs and ducts that participate in the secretion, storage, and delivery of bile make up the biliary tract.

10-64 Bile leaves the liver by the hepatic duct and is taken to the gallbladder for storage until it is needed. The combining form cholecyst(o) often forms part of a term that refers to the gallbladder. **Cholecyst/ic** (ko″lə-sis′tik) means pertaining to the gallbladder.

gallbladder

Cholecysto/gastric (ko″lə-sis″to-gas′trik) pertains to the _____ and the stomach.

duct

10-65 A few words contain the combining form choledoch(o), which means the common bile duct. **Choledoch/al** (ko-led′ə-kəl) means pertaining to the common bile _____.

pancreas

10-66 The pancreas has both digestive and hormonal functions. **Pancreat/ic** (pan″kre-at′ik) means pertaining to the _____.

> ➤ **KEY** POINT <u>Pancreatic juice plays an important role in the digestion of all classes of food.</u> Pancreatic juice contains lipase, amylase, and several other enzymes that are essential to normal digestion. The pancreas also produces hormones (including insulin) that play a primary role in the regulation of carbohydrate metabolism.

10-67 Clusters of cells in the pancreas, the islets of Langerhans, produce glucagon (gloo′kə-gon) and insulin (in′sə-lin). **Glucagon** increases blood glucose levels, and **insulin** lowers blood glucose levels. The two hormones, glucagon and insulin, work together to regulate blood glucose. Secretion of glucagon is stimulated by hypoglycemia. **Hypo/glycemia** (hi″po-gli-se′me-ə) is a decreased level of glucose in the _____. Small amounts of insulin are secreted continuously in the fasting state, but secretion rises in response to an increase in blood glucose levels.

blood

Hyper/glyc/emia (hi″pər-gli-se′me-ə) is a greater than normal amount of sugar in the blood. This condition is most often associated with **diabetes mellitus** (di″ə-be′tēz mel′lĕ-təs, mə-li′tis) (DM). This disorder is primarily a result of insufficient production or improper use of insulin.

EXERCISE 9

Write adjectives that mean pertaining to the following structures.

1. common bile duct _____
2. bile _____
3. gallbladder _____

4. liver _____
5. pancreas _____

EXERCISE 10

Build It! *Use the following word parts to build terms. (Some word parts will be used more than once.)*

extra-, hyper-, hypo-, cholecyst(o), gastr(o), glyc(o), hepat(o), -emia, -ic, -lytic

1. pertaining to the gallbladder and the stomach _____/_____/_____
2. destructive to the liver _____/_____
3. decreased level of blood sugar _____/_____/_____
4. increased level of blood sugar _____/_____/_____
5. situated outside the liver _____/_____/_____

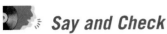 *Say and Check*

Say aloud the terms you wrote for Exercise 10. Use the Companion CD to check your pronunciations.

DIAGNOSTIC TESTS AND PROCEDURES

10-68 Physical assessment of the GI system often begins with an examination of the patient's mouth, pharynx, and abdomen. A systematic assessment of the internal abdominal organs can be made using auscultation, percussion, and palpation (see Figure 3-8). Which of these procedures is usually performed using a stethoscope?

auscultation

_____

10-69 Assessment of the intestinal tract has been greatly facilitated by radiology and endoscopy (direct visualization of internal organs using an endoscope), revealing abnormalities such as masses, tumors, and obstructions. An abdominal x-ray is usually one of the first radiographic studies performed.

    Fluoroscopy (floo-ros'kə-pe) permits both structural and functional visualization of internal body structures and is used to provide visualization of the digestive tract. With the use of contrast media, the motion of a body part can be viewed, and the image can be permanently recorded. The equipment used in fluoro/scopy is a specialized type of x-ray machine called a

fluoroscope

_____ .

10-70 An **esopha/gram** (ə-sof'ə-gram) (or **esophago/gram** [ə-sof'ə-go-gram]) is an x-ray image of the esophagus taken after the patient swallows a liquid barium suspension. This procedure is also called a barium swallow. Being careful with the spelling, write the term that is a shortened version of esophagogram: _____ .

esophagram

10-71 A barium meal (using barium sulfate) is ingested in an upper GI series (UGI), the radiographic examination of the esophagus, stomach, and duodenum. The x-ray image is viewed as the barium passes through the esophagus, stomach, and the first portion of the small intestine. The barium meal, also called barium swallow, is used for an _____ GI study (UGI).

upper

10-72 The lower intestinal tract is studied with a barium enema, a rectal infusion of barium sulfate that is retained in the lower intestinal tract during radiographic studies (see Figure 3-9).

    Structural and functional abnormalities can be seen in a GI series. For example, the emptying time of the stomach can be determined and structural defects of the GI tract can be observed. A barium enema is used in a _____ GI series.

lower

10-73 **Chole/cysto/graphy** (ko″lə-sis-tog'rə-fe) is an x-ray examination of the _____ . Cholecystography is accomplished by rendering the gallbladder and ducts opaque with a contrast medium. In an oral **chole/cysto/gram** (ko″lə-sis'to-gram) the patient is given a contrast agent in tablet form to be taken by _____ . For this reason it is called an oral _____ .

gallbladder

mouth

cholecystogram

    Examine the appearance of several gallstones in Figure 10-10. Oral cholecystograms were the principal method for investigating the presence of gallstones until the advent of ultrasound.

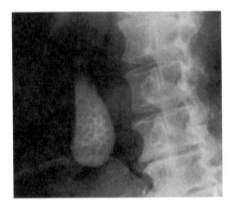

Figure 10-10 Oral cholecystogram. Numerous gallstones are evident on this cholecystogram. In oral cholecystography, radiography of the gallbladder is obtained 12 to 15 hours after ingestion of contrast medium. Because nausea, vomiting, and diarrhea are fairly common with this means of diagnosing biliary disease, it has been largely replaced by ultrasound.

endoscopes

10-74 Computed tomography and endoscopic procedures are also used to detect gallstones. Each of the instruments used in endoscopy is specially designed for the examination of particular organs. The instruments used in endoscopy are called _____.

Other instruments can be inserted through the endoscope to remove small pieces of tissue, to collect samples of tissue for study, to inject agents, or to perform laser surgery.

cholangiography

10-75 Cholangio/graphy (ko-lan″je-og′rə-fe) is radiography of the major bile ducts and is useful in demonstrating gallstones and tumors. One type of cholangiography is performed during surgery to detect residual calculi in the biliary tract, after the gallbladder has been removed. This radiographic procedure is called operative _____, and the contrast material is injected into the common bile duct.

operative

10-76 Operative cholangiography is performed by injecting a contrast medium into the common bile duct through a catheter called a T-tube. This allows residual stones in the bile ducts to be seen. This type of angiography is called _____ cholangiography. It is not unusual for the incision to be closed with the T-tube left temporarily in the common bile duct and extending through the skin. The T-tube allows for drainage and postoperative study.

pancreatography

10-77 Pancreato/graphy (pan″kre-ə-tog′rə-fe) means visualization of the pancreas. This can be accomplished by various means, including CT and sonography. Various methods of imaging of the pancreas are called _____.

10-78 The salivary ducts can also be studied by injecting radiopaque substances into the ducts in a procedure called a **sialography** (si″ə-log′rə-fe). This procedure sometimes demonstrates the presence of calculi in the salivary ducts. Write a word that means salivary calculus: _____.

sialolith (si″al′o-lith)

stomach
gastroscope
(gas′tro-skōp)

10-79 Esophago/gastro/scopy (ə-sof″ə-go-gas-tros′kə-pe) refers to examination of the esophagus and the _____.

Write the name of the instrument used to examine (inside) the stomach: _____.

gastroscopy
(gas-tros′kə-pe)
pylorus

10-80 In an **esophago/gastro/duodeno/scopy** (ə-sof″ə-go-gas″tro-doo″od-ə-nos′kə-pe) (EGD), the esophagus, stomach, and duodenum are examined (Figure 10-11). If the esophagus is the focus of the examination, the procedure is called **esophagoscopy** (ə-sof″ə-gos′ko-pe). If the stomach is the focus, the procedure is called _____.

10-81 Pyloro/scopy (pi″lor-os′kə-pe) is visual inspection of the _____, the pyloric region of the stomach.

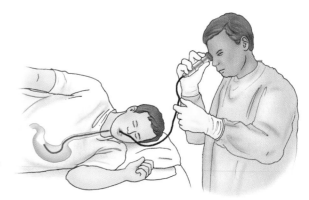

Figure 10-11 Esophagogastroduodenoscopy. If the focus of the examination is the esophagus, the procedure is called esophagoscopy. If the stomach is the focus, the procedure is called gastroscopy.

A
B
C

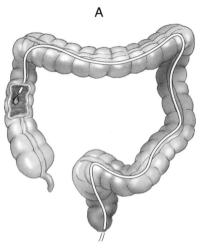
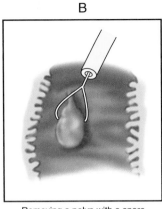
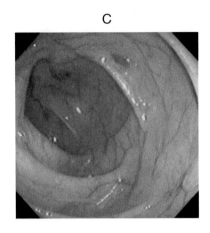

Removing a polyp with a snare

Figure 10-12 Colonoscopy. A, Endoscopic examination of the colon using a flexible colonoscope. **B,** Colonic polyps can often be removed with the use of a snare (wire noose) that fits through the colonoscope. **C,** View of a normal colon through the colonoscope.

duodenum

Duodeno/scopy (doo″o-də-nos´kə-pe) is endoscopic examination of the _____. The fiberoptic instrument used to inspect the duodenum is called a **duodenoscope** (doo″o-de´no-skōp).

colon

10-82 Colono/scopy (ko″lən-os´kə-pe) is visual examination of the mucosal lining of the _____. **Coloscopy** (ko-los´ko-pe) means the same as colonoscopy, but the former is more commonly used in naming this procedure (Figure 10-12). The instrument used is a **colonoscope** (ko-lon´o-skōp). The physician may also obtain tissue biopsy specimens or remove polyps through the colonoscope.
    Procto/sigmoido/scopy (prok″to-sig″moi-dos´kə-pe) is endoscopic examination of the rectum and sigmoid colon. This procedure uses a **sigmoido/scope** (sig-moi´do-skōp) and is also called **sigmoidoscopy** (sig″moi-dos´kə-pe).

EXERCISE 11

Build It! _Use the following word parts to build terms. (Some word parts will be used more than once.)_

cholecyst(o), col(o), esophag(o), fluor(o), gastr(o), sial(o), -gram, -lith, -scopy

1. direct visualization of the large intestine   _____/_____
2. salivary stone   _____/_____
3. visual examination of the esophagus and stomach   _____/_____/_____
4. radiographic record of the gallbladder   _____/_____/_____
5. visual examination using a fluoroscope   _____/_____

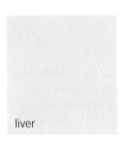 **Say and Check**
Say aloud the terms you wrote for Exercise 11. Use the Companion CD to check your pronunciations.

10-83 Sonography is less invasive than endoscopy and can be used to image soft tissues, such as the liver, the spleen, and the pancreas.
    Nuclear imaging can be used to evaluate the size of organs and vessels as well as to detect the presence of tumors or abscesses. One of the more common tests of this type is a liver scan, which involves intravenous injection of a radioactive compound that is readily absorbed by certain cells of the liver. The radiation emitted by the compound provides information about the size, shape, and consistency of the _____.

liver

10-84 Several blood tests provide information about functions of the liver, and these are aptly named liver function tests (LFTs). Examples include serum bilirubin, alkaline phosphatase, aspartate aminotransferase (AST or SGOT), and alanine aminotransferase (ALT or SGPT). Increases in these laboratory values often indicate liver disease. LFT is an abbreviation for

liver

_____ function test.

10-85 Additional blood tests are helpful in the diagnosis of disorders of the liver as well as other organs of the digestive system. Urine tests and stool examinations are also used.

The presence of blood in the stool is **hematochezia*** (he″mə-to, hem″ə-to-ke′zhə). Using hemat(o), which you know means blood, write the term that means blood in the stool:

hematochezia

_____.

Occult blood is blood that is not obvious on examination but can be detected by chemical tests, guaiac tests (for example, the Hemoccult test). Blood that cannot be seen but can be de-

occult

tected by a chemical test is called _____ blood.

An occult blood test of the stool in healthy individuals is usually negative. The presence of occult blood in the stool may indicate gastrointestinal bleeding, a finding associated with ulcers, ulcerative colitis, or cancer.

10-86 Stool samples are tested for fats as an indication of pancreatic disease or mal/absorption, impaired absorption. Fat is normally absorbed in the small intestine, giving a negative test result for fecal fats. The presence of fat in stool samples is an abnormal finding. Literal translation of

bad

malabsorption is poor or _____ absorption.

Stool samples are also tested for ova and parasites to aid in the diagnosis of parasitic infection.

_____

*Hematochezia (Greek: *haima*, blood +*chezo*, feces).

EXERCISE 12

Match the diagnostic test, procedure, or instrument in the left columns with the digestive structure in the right column that is the focus of study. (Use all terms once.)

_____ 1. cholangiography   _____ 5. gastroscope   A. bile ducts
_____ 2. cholecystography   _____ 6. pancreatography   B. duodenum
                                                                 C. esophagus
_____ 3. duodenoscopy   _____ 7. pyloroscopy   D. gallbladder
                                                                 E. lower region of the stomach
_____ 4. esophagram   _____ 8. sialography   F. pancreas
                                                                 G. salivary ducts
                                                                 H. stomach

PATHOLOGIES

appetite

10-87 Many disturbances of the digestive system can give a feeling of malaise sometimes accompanied by **anorexia** (an″o-rek′se-ə), lack or loss of _____. Basic functions, such as eating, can be severely impaired by problems of the digestive system, but not all eating or nutritional disorders are caused by malfunction of the digestive system. For example, **anorexia nervosa** (an″o-rek′se-ə nur-vo′sə) is a sometimes life-threatening illness that is self-induced starvation. Literal translation of an/orexia is

without

_____ appetite.

This clinical syndrome occurs primarily in females, with onset most often during adolescence. There is often an intense fear of losing control of eating and becoming fat. Unless there is intervention, anorexia nervosa results in **emaciation** (e-ma″she-a′shən), excessive leanness caused by disease or lack of nutrition.

10-88 Bulimia (boo-le′me-ə) is another eating disorder that occurs predominantly in females, with onset usually in adolescence or early adulthood. The derivation of the term bulimia from Greek is *bous*, ox, and *limos*, hunger. This disorder is characterized by episodes of binge eating that often end in purging and depression. Purging is accomplished by self-induced vomiting or

bulimia

the use of laxatives. Dentists sometimes see erosion of the maxillary teeth on the tongue side owing to frequent vomiting (Figure 10-13). The name of this disorder that is characterized by binge eating and purging is ______________________.

poor

10-89 If something interferes with eating or the digestion of food, body cells will lack needed nutrients and malnutrition will result. **Mal/nutrition** (mal″noo-trish′ən) means improper or ______________________ nutrition.

Mal/absorption (mal″əb-sorp′shən) is improper absorption of nutrients into the bloodstream from the intestines. This will eventually result in malnutrition. **Malabsorption syndrome** is subnormal absorption of dietary constituents and can be caused by a number of disorders, including several inborn errors of metabolism, such as celiac disease. Malabsorption is characterized by anorexia, weight loss, abdominal bloating, muscle cramps, and the presence of fat in stool samples.

vomiting

10-90 Excessive vomiting, unless treated with an anti/emetic (an″te-ə-met′ik), can also lead to malnutrition. **Emesis** (em′ə-sis) means vomiting. **Hyper/emesis** (hi″pər-em′ə-sis) is excessive ______________________. Nausea usually accompanies vomiting.

Hemat/emesis (he″mə-tem′ə-sis) is vomiting of blood and indicates upper GI bleeding, such as that caused by an ulcer of the esophagus or stomach.

obesity

10-91 **Obesity** (o-bēs′ĭ-te) is an abnormal increase in the proportion of fat cells of the body, and a person is regarded as medically obese if he or she is 20% above desirable body weight for the person's age, sex, height, and body build. The calculated body mass index (BMI) using weight-to-height ratios is an index of obesity or altered body fat distribution. An abnormal increase in the proportion of fat cells of the body is called ______________________.

Exo/gen/ous (ek-soj′ə-nəs) **obesity** is caused by a greater caloric intake than that needed to meet the metabolic needs of the body. **Endo/gen/ous** (en-doj′ə-nəs) **obesity** originates from within the body, as seen in hormonal disorders such as uncontrolled diabetes.

excessive

10-92 **Poly/phag/ia** (pol″e-fa′jə) means ______________________ eating. Excessive eating over a long period generally leads to weight gain as a result of taking in more calories than the number needed for normal body metabolism. The amount of fuel or energy in food is measured in calories.

difficult

10-93 **Dys/phagia** (dis-fa′je-ə) means difficulty or inability to swallow, although its literal translation is ______________________ eating.

thirst

10-94 **Poly/dips/ia** (pol″e-dip′se-ə) is excessive ______________________. It is characteristic of several different conditions, including those in which there is increased excretion of fluid because of increased urination, which leads to thirst. Polydipsia is a common occurrence in untreated diabetes mellitus. See Chapter 17, Endocrine System, to learn more about this disorder and tests used to diagnose diabetes mellitus.

absence

A/dips/ia (ə-dip′se-ə) is ______________________ of thirst.

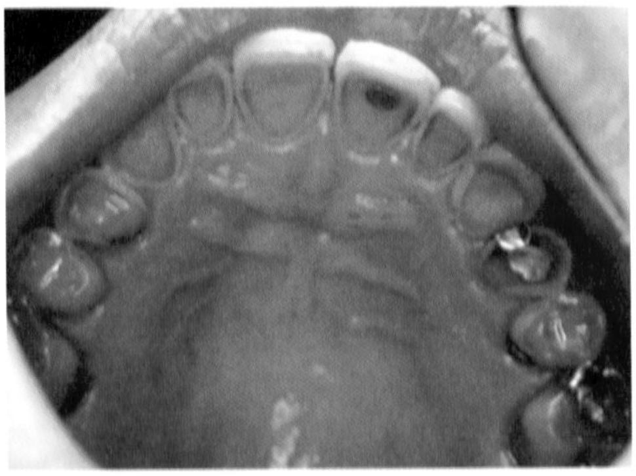

Figure 10-13 **Erosion on the tongue side of the maxillary teeth in bulimia.** This is not an unusual finding in bulimia, owing to frequent contact with regurgitated stomach contents.

difficult

10-95 Literal translation of dys/pepsia (dis-pep´se-ə) is bad or _____ digestion. **Dys/pepsia,** imperfect or painful digestion, is not a disease in itself but symptomatic of other diseases or disorders. It means the same as indigestion. **Eructation*** (ə-rək-ta´shən), or belching, results from the act of drawing up air from the stomach and expelling it through the mouth. Eructation and hiccups sometimes accompany dyspepsia. A hiccup is produced by the involuntary contraction of the diaphragm, followed by rapid closure of the glottis (opening between the vocal cords). Other causes of hiccups include rapid eating and certain types of surgery.

*Eructation (Latin: *eructare,* to belch).

EXERCISE 13

▮▮▮ **Build It!** *Use the following word parts to build terms. (Some word parts will be used more than once.)*

a-, an-, eu-, exo-, hyper-, gen(o), -emesis, -dipsia, -orexia, -ous, -pepsia

1. lack of appetite   _____ / _____

2. excessive vomiting   _____ / _____

3. normal digestion   _____ / _____

4. pertaining to development outside the body   _____ / _____ / _____

5. condition of the absence of thirst   _____ / _____

🔊 **Say and Check**

Say aloud the terms you wrote for Exercise 13. Use the Companion CD to check your pronunciations.

UPPER DIGESTIVE TRACT

eating

10-96 Diseases of the upper digestive tract include those diseases or disorders that affect the mouth, the esophagus, and the stomach.
     Literal translation of a/phag/ia (ə-fa´jə) is absence of _____, but you will need to remember that **aphagia** means an inability to swallow as a result of an organic or psychological cause. This differs from anorexia nervosa, a disorder characterized by self-imposed starvation.

inflammation

10-97 Stomat/itis makes eating difficult because the mouth is painful. **Stomatitis** (sto″mə-ti´tis) is _____ of the mouth.
     Stomato/dynia (sto″mə-to-din´e-ə) means painful mouth. Ulcers (ul´sərs) are defined, craterlike lesions. Ulcerations on the lips are often called cold sores or fever blisters (usually caused by the herpes simplex virus [HSV] type 1) (see Figure 4-10).

mouth

10-98 Any oral disease caused by a fungus is stomatomycosis. **Stomato/myc/osis** (sto″mə-to-mi-ko´sis) is a fungal condition of the _____.
     Candida albicans is a yeast type of fungus that is part of the normal flora of the oral cavity (see Figure 4-14, *B*). Because antibiotic therapy destroys the normal bacteria that usually prevent fungal infections, candidiasis (an infection caused by *Candida,* usually *C. albicans*) can result. Also, patients receiving chemo/therapy often develop candidiasis, because chemotherapy diminishes the ability of the immune system to prevent infection.

lips

10-99 Cheil/osis (ki-lo´sis) is a condition of the _____. In cheilosis there is splitting of the lips and angles of the mouth (Figure 10-14). Cheilosis is a characteristic of riboflavin deficiency in the diet.

cheilitis (ki-li´tis)

10-100 Inflammation of the lip is _____.

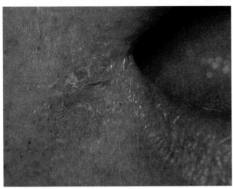

Figure 10-14 Cheilosis. This disorder of the lips and mouth is characterized by splitting of the lips and skin around the mouth.

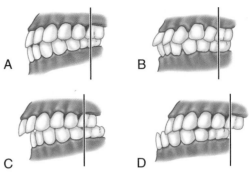

Figure 10-15 Malocclusion. Such malposition and contact of the maxillary and mandibular teeth interfere with the highest efficiency during chewing. **A,** Normal occlusion. **B,** Class I malocclusion. **C,** Class II malocclusion. **D,** Class III malocclusion.

Cheilitis often produces pain when one attempts to eat. Cheilitis and other abnormal conditions of mouth structures can result in poor nutrition.

10-101 Gingivo/stomat/itis (jin″jĭ-vo-sto″mə-ti′tis) is inflammation of the gums and
_____. Inflammation of the gum is **gingiv/itis** (jin″jĭ-vi′tis).

mouth

10-102 Gingiv/algia (jin″jĭ-val′jə) is _____ gums.
Gingivo/gloss/itis (jin″jĭ-vo-glos-i′tis) is inflammation of the tongue and gums.

painful

10-103 Any disease of the tongue is a _____. **Gloss/itis** (glos-i′tis) is inflammation of the tongue. **Glosso/plegia** (glos″o-ple′jə) means paralysis of the tongue.

glossopathy
(glos-op′ə-the)

10-104 Glosso/pyr/osis (glos″o-pi-ro′sis) is an abnormal sensation of pain, burning, and stinging of the tongue without apparent lesions or cause. The combining form pyr(o), which means fire, in glosso/pyr/osis refers to the stinging sensation of the _____.

tongue

10-105 Dent/algia (den-tal′jə) means a toothache. Dentalgia is often caused by caries that have extended into the tooth pulp. **Caries*** (kar′ēz, kar′e-ēz) means decay. Neglected dental caries, over time, invade and inflame pulpal tissues. **End/odont/itis** means inflammation of the endodontium, or the tooth _____.

pulp

10-106 Halitosis† is an offensive breath resulting from poor oral hygiene, dental or oral infections, use of tobacco, ingestion of certain foods such as garlic, or some systemic diseases such as the odor of acetone in diabetes or ammonia in liver disease. Write the term that means bad breath: _____.

halitosis

10-107 Peri/odont/itis (per″e-o-don-ti′tis) is inflammation of the _____, the structure that supports the tooth.
Pyorrhea (pi″o-re′ə) is one type of periodontal disease. Pyorrhea is an inflammation of the gingiva and the periodontal ligament, the fibrous connective tissue that anchors the tooth to the base. Literal interpretation of pyo/rrhea is discharge of _____.

periodontium

pus

10-108 An impacted tooth is one that is unable to erupt because of crowding by adjacent teeth or mal/position of the tooth.
Mal/occlusion (mal″o-kloo′zhən), or improper bite, is abnormal contact of the teeth of the upper jaw, the maxilla, with the teeth of the lower jaw, the mandible (Figure 10-15). Ortho/dontic braces are used to move the teeth into alignment—in other words, to _____ the teeth.

straighten

*Caries (Latin: *decay*).
†Halitosis (Latin: *halitus,* breath).

temporomandibular

10-109 TMJ pain dysfunction syndrome is an abnormal condition that interferes with eating and is believed to be caused by a defective or dislocated **temporo/mandibular** (tem″pə-ro-man-dib´u-lər) **joint** (TMJ), one of a pair of joints connecting the mandible to the skull.

Often called TMJ syndrome, this condition is characterized by facial pain and clicking sounds while chewing. Malocclusion, ill-fitting dentures, and a variety of conditions can cause TMJ syndrome. TMJ refers to the _____ joint.

EXERCISE 14

Word Analysis. *Divide these words into their component parts, and write the meaning of each term.*

1. cheilosis _____

2. gingivalgia _____

3. endodontitis _____

4. glossopyrosis _____

5. pyorrhea _____

6. stomatomycosis _____

cheeks

10-110 The mouth is examined for oral cancer during a routine dental examination. Tumors of the oral cavity can cause pain and change aspects of talking, swallowing, or chewing. Oral tumors can be classified as pre/malignant (precancerous), malignant, or benign.

Leuko/plakia (loo″ko-pla´ke-ə) is a precancerous, slowly developing change in a mucous membrane characterized by white patches with sharply defined edges that are slightly raised. Leukoplakia may occur on the genitals or the lips and buccal mucosa (Figure 10-16). The **buccal mucosa** (buk´əl mu-ko´sə) is the mucous membrane that lines the insides of the _____.

near

10-111 Parot/itis (par″o-ti´tis) is inflammation of the parotid gland. Epidemic or infectious parotitis is another name for mumps, a contagious viral disease that can generally be prevented by immunization.

Mumps is an acute viral infection that is characterized by swelling of the parotid glands and may affect one or both glands. The parotid gland is a salivary gland located _____ the ear.

cleft

10-112 Cleft palate, often associated with cleft lip, is a congenital defect in which there is a division of the palate, resulting from the failure of the two sides of the palate to fuse during development. Cleft lip is one or more clefts in the upper lip (Figure 10-17). Surgical repair beginning in infancy is generally recommended for both of these congenital defects. Failure of the two sides of the palate to fuse during development results in _____ palate.

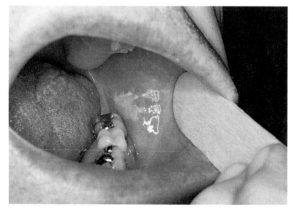

Figure 10-16 **Leukoplakia.** This slowly developing change in a mucous membrane characterized by white, sharply circumscribed patches is a precancerous lesion.

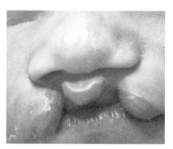

Figure 10-17 **Cleft lip.** This particular cleft in the upper lip is bilateral, but the congenital defect may be unilateral, median, or bilateral and may be accompanied by cleft palate.

10-113 The esophagus is susceptible to a variety of inflammatory, structural, and neoplastic (ne[o], new + -plastic, repair) disorders. A neo/plasm is an abnormal growth of new tissue and can be benign or malignant.

Esophag/itis (ə-sof″ə-ji′tis) is inflammation of the mucosal lining of the esophagus, caused by infection, backflow of gastric juice from the stomach, or irritation from a naso/gastric tube. A nasogastric tube is a tube passed through the nose into the _____ and is used to both remove and introduce substances.

Esophago/malacia (ə-sof″ə-go-mə-la′shə) is a morbid softening of the esophagus. **Esophago/dynia** (ə-sof″ə-go-din′e-ə) is _____ of the esophagus.

10-114 Esophageal achalasia (ak″ə-la′zhə) is an abnormal condition in which the lower esophageal sphincter fails to relax properly. It is characterized by dysphagia. Regurgitation, the return of swallowed food into the mouth, may also occur. Changes in diet and certain drugs may be helpful, but dilation of the esophagus with progressively larger sizes of dilators is also used. Write the name of the condition in which the lower esophageal sphincter fails to relax appropriately in response to swallowing: esophageal _____.

10-115 Esophageal atresia (ə-tre′zhə), usually a congenital abnormality, is an esophagus that ends in a blind pouch or narrows so much that it obstructs continuous passage of food to the stomach. Write this term that is a congenital abnormality that results in a blind pouch or narrowing of the esophagus: esophageal _____. Narrowing may be improved by progressively larger dilators, or corrective surgery may be necessary.

10-116 Esophageal varices (singular, varix) are enlarged and swollen veins at the lower end of the esophagus, which are especially susceptible to hemorrhage. These large and swollen veins are called _____.

Upper gastrointestinal bleeding is usually caused by esophageal varices, gastritis, ulcerations, or cancer of either the esophagus or stomach (Figure 10-18).

10-117 Gastroesophageal reflux disease (GERD) is a dysfunction that involves a backflow of the contents of the stomach into the _____. The cause is often a weak cardiac sphincter. Repeated episodes of reflux can result in esophagitis, stricture (narrowing) of the esophagus, or an esophageal ulcer (craterlike lesion). Treatment of the disorder in its early stages is elevation of the head of the bed, avoidance of acid-stimulating foods, and use of ant/acids or anti/ulcer medications.

(margin answers)
stomach

pain

achalasia

atresia

varices

esophagus

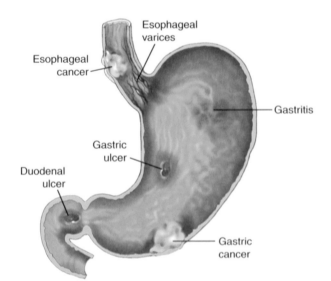

Figure 10-18 Common causes of upper gastrointestinal bleeding.

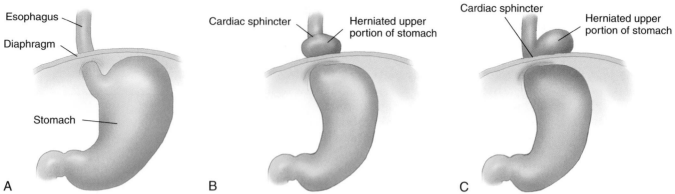

Esophagus
Diaphragm
Stomach

Cardiac sphincter   Herniated upper portion of stomach

Cardiac sphincter   Herniated upper portion of stomach

A   B   C

Figure 10-19 **The normal position of the stomach versus two types of hiatal hernias. A,** Normal position of the stomach. **B,** The sliding type of hiatal hernia accounts for 85% to 90% of hiatal hernias. The upper portion of the stomach slides up and down through the opening in the diaphragm. **C,** The rolling type of hiatal hernia accounts for 10% to 15% of hiatal hernias. The upper portion of the stomach is found above the diaphragm, alongside the esophagus.

hiatal	**10-118** GERD is one of the major symptoms of a **hiatal** (hi-a′təl) **hernia,** protrusion of a portion of the stomach upward through a defect in the diaphragm. Figure 10-19 shows two types of hiatal hernias. As much as 40% of the population may have hiatal hernia, but most are asymptomatic. Diagnosis is generally confirmed by radiology, and surgery is seldom necessary. This type of herniation is called a _____ hernia.
pain	**10-119** **Gastr/itis** (gas-tri′tis), one of the most common stomach disorders, is inflammation of the lining of the stomach. Causes of gastritis include medicines, food allergies, and toxins of microorganisms. *Helicobacter pylori* has been shown to be the cause of most cases of nonerosive gastritis. Chronic gastritis can be a sign of another disease, such as cancer of the stomach or peptic ulcer. Peptic ulcers occur in the stomach, the duodenum, and occasionally the esophagus. The ulcerations are breaks in the continuity of the mucous membrane that comes in contact with the acids of the stomach. They usually occur near the pyloric opening (Figure 10-20). These types of ulcers cause stomachache, also called **gastr/algia** (gas-tral′jə). The literal interpretation of gastralgia is _____ of the stomach.
	10-120 Most peptic ulcers eventually heal, and the pain is controlled with drugs that either neutralize or block secretion of acid. The immediate cause of peptic ulcers remains unknown. A small percentage of patients with ulcers need surgery to remove the affected part of the stomach or to sever a branch of the vagus nerve to reduce the amount of gastric acid produced.
softening cancer	**10-121** Any disease of the stomach is a **gastropathy** (gas-trop′ə-the). **Gastromalacia** (gas″tro-mə-la′shə) means a morbid _____ of the stomach. **Gastromegaly** (gas″tro-meg′ə-le) means abnormal enlargement of the stomach or abdomen. Gastric carcinoma is _____ of the stomach.

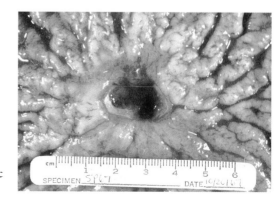

Figure 10-20 **Photograph of a peptic ulcer.** This peptic ulcer is located in the lesser curvature of the stomach.

EXERCISE 15

Build It! *Use the following word parts to build terms. (Some word parts will be used more than once.)*

esophag(o), gastr(o), -algia, -dynia, -eal, -malacia, -pathy

1. pain in the stomach   _____/_____

2. any disease of the stomach   _____/_____

3. pertaining to the stomach and the esophagus   _____/_____/_____

4. morbid softening of the esophagus   _____/_____

5. pain in the esophagus   _____/_____

Say and Check

Say aloud the terms you wrote for Exercise 15. Use the Companion CD to check your pronunciations.

stenosis	**10-122** Pyloric stenosis is narrowing of the pyloric sphincter. The condition is a congenital defect, and it interferes with the flow of food into the small intestine. This condition in which there is narrowing of the pyloric sphincter is pyloric _____.
stretching	**10-123 Gastr/ectasia** (gas-trek-ta´zhe) is abnormal _____ of the stomach. This may be caused by overeating, a hernia, or obstruction of the pyloric opening.
flatulence	**10-124** Some prominent signs and symptoms of gastric dysfunction are pain, excessive belching, flatulence, nausea, vomiting, blood in the stool, and diarrhea. Flatulence is excessive gas in the stomach or intestines. Diarrhea is frequent passage of watery bowel movements, often accompanied by cramping. Write the term that means excessive gas in the stomach or intestines: _____.

EXERCISE 16

Match pathologies of the upper digestive tract in the left columns with their meanings or characteristics in the right column.

_____ 1. dyspepsia	_____ 8. hematemesis	A. enlarged and swollen veins of the esophagus
_____ 2. esophageal achalasia	_____ 9. leukoplakia	B. esophageal sphincter fails to relax properly
_____ 3. esophageal atresia	_____ 10. polydipsia	C. esophagus ends in a blind pouch or narrows
_____ 4. esophageal varices	_____ 11. polyphagia	D. excessive hunger
_____ 5. gastritis	_____ 12. sialadenitis	E. excessive thirst
_____ 6. gingivitis	_____ 13. stomatodynia	F. indigestion
_____ 7. glossitis		G. inflammation of the stomach

A. enlarged and swollen veins of the esophagus
B. esophageal sphincter fails to relax properly
C. esophagus ends in a blind pouch or narrows
D. excessive hunger
E. excessive thirst
F. indigestion
G. inflammation of the stomach
H. inflammation of a salivary gland
I. inflammation of the gums
J. inflammation of the tongue
K. painful mouth
L. precancerous change in a mucous membrane
M. vomiting of blood

LOWER DIGESTIVE TRACT

peritonitis	**10-125** Intestinal disorders can be classified as inflammatory or noninflammatory. Similar symptoms may make it difficult to differentiate inflammatory and infectious disorders. Periton/itis (the "e" in peritone[o] is dropped to facilitate pronunciation) is an acute inflammation of the peritoneum (the lining of the abdominal cavity). Causes of peritonitis include rupture of abdominal organs such as the appendix, peptic ulcers, or perforations of an organ in the GI tract. Without treatment, it becomes a life-threatening illness. A rupture or perforation of an organ in the GI tract may lead to _____.

appendix

intestines

water

colitis

anus

fissure

food

10-126 Three examples of acute inflammatory bowel problems are appendicitis, gastroenteritis, and dysentery. **Appendic/itis** (ə-pen″dĭ-si′tis) is acute inflammation of the vermiform _____.

Gastro/enteritis (gas″tro-en″tər-i′tis) means inflammation of the stomach and _____. It primarily affects the small intestine and can be either viral or bacterial. Intestinal flu (or influenza) is a viral gastroenteritis.

Symptoms of gastroenteritis are anorexia, nausea, vomiting, abdominal discomfort, diarrhea, and possibly fever. The feces may contain blood, mucus, pus, or excessive amounts of fat. Untreated severe diarrhea may lead to rapid dehydration. Dehydration is excessive loss of _____ from body tissues.

Dysentery (dis′ən-ter″e) is an inflammation of the intestine, especially of the colon, that may be caused by bacteria, protozoa, parasites, or chemical irritants. It is characterized by abdominal pain and frequent and bloody stools.

10-127 Literal translation of **col/itis** is inflammation of the large intestine. Ulcerative col/itis, irritable bowel syndrome (IBS), and Crohn disease are three of the more common chronic inflammatory bowel diseases (IBDs). Ulcerative colitis is a chronic inflammatory disorder of the colon or rectum, characterized by profuse, watery diarrhea containing mucus, blood, and pus. The chronic inflammation results in a loss of the mucosal lining and ulceration or abscess formation.

This type of chronic inflammatory bowel disease is called ulcerative _____.

10-128 Crohn disease (krōn dĭ-zēz′) is another inflammatory bowel disease that can affect any part of the GI tract, from the mouth to the anus. As with ulcerative colitis, the cause is unknown. The lesions of Crohn disease are patchy and often extend through all bowel layers.

Abnormal passages between internal organs or abnormal communications leading from internal organs to the body surface are called **fistulas.**[*] Fistulas can occur between the bowel and almost any adjacent structures. An anal fistula (fis′tu-lə) is an abnormal opening near the _____.

10-129 A **fissure** (fish′ər) is a cleft or a groove or a cracklike lesion of the skin. A painful linear ulceration or tear at the anal opening is called an anal _____. Fissures are sometimes associated with constipation, diarrhea, or Crohn disease (Figure 10-21, _A_).

10-130 Parasites and pathogenic bacteria or viruses can invade the GI tract. Food poisoning results when a person ingests toxic substances or infectious organisms in food, but unlike gastroenteritis, food poisoning cannot be passed directly to another person. Mushroom poisoning is a type of _____ poisoning.

[*]Fistula (Latin: _fistula,_ pipe).

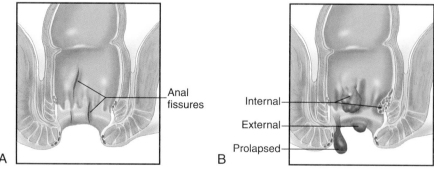

Figure 10-21 Two disorders of the anorectal area. A, Anal fissures. An ulceration or tear of the lining of the anal canal may be caused by excessive tissue stretching. These tears are very tender and tend to reopen when stool is passed. **B,** Hemorrhoids. Three types of hemorrhoids are shown: internal, external, and prolapsed. Internal hemorrhoids lie above the anal sphincter and cannot be seen on inspection of the anal area. External hemorrhoids lie below the anal sphincter and can be seen on inspection of the anal region. Hemorrhoids that enlarge, fall down, and protrude through the anus are called prolapsed hemorrhoids.

Some common types of food poisoning include staphylococcal infection, *Escherichia coli* (commonly called *E. coli*) infection, and botulism. All these types of food poisoning are caused by pathogenic bacteria. Another bacterium, *Salmonella,* causes **salmonell/osis** (sal″mo-nəl-o´sis), and some forms of salmonella infection cause acute gastroenteritis.

duodenum

10-131 A duodenal ulcer, the most common type of peptic ulcer, is one that occurs in the _____. Inflammation of the duodenum is **duodenitis** (doo-od″ə-ni´tis). Inflammation of the ileum is **ileitis** (il″e-i´tis). **Gastro/duoden/itis** (gas″tro-doo″o-də-ni´tis) is inflammation of the _____ and duodenum.

stomach

10-132 Noninflammatory intestinal disorders include malignant diverticulosis, tumors, obstructions, malabsorption, and trauma. Irritable bowel syndrome (IBS), also called spastic colon, spastic bowel, and mucous colitis, is a common chronic noninflammatory intestinal disorder. The cause is unknown, and it primarily involves increased motility of the intestines, diarrhea, and pain in the lower abdomen. Women are affected more than men by a 3:1 ratio.

irritable

This noninflammatory intestinal disorder is called _____ bowel syndrome.

10-133 Rectal bleeding may be indicative of an intestinal disorder. **Hemorrhoids** (hem´ə-roidz), a common cause of rectal bleeding, are masses of dilated veins of the anal canal that lie just inside or outside the rectum. Several types are shown in Figure 10-21, *B*. They are often accompanied by pain, itching, and/or bleeding.

Hemorrhoids are commonly called piles. This condition is aggravated by constipation, difficulty in passing stool, or infrequent passage of hard stools. Constipation, straining to **defecate** (def´ə-kāt), and prolonged sitting contribute to the development of

hemorrhoids

_____.

10-134 Diverticular disease includes diverticul/itis and diverticu/losis. A **diverticulum** (di″vər-tik´u-ləm) is a pouchlike herniation through the muscular wall of a tubular organ. A diverticulum (plural is diverticula) is most commonly present in the colon but also can occur in the esophagus, stomach, or small intestine (Figure 10-22). The combining form diverticul(o) refers to diverticula.

If diverticula are present in the colon without inflammation or symptoms, the condition is called **diverticulosis** (di″vər-tik″u-lo´sis). Diverticula generally do not cause a problem.

inflammation

Diverticul/itis (di″vər-tik″u-li´tis) is _____ of one or more diverticula.

10-135 Common causes of lower gastrointestinal bleeding are shown in Figure 10-23. Colonic polyps, small, tumor-like growths, can arise from the mucosal surface of the colon. They may be seen during a colonoscopy. Some types of colonic polyps are closely linked to colorectal cancer,

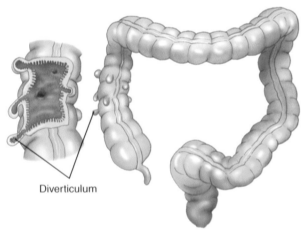

Figure 10-22 Diverticulosis. Several abnormal outpouchings (diverticula) in the wall of the intestine.

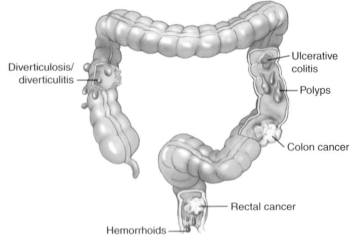

Figure 10-23 Common causes of lower gastrointestinal bleeding.

and for this reason should be removed. **Polyp/ectomy** (pol″ĭ-pek′tə-me), removal of a polyp, can be performed during a colonoscopy.

Small, tumor-like growths on the mucosal surface of the colon are called colonic

polyps _____.

10-136 An accumulation of hardened feces in the rectum or sigmoid colon that the individual cannot expel is **impaction** (im-pak′shən).

Write the term that means the presence of a large or hard fecal mass in the rectum or

impaction colon: _____.

10-137 Impaction leads to colonic stasis, also called **entero/stasis** (en″tər-o-sta′sis). When enterostasis occurs, there is a delay or a stopping of the movement of food in the intestinal tract.

enterostasis Colonic stasis, also called _____, is a stagnation of the normal flow of contents of the colon.

10-138 Intestinal obstruction occurs when intestinal contents cannot pass through the GI tract. The obstruction may be partial or complete and can occur anywhere in the intestinal tract. Figure 10-24 shows several causes of intestinal obstruction. Look closely at the illustration as you read about the different types of bowel obstructions.

Adhesions are bands of scar tissue that bind surfaces that normally are separated. They most commonly form in the abdomen after abdominal surgery, inflammation, or injury. Write the term that means scar tissue that binds surfaces together that are normally separate:

adhesion _____.

10-139 Inguinal hernias develop because of a weakness in the abdominal muscle wall or a widened space at the inguinal ligament (see Figure 6-17, *B*). In a strangulated hernia, the blood vessels become so constricted by the neck of the hernial sac that circulation is stopped in the constricted area. Surgical intervention is necessary. A hernia in which the blood vessels are

strangulated constricted by the neck of the hernial sac is called a _____ hernia.

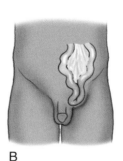
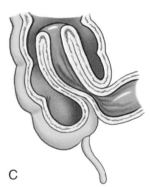
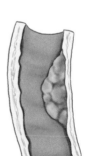
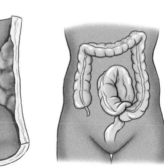
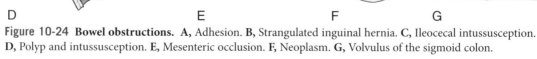

Figure 10-24 **Bowel obstructions. A,** Adhesion. **B,** Strangulated inguinal hernia. **C,** Ileocecal intussusception.
D, Polyp and intussusception. **E,** Mesenteric occlusion. **F,** Neoplasm. **G,** Volvulus of the sigmoid colon.

intussusception	**10-140 Intussusception** (in″tə-sə-sep′shən) is a telescopic folding back of the bowel into itself. Mesenteric occlusion is a binding or closing off of a segment of the intestine by the mesentery, the peritoneum that suspends the intestine from the abdominal wall. A twisting of the bowel is called **volvulus** (vol′vu-ləs), and a folding back of the bowel onto itself is called _____. (Pronounce carefully to aid in the spelling of this term.) Neoplasms or tumors are the most common cause of obstruction of the large intestine. Surgery is usually necessary to correct obstructions of the bowel.
poor fats	**10-141** Mal/absorption syndrome is a disorder in which one or multiple nutrients are not digested or absorbed. Literal translation of mal/absorption is _____ absorption. The nutrient that is not absorbed well depends on which abnormality exists. Various deficiencies can lead to malabsorption of fats, various vitamins, lactose, or iron. **Lipo/penia** (lip″o-pe′ne-ə) is a deficiency of _____.

EXERCISE 17

Build It! *Use the following word parts to build terms. (Some word parts will be used more than once.)*

append(o), duoden(o), enter(o), gastr(o), lip(o), -itis, -penia, -stasis

1. delay or stopping of movement of food in the intestinal tract _____/_____
2. inflammation of the vermiform appendix _____/_____
3. inflammation of the stomach and duodenum _____/_____/_____
4. deficiency of fats _____/_____

Say and Check

Say aloud the terms you wrote for Exercise 17. Use the Companion CD to check your pronunciations.

EXERCISE 18

Write a word in each blank to complete these sentences. The first letter of the word is given as a clue.

1. Inflammation of the stomach and intestines is g_____.
2. Inflammation of the colon that is characterized by abdominal pain and frequent, bloody stools is

   d_____.
3. An abnormal passage between two internal organs is a f_____.
4. The presence of diverticula in the colon without inflammation is called d_____.
5. A painful linear ulceration or tear at the anal opening is an anal f_____.
6. A common noninflammatory intestinal disorder has many names, including spastic bowel, mucous colitis, spastic

   colon, and i_____ bowel syndrome.
7. Masses of dilated veins that are varicose and lie just inside or outside the rectum are h_____.
8. An accumulation of feces that the individual cannot expel is called an i_____.
9. A telescopic folding back of one part of the intestine into itself is i_____.
10. A twisting of the bowel is called v_____.

ACCESSORY ORGANS OF DIGESTION

liver

10-142 The liver is one of the most vital internal organs. Degeneration of the liver may lead to severe consequences, including ascites (accumulation of abdominal fluid), defects in coagulation of the blood, jaundice, neurologic symptoms, and hepatic and renal failure.

Hepato/renal syndrome is a type of kidney failure that is associated with hepatic failure. In hepat/ic failure, the _____ cannot perform its vital functions for the body. Hepatorenal syndrome has a poor prognosis because both the kidneys and liver fail.

enlargement

10-143 Any disease of the liver is **hepato/pathy** (hep″ə-top´ə-the). **Hepato/spleno/megaly** (hep″ə-to-sple″no-meg´ə-le) is _____ of the liver and spleen.

inflammation

10-144 Hepat/itis (hep″ə-ti´tis) is _____ of the liver. It is characterized by jaundice, **hepatomegaly** (hep″ə-to-meg´ə-le), anorexia, abnormal liver function, clay-colored stools, and tea-colored urine.

enlarged

Jaundice (jawn´dis) is a yellow discoloration of the skin, the mucous membranes, and the whites of the eyes, caused by greater than normal amounts of bilirubin in the blood. Bilirubin is the yellow-orange pigment of bile. Hepato/megaly means an _____ liver.

10-145 Hepatitis may result from bacterial or viral infections or other causes, such as medications, toxins, or alcohol. Viral hepatitis is generally one of five major types. Other types of hepatitis are less common or generally have mild symptoms.

> ➤ KEY POINT Five major types of viral hepatitis and their associated viruses are:
> - hepatitis A (hepatitis A virus [HAV])
> - hepatitis B (hepatitis B virus [HBV])
> - hepatitis C (hepatitis C virus [HCV])
> - hepatitis D (hepatitis D virus [HDV])
> - hepatitis E (hepatitis E virus [HEV])

virus

Hepatitis A is caused by HAV, the abbreviation for hepatitis A _____. Hepatitis A and hepatitis E can be acquired by ingestion of contaminated food, but the other types are acquired only by contact with an infected person or infected materials. Most types of viral hepatitis can be acquired by contaminated blood, sexual contact, or the use of contaminated needles and instruments. Immunization is available for some types of hepatitis. Read more about viral hepatitis in the Sexually Transmitted Diseases section of Chapter 13.

liver

10-146 Cirrhosis (sǐ-ro´sis) is a chronic, progressive liver disease that is characterized by degeneration of liver cells with eventual increased resistance to flow of blood through the liver. Cirrhosis is a disease of what organ? _____

Alcoholic cirrhosis occurs in approximately 20% of chronic alcoholics. Unless alcohol is avoided, coma, gastrointestinal hemorrhage, and kidney failure may occur. In addition to alcohol, nutritional deficiencies, poisons, toxic drugs, some types of heart disease, and prior viral hepatitis can lead to cirrhosis.

hepatoma
(hep″ə-to´mə)

10-147 A tumor of the liver is a _____. This term is usually reserved for a specific type of primary liver carcinoma.

carcinoma

Tumors of the liver may be benign or malignant. Cancer of the liver is called hepatic _____. Malignancy in the liver that is spread from another source (metastasis) is many times more common than primary tumor of the liver.

10-148 Bile is produced by the liver, stored in the gallbladder, and released into the duodenum via the common bile duct when needed for digestion. Anything that interferes with the flow of bile interferes with digestion. **Chole/stasis** (ko″lə-sta´sis) is stoppage or suppression of bile flow. Obstruction of bile flow can cause inflammation of the gallbladder, the liver, or the pancreas.

bile

Chol/angitis (ko″lan-ji′tis) is inflammation of a _____
vessel or duct. (Note that the "e" is dropped from chol[e] when it is combined with angi[o].) This
can be caused by bacterial infection or by obstruction of the ducts by calculi or a tumor.

calculus

10-149 Choledoch/itis (ko″lə-do-ki′tis) is inflammation of the common bile duct.
Choledocho/lith/iasis (ko-led″ə-ko-lĭ-thi′ə-sis) is the presence of a _____
in the common bile duct.

gallstones
(or calculi)

10-150 Chole/lith/iasis (ko″lə-lĭ-thi′ə-sis) is the presence of _____
in the gallbladder. Acute **cholecyst/itis**, inflammation of the gallbladder, is usually caused by a
gallstone. If surgery is not performed to remove the gallbladder, a perforation (opening or hole)
in its wall may occur. An abscess may form if the perforation is small, or peritonitis may result if
the perforation is large.

Acute cholecystitis may occur in the absence of gallstones, possibly because of bacterial invasion. A chronic form of cholecystitis, with pain following a fatty meal, may occur when there is
insufficient emptying of bile by the gallbladder.

pancreas

10-151 Both cholangitis and pancreatitis can occur as complications of cholecystitis, resulting
from the backup of bile through the biliary tract. **Pancreat/itis** (pan″kre-ə-ti′tis) is inflammation
of the _____. Acute pancreatitis can be life-threatening,
resulting in destruction of the organ by its own enzymes. Destruction of pancreatic tissue is
pancreatolysis (pan″kre-ə-tol′ĭ-sis).

Several factors that contribute to acute pancreatitis include alcoholism, gallstones, trauma,
tumors, peritonitis, viral infections, and drug toxicity. Chronic pancreatitis may develop after
repeated episodes of acute pancreatitis (particularly that induced by alcohol abuse) or chronic

pus

obstruction of the common bile duct. A pancreatic abscess, a collection of _____
in or around the pancreas, is a serious complication of pancreatitis.

10-152 Stones, tumors, or cysts can cause pancreatic obstructions. **Pancreato/lithiasis**
(pan″kre-ə-to-lĭ-thi′ə-sis) is the presence of calculi in the pancreas or pancreatic duct.

calculus (stone)

Pancreato/lith (pan″kre-at′o-lith) means a pancreatic _____.

Pancreatic carcinoma is one of the most deadly malignancies. The cancer is usually discovered
in the late stages, and prognosis is poor. Pancreatic cancer is not common in North America, but
it ranks fourth as a cause of cancer death because of its extremely low survival rate.

Like pancreatic carcinoma, the prognosis for cancer of the gallbladder is poor. However, cancer of the gallbladder is rare.

10-153 Two of the more likely disorders of the salivary glands are sialadenitis and sialolithiasis.
Tumors of the salivary glands are not common. **Sial/aden/itis** (si″əl-ad″ə-ni′tis),

inflammation

_____ of the salivary glands, can be caused by an infectious
microorganism, an allergic reaction, or irradiation. Sialadenitis due to irradiation may result
from radiation therapy, which causes a very dry mouth, and is treated with substances that stimulate saliva or substitute for saliva.

Sialo/lithiasis (si″ə-lo-lĭ-thi′ə-sis), the presence of salivary stones either within the gland itself or in the salivary ducts, may cause few symptoms unless the duct becomes obstructed.

EXERCISE 19

Match terms in the left columns with their meaning or characteristics in the right column. (Use all choices once.)

_____ 1. ascites   _____ 5. choledocholithiasis   A. accumulation of abdominal fluid

_____ 2. cholangitis   _____ 6. cirrhosis   B. calculus in the common bile duct
                                                            C. chronic degeneration of liver cells
_____ 3. cholecystitis   _____ 7. hepatoma   D. inflammation of a bile duct
                                                            E. inflammation of the common bile duct
_____ 4. choledochitis   _____ 8. jaundice   F. inflammation of the gallbladder
                                                            G. tumor of the liver
                                                            H. yellow discoloration of the skin and increased bilirubin

EXERCISE 20

Build It! *Use the following word parts to build terms. (Some word parts will be used more than once.)*

chol(e), hepat(o), pancreat(o), ren(o), -al, -lith, -lysis, -megaly, -stasis

1. enlargement of the liver   _____/_____

2. suppression of bile flow   _____/_____

3. pertaining to the liver and the kidney   _____/_____/_____

4. destruction of pancreatic tissue   _____/_____

5. a calculus in the pancreas   _____/_____

Say and Check

Say aloud the terms you wrote for Exercise 20. Use the Companion CD to check your pronunciations.

SURGICAL AND THERAPEUTIC INTERVENTIONS
UPPER AND LOWER DIGESTIVE TRACTS

lip

tongue

10-154 Cancer or trauma can affect any structure of the digestive system and may require plastic surgery if there is extensive damage. **Cheilo/plasty** (ki´lo-plas˝te) is surgical repair of the

_____.

    Cheilo/rrhaphy (ki-lor´ə-fe), suture of the lip, and **glosso/rrhaphy** (glos-or´ə-fe), suture of the _____, would probably use nonabsorbable material because of the easy access for removal of the suture.

    Stomato/plasty (sto´mə-to-plas˝te) is surgical repair of the mouth. **Cheilo/stomato/plasty** (ki˝lo-sto-mat´o-plas˝te) is surgical repair of the lips and mouth.

glossoplasty
(glos´o-plas˝te)
gums

10-155 A **gloss/ectomy** (glos-ek´tə-me) is removal of all or part of the tongue, necessary in carcinoma of the tongue.

    Surgical repair of the tongue is called _____.

10-156 **Gingiv/ectomy** (jin˝jĭ-vek´tə-me) is excision of the _____. Gingivectomy is surgical removal of all loose and diseased gum tissue, performed to arrest the progress of periodontal disease. This procedure is performed by a dentist or periodontist.

esophagectomy
(ə-sof˝ə-jek´tə-me)

relax

10-157 Write a term that means surgical excision of all or part of the esophagus: _____. This surgical procedure may be required to treat severe bleeding of the esophagus or esophageal cancer.

    Esophago/myo/tomy (ə-sof˝ə-go-mi-ot´ə-me) is an incision into the muscle of the lower part of the esophagus, performed to expedite the passage of food in esophageal achalasia. You remember from studying this term earlier that achalasia is an abnormal condition characterized by the inability of the muscle to _____.

stomach

opening

10-158 Patients who can digest and absorb nutrients but need nutritional support may receive enteral nutrition. Enteral nutrition is the provision of nutrients through the GI tract when the patient cannot ingest, chew, or swallow food but can digest and absorb nutrients. This is accomplished using an enteral feeding tube. Nasogastric enteral feeding uses a **naso/gastric** (na˝zo-gas´trik) **tube** that is inserted through the nose into the _____.

    Circumstances may require placement of the enteral tube directly into the esophagus, stomach, or jejunum. Terms for surgical procedures to establish this means of feeding are **esophago/stomy** (ə-sof˝ə-gos´tə-me), **gastro/stomy** (gas-tros´tə-me), and **jejuno/stomy** (jĕ˝joo-nos´tə-me), respectively, which mean formation of a new _____ into these structures. Locations for enteral feeding tubes are shown in Figure 10-25.

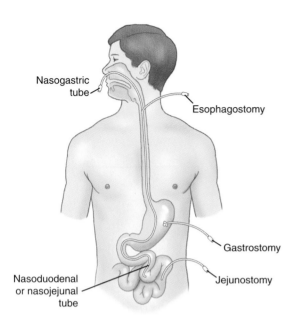

Figure 10-25 **Common placement locations for enteral feeding tubes.**

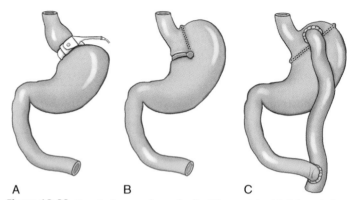

Figure 10-26 **Surgical procedures for limiting nutrient intake.** **A,** Lap-Band system. **B,** Vertical banded gastroplasty. **C,** Gastric bypass.

10-159 **Par/enteral** (pə-ren´tər-əl) means not through the alimentary tract but through some other route; in other words, by injection. **Total parenteral nutrition** (TPN) is the administration of all nutrition through an indwelling catheter into the vena cava or other main vein. This method of feeding has several names, including intravenous alimentation and **hyperalimentation** (hi″pər-al″ĭ-men-ta´shən).

parenteral
    TPN is the abbreviation for total _____ nutrition.

10-160 Alimentation is the process of providing nutrition for the body. Translated literally, hyper/alimentation means _____ nutrition. Hyperalimentation means TPN but has a second meaning of overfeeding, or the ingestion or administration of
excessive
an amount of nutrients that exceeds the demands of the body. Overfeeding on one's own can lead to obesity.

10-161 Conservative approaches to weight loss for obese individuals include restricted food intake and increased exercise. An appetite-suppressing drug is an **anorexiant** (an″o-rek´se-ənt). Alli, an over-the-counter drug, is not an anorexiant but causes weight loss by preventing one's body from breaking down excessive fats in the diet. The treatment effects of excess undigested fat passing out of the body are gas, loose stools, and sometimes diarrhea.
    Surgical approaches for treating extreme obesity, generally tried when conservative methods fail, limit food intake or produce malabsorption by the Lap-Band system, vertical banded gastro/plasty (gas´tro-plas″te) or gastric bypass. The Lap-Band system is an adjustable gastric band that is inserted laparoscopically and considered by many to be the least traumatic of the weight-loss surgeries. The term **gastroplasty** means any surgery performed to reshape or repair
stomach
the _____.
    In vertical banded gastroplasty, the stomach is partitioned into a small upper portion, drastically limiting the stomach's capacity. These three methods are shown in Figure 10-26. In gastric bypass, the stomach size is decreased and an opening is created directly into the jejunum. Variations of this procedure include a procedure commonly called stapling the stomach.

fat

10-162 Two procedures that are performed to remove unsightly flabby folds of fat tissue or to improve body contours are **lipectomy** (lĭ-pek´tə-me) and **liposuction** (lip˝o-suk´shən). Both these procedures are performed for cosmetic reasons rather than weight reduction. Lip/ectomy is excision of subcutaneous _____, and lipo/suction removes fat with a suction pump device.

EXERCISE 21

Word Analysis. *Divide these words into their component parts, and define each term.*

1. cheilorrhaphy   _____

2. cheilostomatoplasty   _____

3. esophagomyotomy   _____

4. esophagostomy   _____

5. gingivectomy   _____

6. glossorrhaphy   _____

7. jejunostomy   _____

8. lipectomy   _____

9. nasogastric   _____

10. stomatoplasty   _____

esophagus

stomach

10-163 Trauma or a tumor in the cardiac region of the stomach sometimes makes it necessary to create a new opening between the esophagus and stomach. **Esophagogastrostomy** (ə-sof˝ə-go-gas-tros´tə-me) means creating a new opening between the _____ and the stomach.

If either the stomach or the esophagus becomes diseased near the cardiac sphincter, an **esophagogastroplasty** (ə-sof˝ə-go-gas´tro-plast˝te) may be performed. This new term means surgical repair of the esophagus and the _____.

fixation

stomach

10-164 **Gastro/pexy** (gas´tro-pek˝se) is surgical _____ of the stomach. Gastropexy involves suturing (sewing) the stomach to the abdominal wall to prevent displacement.

Gastro/rrhaphy (gas-tror´ə-fe), suture of the _____, would probably use absorbable suture material.

gastric

10-165 **Lavage** (lah-vahzh´) is irrigation or washing out of an organ, such as the stomach or bowel. Washing out of the stomach is _____ lavage, performed to remove irritants or toxic substances, and is done before or after surgery on the stomach.

Flushing of the inside of the colon is called colonic irrigation; this is not the same as an enema. Colonic irrigation may be used to remove any material high in the colon, whereas an enema is introduction of a solution into the rectum either for cleansing the rectum or as a treatment for constipation.

excessive

10-166 Some types of ulcers of the stomach, esophagus, and duodenum are caused by a particular bacterium called *Helicobacter pylori* and can be treated with antibiotics. Certain medications can also cause ulcers. Treatment of gastric ulcers can include any of the following: antibiotic, change of a suspected medication, dietary management, and antacids to counteract the acidic gastric contents. An **ant/acid** (ant-as´id) is an agent used to treat gastric **hyper/acidity** (hi˝pər-ə-sid´ĭ-te), _____ acid in the stomach. Gastric hyperacidity may lead to ulcers. (Note the omission of the "i" in antacid.)

10-167 Gastric secretions are controlled by the vagus (va´gəs) nerve, the tenth cranial nerve. **Vago/tomy** (va-got´ə-me) is _____ of certain branches of the vagus nerve to reduce the amount of gastric acid secreted. Vagotomy may be done in such a way that the branches supplying the acid-secreting glands of the stomach are severed without disturbing those branches that supply other abdominal structures.

10-168 **Pyloro/plasty** (pi-lor´o-plas˝te) is surgical repair of the pyloric sphincter. It may be done when other methods of treating peptic ulcers have not been effective. Pyloroplasty consists of surgical enlargement of the pyloric sphincter to facilitate the easy passage of the stomach contents to the duodenum. (Pyloroplasty may be necessary when there is pyloric stenosis, a narrowing of the pyloric sphincter at the outlet of the stomach.)
   Pyloro/tomy (pi˝lor-ot´o-me) is incision of the pylorus. Pylorotomy is often called **pyloromyotomy** (pi-lor˝o-mi-ot´ə-me), which means _____ of the muscles of the pylorus, and is also done to expedite the passage of food from the stomach.

10-169 Persons with ulcers who do not respond to medical treatment or who develop complications (perforation or hemorrhage) may require partial **gastr/ectomy** (gas-trek´tə-me), which is _____ of part of the stomach. A gastrectomy, removal of part or all of the stomach, is done also to remove a malignancy.

10-170 **Anastomosis** (ə-nas˝tə-mo´sis) means a connection between two vessels. It may be created by surgical, traumatic, or pathologic means between two normally distinct organs or spaces. The communication (union) itself is also called an anastomosis. The verb that means to join the structures is **anastomose**˙ (ə-nas´tə-mōs).
   Study the three types of surgical anastomoses of the gastrointestinal tract in Figure 10-27 and write answers in these blanks. A **gastro/entero/stomy** (gas˝tro-en˝tər-os´tə-me) is the simplest of these three anastomoses. In a gastro/entero/stomy, the body of the stomach is joined with some part of the _____ intestine. This term, like the other two terms, begins with the proximal organ (the organ nearest the place where nutrition begins).
   In the two other types of anastomoses, the lower portion of the stomach is removed before the gastric stump is anastomosed to either the duodenum or the jejunum.
   The terms **gastro/duodeno/stomy** (gas˝tro-doo˝o-də-nos´tə-me) and **gastro/jejuno/stomy** (gas˝tro-jə-joo-nos´tə-me) are anastomosis of the gastric stump with the duodenum and _____, respectively. They may also be called **gastro/duodenal** (gas˝tro-doo˝o-de´nəl) **anastomosis** and **gastro/jejunal anastomosis.**

Margin answers: incision; incision; removal; small; jejunum

˙Anastomose (Greek: *anastomoien*, to provide a mouth).

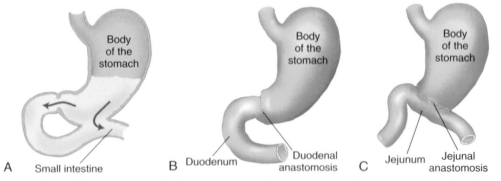

A   Small intestine   B   Duodenum   Duodenal anastomosis   C   Jejunum   Jejunal anastomosis

Figure 10-27 Three types of surgical anastomoses. A, Gastroenterostomy. A passage is created between the stomach and some part of the small intestine, often the jejunum. **B,** Gastroduodenostomy. The lower portion of the stomach is removed, and the remainder is anastomosed to the duodenum. **C,** Gastrojejunostomy. The lower portion of the stomach is removed and the remainder is anastomosed to the jejunum. The remaining duodenal stump is closed.

stomach	**10-171** In extensive gastric cancer, a total gastrectomy with anastomosis of the esophagus to the jejunum is the principal medical intervention. This means that all of the _____ is removed and an esophago/jejuno/stomy (ə-sof-ə-go-je″joo-nos´tə-me) is performed.
esophagus	**Esophagojejunostomy** means surgical anastomosis of the _____ to the jejunum.
duodenum	**10-172** In an **esophago/duodeno/stomy** (ə-sof″ə-go-doo″o-de-nos´tə-me), the anastomosis is between the esophagus and the _____.
ileum	**Jejuno/ileo/stomy** (jə-joo″no-il″e-os´tə-me) is formation of an opening between the jejunum and the _____.

EXERCISE 22

Build It! *Use the following word parts to build terms. (Some word parts will be used more than once.)*

duoden(o), gastr(o), jejun(o), ile(o), pylor(o), vag(o), -pexy, -stomy, -tomy

1. incision of the pylorus _____/_____

2. surgical fixation of the stomach _____/_____

3. formation of an opening between the jejunum
   and the ileum _____/_____/_____

4. severing of vagus nerve branches to reduce
   stomach acid _____/_____

5. anastomosis of the stomach and the duodenum _____/_____/_____

Say and Check

Say aloud the terms you wrote for Exercise 22. Use the Companion CD to check your pronunciations.

ileostomy (il″e-os´tə-me)	**10-173** If the large intestine must be removed, a new opening is made into the ileum through the abdominal wall. Fecal material drains into a bag worn on the abdomen. Formation of an opening into the ileum is _____.
	If all of the colon is removed, an ileostomy is necessary. An ileo/stomy is forming an ileal stoma onto the surface of the abdomen.
colon	**10-174 Col/ectomy** (ko-lek´tə-me) is excision of all, or a part, of the _____. A **hemi/col/ectomy** (hem″e-ko-lek´tə-me) is excision of approximately half of the colon and is sometimes referred to as either left hemicolectomy or right hemicolectomy.
colon	A **colo/stomy** (kə-los´tə-me) is generally performed after partial colectomy. A colostomy is surgical creation of an artificial anus on the abdominal wall by drawing the colon out to the surface or, in other words, creating an artificial opening from the _____ on the abdominal surface. Colostomies may be permanent or temporary, perhaps to divert feces after surgery. Several locations for colostomy and an ileostomy are shown in Figure 10-28.

> ► **KEY** POINT The artificially created opening in a colostomy is called a stoma (sto´mə). The term stoma means any small orifice or opening, and it can refer to the opening established in the abdominal wall by a colostomy or similar surgery or the opening between two portions of the intestine in an anastomosis.

intestine	**10-175** Remembering that lapar(o) means abdominal wall, **laparo/entero/stomy** is formation of an opening through the abdominal wall into the small _____.

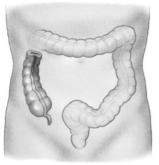
Ascending colostomy

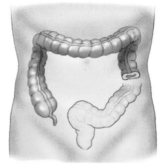
Descending colostomy

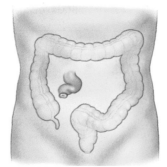
Ileostomy

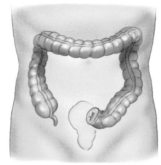
Sigmoid colostomy
single-barreled

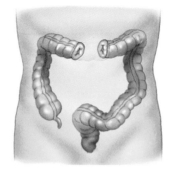
Transverse colostomy
double-barreled

Figure 10-28 Comparison of an ileostomy and several types of col   my procedures. The *lighter section* indicates the portion of the large intestine that is removed.

This procedure is done to install a tube to drain the bowel, or it may be used to supply nutrients to a patient with an upper digestive tract obstruction.

10-176 Jejuno/tomy (jĕ″joo-not´ə-me) is surgical incision of the jejunum. An incision of the duodenum is a **duodeno/tomy** (doo″o-də-not´ə-me). Formation of a new opening into the duodenum is a _____.

duodenostomy
(doo″o-də-nos´tə-me)

10-177 Ceco/ileo/stomy (se″ko-il″e-os´tə-me) is formation of a new opening between the cecum and the ileum.
Using proct(o), write a word that means surgical repair of the rectum and anus: _____.

proctoplasty
(prok´to-plas″te)

10-178 You studied the difference between diverticulosis and diverticulitis earlier in this chapter. **Diverticul/ectomy** (di″vər-tik″u-lek´tə-me), surgical excision of a _____, may be performed if repeated bouts of diverticulitis result in obstruction of the colon.
In cases of acute appendic/itis, an append/ectomy is usually performed. An **append/ectomy** is _____ of the appendix.

diverticulum

removal (excision)

10-179 Nonsurgical management of hemorrhoids is aimed at reducing symptoms without surgery and decreasing the likelihood that the symptoms will recur. Topical anesthetics, application of cold packs, and soaks are used to alleviate hemorrhoid/al pain. **Topi/cal** (top[o], place + -ical, pertaining to) means pertaining to a particular place on the surface area. You have learned that an anesthetic is used to produce a loss of sensation or feeling. The purpose of a topical an/esthetic is to alleviate _____ on a particular area of the skin.
Several surgical methods are available if symptoms persist, and treatment is determined by the type of hemorrhoid. Treatments include elastic band ligation (lĭ-ga´shən) and a **hemorrhoidectomy** (hem″ə-roid-ek´tə-me). In elastic band ligation, the hemorrhoids are bound with

pain

˙Ligation (Latin: *ligare*, to bind).

hemorrhoids

rubber bands, become necrotic, and eventually slough off. A hemorrhoid/ectomy is excision of
_____.

10-180 In addition to those already mentioned, several pharmaceuticals are helpful in the treatment of gastrointestinal problems. Various antibiotics are used, depending on the type of infectious microorganisms that are present.

diarrhea

Anti/diarrheals are used to treat _____, and **anti/emetics** (an″te-ə-met′iks) are used to relieve or prevent vomiting.

Stool softeners are used to prevent constipation. Laxatives cause evacuation of the bowel by a mild action and may be prescribed to correct constipation. Purgatives or cathartics are strong medications used to promote full evacuation of the bowel, as in preparation for diagnostic studies or surgery of the digestive tract.

EXERCISE 23

Build It! *Use the following word parts to build terms. (Some word parts will be used more than once.)*

hemi-, col(o), diverticul(o), enter(o), ile(o), lapar(o), -ectomy, -stomy

1. excision of approximately half of the large colon _____/_____/_____

2. formation of a new opening between the cecum
   and the ileum _____/_____/_____

3. forming an ileal stoma _____/_____

4. formation of an opening through the abdominal
   wall into the small intestine _____/_____/_____

5. surgical excision of a diverticulum _____/_____

Say and Check

Say aloud the terms you wrote for Exercise 23. Use the Companion CD to check your pronunciations.

ACCESSORY ORGANS OF DIGESTION

liver

10-181 Carcinoma that has spread from another site to the liver (metastasized) is more common than primary liver cancer. If the tumor is localized to one portion of the liver, **hepatic lob/ectomy,** excision of a lobe of the _____, may be performed. Other surgeries and chemotherapy are also used, depending on the type of liver cancer.

hepatectomy
(hep″ə-tek′tə-me)

10-182 Surgical incision of the liver is **hepato/tomy** (hep″ə-tot′ə-me). Excision of part of the liver is _____. Liver transplantation may be performed in some cases, usually for liver disease related to chronic viral hepatitis.

pancreatectomy
(pan″kre-ə-tek′tə-me)

10-183 **Pancreato/tomy** (pan″kre-ə-tot′ə-me) is incision of the pancreas. Removal of the pancreas is _____. **Pancreato/lith/ectomy** (pan″kre-ə-to-lĭ-thek′tə-me) is removal of pancreatic stones.

insulin

10-184 Diabetes mellitus results primarily from either a deficiency or lack of insulin secretion by the pancreas or a resistance to insulin. Some forms of diabetes are treated with diet, exercise, and weight control; other forms require glucose-lowering agents (oral agents or insulin by injection). Diabetes mellitus results primarily from a lack of _____ secretion by the pancreas or resistance to insulin.

10-185 Gallstones are a common disorder of the gallbladder and bile ducts and are usually associated with cholecystitis. Several nonsurgical approaches are available, including oral drugs that dissolve stones, **laser lithotripsy** (lith′o-trip″se), and **extracorporeal shock wave lithotripsy** (ESWL).

lithotripsy

lithotriptor

abdominal

cholecystotomy
(ko″lə-sis-tot′ə-me)

opening

jejunum

In ESWL, extracorporeal (outside the body) shock wave _____,
a lithotriptor uses high-energy shock waves to disintegrate the stone. The patient is positioned over a shock wave generator (lithotriptor) by means of a table that moves upward and downward, forward and backward, and side to side. Particles slough off the gallstone as the lithotriptor is fired, and the particles pass through the biliary ducts and are eliminated. The name of the shock wave generator in biliary lithotripsy is a _____ (Figure 10-29).

10-186 **Litho/tripsy** is nonsurgical management of gallstones and can sometimes be an alternative to **cholecyst/ectomy** (ko″lə-sis-tek′tə-me), surgical removal of the gallbladder. The gallbladder stores bile but is not essential for life, because bile is produced continuously.
   Endoscopic removal of biliary stones is called **endoscopic sphinctero/tomy,** because the endoscope is passed to the duodenum, and then the sphincter muscle is incised to reach and retrieve the stone.
   Laparo/scopic cholecystectomy, removal of the gallbladder through four small incisions in the _____ wall, is currently preferred to open cholecystectomy whenever possible. Laparoscopic cholecystectomy is commonly done as an outpatient surgery. The surgical site is exposed through four small portals inserted into the abdominal wall, allowing the gallbladder to be excised and removed easily. The tissue removed is then sent to pathology for histologic examination.

10-187 Write a term that means surgical incision of the gallbladder:
_____. This new term means incision of the gallbladder for the purpose of exploration, drainage, or removal of stones.
   Laparo/cholecysto/tomy (lap″ə-ro-ko″lə-sis-tot′ə-me) means incision into the gallbladder through the abdominal wall.

10-188 **Choledocho/litho/tripsy** (ko-led″ə-ko-lith′o-trip″se) means the crushing of gallstones in the common bile duct. **Choledocho/stomy** (ko-led″ə-kos′tə-me) is surgical formation of an _____ into the common bile duct through the abdominal wall. This is commonly done for temporary drainage of the duct after cholecystectomy.
   Choledocho/jejuno/stomy (ko-led″ə-ko-jə-joo-nos′tə-me) is surgical formation of a new opening between the common bile duct and the _____.

10-189 Treatment of infected salivary glands includes antibiotics and warm compresses. If the flow of saliva is obstructed by a stone, the duct's opening may be dilated and massaged. If these measures fail, surgery may be necessary to remove the stone.
   Tumors of the salivary glands, either benign or malignant, are excised. However, radiation therapy may be used for highly malignant or very large tumors or for recurrence of a tumor after surgery.

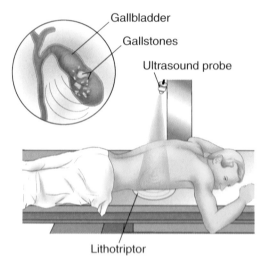

Gallbladder

Gallstones

Ultrasound probe

Lithotriptor

Figure 10-29 Biliary lithotripsy. The gallbladder is positioned over the lithotriptor; then the lithotriptor is fired and particles slough off the gallstones until they are fragmented and can pass through the biliary ducts.

EXERCISE 24

Build It! *Use the following word parts to build terms. (Some word parts will be used more than once.)*

choledocho, hepat(o), lith(o), pancreat(o), -ectomy, -stomy, -tomy, -tripsy

1. surgical crushing of a stone _____/_____

2. incision of the pancreas _____/_____

3. surgical removal of a stone from the pancreas _____/_____/_____

4. surgical incision of the liver _____/_____

5. formation of an opening into the common bile duct _____/_____

Say and Check

Say aloud the terms you wrote for Exercise 24. Use the Companion CD to check your pronunciations.

EXERCISE 25

Match terms in the left columns with their descriptions in the right column.

_____ 1. anastomosis   _____ 6. hyperalimentation   A. a type of gastroplasty
_____ 2. antidiarrheals   _____ 7. lavage   B. administration of all nutrition through an indwelling catheter
_____ 3. diabetes mellitus   _____ 8. liposuction   C. agents to reduce feeling, applied to the mucous membranes or skin
_____ 4. total parenteral nutrition _____ 9. parenteral   D. connection between two vessels
_____ 5. gastric bypass   _____ 10. topical anesthetics E. results primarily from deficiency or lack of insulin
                                                               F. irrigation or washing out of an organ
                                                               G. medications to treat diarrhea
                                                               H. not through the alimentary canal
                                                               I. overfeeding
                                                               J. removal of fat with a suction pump device

CHAPTER ABBREVIATIONS*

ALT	alanine aminotransferase		HSV	herpes simplex virus
AST	aspartate aminotransferase		IBD	inflammatory bowel disease
BMI	body mass index		IBS	irritable bowel syndrome
DM	diabetes mellitus		LFT	liver function tests
EGD	esophagogastroduodenoscopy		RDA	recommended dietary allowance
ESWL	extracorporeal shock wave lithotripsy		SGOT	serum glutamate-oxaloacetic transaminase (enzyme test of heart and liver function, now called AST)
GERD	gastroesophageal reflux disease			
GI	gastrointestinal			
HAV	hepatitis A virus		SGPT	serum glutamate-pyruvate transaminase (enzyme test of liver function, now called ALT)
HBV	hepatitis B virus			
HCV	hepatitis C virus		TMJ	temporomandibular joint
HDV	hepatitis D virus		TPN	total parenteral nutrition
HEV	hepatitis E virus		UGI	upper gastrointestinal (or upper GI) series

*Many of these abbreviations share their meanings with other terms.

▶ CHAPTER 10 REVIEW

Basic Understanding

Labeling

I. *Label the structures (1 through 13) in the diagram with the corresponding combining form. (Write two combining forms for numbers 2 and 6.)*

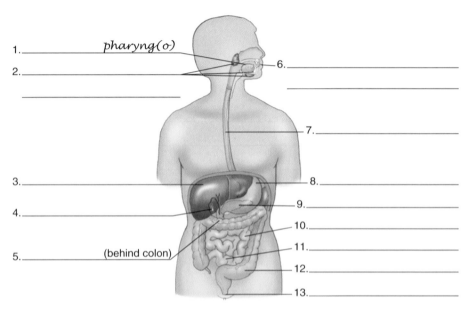

1. _____   *pharyng(o)*
2. _____   6. _____

_____

3. _____   7. _____

4. _____   8. _____

5. _____   (behind colon)   9. _____

                                                10. _____

                                                11. _____

                                                12. _____

                                                13. _____

Matching

II. *Match the major functions of the digestive tract in the left columns with their descriptions in the right column.*

_____ 1. absorption   _____ 3. elimination   A. eating food
_____ 2. digestion   _____ 4. ingestion   B. mechanically and chemically breaking down food
                                                       C. passing nutrient molecules into blood or lymph
                                                       D. removing wastes

III. *Match structures of the digestive system in the left columns with their descriptions in the right column.*

_____ 1. duodenum   _____ 6. liver   A. connects with the cecum
                                                       B. first major site of digestion
_____ 2. esophagus   _____ 7. mouth   C. its lower end connects with the stomach
                                                       D. its upper end connects with the stomach
_____ 3. gallbladder   _____ 8. pancreas   E. midsection of the three parts of the small intestine
                                                       F. part of the large intestine
_____ 4. ileum   _____ 9. stomach   G. produces bile
                                                       H. produces insulin
_____ 5. jejunum   _____ 10. transverse colon I. stores bile
                                                       J. where the buccal cavity is located

IV. *Match pathologies in the left columns with meanings on the right.*

_____ 1. caries   _____ 6. fistula

_____ 2. fissure   _____ 7. hernia

_____ 3. esophageal atresia   _____ 8. malocclusion

_____ 4. esophageal achalasia   _____ 9. sialadenitis

_____ 5. esophageal varices   _____ 10. ulcer

A. abnormal passage
B. cleft or cracklike lesion
C. decay
D. improper bite
E. inflammation of a salivary gland
F. enlarged and swollen veins at the lower end of the esophagus
G. lower esophageal sphincter fails to relax properly
H. esophagus ends in a blind pouch or is too narrow
I. open sore or lesion
J. protrusion of an organ through the wall of a cavity

Listing

V. *List the three classes of nutrients and explain their functions.*

1. _____

2. _____

3. _____

VI. *List the four accessory organs of digestion and write their combining form(s).*

1. _____ = _____

2. _____ = _____

3. _____ = _____

4. _____ = _____

Photo ID

VII. *Build words to label these illustrations.*

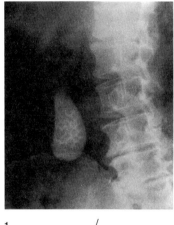

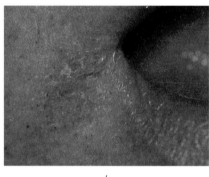

1. _____ / _____
   (gallbladder)   (record)

2. _____ / _____
   (lip)   (condition)

Gallbladder
Gallstones
Ultrasound probe
Lithotriptor

3. _____ / _____
(bile)   (pertaining to)

_____ / _____
(stone)   (surgical crushing)

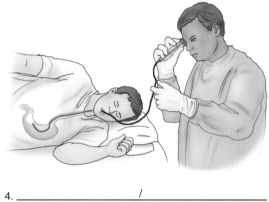

4. _____ / _____
(stomach)   (visual examination)

Word Analysis

VIII. *Divide these words into their component parts, and write the meanings of the terms.*

1. ileocecal _____

2. choledocholithotripsy _____

3. cholestasis _____

4. esophagomyotomy _____

5. gastroduodenostomy _____

6. gingivostomatitis _____

7. glossoplegia _____

8. nasogastric _____

9. sialolithiasis _____

10. stomatoplasty _____

Say and Check

Say aloud the terms in Exercise VIII. Use the Companion CD to check your pronunciations.

Multiple Choice

IX. *Circle the correct answer for each of the following multiple choice questions.*

1. Mrs. Vogel's physician tells her that she needs to see a specialist for the problem that she's been having with her colon. What is the name of the specialty practiced by the physician Mrs. Vogel should see?
(cardiology, gastroenterology, gynecology, urology)

2. Cal Stone undergoes radiography of the gallbladder. What is the name of this diagnostic test?
(barium enema, barium meal, cholecystography, esophagogastroscopy)

3. Tests show that Cal Stone has a gallstone in the common bile duct. Which of the following is a noninvasive conservative procedure to alleviate Cal's problem?
(cholecystostomy, choledochostomy, choledochojejunostomy, extracorporeal shock wave lithotripsy)

4. Linda M., a 16-year-old girl, is diagnosed as having self-induced starvation. Which of the following is the name of the disorder associated with Linda's problem? (anorexia nervosa, aphagia, malaise, polyphagia)

5. Unless there is intervention for Linda's self-induced starvation, which condition is likely to result?
(adipsia, atresia, emaciation, volvulus)

6. A 70-year-old man is diagnosed with cancer of the colon. Which term indicates a surgical intervention for this condition? (colectomy, colonoscopy, colonic irrigation, colonic stasis)

7. Baby Jake is born with a narrowing of the muscular ring that controls the outflow of food from the stomach. What is the name of this disorder? (pyloric sphincter, pyloric stenosis, pyloroplasty, pyloromyotomy)

8. What is the name of the valve that regulates movement of intestinal contents from the small intestine into the large intestine? (cecorectal valve, ileocecal valve, jejunocecal valve, pyloric valve)

9. Mary suffers from GERD. The physician explains to her that radiography indicates that a portion of the stomach is protruding upward through the diaphragm. What is the name of this disorder? (caries, cholelith, hiatal hernia, varices)

10. Jane is scheduled for a cheilostomatoplasty. What structures are involved in her surgery? (gums and mouth, lips and mouth, mouth and stomach, tongue and mouth)

11. A 70-year-old woman has an obstruction that has led to stagnation of the normal movement of food in the intestinal tract. What is the name of this condition? (duodenitis, enterostasis, peptic ulcer, peristalsis)

12. Which of the following is an instrument designed for passage into the stomach to permit examination of its interior? (gastric lavage, gastroscope, gastrotome, gastrorrhaphy)

13. Which of the following is the main source of energy for body cells? (fats, glucose, lactose, starches)

14. Which of the following is a disorder characterized by episodes of binge eating that are terminated by abdominal pain, sleep, self-induced vomiting, or purging with laxatives? (anorexia nervosa, bulimia, Crohn disease, malabsorption syndrome)

15. Which of the following is the name of the procedure in which the stomach is anastomosed with the small intestine? (gastrectasis, gastrectomy, gastroenterostomy, gastropexy)

Writing Terms

X. *Write a term for each of the following.*

1. absence of thirst   _____

2. any disease of the stomach   _____

3. enzyme that breaks down starch _____

4. excessive vomiting   _____

5. excision of the gallbladder   _____

6. incision of the vagus nerve   _____

7. inflammation of the stomach   _____

8. pertaining to the throat   _____

9. poor digestion   _____

10. visual inspection of the duodenum _____

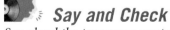 **Say and Check**

Say aloud the terms you wrote for Exercise X. Use the Companion CD to check your pronunciations.

Greater Comprehension

Health Care Reports

XI. Read this operative report and answer the questions that follow it. Although you may be unfamiliar with some of the terms, you should be able to decide their meaning by determining the word parts.

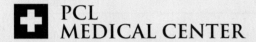

PCL MEDICAL CENTER

7700 Lexicon Way
St. Louis, MO 63146

Phone (555) 437-0000 • Fax (555) 437-0001

OPERATIVE REPORT

Patient Name: Gloria Rush   **ID No.:** 010-4001   **Date of Surgery:** Jan 12, ----
PREOPERATIVE DIAGNOSIS: Suspected neoplasm of the distal rectum
POSTOPERATIVE DIAGNOSIS: Suspected neoplasm of the distal rectum
SURGEON: James Miller, M.D.
ANESTHESIOLOGIST: Harvey Bell, M.D.   **ANESTHESIA:** Propofol
OPERATIVE PROCEDURE: Colonoscopy to cecum; multiple biopsies of rectal mass
INDICATIONS: This 55-year-old woman has experienced progressive constipation and hematochezia ×3 weeks. Has also had pelvic and rectal pressure. A sonogram showed a large pelvic mass between the rectum and the vagina. She also has a history of diverticulitis. Cholecystectomy 2 years ago.
PROCEDURE IN DETAIL: The patient was brought to the GI lab, sedated with Propofol, and the colonoscope was passed per anus to what appeared to be the cecum. It appeared that the ileocecal valve was seen; because of poor preparation, the appendiceal orifice could not be identified. A hard mass was seen in the distal rectum. Multiple biopsies were taken of numerous small lesions in the ascending, transverse, descending, sigmoid, and rectosigmoid colon.
PLAN: Biopsy results pending. Patient requires an urgent exploratory laparotomy with probable colectomy and ileostomy.

P. J. Posey, MD
P. J. Posey, MD, Gastroenterologist

Circle one answer for each of these questions.

1. To which body structure does the diagnosis pertain? (gallbladder, large intestine, small intestine, stomach)

2. Which of the following describes the rectum in the preoperative diagnosis?
   (abnormal new growth, enlarged, inflamed, impacted with feces).

3. The patient has a history of cholecystectomy. Which organ is removed in a cholecystectomy?
   (colon, gallbladder, liver, small intestine)

4. What structure is incised in a laparotomy? (abdominal wall, cecum, ileum, umbilicus)

5. All or part of which structure is excised in a colectomy? (large intestine, small intestine, stomach, umbilicus)

6. Where is the stoma created in an ileostomy? (abdomen, anus, colon, umbilicus)

Write T for True or F for False for each of these statements.

7. The procedure involved a visual inspection of the large intestine. _____

8. The procedure involved excising tissue from a visible hard mass. _____

9. The patient has a history of hematochezia, which means she experienced bloody vomitus. _____

10. The patient has a history of diverticula with accompanying inflammation. _____

11. The surgeon identified the opening to the appendix. _____

12. The surgeon examined most of the small intestine. _____

XII. *Read this consultation report and answer the questions that follow it. Although you may be unfamiliar with some of the terms, you should be able to decide their meanings by determining the word parts.*

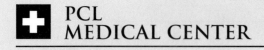

PCL
MEDICAL CENTER

7700 Lexicon Way
St. Louis, MO 63146

Phone (555) 437-0000 • Fax (555) 437-0001

GASTROINTESTINAL CONSULT

Patient Name: Gregory Harper   **ID No:** 010-4002   **DOB:** Dec 29, ----
REASON FOR CONSULTATION: Severe colitis
CHIEF COMPLAINT: Bloody diarrhea and abdominal pain
HISTORY OF PRESENT ILLNESS: 35-year-old man with history of ulcerative colitis. The patient had an exacerbation that required treatment with steroids 5 years ago. He underwent an endoscopy in May that showed active colitis with both acute and chronic inflammation throughout most of the colon with abscess formation. He has had persistent symptoms despite increasing doses of steroids.
PAST MEDICAL HISTORY: Depression/anxiety. Recent gastroenteritis.
FAMILY HISTORY: Father with Crohn disease and colorectal carcinoma
PHYSICAL EXAM: Vital signs stable. Lungs: Clear to auscultation. Heart: Regular rate and rhythm. Abdomen: Soft with hyperactive bowel sounds. No hepatosplenomegaly. Tenderness to palpation in both right and left lower quadrants. Rectal: Good tone but exam painful. No stool in the vault.
LABS: LFTs elevated. Albumin 3.2. Sed rate elevated at 38. Hemoccult positive.
CURRENT MEDICATIONS: Prednisone, multivitamins
ASSESSMENT: Toxic colitis with distended transverse colon
TREATMENT PLAN: Patient requests conservative treatment. He will be treated with IV antibiotics and IV steroids. Dietary intake limited for a few days.

Timothy Lind, MD
Timothy Lind, MD

D: Dec 29, ----
T: Dec 30, ----

Circle the correct answer in the following questions.

1. Which structure is the focus of the consultation? (gallbladder, large intestine, liver, small intestine)

2. Which adjective describes the patient's ulcerative colitis? (acute, cancerous, chronic, noninflammatory)

3. To which category does the term endoscopy belong? (anatomy, diagnostic procedure, radiology, therapy)

4. Which of the following terms is associated with the presence of an abscess? (anorexia, emesis, malaise, pus)

5. Which of the following is *not* included in the family history?
   (cancer of the lower GI tract, colonic obstruction, Crohn disease, inflammatory bowel disease)

Define these terms.

6. ulcerative colitis _____

7. endoscopy _____

8. gastroenteritis _____

9. Crohn disease _____

10. Hemoccult _____

XIII. *Read the following operative report, and write the definitions of the underlined words. Although you may be unfamiliar with some of the terms, you should be able to decide their meanings by determining the word parts.*

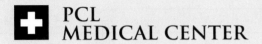 **PCL**
MEDICAL CENTER

7700 Lexicon Way
St. Louis, MO 63146

Phone (555) 437-0000 • Fax (555) 437-0001

OPERATIVE REPORT

Patient Name: Betty Carter   **ID No:** 010-4003   **Date:** Jul 11, ----
PREOPERATIVE DIAGNOSIS: Status post right <u>hemicolectomy</u> with subsequent <u>dehiscence</u>
POSTOPERATIVE DIAGNOSIS: Status post right hemicolectomy with subsequent dehiscence
OPERATION PERFORMED: Abdominal washout
Complications: None
Estimated blood loss: Approximately 50 mL
DESCRIPTION OF OPERATION:
Patient was taken to the operating room, where her vacuum-packed dressing was removed except for the sterile inner towels. She was prepped and draped in the usual sterile fashion. Towels were removed. At the beginning of the procedure, a right subclavian triple lumen catheter was placed by anesthesia. A left subclavian <u>dialysis</u> catheter was placed by anesthesia.

All the <u>pericolic</u> gutters in the four quadrants were inspected and irrigated. Her small bowel was run and irrigated. It looked fairly healthy; however, her <u>transverse colon</u> was noted to be very <u>distended</u> once we thoroughly irrigated. There was a little bleeding from the edge of her liver anteriorly, which was packed with Surgicel. Pressure was held, and <u>hemostasis</u> was obtained.

Vacuum-packed dressing was then replaced. Chest tube with Heimlich valve and two more towels, then an Ioban dressing placed. Patient was placed to suction. Patient tolerated the procedure well. No complications. She was awakened in the PAR and will be transferred to ICU for observation overnight, then back to the GI Unit.

Benjamin Cho, MD
Benjamin Cho, MD
General Surgery

BC:pai
D: Jul 11, ----
T: Jul 12, ----

Define:

1. hemicolectomy _____

2. dehiscence _____

3. dialysis _____

4. pericolic _____

5. transverse colon _____

6. distended _____

7. hemostasis _____

Spelling

XIV. *Circle all misspelled terms and write their correct spelling.*

emaciation   enteral   glossorhaphy   nasogastrik   varaces

Interpreting Abbreviations

XV. *Write the meaning of these abbreviations.*

1. BMI _____

2. GI _____

3. HBV _____

4. HSV _____

5. TPN _____

Pronunciation

XVI. *The pronunciation is shown for several medical words. Indicate which syllable has the primary accent by marking it with an ´.*

1. cholecystogastric (ko lə sis to gas trik)

2. choledochal (ko led ə kəl)

3. dysentery (dis ən ter e)

4. fistula (fis tu lə)

5. hemorrhoidectomy (hem ə roid ek tə me)

Say and Check

Say aloud the five terms in Exercise XVI. Use the Companion CD to check your pronunciations. In addition, be prepared to pronounce aloud these terms in class:

achalasia	duodenal	hemicolectomy	pyloric sphincter
anastomosis	esophagogastroscopy	intussusception	sialography
bulimia	eupepsia	liposuction	stomatomycosis
cheilitis	glossopathy	polypectomy	temporomandibular
choledochojejunostomy	hematemesis	postesophageal	ulcerative colitis

Categorizing Terms

XVII. *Classify the terms in the left columns (1 to 10) by selecting A, B, C, D, or E.*

_____ 1. achalasia

_____ 2. antiemetics

_____ 3. cholecystogram

_____ 4. choledochal

_____ 5. diverticulosis

_____ 6. esophagogram

_____ 7. esophagoduodenostomy

_____ 8. gingivoglossitis

_____ 9. jaundice

_____ 10. sialolithiasis

A. anatomy
B. diagnostic test or procedure
C. pathology
D. surgery
E. therapy

Challenge

XVIII. *Break these words into their component parts, and write their meanings. Even if you have not seen these terms before, you may be able to break them apart and determine their meanings.*

1. cecocolostomy _____

2. esophagogastrectomy _____

3. hemigastrectomy _____

4. sialogenous _____

5. sigmoidosigmoidostomy _____

PRONUNCIATION LIST

Use the practice CD to review the terms that have been presented. Look closely at the spelling of each term as it is pronounced and be sure you know the meaning of each term.

absorption
adipsia
alimentary tract
alimentation
amylase
amylolysis
anal
anastomose
anastomosis
anorexia
anorexia nervosa
anorexiant
antacid
antidiarrheal
antiemetics
anus
aphagia
appendectomy
appendicitis
appendicular
bicuspids
biliary
bolus
buccal cavity
buccal mucosa
bulimia
cardiac region
caries
cecoileostomy
cecum
cheilitis
cheiloplasty
cheilorrhaphy
cheilosis
cheilostomatoplasty
cholangiography
cholangitis
cholecystectomy
cholecystic
cholecystitis
cholecystogastric
cholecystogram
cholecystography
cholecystotomy
choledochal
choledochitis
choledochojejunostomy
choledocholithiasis
choledocholithotripsy
choledochostomy

cholelithiasis
cholestasis
chyme
cirrhosis
colectomy
colic
colitis
colon
colonoscope
colonoscopy
colorectal
coloscopy
colostomy
cuspids
defecate
defecation
dental
dentalgia
dentilingual
denture
diabetes mellitus
digestion
diverticulectomy
diverticulitis
diverticulosis
diverticulum
duodenal
duodenitis
duodenoscope
duodenoscopy
duodenostomy
duodenotomy
duodenum
dysentery
dyspepsia
dysphagia
elimination
emaciation
emesis
endodontics
endodontist
endodontitis
endodontium
endogastric
endogenous obesity
endoscopic sphincterotomy
enteral
enteric
enteritis
enterostasis

eructation
esophageal
esophageal achalasia
esophageal atresia
esophageal varices
esophagectomy
esophagitis
esophagoduodenostomy
esophagodynia
esophagogastroduoden-
    oscopy
esophagogastroplasty
esophagogastroscopy
esophagogastrostomy
esophagogram
esophagojejunostomy
esophagomalacia
esophagomyotomy
esophagoscopy
esophagostomy
esophagram
esophagus
eupepsia
exogenous obesity
extracorporeal shock wave
    lithotripsy
extrahepatic
feces
fissure
fistula
fundus
gastralgia
gastrectasia
gastrectomy
gastric
gastritis
gastroduodenal anasto-
    mosis
gastroduodenitis
gastroduodenostomy
gastroenteritis
gastroenterology
gastroenterostomy
gastrointestinal
gastrojejunal anastomosis
gastrojejunostomy
gastromalacia
gastromegaly
gastropathy
gastropexy

gastroplasty
gastrorrhaphy
gastroscope
gastroscopy
gastrostomy
gerodontics
gerodontist
gingiva
gingival
gingivalgia
gingivectomy
gingivitis
gingivoglossitis
gingivostomatitis
glossal
glossectomy
glossitis
glossopathy
glossopharyngeal
glossoplasty
glossoplegia
glossopyrosis
glossorrhaphy
glucagon
glucose
glycolysis
halitosis
hematemesis
hematochezia
hemicolectomy
hemorrhoid
hemorrhoidectomy
hepatectomy
hepatic
hepatic lobectomy
hepatitis
hepatolytic
hepatoma
hepatomegaly
hepatopathy
hepatorenal syndrome
hepatosplenomegaly
hepatotomy
hepatotoxic
hiatal hernia
hyperacidity
hyperalimentation
hyperemesis
hyperglycemia
hypoglossal

Continued

hypoglycemia
ileac
ileal
ileitis
ileocecal valve
ileostomy
ileum
impaction
incisors
ingestion
insulin
interdental
intestinal
intussusception
jaundice
jejunal
jejunoileostomy
jejunostomy
jejunotomy
jejunum
laparocholecystotomy
laparoenterostomy
laparoscopic cholecys-
    tectomy
laser lithotripsy
lavage
leukoplakia
lingual
lipase
lipectomy
lipids
lipoid

lipopenia
liposuction
lithotripsy
lithotriptor
malabsorption syndrome
malnutrition
malocclusion
mandible
mandibular
maxilla
maxillary
metabolism
molars
mucoid
mucosa
mucous
nasogastric tube
obesity
oral
oropharyngeal
orthodontics
orthodontist
palatine
pancreatectomy
pancreatic
pancreatitis
pancreatography
pancreatolith
pancreatolithectomy
pancreatolithiasis
pancreatolysis
pancreatotomy

parenteral
parotid gland
parotitis
pedodontics
pedodontist
pericolic
periodontal
periodontics
periodontist
periodontitis
periodontium
peristalsis
pharyngeal
pharynx
polydipsia
polypectomy
polyphagia
postesophageal
proctologist
proctoplasty
proctosigmoidoscopy
protease
proteinase
proteolysis
pyloric region
pyloromyotomy
pyloroplasty
pyloroscopy
pylorotomy
pylorus
pyorrhea
rectal

rectum
retrocecal
retrocolic
rugae
salmonellosis
serosa
sialadenitis
sialography
sialolith
sialolithiasis
sigmoid colon
sigmoidoscope
sigmoidoscopy
sphincter
stomatitis
stomatodynia
stomatomycosis
stomatoplasty
sublingual
sublingual gland
submandibular glands
suprahepatic
temporomandibular joint
topical
total parenteral nutrition
vagotomy
vermiform appendix
villi
volvulus

Español — ENHANCING SPANISH COMMUNICATION

English	Spanish (pronunciation)
appetite	apetito (ah-pay-TEE-to)
belch	eructo (ay-ROOK-to)
chew, to	masticar (mas-te-CAR)
constipation	estreñimiento (es-tray-nye-me-EN-to)
defecate	evacuar (ay-vah-coo-AR)
dentist	dentista (den-TEES-tah)
diabetes	diabetes (de-ah-BAY-tes)
digestion	digestión (de-hes-te-ON)
enzyme	enzima (en-SEE-mah)
esophagus	esófago (ay-SO-fah-go)
excretion	excreción (ex-cray-se-ON)
feces	excremento (ex-cray-MEN-to)
gallbladder	vesícula biliar (vay-SEE-coo-la be-le-AR)
gallstone	cálculo biliar (CAHL-coo-lo be-le-AR)
glucose	glucosa (gloo-CO-sah)
gum, gingiva	encía (en-SEE-ah)
hunger	hambre (AHM-bray)
insulin	insulina (in-soo-LEE-nah)
laxative	purgante (poor-GAHN-tay)
lips	labios (LAH-be-os)
milk	leche (LAY-chay)
mouth	boca (BO-cah)
orthodontist	ortodóntico (or-to-DON-te-co)
pancreas	páncreas (PAHN-cray-as)
rectum	recto (REK-to)
saliva	saliva (sah-LEE-vah)
starch	almidón (al-me-DON)
swallow	tragar (trah-GAR)
teeth	dientes (de-AYN-tays)
thirst	sed (sayd)
tongue	lingua (LEN-goo-ah)

Urinary System 11

FUNCTION FIRST

The urinary system plays an important role in maintaining homeostasis by constantly filtering the blood to remove urea and other waste products, maintaining the proper balance of water, salts, and other substances by removing or reabsorbing them as needed, and excreting the waste products via the urine. Other less known roles are production of renin, erythropoietin, and prostaglandins, as well as degrading insulin and metabolizing vitamin D to its active form.

ANATOMY AND PHYSIOLOGY

11-1 There are several **excretory** (eks´krə-tor-e) routes through which the body eliminates wastes. The lungs eliminate carbon dioxide. The digestive system provides a means of expelling solid wastes. The skin serves as an excretory organ by eliminating wastes in the form of perspiration. Another important mode of **excretion** (eks-kre´shən) is performed by the kidneys, which are part of the urinary system.

The combining form urin(o) means urine. **Urin/ary** (u´rĭ-nar″e) means pertaining to

urine

_____. The organs and ducts that are involved in the secretion and excretion (elimination) of urine from the body are referred to as the **urinary tract.**

ANATOMY OF MAJOR URINARY STRUCTURES

11-2 You learned in an earlier chapter that ur(o) means urinary system or urine. In terms that use the combining form ur(o), you will use your critical thinking skills to decide which meaning is intended.

The urinary system consists of paired kidneys, one on each side of the spinal column, a ureter (u-re´tər, u´rə-tər) for each kidney, a bladder, and a urethra (u-re´thrə). The terms ureter and urethra are often confused, but note the difference in their spelling and their pronunciation. Remember, the body has two kidneys, two ureters, one bladder, and only one

urethra

_____.

11-3 Figure 11-1 shows the location of these structures in the body. Read all the information that accompanies Figure 11-1. Complete the blank lines 1 through 4 by reading the following information.

Urine is formed in the kidneys. Label the left kidney *(1)*. The **ureters** carry the urine to the urinary bladder. Label the left ureter *(2)*. The **bladder** *(3)* is a temporary reservoir for the urine until it is excreted via the **urethra** *(4)*. The external opening of the urethra is called the **urinary meatus** (me-a´təs).

The information that accompanies Figure 11-1 explains that blood is transported to the kidneys by vessels of the cardio/vascular (cardi[o], heart + vascul[o], vessel + -ar, pertaining to) system. These vessels that carry blood to the kidneys are **renal** _____.

arteries

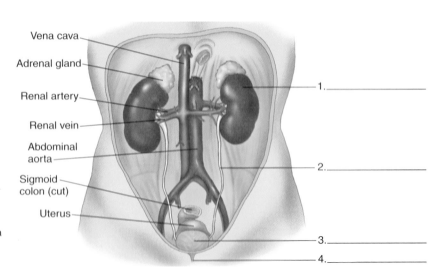

Figure 11-1 The urinary system. Adjacent vessels of the cardiovascular system are also shown. The right and left renal arteries branch off the abdominal aorta to transport blood to the kidneys. Urine, formed in the kidneys, leaves by way of the ureters and passes to the bladder, where it is stored. When voluntary control is removed, urine is expelled through the urethra. When blood is filtered, wastes are removed, but much of the water and other substances are reabsorbed. They enter the renal vein and are returned to the bloodstream via the inferior vena cava.

Vena cava
Adrenal gland
Renal artery
Renal vein
Abdominal aorta
Sigmoid colon (cut)
Uterus

1._____
2._____
3._____
4._____

Learn the following word parts for major structures of the urinary system.

Word Parts: Urinary Structures

Word Part	Meaning	Word Part	Meaning
ur(o)	urine, urinary tract	**Internal Structures of the Kidneys**	
urin(o)	urine	glomerul(o)	glomerulus
-uria	urine or urination	pyel(o)	renal pelvis
Major Urinary Structures		**Other**	
cyst(o)	bladder (also cyst or fluid-filled sac)	gon(o)	genitals or reproduction
nephr(o), ren(o)	kidney	thromb(o)	thrombus (internal blood clot)
ureter(o)	ureter		
urethr(o)	urethra		
vesic(o)	bladder or blister		

11-4 Most of the work of the urinary system takes place in the kidneys. The average adult kidney is about 11 cm long by 6 cm wide (about 4 ½ by 2 ⅓ inches) and weighs about 145 grams (less than half a pound).

➤ **KEY** POINT The kidneys have several functions. Although the **kidneys** are best known for their life-maintaining functions of filtering the blood and regulating the volume and composition of blood plasma, they also do the following:
- produce renin (assists regulation of blood pressure)
- produce erythropoietin (ə-rith″ro-poi′ə-tin) (erythrocyte production)
- produce prostaglandins (pros″tə-glan′dinz) (affect many organs)
- help degrade insulin and metabolize vitamin D

red

Erythr(o) means _____, and -poietin means that which causes production. **Erythropoietin** is a substance that causes the production of red blood cells.

11-5 Ren/al (re′nəl) means pertaining to the kidney. Use supra- to write a term that means above a kidney: _____.

suprarenal
(soo″prə-re′nəl)

Inter/renal (in″tər-re′nəl) means between the kidneys.

11-6 Urine leaves the kidney by way of the right and left ureters, which take it to the bladder. **Ureter/al** (u-re′tər-əl) means pertaining to a ureter. A **ureteral dysfunction** is a disturbance of the normal flow of urine through one or both _____.

ureters

11-7 The combining form cyst(o) means cyst, bladder, or fluid-filled sac. The term **cystic** (sis′tik) pertains to a cyst, the gallbladder, or the urinary _____.
Extra/cystic (eks″trə-sis′tik) means outside a cyst or outside the bladder.

bladder

Vesic/al (ves′ĭ-kəl) means pertaining to a fluid-filled sac, usually the urinary bladder. **Vesico/ureter/al** (ves″ĭ-ko-u-re′ter-al) means pertaining to the urinary bladder and a _____. **Vesico/vaginal** (ves″ĭ-ko-vaj′ĭ-nəl) means pertaining to the urinary bladder and the vagina.

ureter

11-8 Urine leaves the bladder by way of the urethra and is expelled from the body. **Urethr/al** (u-re′thrəl) means pertaining to the _____.
The urethra is about 3 cm long in women and lies anterior to the vagina. In men the urethra is about 20 cm long and serves as a passageway for semen and as a canal for urine.

urethra

11-9 Anatomic features of the kidney are shown in Figure 11-2. The kidney is encased in a fibrous (fibr[o], fiber + -ous, characterized by) (fi′brəs) capsule. **Fibrous** means consisting mainly of fibers. The fibrous capsule provides protection for the delicate internal parts of the kidney. The ribs and muscle also provide protection from direct trauma.

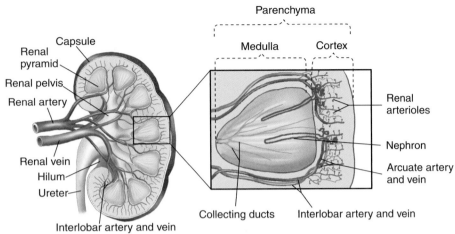

Figure 11-2 **The kidney (sectioned).** The kidney has a convex contour with the exception of the hilum, a notch on the inner border. A longitudinal section shows two distinct regions: the outer cortex and the inner medulla. The medulla has 10 to 15 triangular wedges called renal pyramids, made up of collecting ducts, lymphatics, and blood vessels. Cortical and medullary regions of each kidney contain approximately one million nephrons, the functioning units. A normal person can survive, although with difficulty, with less than 20,000 functioning nephrons.

pyel(o)

The notch or depression on the inner border of the kidney where the renal artery, renal vein, lymphatics, and nerves enter or leave the kidney is called the **hilum** (hi´ləm).

The renal pelvis is a funnel-shaped structure located in the center of each kidney. The combining form for renal pelvis is _____.

EXERCISE 1

Name the four major structures that make up the urinary system.

1. _____   3. _____

2. _____   4. _____

EXERCISE 2

Build It! *Use the following word parts to build terms. (Some word parts will be used more than once.)*

extra-, inter-, cyst(o), ren(o), urethr(o), urin(o), vesic(o), -al, -ary, -ic

1. pertaining to the urethra   _____/_____

2. pertaining to urine   _____/_____

3. between the kidneys   _____/_____/_____

4. pertaining to outside the bladder   _____/_____/_____

5. pertaining to the bladder and the ureters   _____/_____/_____

Say and Check

Say aloud the terms you wrote for Exercise 2. Use the Companion CD to check your pronunciations.

FORMATION AND EXCRETION OF URINE

nephr(o)

11-10 Normal kidney function requires constant filtering of the blood, selective reabsorption, and formation of urine. About 1 million **nephrons** serve as the functional units of each kidney.

The nephron (nef´ron) is named for the combining form _____, which means kidney. A nephron is shown in Figure 11-3. Its components are a **glomerulus** (glo-mer´u-ləs) and **tubules** (too´būlz).

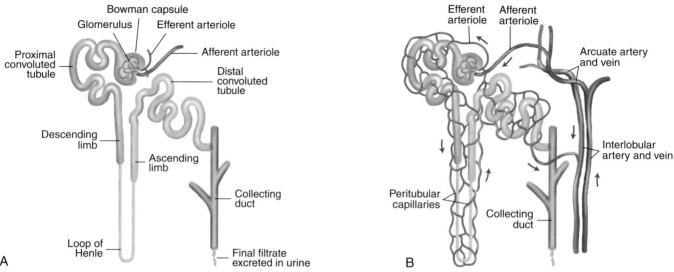

Figure 11-3 A nephron and surrounding capillaries. A, Nephron. Resembling a microscopic funnel with a long stem and tubular sections, a nephron consists of a renal corpuscle (nephron and Bowman's capsule) and renal tubules. The final filtrate that is formed is urine. **B,** Nephron shown with peritubular capillaries. The renal arteries arise from the abdominal aorta. Each renal artery branches as it enters the hilum and after branching several times, gives rise to the afferent arteriole, eventually terminating in capillary tufts called glomeruli. Blood leaves a glomerulus through the efferent arteriole, which subdivides into peritubular capillaries. As the glomerular filtrate flows through the tubules, most of its water and varying amounts of solutes are reabsorbed into the peritubular capillaries. These capillaries join others and become the arcuate vein and eventually the renal vein, whereby blood leaves the kidney.

11-11 Each glomerulus (plural, glomeruli) is a cluster of blood vessels surrounded by a structure called a **Bowman capsule. Glomerular** (glo-mer´u-lər) **filtration** is the initial process in the formation of urine. The glomerulus allows water, salts, wastes, and practically everything except blood cells and proteins to pass through its thin walls. The Bowman capsule collects the substances that filter through the glomerular walls and passes them to the long, twisted tube, the tubule.

The **proxim/al tubule** is that part of the tubule near the glomerulus. You learned that proxim(o) means near. That part of the renal tubule that is near the glomerulus and Bowman capsule is the _____ tubule.

proximal

11-12 Follow the long, twisting tubule. Notice that a tubule consists of a proximal tubule, a **loop of Henle,** and a **distal tubule** that opens into a collecting duct.

As fluid passes through the tubules, substances that the body conserves, such as sugar and much of the water, are reabsorbed into the blood vessels surrounding the tubules. This second process is known as **reabsorption.** The water and other substances remaining in the tubule become urine. **Anti/diuretic** (an˝te-, an˝ti-di˝u-ret´ik) **hormone** (ADH) increases the reabsorption of water by the renal tubules, thus decreasing the amount of urine produced. ADH is secreted by the brain and released as needed. The nephron functions in filtering of the blood, reabsorption of substances that the body conserves, and secretion of other substances, such as potassium, hydrogen ions, and certain drugs, into the urine to be excreted from the body (Figure 11-4). Filtering occurs in what part of the nephron? _____

glomerulus

tubule

In what part of the nephron does reabsorption occur? _____

The third process in urine formation, called tubular secretion, is the secretion of some substances from the bloodstream into the renal tubule (waste products of metabolism that become toxic if they are not excreted and certain drugs, such as penicillin).

> ➤ **KEY** POINT What does urine have to do with math?
> Substances that are filtered by the glomerulus
>   − substances that are reabsorbed
>   + substances that are added by tubular secretion
>   = URINE

A schematic diagram of the forming and expelling of urine is included in Figure 11-5.

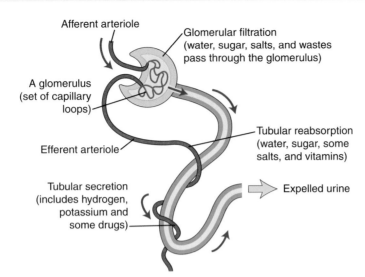

Figure 11-4 **Functions of the nephron: glomerular filtration, tubular reabsorption, and tubular secretion.**

11-13 Waste products and some of the water remaining in the tubules after reabsorption combine to become **urine,** which passes to the collecting duct. Thousands of collecting ducts deposit urine in the renal pelvis, the large central reservoir of the kidney.

After urine collects in the **renal pelvis,** it drains to the bladder by passing through a tube called the _____.

ureter

The urinary bladder is a collapsible muscular bag that serves as a reservoir for urine until it is expelled. It has a storage capacity in health of about 500 mL (1 pint) or more. **Micturition** (mik″tu-ri´shən), or **voiding,** means **urination,** expelling urine from the bladder.

11-14 The **glomerular filtration rate** (GFR) is a calculated volume of fluid filtered by the glomeruli. GFR decreases with advancing age, and the decline in the filtration rate is more rapid in persons with diabetes or hypertension (elevated blood pressure). GFR forms the basis of a test for how well the kidneys are functioning.

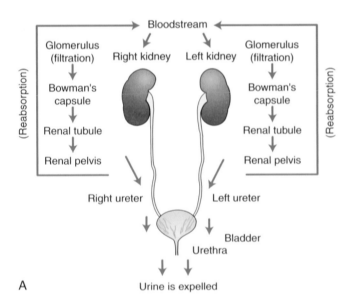

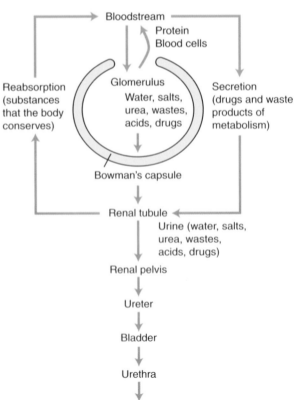

Figure 11-5 **Forming and expelling of urine. A,** Diagram of forming and expelling urine. **B,** Schematic of filtration of the blood, the processes of reabsorption and secretion, and expelling urine.

glomerular

This calculated volume of fluid filtered by the glomeruli is called _____ filtration rate.

11-15 Decide which meaning of cystic is implied in the term **abdomino/cystic** (ab-dom″ĭ-no-sis′tik), which means pertaining to the abdomen and the urinary _____.

bladder

This term means the same as **abdomino/vesical** (ab″dom″ĭ-no-ves′ĭ-kəl).

Filling of the bladder with urine stimulates receptors, producing the desire to urinate. Voluntary control prevents urine from being released. When the control is removed, urine is expelled through the urethra.

urethra

11-16 **Recto/urethr/al** (rek″to-u-re′thrəl) pertains to the rectum and the _____. **Urethro/rect/al** (u-re″thro-rek′təl) also means pertaining to the urethra and rectum; however, not all words can be reversed like this!

Urethro/vaginal (u-re″thro-vaj′ĭ-nəl) means pertaining to the urethra and the vagina. **Genito/urinary** (jen″ĭ-to-u′rĭ-nar-e) (GU) or **uro/genital** (u″ro-jen′ĭ-təl) pertains to the genitals as well as to the urinary organs.

EXERCISE 3

Write the names of the structures to complete these sentences.

1. The cavity in the kidney that collects urine from many collecting ducts is the renal _____.

2. A tube that carries urine to the bladder is a/an _____.

3. The tube that carries urine from the bladder is the _____.

4. The _____ is the functional unit of the kidney.

5. The _____ is the reservoir for urine until it is expelled.

6. The filtering structure of the kidney is the _____.

7. Reabsorption occurs in structures called the _____.

8. The external opening of the urethra is the urinary _____.

DIAGNOSTIC TESTS AND PROCEDURES

palpation

11-17 Physical assessment of the kidneys, ureters, and bladder (KUB) includes abdominal inspection, auscultation, palpation, and percussion (see Figure 3-8). Which of these procedures makes use of the examiner's hands to assess the texture, size, consistency, and location of the kidneys and bladder? _____ Laboratory tests, biopsies, radiography, and endoscopy are helpful in diagnostic assessment of the urinary system.

A 24-hour record of **intake and output** (I&O) often provides valuable information regarding fluid and/or electrolyte problems. Intake should include oral, intravenous, and tube feedings. A major source of fluid output is urine, but other output to record includes excess perspiration, vomitus, and diarrhea. I&O is the abbreviation for intake and _____.

output

LABORATORY TESTS

urinalysis

11-18 Several urine tests are used to evaluate the status of the urinary system. A **urinalysis** (u″rĭ-nal′ĭ-sis) is usually part of a physical examination but is particularly useful for patients with suspected urologic disorders. The urin/alysis is an examination of urine. Urinalysis was originally called urine analysis. It is often abbreviated UA or U/A. Examination of the urine is called

_____.

The complete urinalysis generally includes a physical, chemical, and microscopic examination performed in the clinical laboratory.

11-19 The urine specimen is physically examined for color, turbidity, and specific gravity. Ideally the urine is collected at the first morning's voiding. Freshly voided urine is normally clear and straw-colored. Changes in the color of urine may indicate dilute or concentrated urine. Dark red or brown urine may indicate blood in the urine; other color changes may result from diet or medications. In a urinalysis the **specific gravity** is the density of urine compared with the density of water. The specific gravity of water is 1.0, and urine is normally 1.010 to 1.025. Dilute urine has a low specific gravity, and concentrated urine has a high specific gravity.

Specific gravity can be measured by various means, including the use of a **chemical dipstick** or a **urino/meter** (u″rĭ-nom´ə-tər), an instrument that measures the specific gravity of

urine

_____ (Figure 11-6, *A*).

11-20 Chemical analysis of urine may be performed to measure the pH (potential of hydrogen; the numeric pH value indicates the relative concentration of hydrogen ions in a solution) and to identify and measure the levels of ketones (ke´tōnz), sugar, protein, blood components, and many other substances. Urea (u-re´ə), ammonia, creatinine (kre-at´ĭ-nin), and salts are important waste products in urine. **Urea** is a nitrogen compound that is the final product of protein metabolism.

Several substances are not present in normal urine, and their presence indicates various pathologic states. Some abnormal components of urine are sugar, **albumin** (main protein found in urine), ketones, and blood. The presence of these substances can be detected in which part of the urinalysis:

chemical

the physical, chemical, or microscopic part? The _____ part. Learn the meaning of the following word parts.

Word Parts: Urine

Word Part	Meaning	Word Part	Meaning
urin(o)	urine	**Abnormal Substances in Urine**	
		albumin(o)	albumin
Other		glyc(o), glycos(o)	sugar
noct(i), nyct(o)	night	ket(o), keton(o)	ketone bodies
olig(o)	few, scanty	prote(o), protein(o)	protein

11-21 Sugar in the urine is **glycos/uria** (gli″ko-su´re-ə). The combining forms glyc(o) and glycos(o) mean sweet or sugar. Remember that glycos(o) is combined with -uria. Sugar should not be detected in the chemical testing of urine (Figure 11-6, *B*), because glucose is generally reabsorbed in the renal tubules. When the blood glucose rises above a certain level, the **renal threshold** for reabsorption is exceeded, and glucose is excreted in the urine. Glycosuria may indicate diabetes and re-

sugar

quires further testing. Glycosuria means _____ in the urine.

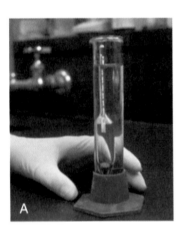
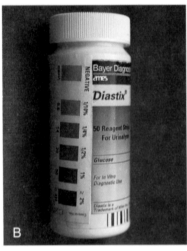
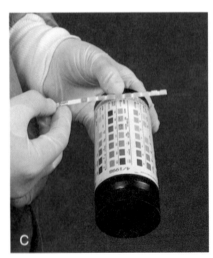

Figure 11-6 Simple urine tests. A, A urinometer is used to determine the specific gravity, the degree of concentration of a sample of urine. **B,** Glucose test strips provide a means of screening for the presence of glucose in the urine. **C,** Testing urine with a Multistix, a plastic strip on which there are reagent areas for testing various chemical constituents that may be present in the urine. These reagent strips are considered qualitative tests and a positive result for an abnormal substance in the urine generally requires further testing.

blood

11-22 Hemat/uria (he″mə-, hem″ə-tu´re-ə) means _____ in the urine. Blood should not be present in the urine, so hematuria is considered an abnormal condition. (Of course, urine can be contaminated by blood in voided urine of menstruating women.)

protein

11-23 Protein/uria (pro″te-nu´re-ə) is _____ in the urine, usually albumin. **Albumin/uria** (al″bu-mĭ-nu´re-ə) is albumin in the urine.

Ketone bodies are end products of lipid (fat) metabolism in the body. Excessive production of ketone bodies, however, leads to urinary excretion of **ketones.** Under normal conditions, ketones are not present in urine (Figure 11-6, C). **Keton/uria** (ke″to-nu´re-ə) is the presence of ketones

urine

in the _____.

Ketone bodies are acids, and ketones are found in the urine when the body's fat stores are metabolized for energy, thus providing an excess of metabolic end products. This can occur in uncontrolled diabetes mellitus because of a deficiency of insulin. **Keto/acid/osis** (ke″to-as″ĭ-do´sis) means acidosis accompanied by an accumulation of ketones in the body and results from faulty carbohydrate metabolism. It occurs primarily as a complication of diabetes mellitus. Write this

ketoacidosis

term that means acidosis accompanied by an accumulation of ketones: _____.

11-24 A microscopic study is generally part of a complete urinalysis. Body cells, crystals, and bacteria are some of the particles present in a microscopic study (Figure 11-7). These are gener-

high

ally reported as number/high power field (HPF). HPF means a microscopic _____ power field.

A healthy urine sample contains very few white blood cells. The presence of a large number of white blood cells may be indicative of an infectious or inflammatory process somewhere in the urinary tract. For example, there is usually a large number of white blood cells/HPF in most urinary tract infections.

Pus cells, necrotic white blood cells, are a major component of pus. **Py/uria** (pi-u´re-ə)

urine

means the presence of pus in the _____.

11-25 Only a few red blood cells are normally present in urine. If several red blood cells/HPF are present, it may indicate a variety of abnormalities, including a tumor, urinary stones, infection, or a bleeding disorder.

Urinary casts are gelatinous structures that take the shape of the renal tubules. Casts are described by the type of element in the structure (for example, WBC cast, RBC cast, granular cast, waxy cast). There are usually few to no casts, so the presence of several casts in urine generally indi-

kidney

cates renal disease or urinary calculi. Renal disease means disease of a _____. Study the summary of routine laboratory tests for renal function in Table 11-1.

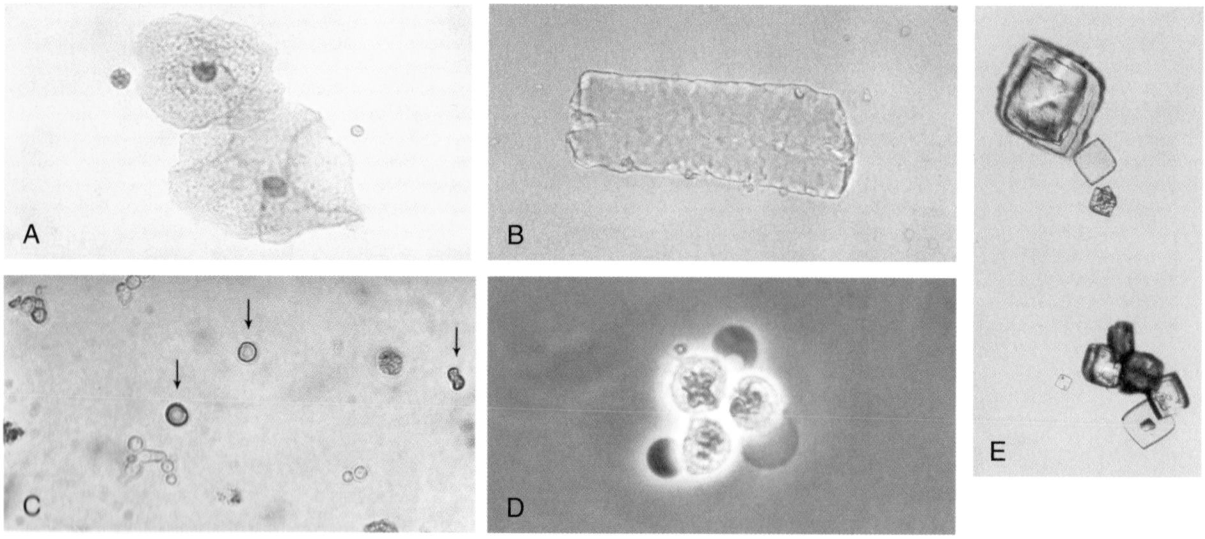

Figure 11-7 Structures seen in a microscopic examination of urine. A, Squamous epithelial cells. **B,** Waxy cast. **C,** Red blood cells *(arrows).* **D,** White blood cells (the nucleated cells shown). **E,** Uric acid crystals.

TABLE 11-1	Routine Laboratory Renal Function Tests
Type of Test	**Indications**
Blood Studies	
Blood urea nitrogen (BUN)	Increased level may indicate liver or kidney disease; other causes include dehydration, infection, stress, and/or steroid use
Serum creatinine	Increased level indicates renal impairment; decreased level may be caused by muscle mass loss
Urinalysis	**Normal**
Appearance	
Color	Usually pale straw
Odor	Aromatic, similar to ammonia (ingestion of certain foods may cause foul smell)
Turbidity	Clear
Specific gravity	1.005-1.030
Chemical	
pH	6 (possible range 4.6-8)
Glucose	None
Ketones	None
Protein	None
Bilirubin (urobilinogen)	None
Leukoesterase	None
Nitrites	None
Microscopic	
Crystals	None
RBCs	0-2/HPF (increased RBCs are seen with indwelling or intermittent catheterization and/or menstruation)
WBCs	Females 0-5/HPF; males 0-3/HPF
Bacteria	None or few per HPF (less than 1000 colonies/mL)
Parasites	None
Casts	Few to none

HPF, High-power field; *RBCs,* red blood cells; *WBCs,* white blood cells.

11-26 Few bacteria reside in freshly collected urine. The presence of many bacteria may indicate a urinary tract infection. If the patient has symptoms of a urinary tract infection, a **urine culture** is used to determine the types of pathogenic bacteria present. When bacteria are present in significant numbers, another test (an **antibiotic sensitivity test**) is used to determine which antibiotics are effective against that particular pathogen.

culture

The test is ordered as a culture and sensitivity (C&S). The cultivation of microorganisms in the laboratory on special culture medium is called a _____.

11-27 Urine specimens are collected according to the laboratory or physician's instructions. A

voids (or urinates)

voided specimen is one in which the patient _____ into a container supplied by the laboratory or physician's office. Because improperly collected urine may yield incorrect test results, voided urine should always be collected using the clean-catch midstream technique. This technique is based on the concept that the tissues adjacent to the urethral meatus must be cleansed before collection to avoid contamination of the specimen, and only the middle portion of the urine stream (**clean-catch specimen**) is collected.

A **catheterized urine specimen** is obtained by placing a catheter (kath´ə-tər) into the bladder and withdrawing urine. This may be necessary to obtain an uncontaminated urine specimen.

11-28 Creatinine is a substance formed in normal metabolism and is commonly found in blood, urine, and muscle tissue. Creatinine is measured in blood and urine as an indicator of kidney function. A serum creatinine test is a measurement of the creatinine level in the blood. A **creatinine**

creatinine

clearance test is a diagnostic test that measures the rate at which creatinine is cleared from the blood by the kidney. This kidney function test is called a _____ clearance test, one example of a renal clearance test. **Renal clearance tests** determine the efficiency with which the kidneys excrete particular substances.

A 24-hour urine collection is collection of all of the urine voided in a 24-hour period. This type of collection may be ordered to measure levels of various substances in the urine, such as calcium or creatinine.

11-29 In addition to blood creatinine levels, **blood urea nitrogen** (BUN) is directly related to the metabolic function of the liver and the excretory function of the kidney. BUN is a measure of the amount of urea in the blood. Urea forms in the liver as the end product of protein metabolism and is excreted by the kidneys in urine. A critically elevated BUN level indicates serious impairment of renal function.

BUN, a blood test that measures the excretory function of the kidney, means blood

urea

_____ nitrogen.

EXERCISE 4

 Build It! *Use the following word parts to build terms. (Some word parts will be used more than once.)*

glycos(o), keton(o), protein(o), py(o), urin(o), -meter, -uria

1. protein in the urine   _____/_____

2. sugar in the urine   _____/_____

3. instrument to measure the specific gravity of urine   _____/_____

4. pus in the urine   _____/_____

5. presence of the end products of fat metabolism in the urine   _____/_____

Say and Check

Say aloud the terms you wrote for Exercise 4. Use the Companion CD to check your pronunciations.

URINARY CATHETERIZATION

11-30 In **urinary catheterization** (kath´ə-tur-ĭ-za´shən), a catheter is inserted through the urethra and into the bladder for temporary or permanent drainage of urine. Urinary catheterization may be done to collect a urine specimen, and for other reasons, including urinary testing, instillation of medications into the bladder, and drainage of the bladder during many types of surgeries or in cases of urinary obstruction or paralysis.

Catheters are hollow, flexible tubes that can be inserted into a vessel or cavity of the body. They vary in type and size, and the type that is used varies with the size of the individual and the purpose of catheterization. The hollow tube that is used in catheterization is a

catheter

_____.

11-31 An **indwelling catheter** is designed to be left in place for a prolonged period. A **Foley catheter** is held securely in place by a balloon tip that is filled with a sterile liquid after the catheter has been placed in the bladder (Figure 11-8). This type of catheter is used when continuous

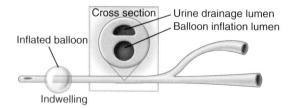

Figure 11-8 Foley catheter. This type of catheter has a balloon tip to be filled with a sterile liquid after it has been placed in the bladder. This is a type of indwelling catheter and is used when continuous drainage is desired.

drainage of the bladder is desired, such as in surgery, or when repeated urinary catheterization would be necessary if an indwelling catheter were not used.

An indwelling catheter that has a balloon tip and is left in place in the bladder is a _____ catheter.

Foley

Ureteral catheters are usually passed into the distal ends of the ureters from the bladder via a cystoscope and may be threaded up the ureters into the renal pelves (plural for pelvis). A ureteral catheter may also be surgically inserted through the abdominal wall into a ureter. Placement of catheters through the urethra into a ureter is _____ **catheterization**.

ureteral

Ureteral catheters may be placed temporarily as part of a diagnostic procedure called a retrograde urogram or pyelogram, which permits visualization of the renal collecting system in patients whose renal function is too limited for adequate visualization with intravenous urography.

11-32 Four methods are used for urinary tract catheterizations. They are urethral, ureteral, and suprapubic (soo″prə-pu′bik) and nephrostomy (nə-fros′tə-me). The four types of urinary catheterization are shown in Figure 11-9.

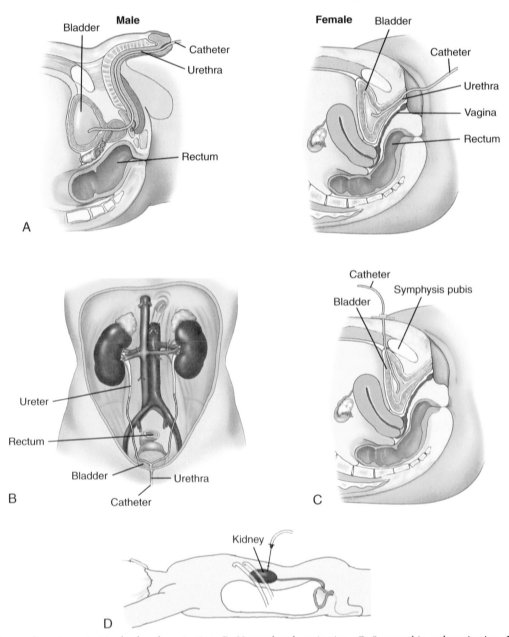

Figure 11-9 Urinary diversion. A, Urethral catheterization. **B,** Ureteral catheterization. **C,** Suprapubic catheterization. **D,** Percutaneous nephrostomy.

urethral

The most common means is insertion of the catheter through the external meatus into the urethra and then to the bladder. Insertion of the catheter through the urethra and into the bladder is _____ **catheterization.**

11-33 If disease or obstruction does not allow urethral catheterization, a **supra/pubic catheter** can be placed into the bladder through a small incision or puncture of the abdominal wall about 1 inch above the symphysis pubis, the bony eminence that lies beneath the pubic hair. **Supra/pubic** means pertaining to a location _____ the symphysis pubis.

above

The fourth means of urinary catheterization is using a **nephrostomy catheter,** which is inserted on a temporary basis into the renal pelvis when a complete obstruction of the ureter is present. This procedure is a **per/cutaneous nephro/stomy,** which means formation of a new opening into the renal pelvis through the overlying skin.

11-34 Urodynamic studies measure various aspects of the process of voiding and are used along with other procedures to evaluate problems with urine flow. Types of urodynamic studies include cystometrography, electromyography, and urethral pressure profile.

Cysto/metro/graphy (cyst[o], bladder + metr[o], to measure + -graphy, process of recording) (sis″to-mə-trog′rə-fe) provides information about the effectiveness of the bladder wall muscle. This procedure may incorporate the use of a urinary catheter with an attached **cysto/meter** ([sis-tom′ə-tər -meter], instrument for measuring) that measures bladder capacity in relation to changing urine pressure. Looking at its word parts, it is noted that a cysto/meter is an instrument that measures aspects of the _____.

bladder

Electro/myo/graphy (electr[o], electricity + my[o], muscle + -graphy) (EMG) can be used to evaluate the strength of the muscles used in voiding (the **perineal** [per″ĭ-ne′əl] **muscles**). The **perineum** supports and surrounds the distal parts of the uro/genital and gastro/intestinal tracts of the body. Electromyography is the electrical recording of _____ action, in this case, the strength of the perineal muscles. This test can be used to evaluate urinary incontinence, the inability to control urination.

muscle

Urethral pressure profile provides information about the nature of urinary incontinence or retention (accumulation of urine in the bladder that results from inability to urinate).

EXERCISE 5

Word Analysis. *Divide these words into their component parts and write the meaning of each term.*

1. cystometrography _____

2. nephrostomy _____

3. cystometer _____

4. electromyography _____

Say and Check

Say aloud the terms in Exercise 5. Use the Companion CD to check your pronunciations.

URINARY RADIOGRAPHY

11-35 Several special radiologic procedures are used to diagnose abnormalities of the urinary system, and plain abdominal x-ray images are used to show obvious aspects of the kidneys, ureters, and bladder (KUB).

> ➤ **KEY** POINT Many noninvasive radiologic tests are available. Plain x-ray images, nephro-sonography, nephrotomography, and MRI along with urine and blood studies provide a great deal of diagnostic information about the urinary system. Bladder scans are particularly useful in determining bladder volume as well as postvoid residual volume.

nephrotomogram
(nef″ro-to′mo-gram)

Nephro/sono/graphy (nef″ro-so-nog′rə-fe) is ultrasonic scanning of the kidney. Very large or very small kidneys, cysts, and kidney stones can be diagnosed using nephrosonography. **Nephro/tomo/graphy** (nef″ro-to-mog′re-fe) means tomography of the kidney. The film produced by nephrotomography is a _____ (Figure 11-10).

11-36 Intra/venous (in″trə-ve′nəs) **uro/graphy** (u-rog′rə-fe) is the making of x-ray images of the entire urinary system or part of it after the urine has been rendered opaque by a contrast medium that is injected intravenously. Various structural features can be seen on the resulting radiographs, as well as tumors or stones. Various functional abnormalities may also be diagnosed with this technique. The renal pelves and ureters are clearly visible in the normal **urogram** (u′ro-gram) shown in Figure 11-11.

urogram
(or **pyelogram**)
(pi′ə-lo-gram)

Intravenous urography is also called **intravenous pyelography** (pi″ə-log′rə-fe), IVP, and the resulting radiograph is called a _____.

urethra

11-37 Cysto/graphy (sis-tog′rə-fe) is radiography of the bladder, and **urethrography** (u″rə-throg′rə-fe) is radiography of the urethra after introduction of a radiopaque contrast medium. In **cysto/urethro/graphy** (sis″to-u″rə-throg′rə-fe), both the bladder and _____ are studied. A urinary catheter is used to instill the contrast medium.

In a **voiding cysto/urethro/gram** (sis″to-u-re′thro-gram) (VCUG), radiographs are made before, during, and after voiding (urination). It allows observation of the bladder as it empties and checks for reflux of urine into the ureters.

11-38 Adequate blood circulation is essential for normal renal function. Anything that interferes with the normal circulation significantly reduces renal capabilities. **Renal angio/graphy** (renal arteriography) is a radiographic study to assess the arterial blood supply to the

kidneys

_____.
This procedure requires injection of a radiopaque contrast agent into the renal arteries via a catheter that is inserted into a major artery, usually a femoral artery, and threaded up the aorta under fluoroscopic control to the point where the renal arteries branch off from the aorta.

arteriogram

A **renal** _____ is the record of the arterial blood supply to the kidneys (Figure 11-12).

11-39 A **kidney scan** also provides information about renal blood flow. In this procedure, radioactive material is intravenously injected and is absorbed by kidney tissue. Special equipment measures, records, and produces an image of the low-level radioactivity that is emitted.

kidney

Reno/graphy (re-nog′rə-fe) means the same as a kidney scan, because the literal translation of reno/graphy is the process of recording the _____.

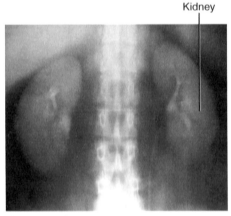

Figure 11-10 Nephrotomogram. The procedure, nephrotomography, is helpful in assessing various planes of kidney tissue for tumors, cysts, or stones.

Kidney

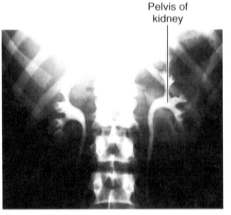

Figure 11-11 Intravenous urogram. The x-ray image was taken as the contrast medium was cleared from the blood by the kidneys. The renal pelvis and ureters are clearly visible and indicate normal findings.

Pelvis of kidney

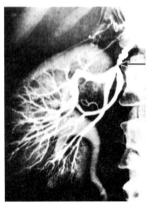

Figure 11-12 Renal arteriogram showing stenosis (*arrow*) **of the right renal artery.**

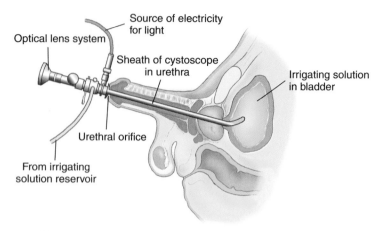

Figure 11-13 **A cystoscope in place inside the male bladder.**

ENDOSCOPY

cystoscopy
(sis-tos′kə-pe)

11-40 Write a term for direct visual examination of the bladder: _____.
In this type of examination, a hollow metal tube is passed through the urethra and into the bladder. By means of a light, special lenses, and mirrors, the bladder mucosa is examined (Figure 11-13).

The instrument used in cystoscopy is a **cystoscope** (sis′to-skōp″). In addition to examining the interior of the bladder, cystoscopy is used to obtain biopsy specimens of tumors or other growths, to remove polyps (growths protruding from the lining of the bladder) or stones, and to pass catheters into the ureters.

11-41 Urethro/scopy (u″rə-thros′kə-pe) is visual examination of the urethra. If this also involves the bladder, it is referred to as cysto/urethro/scopy (sis″to-u″re-thros′kə-pe).

ureter

Uretero/scopy (u-re-tər-os′kə-pe) is examination of a _____.

11-42 Nephro/scopy (nə-fros′kə-pe) allows visualization of the kidney using a fiberoptic instrument. A major use of this procedure is to remove or crush renal calculi. Nephroscopy requires the use of an instrument that is inserted through the skin into a small incision in the renal pelvis, allowing the urologist to view inside the kidney (Figure 11-14).

nephroscope
(nef′ro-skōp)

The instrument for nephroscopy is called a _____.
Common radiologic and special diagnostic tests in this section are summarized in Table 11-2.

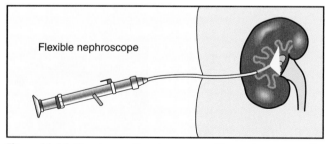

Flexible nephroscope

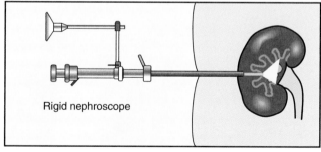

Rigid nephroscope

Figure 11-14 **Two types of nephroscopes.** The nephroscope, a fiberoptic instrument, is inserted percutaneously into the kidney. Additional instruments can be introduced through the scope, for example, to remove or break up calculi.

TABLE 11-2 Common Renal and Urinary Diagnostic Tests	
Noninvasive	**Others**
Plain radiography of the kidneys, ureters, and bladder	Cystography and cystoscopy
Magnetic resonance imaging	Intravenous urography
Nephrotomography	Renal arteriography
Ultrasonography	Renal scan
	Nephroscopy (not as common)

EXERCISE 6

Circle the correct answer for each of the following questions.

1. Which of the following is an examination of urine that is usually part of a routine physical examination? (BUN, creatinine clearance test, renal clearance test, urinalysis)

2. Which of the following is a normal component of urine? (ketone, protein, sugar, urea)

3. Which of the following is not a means of urinary tract catheterization? (cystometrography, ureteral, urethral, suprapubic)

4. Which term means a kidney scan? (cystourethrogram, renography, nephroscopy, nephrostomy)

5. Which term means a radiographic procedure that produces layered images as if the kidney had been sliced in a plane? (intravenous urography, nephrosonography, nephrostomy, nephrotomography)

PATHOLOGIES

urinary

vessels

11-43 A **uro/pathy** (u-rop´ə-the) is any disease or abnormal condition of the _____ tract. Uropathies include inflammatory, hereditary, obstructive, and renovascular disorders. In addition, some uropathies are the result of metabolic disease processes that affect renal function. **Reno/vascular disorders** are those affecting the blood _____ of the kidneys.

difficult

many

11-44 Discomfort during urination and unexplained change in the volume of urine are sometimes the earliest indications of a urinary problem. **Dys/uria** (dis-u´re-ə) is _____ or painful urination and can be caused by a bacterial infection or an obstruction of the urinary tract.
   Poly/uria (pol″e-u´re-ə) is excretion of an abnormally large quantity of urine. Literal translation of polyuria is _____ urines or urinations. You will need to remember that polyuria means excretion of an abnormally large quantity of urine. This can be brought about by excessive intake of fluids or the use of medications. Two pathologies in which polyuria is common are diabetes insipidus and diabetes mellitus. Both are described later in this section.

urination

oliguria

11-45 Literal translation of an/uria (an-u´re-ə) is absence of _____. The full meaning of **anuria** is a urinary output of less than 100 mL per day. The patient who has less than 100 mL of urine output per day is described as **anur/ic** (an-u´rik).
   Compare anuria and **olig/uria** (ol″ĭ-gu´re-ə), which means diminished capacity to form urine, excreting less than 500 mL of urine per day. The combining form olig(o) means few or scanty. Write this term that means diminished urine production of less than 500 mL per day: _____.

> ➤ **KEY** POINT Be sure you can distinguish these terms ending in -uria.
> Polyuria is excretion of an abnormally large quantity of urine.
> Dysuria is difficult or painful urination.
> Oliguria is excreting less than 500 mL of urine per day.
> Anuria is excreting less than 100 mL of urine per day.

retention

11-46 Urgency, frequency, and hesitancy are terms that are often used to describe urination patterns. **Urgency** is a sudden onset of the need to urinate immediately. Increased **frequency** is a greater number of urinations than expected in a given time. **Hesitancy** is difficulty in beginning the flow, often with a decrease in the force of the urine stream.
   Retention (re-ten´shən) means holding in place or persistent keeping within the body of matter that is normally excreted. Incomplete emptying of the bladder is called **urinary** _____. **Urinary reflux** is an abnormal backward or return flow of urine from the bladder into the ureters.

11-47 Continence* (kon´tĭ-nəns) is the ability to control bladder or bowel function. **Urinary incontinence** (in-kon´tĭ-nəns) is inability to control urination. This is loss of control of the passage of urine from the bladder. There are many causes of incontinence, such as loss of muscle tone, obesity, or unconsciousness. For the latter reason, indwelling catheters are used when patients are anesthetized.

   Enuresis (en″u-re´sis) also means the inability to control urination, and the term is applied especially to nocturnal bed-wetting. Nocturnal means pertaining to or occurring at night.

11-48 **Noct/uria** (nok-tu´re-ə), also called **nyct/uria** (nik-tu´re-ə), is excessive urination at night. Both noct(i) and nyct(o) mean night. Although nocturia may be a symptom of disease, it also can occur in people who drink excessive amounts of fluids before bedtime or when nearby structures put pressure on the bladder. An example of the latter is pressure on the bladder by a prolapsed uterus.

night

   Both nocturia and nycturia mean excessive urination at _____, sometimes interfering with sleep because of the need to urinate several times during the night.

11-49 When one kidney is removed, the other kidney becomes enlarged. Enlargement of the kidney is **nephro/megaly** (nef″ro-meg´ə-le).

one

   Kidney enlargement may involve one or both kidneys. Uni/lateral nephromegaly is enlargement of _____ kidney; bi/lateral nephromegaly involves both kidneys.

11-50 Some renal disorders are hereditary. **Poly/cyst/ic** (pol″e-sis´tik) **kidney disease,** one of the more common hereditary renal disorders, is characterized by enlarged kidneys containing many cysts. Poly/cystic means containing many cysts. See Figure 11-15 for comparison of a polycystic kidney and a normal kidney.

11-51 Because the urinary system is responsible for removing harmful waste products from the blood, anything that interferes with excretion of wastes can be dangerous. **Uremia** (u-re´me-ə) is an accumulation of toxic products in the blood. This occurs when the kidneys fail to function properly. The meaning of ur/emia (ur[o], urine + -emia, blood) is implied.

uremia

   Write this term that means an accumulation of waste products in the blood resulting from inadequate functioning of the urinary system: _____.

➤ **KEY** POINT Note the difference in uremia and hematuria. Uremia is an accumulation of waste products in the blood. Hematuria is the presence of blood in urine.

11-52 Inability of the kidneys to excrete wastes, concentrate urine, and function properly is **renal failure.** It may be acute or chronic. Acute renal failure (ARF) has symptoms that are more severe than those of _____ renal failure (CRF).

chronic

   Acute renal failure is characterized by oliguria and by the rapid accumulation of nitrogenous wastes in the blood, indicated by a higher than normal amount of blood urea nitrogen. Acute renal failure may be caused by nephr/itis (inflammation of the kidney), interference in blood flow to the kidney, or conditions that disrupt urinary output.

   Acute renal failure can often be reversed after the cause has been identified (for example, removal of an obstruction in the urinary tract). However, chronic renal failure may lead to the need for dialysis (di-al´ə-sis) if all other medical measures have not alleviated the problem.

11-53 A substance that is **nephro/toxic** (nef´ro-tok″sik) is toxic or destructive to kidney cells. Build a word that means destruction of the kidney by combining nephr(o) with the suffix for destruction: _____.

nephrolysis
(nə-frol´ə-sis)

   Nephrolysis also means freeing of a kidney from adhesions, bands of scar tissue that bind together surfaces that are normally separate.

   Nephro/malacia (nef″ro-mə-la´shə) is abnormal softening of the kidney.

11-54 A polyp (pol´ip) is any growth or mass protruding from a mucous membrane. A **bladder polyp** is a growth protruding from the lining of the bladder. This abnormality is one of the con-

*Continence (Latin: *continere,* to contain).

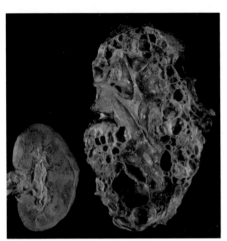

Figure 11-15 Comparison of polycystic kidney with a normal kidney. Note the diseased kidney's enlargement and the replacement of normal tissue by numerous fluid-filled cysts.

Cancerous tumor

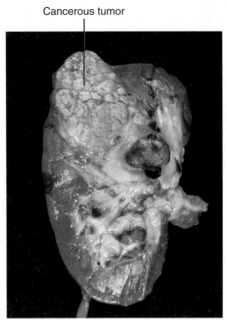

Figure 11-16 Kidney cancer. Note the large tumor in this adult kidney that has been excised.

ditions that may be detected during cystoscopy. Polyps may occur anywhere there is mucous membrane, such as the urethra.

Polyps are removed and the tissue is studied microscopically, even though cancer may not be suspected.

11-55 Bladder cancer is the most common malignancy of the urinary tract and occurs more than twice as frequently in men than women. Bladder-wash specimens and bladder biopsies (obtained during cystoscopy) are often used to diagnose cancer of the bladder. The most common malignancy of the urinary tract is _____ cancer.

| bladder

Kidney cancer is a malignant neoplasm of the renal parenchyma (Figure 11-16) or the renal pelvis. **Wilms tumor** is a malignant neoplasm of the kidney occurring in young children.

11-56 Urethrorrhagia (u-re″thro-ra´jə) means urethral hemorrhage. **Urethro/rrhea** (u-re″thro-re´ə) means _____ from the urethra.

| discharge

EXERCISE 7

Build It! *Use the following word parts to build terms. (Some word parts will be used more than once.)*

nephr(o), noct(i), tox(o), urethr(o), -ic, -malacia, -megaly, -rrhagia, -uria

1. abnormal softening of the kidney   _____ / _____

2. hemorrhage from the urethra   _____ / _____

3. excessive urination at night   _____ / _____

4. enlargement of the kidney   _____ / _____

5. pertaining to being destructive to the kidney   _____ / _____ / _____

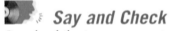 *Say and Check*

Say aloud the terms you wrote for Exercise 7. Use the Companion CD to check your pronunciations.

EXERCISE 8

Match terms in the left columns with their descriptions in the right column.

_____ 1. anuria   _____ 6. polyp   A. a decrease in the force of the urine stream
                                             B. a mass protruding from a mucous membrane
_____ 2. dysuria   _____ 7. polyuria   C. difficult or painful urination
_____ 3. hesitancy   _____ 8. urgency   D. excessive urination at night
                                             E. excretion of an abnormally large volume of urine
_____ 4. nycturia   _____ 9. urinary incontinence   F. excretion of less than 100 mL of urine a day
_____ 5. oliguria   _____ 10. urinary retention   G. excretion of less than 500 mL of urine a day
                                             H. incomplete emptying of the bladder
                                             I. loss of control of the passage of urine from the bladder
                                             J. the sense of the need to urinate immediately

11-57 Bacterial infection is the most common cause of inflammation of the urinary tract, but inflammation may be attributed to other disorders, such as the presence of a stone.

A **urinary tract infection** (UTI), an infection of one or more structures in the urinary system, is one of the more common disorders of the urinary tract. A UTI may be asymptomatic but is usually characterized by urinary frequency and possibly discomfort during urination. Other signs and symptoms, particularly in severe infections, include backache, fever, and blood and/or pus in the urine. It is important to diagnose and treat urinary tract infections to prevent their spreading to another part of the body, such as the blood. **Septic/emia** (sept[o], infection + -emia, blood) is a systemic infection in which pathogens are present in the circulating blood, having spread from an infection in another part of the body, such as the urinary tract.

infection

UTI means urinary tract _____.

11-58 Urinary tract infections can include cyst/itis (sis-ti´tis), urethritis (u″rə-thri´tis), and pyelonephritis (pi″ə-lo-nə-fri´tis). Most urinary infections are caused by bacteria (especially *Escherichia coli*), but certain fungi *(Candida)* can also cause infection. When UTIs are caused by bacteria, they are treated with an antibiotic.

> ➤ **KEY** POINT   Most of the time, UTIs are caused by ascending infection. The anus serves as a reservoir for bacteria, and organisms spread directly from the anal area (occasionally the vagina) to the urethral meatus, where they multiply and can ascend throughout the urethra to the bladder and eventually the kidney in some cases. Infection is more likely in females than in males because of the short distance separating the anus and the urethra, as well as a shorter urethra. Both catheterization and sexual intercourse promote the ascent of bacteria. Urinary tract infections are also more common in persons with structural abnormalities or lowered immunity and are a major type of hospital-acquired infections.

urethritis

Write the term that means inflammation of the urethra: _____.
This condition is characterized by dysuria. It may result from minor trauma or from infection. **Urethro/cyst/itis** (u-re″thro-sis-ti´tis) is inflammation of the urethra and bladder. This means the same as **cysto/urethr/itis** (sis″to-u″re-thri´tis).

cystitis

Write the term that means inflammation of the bladder: _____.

11-59 Cystitis often involves inflammation of the ureters. Write a term that means inflammation

ureteritis
(u-re″tər-i´tis)

of a ureter: _____. Ureteritis may also be caused by the mechanical irritation of a stone. **Ureteropathy** (u-re″tər-op´ə-the) means any disease of a ureter.

Uretero/pyelo/nephritis (u-re″tər-o-pi″ə-lo-nə-fri´tis) means inflammation of a ureter, renal pelvis, and kidney. Write a word that means inflammation of the renal pelvis:

pyelitis (pi″ə-li´tis)

_____.

Pyelonephritis means inflammation of the kidney and its renal pelvis. Acute pyelonephritis is usually the result of spreading of an infection from the lower urinary tract and has a rapid onset. Chronic pyelonephritis can develop after bacterial infection of the kidney that is either untreated or resistant to treatment.

inflammation

11-60 Nephr/itis (nə-fri´tis) is one of a large group of kidney diseases that is characterized by _____ and abnormal function. The most usual form is **glomerulo/nephritis** (glo-mer″u-lo-nə-fri´tis), in which glomeruli within the kidney are inflamed. Glomeruli (glo-mer´u-li) are clusters of capillaries that act as filters. In glomerulonephritis there is impairment of the filtering process. Inflammation of the kidney may be caused by microorganisms or their toxins or even by toxic drugs or alcohol.

Glomerul(o) is a combining form that means glomerulus. Write a word that means any disease of the glomeruli: _____.

glomerulopathy
(glo-mer″u-lop´ə-the)

11-61 Interstitial nephritis is inflammation of the interstitial tissue of the kidney, including the tubules. This type of nephritis can be acute or chronic. When acute interstitial nephritis is an adverse immunologic reaction to a drug, normal kidney function is generally regained when the offending drug is discontinued. In interstitial nephritis, there is inflammation of the _____ tissue of the kidney.

interstitial

11-62 Nephrotic (nə-frot´ik) **syndrome** is an abnormal condition of the kidney characterized by marked proteinuria and edema. It occurs as a complication of many systemic diseases, such as diabetes mellitus.

Diabetes mellitus (di″ə-be´tēz mel´lĭ-təs, mə-li´təs) is a complex disorder of carbohydrate, fat, and protein metabolism that is primarily a result of a deficiency or lack of insulin secretion by the pancreas or a resistance to insulin.

Diabetic nephro/pathy (nə-frop´ə-the) is a disease of the _____ resulting from diabetes mellitus. Chronic hyperglycemia and increased blood pressure accelerate the progression of the disorder. **Hyper/glycemia** means excessive glucose in the _____.

kidneys

blood

Diabetes mellitus is a major cause of end-stage renal disease in the United States and can result from either type 1 or type 2 diabetes mellitus. See Chapter 17 for additional information about this disorder.

11-63 Obstructive nephropathies are conditions that block or interfere with the flow of urine. Several causes are illustrated in Figure 11-17 and include prolapsed adjacent structures, tumors (benign or malignant), stones, narrowing of the ureters or urethra, and dysfunctions of the bladder that result from spinal cord injury or a lesion of the nervous system (neurogenic bladder).

Try to remember that **neuro/genic bladder** is a dysfunction of the bladder caused by a lesion of the _____ system.

nervous

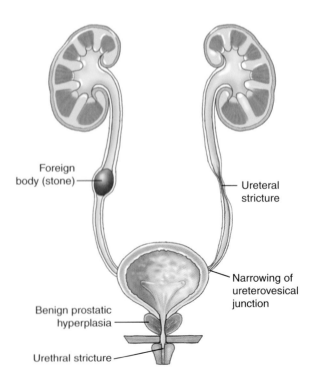

Foreign body (stone)

Ureteral stricture

Narrowing of ureterovesical junction

Benign prostatic hyperplasia

Urethral stricture

Figure 11-17 **Five common causes of urinary tract obstruction are illustrated.**

urolithiasis
(u″ro-lĭ-thi′ə-sis)

kidney

ureterolith
(u-re′tər-o-lith)

water

ureter

ureter

urethrocele
(u-re′thro-sēl)

cystocele (sis′to-sēl)

benign

11-64 Knowing that lith(o) means stone, build the word that means formation of urinary calculi by using ur(o), lith(o), and -iasis: _____.

Urinary stones are often named according to their location: kidney, ureter, or bladder. They vary greatly in size, from small enough to pass through the ureter, to large stones that occupy the entire renal pelvis and have roughly the shape of a deer antler (staghorn calculi). **Nephro/lith/iasis** (nef″ro-lĭ-thi′ə-sis) is a condition marked by the presence of _____ stones. A kidney stone is also called a renal calculus or a **nephro/lith** (nef′ro-lith).

Uretero/lith/iasis (u-re″tər-o-lĭ-thi′ə-sis) is the presence of a ureteral stone. If a nephro/lith is a kidney stone, build a word that means stone in a ureter: _____. A **cystolith** (sis′to-lith) means a calculus in the urinary bladder.

11-65 **Hydro/nephrosis** (hi″dro-nə-fro′sis) is distension (or distention) of the renal pelvis and kidney by urine that cannot flow past an obstruction in a ureter. The literal translation of hydro-nephrosis is a condition of _____ in the kidney. Remember that hydronephrosis means distension of the renal pelvis with urine as a result of an obstruction in the upper part of a ureter.

If a stone or another obstruction occurs in the lower part of the ureter, the condition that results is called **hydroureter** (hi″dro-u-re′tər), abnormal distension of a _____ with urine or watery fluid. See Figure 11-18 for comparison of hydronephrosis and hydroureter.

11-66 Uterine prolapse, the loss of support that anchors the uterus, can result in pressure on the bladder and lead to urinary frequency.

Prolapse can also occur in the urinary structures themselves. **Uretero/cele** (u-re′tər-o-sēl″) is a prolapse or herniation of a _____. This condition may lead to obstruction of the flow of urine and hydronephrosis.

Herniation of the urethra is a _____. This is characterized by a protrusion of the female urethra through the urethral opening or encroachment of a segment of the urethral wall upon the vaginal canal.

Using -cele, write a word that means herniation of the bladder: _____. In a cystocele, the bladder hernia protrudes into the vagina (Figure 11-19).

11-67 Enlargement of a nearby structure (for example, the prostate) also puts pressure on urinary structures. The prostate is a gland in men that surrounds the neck of the bladder. **Benign prostatic hyperplasia** (BPH) is a nonmalignant, noninflammatory enlargement of the prostate that is common among men over 50 years of age. It may lead to urethral obstruction and interference with urine flow, causing frequency, dysuria, nocturia, and urinary tract infections (Figure 11-20).

Prostatic hyperplasia results in enlargement of the prostate. This is not a malignant disease, as noted by its name, _____ prostatic hyperplasia.

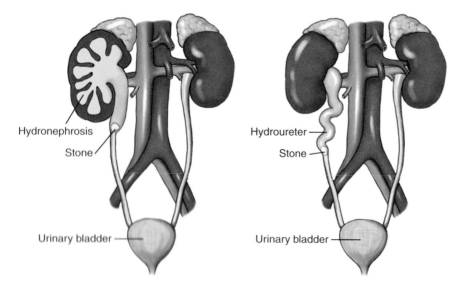

Figure 11-18 **Hydronephrosis and hydroureter.** Hydronephrosis is caused by obstruction in the upper part of the ureter. Hydroureter is caused by obstruction in the lower part of the ureter.

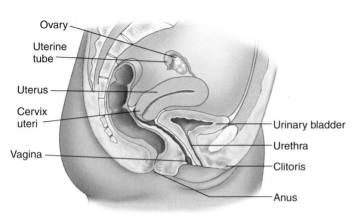

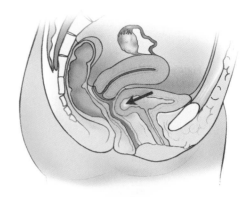

Figure 11-19 Comparison of a cystocele with the normal position of the urinary bladder. A large cystocele displaces the bladder downward, resulting in a bulging of the anterior vaginal wall.

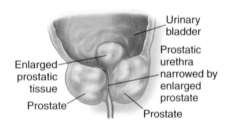

Figure 11-20 Benign prostatic hyperplasia. This nonmalignant enlargement of the prostate is common among men over 50 years of age. As the prostate enlarges, it extends upward into the bladder and inward, obstructing the outflow of urine from the bladder.

11-68 A **ureteral** or **urethral stricture** is a narrowing of the lumen (inner space) of the ureter or urethra. A narrowing can also occur at the place where the ureter joins the bladder. This is called narrowing of the uretero/vesical junction. **Uretero/vesical** pertains to the ureter and the

bladder

_____.

stricture
(narrowing)

Urethro/stenosis (u-re″thro-stə-no´sis) is a stricture of the urethra, and **uretero/stenosis** (u-re″tər-o-stə-no´sis) is a _____ of a ureter. Stenosis is narrowing of an opening or passageway of a vessel.

These strictures may lead to urinary stasis or reflux, oliguria, and eventually anuria. In some cases the stricture is relieved or corrected by balloon or catheter dilation.

11-69 Reno/vascular disease, problems of the blood vessels of the kidney, include nephrosclerosis (nef″ro-sklə-ro´sis), stenosis of the renal artery, and thrombosis of the renal vein.

Nephro/sclerosis is hardening of the small arteries of the kidney and results in decreased blood flow and eventually necrosis of kidney cells. This condition occurs in a small number of persons with hypertension (elevated blood pressure). Treatment of nephrosclerosis is the use of medications to lower the blood pressure. Write this term that means hardening of the arteries of

nephrosclerosis

the kidney: _____.

Renal artery stenosis is partial or complete blocking of one or both renal arteries. The pathologic changes to the renal arteries result in drastically reduced blood flow through the kidneys and lead to hypertension and damage to the kidneys. Hypertension resulting from renal artery stenosis or other kidney disorders is called **renal hypertension.**

A blood clot in the renal vein is called **renal vein thrombosis.** The cause of the blood clot (the thrombus) includes compression by a nearby tumor, renal carcinoma, or renal trauma. The

thrombosis

presence of a thrombus in the renal vein is called renal vein _____.

11-70 The characteristics of diabetes mellitus were described earlier. Another disorder that shares the name diabetes is diabetes insipidus (di-ə-be´tēz in-sĭ´pə-dəs). The disorder is not related to diabetes mellitus but was so named because of the large quantity of urine excreted.

Unlike diabetes mellitus, **diabetes insipidus** is not related to the body's use of insulin. Its cause may be hormonal or renal, and the disorder refers to several types of polyuria in

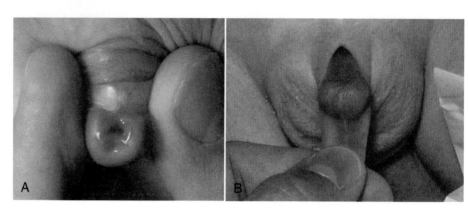

Figure 11-21 Two developmental defects of the urinary meatus in male infants. A, Hypospadias. Note the location of the urinary meatus below its usual location. **B,** Epispadias. Note the urethral opening on the upper side of the penis.

insipidus

which the urinary output exceeds 3000 mL a day. Write the name of this disorder: diabetes _____.

urinary

11-71 Genitourinary infections are those affecting both the genital and _____ structures.

A **sexually transmitted disease** (STD) is one that may be acquired as a result of sexual contact with a person who has the disease or with secretions containing the suspected organism. Sexually transmitted diseases were formerly called **venereal** (və-nēr′e-əl) **diseases** (VDs).

11-72 You have learned that -rrhea means flow or discharge, and you probably have heard of **gono/rrhea** (gon″o-re′ə), a sexually transmitted disease. Gonorrhea is derived from gon(o), which means the genitals or reproduction. This sexually transmitted disease, caused by the bacterium *Neisseria gonorrhoeae,* is characterized by a heavy discharge from the vagina in females or from the urethra in either males or females. The discharge may be accompanied by urethritis and dysuria. See Chapter 13 for more information about gonorrhea.

Write the name of the sexually transmitted disease that can cause urethritis:

gonorrhea

_____.

11-73 The absence of both kidneys in a developing fetus is not compatible with life outside the uterus, but less severe congenital defects of the urinary system do occur. Hypo/plasia may affect only one kidney or both kidneys and is a common cause of hypertension in the first decade of life. High blood pressure resulting from any type of renal disorder is called

renal

_____ hypertension.

11-74 Two anomalies of the urethra are hypospadias (hi″po-spa′de-əs) and epispadias (ep″ĭ-spa′de-əs). **Hypo/spadias** is a congenital defect in which the urinary meatus is located below its usual location (usually seen in males with the opening on the underside of the penis). **Epi/spadias** is a developmental defect in which the urinary meatus is located above its usual location (usually seen in males with the opening on the upper surface of the penis). Epispadias occurs as a groove or cleft without a covering and not in its usual location. Remember that in

below

hypo/spadias the urinary meatus is usually located _____ its normal location, and above its normal location in epispadias. Compare these two anomalies (Figure 11-21).

EXERCISE 9

Build It! *Use the following word parts to build terms. (Some word parts will be used more than once.)*

lith(o), nephr(o), pyel(o), ureter(o), urethr(o), -iasis, -itis, -pathy, -sclerosis

1. inflammation of the urethra and the bladder   _____/_____/_____

2. any disease of the kidney   _____/_____

3. inflammation of a ureter, the
   renal pelvis, and the kidney   _____/_____/_____/_____

4. presence of a stone in the ureter   _____/_____/_____

5. hardening of the small arteries of the kidneys   _____/_____

EXERCISE 10

Write a word in each blank to complete these sentences. The first letter of each answer is given as a clue.

1. Enlargement of both kidneys is called b_____ nephromegaly.

2. An accumulation of toxic products in the blood is u_____.

3. Abnormal softening of the kidney is n_____.

4. Discharge from the urethra is u_____.

5. Disorders that affect the blood vessels of the kidneys are r_____ disorders.

6. Inflammation of the bladder is c_____.

7. Inflammation of the kidney and its renal pelvis is p_____.

8. A hereditary disorder characterized by enlarged kidneys containing many cysts is called

    p_____ kidney disease.

9. Inflammation of the renal glomeruli is called g_____.

10. A complex disorder of carbohydrate, fat, and protein metabolism that is primarily a result of deficiency of insulin

    or a resistance to insulin is diabetes m_____.

11. Distension of the renal pelvis with urine, resulting from an obstruction in the upper part of a ureter,

    is h_____.

12. Distension of a ureter with urine or a watery fluid is h_____.

13. Hernial protrusion of the bladder into the vagina is a c_____.

14. A nonmalignant, noninflammatory enlargement of the prostate is called benign prostatic h_____.

15. A condition marked by the presence of kidney stones is n_____.

16. A hormonal or renal disorder in which the urinary output exceeds 3000 mL a day is diabetes i_____.

17. Partial or complete blocking of one or both renal arteries is renal artery s_____.

18. Blood clot in the renal vein is renal vein t_____.

19. A congenital defect in which the urinary meatus is located below its usual location is h_____.

20. A congenital defect in which the urinary meatus is located above its usual location is e_____.

Say and Check

Say aloud the terms you wrote for Exercises 9 and 10. Use the Companion CD to check your pronunciations.

SURGICAL AND THERAPEUTIC INTERVENTIONS

blood

11-75 Kidney dialysis (di-al´ə-sis) is required when the kidneys fail to remove waste products from the blood. This is also called **hemo/dialysis** (he″mo-di-al´ə-sis), which means dialysis of the _____. Kidney dialysis or hemodialysis is the process of diffusing blood through a semipermeable membrane for the purpose of removing toxic materials and maintaining the acid-base balance in cases of impaired kidney function (Figure 11-22).

   Peritoneal dialysis is dialysis through the peritoneum, with the solution being introduced into and removed from the peritoneal cavity. Sometimes this type of dialysis is done as an alternative to hemodialysis.

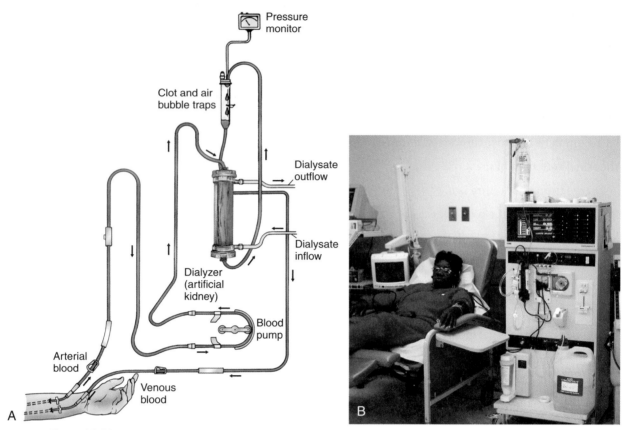

Figure 11-22 Hemodialysis. **A,** A hemodialysis circuit. **B,** Patient receiving hemodialysis in a dialysis center.

nephrectomy
(nə-frek′tə-me)
ureter

11-76 In a **renal transplant** the patient (recipient) receives a kidney from a suitable donor. The donated kidney is surgically removed from the donor. Build a word that means surgical excision of a kidney, using nephr(o) and the suffix for excision: _____.
Nephroureterectomy (nef″ro-u-re″tər-ek′tə-me) means surgical excision of a kidney with the _____. Selected situations may allow **laparo/scopic** (lap″ə-ro-skop′ik) **nephrectomy,** removal of the kidney through several small incisions in the abdominal wall, rather than an open surgical excision.

Immuno/suppressive therapy, the administration of agents that significantly interfere with the immune response of the recipient, are provided after renal transplantation to prevent rejection of the donor kidney.

kidney

11-77 Either removal of the diseased kidney or radiation therapy can be used to treat renal carcinoma. **Ren/al carcinoma** is cancer of a _____.

Treatment for bladder cancer depends on several factors, including the size of the lesion. Tests of the urine may show atypical cells or the presence of factors associated with cancer, but cystoscopy and biopsy are generally used for confirmation. Radiation therapy, laser eradication of small lesions, chemotherapy, and cystectomy may be used. Chemotherapy can be given systemically, or in some cases the chemical treatment is instilled directly into the bladder through a catheter.

bladder

Cyst/ectomy (sis-tek′tə-me) is surgical excision of the _____.
It may be a partial cystectomy, in which only a portion of the bladder is removed, or the cystectomy may be radical, in which all of the bladder is removed along with selected adjacent organs (the prostate and seminal vesicles in males; the uterus, cervix, ovaries, and urethra in females).

11-78 Various surgical procedures may be performed for urinary diversion if the bladder is removed. The ureters must be diverted into some type of collecting reservoir, opening either onto the abdomen or into the large intestine so that urine is expelled with bowel movements.

Formation of a new opening through which a ureter empties is called a **ureterostomy** (u-re″tər-os′tə-me) (Figure 11-23). In a bilateral or double ureterostomy, there are two pouches on the abdominal surface, one for each ureter, to receive drainage of the urine.

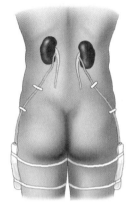
A   Nephrostomy

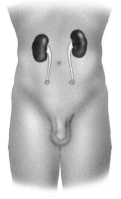
B   Bilateral ureterostomy

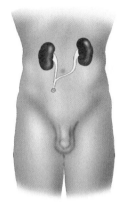
C   Transureteroureterostomy

Figure 11-23 Comparing nephrostomy and two ureterostomies. A, Nephrostomy. Percutaneous openings are made into the renal pelvis and urine is diverted to bags. **B,** Bilateral ureterostomy. Both ureters are brought out onto the skin for drainage of urine into bags. **C,** Transureteroureterostomy. One ureter is surgically attached to the other ureter, which is brought out onto the skin for drainage of urine into a bag.

---

ureter

Surgical connection of one ureter to another is called **trans/ureteroureterostomy** (trans″u-re″tər-o-u-re″tər-os´tə-me). In other words, one ureter is brought across and joined to the other _____. The latter results in only one opening on the abdominal surface that serves both ureters.

skin

11-79 Percutaneous nephro/stomy (nə-fros´tə-me) is a surgical procedure in which the skin is punctured so that a catheter can be inserted into the renal pelvis. Literal translation of nephro/stomy is formation of a new opening into the kidney. Percutaneous tells us that the _____ is punctured to gain access to the renal pelvis. This procedure allows for drainage, drug instillation, and selected surgical procedures, including removal of calculi (Figure 11-24, *B*) or dilation of a stenosed ureter (Figure 11-24, *A*).

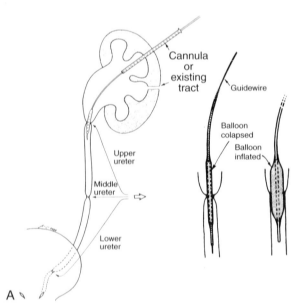

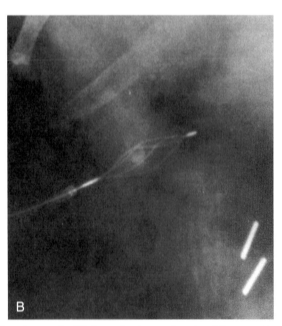

Figure 11-24 Two procedures that can be performed after percutaneous nephrostomy. A, Dilation of a stenosed ureter. After percutaneous nephrostomy, a collapsed balloon catheter is introduced. After reaching the area of stenosis, the balloon is inflated to stretch the stenosed area, then the balloon catheter is withdrawn. **B,** Removal of a kidney stone. This radiograph shows a renal calculus that has been caught in a stone basket and is ready for removal. After percutaneous nephrostomy, the stone basket is maneuvered to engage the renal calculus, then both are removed through the cannula.

A nephrostomy may be performed on one or both kidneys and may be temporary or permanent. If both ureters are removed, a nephrostomy is necessary. Compare nephrostomy and the two types of ureterostomies described in the previous frame.

Cancer is one reason for urinary diversion. An obstruction lower in the urinary tract could also require formation of a new opening through which the ureter could discharge its contents.

11-80 Stones in the urinary tract are sometimes passed out through the urethra, but many either are too large or do not dissolve. Stones can cause urinary obstruction, which interferes with function and can be very painful. There are several methods of dealing with stones, including lithotripsy and open surgery to remove a large stone if it cannot be broken up or removed by other means.

Litho/tomy (lĭ-thot´ə-me) is the incision of an organ or duct for removal of a calculus, especially one from the urinary tract. The suffix -tomy means incision, so the meaning of lithotomy is implied. Write this term that means an incision of an organ or duct for removal of a calculus:

lithotomy

_____. Be aware that the term lithotomy is also used to mean the lithotomy position, often used in obstetrics and gynecology. In the lithotomy position, the patient lies on the back with the hips and the knees flexed and the thighs rotated outward.

stone

11-81 **Litho/tripsy** (lith´o-trip˝se) is the crushing of a _____ within the body, followed by the washing out of the fragments. This was originally done by surgical removal, but noninvasive methods such as high-energy shock waves or lasers often eliminate the need for surgery. This is called **extracorporeal shock wave lithotripsy** (ESWL). Extra/corpor/eal means outside the body. Extracorporeal shock wave lithotripsy uses ultrasonic energy from a source outside the body (Figure 11-25). This technique is used on stones that resist passage and is far less incapacitating than a full-scale operation, even laparoscopic surgery.

extracorporeal

Write the name of the procedure that uses ultrasonic energy from a source outside the body to break up a stone: _____ shock wave lithotripsy.

11-82 Invasive lithotripsy may be successful with small stones in the bladder. This type of lithotripsy is accomplished by inserting a catheter through the urethra. The stone is then crushed with an instrument called a **lithotrite** (lith´o-trīt). The fragments may then be expelled or washed out. Write the name of the instrument that is used in conjunction with a catheter to

lithotrite

crush stones in the bladder: _____.

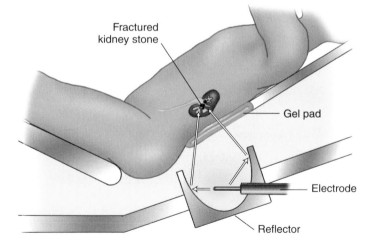

Figure 11-25 Lithotripsy, crushing of a kidney stone (calculus). Extracorporeal shock wave lithotripsy, illustrated here, is used to crush certain types of urinary stones. The reflector focuses a high-energy shock wave on the stone. The stone disintegrates into particles and is passed in the urine.

EXERCISE 11

![icon] ***Build It!*** *Use the following word parts to build terms. (Some word parts will be used more than once.)*

trans-, cyst(o), lith(o), nephr(o), ureter(o), -ectomy, -stomy, -tomy, -tripsy

1. surgical connection of one ureter to another:

   _____/_____/_____/_____

2. surgical crushing of a stone   _____/_____

3. excision of the bladder   _____/_____

4. excision of a kidney with its
   ureter   _____/_____/_____

5. incision of an organ for
   removal of a stone   _____/_____

![icon] ***Say and Check***

Say aloud the terms you wrote for Exercise 11. Use the Companion CD to check your pronunciations.

calculi (or stones)	**11-83 Nephro/litho/tomy** (nef″ro-lĭ-thot′ə-me) is removal of renal _____ by cutting through the body of the kidney. Notice that -tomy is used rather than -ectomy, because -tomy refers to incision of the kidney, and removal of the stone is only implied. Nephrolithotomy is necessary if the stone is too large to pass or break up or if it will not dissolve.
	Pyelo/lithotomy (pi″ə-lo-lĭ-thot′ə-me) is surgical removal of a stone from the renal
pelvis	_____. Literal translation of this term is incision of the renal pelvis for stones, and it is understood that the procedure is done for this purpose. Write the
pyelolithotomy	term: _____.
	Ureterolithotomy (u-re″tər-o-lĭ-thot′ə-me) and **cysto/litho/tomy** (sis″to-lĭ-thot′ə-me) are procedures for surgical removal of a stone or stones from the ureter and the
bladder	_____, respectively. It is important that the patient have a high fluid intake after a stone is removed to prevent the formation of another stone. Stones are routinely analyzed in the laboratory to determine their chemical makeup.
	11-84 Renal artery stenosis, partial blocking of one or both renal arteries, is treated by **percutaneous transluminal renal angio/plasty** or by using another major artery to route blood to the kidney. In percutaneous angio/plasty, the repair of the renal artery is via an incision of the
skin	_____.
	Anticoagulant therapy is used in renal vein thrombosis, a blood clot in the renal vein. A thromb/ectomy may also be performed, which means surgical excision of the
thrombus	_____.
	11-85 Catheter dilation is useful in treating strictures of the ureter (see Figure 11-24, *A*) or urethra. Severe stricture that does not respond to dilation may require **ureter/ectomy** (u-re″tər-ek′tə-me), partial or complete surgical excision of the ureter.
	The section of the ureter that remains after ureterectomy is attached to a different site on the bladder. This surgical procedure is called **ureterocystostomy** (u-re″tər-o-sis-tos′tə-me). This involves surgical transplantation of the ureter to a different site on the bladder and is called **uretero/cysto/neo/stomy** (u-re″tər-o-sis″to-ne-os′tə-me).
	11-86 Ureteroplasty (u-re′tər-o-plas″te) means surgical repair of a ureter. Write a term that
pyeloplasty (pi′ə-lo-plas″te)	means surgical repair of the renal pelvis: _____.
cystoplasty (sis′to-plas″te)	**11-87** Write another term that means surgical repair of the bladder: _____.

bladder

Cystostomy (sis-tos´tə-me) means formation of a new opening into the bladder. **Suprapubic cystotomy** is surgical incision of the _____ via an incision just above the symphysis pubis. **Cystotomy** (sis-tot´ə-me) means incision of the bladder.

urethrotomy
(u˝rə-throt´ə-me)
urethra

11-88 Surgical incision of the urethra is _____.

Remembering that trans- means through or across, **trans/urethral** (trans˝u-re´thrəl) means through the _____. Transurethral surgery is performed by inserting an instrument through or across the wall of the urethra and makes it possible to perform surgery on certain organs that lie near the urethra without having an abdominal incision. In **transurethral resection** (TUR), small pieces of tissue from a nearby structure are removed through the wall of the urethra.

11-89 One surgery of this type is a **transurethral resection of the prostate** (TURP). In a TURP, surgery is performed on the prostate gland by means of an instrument passed through the wall of the urethra and is sometimes done to alleviate the problems of benign prostatic hyperplasia.

transurethral

In a TURP (Figure 11-26), an abdominal incision is not involved, since the surgeon approaches the prostate through the urethra. Small pieces of the prostate are removed with a special instrument called a resectoscope (re-sek´to-skōp). Because this surgery is performed by passing the instrument through the urethra, it is called _____ resection of the prostate.

nephropexy
(nef´ro-pek˝se)

11-90 Use nephr(o) and -pexy to write a word that means surgical fixation of the kidney: _____. This type of surgery is often used to correct **nephroptosis** (nef˝rop-to´sis, nef˝ro-to´sis), also called floating kidney.

Nephroptosis is a gradual downward displacement of the kidney and is also called floating, hypermobile, or wandering kidney. It can occur when the kidney supports are weakened by sudden strain or a blow, or it may be present at birth (congenital).

11-91 There are several types of urinary incontinence, and treatment depends on the cause. One of the more common types, stress incontinence (leakage of urine when coughing, sneezing, or straining), is sometimes helped with the use of **Kegel exercises** to strengthen the pelvic muscles. Also, weight loss in overweight persons, drug therapy, and/or surgery can be helpful. Incontinence resulting from spinal cord injury necessitates use of an indwelling catheter. Urinary incontinence means the inability to control _____.

urination

Urinary retention may require catheterization, either intermittent or indwelling. Certain medications are also helpful.

11-92 Treatment of urinary tract infections includes antibiotics, analgesics, and increased intake of water.

Increased or excessive urination is polyuria or **diuresis** (di˝u-re´sis). Sometimes **diuretics** (di˝u-ret´ikz) are prescribed to increase urination. An agent that causes the body to eliminate more water in the form of urine is called a _____.

diuretic

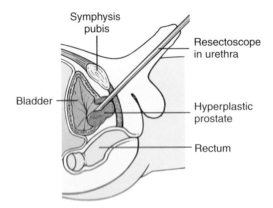

Figure 11-26 Transurethral resection of the prostate. This surgical procedure involves passing a resectoscope through the urethra, then excising pieces of the obstructing prostatic tissue.

urethrospasm
(u-re´thro-spaz-əm)
against

11-93 Write a term that means spasm of the urethra (actually, the muscular tissue of the urethra): _____.
    This may occur after certain surgical procedures, such as transurethral resection of the prostate. Literal interpretation of anti/spasmodics is _____ spasms.
Antispasmodics (an″te-, an″ti-spaz-mod´ikz) are drugs or other agents that prevent muscle spasms.

EXERCISE 12

Circle the correct answer for the following questions.

1. Which term means excision of a kidney? (nephrectomy, nephroscopy, nephrostomy, nephrotomy)

2. Which of the following terms is a type of urinary diversion?
   (cystometrography, glomerular filtration, hemodialysis, ureterostomy)

3. Which of the following is least likely to cause a urinary obstruction? (infection, stone, tumor, ureterolith)

4. Which of the following is not a likely treatment of a stone located in the bladder?
   (cystolithotomy, ESWL, lithotripsy, pyelolithotomy)

5. Which of the following may be used to treat renal vein thrombosis?
   (anticoagulant therapy, cystoplasty, nephropexy, shock wave lithotripsy)

6. Which term means a procedure that is performed by inserting an instrument through or across the wall of the urethra? (nephroptosis, transurethral resection, ureterocystostomy, urinary retention)

CHAPTER ABBREVIATIONS*

ADH	antidiuretic hormone	IVP	intravenous pyelography
ARF	acute renal failure	KUB	kidneys, ureters, and bladder
BPH	benign prostatic hyperplasia	pH	potential of hydrogen; symbol for hydrogen
BUN	blood urea nitrogen		ion concentration
C&S	culture and sensitivity	STD	sexually transmitted disease
CRF	chronic renal failure	TUR	transurethral resection
EMG	electromyography	TURP	transurethral resection of the prostate
ESWL	extracorporeal shock wave lithotripsy	UA, U/A	urinalysis
GFR	glomerular filtration rate	UTI	urinary tract infection
GU	genitourinary	VCUG	voiding cystourethrogram
I&O	intake and output	VD	venereal disease

*Many of these abbreviations share their meanings with other terms.

Be Careful with These!

Prostate is a frequently misspelled term.

Note the difference in spelling of prostate and prostrate, which means lying in a face-down, horizontal position.

▶ CHAPTER 11 REVIEW

Basic Understanding

Labeling
I. *Label the numbered structures with their corresponding combining form. Number 1 has two answers.*

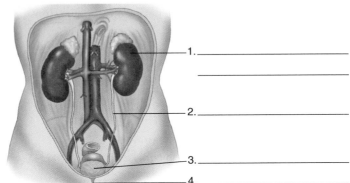

1. _____

_____

2. _____

3. _____

4. _____

Matching
II. *Match structures in the left columns with their functions in the right column.*

_____ 1. bladder   _____ 4. ureter   A. cavity in the kidney that collects urine from many collecting ducts
                                              B. carries urine from the bladder
_____ 2. nephron   _____ 5. urethra   C. carries urine to the bladder
                                              D. functional unit of the kidney
_____ 3. renal pelvis   E. reservoir for urine until it is expelled

Listing
III. *List three major functions of the urinary system.*

1. _____

2. _____

3. _____

True or False
IV. *Several urinary substances are listed. Write T for those substances that are normally detected in urine and F for those substances that are not normally detected.*

1. albumin   _____   5. ketones   _____

2. blood   _____   6. protein   _____

3. creatinine _____   7. sugar   _____

4. glucose   _____   8. urea   _____

V. *Divide these terms into their component parts, and define the terms.*

1. anuric _____

2. lithotomy _____

3. nocturia _____

4. oliguria _____

5. transurethral _____

Photo ID

VI. *Use word parts to build terms to label these illustrations.*

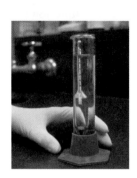

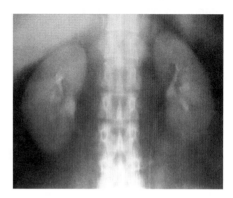

1. _____/_____
   (urine)   (instrument used
                    to measure)

2. _____/_____/_____
   (kidney)   (to cut)   (a record)

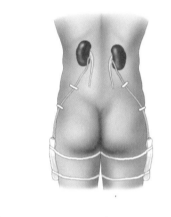

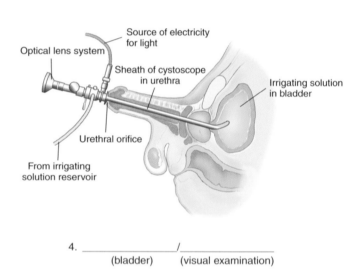

Source of electricity for light

Optical lens system

Sheath of cystoscope in urethra

Irrigating solution in bladder

Urethral orifice

From irrigating solution reservoir

3. _____/_____
   (kidney)   (formation of
                    a new opening)

4. _____/_____
   (bladder)   (visual examination)

Multiple Choice

VII. *Circle the correct answer for each of the following multiple choice questions.*

1. Which of the following is the filtering structure of the kidney? (glomerulus, tubule, ureter, urethra)

2. Which of the following means excision of a renal calculus from the pelvis of the kidney?
   (cystolithectomy, lithotripsy, pyelolithotomy, pyelostomy)

3. Which of the following means the same as nephromegaly?
   (floating kidney, kidney dialysis, renal enlargement, renal stone)

4. Which of the following is not a method of collecting a urine sample? (catheterization, lithotripsy, urinating, voiding)

5. Which of the following terms means making radiographic images of the urinary system after the urine has been rendered opaque by a contrast medium? (cystoscopy, cystoureteroscopy, intravenous pyelography, nephrotomography)

6. Which of the following is indicated if the blood urea nitrogen is elevated?
   (pyelostomy, pyuria, renal clearance, renal failure)

7. Which term means an inability to control urination? (frequency, hesitancy, incontinence, retention)

8. Which term means excretion of an abnormally large quantity of urine? (anuria, dysuria, oliguria, polyuria)

9. Which of the following is not a type of urinary tract catheterization?
   (endoscopy tube, nephrostomy tube, suprapubic tube, urethral tube)

10. Which of the following involves an instrument being passed through the urethra in order to remove small pieces of the prostate gland? (intravenous pyelogram, retrograde pyelography, transurethral resection, urethrography)

11. Which of the following is a toxic condition of the body that occurs when the kidneys fail to function properly? (nephromalacia, nephrolithiasis, uremia, urography)

12. What does pyuria indicate about a urine specimen? (excessive sugar, excessive number of white cells, increased creatinine, increased protein)

13. Which of the following terms means distension of a ureter with urine or watery fluid? (hydronephrosis, hydroureter, ureteral stricture, ureterolithiasis)

14. Which term describes partial or complete blocking of a blood vessel? (herniation, sclerosis, stenosis, thrombosis)

15. Which term means inflammation of the kidney and renal pelvis? (pyelography, pyelonephritis, pyelolithotomy, pyelostomy)

Writing Terms

VIII. *Write a term for each of the following:*

1. any disease of the urinary tract _____

2. between the kidneys _____

3. blood in the urine _____

4. herniation of the urethra _____

5. inflammation of the renal glomeruli _____

6. inflammation of the renal pelvis _____

7. kidney dialysis _____

8. outside the urinary bladder _____

9. radiography of the bladder _____

10. surgical crushing of a stone _____

 Say and Check

Say aloud the terms you wrote for Exercise VIII. Use the Companion CD to check your pronunciations.

Greater Comprehension

Labeling

IX. *Choose from the following list to label parts of the nephron shown (1 to 5):*

afferent arteriole, distal convoluted tubule, glomerulus, Bowman capsule, efferent arteriole, proximal convoluted tubule, collecting duct

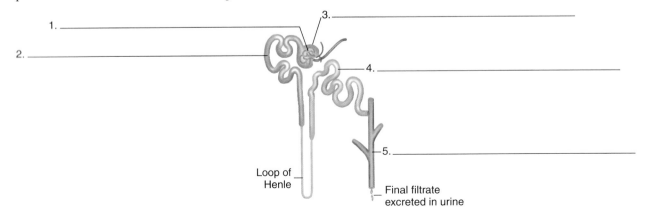

1. _____
2. _____
3. _____
4. _____
5. _____

Loop of Henle

Final filtrate excreted in urine

Health Care Reports

X. *Read the urology clinic note, and answer the questions that follow.*

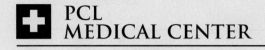

PCL MEDICAL CENTER

7700 Lexicon Way
St. Louis, MO 63146

Phone (555) 437-0000 • Fax (555) 437-0001

UROLOGY CLINIC NOTE

Patient Name: Wayne Emerson   **Date of Exam:** Aug 1, ----

CHIEF COMPLAINT: Feels uncomfortable when urinating

HISTORY: This 43-year-old male patient, well known to me, reports having dysuria for the past week. He has a history of cystitis and nephritis.

FAMILY HISTORY: Father is age 65 with history of BPH. Mother is age 64 with a history of renal calculi and pyelonephritis. One sibling who lives out of state is L&W.

SOCIAL HISTORY: Denies ×3. No unprotected sexual encounters.

PHYSICAL EXAM: Vitals show BP 108/72, pulse 76, temp 98F. In no acute distress. WD, WN, divorced white male, A&O ×3. Testes nontender, both descended. No masses. Penis is circumcised. There is no drainage, no lesions. Penis is nontender. Prostate is not enlarged. Brown stool on examining glove.

DIAGNOSTIC STUDIES: KUB and IV urography show three small calculi in the right ureter. CBC: WBCs 6.3, Hgb 13.3, Hct 39.8, plts 219,000. UA with trace blood. Culture no growth. PSA is WNL. Hemoccult test result is negative.

DIAGNOSIS: Ureteral urolithiasis

PLAN: Ureteroscopy to be done with possible lithotripsy.

Circle one answer for each of the following.

1. Mr. Emerson's dysuria indicates what aspect of urine or urination?
   (blood, decreased output, difficult or painful, protein)

2. What does his history indicate? (bladder and kidney stones, inflammation of the bladder and kidney, inflammation caused by trauma, frequent urinary infections)

3. His father's history indicates problems with which of the following? (bladder, kidney, prostate, urethra)

4. Which of the following is indicated in his mother's history?
   (kidney stones, polycystic kidney, renal vein thrombosis, renovascular disease)

5. Which of the following is Mr. Emerson's diagnosis?
   (narrowing of the ureter, obstruction of the ureter, stone in the ureter, urinary infection)

6. According to the plan, what is the next step that is suggested for this patient?
   (a surgical procedure, examination of the ureter, evaluation for an STD, referral to a radiologist)

Write the meanings of the following abbreviations.

7. BPH _____

8. KUB _____

9. IV _____

10. UA _____

XI. Read the urology clinic note and answer the questions that follow.

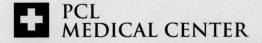

PCL
MEDICAL CENTER

7700 Lexicon Way
St. Louis, MO 63146

Phone (555) 437-0000 • Fax (555) 437-0001

UROLOGY CLINIC NOTE

Patient Name: Leroy R. Schmitt   **Date of Exam:** Aug 3, ----
CHIEF COMPLAINT: Trouble going to the bathroom, going often
HISTORY: This 65-year-old man has complaints of nocturia, frequency, urgency, interruption of urinary stream, dribbling, fatigue, frequent UTIs—ongoing problems.
FAMILY HISTORY: Father died at age 80 from CA of the prostate with mets to the bone; he also had nephrolithiasis. Mother is age 84 with history of IDDM, hypertension, and renal failure, currently on hemodialysis. Married with no children, patient's mother lives with them.
PHYSICAL EXAM: Vital signs are WNL except for weight of 275 lb on a 5'7" frame. Alert and oriented white man in no acute distress. Normal male genitalia, circumcised. Rectal exam demonstrates large, rubbery prostate. No stool on the examining glove.
DIAGNOSTIC STUDIES: UA: Clear yellow urine with specific gravity 1.006, pH 5.0, negative glucose, negative blood. PSA 2.0 (normal: 0 to 4.0 ng/mL). Cystoscopy demonstrated a normal bladder and urethra. Utrasound and biopsy of the prostate: Benign hypertrophy.
DIAGNOSIS:
1. Benign prostatic hypertrophy   2. Obesity
Plan: Conservative treatment with Proscar and Flomax. Will eventually need to have surgical intervention with TURP. Counseled patient on his obesity and the fact that he should lose weight prior to any surgical procedure. Will set up a consult with the dietitian/nutritionist.

Murray A. Stewart, MD
Murray A. Stewart, MD, Urologist

Circle one answer for each of the following questions.

1. Mr. Schmitt's symptom of nocturia indicates which of the following about urination?
   (nighttime frequency, incontinence, painful, retention)

2. His father's history indicates which of the following?
   (diabetes insipidus, diabetes mellitus, frequent urinary tract infections, kidney stones)

3. His mother's health condition indicates a deficiency or improper use of which of the following?
   (ADH, carbohydrates, diuretics, insulin)

4. Which instrument was used for Mr. Schmitt's diagnostic study? (catheter, cystoscope, nephroscope, ultrascope)

What do these abbreviations mean?

5. CA   _____

6. UTI   _____

7. TURP   _____

XII. *Read the following partial operative report and answer the questions that follow.*

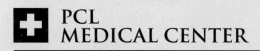

PCL MEDICAL CENTER

7700 Lexicon Way
St. Louis, MO 63146

Phone (555) 437-0000 • Fax (555) 437-0001

OPERATIVE REPORT

Patient Name: Juan S. Pedro **ID No.:** 011-0004 **Date of Surgery:** May 4, ----
Surgeon: Murray A. Stewart, MD **Assistant:** Barbara Richards, MD
Anesthetist: Ron DeVittore, MD **Anesthetic:** General endotracheal with caudal block
PREOPERATIVE DIAGNOSES
1. Possible hypospadias 2. Physiologic phimosis 3. Meatal stenosis
POSTOPERATIVE DIAGNOSES
1. Hypospadias 2. Meatal stenosis
OPERATIONS PERFORMED
1. Repair of hypospadias 2. Repair of meatal stenosis
ESTIMATED BLOOD LOSS: 5 mL
COMPLICATIONS: None
INDICATIONS: This 10-month-old male was noted to have some redundant dorsal foreskin at the time of evaluation by his pediatrician. Patient was referred to Urology for evaluation and was seen by Dr. Stewart. Patient was thought to have at the minimum physiologic phimosis and meatal stenosis, but this was difficult to assess owing to the degree of his phimosis. His parents therefore consented to possible hypospadias repair, meatoplasty, and circumcision.

1. What is hypospadias? _____

2. What is meatal stenosis? _____

3. What is meatoplasty? _____

Spelling
XIII. *Circle all misspelled terms and write their correct spelling.*

antispasmodic   catheterization   hydronefrosis   ketoacidosis   gonorhea

Interpreting Abbreviations
XIV. *Write the meaning of these abbreviations.*

1. ARF _____

2. EMG _____

3. BUN _____

4. ESWL _____

5. VCUG _____

Pronunciation
XV. *The pronunciation is shown for several terms. Indicate which syllable has the primary accent by marking it with an ´.*

1. diuresis (di u re sis)

2. lithotripsy (lith o trip se)

3. nephrolithiasis (nef ro lĭ thi ə sis)

4. pyelogram (pi ə lo gram)

5. ureteroplasty (u re tər o plast te)

 Say and Check

Say aloud the five terms in Exercise XV. Use the Companion CD to check your pronunciations.

In addition, be prepared to pronounce aloud these terms in class:

antispasmodics	epispadias	ketoacidosis	septicemia
anuric	excretory	lithotomy	ureteroscopy
cystography	glomerulopathy	nephrostomy	ureterovesical
cystometer	hypospadias	nycturia	urinary catheterization
diabetes mellitus	interstitial nephritis	perineum	vesicoureteral

Categorizing Terms

XVI. *Classify the terms in the left columns (1 to 10) by selecting A, B, C, D, or E from the right column.*

_____ 1. cystourethrography   _____ 6. nephrectomy

_____ 2. diuretics   _____ 7. nephrosclerosis

_____ 3. genitourinary   _____ 8. nephrosonography

_____ 4. glycosuria   _____ 9. tubule

_____ 5. hemodialysis   _____ 10. ureterocele

A. anatomy
B. diagnostic test or procedure
C. pathology
D. surgery
E. therapy

Challenge

XVII. *Break these words into their component parts, and write their meanings. Even if you have not seen these terms before, you may be able to break them apart and determine their meanings.*

1. cystorrhagia _____

2. ketonemia _____

3. nephrotoxic _____

4. perineocele _____

5. urogenital _____

(Use Appendix VI to check your answers.)

 PRONUNCIATION LIST

Use the Companion CD to review the terms that have been presented. Look closely at the spelling of each term as it is pronounced and be sure you know the meaning of each term.

abdominocystic	clean-catch specimen	diabetic nephropathy	glomerulonephritis
abdominovesical	creatinine	distal tubule	glomerulopathy
albumin	creatinine clearance test	diuresis	glomerulus
albuminuria	cystectomy	diuretics	glycosuria
antibiotic sensitivity test	cystic	dysuria	gonorrhea
antidiuretic hormone	cystitis	electromyography	hematuria
antispasmodics	cystocele	enuresis	hemodialysis
anuria	cystography	epispadias	hesitancy
anuric	cystolith	erythropoietin	hilum
benign prostatic	cystolithotomy	excretion	hydronephrosis
hyperplasia	cystometer	excretory	hydroureter
bladder	cystometrography	extracorporeal shock wave	hyperglycemia
bladder cancer	cystoplasty	lithotripsy	hypospadias
bladder polyp	cystoscope	extracystic	indwelling catheter
blood urea nitrogen	cystoscopy	fibrous	intake and output
Bowman capsule	cystostomy	Foley catheter	interrenal
catheter dilation	cystotomy	frequency	interstitial nephritis
catheterized urine	cystourethritis	genitourinary	intravenous pyelography
specimen	cystourethrography	genitourinary infections	intravenous urography
catheters	diabetes insipidus	glomerular filtration	Kegel exercises
chemical dipstick	diabetes mellitus	glomerular filtration rate	ketoacidosis

ketone
ketonuria
kidney dialysis
kidney scan
kidneys
laparoscopic nephrectomy
lithotomy
lithotripsy
lithotrite
loop of Henle
micturition
nephrectomy
nephritis
nephrolith
nephrolithiasis
nephrolithotomy
nephrolysis
nephromalacia
nephromegaly
nephrons
nephropexy
nephroptosis
nephrosclerosis
nephroscope
nephroscopy
nephrosonography
nephrostomy catheter
nephrotic syndrome
nephrotomogram
nephrotomography
nephrotoxic
nephroureterectomy
neurogenic bladder
nocturia
nycturia
obstructive nephropathies
oliguria
percutaneous nephrostomy

percutaneous transluminal
    renal angioplasty
perineal muscles
perineum
peritoneal dialysis
polycystic kidney disease
polyuria
proteinuria
proximal tubule
pus cells
pyelitis
pyelogram
pyelolithotomy
pyelonephritis
pyeloplasty
pyuria
reabsorption
rectourethral
renal
renal angiography
renal arteries
renal arteriogram
renal artery stenosis
renal carcinoma
renal clearance tests
renal failure
renal hypertension
renal pelvis
renal threshold
renal transplant
renal vein thrombosis
renography
renovascular disorders
septicemia
sexually transmitted
    disease
specific gravity
suprapubic

suprapubic catheter
suprapubic cystotomy
suprarenal
transureteroureterostomy
transurethral
transurethral resection
transurethral resection of
    the prostate
tubules
urea
uremia
ureter
ureteral
ureteral catheterization
ureteral dysfunction
ureteral stricture
ureterectomy
ureteritis
ureterocele
ureterocystoneostomy
ureterocystostomy
ureterolith
ureterolithiasis
ureterolithotomy
ureteropathy
ureteroplasty
ureteropyelonephritis
ureteroscopy
ureterostenosis
ureterostomy
ureterovesical
urethra
urethral
urethral catheterization
urethral stricture
urethritis
urethrocele
urethrocystitis

urethrography
urethrorectal
urethrorrhagia
urethrorrhea
urethroscopy
urethrospasm
urethrostenosis
urethrotomy
urethrovaginal
urgency
urinalysis
urinary
urinary casts
urinary catheterization
urinary incontinence
urinary meatus
urinary reflux
urinary retention
urinary tract
urinary tract infection
urination
urine
urine culture
urinometer
urodynamic studies
urogenital
urogram
urolithiasis
uropathy
venereal diseases
vesical
vesicoureteral
vesicovaginal
voided specimen
voiding
voiding cystourethrogram
voids
Wilms tumor

Español ENHANCING SPANISH COMMUNICATION

English	Spanish (pronunciation)
acidity	acidez (ah-se-DES)
catheter	catéter (cah-TAY-ter)
dialysis	diálisis (de-AH-le-sis)
excretion	excreción (ex-cray-se-ON)
renal artery	arteria renal (ar-TAY-re-ah ray-NAHL)
renal calculus	cálculo renal (CAHL-coo-lo ray-NAHL)
urea	urea (oo-RAY-ah)
urinalysis	urinálisis (oo-re-NAH-le-sis)
urinary	urinario (oo-re-NAH-re-o)
urinate	orinar (o-re-NAR)
urination	urinación (oo-re-nah-se-ON)
voiding	urinar (oo-re-NAR)

Reproductive System

12

LEARNING GOALS

Basic Understanding
In this chapter you will learn to do the following:
1. State the function of the female reproductive system, and analyze associated terms.
2. Write the meanings of the word parts associated with the female reproductive system, and use the word parts to build and analyze terms.
3. Write the names of the structures of the female reproductive system when given their descriptions, define the terms associated with these structures, and label the structures.
4. Sequence the reproductive cycle.
5. Write the names of the diagnostic tests and procedures for assessment of the female reproductive system when given descriptions of the procedures, or match the procedures with their descriptions.
6. Write the names of pathologies of the female reproductive system when given their descriptions, or match them with their descriptions.
7. Label uterine displacements.
8. Match surgical and therapeutic interventions for female reproductive system pathologies with descriptions of the interventions, or write the names of the interventions when given their descriptions.
9. State the function of the male reproductive system, and analyze associated terms.
10. Write the meanings of the word parts associated with the male reproductive system, and use the word parts to build and analyze terms.
11. Write the names of the structures of the male reproductive system when given their descriptions, define the terms associated with these structures, and label the structures.
12. Describe the production of sperm.
13. Write the names of the diagnostic tests and procedures for assessment of the male reproductive system when given descriptions of the procedures, or match diagnostic tests and procedures with their descriptions.
14. Write the names of pathologies of the male reproductive system when given their descriptions, or match them with their descriptions.
15. Match surgical and therapeutic interventions for male reproductive system pathologies with descriptions of the interventions, or write the names of the interventions when given their descriptions.

Greater Comprehension
16. Use word parts from this chapter to determine the meaning of terms in a health care report.
17. Spell the terms accurately.
18. Pronounce the terms correctly.
19. Write the meanings of the abbreviations.
20. Categorize terms as anatomy, diagnostic test or procedure, pathology, surgery, or therapy.

MAJOR SECTIONS OF THIS CHAPTER:

❏ **FEMALE REPRODUCTIVE SYSTEM**
   Anatomy and Physiology
   Diagnostic Tests and Procedures
   Pathologies
   Surgical and Therapeutic Interventions

❏ **MALE REPRODUCTIVE SYSTEM**
   Anatomy and Physiology
   Diagnostic Tests and Procedures
   Pathologies
   Surgical and Therapeutic Interventions

FUNCTION FIRST

Reproduction is the process by which genetic material is passed from one generation to the next. The major function of the reproductive system is to produce offspring. The male and female reproductive systems can be broadly organized by organs with different functions. For example, the testes and ovaries function in the production of spermatozoa (sperm) or ova (eggs), and they secrete important hormones. Ducts transport and receive eggs or sperm and important fluids. Still other reproductive organs produce materials that support the sperm and ova.

FEMALE REPRODUCTIVE SYSTEM
ANATOMY AND PHYSIOLOGY

12-1 The female reproductive system aids in the creation of new life and provides an environment and support for the developing child. After birth, the female breasts produce milk to feed the child. Information about the breasts, often considered a part of this system, is found in Chapter 17, which covers hormones and the endocrine system.

The female reproductive system includes the ovaries, fallopian tubes, uterus, vagina, accessory glands, and external genital structures. The ovaries are the female gonads. A **gonad** (go´nad) produces the reproductive cells.

genitalia

The reproductive organs, whether male or female, are called the genitals or **genitalia** (jen″ĭ-tāl´e-ə). The combining form genit(o) refers to organs of reproduction. The genitalia include both external and internal organs. Another name for genitals is _____.

Knowing that ur(o) means pertaining to urine or the urinary system, **uro/genit/al** (u″ro-jen´ĭ-təl) or **genito/urinary** (jen″ĭ-to-u´rĭ-nar-e) (GU) means pertaining to the urinary and the reproductive systems.

12-2 The combining form that means woman or female is gynec(o). The medical specialty that treats diseases of the female reproductive organs is **gynecology.**

females

Gyneco/logic (gi″nə, jin″ə-kə-loj´ik) means pertaining to gynecology (Gyn) or study of diseases that occur only in _____.

internal

12-3 Examine Table 12-1, which lists the internal and external structures of the female genitalia. Note that the ovaries, uterus, vagina, and several glands make up the _____ structures of the female genitalia.

Vulva refers to the external genitalia in the female, and the combining form is vulv(o).

vulva

Vulv/ar (vul´vər) and **vulv/al** (vul´vəl) mean pertaining to the _____.

12-4 The structures that comprise the vulva are external to the vagina. Label the structures as you read the material that accompanies Figure 12-1.

TABLE 12-1   The Female Genitalia

Internal Structures	External Structures (Vulva)
Left ovary and associated left uterine tube	Mons pubis
Right ovary and associated right uterine tube	Labia majora
Uterus	Labia minora
Vagina	Clitoris
Special glands	Prepuce
	Openings for glands

The **mons*** **pubis** (monz pu´bis) is a pad of fatty tissue and thick skin that overlies a bone called the symphysis pubis. The pubis is the anterior portion of the hipbones. After puberty, the mons pubis is covered with hair.

---

*Mons (Latin: *mons,* mountain).

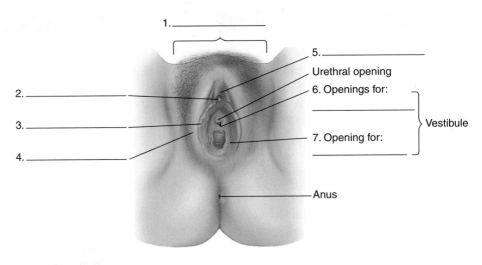

Figure 12-1 Female external genitalia. These structures are external to the vagina and are called the vulva. The mons pubis *(1)* is a pad of fatty tissue and thick skin that overlies the front of the pubic bone. The clitoris *(2)* is a small mass of erectile tissue and nerves. Two pairs of skin folds protect the vaginal opening. The smaller pair is called the labia minora *(3)*, and the larger pair is called the labia majora *(4)*. The retractable cover around the clitoris is the prepuce *(5)*. The para-urethral glands *(6)* and the vestibular glands *(7)* are also shown.

The **clitoris** (klit´ə-ris, kli´tə-ris, klĭ-tor´is) is a small mass of erectile tissue and nerves that has similarities to the male penis. This small mass of erectile tissue becomes erect in response to sexual stimulation.

Two pairs of skin folds, the **labia** (la´be-ə) **majora** and the **labia minora,** protect the vaginal opening.

> ➤ **KEY** POINT Note the singular vs. the plural forms of the terms labium majus and labium minus.
>
> | Singular | Plural |
> |----------|--------|
> | labium | labia |
> | majus | majora |
> | minus | minora |

minora

majora

The smaller pair of skin folds is called the labia _____.
The larger pair of skin folds is called the labia _____.
The labia minora merge and form a hood over the clitoris. This fold of skin that forms a retractable cover is called the **prepuce** (pre´pūs).
The name of the **para/urethral** (par″ə-u-re´thrəl) **glands** tells us they are located

near

_____ the urethra.
Other glands, the **vestibular glands,** lie adjacent to the vaginal opening.

12-5 Vestibule (ves´tĭ-būl) is any space or cavity at the entrance to a canal. The vaginal vestibule is the space between the two labia minora into which the urethra and vagina open. The greater vestibular glands (**Bartholin glands**) produce a mucus-like secretion for lubrication during sexual intercourse.

Another important locational term is **perineum** (per″ĭ-ne´əm), the area between the vaginal

perineum

opening and the anus. **Perine/al** means pertaining to the _____.

12-6 Label the internal structures as you read the material that accompanies Figure 12-2. The right **ovary** (o´və-re) and left ovary are the primary reproductive structures because they produce **ova** (eggs) and hormones. The singular form of ova is ovum. The drawing in Figure 12-2, *A* is a midsagittal view of the internal genitalia, so only one ovary is shown. An ovary is about the size and shape of an almond.

One **fallopian tube** is associated with each ovary. These tubes are also called **uterine tubes**

uterus

because they extend laterally from the upper portion of the _____ to the region of the ovary. There is no direct connection between the ovary and the finger-like projections of the fallopian tube, the **fimbriae.** When an ovum is produced, the fimbriae create

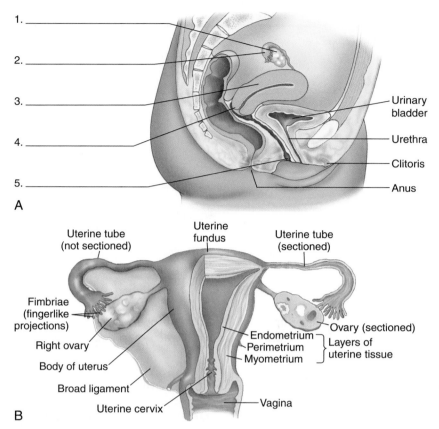

1. _____
2. _____
3. _____
4. _____
5. _____

Urinary bladder
Urethra
Clitoris
Anus

A

Uterine tube (not sectioned)
Uterine fundus
Uterine tube (sectioned)

Fimbriae (fingerlike projections)
Right ovary
Body of uterus
Broad ligament
Uterine cervix

Endometrium
Perimetrium   } Layers of
Myometrium   uterine tissue

Ovary (sectioned)

Vagina

B

Figure 12-2 Female genitalia, midsagittal and anterior views. A, Midsagittal section. Write the names of the structures on the numbered lines as you read the following. Each ovary *(1)* produces ova and hormones. One uterine tube *(2)* is associated with each ovary. The uterus *(3)* is the muscular organ that prepares to receive and nurture the fertilized ovum. The lower and narrower part that has the outlet from the uterus is the cervix uteri *(4)*. The vagina *(5)* is the connection between the internal genitalia and the outside. **B,** Anterior view of the organs of the female reproductive system. The left ovary, left uterine tube, and the left side of the uterus are sectioned to show their internal structure.

currents that sweep the ovum into the tube, and it is then carried along toward the uterus over the next 5 to 7 days. The fallopian tube is the most common site of fertilization of the ovum, which disintegrates or dies within 24 to 48 hours if it is not fertilized.

> ➤ **KEY** POINT The **uterus** (u´tər-əs) is a muscular organ that prepares to receive and nurture the fertilized ovum. The uterus is hollow and pear shaped. The lower and narrower part that has the outlet from the uterus is the cervix uteri (sur´viks u´tər-i), commonly called the uterine cervix (Cx). When used alone, the term cervix often means the cervix uteri.

The **vagina** (və-ji´nə), commonly called the birth canal, is muscular and capable of sufficient expansion for passage of the child during childbirth. It also serves as the repository for sperm during intercourse. The vagina is the connection between the internal genitalia and the outside through its opening called the vaginal orifice (opening). Note that there is one uterus but two ovaries and two _____ tubes.

uterine or fallopian

Learn the following word parts that are used to write terms about the female genitalia.

Word Parts: Female Genitalia

Word Parts	Meaning	Other Word Parts	Meaning
cervic(o)	neck; uterine cervix	lapar(o)	abdominal wall
colp(o), vagin(o)	vagina	men(o)	month
genit(o)	organs of reproduction	o(o)	egg (ovum)
hyster(o), uter(o)	uterus	top(o)	place or position
metr(o)	measure; uterine tissue	-tropin	that which stimulates
oophor(o), ovari(o)	ovary		
perine(o)	perineum		
salping(o)	fallopian tube		
vulv(o)	vulva		

EXERCISE 1

Write word parts or meanings as indicated in the following blanks.

Combining Form　　　**Meaning**

1. colp(o) _____

2. genit(o) _____

3. hyster(o) _____

4. men(o) _____

5. metr(o) _____

6. o/o _____

7. oophor(o) _____

8. ovari(o) _____

9. uter(o) _____

10. vagin(o) _____

11. _____ perineum

12. _____ cervix uteri or neck

13. _____ fallopian tube

14. _____ vulva

ovary

salping(o)

uterus

12-7 Two word parts mean ovary: ovari(o) and oophor(o). The combining form ovari(o) is generally used to write terms that describe the structure of the ovary. **Ovari/an** (o-var´e-ən) means pertaining to the _____.

12-8 Write the combining form that is used to write terms about the uterine tubes: _____.
　　Two combining forms that mean uterus are uter(o) and hyster(o). You have already used the term **uterine** (u´tər-in), which means pertaining to the _____.
　　Write any word that you know that begins with hyster(o): _____.

> ➤ **KEY** POINT Hysterics, hysterical, or hysterectomy use the combining form hyster(o), which means uterus. The use of hyster(o) as a combining form may have originated with the ancient Greeks, who believed that women were especially susceptible to emotional disorders that arose from the womb. The Greeks used the word *hysterikos* to refer to suffering in the womb and the emotional upheaval caused by this suffering.

vagina

vagina

12-9 The vagina is the birth canal, the receptacle for receiving sperm, and the passageway for menstrual flow. Both vagin(o) and colp(o) mean vagina. **Vaginal** (vaj´ĭ-nəl) is an adjective and refers to the _____.
　　Knowing that cyst(o) means bladder, **colpo/cyst/itis** is inflammation of the _____ and the urinary bladder.

12-10 The uterus is the normal site where a fertilized ovum implants and develops. Examine the anterior view of the female genitalia in Figure 12-2, *B*.
　　The uterus consists of an upper portion, a large main portion, and a narrow region that connects with the vagina. The upper, bulging surface of the uterus, above the entrance of the uterine tubes, is called the uterine _____.
　　The large, main portion is called the body of the uterus, and the narrow region is the uterine _____.

fundus (fun´dəs)

cervix

uteri

uteri

12-11 The word **cervix** refers to the neck itself or part of an organ that resembles a neck. The **cervix uteri** specifically means the lower, necklike portion of the uterus, although it is common to see cervix written alone and meaning the cervix uteri. The proper name of the uterine cervix is the cervix _____.
　　The combining form cervic(o) means neck or cervix uteri. Look at other parts of a term to decide which meaning of cervic(o) is intended. **Cervico/colp/itis** (sur″vĭ-ko-kol-pi´tis) is inflammation of the cervix _____ and the vagina.

uterine uterine	**12-12** You have learned that uter(o) and hyster(o) mean uterus. A third combining form, metr(o), also means the uterus, and occasionally metr(o) means measure. Whenever you see metr(o) used in a word, use your critical thinking skills to decide if it means measure or _____ tissue. It is not as difficult as it might seem. For example, **metr/itis** (mə-tri′tis) could only refer to inflammation of _____ tissue.
uterine endometrium	**12-13** The uterus consists of three layers of tissue. From the outermost layer to the innermost layer, the layers are called perimetrium (per″ĭ-me′tre-əm), myometrium (mi-o-me′tre-əm), and endometrium (en″do-me′tre-əm). Find these three layers of uterine tissue in Figure 12-2, *B*. The outer layer is **visceral peritoneum** and is called **peri/metr/ium.** Analyzing its word parts, peri- means around, metr(o) means _____ tissue, and -ium means membrane. In other words, perimetrium is a membrane that surrounds the uterus. The **myo/metr/ium** (my[o] means muscle) is the thick muscular wall of the uterus. The inner layer, the **endo/metr/ium,** is a mucous membrane. Write the name of this mucous membrane that lines the uterus: _____.

EXERCISE 2

Match terms in the left columns with definitions or descriptions in the right column.

_____ 1. ovary   _____ 4. fallopian tube

_____ 2. ovum   _____ 5. vagina

_____ 3. uterus

A. a gonad
B. its endometrium sloughs off in menstruation
C. receives the sperm during intercourse
D. reproductive cell
E. usual site of fertilization

EXERCISE 3

Build It! *Use the following word parts to build terms. (Some word parts will be used more than once.)*

endo-, intra-, peri-, cervic(o), metr(o), my(o), ovari(o), uter(o), -al, -an, -ine, -ium

1. pertaining to the cervix   _____/_____

2. pertaining to the ovary   _____/_____

3. pertaining to within the uterus   _____/_____/_____

4. a membrane that surrounds the uterus _____/_____/_____

5. thick muscular wall of the uterus   _____/_____/_____

6. inner layer of the uterus   _____/_____/_____

Say and Check

Say aloud the terms you wrote for Exercise 3. Use the Companion CD to check your pronunciations.

OVARIAN AND UTERINE CYCLES

menstrual	**12-14** During much of a woman's life, the endometrium goes through a monthly cycle of growth and discharge known as the **menstrual cycle.** Reproductive cycles normally occur in females from shortly after the onset of menstruation to menopause. The monthly cycle of growth and discharge of the endometrium is called the _____ cycle.
	12-15 The hypothalamus (part of the brain) and the pituitary gland, located just beneath the brain, have significant roles in the control of reproductive functions.

> ➤ KEY POINT <u>The hormones produced by these structures act on the ovaries to bring about two important functions:</u> The production of ova and additional hormones, **estrogen** (es´trə-jen) and **progesterone** (pro-jes´tə-rōn).

Female reproductive cycles begin at puberty (pu´bər-te) and continue for about 40 years until menopause (men´o-pawz). **Puberty** is that stage of development when genitalia reach maturity and secondary sex characteristics appear. The external characteristics of sexual maturity include adult distribution of hair and development of the penis or breasts and the labia. The onset of puberty normally occurs in girls between 9 and 13 years of age with the development of breasts and menarche (mə-nahr´ke). **Menarche** is the first occurrence of **menstruation** (men″stroo-a´shən), the periodic bloody discharge caused by the shedding of the endometrium from the nonpregnant uterus. Write this term that means the first menstruation: _____.

> menarche

Menopause, also called the **climacteric** (kli-mak´tər-ik), is the natural cessation of reproductive cycles and menstruation with the decline of reproductive hormones in later years. Menopause may occur earlier as a result of illness or surgical removal of the uterus or both ovaries. Write the term that means menopause: _____.

> climacteric

The date of the last menstrual period (LMP) is important information, particularly when pregnancy is suspected or menopause is being investigated.

12-16 Paying particular attention to its pronunciation and its spelling, write the term that means the periodic (generally monthly) bloody discharge from the shedding of the endometrium: _____.

> menstruation

The secretion of female reproductive hormones follows monthly cyclic patterns that affect the ovaries and uterus. Together, these cycles, called the ovarian cycle and the menstrual (uterine) cycle, make up the female reproductive cycle. The ovarian cycle reflects the changes that occur within the _____. The uterine (menstrual) cycle reflects the changes that take place in the _____. See Figure 12-3 for the correlation of events in the ovarian and uterine cycles.

> ovaries
> uterus

12-17 The ovarian and uterine cycles begin at puberty when certain unknown stimuli cause the hypothalamus to start secreting a hormone that acts on the pituitary gland. The pituitary gland then begins to secrete two hormones, **follicle-stimulating hormone** (FSH) and **luteinizing hormone** (LH). Looking at Figure 12-3, you see that FSH and LH act on follicles in the _____.

> ovaries

The **graafian follicle** is a small ovarian recess or pit that contains fluid and surrounds an ovum (egg). Generally one ovum is released each month. The follicle produces hormones and grows in preparation for release of the ovum. These changes in the follicle are classified as the follicular phase, which is followed by the luteal phase. Find these two phases in the upper part of Figure 12-3. The follicular changes are represented by follicle development, _____, and corpus luteum.

> ovulation

> ➤ KEY POINT <u>**Ovulation** (ov″u-la´shən) is the release of the ovum from the follicle.</u> After the ovum is released, the ruptured follicle enlarges, takes on a yellow appearance, and is called the **corpus luteum** (kor´pəs loo´te-um)**,** meaning yellow body.

The luteal phase is named after the yellowish structure called the corpus _____.

> luteum

12-18 Two important hormones that are secreted by the follicles influence the uterine cycle. During the follicular phase, increasing amounts of estrogen are secreted and stimulate repair of the endometrium. Estrogen reaches its peak near the middle of the cycle, then decreases until the next month. The corpus luteum secretes another important hormone, progesterone, which causes continued growth and thickening of the endometrium with additional preparatory activities to support a potential embryo. If fertilization (union of the ovum and sperm) does not occur, the corpus luteum begins to degenerate and the cycle starts again.

The initial hormone secreted by the ovarian follicle that causes the endometrium to thicken is _____.

> estrogen

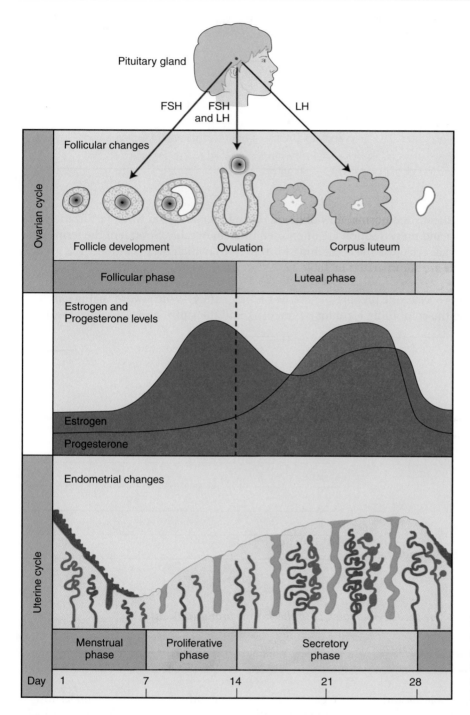

Pituitary gland

FSH   FSH   LH
      and LH

Ovarian cycle

Follicular changes

Follicle development   Ovulation   Corpus luteum

| Follicular phase | Luteal phase | |

Estrogen and
Progesterone levels

Estrogen

Progesterone

Uterine cycle

Endometrial changes

| Menstrual phase | Proliferative phase | Secretory phase | |

Day   1   7   14   21   28

Figure 12-3 Correlation of events in the ovarian and uterine cycles. These two cycles make up the female reproductive cycle, with an average length of 28 days from the first day of bleeding of one cycle to the first day of bleeding of the next cycle.

This is the same hormone that brings about development of the female secondary sex characteristics, the external physical signs of sexual maturity, such as the development of breasts and pubic hair.

A second hormone is secreted by the corpus luteum. That hormone is called

progesterone

_____.

12-19 The uterine cycle occurs simultaneously with the ovarian cycle and is the result of estrogen and progesterone secretion by the ovaries. Looking again at Figure 12-3, write down the phases of the uterine cycle: the menstrual phase, the proliferative phase, and the _____ phase.

secretory

The menstrual phase begins on day 1 of the cycle and continues for 3 to 5 days. The proliferative phase lasts for about 8 days. The name of this phase refers to the growth of the endometrium as it thickens and as glands and blood vessels develop in the new tissue. The endometrium continues to grow and thicken in the secretory phase and in addition begins to secrete glycogen, which will nourish a developing embryo if fertilization occurs.

TABLE 12-2	The Reproductive Cycle	
Days	**Ovarian Phase**	**Uterine (Menstrual) Phase**
1-5	Follicular phase. Growth of the follicle. Secretion of estrogen.	Menses. Blood is shed from the vagina.
6-12	Follicular phase continues.	Proliferative phase. Growth of the endometrium.
13-14	Ovulation. Ovum is released by the follicle.	Proliferative phase continues.
15-28	Luteal phase. Follicle becomes corpus luteum. Secretes progesterone.	Secretory phase. Continued growth of endometrium, secretion of glycogen.

The term **menses** means the normal flow of blood during menstruation when fertilization has not occurred. Menses and menstruation are often used interchangeably. Several of the terms pertaining to the menstrual cycle use the combining form men(o), which means month. The events of the menstrual cycle are summarized in Table 12-2.

12-20 Estrogen and progesterone prepare the uterus for pregnancy. Write a word that means formation of ova, using the combining form for ovum, o(o), and the suffix -genesis, which means origin or beginning: _____.

oogenesis
(o″o-jen′ə-sis)

EXERCISE 4

Write a term for each description or definition.

1. another term for menses   _____

2. another term for menopause   _____

3. first occurrence of menstruation   _____

4. release of an ovum from the ovarian follicle   _____

5. initial hormone that causes thickening of the endometrium _____

 Say and Check

Say aloud the terms you wrote for Exercise 4. Use the Companion CD to check your pronunciations.

DIAGNOSTIC TESTS AND PROCEDURES

12-21 Gynecologic problems and obstetric care account for one fifth of all visits by females to physicians. Many diagnostic procedures and treatments are available to females with gynecologic disorders.

The physical assessment of the female reproductive system includes examination of the breasts, the external genitalia, and the pelvis. A **vaginal speculum** (spek′u-ləm) is an instrument that can be pushed apart after it is inserted into the vagina to allow examination of the cervix and the walls of the vagina (Figure 12-4).

A speculum is an instrument for examining body orifices (openings) or cavities. A speculum that is used to examine the vagina is a _____ speculum.

vaginal

12-22 Specimens (scrapings) for cytology can be collected during the pelvic examination. **Cyto/logy** means the study of _____. Both Pap smears and endo/metrial biopsies are performed to detect cancer of the cervix.

cells

Pap smear is an abbreviated way of saying **Papanicolaou** smear or **test**. In a Pap smear, material is collected from areas of the body that shed cells. The cells are then studied microscopically. A shortened way of saying Papanicolaou smear is _____ smear.

Pap

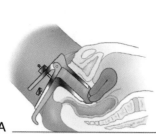 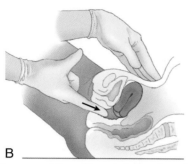 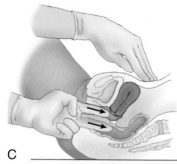

A _____ B _____ C _____

Figure 12-4 **The gynecologic examination.** **A,** Proper position of inserted speculum. **B,** The bimanual examination. The abdominal hand presses the pelvic organs toward the intravaginal hand. **C,** Rectovaginal examination. The examiner's index finger is placed in the vagina and the middle finger is inserted into the rectum. The gynecologic inspection consists of four parts: (1) Inspection of the external genitalia. (2) The speculum examination. The vaginal walls and cervix are inspected. Smears (Pap smear for cytologic examination) are obtained. (3) Bimanual examination assesses the location, size, and mobility of the pelvic organs. (4) The rectovaginal examination is not always performed. In this examination, the posterior aspect of the genital organs and rectal tissue can be evaluated.

12-23 The term Pap smear may refer to collection of material from other surfaces that shed cells, but it usually refers to collection and examination of cells from the vagina and cervix (Figure 12-5). Early diagnosis of cancer of the cervix is possible with the Pap test. When the Pap smear is examined microscopically, malignant cells have a characteristic appearance that indicates cancer, sometimes before symptoms appear.

Cancer of the uterus may begin with a change in shape, growth, and number of cells, called **dysplasia** (dis-pla´zhə). The dysplasia (dys-, bad or difficult + -plasia, development) is not cancer, but cells of this type tend to become malignant. This abnormality, which can be detected before cancer occurs, is called _____.

> dysplasia

It is standard practice to grade Pap smears as class I, II, III, IV, or V. Class I is normal, and class V is definitely cancer. Most physicians recommend having Pap smears done on a routine basis. Regular Pap smears are an excellent method for early detection of cervical cancer, when it is possible that the lesion can be excised, thus preventing spread of cancer to other organs.

12-24 Specimens of vaginal or cervical discharge are collected and tested for the presence of microorganisms using several techniques. Wet mounts, the direct microscopic examination of the fluid, aid in diagnosis of infections with yeast or **Trichomonas,** a vaginal and urethral parasite. Gram stain, a slide-staining technique that aids in classification and identification of bacteria, is especially useful for vaginal smears if **gonorrhea** is suspected. Bacterial or fungal cultures may also be helpful in identifying the cause of infections.

The Venereal Disease Research Laboratories (VDRL) test and the **rapid plasma reagin (RPR) test** are blood tests to detect and monitor **syphilis.**

Levels of hormones in the blood and urine are helpful in determining the function of the ovaries, particularly in fertility studies and pregnancy. **Human chorionic gonadotropin** (go˝nə-do-tro´pin) (HCG) is present in body fluids of pregnant females, and blood or urine is tested to determine if pregnancy exists. Chorion/ic pertains to the chorion, a membrane that develops around a fertilized embryo. **Gonado/tropin** (gonad(o) + -tropin, that which stimulates) is a hormonal substance that stimulates the _____—in this case, the ovaries.

> gonads

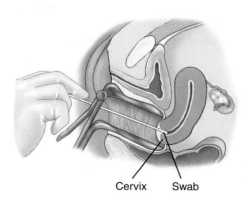

Cervix Swab

Figure 12-5 Obtaining a cervical Pap smear.

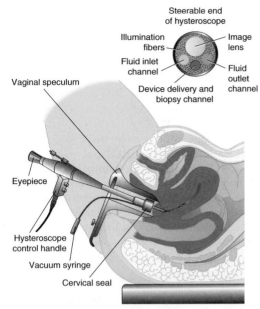

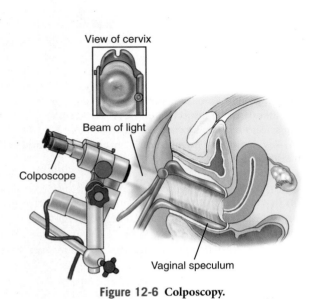

Figure 12-6 Colposcopy.

Figure 12-7 Hysteroscopy. Direct visual examination of the cervical canal and uterine cavity using a hysteroscope is performed to examine the endometrium to obtain a specimen for biopsy, to excise cervical polyps, or to remove an intrauterine device.

gonadotropin

HCG can be detected long before other signs of pregnancy appear. This test may also be used to detect rare forms of tumors in either men or women, but more often the test is performed to ascertain pregnancy. Write the name of the hormone that is tested for in pregnancy tests: human chorionic _____.

12-25 Colposcopy (kol-pos´kə-pe) involves the use of a low-powered microscope to magnify the mucosa of the vagina and the cervix. The instrument used is a _____ (Figure 12-6).

colposcope
(kol´po-skōp)

Suspicious cervical or vaginal lesions may be seen during colposcopy. Some findings indicate the need for a cervical or endometrial biopsy. A **cervical biopsy** is removal of tissue from the _____. An **endometrial biopsy** requires collection of tissue

cervix
uterus

from the lining of the _____.

12-26 Hysteroscopy (his″tər-os´kə-pe) is direct visual inspection of the cervical canal and uterine cavity, using an endoscope passed through the vagina (Figure 12-7). Change the suffix of hysteroscopy to write the name of the endoscope: _____.

hysteroscope
(his´tər-o-skōp″)

12-27 Pelvic ultrasonography may be helpful in detecting masses, such as ovarian cysts. Computed tomography may be used to detect a tumor within the pelvis.

Hystero/salpingo/graphy (his″tər-o-sal″ping-gog´rə-fe) is radiologic examination of the uterus and the _____ tubes after an injection of radiopaque material into those organs (Figure 12-8). It allows evaluation of the size, shape, and position of the organs, including tumors and certain other abnormalities, as well as obstruction of a uterine tube.

uterine (or fallopian)

A **hysterosalpingogram** (his″tər-o-sal-ping´go-gram) is the _____ that is produced in hysterosalpingography.

record

12-28 Laparo/scopy (lap″ə-ros´kə-pe) is the examination of the abdominal cavity with a **laparoscope** (lap´ə-ro-skōp″) through one or more small incisions in the abdominal wall. This surgical procedure is especially useful for inspection of the ovaries and other structures within the pelvic cavity, as well as collection of biopsy specimens or performance of tubal ligation to prevent pregnancy (Figure 12-9). Write the name of the instrument used in laparoscopy: _____.

laparoscope

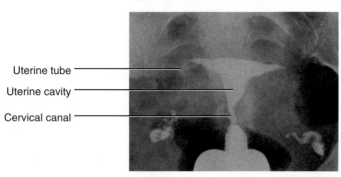

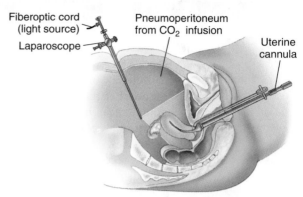

Uterine tube
Uterine cavity
Cervical canal

Figure 12-8 Hysterosalpingogram. This x-ray image of the uterus and uterine tubes was made after the introduction of a radiopaque substance through the cervix.

Figure 12-9 Laparoscopy. Using the laparoscope with a fiberoptic light source, the surgeon can view the pelvic cavity and the reproductive organs. Further instrumentation, for example, for tubal sterilization, is possible through a second small incision. The purpose of the uterine cannula is to allow movement of the uterus during laparoscopy.

EXERCISE 5

Write a term in each of the blanks to complete the sentences. The first letter of each term is given as a clue.

1. An instrument used to examine the vagina and cervix walls is a s_____.

2. The study of cells in a Pap test is called c_____.

3. In a Pap smear, an alteration in the shape, growth, or number of cells that is not a sign of cancer but indicates a tendency of the cells to become malignant is called d_____.

4. A hormone that is tested to ascertain pregnancy is human chorionic g_____.

5. Using low-powered microscopy to examine the vaginal mucosa and cervix is called
   c_____.

6. Direct visualization of the uterus with a hysteroscope is h_____.

7. A radiographic examination of the uterus and the uterine tubes after an injection of a radiopaque contrast medium is called h_____.

8. Examining the pelvic cavity after making one or more small abdominal incisions is l_____.

Say and Check

Say aloud the terms you wrote for Exercise 5. Use the Companion CD to check your pronunciations.

EXERCISE 6

Match descriptions in the left column with the correct terms in the right column.

_____ 1. membrane that develops around the fertilized embryo

_____ 2. blood test to detect and monitor syphilis

_____ 3. slide-staining technique that helps identify bacteria

_____ 4. collection and examination of cells from the vagina and cervix

_____ 5. direct microscopic examination of fluid

A. Pap smear
B. rapid plasma reagin
C. wet mounts
D. Gram stain
E. chorion

PATHOLOGIES

12-29 Menstrual disorders include painful menstruation, heavy or irregular flow, spotting, absence of or skipping periods, and premenstrual syndrome.

menorrhea
(men″ə-re′ə)

Build a word by combining men(o) and -rrhea (flow or discharge): _____.
Menorrhea means either normal menstruation or too profuse menstruation. Because of the double meaning of menorrhea, it would be clearer to use either of the following terms to mean

menstruation

the normal monthly flow of blood from the genital tract: _____
or menses.

The second meaning of menorrhea is profuse menstruation. Build a word that is a synonym for this meaning by using the combining form for month and the suffix for hemorrhage:

menorrhagia
(men″ə-ra′jə)

_____.
Menorrhagia is abnormally heavy or long menstrual periods.

12-30 Metrorrhagia (me″tro-ra′jə) is uterine bleeding other than that caused by menstruation. It may occur as spotting or outright bleeding, the period of flow sometimes being prolonged.

hemorrhage

The literal translation of metro/rrhagia is _____ of the uterus.
Metrorrhagia may be caused by uterine tumors, benign or malignant, and especially cervical cancer.

absence

12-31 A/menorrhea (ə-men″o-re′ə) is _____ of menstruation. Amenorrhea is normal before puberty, after menopause, and during pregnancy. Underdevelopment of the reproductive organs or hormonal disturbances can cause absence of the onset

amenorrhea

of menstruation at puberty. This absence of menstruation is called _____.
When menstruation has begun but then ceases, this is also called amenorrhea.

menstruation

12-32 Dys/menorrhea (dis-men″ə-re′ə) is painful or difficult _____.
Mittelschmerz[*] (mit′əl-shmertz) means abdominal pain in the region of an ovary during ovulation. It is helpful in pinpointing the fertile period of the ovarian cycle.

12-33 Premenstrual syndrome (PMS) is nervous tension, irritability, edema, headache, and painful breasts that can occur the last few days before the onset of menstruation. Various studies indicate that many females experience some degree of PMS, but fewer than half experience

premenstrual

symptoms that disrupt their lives. PMS means _____ syndrome.

12-34 Cervic/itis (sur″vĭ-si′tis) refers specifically to inflammation of the cervix uteri. Acute cervicitis is infection of the cervix marked by redness, bleeding on contact, and often pain, itching, or burning, and a foul-smelling discharge from the vagina. Acute cervicitis may be caused by several species of bacteria, *Chlamydia* (specialized bacteria), *Candida albicans* (yeast), or the parasite *Trichomonas vaginalis*. Some sexually transmitted diseases (STDs)—for example, gonorrhea—cause cervicitis. Diagnosis of gonorrhea can often be made by examination of a stained smear and is confirmed by culture.

cervicitis

Persistent inflammation of the cervix is called chronic _____.

12-35 Vagin/itis (vaj″ĭ-ni′tis) is inflammation of the vaginal tissues. This may be accompanied by itching, burning or discomfort during urination, and vaginal discharge; however, some infections are asymptomatic. Many of these lower genital tract infections are related to sexual intercourse, which can irritate vaginal tissues and transmit microorganisms. Vaginal infections are sometimes considered a sexually transmitted disease, but infection can also occur following childbirth or after taking antibiotics that produce changes in the vaginal tissues that allow overgrowth of normal bacterial flora such as *C. albicans*.

vaginitis

Write this term that means infection of the vagina: _____.
This is the same as **colp/itis** (kol-pi′tis).

vulva

12-36 Vulv/itis (vəl-vi′tis) is inflammation of the _____ and is associated with itching and burning. This can be caused by infection, contact with irritants, or systemic conditions.

---

[*]Mittelschmerz (German: *mittel,* mid, middle + *schmerz,* pain, suffering).

Irritants such as soaps and detergents or allergens can cause vulvitis as well as dryness of the tissues and hormonal changes, particularly associated with aging. Sexually transmitted diseases should be considered, particularly if lesions are present such as venereal warts or the blisters that occur with genital herpes. See information about sexually transmitted diseases in Chapter 13.

12-37 Vulvo/vaginitis (vul″vo-vaj″ĭ-ni′tis) is inflammation of the vulva and vagina. Vulvar infections can be extensions of vaginal infections. Vulvo/vagin/al candidiasis is infection of the vagina and vulva with *C. albicans.* An infection caused by *Candida* is called **candidiasis** (kan″dĭ-di′ə-sis). Remembering that -iasis means condition, write this term that means a condition caused by *C. albicans:* _____.

candidiasis

12-38 Practice using oophor(o) to write pathologies of the ovaries. **Oophoropathy** (o-of″ə-rop′ə-the) is any _____ of an ovary.

disease   Inflammation of an ovary is _____.
oophoritis   **Oophor/algia** (o″of-ər-al′jə) is also called ovarian pain.
(o″of-ə-ri′tis)   **Oophoro/salping/itis** (o-of″ə-ro-sal″pin-ji′tis) is inflammation of an _____
ovary   and a fallopian tube.

12-39 An/ovulation (an″ov-u-la′shən), absence of ovulation, is failure of the ovaries to produce, mature, or release ova. Its causes include altered ovarian function or dysfunction, side effects of medications, and stress or disease. Write this term that means lack of ovulation:

anovulation   _____.
   Polycystic ovary syndrome is a hormonal disturbance characterized by anovulation, amenorrhea, and infertility. It is caused by increased levels of testosterone (male hormone), estrogen, and luteinizing hormone and decreased secretion of FSH. Numerous cysts may develop, with the affected ovary sometimes doubling in size.

12-40 Polycystic ovary syndrome differs from what is usually meant by the term **ovarian cyst,** which is a globular sac filled with fluid or semisolid material that develops in or on the ovary. This type of ovarian cyst may be transient or pathologic. Benign cysts are common and may be asymptomatic, or they may cause pelvic pain and menstrual irregularities. If a female is a/symp-

without   tomatic, this means that she is _____ symptoms.
   Ovarian cancer is the leading cause of death from reproductive cancers because the disease has usually spread to other organs by the time it is discovered. Sonography and CT may detect the ovarian mass, but diagnosis generally requires surgical exploration and pathologic confirmation of the diagnosis. Compare a benign ovarian cyst and a malignant ovarian tumor (Figure 12-10).

fallopian (or uterine)   **12-41 Salpingo/cele** (sal-ping′go-sēl) is hernial protrusion of a _____ tube.
salpingitis   Inflammation of a fallopian tube is _____.
(sal″pin-ji′tis)

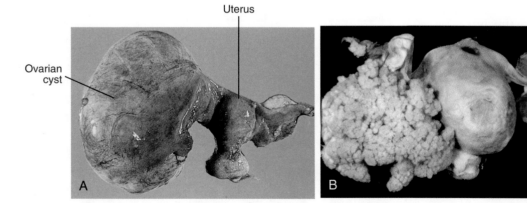

Figure 12-10 An ovarian cyst vs. ovarian carcinoma. A, Ovarian cyst. This very large benign cyst is soft and surrounded by a thin capsule. Ovarian masses are often asymptomatic until they are large enough to cause pressure in the pelvis. **B,** Carcinoma of the ovary. The ovary is enormously enlarged by the tumor. Ovarian cancer is often far advanced when diagnosed.

> ➤ **KEY** POINT An **ectopic** (ek-top´ik) **pregnancy** is one in which a fertilized ovum implants somewhere outside the uterine cavity. Ectopic (ect[o], outside + top[o], position + -ic, pertaining to) means situated in an unusual place, away from its normal location. The abnormal implantation site is usually in the fallopian tube, and this is called a **tubal pregnancy.** Treatment is generally removal of the pregnancy, often with removal of the fallopian tube.

12-42 The fallopian tubes are usually infected in **pelvic inflammatory disease** (PID). Without treatment, the tubes can become obstructed and cause infertility. Pelvic inflammatory disease is any infection that involves the upper genital tract beyond the cervix. Untreated gonococcal or staphylococcal infections, for example, can spread along the endometrium to the fallopian tubes and cause an acute salpingitis. If untreated or treated inadequately, the tubes can become

pelvic

obstructed. PID stands for _____ inflammatory disease.

Septicemia (sept[o], infection + -emia, blood) and other severe complications rarely occur in PID as they do in **toxic shock syndrome** (TSS). A sudden high fever, headache, confusion, acute renal failure, and abnormal liver function are characteristic of TSS. This acute disease is caused by a type of *Staphylococcus* species and is most common in menstruating women who use tampons.

12-43 Cancer can occur in any of the reproductive structures and spread to other organs. The stage of **uterine cancer** is identified by the extent to which it has spread to other organs (Figure 12-11). Early removal of cancerous tissue is vital for preventing the spread of cancer.

hysteropathy
(his˝tə-rop´ə-the)

Write a word that means any disease of the uterus: _____.

12-44 The uterus is normally held in its proper alignment with the vagina and the uterine tubes by ligaments that hold each structure in its proper place. Weakening of the ligaments causes a prolapsed uterus. Using -ptosis, write a word that means uterine prolapse:

hysteroptosis
(his˝tər-op-to´sis)

_____.

A prolapsed uterus can be congenital or caused by heavy physical exertion. It is classified according to its severity (Figure 12-12).

12-45 The uterus normally lies midline in the pelvis; however, some variations, called **uterine displacements,** occur (Figure 12-13). Mild degrees of these four types of displacements are common, may or may not cause symptoms, and may be determined by the position of the cervix when the pelvic examination is performed. Use the information in Figure 12-13 to complete these sentences.

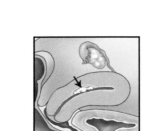
Stage I

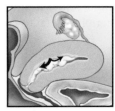
Stage II

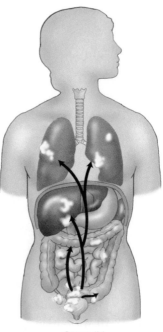
Stage IV

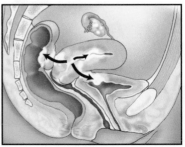
Stage III

Figure 12-11 **Staging uterine cancer.** Stage I: Tumor is confined to the uterine corpus. Stage II: The cancer has invaded the cervix also. Stage III: The cancer has spread beyond the uterus but remains confined to the pelvis, such as in the bladder or rectum. Stage IV: The highest level of invasiveness; the cancer has spread beyond the pelvis, causing metastatic disease and large masses, such as in the liver or lungs.

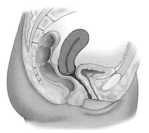 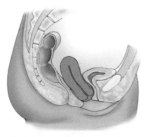 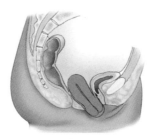

1st degree uterine prolapse
A

2nd degree uterine prolapse
B

3rd degree uterine prolapse
C

Figure 12-12 Three stages of uterine prolapse of increasing severity. Uterine prolapse may be congenital or may be caused by heavy physical exertion or other situations that weaken the pelvic supports. **A,** The uterus bulges into the vagina but does not protrude through the entrance. **B,** The uterus bulges farther into the vagina and the cervix protrudes through the entrance. **C,** The body of the uterus and the cervix protrude through the entrance to the vagina.

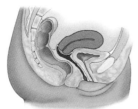 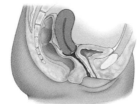 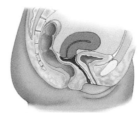 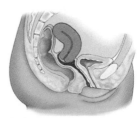

A Anteversion B Retroversion C Anteflexion D Retroflexion

Figure 12-13 Abnormal (forward or backward) displacements of the uterus. A, Anteversion, forward displacement of the body of the uterus toward the pubis, with the cervix tilted up. **B,** Retroversion, tipped backward, the opposite of anteversion. **C,** Anteflexion, bending forward. **D,** Retroflexion, bending backward.

---

anteversion
(an″te-vur´zhən)
backward
anteflexion
(an-te-flek´shən)

A forward displacement of the body of the uterus toward the pubis, the anterior portion of the hipbone, is _____.

Retro/version (ret″ro-vur´zhən) is a common condition in which the uterus is tipped _____ and is the opposite of anteversion.

A bending forward of the uterus is called _____, and a bending backward of the uterus is **retroflexion** (ret″ro-flek´shən).

12-46 A **uterine leiomyoma** (leio-, smooth + my[o], muscle + -*oma*, tumor) (li″o-mi-o´mə) is a benign tumor occurring in the uterus and is also called a uterine fibroid. Large tumors may cause a general enlargement of the lower abdomen. Write the name of this type of uterine tumor: _____.

leiomyoma

Cervical polyps are benign lesions attached to the cervix, often by a stalk, and can sometimes be seen in a gynecologic examination.

myometritis
(mi″o-mə-tri´tis)

12-47 Write a term that means inflammation of the myometrium: _____.

12-48 **Endometritis** (en″do-me-tri´tis) is inflammation of the endometrium and is generally produced by bacterial invasion of the endometrium.

Endometriosis (en″do-me″tre-o´sis), however, is an abnormal condition in which tissue that contains typical endometrial elements is present outside the uterus, usually within the pelvic cavity. See the common sites of endometriosis in Figure 12-14.

Endometrial tissue that is located outside the uterine lining responds to hormonal changes and goes through cyclic changes of bleeding and proliferation. Scarring and adhesions result. An adhesion is an abnormal adherence of structures that are not normally joined. A condition in which endometrium occurs in other places besides the uterus is called _____.

endometriosis

12-49 **Leuko/rrhea** (loo″ko-re´ə) normally occurs in the adult female and is somewhat increased before and after the menstrual period. It may be abnormal if there is either an increase in amount or a change in color or odor.

white

Literal translation of leuko/rrhea is _____ discharge. This new term specifically refers to a white, viscid discharge from the vagina and the uterine cavity.

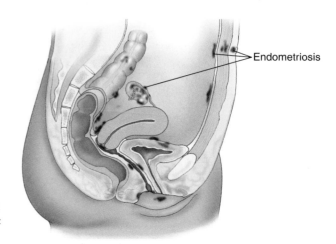

Figure 12-14 Common sites of endometriosis. The abnormal location of endometrial tissue is often the ovaries and less commonly other pelvic structures.

vagina
colporrhagia
(kol″po-ra′jə)
 	
urethra
 	
bladder
 	
cystocele
	12-50 Colpo/dynia (kol″po-din′e-ə) is pain of the _____.
	    Use colp(o) to write a word that means hemorrhage from the vagina: _____.
	
	12-51 Vaginal **fistulas** are abnormal openings between the vagina and the urethra, the bladder, or the rectum. **Urethro/vaginal** (u-re″thro-vaj′ĭ-nəl) fistulas occur between the _____ and the vagina. A **rectovaginal** (rek″to-vaj′ĭ-nəl) fistula is one that occurs between the rectum and the vagina.
	    Knowing that vesic(o) means bladder, a **vesicovaginal** (ves″ĭ-ko-vaj′ĭ-nəl) fistula occurs between the urinary _____ and the vagina. (See the locations of these types of fistulas in Figure 12-15.)
	
	12-52 A **cysto/cele** (cyst[o], bladder + -cele, herniation) (sis′to-sēl), protrusion of the urinary bladder through the wall of the vagina, occurs when support is weakened between the two structures. A **recto/cele** (rect[o], rectum) occurs from a weakening between the vagina and rectum. Both problems are common and often asymptomatic. A large cystocele can interfere with emptying the bladder, and a large rectocele can interfere with emptying the rectum. (Compare these two types of herniations in Figure 12-16.)
	    Herniation of the urinary bladder through the wall of the vagina is called a _____.

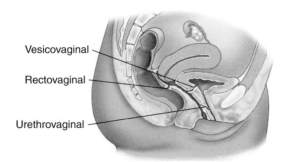

Vesicovaginal

Rectovaginal

Urethrovaginal

Figure 12-15 Sites of vaginal fistulas. Abnormal openings between the vagina and the bladder, rectum, and urethra are shown. These abnormal openings are called vesicovaginal fistula, rectovaginal fistula, and urethrovaginal fistula, respectively.

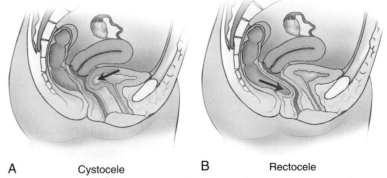

A   Cystocele   **B**   Rectocele

Figure 12-16 Comparison of a cystocele and a rectocele. A, Cystocele. The urinary bladder is displaced downward, causing bulging of the anterior vaginal wall. **B,** Rectocele. The rectum is displaced, causing bulging of the posterior vaginal wall.

EXERCISE 7

Match menstrual disorders in the left columns with their descriptions in the right column.

_____ 1. amenorrhea _____ 3. menorrhagia A. abnormally heavy or long menstrual periods
_____ 2. dysmenorrhea _____ 4. metrorrhagia B. absence of menstruation
 C. painful or difficult menstruation
 D. uterine bleeding other than menstruation

EXERCISE 8

Write words in the blanks to complete these sentences.

1. PMS means _____ syndrome.

2. Mittelschmerz means pain in the region of the ovary during _____.

3. Failure of the ovaries to produce, mature, or release ova is _____.

4. The leading cause of death from reproductive cancer is _____ carcinoma.

5. PID means _____ inflammatory disease.

6. Weakening of the ligaments that hold the uterus in place is uterine _____.

7. A common uterine condition in which it is tipped backward is _____.

8. A uterine fibroid is also called a/an _____.

9. An abnormal opening between the rectum and the vagina is called a rectovaginal _____.

10. Herniation of the urinary bladder through the wall of the vagina is a/an _____.

EXERCISE 9

Word Analysis. *Break these words into their component parts by placing a slash between the word parts. Then write the meaning of each term.*

1. salpingocele _____

2. oophoropathy _____

3. cervicitis _____

4. colpodynia _____

5. endometritis _____

Say and Check

Say aloud the terms you wrote for Exercise 9. Use the Companion CD to check your pronunciations.

SURGICAL AND THERAPEUTIC INTERVENTIONS

12-53 **Contra/ceptives** (contra-, against) are used to prevent conception—in other words, pregnancy. Read about the various methods of preventing pregnancy in Chapter 13.

Some of the most common gynecologic problems for which females seek treatment are vaginal discharge, bleeding, and pain. Dysmenorrhea, painful _____

menstrual

flow, is caused by uterine cramping and can usually be alleviated with aspirin or antiinflammatory drugs such as ibuprofen. Advil is a common over-the-counter brand of ibuprofen.

Other medications and changes in diet may be recommended for premenstrual syndrome.

12-54 After the cause of amenorrhea is established, it can be treated by surgical and pharmaceutical means (hormone replacement and stimulation of the ovaries, for example).

Menopause, though, is a natural termination of menstruation, and many women experience few if any unpleasant symptoms of hot flashes and night sweats. Hormone replacement therapy

(HRT), a combination of estrogen and progesterone, is the primary intervention for women who experience the symptoms of transition or those at high risk for osteoporosis (abnormal loss of bone density) and deterioration of bone tissue. There is no agreement on the value versus risk of HRT: prevention of osteoporosis, heart disease, and Alzheimer disease (progressive mental deterioration) versus the risks of breast and endometrial cancer. HRT means _____ replacement therapy.

hormone

12-55 Treatment of vulvitis can sometimes be as simple as avoiding contact with irritants, such as soaps or detergents. Therapeutic interventions for infections of the vulva, vagina, and cervix depend on the causative organism. Oral or topical antibiotics, vaginal creams, and suppositories (sə-poz´ĭ-tor-ēz) are prescribed according to the type of infection. Oral antibiotics are taken by _____. Topical (top[o], position or place) medications, such as antibiotic ointments or gynecologic creams, are applied directly to the affected area. Vaginal suppositories are easily melted medicated materials that are inserted into the vagina.

mouth

Laser therapy may be performed for persistent vulvitis. **Vulv/ectomy** (vəl-vek´tə-me), _____ of the vulva, is characteristically used to treat cancer of the vulva (Figure 12-17).

excision

12-56 Vaginal and vulvar cancer are not common and occur mainly in women older than 50 years. Two terms that mean the removal of all or a part of the vagina are **vaginectomy** (vaj˝ĭ-nek´tə-me) and _____. (In vaginal cancer, this surgical procedure may be part of a radical hysterectomy—removal of ovaries, fallopian tubes, lymph nodes, and lymph channels, as well as the uterus and cervix.)

colpectomy
(kol-pek´tə-me)

Remembering that -rrhaphy means suture, **colporrhaphy** (kol-por´ə-fe) is _____ of the vagina.

suture

Surgical repair of the vagina is _____.

colpoplasty
(kol´po-plas˝te)

12-57 The combining form oophor(o) is used to write most surgical terms concerning the ovaries. Using oophor(o), write a word that means surgical fixation to correct an ovary that has lost its normal support: _____.

If benign ovarian cysts become large enough to cause pressure in the pelvis, they produce variable symptoms, including pain, menstrual irregularities, and urinary frequency. The cysts may be removed surgically, using either a laparoscope or open (abdominal) surgery.

oophoropexy
(o-of´ə-ro-pek˝se)

Removal of an adult woman's ovaries prohibits reproduction and prevents further production of ovarian hormones. **Oophor/ectomy** (o˝of-ə-rek´tə-me) is surgical _____ of one or both ovaries. **Laparoscopic oophorectomy** is selected whenever possible and greatly reduces the recovery time required for an abdominal oophorectomy.

excision

12-58 Treatment of ovarian cancer includes a combination of surgical removal of the uterus, ovaries, and uterine tubes, either preceding or following chemotherapy. A **hyster/ectomy** (his˝tər-ek´tə-me) is removal of the _____. A hysterectomy

uterus

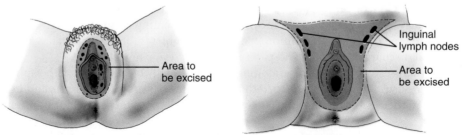

A. Simple vulvectomy   **B.** Radical vulvectomy

Figure 12-17 Vulvectomy. A, Simple vulvectomy includes the removal of the skin of the labia minora, labia majora, and clitoris. **B,** Radical vulvectomy is excision of the labia majora, labia minora, clitoris, surrounding tissues, and pelvic lymph nodes.

and bilateral **oophorosalpingectomy** (o-of″ə-ro-sal″pin-jek′tə-me) is removal of the uterus, both ovaries, and both _____ tubes. **Salpingo-oophorectomy** (sal-ping″go-o-of″ə-rek′tə-me) is removal of an ovary and its uterine tube.

When the uterus is removed through an incision in the abdominal wall, it is called an **abdominal hysterectomy.**

12-59 Oophoro/hyster/ectomy (o-of″ə-ro-his″tər-ek′tə-me) is removal of the _____ and the _____.

> ➤ **KEY** POINT   <u>A hysterectomy can be done laparoscopically, vaginally, or via open abdominal surgery, depending on the individual's needs.</u> The abdominal route is used when the pelvic cavity is to be explored or when the ovaries and uterine tubes are to be removed at the same time. A subtotal hysterectomy, rarely done, is removal of the uterus without removing the cervix. A total hysterectomy is removal of the uterus and cervix. A total abdominal hysterectomy is abbreviated TAH. Compare four types of hysterectomies (Figure 12-18).

Pelvic exenteration (ek″sen″tər-a′shən), removal of all pelvic organs, is done when other forms of therapy are ineffective in controlling the spread of cancer and no metastases have been found outside the pelvis. This radical surgery usually involves removal of the uterus, ovaries, uterine tubes, vagina, bladder, urethra, and pelvic lymph nodes.

12-60 Removal of the uterus is also commonly performed for large fibroids. Symptoms and treatment of fibroids vary widely. When a hyster/ectomy is performed, the uterus is _____.

In cases other than cancer, a hysterectomy is performed in one of three ways: abdominally, vaginally, or laparoscopically. A **colpo/hyster/ectomy** (kol″po-his″tər-ek′tə-me) is removal of the uterus by way of the vagina. In a colpohysterectomy, an abdominal incision is not required because the uterus is removed through the vagina. This is also called a _____ **hysterectomy.**

Left margin answers:
fallopian (uterine)

ovaries; uterus

removed

vaginal

A. Subtotal hysterectomy

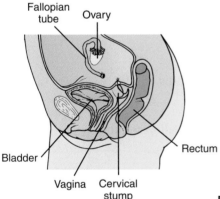

Fallopian tube
Ovary
Bladder
Rectum
Vagina   Cervical stump

B. Total hysterectomy

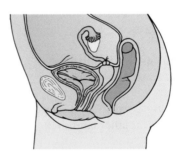

C. Vaginal hysterectomy

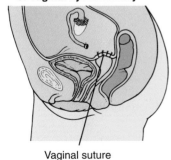

Vaginal suture line

D. Total hysterectomy, salpingectomy, and oophorectomy

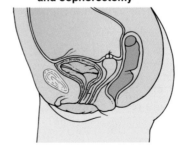

Figure 12-18 Types of hysterectomies. A, In a subtotal hysterectomy, the uterus is removed without the cervix. This surgery is rarely done. **B,** Total hysterectomy is removal of the uterus and cervix. **C,** In a vaginal hysterectomy the uterus is removed through the vagina. **D,** In a total hysterectomy with salpingo-oophorectomy the uterus and both ovaries and uterine tubes are removed.

abdominal

uterine

opening

cervix
endometrium

cold

hysteropexy
(his´tər-o-pek˝se)
salpingorrhaphy
(sal˝ping-gor´ə-fe)

In some cases the uterus can be removed laparoscopically. A **laparo/hyster/ectomy** (lap˝ə-ro-his˝tə-rek´tə-me) is removal of the uterus through small openings in the _____ wall.

12-61 Salpingectomy (sal˝pin-jek´tə-me) is surgical removal of one or both _____ tubes, and one must state which uterine tube is removed or if it is bilateral removal. It is performed for removal of a tumor or cyst, or as a method of sterilization, and is included in a hysterectomy and oophorectomy.

A **tubal ligation** (li-ga´shən) is one of several sterilization procedures in which both uterine tubes are constricted, severed, or crushed to prevent conception. The procedure originally involved the use of a ligature (a substance that tied or constricted), hence its name. This is now most often performed laparoscopically. Tubal ligation can be reversed in some cases by making a new opening to restore patency (condition of being open), but this is not always successful. **Salpingostomy** (sal˝ping-gos´tə-me), making a new _____ into a uterine tube, may be performed also for the purpose of drainage if a uterine tube is obstructed by infection or scar tissue.

12-62 A common surgical procedure that is performed for either diagnosis or treatment is **dilation and curettage** (ku˝rə-tahzh´) (D&C). In this procedure the cervix is dilated to allow the insertion of a curet into the uterus. The **curet** is a surgical instrument shaped like a spoon or scoop and is used for scraping and removal of material from the endometrium. In this procedure, called D&C, what structure is dilated? _____ What structure is scraped? _____

This surgical procedure is done to assess disease of the uterus, to correct heavy or prolonged vaginal bleeding, to empty the uterus of residue after childbirth, and/or to remove the products of conception.

12-63 Cryo/therapy (kri˝o-ther´ə-pe), also called **cryosurgery** (kri˝o-sur´jər-e), is a treatment that uses a subfreezing temperature to destroy tissue. Cryosurgery and laser surgery are especially useful in the treatment of lesions of **condyloma acuminatum,** commonly called genital warts. In cryotherapy, cry(o) means cold, and -therapy is a suffix that means treatment. The literal interpretation of cryotherapy is treatment using _____ temperatures.

To burn tissues by laser, hot metal, electricity, or another agent with the objective of destroying tissue is **cauterization** (kaw´tər-ĭ-za´shən). The verb is **cauterize** (kaw´tər-īz). For example, tissue is cauterized in cauterization.

12-64 Build a word that means surgical fixation of a displaced uterus by adding -pexy to the combining form that means uterus: _____.

12-65 Salpingopexy (sal-ping´go-pek˝se) is surgical fixation of a fallopian tube.
Write the term for suture of a fallopian tube: _____.

EXERCISE 10
_____

Write a word in each blank to complete these sentences.

1. A pharmaceutical intervention for treating the symptoms of menopause is _____

   replacement therapy.

2. Excision of the vulva is _____.

3. Surgical fixation of an ovary is _____.

4. When the ovaries, uterus, and fallopian tubes are removed, this surgery is called a total abdominal

   _____.

5. Removal of the uterus through a small opening in the abdominal wall is _____.

6. Removal of a fallopian tube is _____.

7. The sterilization procedure in which both fallopian tubes are constricted, severed, or crushed is called tubal

   _____.

8. Forming a new opening into a fallopian tube is _____.

9. Dilation of the cervix and removal of material from the endometrium is called dilation and

   _____.

10. Treatment using subfreezing temperature to destroy tissue is _____.

EXERCISE 11

Build It! *Use the following word parts to build terms. (Some word parts will be used more than once.)*

colp(o), hyster(o), lapar(o), oophor(o), salping(o), -ectomy, -pexy, -rrhaphy, -scope

1. suture of the vagina _____/_____

2. surgical fixation of a fallopian tube _____/_____

3. surgical removal of the ovaries and uterus _____/_____/_____

4. surgical fixation of the uterus to the abdominal wall _____/_____

5. instrument to visualize the abdomen _____/_____

Say and Check

Say aloud the terms you wrote for Exercise 11. Use the Companion CD to check your pronunciations.

MALE REPRODUCTIVE SYSTEM
ANATOMY AND PHYSIOLOGY

12-66 The male reproductive system produces, sustains, and transports spermatozoa; introduces them into the female vagina; and produces hormones. The testes are responsible for production of both spermatozoa and hormones. Testes is the plural form of testis, which means the same as testicle.

All other organs, ducts, and glands in this system transport and sustain the spermatozoa, the male sex cells, often shortened to sperm (singular, spermatozoon, or sperm).

The male gonads are the testes (tes´tēz), the primary organs of the male reproductive system. The _____ are the male gonads. Learn the following word parts that pertain to the male reproductive system.

testes

Word Parts: Male Reproductive System

Word Parts	Meaning	Other Word Parts	Meaning
Male Reproductive Structures		rect(o)	rectum
balan(o)	glans penis	semin(o)	semen
epididym(o)	epididymis	sperm(o), spermat(o)	spermatozoa
orchi(o), orchid(o), test(o), testicul(o)	testicle	urethr(o)	urethra
pen(o)	penis		
prostat(o)	prostate		
scrot(o)	scrotum		
vas(o)	vessel; ductus deferens		

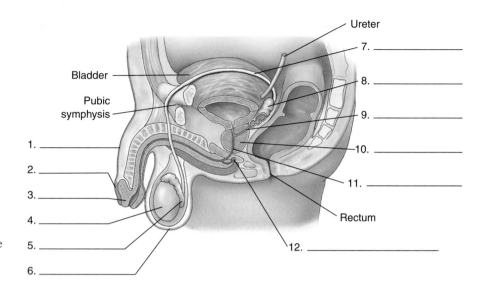

Labels on figure: Ureter, Bladder, Pubic symphysis, Rectum

7. _____

8. _____

9. _____

10. _____

11. _____

1. _____
2. _____
3. _____
4. _____
5. _____
6. _____

12. _____

Figure 12-19 Structures of the male reproductive system. The structures that are already labeled lie near, but are not part of, the male reproductive system.

12-67 Study Figure 12-19 and write the names of the structures in the blank lines as you read the following information. Label the penis on line l. A loose fold of skin, the **prepuce** (foreskin, line 2), covers the glans penis (line 3).

Figure 12-19 is a midsagittal section, so only one testis is shown. Label the **testis** (line 4). Sperm leave the testes through ducts that enter the **epididymis** (ep″ĭ-did′ə-mis), a tightly coiled comma-shaped organ located along the superior and posterior margins of the testes. Label the epididymis (line 5). The testes and epididymides are contained in a pouch of skin that is posterior to the penis. This pouch of skin is called the **scrotum** (skro′təm). Label the scrotum (line 6).

Each **ductus deferens** (line 7), also called the **vas deferens,** begins at the epididymis, continues upward, and then enters the abdominopelvic cavity. Each ductus deferens joins a duct from the seminal vesicle (line 8) to form a short **ejaculatory** (e-jak′u-lə-to″re) **duct.** Label the ejaculatory duct (line 9), which passes through the prostate (pros′tāt) gland and then empties into the urethra. Label the **prostate** (line 10) and the urethra (line 11). Paired **bulbourethral glands** contribute an alkaline mucus-like fluid to the semen. Label the bulbourethral gland (line 12). **Ejaculation** (e-jak″u-la′shən) is the expulsion of semen (se′mən) from the urethra.

12-68 The **penis** (pe′nis), the male organ for copulation, transfers sperm to the vagina. The combining form pen(o) means penis. **Pen/ile** means pertaining to the penis.

The conical tip of the penis is the **glans penis.** Write the combining form that means glans penis: _____.

balan(o)

Sexual intercourse refers to physical contact involving stimulation of the genitals between persons of the same or opposite gender. However, the medical definition of **copulation** (kop″u-la′shən), also called **coitus** (ko′ĭ-təs) (Latin: *coitio,* a coming together, meeting), is sexual union between male and female during which the penis is inserted into the vagina.

coitus

Write this word that means the same as copulation: _____.

12-69 In labeling Figure 12-19, you read that the scrotum is a pouch of loose skin that contains the two testes and their accessory organs. The combining form scrot(o) means scrotum. Use the suffix -al to write a term that means pertaining to the scrotum: _____.

scrotal (skro′təl)

Four combining forms are used to write words about the testes: orchi(o), orchid(o), test(o), and testicul(o). **Testicul/ar** (tes-tik′u-lər) means pertaining to a _____, but most diagnostic and surgical terms will use either orchi(o) or orchid(o). Practice in later frames will help you remember which combining form to use.

testicle or testis

The combining form epididym(o) means epididymis.

12-70 Each testicle is suspended in the scrotum by the spermat/ic cord, which is made up of arteries, veins, lymphatic vessels, nerves, and the ductus deferens. **Spermatic** (spər-mat′ik) has two meanings, either pertaining to _____ or pertaining to semen.

sperm

prostatic (pros-tat´ik)

12-71 The ductus deferens is a long duct that begins at the epididymis, enters the abdominal cavity, and connects with other structures of the internal reproductive tract. The combining form for ductus deferens is vas(o), which also means vessel. It will mean the ductus deferens most of the time in this chapter.

The combining form prostat(o) means the prostate. Using the suffix -ic, write a term that means pertaining to the prostate: _____.

The prostate, the **seminal vesicles,** and the bulbourethral glands produce fluids that contribute to the semen and are necessary for the survival of the sperm. Semen is the secretion of the male reproductive organs that is discharged from the **urethra** (u-re´thrə) during ejaculation.

seminal

Combine semin(o) and -al to write a word that means pertaining to semen: _____.

EXERCISE 12

Write the meaning of the following combining forms.

1. epididym(o) _____
2. orchi(o) _____
3. rect(o) _____

4. urethr(o) _____
5. vas(o) _____

EXERCISE 13

Write adjectives (words that mean pertaining to) for these structures.

1. penis _____
2. prostate _____
3. scrotum _____

4. semen _____ (or spermatic)
5. testicle _____

SPERMATOGENESIS

production
(or formation)

12-72 Each testis is capable of producing sperm and male hormones. **Spermato/genesis** (sper″mə-to-jen´ə-sis) is the _____ of mature, functional sperm capable of participating in conception, the union of a sperm with an ovum.

12-73 Sperm production requires a temperature slightly lower than normal body temperature. Because the scrotum is outside the body cavity, it provides the proper environment.

The testes are paired oval glands. In Figure 12-20, *A,* note that a testis is divided into several compartments called lobules, and each lobule contains convoluted **seminiferous** (sem″ĭ-nif´ər-əs) **tubules.** Sperm are produced in these tubules. Lying just posterior to the testis is the epididymis, where sperm are stored until they are released. The duct leading from the epididymis is the vas

deferens

_____.

A cross-section of a seminiferous tubule (Figure 12-20, *B*) shows that seminiferous tubules are surrounded by cells called **interstitial cells of Leydig.** These cells produce a major male sex hormone, **testosterone** (tes-tos´tə-rōn).

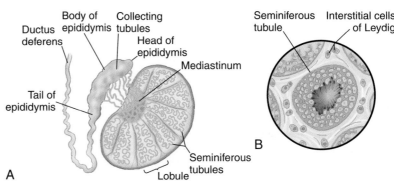

Figure 12-20 Sectional view of a testis. A, Each testis has about 250 lobules that contain as many as four seminiferous tubules where sperm are produced. **B,** Cross-section of a seminiferous tubule. The tubule is surrounded by interstitial cells, which are responsible for the production of testosterone.

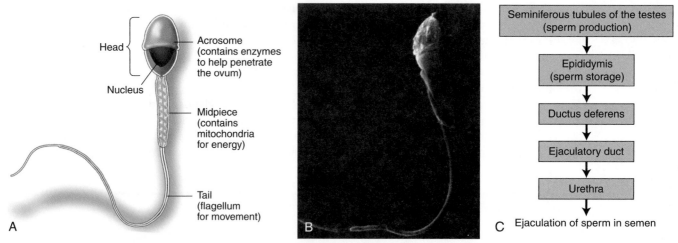

A

B

C Ejaculation of sperm in semen

Figure 12-21 The human spermatozoon and passageway of sperm. A, A sperm in cross-section. The nucleus contains the chromosomes and is located in the head. The tip of the head is covered by an acrosome, which contains enzymes that help the sperm penetrate the ovum. The midpiece contains mitochondria that provide energy, and the tail is a typical flagellum. **B,** Spermatozoon as seen using a scanning electron microscope. **C,** The passage of sperm from where they are produced in the testes to ejaculation in semen.

spermatozoon

12-74 Sperm are produced within the seminiferous tubules. In the development of mature sperm, early spermatocytes (spər-mat´o-sītz) undergo a process called meiosis, which eventually results in mature, functional spermatozoa (Figure 12-21 *A, B*). Write the singular form of spermatozoa: _____.

There are usually millions of sperm each time semen is ejaculated, and although only one sperm fertilizes an ovum, it takes millions of sperm to ensure that fertilization will take place. Be sure you understand the route of sperm from the time of production to when they are ejaculated in semen (Figure 12-21, *C*).

12-75 The hypothalamus in the brain, the pituitary gland, and the testes produce hormones that influence spermatogenesis (Figure 12-22).

FSH and testosterone produced by the testes stimulate spermatogenesis. LH acts on interstitial cells in the testes to produce testosterone. Testosterone also brings about male secondary sex

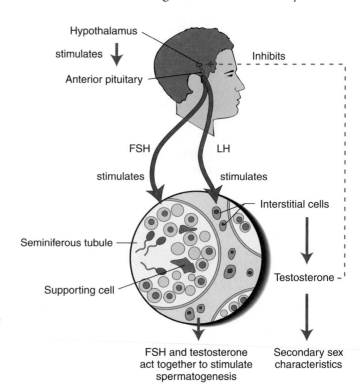

Figure 12-22 Hormonal control of the testes. The hypothalamus produces hormones that stimulate the anterior pituitary to produce follicle-stimulating hormone (FSH) and luteinizing hormone (LH). Luteinizing hormone stimulates the interstitial cells of the testes to secrete testosterone. Acting together, FSH and testosterone stimulate spermatogenesis.

characteristics—for example, enlarging of the sex organs, distribution of hair, deepening of the voice, and increased muscular development. Write the name of this hormone, which is often called the masculinizing hormone: _____.

testosterone

12-76 Spermatogenesis begins at puberty and normally continues throughout life, showing a decline in later years. **Semen,** also called seminal fluid, is a mixture of sperm cells and secretions from the accessory glands (prostate, seminal vesicles, and bulbourethral glands). The combining form semin(o) means semen. Write the other name for semen that uses this combining form: _____ fluid.

seminal

EXERCISE 14

Write a term in each blank.

1. The production of sperm is called _____.

2. The structure that is responsible for sperm production is the _____.

3. Sperm are produced within the _____ tubules.

4. The major male sex hormone produced by the testicles is _____.

5. Two important hormones that stimulate sperm production are follicle-stimulating hormone and _____ hormone.

Say and Check

Say aloud the terms you wrote for Exercise 14. Use the Companion CD to check your pronunciations.

DIAGNOSTIC TESTS AND PROCEDURES

12-77 Three important parts of a routine examination of the male genitalia are inspection of the external genitalia, palpation for inguinal hernias, and examination of the rectum digitally.

The external genitalia are examined for the descent and size of the testicles, abnormalities of the scrotum and penis, and the presence of urethral discharge. **Urethr/al discharge** means secretions from the _____. Smears of the secretions are stained and examined microscopically if gonorrhea is suspected. Material may be collected for bacterial or fungal culture.

urethra

Lesions or ulcers on the penis may indicate a sexually transmitted disease such as genital herpes, which produces blisters, or a **chancre,** a lesion that indicates the first stage of syphilis. The VDRL and the RPR tests are blood tests to detect and monitor syphilis.

12-78 Remember from a previous chapter that palpation is a technique in which the examiner uses the _____ to feel the size and location of internal structures. An inguinal hernia is one in which a loop of intestine enters the inguinal canal, the passageway in the lower muscular layers of the abdominal wall that is a common site for hernias. An inguinal hernia in a male sometimes fills the entire scrotal sac.

hands

12-79 The digital rectal examination is an assessment of the prostate gland and the _____. The examiner inserts a lubricated, gloved finger (a digit—hence, the name of the procedure) into the rectum, and the size and consistency of the prostate gland are assessed.

rectum

12-80 The **prostate-specific antigen** (PSA) test is a blood test used to screen for prostatic cancer and to monitor the patient's response to treatment. Elevated PSA levels are associated with prostatic cancer.

The antigen that is a tumor marker for prostatic cancer is called _____ -specific antigen.

prostate

testicles

12-81 Testicular self-examination is a procedure recommended by the National Institutes of Health (NIH) for detecting tumors or other abnormalities of the _____.
The presence of swelling or a small lump on either testicle should be reported to one's physician.

12-82 Needle biopsy of the prostate is generally performed if cancer of the prostate is suspected. In a needle biopsy a small amount of tissue is removed using a needle inserted from the outside. In this case the needle is inserted through the rectal mucosa to the prostate. Cyto/logy is performed on the tissue, examining the cells microscopically for the presence of cancer cells.

cells

Cyto/logy is the study of _____.

12-83 The sperm count is a test for male fertility. In a sperm count the number, appearance, and motility of the sperm in a collected sample of semen are examined. The test that evaluates the

sperm

number and health of spermatozoa is called a _____ count.

EXERCISE 15

Match the diagnostic tests in the left columns with their descriptions in the right column.

_____ 1. needle biopsy   _____ 3. RPR   A. blood test for prostatic cancer
                                                                B. blood test for syphilis
_____ 2. PSA   _____ 4. sperm count   C. removal of tissue for microscopic study
                                                                D. test of semen

PATHOLOGIES

12-84 Uro/logy (u-rol´ə-je) is the branch of medicine that specializes in the male and female urinary tract and also includes male reproductive structures.

    Statistically testicular cancer occurs most often in younger men, and prostatic cancer is common in older men. Which type of cancer is more common in younger men?

testicular

_____ cancer

    Learn these word parts that are used to describe pathologies of the male reproductive system.

Word Parts: Male Reproductive Pathologies

Word Parts	Meaning
crypt(o)	hidden
olig(o)	few
varic(o)	twisted and swollen

12-85 Torsion means twisting. Torsion of the testis, axial rotation of the spermatic cord, cuts off the blood supply to the testicle and can lead to loss of the testicle. Surgical correction within a few hours of the injury is required in most cases to save the testicle. Torsion of the testicle can

testicular

also be called _____ **torsion.**

12-86 **Oligo/sperm/ia** (ol″ĭ-go-spur´me-ə) means insufficient sperm in the semen. **A/spermia**

absence

(ə-spər´me-ə) or **a/spermato/genesis** (ə-spur″mə-to-jen´ə-sis) is _____
of sperm. **A/zoo/spermia** (a-zo″ə-spur´mə-ə) is absence of living sperm. Literal interpretation of the word parts of azoospermia is that a- means not, zo(o) means animal, and spermia means a condition of the sperm. But you need to remember that azoospermia means the absence of

living

_____ sperm.

    In addition to sufficient numbers, sperm must be actively motile and live long enough to reach the ovum. There are many causes of infertility besides insufficient sperm; therefore it is best that the partners be treated together.

12-87 **Erection** is the condition of swelling, rigidity, and elevation of the penis, and to a lesser degree in the clitoris of the female, caused by sexual arousal. It can also occur during sleep. Erection is necessary for the introduction of the penis into the vagina and for the emission of semen.

The inability to achieve penile erection, alternating periods of normal function and dysfunction, or inability to ejaculate after achieving an erection is called **erectile dysfunction,** also known as male impotence.

Poor health, certain drugs, fatigue, and vascular problems can cause sexual dysfunction. Males can often be treated medically or by changing the drugs that are causing erectile

dysfunction

_____.

12-88 The production of sperm outside the body cavity is necessary for the production of viable sperm. The testes develop in the abdominal cavity of the fetus and normally descend through the inguinal canal into the scrotum shortly before birth (sometimes shortly after birth). This provides a temperature about 3° F below normal body temperature.

Crypt/orchid/ism (krip-tor´kĭ-diz″əm) is a developmental defect characterized by the failure of one or both testes to descend into the scrotum (Figure 12-23). The combining form crypt(o) means hidden. The "o" in crypt(o) is usually omitted when the word part is joined to a combining form that begins with a vowel. Translated literally, crypt/orchid/ism means a condition of

hidden

_____ testicle or testes.

Cryptorchidism is the same as undescended testicle. If the testes do not descend spontaneously or with hormonal injections, surgery is usually performed. Write the word that means the same as undescended testicle: _____.

cryptorchidism

12-89 **Test/algia** (tes-tal´jə), **orchi/algia** (or″ke-al´jə), and **orchid/algia** (or″kĭ-dal´jə) mean testicular _____.

pain
orchiopathy
(or″ke-op´ə-the)

Write a word using orchi(o) that means any disease of the testes: _____.

Both **anorchidism** (an-or´kĭ-diz″əm) and **an/orchism** (an-or´kiz-əm) mean a congenital absence of the testis, which may occur unilaterally or bilaterally.

Both **orchiditis** (or″kĭ-di´tis) and **orchitis** (or-ki´tis) mean _____ of a testis, marked by pain, swelling, and a feeling of weight.

inflammation

12-90 **Epididym/itis** (ep″ĭ-did″ə-mi´tis) is inflammation of the _____.

Orchi/epididymitis (or″ke-ep″ĭ-did″ĭ-mi´tis) is inflammation of a testicle and its epididymis.

epididymis

12-91 Several less severe problems occur within the scrotum, including hydrocele, spermatocele, and varicocele. You have learned that -cele means hernia, but in these three terms -cele is used to mean a swelling. See Figure 12-24 for these three disorders as well as testicular torsion.

A **hydro/cele** (hi´dro-sēl) is a mass, usually filled with a straw-colored fluid. For this reason, its name incorporates the combining form hydr(o), which means _____. In this term, hydr(o) may help you remember that the swelling contains a straw-colored fluid. A hydrocele in the scrotum may be the result of orchitis, epididymitis, or venous or lymphatic obstruction.

water

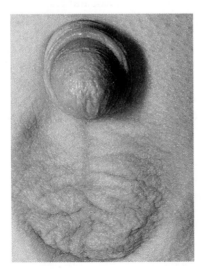

Figure 12-23 Cryptorchidism. In this illustration both testes have failed to descend into the scrotum. If the testes do not descend spontaneously, hormonal injections may be given. If injections are unsuccessful, surgery is usually performed before age 3.

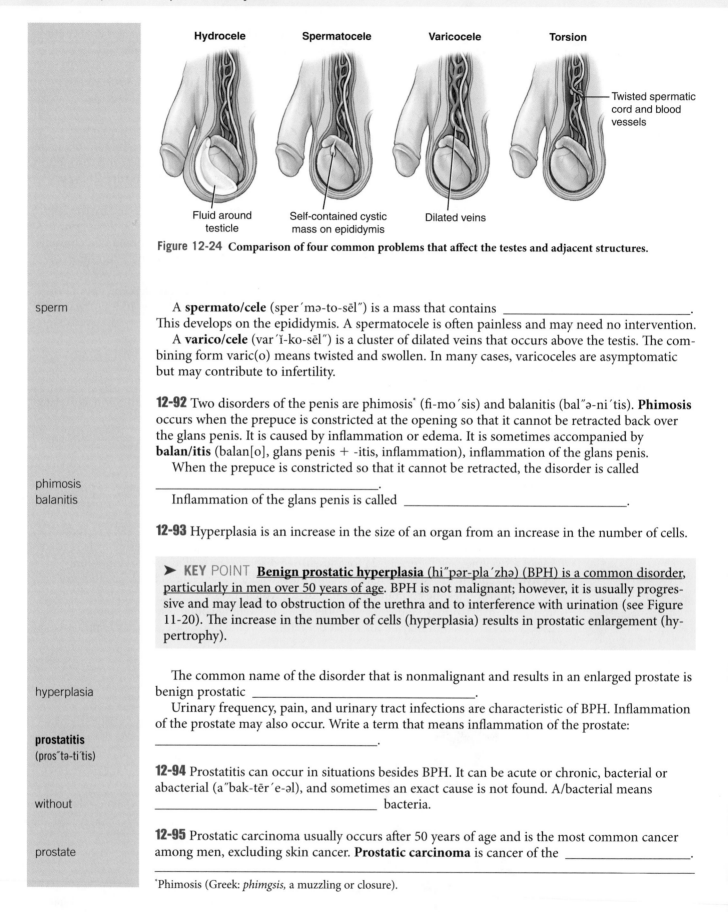

Hydrocele **Spermatocele** **Varicocele** **Torsion**

Twisted spermatic cord and blood vessels

Fluid around testicle

Self-contained cystic mass on epididymis

Dilated veins

Figure 12-24 Comparison of four common problems that affect the testes and adjacent structures.

sperm

A **spermato/cele** (sper´mə-to-sēl″) is a mass that contains _____. This develops on the epididymis. A spermatocele is often painless and may need no intervention.

A **varico/cele** (var´ĭ-ko-sēl″) is a cluster of dilated veins that occurs above the testis. The combining form varic(o) means twisted and swollen. In many cases, varicoceles are asymptomatic but may contribute to infertility.

12-92 Two disorders of the penis are phimosis* (fi-mo´sis) and balanitis (bal″ə-ni´tis). **Phimosis** occurs when the prepuce is constricted at the opening so that it cannot be retracted back over the glans penis. It is caused by inflammation or edema. It is sometimes accompanied by **balan/itis** (balan[o], glans penis + -itis, inflammation), inflammation of the glans penis.

When the prepuce is constricted so that it cannot be retracted, the disorder is called

phimosis
balanitis

_____.

Inflammation of the glans penis is called _____.

12-93 Hyperplasia is an increase in the size of an organ from an increase in the number of cells.

> ➤ KEY POINT <u>Benign prostatic hyperplasia (hi″pər-pla´zhə) (BPH) is a common disorder,</u> <u>particularly in men over 50 years of age.</u> BPH is not malignant; however, it is usually progressive and may lead to obstruction of the urethra and to interference with urination (see Figure 11-20). The increase in the number of cells (hyperplasia) results in prostatic enlargement (hypertrophy).

hyperplasia

The common name of the disorder that is nonmalignant and results in an enlarged prostate is benign prostatic _____.

Urinary frequency, pain, and urinary tract infections are characteristic of BPH. Inflammation of the prostate may also occur. Write a term that means inflammation of the prostate:

prostatitis
(pros″tə-ti´tis)

_____.

12-94 Prostatitis can occur in situations besides BPH. It can be acute or chronic, bacterial or abacterial (a″bak-tēr´e-əl), and sometimes an exact cause is not found. A/bacterial means

without

_____ bacteria.

12-95 Prostatic carcinoma usually occurs after 50 years of age and is the most common cancer among men, excluding skin cancer. **Prostatic carcinoma** is cancer of the _____.

prostate

---

*Phimosis (Greek: *phimgsis,* a muzzling or closure).

EXERCISE 16

Write a word in each blank to complete the sentences.

1. The branch of medicine that specializes in the male and female urinary tract and also includes male reproductive

   structures is _____.

2. Axial rotation of the spermatic cord is testicular _____.

3. Insufficient sperm in the semen is _____.

4. A developmental defect characterized by the failure of one or both testes to descend into the scrotum is

   _____.

5. Inflammation of the epididymis is _____.

6. A mass in the scrotum that contains straw-colored fluid is called _____.

7. A cluster of dilated veins above the testis is _____.

8. Tightness of the prepuce that prevents the retraction of the foreskin over the glans penis is

   _____.

9. Inflammation of the glans penis is _____.

10. A nonmalignant increase in the size of the prostate is benign prostatic _____.

Say and Check

Say aloud the terms you wrote for Exercise 16. Use the Companion CD to check your pronunciations.

EXERCISE 17

Word Analysis. *Break these words into their component parts by placing a slash between the word parts. Write the meaning of each term.*

1. azoospermia   _____

2. orchidalgia   _____

3. prostatitis   _____

4. anorchism   _____

5. hypertrophy   _____

SURGICAL AND THERAPEUTIC INTERVENTIONS

excision

12-96 Testicular cancer is often curable. Some men choose semen storage as soon as possible after diagnosis. Semen storage is a special processing, freezing, and storage of sperm by a sperm bank for future use. Depending on the type of cancer, chemo/therapeutic agents may save the testis. Otherwise, orchi/ectomy may be necessary. **Orchi/ectomy** is _____ of the testis. Removal of both testes results in infertility. Radiation therapy is sometimes used after surgery.

Stem-cell transplantation is sometimes used after high-dose chemotherapy. In stem-cell transplantation, the patient's stem cells are removed from the bone marrow and preserved by freezing for later transplantation.

orchioplasty
(or′ke-o-plas′te)

12-97 When torsion, twisting of the spermatic cord, has occurred, loss of blood supply to a testicle for more than a few hours will result in deterioration of the testicle. Surgical correction soon after the injury is important to prevent loss of the testicle. Write a term using orchi(o) that means surgical repair of a testicle: _____.

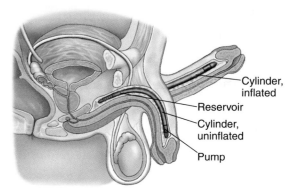

Figure 12-25 A penile prosthesis. One of several types of prostheses, this self-contained type consists of a pump, a cylinder filled with fluid, and a reservoir, all in one unit. The patient squeezes the pump just below the head of the penis to fill the cylinder and achieve erection. When an erection is no longer desired, the patient presses a release valve located behind the pump.

Cylinder, inflated
Reservoir
Cylinder, uninflated
Pump

Orchio/tomy (or″ke-ot′ə-me) is incision (and drainage) of a testis. **Orchio/rrhaphy** (or″ke-or′ə-fe) is suture of a testicle.

12-98 Drugs such as sildenafil (Viagra) or tadalafil (Cialis) are used to treat erectile dysfunction, particularly when the problem is inability to sustain an erection.

In some cases, treatment may include correction of the cause of the problem, such as restoration of the flow of blood to the penis or modification of medications that interfere with sexual activity. Surgical treatment includes injections and surgical implantation of a **penile prosthesis** (pros-the′sis). The term prosthesis means an artificial replacement for a body part (for example, an artificial arm or leg) or a device designed to improve function (for example, a hearing aid). The prosthesis that is designed to treat an erectile dysfunction is called a _____ prosthesis (Figure 12-25).

penile

12-99 **Orchio/pexy** (or′ke-o-pek″se) is corrective surgery for cryptorchidism. Orchiopexy, sometimes called **orchidopexy** (or′kĭ-do-pek″se), is the attachment of the previously undescended testis to the wall of the scrotum.

12-100 A hydrocele in a newborn may resolve spontaneously. In an adult a hydrocele may become large and uncomfortable and require surgical incision of the scrotum and removal of the hydrocele, because aspiration of the fluid with a needle is a temporary measure and may induce infection.

A **hydrocel/ectomy** (hi″dro-se-lek′tə-me) is surgical removal of a _____.

hydrocele

12-101 The tightness of the prepuce in phimosis can usually be corrected by circumcision (sur″kəm-sizh′ən). **Circumcision** is surgical removal of the end of the prepuce and is commonly performed on the male infant at birth. Write this term that means surgical removal of the end of the prepuce: _____.

circumcision

12-102 In prostatitis, inflammation is often the result of infection and is treated with antibiotics. When the prostate gland is so enlarged (BPH) that it interferes with urination or causes frequent infection, a **transurethral resection prostatectomy** or transurethral resection of the prostate (TURP) may be necessary. A trans/urethral resection is a surgical procedure that is performed through the _____. In a TURP, small pieces of the enlarged prostate are excised (see Figure 11-26).

urethra

Several less invasive technologies are available for treatment of obstructive BPH, particularly in the early stages of the disease. **Transurethral microwave thermo/therapy** (TUMT) uses microwave energy to raise the temperature of the prostatic tissue, and **transurethral needle ablation** (TUNA) uses low-level radio frequency energy. **Ablation** (ab-la′shən) means removal or excision of a growth on any part of the body. In both of these procedures, the heat causes necrosis and death of the prostatic tissue, thus relieving the obstruction. Because trans/urethral is part of their names, you know that the procedures are performed through the _____.

urethra

A variety of laser procedures are available, sometimes referred to as laser prostatectomy.

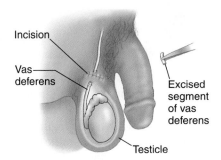

Incision

Vas deferens

Excised segment of vas deferens

Testicle

Figure 12-26 Vasectomy. This elective surgical procedure is performed as a permanent method of contraception (although it sometimes can be surgically reversed). It can be performed under local anesthesia. A small incision is made in the scrotum, and a piece of the vas deferens is removed.

excision

12-103 There are several treatments for prostatic (pros-tat´ik) carcinoma, including radiation, hormonal therapy, and prostatectomy (pros˝tə-tek´tə-me). A **prostat/ectomy** is _____ of all or part of the prostate gland.

excision

incision

12-104 A **vas/ectomy** (və-sek´tə-me) is _____ of a portion of the vas deferens (Figure 12-26). Bilateral vasectomy results in sterility.
   Vaso/tomy (va-zot´ə-me) is _____ of the vas deferens. A **vasostomy** (va-zos´, vas-os´tə-me) is surgical formation of a new opening into the vas deferens, but the term is sometimes used as a synonym for vasotomy.
   A **vaso/vaso/stomy** (vas˝o, va˝zo-va-zos´tə-me) can sometimes be used to correct an obstruction or to restore the severed ends of the vas deferens. The latter procedure is used to reverse a vasectomy.

EXERCISE 18

Match the procedures listed in the left columns with their descriptions in the right column.

_____ 1. chemotherapy   _____ 5. orchioplasty
_____ 2. circumcision   _____ 6. penile prosthesis
_____ 3. orchiectomy   _____ 7. TURP
_____ 4. orchiopexy   _____ 8. vasectomy

A. chemical treatment for cancer
B. removal of small pieces of the prostate via the urethra
C. surgical repair of a testicle
D. surgical excision of a testicle
E. surgical fixation of a testicle
F. surgical implantation to correct erectile dysfunction
G. surgical removal of the end of the prepuce
H. surgical excision of a portion of the vas deferens

EXERCISE 19

Build It! *Use the following word parts to build terms. (Some word parts will be used more than once.)*

trans-, orchi/o, prostat/o, urethr/o, vas/o, -al, -ectomy, -stomy, -tomy

1. incision of a testis   _____/_____

2. creation of a new opening in the vas deferens   _____/_____

3. pertaining to through the urethra   _____/_____/_____

4. surgical excision of the prostate gland   _____/_____

Say and Check

Say aloud the terms you wrote for Exercise 19. Use the Companion CD to check your pronunciations.

CHAPTER ABBREVIATIONS*

BPH	benign prostatic hyperplasia	PID	pelvic inflammatory disease
Cx	cervix	PMS	premenstrual syndrome
D&C	dilation and curettage	PSA	prostate-specific antigen
FSH	follicle-stimulating hormone	RPR	rapid plasma reagin test (for syphilis)
GU	genitourinary	STD	sexually transmitted disease
GYN, Gyn, gyn	gynecology	TAH	total abdominal hysterectomy
hCG, HCG	human chorionic gonadotropin	TSS	toxic shock syndrome
HRT	hormone replacement therapy	TUMT	transurethral microwave thermotherapy
LH	luteinizing hormone	TUNA	transurethral needle ablation
LMP	last menstrual period	TURP	transurethral resection of the prostate
NIH	National Institutes of Health	VDRL	Venereal Disease Research Laboratories
Pap	Papanicolaou smear, stain, or test		

*Many of these abbreviations share their meanings with other terms.

▶ CHAPTER 12 REVIEW

Basic Understanding

Labeling

I. *Label the diagram with the following combining forms that correspond to numbered lines 1 through 5 (the first one is done as an example):* cervic(o), colp(o), hyster(o), oophor(o), salping(o).

1. *oophor(o)*

2. _____

3. _____

4. _____

5. _____

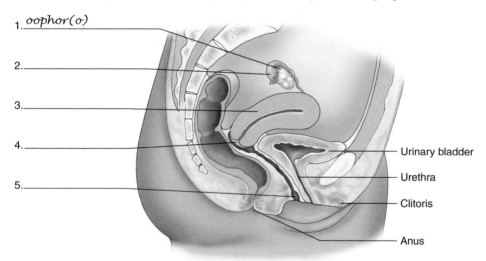

Urinary bladder

Urethra

Clitoris

Anus

II. *Label the diagram with the following combining forms that correspond to numbered lines 1 through 7 (the first one is done as an example):* epididym(o), orchi(o), pen(o), prostat(o), scrot(o), urethr(o), vas(o).

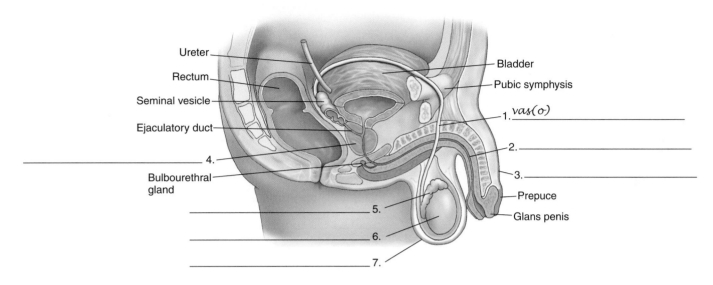

Matching

III. *Names of the three types of uterine tissue are in the left column. Match them with their locations in the uterus (A through C):*

_____ 1. endometrium

_____ 2. myometrium

_____ 3. perimetrium

A. innermost
B. middle
C. outermost

IV. *Match terms in the left columns with descriptions in the right column. (Selections A through F may be used more than once.)*

_____ 1. ovary

_____ 2. ovum

_____ 3. sperm

_____ 4. testis

_____ 5. uterus

_____ 6. uterine tube

_____ 7. vagina

A. gonad
B. female sex cell
C. male sex cell
D. normal site of implantation
E. receives the sperm during intercourse
F. usual site of fertilization

Photo ID

V. *Label the illustrations using word parts you have learned.*

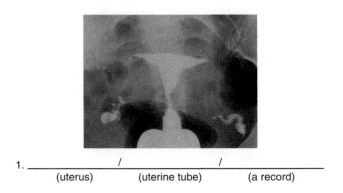

1. _____ / _____ / _____
   (uterus)   (uterine tube)   (a record)

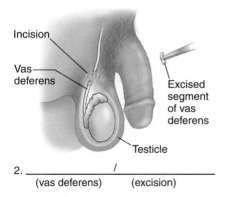

2. _____ / _____
   (vas deferens)   (excision)

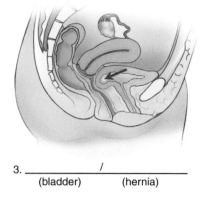

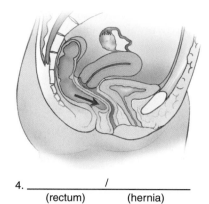

3. _____ / _____
   (bladder)   (hernia)

4. _____ / _____
   (rectum)   (hernia)

Word Analysis

VI. *Divide the following words into their component parts, and write the meaning of each term.*

1. hysteroscope _____

2. salpingitis _____

3. oophorectomy _____

4. spermatogenesis _____

5. vasovasostomy _____

Multiple Choice

VII. *Circle one answer for each of the following questions.*

1. Which term means difficult or painful menstruation? (amenorrhea, dysmenorrhea, metrorrhagia, menorrhea)

2. Which of the following instruments is commonly used in a gynecologic examination?
   (curet, hysterosalpingograph, hysteroscope, speculum)

3. Which examination of the abdominal cavity uses an instrument that is inserted through one or more small incisions in the abdominal wall? (dilation and curettage, hysteroscopy, laparoscopy, ultrasonography)

4. Which term means inflammation of an ovary? (cervicitis, oophoritis, salpingitis, vulvitis)

5. Which term means the first occurrence of menstruation? (amenorrhea, dysmenorrhea, menarche, mittelschmerz)

6. Which term means surgical fixation of a prolapsed uterus?
   (cervicectomy, hysterectomy, hysteropexy, leiomyomectomy)

7. Which term means a white, viscid discharge from the vagina and uterine cavity?
   (leukorrhea, occult blood, mittelschmerz, trichomoniasis)

8. Which term means a condition in which tissue that contains typical endometrial elements is present outside the uterus? (endometriosis, endometritis, hysteropathy, salpingopathy)

9. Which term means surgical repair of the vagina? (colpectomy, colpoplasty, colporrhaphy, oophorectomy)

10. Which term means absence of a testis? (anorchidism, aspermia, oligospermia, orchidectomy)

11. Which of the following results is expected following a bilateral vasectomy?
    (impotence, increased PSA, oligospermia, sterility)

12. What is surgically removed in a circumcision? (glans penis, prepuce, prostate, testes)

13. What is a term for undescended testicle? (cryptorchidism, orchidism, orchidorrhaphy, testalgia)

14. What is the term for twisting of the spermatic cord that results in cutting off the blood supply to the testicle?
    (hydrocele, spermatocele, torsion, varicocele)

15. Which term means testicular pain? (orchialgia, orchidism, orchiopathy, orchiotomy)

Fill in the Blanks

VIII. *Write a word in each blank to complete this paragraph.*

The female reproductive cycle is composed of two cycles that occur simultaneously. The

(1) _____ cycle reflects the changes that occur in the ovaries. The changes in the

ovarian follicle are called follicle development, (2) _____ , and the corpus luteal

stage. Two important hormones secreted by the follicles are (3) _____ and pro-

gesterone. The (4) _____ cycle is also called the menstrual cycle. In this cycle,

the endometrium thickens and prepares for a developing embryo. If fertilization does not occur, the endometrial lining

is shed, a process that is called (5) _____ .

Labeling

IX. *The following diagrams represent displacements of the uterus. Label each as anteflexion, anteversion, retroflexion, or retroversion.*

1._____   2._____   3._____   4._____

Writing Terms

X. *Write a term for each of the following phrases.*

1. excision of the uterus   _____

2. heavy or long menstrual periods   _____

3. herniation of a fallopian tube   _____

4. incision of the vas deferens   _____

5. inflammation of the cervix uteri   _____

6. inflammation of the vulva and vagina   _____

7. insufficient sperm in the semen   _____

8. surgical fixation of a fallopian tube   _____

9. viewing the vagina and cervix with magnification   _____

10. excision of the prostate   _____

Say and Check

Say aloud the terms you wrote for Exercise X. Use the Companion CD to check your pronunciations.

Greater Comprehension

Pronunciation

XI. *The pronunciation is shown for several medical words. Indicate which syllable has the primary accent by marking it with an ´.*

1. perimetrium (per ĭ me tre əm)

2. perineum (per ĭ ne əm)

3. progesterone (pro jes tə rōn)

4. testicular (tes tik u lər)

5. spermatogenesis (sper mə to jen ə sis)

 Say and Check

Say aloud the five terms in Exercise XI. Use the Companion CD to check your pronunciations. In addition, be prepared to pronounce aloud these terms in class:

cauterization	human chorionic gonadotropin	menorrhagia	perineal
cervicocolpitis	hydrocelectomy	mittelschmerz	seminiferous tubule
colpocystitis	hysterosalpingography	oligospermia	spermatozoon
dilation and curettage	hysteroscopy	oophorosalpingectomy	transurethreal needle ablation
endometrial biopsy	menarche	penile prosthesis	uterine leiomyoma

Health Care Reports

XII. *Read the following history and physical report and answer the questions.*

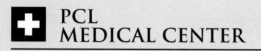 **PCL MEDICAL CENTER**

7700 Lexicon Way
St. Louis, MO 63146

Phone (555) 437-0000 • Fax (555) 437-0001

PREADMISSION HISTORY AND PHYSICAL EXAM

Patient Name: Joan Martin   **DOB:** 5/21/----   **Date of Exam:** Jul 22, ----

HISTORY: This 32-year-old black woman complains of low back and pelvic pain. No history of uterine pathology. She has midline pelvic pain as well as low back pain. Denies dysuria, urgency, or frequency of urination. No unusual vaginal bleeding or other GYN complaints. Hysteroscopy showed no uterine pathology. Low-grade temperature. Completed a 7-day cycle of Cipro with no relief. UA negative.

ALLERGIES: Penicillin

PAST MEDICAL HISTORY: Carcinoma of the right breast 2 years ago with lymphadenopathy. Lumpectomy done at that time. Left ovarian cyst with oophorectomy. D&C last year.

GYNECOLOGIC HISTORY: Gravida 2, para 2. Menarche at age 13, LMP 6/20/——, WNL.

LABS: Admission CBC, chem panel, chest x-ray to be done stat.

PHYSICAL EXAMINATION: Vitals show temp of 99.8. Chest: Lungs clear to auscultation bilaterally. Heart: RRR. Abdominal exam: Tender over midpelvis. Bowel sounds present. Vaginal exam: Deferred owing to pain.

IMPRESSION: Endometritis

PLAN: Admit for triple IV antibiotics ×5 days; control pain; consider for possible repeat D&C. Set up consult with patient's Hem/Onc physician.

Emma Stevens, MD

Emma Stevens, MD
Obstetrics/Gynecology

ES:pai
D: Jul 22, ----
T: Jul 22, ----

Circle the correct answer for each of these questions.

1. This patient's history indicates removal of which organ? (breast, ovary, uterus, vagina)

2. Hysteroscopy is direct visualization of which organ? (breast, ovary, uterus, vagina)

3. Endometritis is inflammation of which of the following? (inner lining of the uterus, lower part of the uterus, muscle of the uterus, outer layer of the uterus)

Write the meaning of these abbreviations:

4. D&C   _____

5. LMP   _____

6. GYN   _____

7. Hem/Onc   _____

XIII. *Read the following history and physical report, and define the terms that are underlined.*

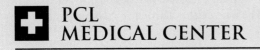

PCL MEDICAL CENTER

7700 Lexicon Way
St. Louis, MO 63146

Phone (555) 437-0000 • Fax (555) 437-0001

PREADMISSION HISTORY AND PHYSICAL EXAM

Patient Name: Mary Lou Garcia   **DOB:** 16/Nov ----   **Date of Exam:** Jun 7, ----

CHIEF COMPLAINT: Pelvic pressure

HISTORY: This 61-year-old Hispanic woman, gravida 6, para 5, abortus 1, is experiencing pelvic pressure. She is status post <u>ectopic pregnancy</u>, <u>vaginal hysterectomy</u>, and bilateral <u>oophorosalpingectomy</u>.

FAMILY HISTORY: Mother deceased at age 68 with history of carcinoma of the cervix with metastasis to the colon. Father age 85 with high blood pressure and <u>benign prostatic hyperplasia</u>. Married with five children, all L&W.

PHYSICAL EXAM: Bladder, rectum, and part of colon herniating into vagina with vagina prolapsing

LAB WORK: Admission CBC, chem panel, chest x-ray stat

DIAGNOSIS: <u>Cystocele</u>, <u>rectocele</u>, and <u>vaginal prolapse</u>

PLAN: patient to be admitted for surgery, to include cystocele and rectocele repairs, <u>perineoplasty</u>, and <u>colpopexy</u>. Will call admitting office first thing tomorrow morning.

Define:

1. ectopic pregnancy   _____

2. vaginal hysterectomy   _____

3. oophorosalpingectomy   _____

4. benign prostatic hyperplasia _____

5. cystocele   _____

6. rectocele   _____

7. vaginal prolapse   _____

8. perineoplasty   _____

9. colpopexy   _____

XIV. Read the following partial report of an emergency department record, and define the terms that are indicated.

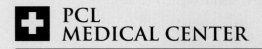

PCL
MEDICAL CENTER

7700 Lexicon Way
St. Louis, MO 63146

Phone (555) 437-0000 • Fax (555) 437-0001

EMERGENCY DEPARTMENT RECORD

Patient Name: George L. White   **ID No.:** 012-0003   **Date:** Jun 18, ----
CHIEF COMPLAINT: Penile discharge
HISTORY OF PRESENT ILLNESS: This 19-year-old white male Airman states that approximately 2 or 3 days ago he was masturbating and noticed a brownish discoloration to his ejaculate. Patient states this was not painful, and he knows of no history of prior incidences of this; however, he does state that when he came into basic training in late April or early May he was diagnosed with *Chlamydia* and was given azithromycin for that. Patient states he was given no other antibiotics to include no other antibiotic injections and no other medication at that time. He completed his course of azithromycin and had no follow-up. Patient states that he has had no dysuria, hematuria, abdominal pain, testicular pain, or penile discharge with the exception of that noted above. No dysuria, hematuria, back pain, fevers, chills, or rashes. Patient states he was sexually active before coming into the military, but he has not been sexually active since April or May.

Define:

1. ejaculate _____

2. testicular _____

3. penile _____

Spelling
XV. *Circle all misspelled terms and write their correct spelling.*

colpectomy   displasia   ginecology   salpingorhaphy   seminiferous

Interpreting Abbreviations
XVI. *Write the meanings of these abbreviations.*

1. BPH   _____

2. FSH   _____

3. HCG   _____

4. Pap   _____

5. TUNA   _____

Categorizing Terms
XVII. *Classify the terms in the left columns (1 through 10) by selecting A, B, C, D, or E from the right column.*

_____ 1. anorchidism   _____ 6. orchidalgia   A. anatomy
                                                        B. diagnostic test or procedure
_____ 2. balanitis   _____ 7. scrotum   C. pathology
_____ 3. colpodynia   _____ 8. speculum   D. surgery
                                                        E. therapy
_____ 4. curettage   _____ 9. tubal ligation

_____ 5. hysterosalpingography   _____ 10. vestibule

Challenge

XVIII. *Break these words into their component parts and write their meanings. Even if you haven't seen the terms before, you may be able to break them apart and determine their meanings.*

1. balanoplasty _____

2. epididymoorchitis _____

3. gonadal shield _____

4. leiomyofibroma _____

5. oosperm _____

(Use Appendix VI to check your answers.)

PRONUNCIATION LIST

Use the Companion CD to review the terms that have been presented. Look closely at the spelling of each term as it is pronounced and be sure you know the meaning of each term.

abdominal hysterectomy	colporrhaphy	genitourinary	metritis
ablation	colposcope	glans penis	metrorrhagia
amenorrhea	colposcopy	gonad	mittelschmerz
anorchidism	condyloma acuminatum	gonadotropin	mons pubis
anorchism	contraceptives	gonorrhea	myometritis
anovulation	copulation	graafian follicles	myometrium
anteflexion	corpus luteum	gynecologic	oligospermia
anteversion	cryosurgery	gynecology	oogenesis
aspermatogenesis	cryotherapy	human chorionic gonado-	oophoralgia
aspermia	cryptorchidism	tropin	oophorectomy
azoospermia	curet	hydrocele	oophoritis
balanitis	cystocele	hydrocelectomy	oophoropathy
Bartholin gland	cytology	hysterectomy	oophoropexy
benign prostatic hyperplasia	dilation and curettage	hysteropathy	oophorosalpingectomy
bulbourethral gland	ductus deferens	hysteropexy	oophorosalpingitis
candidiasis	dysmenorrhea	hysteroptosis	orchialgia
cauterization	dysplasia	hysterosalpingogram	orchidalgia
cauterize	ectopic pregnancy	hysterosalpingography	orchiditis
cervical biopsy	ejaculation	hysteroscope	orchidopexy
cervical polyp	ejaculatory duct	hysteroscopy	orchiectomy
cervicitis	endometrial biopsy	interstitial cells of Leydig	orchiepididymitis
cervicocolpitis	endometriosis	labia majora	orchiopathy
cervix	endometritis	labia minora	orchiopexy
cervix uteri	endometrium	laparohysterectomy	orchioplasty
chancre	epididymis	laparoscope	orchiorrhaphy
circumcision	epididymitis	laparoscopic oophorectomy	orchiotomy
climacteric	erectile dysfunction	laparoscopy	orchitis
clitoris	erection	leukorrhea	ova
coitus	estrogen	luteinizing hormone	ovarian
colpectomy	fallopian tube	menarche	ovarian cancer
colpitis	fimbria	menopause	ovarian cyst
colpocystitis	fistula	menorrhagia	ovary
colpodynia	follicle-stimulating	menorrhea	ovulation
colpohysterectomy	hormone	menses	Pap smear
colpoplasty	fundus	menstrual cycle	Papanicolaou test
colporrhagia	genitalia	menstruation	paraurethral gland

pelvic exenteration
pelvic inflammatory
   disease
penile
penile prosthesis
penis
perimetrium
perineal
perineum
phimosis
polycystic ovary syndrome
premenstrual syndrome
prepuce
progesterone
prostate
prostate-specific antigen
prostatectomy
prostatic
prostatic carcinoma
prostatitis
puberty
rapid plasma reagin test
rectocele

rectovaginal
retroflexion
retroversion
salpingectomy
salpingitis
salpingo-oophorectomy
salpingocele
salpingopexy
salpingorrhaphy
salpingostomy
scrotal
scrotum
semen
seminal
seminal vesicles
seminiferous tubule
spermatic
spermatocele
spermatogenesis
spermatozoon
syphilis
testalgia
testicular

testicular torsion
testis
testosterone
toxic shock syndrome
transurethral microwave
   thermotherapy
transurethral needle
   ablation
transurethral resection
   prostatectomy
Trichomonas
tubal ligation
tubal pregnancy
urethra
urethral discharge
urethrovaginal
urogenital
urology
uterine
uterine cancer
uterine displacement
uterine leiomyoma
uterine tube

uterus
vagina
vaginal
vaginal hysterectomy
vaginal speculum
vaginectomy
vaginitis
varicocele
vas deferens
vasectomy
vasostomy
vasotomy
vasovasostomy
vesicovaginal
vestibular glands
vestibule
visceral peritoneum
vulva
vulval
vulvar
vulvectomy
vulvitis
vulvovaginitis

Español ENHANCING SPANISH COMMUNICATION

English	Spanish (pronunciation)
circumcision	circuncisión (ser-coon-se-se-ON)
conception	concepción (con-sep-se-ON)
erection	erección (ay-rec-se-ON)
feminine	femenina (fay-may-NEE-na)
hormone	hormona (or-MOH-nah)
impotency	impotencia (im-po-TEN-se-ah)
intercourse, sexual	cópula (CO-poo-lah)
masculine	masculino (mas-coo-LEE-no)
menopause	menopausia (may-no-PAH-oo-se-ah)
menstruation	menstruación (mens-troo-ah-se-ON)
ovarian	ovárico (o-VAH-re-co)
ovary	ovario (o-VAH-re-o)
penis	pene (PAY-nay)
prostate	próstata (PROS-ta-tah)
prostatic	prostático (pros-TAH-te-co)
prostatitis	prostatitis (pros-ta-TEE-tis)
sexual	sexual (sex-soo-AHL)
testicle	testículo (tes-TEE-coo-lo)
uterus	útero (OO-tay-ro)
vagina	vagina (vah-HEE-nah)

Reproduction and Sexually Transmitted Diseases

Basic Understanding

In this chapter you will learn to do the following:

1. State the function of reproduction, and analyze associated terms.
2. Write the meaning of the word parts associated with reproduction, and use them to build and analyze terms.
3. Select the correct terms to match descriptions of fertilization, implantation, and growth of the embryo, and label the structures that surround the embryo.
4. Define or select the correct meaning of terms related to pregnancy, labor, and the newborn.
5. Write the names of the diagnostic tests and procedures used to monitor reproduction when given descriptions of the procedures, or match the procedures with their descriptions.
6. Write the names of reproductive pathologies when given their descriptions, or match them with their descriptions.
7. Match reproductive surgical and therapeutic interventions with descriptions of the interventions, or write the names of the interventions when given their descriptions.
8. Match sexually transmitted diseases with their characteristics, or write the names of the diseases when given their descriptions.

Greater Comprehension

9. Use word parts from this chapter to determine the meaning of terms in a health care report.
10. Spell the terms accurately.
11. Pronounce the terms correctly.
12. Write the meanings of the abbreviations.
13. Categorize terms as anatomy, diagnostic test or procedure, pathology, surgery, or therapy.

MAJOR SECTIONS OF THIS CHAPTER:

- ❑ **REPRODUCTION**
- ❑ **PREGNANCY AND CHILDBIRTH**
  Diagnostic Tests and Procedures
  Pathologies

Surgical and Therapeutic Interventions
- ❑ **SEXUALLY TRANSMITTED DISEASES**

FUNCTION FIRST

Sexual reproduction is the way in which genetic material is passed from one generation to the next. Sexually transmitted diseases are passed from one person to another by anal, oral, or vaginal contact, but some are transmitted by contact with contaminated materials. Sexually transmitted diseases may infect the fetus or the infant at birth.

REPRODUCTION

gonad

13-1 The **gonads** (go´nads), ovaries, and testes produce ova and sperm as well as hormones necessary for proper functioning of the reproductive organs. Write this term that means an organ that produces ova or sperm: _____.

ovum

13-2 A **gamete** (gam´ēt) is a reproductive cell (ovum or spermatozoon), and the union of the ovum and sperm is necessary in sexual reproduction to initiate the development of a new individual. The **ovum** (o´vəm), also called the egg, lives only a few days. The sperm have about the same time or less before they die after being discharged into the vagina. The gametes of reproduction are the _____ and the sperm.

13-3 **Ovulation** (ov″u-la´shən) is the release of an ovum from the ovary. Fertilization, or **conception,** is the union of the sperm cell nucleus with an egg cell nucleus. This usually occurs in the uterine tube.

The fertilized ovum undergoes a series of cell divisions as it moves along the uterine tube and then enters into the uterine cavity. About the seventh day after ovulation, the fertilized ovum attaches to the endometrium. This is called **implantation.**

uterus

The **endo/metr/ium** (endo-, inside + metr[o], uterine tissue + -ium, membrane) is the inner lining of the _____.

13-4 The product of fertilization is the **zygote** (zi´gōt), which undergoes rapid cell divisions. The zygote is known by different names at various stages. Some of these stages between fertilization and implantation are shown in Figure 13-1. The product of fertilization is called a

zygote

_____.

13-5 It is usually at the beginning of the third week that the developing offspring is called an embryo. It is during the embryonic stage that all the organ systems form, making this the most critical time in development. This is also when the extraembryonic (eks″trə-em″bre-on´ik) membranes form. Knowing that embryonic refers to the embryo, extra/embryonic means

outside

_____ the embryo. Look at Figure 13-2, and locate two **extraembryonic membranes,** the **amnion** (am´ne-on) and the **chorion** (kor´e-on), that surround the embryo. The amnion and chorion are membranes that provide protection by surrounding the embryo with amniotic fluid. Although **amnion/ic** (am″ne-on´ik) has the same meaning as **amniotic** (am″ne-ot´ik), the latter is more commonly used. The embryo is called a **fetus** after the eighth week. The combining form fet(o) means fetus, so **fet/al** means pertaining

fetus

to the _____.

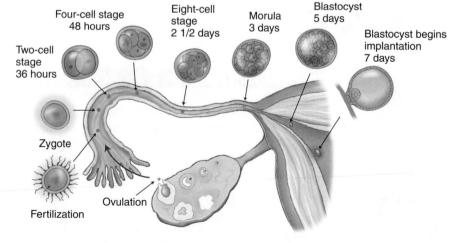

Figure 13-1 Fertilization, implantation, and growth of the embryo. A mature ovum is released in ovulation. The ovum is fertilized by a sperm, and the product of fertilization, the zygote, undergoes rapid cell division known by these stages: two-cell stage, four-cell stage, eight-cell stage, morula, and blastocyst. The blastocyst implants in the endometrium.

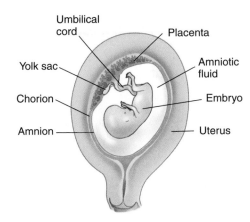

Figure 13-2 The embryo in utero at approximately 7 weeks. The placenta and extra-embryonic membranes (the amnion and the chorion) form and surround the embryo, providing nourishment and protection. The human embryonic stage begins about 2 weeks after conception and lasts until about the end of the eighth week, after which time the fetal stage begins.

Learn the following word parts and their meanings.

Principal Word Parts: Reproduction

Combining Forms	Meaning	Suffix	Meaning
amni(o)	amnion	-blast	embryonic or immature
chori(o)	chorion		
fet(o)	fetus		
gonad(o)	gonad		
o(o)	ovum		
spermat(o)	sperm		

ovum

13-6 The combining form o(o) means ovum. An **ooblast** (o´o-blast) is an immature _____. (The suffix -blast means embryonic or early form.)

sperm

13-7 Use spermat(o) to write terms about **spermatozoa** (sper″mə-to-zo´ə) or sperm. A **spermato/blast** (sper´mə-to-blast″) is an immature form of _____.

chorionic

amnion

13-8 Use chori(o) to write words about the chorion. Join chorion and -ic to write a word that means pertaining to the chorion: _____.
    Amnio/chorionic (am″ne-o-kor″e-on´ik) pertains to two membranes, the _____ and the chorion. **Amnio/chorial** (am″ne-o-kor´e-əl) is another word that means pertaining to the amnion and chorion.

13-9 The **placenta,** formed in the embryonic stage, is a highly vascular structure that nourishes the fetus.

> ➤ **KEY** POINT <u>Membranes normally keep the fetal and maternal blood from actually mixing.</u> Oxygen, nutrients, and antibodies diffuse from the mother to fetal blood vessels, and fetal wastes diffuse from the fetal blood into the maternal blood. Maternal means from the mother.

progesterone

The placenta also secretes large amounts of **progesterone** (pro-jes´tə-rōn), which is necessary for maintaining the uterus during pregnancy. The hormone that is responsible for maintaining the uterus throughout pregnancy is _____. Along with the placenta, the amnion and chorion are called the afterbirth and are shed shortly after birth.

Write a word in each blank space to complete these sentences.

1. An organ that produces ova or sperm is called a/an _____.

2. An ovum or sperm is called a/an _____.

3. The product of fertilization is called a/an _____.

4. The release of an ovum from the ovary is called _____.

5. Another name for fertilization is _____.

6. Attachment of the fertilized ovum to the endometrium is called _____.

7. After the eighth week, the developing individual is called a/an _____.

8. Two extraembryonic membranes are the amnion and the _____.

9. An embryonic sperm is called a/an _____.

10. The placenta secretes large amounts of the hormone _____, which is necessary for maintaining the uterus during pregnancy.

PREGNANCY AND CHILDBIRTH

parturition

13-10 **Pregnancy** is the process of growth and development of a new individual from conception through the embryonic and fetal periods to birth. The birth of the baby is **parturition** (pahr″tu-rĭ′shən). Write this term that means childbirth: _____.

obstetrics
(ob-stet′riks)

13-11 An **obstetrician** (ob″stə-trĭ′shən) specializes in _____, the medical specialty that is concerned with pregnancy and childbirth, and includes the time immediately after childbirth. OB is the abbreviation for obstetrics.

A nurse midwife has advanced education and clinical experience in obstetric care and care of the newborn. The nurse midwife manages care of women having a normal pregnancy, labor, and childbirth. A midwife is a person who assists women in childbirth.

Learn the meanings of the following terms.

Word Parts: Pregnancy and Childbirth

Combining Forms	Meaning	Suffixes	Meaning
nat(o)	birth	-cyesis	pregnancy
par(o)	bearing offspring	-gravida	pregnant female
Prefix	**Meaning**	-para	woman who has given birth
pseudo-	false	-tropin	that which stimulates

before

13-12 **Gestation** (jes-ta′shən) is another name for pregnancy. This is also called the prenatal (pre-na′təl) period. Knowing that nat(o) means birth, **pre/natal** is that time _____ birth.

You saw in the previous section that the developing human individual is called an embryo at the beginning of the third week. By the end of the eighth week after fertilization, the developing individual is called a fetus, because by this time there are recognizable human features. Look at the timetable of prenatal development (Figure 13-3) and see the age when different features are present. **Quickening,** the first recognizable movements of the fetus in the uterus, occurs at about 18 to 20 weeks in a first pregnancy and slightly sooner in later pregnancies.

13-13 The average period of gestation is about 266 days from the date of fertilization, but it is clinically considered to last 280 days from the first day of the last menstrual period (LMP). The expected date of delivery (EDD) is usually calculated on the latter basis.

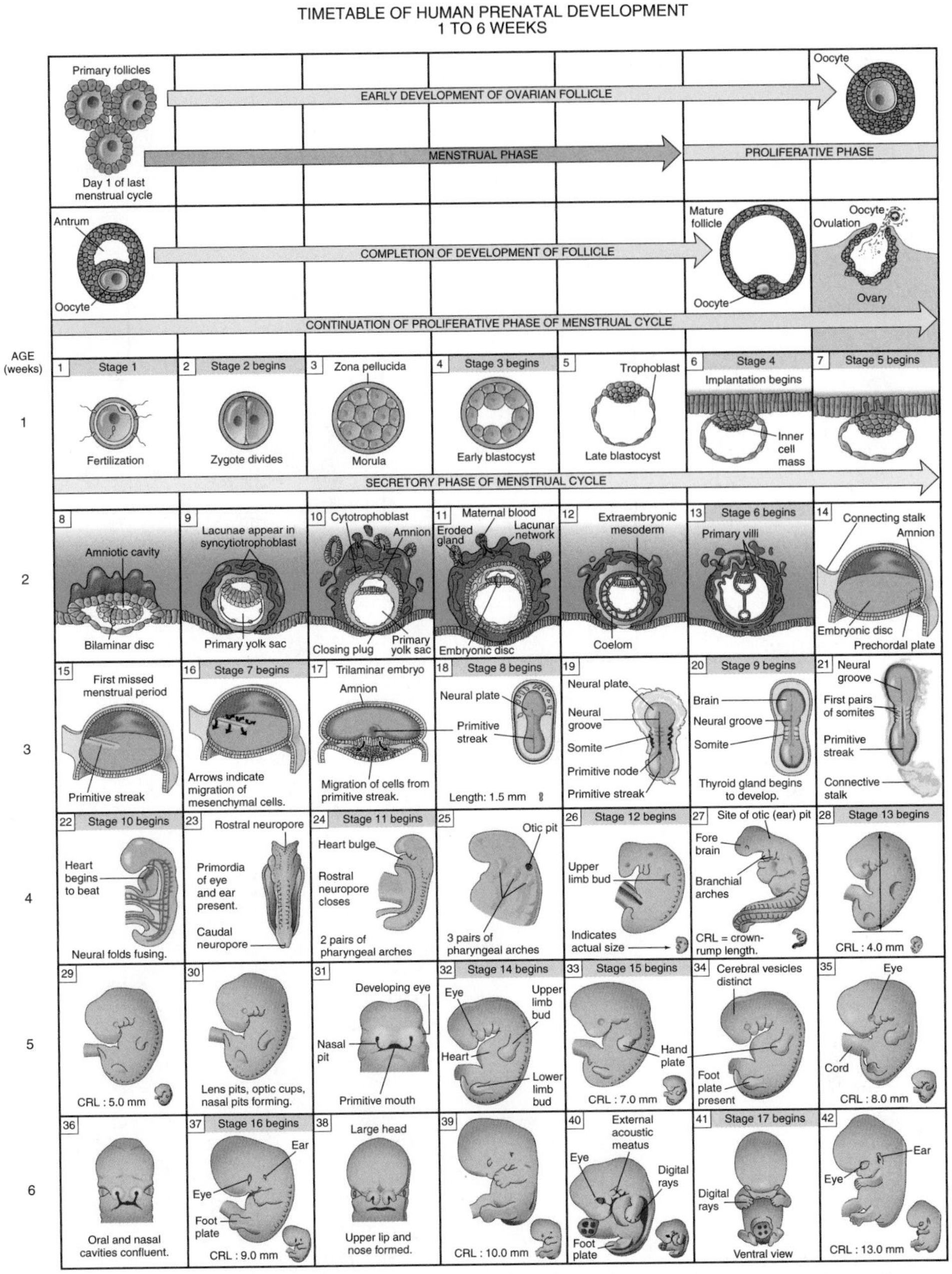

TIMETABLE OF HUMAN PRENATAL DEVELOPMENT
1 TO 6 WEEKS

Figure 13-3 Timetable of prenatal development. Several significant events in the process of growth, maturation, differentiation, and development are shown in the timetable: three germ layers develop; heart begins beating; fingers, eyelids, toes, and external genitalia are visible, and face has human appearance.

Continued

➤ **KEY** POINT For convenience, pregnancy is discussed in terms of the first, second, and third trimesters. A **trimester** is one of the three periods of approximately 3 months into which pregnancy is divided.

The time from the first day of the last menstrual period to the end of 12 weeks is the first

trimester _____.

13-14 Gravid (grav´id) means pregnant (G), and **gravida** (grav´ĭ-də) refers to a pregnant female.

pregnant If a female is gravid, she is _____.

The female may be identified more specifically as gravida I or 1, if pregnant for the first time,

second or gravida II or 2, if pregnant for the _____ time.

TIMETABLE OF HUMAN PRENATAL DEVELOPMENT
7 to 38 weeks

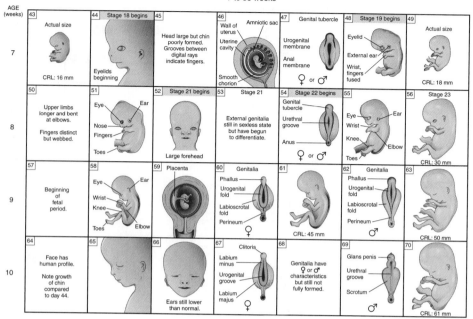

Eleventh Week to Full Term

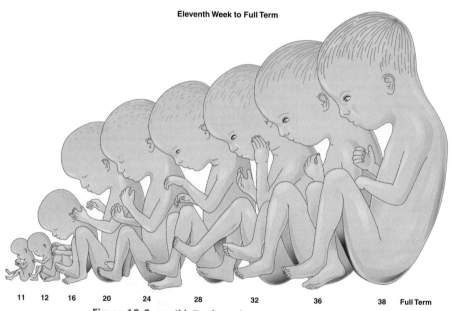

11 12 16 20 24 28 32 36 38 **Full Term**

Figure 13-3, cont'd For legend, see opposite page.

---

gravida 3 (or III)

A designation for a female who has been pregnant three times is _____.

13-15 The suffix -gravida also refers to a pregnant female and is combined with various prefixes that designate the number of pregnancies. Because the prefix primi- means first, a **primi/gravida** (pri″mĭ-grav´ĭ-də) is a female during her _____ pregnancy.

first

This is the same as gravida 1.

    The prefix multi- means many, and **multi/gravida** (mul″te-grav´ĭ-də) means a female who has been pregnant more than one time.

13-16 A term that is used for a female who has produced viable offspring is para. A **viable offspring** is defined as one that has reached a stage of development that it can live outside the uterus and usually means a fetus that weighs at least 500 grams (just over 1 pound) and has reached a gestational age of 24 weeks. The term is used with numerals to indicate the number of pregnancies carried to more than 20 weeks' gestation, such as para III or 3, indicating three pregnancies, regardless of the number of offspring produced in a single pregnancy or the number of stillbirths after 20 weeks.

The combining form par(o) means producing or bearing viable offspring. **Par/ous** (par´əs) refers to producing viable _____.

13-17 The suffix -para refers to a female who has given birth, specifically one who has produced viable offspring.

Determine the designation, para I or 1, para II or 2, or para III or 3, for the following females. In each case, the pregnancies lasted more than 20 weeks.

What is the para designation for a female who has one living child and has had no other pregnancies? _____

The para status of a female who has twins and has had no other pregnancies is para 1. What is the para status of a female who has four children that resulted from three pregnancies and has had no additional pregnancies? _____

13-18 A female who is designated as para 1 is also called a **primi/para** (pri-mip´ə-rə), which means that she has produced _____ viable offspring. (The number is implied from the prefix primi-, which means first.)

Because the number or prefix indicates how many pregnancies, a multiple birth counts as just one in the calculation. **Secundipara*** (se″kən-dip´ə-rə), or para 2, designates that a woman has had two pregnancies that produced viable offspring. Additional successful pregnancies are designated as **tripara** (trip´ə-rə) for _____ and **quadripara** (kwod-rip´ə-rə) for four successful pregnancies. The prefix quadri- means four.

The prefix nulli- refers to none. How many viable offspring have been produced by a **nulli/para** (nə-lip´ə-rə)? _____ This is the same as para 0. Translated literally, a **multi/para** (məl-tip´ə-rə) has produced many viable offspring, but the term is used to indicate a woman who has delivered more than one viable offspring.

13-19 Using -rrhexis, write a new word that means rupture of the amnion: _____. Amniorrhexis occurs before the child is born and sometimes is the mother's first sign of impending labor. The "water breaks" or the "bag of water breaks" are common sayings that mean **amniorrhexis.**

13-20 **Labor,** the process by which the child is expelled from the uterus, is that time from the beginning of cervical dilation to the delivery of the placenta. Look closely at the term dilation and its three-syllable pronunciation: di-la´shən. A synonym for dilation is **dilatation** (dil″ə-ta´shən). **Cervical dilation** is enlargement of the diameter of the opening of the uterine cervix in labor. The uterine cervix is the neck of the _____.

Dilatation is the condition of being dilated or stretched beyond the normal dimensions. Cervical dilatation is the dilation or stretching of the cervical opening. The shortening and thinning of the cervix during labor is called **effacement** (ə-fās´mənt). This term describes how the constrictive neck of the uterus is obliterated or effaced.

Shortening and thinning of the cervix during labor is called _____. When this occurs, the mucous plug that fills the cervical canal dislodges.

13-21 Labor may be divided into three (or sometimes four) stages: cervical dilatation, expulsion, placental, and postpartum (pōst-pahr´təm) stages (Figure 13-4). Not everyone recognizes the postpartum stage as a stage of labor, because it occurs after childbirth. The first stage (cervical dilatation) begins with the onset of regular uterine contractions and ends when the _____ opening is completely dilated.

The second stage **(expulsion)** extends from the end of the first stage until complete _____ of the infant. During this stage the amniotic sac ruptures if that has not occurred already.

The third stage, the **placental stage,** extends from the expulsion of the child until what structure and the membranes are expelled? _____

*Secundipara (Latin: *secundus,* following; *parere,* to bring forth).

Margin answer column (left):

offspring

para I or 1

para III or 3

one

three

zero

amniorrhexis
(am″ne-o-rek´sis)

uterus

effacement

cervical

expulsion

placenta

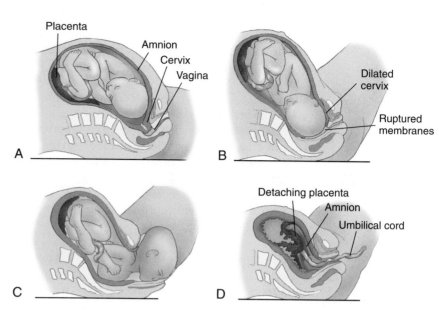

Figure 13-4 The fetus in utero before labor compared with three stages of labor. A, The normal position of the fetus shortly before labor begins. **B,** The first stage of labor (cervical dilatation) begins with the onset of regular uterine contractions and ends when the cervical opening is completely dilated. **C,** The second stage (expulsion) results in expulsion of the infant. **D,** The third stage (placental) ends when the placenta and membranes are expelled. A fourth stage (not shown) is sometimes identified as the hour or two after delivery, when uterine tone is established.

The fourth stage (**postpartum**) is the hour or two after delivery, when uterine tone is established. Study Figure 13-4 and try to determine the stage of labor for each drawing. Notice how the fetal head turns in order to pass through the vaginal opening. The fourth and final stage of labor is not shown.

13-22 The events just described are the stages of a vaginal delivery. A cesarean (sə-zar′e-ən) section or cesarean birth is performed when abnormal fetal or maternal conditions make vaginal delivery hazardous. A **cesarean section** (CS) is a surgical procedure in which the abdomen and uterus are incised and the baby is removed from the uterus. Write this term that means removing the baby from the uterus after incision of the abdomen and uterus: _____ birth.

cesarean

after

before

13-23 Post/partum means after childbirth because the prefix post- means _____.
You have learned that the prefixes ante- and pre- mean before. Prenatal and **ante/natal** (an″te-na′təl) both refer to the time _____ birth.
The prefix ante- is not always joined to the word, and sometimes there are two acceptable ways to write the same word. Either **antepartum** (an″te-pahr′təm) or ante partum is acceptable and means before _____.

parturition (childbirth)
birth

13-24 Postnatal (pōst-na′təl) means the time after _____.
The prefix neo- means new. A **neonate** (ne′o-nāt) is a newborn child. **Neo/natal** (ne″o-na′təl) is a specific term that refers to the period covering the first 28 days after birth. Neonatal also means pertaining to the newborn child. **Neonatology** (ne″o-na-tol′ə-je) is the branch of medicine that specializes in the care of the newborn. Write the term for a physician who specializes in neonatology: _____.

neonatologist (ne′o-na-tol′ ə-jist)

EXERCISE 2

Complete the table by writing a word part or its meaning in each blank.

Combining Form	Meaning	Suffixes	Meaning
1. _____	birth	4. -cyesis	_____
2. _____	bearing offspring	5. -gravida	_____
		6. -tropin	_____

Prefix	Meaning
3. pseudo-	_____

Word Analysis
Break these words into their component parts and write the meaning of each term.

1. postnatal _____

2. amniorrhexis _____

3. primigravida _____

4. quadripara _____

5. neonatologist _____

Say and Check
Say aloud the terms in Exercise 3. Use the Companion CD to check your pronunciations.

DIAGNOSTIC TESTS AND PROCEDURES

stimulates

13-25 Within a few days after conception, the chorion starts producing a hormone, **human chorionic gonadotropin** (go″nə-do-tro′pin) (HCG). Gonado/tropin means a substance (hormone) that _____ the gonads. HCG is present in body fluids (urine, blood) of pregnant females, and blood or urine is tested to determine if pregnancy exists (Figure 13-5). HCG can be detected long before other signs of pregnancy appear. The hormone that is tested for in pregnancy tests is HCG, or human chorionic _____.

gonadotropin

measurement

13-26 Literal translation of pelvi/metry (pel-vim′ə-tre) is _____ of the pelvis. This procedure is usually performed by the obstetrician during the first prenatal examination of a pregnant woman or may be used if problems arise during labor. Clinical **pelvimetry** is vaginal palpation of specific bony landmarks and is used to estimate the size of the birth canal.

A **cephalo/pelvic** (sef″ə-lo-pel′vik) **disproportion** (CPD) is a condition in which a baby's head is too large or the mother's birth canal is too small to permit normal labor or birth. If the disproportion is too great, a cesarean delivery will be necessary. X-ray pelvimetry can be performed but is not generally used because of the risk of radiation exposure to the fetus.

fetus

13-27 Other diagnostic tools, such as sonography, provide a great deal of information about the fetus with less apparent risk. Fetal sonography is a noninvasive procedure that is used to assess structural abnormalities and monitor development of the _____ (Figure 13-6). The gender of the fetus can sometimes be determined by sonography.

13-28 Amnio/centesis (amni[o], amnion + -centesis, surgical puncture) (am″ne-o-sen-te′sis) is a surgical procedure in which a needle is passed through the abdominal and uterine walls to obtain a small amount of amniotic fluid for laboratory analysis (Figure 13-7). The procedure is usually performed to aid in the assessment of fetal health and diagnosis of genetic defects or other abnormalities. Fetal cells in the fluid can be cultured (grown in the laboratory), and

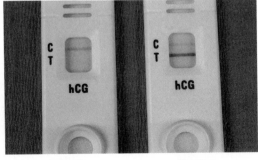

Negative   Positive

Figure 13-5 Urine pregnancy test. The positive test has a *red line* near the label hCG (human chorionic gonadotropin) and a *light blue line*. The negative test lacks the red band of color near the hCG.

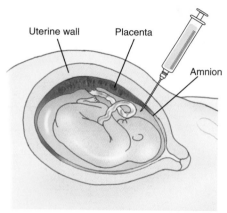

Figure 13-7 **Amniocentesis.** Transabdominal puncture of the amniotic sac is done to remove fluid for diagnostic study.

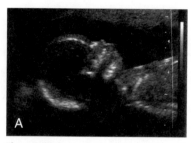

Figure 13-6 Ultrasound imaging of a fetus in the second trimester. **A,** Sonogram. **B,** Drawing.

amniocentesis

biochemical and cytologic studies may be performed. Write the name of this procedure in which a needle is passed trans/abdominally to collect amniotic fluid: _____.

13-29 Chorionic villi (vil´i) are the tiny finger-like projections of the chorion that infiltrate the endometrium and help form the placenta. **Chorionic villus sampling** is sampling of these villi (placental tissue) for prenatal diagnosis of potential genetic defects and is usually performed between the eighth and twelfth weeks of pregnancy (Figure 13-8). This test is called _____ villus sampling.

chorionic

13-30 Looking again at the information in Figure 13-3, see how early the heart begins to beat. A **feto/scope** (fe´to-skōp) is a stethoscope for assessing the fetal heart rate (FHR) through the mother's abdomen (Figure 13-9). It may be used during prenatal visits to the doctor and during labor, when it also gives information about uterine contractions. Write the name of this special type of stethoscope that is used to monitor the fetal heartbeat: _____.

fetoscope

13-31 An electronic fetal monitor (EFM) may be used during labor to monitor the fetal heart and record the fetal heart rate and the maternal uterine contractions. The EFM may be applied either internally or externally. EFM means an electronic _____ monitor.

fetal

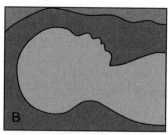

Figure 13-8 Chorionic villus sampling. Two types of chorionic tissue sampling are illustrated. One type of villus sample is obtained by insertion of a needle through the mother's abdominal and uterine walls. Another method is aspiration by catheter through the cervix. Both methods are performed using ultrasonic guidance.

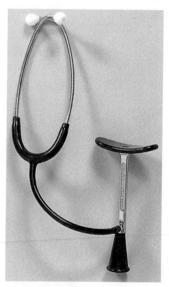

Figure 13-9 Fetoscope. A fetoscope is a special stethoscope for monitoring the fetal heartbeat.

Write a word in each blank to complete these sentences.

1. HCG is the hormone that is tested for in _____ tests.

2. An estimation of the size of the birth canal to determine if the baby's head is too large to permit normal birth is

   called _____.

3. Surgical puncture of the amnion to obtain amniotic fluid for testing is _____.

4. A sampling of placental tissue early in pregnancy to determine potential genetic defects is called

   _____ villus sampling.

5. A stethoscope for assessing the fetal heart rate is a/an _____.

PATHOLOGIES

13-32 Whenever a fertilized ovum implants anywhere other than the uterus, this is an **ectopic** (ek-top´ik) **pregnancy.** The prefix ecto- means situated on or outside. The combining form top(o) refers to place. When ecto- and top(o) are combined, as in ectopic, it means outside the usual place. If the ovum implants in a fallopian tube, this is called a tubal pregnancy or an

ectopic

_____ pregnancy.

13-33 An ectopic pregnancy could also be called an **extra/uterine** (eks″trə-u´tər-in) **pregnancy,** because extra- means outside. Extrauterine means pertaining to _____

outside

the uterus.

  Ectopic pregnancy implantation sites include various places in the uterine tube, the ovary, the cervix, and the abdominal cavity. Sonography and radiography are important in diagnosing these abnormal pregnancies, and the products of fertilization are removed by surgery.

13-34 The prefix pseudo- means false and -cyesis means pregnancy. **Pseudo/cyesis** (soo″do-si-e´sis) is a term for false _____. This is also called **pseudopregnancy**

pregnancy

(soo″do-preg´nən-se), in which certain signs and symptoms suggest pregnancy, such as the absence of menstruation. Pseudocyesis is the presence of one or more of these signs or symptoms when conception has not occurred. The condition may be psycho/genic, or it may be caused by a physical disorder.

13-35 **Pre/eclampsia** (pre″e-klamp´se-ə) is one of several complications of pregnancy. This condition is characterized by the onset of acute high blood pressure after the twenty-fourth week of gestation. **Protein/uria** (pro″te-nu´re-ə), protein in the urine, and edema may also be present. Write the name of this complication of pregnancy characterized by acute high blood pressure:

preeclampsia

_____.

  Preeclampsia may progress to **eclampsia** (ə-klamp´se-ə), the gravest form of pregnancy-induced high blood pressure. The latter, characterized by seizures, coma, high blood pressure, proteinuria, and edema, leads to convulsions and death if untreated.

13-36 A second complication of pregnancy is **abruptio placentae** (ab-rup´she-o plə-sen´te). This condition is a separation of the placenta from the uterine wall after 20 weeks or more or during labor, and it often results in severe hemorrhage. Fetal death results if there is complete separation of the placenta from the uterine wall, so cesarean sections are performed in severe cases. Labor and normal delivery may be possible if only partial separation exists. This complication of separation of

abruptio

the placenta from the uterine wall is called _____ placentae.

13-37 **Placenta previa** (pre´ve-ə) is a condition in which the placenta is implanted abnormally in the uterus so that it impinges on or covers the **internal os** (opening at the upper end of the uterine cervix). This is one of the most common reasons for painless bleeding in the last

Figure 13-10 Comparison of two complications of pregnancy. A, Abruptio placentae. Separation of the placenta implanted in a normal position in a pregnancy of 20 weeks or more, or during labor before delivery of the fetus. This causes severe maternal hemorrhage that may be evident externally *(as shown in this example),* or the hemorrhage may be concealed within the uterus. **B,** Placenta previa. Abnormal implantation of the placenta too low in the uterus. Even slight dilation of the cervical opening can cause separation of an abnormally implanted placenta. This is the most common cause of painless bleeding in the third trimester.

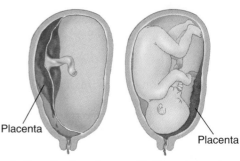

Placenta

Placenta

A. Abruptio placentae   **B.** Placenta previa

previa

trimester. Cesarean section is required if severe hemorrhage occurs. This condition in which the placenta is implanted abnormally in the uterus is called placentae, _____ _. Study Figure 13-10 and compare placenta previa with abruptio placentae, which was described in the previous frame.

stillbirth

13-38 Stillbirth is the birth of a fetus that died before or during delivery. A fetus that is born dead is also called a _____.

difficult

13-39 Abnormal or difficult labor is called **dystocia***. Literal translation of dys/tocia (dis-to´shə) is _____ labor. It may be caused either by an obstruction or constriction of the birth passage or by an abnormal shape, size, position, or condition of the fetus.

Down

13-40 One of the genetic disorders that can be detected by study of the amniotic fluid is **Down syndrome.** Patients with Down syndrome have an extra chromosome, usually number 21, and have moderate to severe mental retardation. This chromosomal aberration, also called trisomy 21 (tri- means three), is most often associated with late maternal age (Figure 13-11). The name of this genetic disorder, usually associated with trisomy of chromosome number 21, is _____ syndrome.

hemolytic

13-41 Another condition that may be diagnosed by means of amniocentesis is **hemolytic disease of the newborn,** an anemia of newborns characterized by premature destruction of red blood cells and resulting from maternal-fetal blood group incompatibility, especially involving the Rh factor and the ABO blood groups. In Rh incompatibility, the hemolytic reaction occurs because the mother is Rh negative and the infant is Rh positive. The name of the disease, _____ disease of the newborn, describes the destruction of the red blood cells. This is also called **erythro/blast/osis fetalis** (ə-rith″ro-blas-to´sis fĕ-tă´lis). An

*Dystocia (*dys-* + Greek: *tokos,* birth).

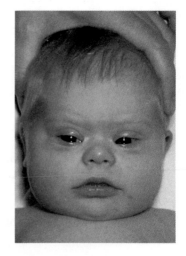

Figure 13-11 Typical facial characteristics of Down syndrome. This congenital condition, usually caused by an extra chromosome 21, is characterized by varying degrees of mental retardation and multiple defects. It can be diagnosed prenatally by amniocentesis. Infants with the syndrome generally have a small, flattened skull, flat-bridge nose, and eyes with the mongoloid slant shown here. Down syndrome was formerly called mongolism.

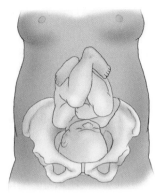 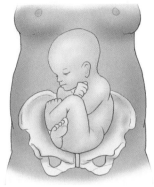 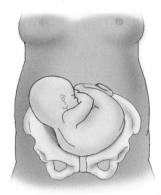

A   Normal presentation   **B**   Breech presentation   **C**   Shoulder presentation

Figure 13-12 Fetal presentation. A, Cephalic presentation, the normal presentation of the top of the head, the brow, the face, or the chin at the cervical opening. **B,** Breech presentation. **C,** Shoulder presentation.

erythro/blast (erythr[o], red + -blast, embryonic form) is an immature form of a red blood cell that is present in the blood of newborns with this type of anemia.

The first pregnancy usually does not present a serious problem, and complications in a future pregnancy can generally be prevented by injection of the mother shortly after delivery with RhoGAM or a similar immune globulin. Otherwise, abortion of an Rh positive fetus may occur.

When hemolytic disease of the newborn is suspected, prenatal diagnosis of the disease is confirmed by high levels of bilirubin in the amniotic fluid, obtained by amniocentesis. Intra/uterine transfusion or immediate exchange transfusions after birth may be necessary. Intra/uterine transfusion is transfusion of the fetus while it is still within the uterus. Another name for hemolytic disease of the newborn is _____ fetalis.

erythroblastosis

13-42 Fetal presentation describes the part of the fetus that is touched by the examining finger through the cervix or has entered the mother's lesser pelvis during labor. **Cephalic presentation** is expected, which means that the top of the head, the brow, the face, or the chin presents itself at the cervical opening during labor. To help you remember cephalic presentation, remember the meaning of cephalic, which is pertaining to the _____.

head

A **breech presentation** is one in which the buttocks, knees, or feet are presented. It occurs in approximately 3% of labors. Because the head is generally larger than the rest of the body, it may become trapped. If the buttocks or feet are felt by the examining finger during labor, it is called _____ presentation.

breech

Shoulder presentation is one in which the long axis of the baby's body is across the long axis of the mother's body, and the shoulder is presented at the cervical opening. This type of presentation is also called **transverse presentation.** Vaginal delivery is impossible unless the baby turns spontaneously or is turned in utero. Compare the different types of presentations shown in Figure 13-12.

EXERCISE 5

Match terms in the left columns with their descriptions in the right column.

_____ 1. abruptio placentae   _____ 4. placenta previa   A. abnormal or difficult labor
_____ 2. dystocia   _____ 5. pseudocyesis   B. false pregnancy
_____ 3. ectopic pregnancy   C. fertilized egg implants outside the uterus
                                                                   D. placenta covers the internal os
                                                                   E. separation of the placenta from the uterine wall

SURGICAL AND THERAPEUTIC INTERVENTIONS

amniotomy
(am″ne-ot′ə-me)

uterus

episiotomy

abdominal

laparorrhaphy
(lap″ə-ror′ə-fe)

against

mouth

uterus

sperm

13-43 The word for deliberate rupture of the fetal membranes to induce labor is translated literally as incision of the amnion. Write this new term: _____.

    Oxytocin (ok″se-to′sin) is a hormone that is produced by the pituitary gland and stimulates uterine contraction. Oxytocin (Pitocin is the trademark for the generic drug oxytocin) is also used as a drug to induce or augment uterine contractions. Other drugs, uterine relaxants, slow or stop labor by slowing or stopping contractions of the _____.

13-44 An episiotomy* (ə-piz″e-ot′o-me) facilitates delivery if the vaginal opening is too small. An **episio/tomy** is a surgical procedure in which an incision is made in the female perineum to enlarge the vaginal opening for delivery. The suffix -tomy will help you remember that an episiotomy involves an incision. Write this new term that means an incision that enlarges the vaginal opening to facilitate delivery: _____.

13-45 A **laparotomy** (lap″ə-rot′ə-me) is necessary in cesarean sections and in all other abdominal surgeries that require opening of the abdominal cavity. Because lapar(o) means abdominal wall, laparo/tomy is incision of the _____ wall.

    If the abdominal wall is incised, it must be sutured (or stapled). Suturing of the abdominal wall is _____.

13-46 A pregnant woman does not ovulate because high levels of estrogen and progesterone prevent ova from maturing. Knowledge of the interaction of hormones that prevent ovulation forms the basis of some types of contraception. Literal translation of contra/ception is _____ conception. In other words, **contraception** is birth control, a process or technique for preventing pregnancy.

13-47 **Contra/ceptives** diminish the likelihood of or prevent conception. Oral contraceptives, contraceptive implants, contraceptive patches, and injectable contraceptives are methods that use hormones to prevent ovulation. Oral contraceptive is what is meant when someone says she is "on the pill." The word oral in the name tells us that the medication is taken by _____.

13-48 An **intrauterine** (in″trə-u′tər-in) **device** (IUD) is inserted into the _____ by a physician (Figure 13-13). It can be removed when the woman wishes to become pregnant.

13-49 Sometimes sperm(i) is used instead of spermat(o) to write words about sperm. A **spermi/cide** (sper′mĭ-sīd) is a chemical substance that kills _____. Spermicides are placed in the vagina before intercourse to kill sperm, but they are not as effective as several other contraceptive methods. Spermicides are also used with other devices that are placed in the vagina to prevent sperm from reaching the uterus. Read about the different contraceptive methods in Table 13-1.

---

*Episiotomy (Greek: *epision*, pubic region + *-tomy*, incision).

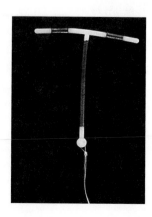

Figure 13-13 Intrauterine device (IUD) used to prevent pregnancy. There are several types, but these are essentially a bent strip of radiopaque plastic. Progesterone-filled IUDs are also available. The tail string of the IUD is left projecting a few centimeters from the cervix, so the person wearing it can feel the string with her finger to ensure the device is still in place. The string also provides a hold for removing the IUD.

TABLE 13-1	Selected Contraceptive Methods*	
Method	**Protection from STDs†**	**Action**
100% Effective		
Abstinence	Most successful	Refraining from sexual intercourse
Very Effective		
Injectable contraceptive	No	Hormonal injection on a specific schedule prevents ovulation
Implant (Norplant)	No	Capsules surgically implanted under the skin slowly release a hormone that blocks the release of ova
Contraceptive patch	No	Transdermal patch worn on the skin
Postcoital contraceptive	No	Pill that must be taken within 72 hours of unprotected intercourse
Effective		
Intrauterine device	No	Small plastic or metal device placed in the uterus; cause of effectiveness is not known but may prevent fertilization or implantation; some release hormones
Contraceptive patch	No	Skin patch that releases the hormones progestin and estrogen into the bloodstream
Oral contraceptives	No	Hormones, usually progestin and estrogen, which prevent ovulation
Vaginal contraceptive ring	No	Ring that is inserted into the vagina and releases progestin and estrogen; worn 3 weeks out of every 4 weeks
Less Effective		
Douche	No	Washing out the vagina immediately after intercourse
Spermicides	No	Vaginal foams, creams, or jellies that are inserted into the vagina before intercourse to destroy the sperm
Coitus interruptus	No	Withdrawal of the penis before ejaculation
Diaphragm with spermicide	No	Soft rubber cup that covers the uterine cervix and prevents sperm from reaching the egg
Condom	Male: fairly successful Female: less successful	Thin sheath (usually latex) worn over the penis or in the vagina to collect semen
Cervical cap with spermicide	No	Similar to diaphragm, but smaller and covers cervix closely
Sponge with spermicide	No	Acts as barrier to the sperm and releases spermicide
Calendar or rhythm method (periodic abstinence)	No	Determine fertile period and practice abstinence (voluntarily avoiding sexual intercourse) during "unsafe" days
Basal body temperature (BBT)	No	Ovulation is determined by drop and subsequent rise in BBT; abstinence is practiced during fertile periods
Cervical mucus	No	Ovulation is determined by observing the changes in the cervical mucus; abstinence is practiced during fertile period
Symptothermal	No	Combination of observing symptoms and increase in body temperature (cervical mucus and BBT); abstinence is practiced on fertile days

*Tubal ligation and vasectomy are not included here because they are forms of sterilization, often permanent.
†STD, Sexually transmitted disease.

Abstinence, refraining from sexual intercourse, is the only means of contraception that is 100% effective. **Coitus interruptus** (ko´ĭ-təs in˝tər-rup´təs) is withdrawal of the penis before ejaculation. Male **condoms** are informally called rubbers; there are also female condoms. A contraceptive **diaphragm** (di´ə-fram) (a molded rubber or other soft plastic material) is placed over the cervix uteri before intercourse. In periodic abstinence, sexual intercourse is avoided during what are considered unsafe days; this is sometimes called the rhythm method. Another version of periodic abstinence is **symptothermal** (simp˝to-thur´məl) abstinence, where abstinence is practiced on what are considered fertile days.

EXERCISE 6

Match the contraceptive methods in the left columns with their descriptions in the right column.

_____ 1. coitus interruptus   _____ 4. Norplant

_____ 2. condom   _____ 5. spermicide

_____ 3. diaphragm

A. rubber cup that covers the uterine cervix
B. thin sheath that collects semen
C. substance placed in the vagina to destroy the sperm
D. surgically implanted capsules that prevent ovulation
E. withdrawal of the penis before ejaculation

13-50 Tubal ligation (too´bəl li-ga´shən) and **vasectomy** (və-sek´tə-me) are sterilization procedures. Tubal ligation is one of several sterilization procedures accomplished by constricting, severing, or crushing both fallopian _____ (Figure 13-14).

tubes

> ➤ **KEY** POINT <u>Tubal ligation is generally done laparoscopically</u>. Many techniques are used for tubal ligation, all for the purpose of interrupting the continuity of the uterine tubes. A method of tying off a loop of uterine tube, cutting the loop in half, and burning or tying off the ends is sometimes done after a cesarean section when no more pregnancies are wanted. Burning to seal the cut ends of the tube is accomplished by several means, including laser and cauterization. Most tubal ligations are done laparoscopically, sometimes called the "belly button" surgery. In general, some combination of severing, burning, clips, or bands are used to close off the uterine tubes. A less common vaginal tubal ligation is performed through the vagina with a local anesthetic, and blocks the fallopian tubes from the inside. Although surgery to rejoin the separated ends of the uterine tubes by suture (**tubal ligation reversal**) is available, all methods of tubal ligation should be considered permanent means of sterilization, especially vaginal tubal ligation.

A vas/ectomy is bilateral excision of the vas deferens (vas def´ər-enz), the duct that transports sperm (see Figure 12-26). It also should be considered a permanent means of sterilization because it is not always reversible. The surgical procedure in which the function of the vas deferens on each side of the testes is restored after a vasectomy is a **vaso/vaso/stomy** (va˝zo-, vas˝o-va-zos´tə-me). Note that this term uses vas(o) twice. Write this term that means a surgical procedure that is used to reverse a vasectomy: _____.

vasovasostomy

Conception cannot occur after a hysterectomy (surgical removal of the uterus); however, hysterectomy is not done for the purpose of contraception.

13-51 Infertility is the condition of being unable to produce offspring. It may be present in one or both sex partners and may be temporary and reversible, as in the performance of a vasovasos-

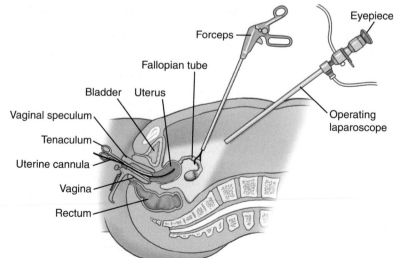

Figure 13-14 Laparoscopic tubal ligation. Both uterine tubes are blocked to prevent conception. A laparoscope is an illuminated tube with an optical system. Forceps are used to grasp the uterine tubes or other tissue. The vaginal speculum keeps the vaginal cavity open. The tenaculum is a hooklike instrument for seizing and holding the uterine cervix, and the uterine cannula is used to manipulate the uterus.

not

tomy. Administration of hormones, use of vaginal medications, surgery, and counseling are some of the treatments used in correcting infertility, depending on the cause. In/fertility is the condition of _____ being able to produce offspring.

In vitro fertilization (IVF) may be successful when failure to conceive is caused by insufficient numbers of sperm. In vitro fertilization is a method of fertilizing the ova outside the body by collecting mature ova and placing them in a dish with spermatozoa. Fertilized ova are then placed in the uterus for implantation.

abortion

13-52 Termination of pregnancy before the fetus is capable of survival outside the uterus is an **abortion.** In lay language, a spontaneous or natural loss of the fetus is called a miscarriage, and abortion most often refers to a deliberate interruption of pregnancy. In the medical sense, both spontaneous loss and deliberate interruption of pregnancy are called abortion. A miscarriage is a spontaneous _____.

EXERCISE 7

Write a word in each blank to complete these sentences.

1. Bilateral excision of the vas deferens is a/an _____.

2. Constricting, severing, or crushing the fallopian tubes is called a tubal _____.

3. In vitro _____ is a method of fertilizing the ova outside the body, then placing them in the uterus for implantation.

4. Termination of pregnancy before the fetus is capable of survival outside the uterus is a/an _____.

5. A surgical procedure to enlarge the vaginal opening for delivery is a/an _____.

EXERCISE 8

Build It! *Use the following word parts to build terms. (Some word parts will be used more than once.)*

amni(o), blast(o), erythr(o), lapar(o), -osis, -rrhaphy, -rrhexis, -tomy

1. incision into the abdomen   _____/_____

2. rupture of the inner membrane surrounding the fetus   _____/_____

3. condition of immature form of a red blood cell   _____/_____/_____

4. suturing of the abdominal wall   _____/_____

SEXUALLY TRANSMITTED DISEASES

sexually

13-53 Sexually transmitted diseases (STDs) are usually caused by infectious organisms that have been passed from one person to another through anal, oral, or vaginal intercourse. Abstinence is the only 100% reliable means of preventing infection with an STD by sexual activity. Latex condoms are the only other recommended means. Some of the organisms that cause STDs are transmitted only through sexual intercourse, but others are transmitted also by infected blood or needles, by intrauterine transmission to the fetus, or by infection of the infant during birth. STDs were formerly called **venereal** (və-nēr´e-əl) **diseases** (VDs), named for Venus, goddess of love. These diseases are now called _____ transmitted diseases. Most STDs start as lesions on the genitalia and other sexually exposed mucous membranes. A person who already has one STD can become infected with another STD. Different STDs are caused by specific types of viruses, bacteria, protozoa, fungi, and parasites. Without treatment, they can contribute to infertility, ectopic pregnancy, cancer, and death.

13-54 One sexually transmitted disease, gonorrhea, was discussed in Chapter 11, the Urinary System. **Gonorrhea** (gon[o], genitals + -rrhea, discharge) (gon″o-re′ə) is caused by the **gono/coccus** (gon″o-kok′əs) (GC), a gram-negative intracellular diplococcus. Intra/cellular means that the bacteria are located _____ the cells (in this case, white blood cells).

within

Gonorrhea causes a heavy urethral discharge in males, but females may be asymptomatic. See Figure 13-15 for a common sign of gonorrhea and a stained urethral smear that is indicative of the disease. The disease can usually be treated with penicillin or with another antibiotic in penicillin-sensitive persons.

13-55 Many of the words in the medical dictionary that begin with gon(o) pertain to the gono/coccus, the type of bacteria that causes gonorrhea.

Write the name of the microorganism that causes gonorrhea: _____.

gonococcus

The gonococcus that causes gonorrhea, *Neisseria gonorrhoeae,* is a bacterium. Gram stain is a special staining technique that serves as a primary means of identifying and classifying bacteria. The presence of gram-negative intracellular diplococci is generally followed by a bacterial culture to confirm that the organisms are gonococci. This technique of growing microorganisms, done for the purpose of identifying the pathogen, is called _____.

culturing

13-56 The origin of **syphilis** (sif′ĭ-lis) is not clear, but the disease occurred throughout Europe shortly after the return of Christopher Columbus and his crew from the New World in 1493. Write the name of this sexually transmitted disease: _____.

syphilis

The first stage of syphilis is characterized by swollen lymph nodes and the appearance of a painless sore called a **chancre** (shang′kər) (Figure 13-16). Do not confuse chancre with the word canker (kang′kər), which is an ulceration of the oral mucosa. The painless sore of syphilis that occurs usually on the genitals is called a _____.

chancre

Material from a chancre may be examined for the **spirochete** that causes syphilis (see Figure 4-13). Syphilis can be spread to another person through sexual contact.

13-57 If the disease is not treated with penicillin or another antibiotic, the second stage of syphilis occurs 2 weeks to 6 months after the chancre disappears. The results of blood tests for syphilis (Venereal Disease Research Laboratories [VDRL] or rapid plasma reagin [RPR] tests) are gener-

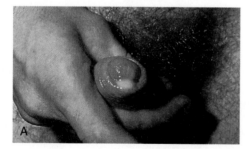
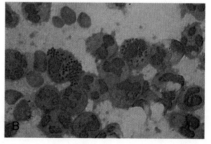

Figure 13-15 Gonorrhea and a stained smear that is indicative of the disease in a male. A, Gonococcal urethritis. Profuse, purulent drainage from the urethra. **B,** Gram-negative intracellular diplococci. The presence of gram-negative intracellular diplococci in a urethral smear is usually indicative of gonorrhea in males. The same finding in females is considered presumptive and is generally followed by culture to confirm the diagnosis. Note also the presence of many extracellular diplococci.

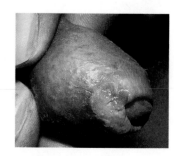

Figure 13-16 Syphilitic chancre. The lesion of primary syphilis generally occurs about two weeks after exposure. It is not commonly located on the glans penis but can be located on the foreskin. Scrapings from the ulcer show spirochetes, the causative organism of syphilis, when examined microscopically using dark-field illumination (see Figure 4-13).

rash

ally positive at this time but should be confirmed by additional tests. The disease becomes systemic as organisms spread throughout the body, and a generalized rash appears. It can affect many organs. The outward sign that is characteristic of the second stage of syphilis is the _____. The second stage lasts 2 to 6 weeks and is followed by a fairly asymptomatic latent stage. Transmission of the disease can occur by blood transfer to another person during the latent stage.

Only about one third of untreated individuals progress to the third stage, which has irreversible complications, including changes in the cardiovascular and nervous system and soft rubbery tumors, called **gummas** (gum´əz), on any part of the body.

13-58 Before the problems of the third stage of syphilis were recognized, some "psychotic" patients in mental hospitals may have been suffering from **neuro/syphilis** (noor″o-sif´ĭ-lis), a complication of late syphilis. Fever therapy (such as intentional infection with malaria, a disease characterized by chills and fever) was used to treat mental illness in past times. Syphilitic patients who were infected with malaria developed high fever and improved. The organisms that cause syphilis, like many others, are adversely affected by high temperatures (sometimes a rise of as little as only 1° or 2° F).

syphilis

13-59 Congenital syphilis is acquired by the fetus in utero. The bacteria that cause syphilis can cross the placenta of an infected female and cause congenital _____.
Infants who are born with congenital syphilis may have severe physical and mental defects and die within a few weeks after birth.

Several of the organisms that cause STDs can cross the placenta and infect the fetus, sometimes causing physical and mental defects or stillbirth. Others may infect the infant during childbirth. In the latter cases, a cesarean section is usually performed when the mother is known to be infected.

The stages of syphilis and information about additional STDs are summarized in Table 13-2.

13-60 Chlamydial (klə-mid´e-əl) infection, **chlamyd/iosis** (klə-mid″e-o´sis), is a treatable bacterial disease transmitted by intimate sexual contact and is the most common sexually transmitted disease in the United States. Antibiotics are used to treat chlamydiosis. Undetected and untreated cases can progress to scarring and ulcerations of the epididymis in males or the uterine tubes in females, causing infertility.

Read and answer questions about the characteristics of sexually transmitted diseases using the information in Table 13-2.

ulceration

13-61 Chancroid is another STD caused by a bacterium. As shown in the table, the major characteristic of chancroid (shang´kroid) is _____ of the genitals. Unlike the painless chancre of syphilis, the ulceration of chancroid is painful. Like other sexually transmitted diseases that are caused by bacteria, it can be treated with an antibiotic.

13-62 Nonspecific genital infections are caused by a variety of microorganisms. **Non/gonococcal urethritis** (u″rə-thri´tis) is inflammation of the urethra by an organism other than the gonococcus, the bacteria that causes _____.

gonorrhea

13-63 Four general types of viral STDs are acquired immunodeficiency (im″u-no-də-fish´ən-se) syndrome, genital herpes, genital warts, and several types of hepatitis (hep″ə-ti´tis).

immunodeficiency

The abbreviation AIDS means **acquired** _____ **syndrome.**
As a result of the deficiency of antibodies, the immune response does not adequately protect the person from malignancies or opportunistic infections, infections that are caused by normally nonpathogenic organisms in someone whose resistance is decreased.

AIDS is caused by the human immunodeficiency virus (HIV) and is spread by sexual intercourse or exposure to contaminated blood, semen, breast milk, or other body fluids of infected persons. The virus has a long incubation period (time between exposure and the onset of symptoms), and the disease we recognize as AIDS is the late, fatal stage of infection. Some persons with AIDS are susceptible to opportunistic infections and malignant neoplasms (tumors), especially **Kaposi sarcoma** (kah´po-she, kap´o-se, sahr-ko´mə) (Figure 13-17).

TABLE 13-2	Sexually Transmitted Diseases and Their Causes	
Disease of the Genitals*	**Causative Agent**	**Characteristics**
Bacterial		
Gonorrhea	*Neisseria gonorrhoeae*	Males: Urethral discharge, dysuria Females: Often asymptomatic
Syphilis	*Treponema pallidum* (a spirochete)	Primary stage: painless chancre Secondary stage: Rash Late: Only about one third of untreated cases progress to syphilitic involvement of the viscera, the cardiovascular system, and the central nervous system
Chlamydial infection	*Chlamydia trachomatis*	Males: Urethritis, dysuria, and frequent urination Females: Mild symptoms to none; one of the most common STDs in North America, often the cause of pelvic inflammatory disease, and a common cause of sterility
Chancroid (nonsyphilitic venereal ulcer)	*Haemophilus ducreyi*	Painful ulceration of the genitals
Nonspecific genital infection	Various organisms, not all of which are bacteria	Males: Nongonococcal urethritis Females: Pelvic inflammatory disease, cervicitis
Viral		
Acquired immunodeficiency syndrome	Human immunodeficiency virus	A fatal late stage of infection with HIV that involves profound immunosuppression. To be diagnosed as having AIDS, one must be infected with HIV and have a clinical disease that indicates cellular immunodeficiency or have a specified level of CD4 and T-lymphocytes (T4). Characterized by opportunistic infections and malignant neoplasms that rarely affect healthy individuals, especially Kaposi sarcoma. Transmitted by infected body fluids (sexual contact, blood and blood products, breast milk).
Herpes genitalis (genital herpes)	Herpes simplex virus type 2 (HSV-2)	Blisters and ulceration of the genitalia, fever, and dysuria
Condyloma acuminatum (genital warts)	Human papillomavirus (HPV)	Cauliflowerlike genital and anal warts; infection puts females at high risk for cervical cancer; a vaccine that prevents infection with the two types of HPV responsible for most cervical cancer cases is available
Hepatitis B	Hepatitis B virus (HBV)	Disease varies from mild symptoms to serious complications; transmitted by contaminated blood or needles and sexual contact (hepatitis B vaccine is available for those at high risk; HBIG, hepatitis B immune globulin, provides postexposure passive immunity)
Hepatitis C	Hepatitis C virus (HCV)	Symptoms are generally mild; about 50% of patients progress to chronic hepatitis; transmitted mainly by blood products, sharing needles or straws for inhaling cocaine; transmitted less commonly by sexual intercourse
Hepatitis D	Hepatitis D virus (HDV)	Occurs only in patients infected with HBV; usually develops into a chronic state; transmitted through sexual contact and needle sharing; prevention of hepatitis B with vaccine prevents hepatitis D
Protozoal		
Trichomoniasis	*Trichomonas vaginalis*	Females: Frothy discharge of varying severity Males: Often asymptomatic
Fungal		
Candidiasis	*Candida albicans*	Vulvovaginitis: White patches, cheeselike discharge
Parasitic		
Pubic lice	*Phthirus pubis*	Severe itching and erythema

*Although diseases of the genitals are given emphasis here, many of the organisms can infect other organs.

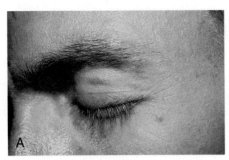
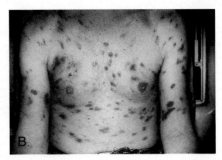

Figure 13-17 Kaposi sarcoma. A, An early lesion of Kaposi sarcoma. **B,** Advanced lesions of Kaposi sarcoma. Note widespread hemorrhagic plaques and nodules.

genital

13-64 Herpes genitalis (hur´pēz jen-ĭ-tal´is), a viral infection caused by the **herpes simplex virus (HSV-2)**, is also known as _____ **herpes.** Painful genital blisters and ulcerations are characteristic of this disease (Figure 13-18). The causative organism enters through the mucous membranes or breaks in the skin during contact with an infected person. Anti/viral agents may lessen the severity and duration of the symptoms. Active infection during pregnancy can lead to spontaneous abortion, stillbirth, or congenital birth defects. Delivery of the infant is often by cesarean section to prevent infection of the infant at the time of delivery.

warts

13-65 Looking at Table 13-2, you see that **condyloma acuminatum** (kon˝də-lo´mə ə-ku˝mĭ-nāt´əm) is commonly called **genital** _____, which also describes its major characteristic (Figure 13-19). Persons who have had genital warts are at greater risk for genital malignancy, especially cervical cancer.

> ➤ **KEY** POINT <u>Genital warts is the only sexually transmitted disease, as well as the only cancer, for which a vaccine is available.</u> The vaccine prevents infection against the two types of HPV responsible for the majority of cervical cancer cases. To further reduce the risk of cervical cancer, it is recommended that women practice safe sex (using condoms) and limit their number of sexual partners, avoiding partners who participate in high-risk sexual activities. Cervical cancer is the third most common type of cancer in women worldwide.

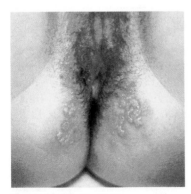

Figure 13-18 Genital herpes. These unruptured vesicles of HSV-2 appear in the vulvar area.

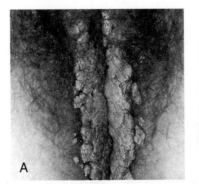
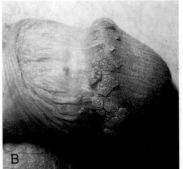

Figure 13-19 Genital warts. A, Severe vulvar warts. Minor trauma during intercourse can cause abrasions that allow the human papillomavirus to enter the body. **B,** Multiple genital warts of the glans penis.

cold

Treatment to destroy the genital warts includes destruction with acid, laser, or cryo/therapy (cry[o], cold + -therapy, treatment). **Cryo/therapy** is destruction of the lesions using very _____ temperatures.

liver

13-66 Viral hepatitis is an inflammatory condition of the _____ caused by one of the hepatitis viruses, A, B, C, D, or E. Hepatitis A and E are not considered sexually transmitted diseases because transmission is generally through direct contact with contaminated food or water.

blood

Hepatitis B is transmitted by sexual contact, _____ products, and contaminated needles. Hepatitis B vaccine is available, required by various educational institutions, and recommended for health care workers and others at greater than usual risk.

Hepatitis C is primarily transmitted by blood products, shared needles, or shared straws for inhaling cocaine. It is transmitted less commonly by sexual intercourse. This type of hepatitis has a high likelihood of progressing to chronic hepatitis.

hepatitis

Hepatitis D occurs only in patients who are infected with _____ B. It is transmitted by sexual contact and needle sharing.

Hepatitis B, C, and D are caused by hepatitis viruses B, C, and D, respectively. These viruses are abbreviated HBV, HCV, and HDV.

Trichomonas

13-67 Trichomon/iasis (trik″o-mo-ni´ə-sis) is an infection caused by _____ *vaginalis,* a protozoon. Diagnosis is by microscopic examination of fresh urethral or vaginal secretions (see Figure 4-15). Symptoms of trichomoniasis include a frothy discharge with a bad odor in females; symptoms are minor or absent in males.

13-68 Candid/iasis (kan″dĭ-di´ə-sis) is a fungal infection that is not limited to the genitals but can cause vulvo/vaginitis (vul″vo-vaj″ĭ-ni´tis), which means inflammation of the

vulva

_____ and the vagina. The infection is usually caused by *Candida albicans,* a yeast-type fungus (see Figure 4-14, *A*), and it sometimes occurs after administration of antibiotics for a bacterial infection or when immunity is suppressed.

mouth

The fungus can be seen microscopically in urethral or vaginal secretions and can be treated with oral and topical anti/fungal medications. Oral medications are taken by _____, and topical ones are applied directly to the affected area. *C. albicans* is also called **Monilia** (mo-nil´e-ə), and the infection is sometimes called **moniliasis** (mon-ĭ-li´ə-sis).

13-69 Pubic (pu´bik) **lice** are external parasites and are sometimes included with STDs because they can be transmitted by sexual contact. They are also transmitted by close contact with contaminated objects, such as linens. They are commonly called crab lice and primarily infest the pubic region but are also found in armpits, beards, eyebrows, and eyelashes. Observe in Table 13-2 that

itching

characteristic symptoms of pubic lice are severe _____ and redness. The use of topical agents and particular attention to hygiene is used in treating lice.

13-70 The physician uses the patient's sexual history and symptoms to decide which diagnostic tests will be helpful in establishing the diagnosis of a sexually transmitted disease. At times the patient has classic symptoms (such as the blisters of genital herpes) and is treated without a positive diagnostic test. After the diagnosis of a sexually transmitted disease, blood tests for syphilis as well as cervical or urethral cultures for gonorrhea and chlamydia are often recommended. Read the information in Table 13-3 to learn more about diagnostic tests that are used to diagnose sexually transmitted diseases.

EXERCISE 9

Match sexually transmitted diseases in the left columns with their characteristics in the right column.

_____ 1. AIDS

_____ 2. genital herpes

_____ 3. gonorrhea

_____ 4. hepatitis B

_____ 5. syphilis

A. fatal late stage of infection with HIV
B. blisters and ulcerations of the genitals
C. caused by gram-negative intracellular diplococci
D. caused by HB virus
E. one sign is a painless chancre

TABLE 13-3   Diagnostic Tests for Selected Sexually Transmitted Diseases

STD	Diagnostic Tests*
Bacterial	
Gonorrhea	Gram stain and culture
Syphilis	Darkfield microscopic examination of material from chancre (if present); blood test: RPR (recheck later if all test results are negative); if in late stage: darkfield microscopic examination of material from gummas, if present
Chlamydiosis	Gram stain of cervical or urethral discharges, sometimes cultures; direct fluorescent antibody (DFA) tests; enzyme immunoassay (EIA); DNA amplification (can be used with urine samples rather than urethral and cervical swabs)
Viral	
AIDS	HIV-antibody positive is reported when blood is reactive in all of several tests; HIV-specific antibody test is performed, but the test result is sometimes negative even when the person has HIV infection; if enzyme-linked immunosorbent assay (ELISA) is positive for HIV, diagnosis is confirmed by Western blot analysis or immunofluorescent assay (IFA), more expensive and sophisticated tests; many laboratory tests—some common types as well as uncommon (viral load testing)—help monitor the disease; biopsy of lesions of Kaposi sarcoma is positive for the virus
Genital herpes	Often diagnosed based on the history and physical examination and the appearance of the lesions; cultures are most accurate if obtained within 48 hours of the first outbreak
Genital warts	Diagnosis is made by appearance of the lesions; Pap smear is obtained to assess for cervical dysplasia; for confirmation of diagnosis, HPV can usually be detected in swab specimens of infected genitals using DNA probe (test involving special collection of cervical swabs and finding a specific sequence of nucleotides in a DNA molecule)
Hepatitis	Symptoms usually indicate laboratory assessment of serum enzyme levels; liver biopsy; several tests help determine type of hepatitis, including serologic testing to confirm the presence of specific types of hepatitis antigen-antibody systems, and ELISA
Protozooal	
Trichomoniasis	Microscopic examination of wet mount slide preparation
Fungal	
Candidiasis	Microscopic examination of body fluid

*To rule out the presence of other infections, blood tests for syphilis and cervical or urethral cultures for gonorrhea and chlamydia are often recommended.

CHAPTER ABBREVIATIONS*

AIDS	acquired immunodeficiency syndrome	HCV	hepatitis C virus
BBT	basal body temperature	HDV	hepatitis D virus
CPD	cephalopelvic disproportion	HIV	human immunodeficiency virus
CS or C-section	cesarean section	HPV	human papillomavirus
DFA	direct fluorescent antibody	HSV-2	herpes simplex virus type 2 (genital herpes)
EDD	expected delivery date	IFA	immunofluorescent assay
EFM	electronic fetal monitor	IUD	intrauterine device
EIA	enzyme immunoassay	IVF	in vitro fertilization
ELISA	enzyme-linked immunosorbent assay	LMP	last menstrual period
FHR	fetal heart rate	OB	obstetrics
G	gravida (pregnant)	RPR	rapid plasma reagin
GC	gonococcus	STD	sexually transmitted disease
HBV	hepatitis B virus	VD	venereal disease
hCG, HCG	human chorionic gonadotropin	VDRL	Venereal Disease Research Laboratories

*Many of these abbreviations share their meanings with other terms.

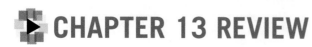

CHAPTER 13 REVIEW

Basic Understanding

Labeling

I. *Label the following structures in the drawing: amnion, amniotic fluid, chorion, placenta, umbilical cord, uterus.*

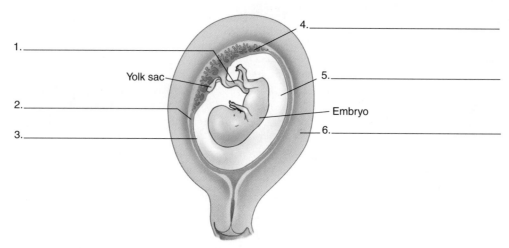

Matching

II. *Match terms in the left columns with their descriptions in the right column.*

_____ 1. gamete   _____ 4. progesterone   A. afterbirth

_____ 2. gonad   _____ 5. zygote   B. important hormone of pregnancy

_____ 3. placenta   C. ovary or testis

                                                               D. ovum or spermatozoon

                                                               E. product of fertilization

III. *Match the following pathologies of pregnancy with their descriptions.*

_____ 1. abruptio placentae   _____ 4. preeclampsia   A. abnormal implantation of the placenta in the uterus

_____ 2. ectopic pregnancy   _____ 5. pseudocyesis   B. onset of acute high blood pressure after the twenty-fourth week

_____ 3. placenta previa   C. false pregnancy

                                                               D. implantation of a fertilized ovum outside the uterus

                                                               E. premature separation of the placenta from the uterine wall

Word Analysis

IV. *Divide these words into their component parts, then define each term.*

1. endometrium   _____

2. erythroblastosis _____

3. laparorrhaphy   _____

4. neonatology   _____

5. proteinuria   _____

 Say and Check

Say aloud the terms you wrote for Exercise IV. Use the Companion CD to check your pronunciations.

Photo ID

V. *Use word parts to label these illustrations.*

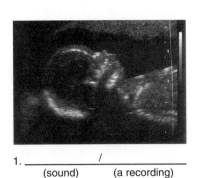
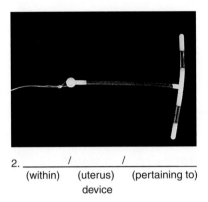
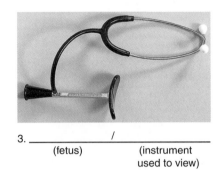

1. _____ / _____
   (sound)   (a recording)

2. _____ / _____ / _____
   (within) (uterus) (pertaining to)
              device

3. _____ / _____
   (fetus)   (instrument
              used to view)

Multiple Choice

VI. *Circle the correct answer in each of the following.*

1. Which of the following is the hormone tested for in a pregnancy test? (CPD, EFM, HCG, LMP)

2. Which of the following is an estimation of the size of the birth canal?
   (amniocentesis, cephalopelvic disproportion, chorionic villus sampling, pelvimetry)

3. Which term means abnormal or difficult labor? (abortion, dystocia, eclampsia, stillbirth)

4. Which of the following is a genetic disorder in which the fetus has an extra chromosome?
   (Down syndrome, erythroblastosis fetalis, hemolytic anemia, implantation)

5. Which term means the same as pregnancy? (embryonic, gestation, ovulation, parturition)

6. Which of the following is the normal presentation of the fetus during labor? (breech, cephalic, shoulder, transverse)

7. Which contraceptive acts by killing the sperm? (hormonal implant, IUD, oral contraceptive, spermicide)

8. Which of the following is a primipara? (para 1, para 2, para 3, para 4)

9. Which of the following is the common name for condyloma acuminatum?
   (genital herpes, genital warts, moniliasis, venereal ulcer)

10. Which of the following sexually transmitted diseases is caused by a fungus?
    (candidiasis, chancroid, chlamydiosis, trichomoniasis)

Writing Terms

VII. *Write a term for each of the following.*

1. a newborn _____

2. a woman who has produced many viable offspring _____

3. an embryonic form of spermatozoa _____

4. attachment of a fertilized ovum to the endometrium _____

5. deliberate rupture of the fetal membranes to induce labor _____

6. incision made to enlarge the vaginal opening for delivery _____

7. painless sore of syphilis _____

8. pertaining to the amnion and the chorion _____

9. pertaining to the fetus _____

10. release of an ovum from the ovary _____

Say and Check

Say aloud the terms you wrote for Exercise VII. Use the Companion CD to check your pronunciations.

Greater Comprehension

Health Care Reports

VIII. *Read the operative report. Then write the meaning of the underlined words or phrases as they are used in this report.*

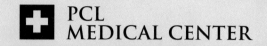 **PCL
MEDICAL CENTER**

7700 Lexicon Way
St. Louis, MO 63146

Phone (555) 437-0000 • Fax (555) 437-0001

OPERATIVE REPORT

Patient Name: Marie Aaron   **ID No:** 013-0003   **Date of Surgery:** Feb. 23, ----
Surgeon: Oscar M. Gonzales   **Assistant:** Barbara Richards, MD
Anesthetist: Ron DeVittore   **Anesthesia:** General endotracheal
PREOPERATIVE DIAGNOSIS: Rule out <u>ectopic pregnancy</u>
POSTOPERATIVE DIAGNOSES
1. Right corpus luteum cyst   3. Right indirect inguinal hernia
2. Abdominal adhesive disease   4. Threatened abortion
Intravenous fluids: 1600 mL
Urine output: 350 mL clear urine at end of procedure
Estimated blood loss: Minimal
Complications: None
Condition: Stable
OPERATIVE PROCEDURES
1. Exam under anesthesia   2. <u>Diagnostic laparoscopic exam</u>   3. <u>Adhesiolysis</u>
FINDINGS: Mobile uterus. Dense adhesive disease in the pelvis. Indirect right inguinal hernia. Right corpus luteum cyst. Normal tubes bilaterally.
DESCRIPTION OF OPERATION: Patient was taken to the operating room where general endotracheal anesthesia was found to be adequate. She was prepped and draped in the usual sterile fashion in the dorsal lithotomy position. The 10-mm scope was then entered through the umbilicus under direct visualization and confirmed to be in the abdomen. Abdomen was insufflated. A 5-mm port was placed in the left lower quadrant 2 cm superior and medial to the anterior superior iliac crest. This was placed under direct visualization. Dense adhesive disease was noted in the pelvis. Thorough inspection of the abdomen revealed no trauma from the port placements.

Thorough survey of the pelvis revealed normal anterior cul-de-sac. The left adnexa was grossly normal. Right adnexa showed an indirect inguinal hernia. Grossly normal otherwise. Posterior cul-de-sac was normal. There was a globally enlarged uterus, but no abnormalities seen otherwise. <u>Bilateral tubes</u> were thoroughly inspected from the cornua to the fimbria with no masses seen. The liver edge was seen and was within normal limits. Gallbladder was seen and was within normal limits. An adhesion from the omentum to the anterior abdominal wall was taken down under electrocautery dissection.

The 5-mm port was removed under direct visualization with excellent hemostasis. The 10-mm port was removed and the abdomen was relieved of gas. The port sites were closed with 3-0 Monocryl and covered with Steri-Strips. Excellent <u>hemostasis</u> was noted at the end of the procedure. Patient tolerated the procedure well. Sponge lap and needle counts correct ×2.

Write the meanings of the following terms.

1. ectopic pregnancy   _____

2. diagnostic laparoscopic exam   _____

3. adhesiolysis   _____

4. bilateral tubes   _____

5. hemostasis   _____

IX. *Imagine you are a health care worker. Read the following surgical pathology report. Then define the underlined terms or phrases. (Although some of the terms may be new, use your critical thinking skills to determine their meanings.)*

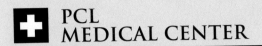 **PCL**
MEDICAL CENTER

7700 Lexicon Way
St. Louis, MO 63146

Phone (555) 437-0000 • Fax (555) 437-0001

SURGICAL PATHOLOGY REPORT

Patient Name: W. Mary Ricks **ID No:** 013-0002 **Report Date:** June 1, ----
DOB: 10/18/---- **Age:** 45 **Specimen Rec'd:** 5/31/——

GROSS DESCRIPTION
Specimen #1 at 6 o'clock labeled "cervical biopsy" received in formalin solution and consisted of portions of tissue measuring 0.4 × 0.4 × 0.2 cm. Specimen submitted in toto.
Specimen #2 at 11 o'clock labeled "cervical biopsy" received in formalin solution and consisted of portions of tissue measuring 0.4 × 0.3 × 0.2 cm. Specimen submitted in toto.
Specimen #3 labeled "endocervical curettings" received in formalin solution and consisted of portions of tissue measuring 0.5 × 0.4 × 0.2 cm. Specimen submitted in toto.

RR:pai
D/T: 5/31/——

MICROSCOPIC DESCRIPTION
Cervical biopsy at 6 o'clock: Low-grade cervical intraepithelial neoplasia
Cervical biopsy at 11 o'clock: Low-grade cervical intraepithelial neoplasia with gland involvement
Endocervical curettings: Fragments of negative endocervix
MICROSCOPIC DIAGNOSES
Epithelial cell abnormalities
Low-grade squamous intraepithelial lesion consistent with carcinoma in situ, grade 1, or condyloma.

Ronald Richart, MD
Ronald Richart, MD

RR:pai
D: June 1, ——
T: June 1, ——

Define:

1. gross description _____

2. 6 o'clock _____

3. cervical biopsy _____

4. in toto _____

5. 11 o'clock _____

6. endocervical curettings _____

7. microscopic description _____

8. intraepithelial neoplasia _____

9. negative endocervix _____

10. microscopic diagnoses _____

11. carcinoma in situ, grade 1 _____

12. condyloma _____

X. *Answer the questions after reading the following report.*

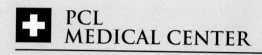

PCL MEDICAL CENTER

7700 Lexicon Way
St. Louis, MO 63146

Phone (555) 437-0000 • Fax (555) 437-0001

LABORATORY REPORT

Patient Name: Esra Esselman   **ID No:** 013-0001   **Report Date:** Feb 2, ----
DOB: 9/26/----   **Age:** 23   **Specimen Rec'd:** 2/1/----
SPECIMEN RECEIVED: Vaginal swab
FINDINGS: Gram stain of the material shows the presence of both intracellular and extracellular gram-negative diplococci. *Neisseria gonorrhoeae* grown in culture.

REVIEWED BY: Ronald Richart, MD
(Electronic Signature)

Vanessa Gale, MT, ASCP
Laboratory Technologist

1. Name and describe the type of specimen received by the laboratory: _____
   _____

2. What is meant by intracellular and extracellular diplococci? _____
   _____

3. What is the name of the sexually transmitted disease that is implied? _____
   _____

4. What is the name of the organism that causes this disease? _____
   _____

5. How is this disease usually treated?_____
   _____

Spelling
XI. *Circle all misspelled terms and write their correct spellings.*

amniosentesis   antenatal   contraseptive   extraembryonic   parturition

Interpreting Abbreviations
XII. *Write the meanings of these abbreviations.*

1. AIDS _____

2. CPD _____

3. FHR _____

4. GC _____

5. IUD _____

Pronunciation

XIII. *The pronunciation is shown for several medical words. Indicate which syllable has the primary accent by marking it with an ´.*

1. amnion (am ne on)

2. chancre (shang kər)

3. gamete (gam ēt)

4. immunodeficiency (im u no də fish ən se)

5. secundipara (se kən dip ə rə)

 Say and Check

Say aloud the five terms in Exercise XIII. Use the Companion CD to check your pronunciations. In addition, be prepared to pronounce aloud these terms in class:

abruptio placentae
amniochorionic
candidiasis
cephalopelvic disproportion
chancroid

chlamydiosis
condyloma acuminatum
dystocia
effacement
episiotomy

Kaposi sarcoma
laparorrhaphy
moniliasis
nullipara
oxytocin

preeclampsia
spermatoblast
trichomoniasis
tubal ligation
zygote

Categorizing Terms

XIV. *Classify the terms in the left columns by selecting A, B, C, D, or E.*

_____ 1. cesarean section

_____ 2. antifungals

_____ 3. antivirals

_____ 4. chorion

_____ 5. episiotomy

_____ 6. fetoscope use

_____ 7. hepatitis C

_____ 8. laparorrhaphy

_____ 9. preeclampsia

_____ 10. trichomoniasis

A. anatomy
B. diagnostic test or procedure
C. pathology
D. surgery
E. therapy

Challenge

XV. *Write the meaning of these terms. Even if you haven't seen the terms before, you may be able to divide the words into their component parts and determine their meanings.*

1. amnioinfusion _____

2. fetoscopy _____

3. gonococcal pyomyositis _____

4. oocyte donation _____

5. spermatopathia _____

(Check your answers with the solutions in Appendix VI.)

PRONUNCIATION LIST

Use the Companion CD to review the terms that have been presented. Look closely at the spelling of each term as it is pronounced and be sure you know the meaning of each term.

abortion
abruptio placentae
abstinence
acquired
    immunodeficiency
    syndrome
amniocentesis

amniochorial
amniochorionic
amnion
amnionic
amniorrhexis
amniotic
amniotomy

antenatal
antepartum
breech presentation
candidiasis
cephalic presentation
cephalopelvic
    disproportion

cervical dilation
cesarean section
chancre
chancroid
chlamydial
chlamydiosis
chorion

chorionic
chorionic villi
chorionic villus sampling
coitus interruptus
conception
condom
condyloma acuminatum
congenital syphilis
contraception
contraceptives
cryotherapy
diaphragm
dilatation
Down syndrome
dystocia
eclampsia
ectopic pregnancy
effacement
endometrium
episiotomy
erythroblastosis fetalis
expulsion
extraembryonic membrane
extrauterine pregnancy
fetal
fetal presentation
fetoscope
fetus

gamete
genital herpes
genital warts
gestation
gonad
gonococcus
gonorrhea
gravid
gravida
gummas
hemolytic disease
    of the newborn
herpes genitalis
herpes simplex virus
human chorionic
    gonadotropin
implantation
in vitro fertilization
infertility
internal os
intrauterine device
Kaposi sarcoma
labor
laparorrhaphy
laparotomy
Monilia
moniliasis
multigravida

multipara
neonatal
neonate
neonatologist
neonatology
neurosyphilis
nongonococcal urethritis
nullipara
obstetrician
obstetrics
ooblast
ovulation
ovum
oxytocin
parous
parturition
pelvimetry
placenta
placenta previa
placental stage
postnatal
postpartum
preeclampsia
pregnancy
prenatal
primigravida
primipara
progesterone

proteinuria
pseudocyesis
pseudopregnancy
pubic lice
quadripara
quickening
secundipara
shoulder presentation
spermatoblast
spermatozoa
spermicide
spirochete
stillbirth
symptothermal
syphilis
transverse presentation
trichomoniasis
trimester
tripara
tubal ligation
tubal ligation reversal
vasectomy
vasovasostomy
venereal diseases
viable offspring
viral hepatitis
zygote

Español ENHANCING SPANISH COMMUNICATION

English	Spanish (pronunciation)
birth	nacimiento (nah-se-me-EN-to)
childbirth	parto (PAR-to)
condom	condón (con-DON)
contraception	contracepción (con-trah-cep-se-ON)
cream	crema (CRAY-mah)
diaphragm	diafragma (de-ah-FRAHG-mah)
fetus	feto (FAY-to)
foam	espuma (es-POO-mah)
newborn	recién nacida (ray-se-EN nah-SEE-dah)
parturition	parto (PAR-to)
pregnancy	embarazo (em-bah-RAH-so)
pregnant	embarazada (em-bah-rah-SAH-dah)
reproduction	reproducción (ray-pro-dooc-se-ON)
rhythm method	método de ritmo (MAY-to-do day REET-mo)

Musculoskeletal System

14

LEARNING GOALS

Basic Understanding

In this chapter you will learn to do the following:

1. State the function of the musculoskeletal system, and analyze associated terms.
2. Write the meanings of the word parts associated with the musculoskeletal system, and use them to build and analyze terms.
3. Label the major bones of the body, and match them with their common names.
4. Name the four types of connective tissue and their functions.
5. List the three types of muscle tissue, and describe their functions.
6. Write the names of the diagnostic tests and procedures for assessment of the musculoskeletal system, or write the names of the procedures when given descriptions.
7. Write the names of musculoskeletal pathologies when given their descriptions, or match them with their descriptions.
8. Match surgical and therapeutic interventions with their descriptions, or write the names of the interventions when given their descriptions.

Greater Comprehension

9. Use word parts from this chapter to determine the meanings of terms in a health care report.
10. Spell the terms accurately.
11. Pronounce the terms correctly.
12. Write the meanings of the abbreviations.
13. Categorize terms as anatomy, diagnostic test or procedure, pathology, surgery, or therapy.

MAJOR SECTIONS OF THIS CHAPTER:

❏ **ANATOMY AND PHYSIOLOGY**
  Characteristics of Bone
  Bones of the Skeleton
  Joints, Tendons, and Ligaments
  Muscles
❏ **DIAGNOSTIC TESTS AND PROCEDURES**

❏ **PATHOLOGIES**
  Stress and Trauma Injuries
  Infections
  Tumors and Malignancies
  Metabolic Disturbances
  Congenital Defects
  Arthritis and Connective Tissue Diseases
  Muscular Disorders
❏ **SURGICAL AND THERAPEUTIC INTERVENTIONS**

FUNCTION FIRST

The most widely known function of the skeletal system is that of support, providing form and shape for the body. Additional functions are protection of soft body parts, movement, blood cell formation, and storage. Bones provide a place for muscles and supporting structures to attach. Muscles function in the movement of body parts by contraction and relaxation of muscle fibers.

ANATOMY AND PHYSIOLOGY

muscles

14-1 Musculo/skeletal (mus″ku-lo-skel′ə-təl) means pertaining to the _____ and the skeleton. Because of the close association of the body's skeleton and muscles, the two systems are often referred to as one, as in musculoskeletal disorders. The muscular system is also closely associated with the nervous system, as indicated by the term neuromuscular, because a muscle fiber must first be stimulated by a nerve impulse before it can contract.

Cells of the musculoskeletal system are derived from stem cells that mature and then begin to function as bone cells, muscle cells, and so on. This is not unlike cells of other body systems.

CHARACTERISTICS OF BONE

yellow

14-2 Bone marrow is the soft tissue that fills the cavities of the bones. Red bone marrow functions in the formation of red blood cells, white blood cells, and platelets. In addition, bones store and release minerals, especially calcium, and are essential parts of mineral balance in the body. Fat is stored in the yellow bone marrow. The two types of bone marrow are red and _____ marrow.

calcium

14-3 The intercellular substance of bone contains an abundance of mineral salts, primarily calcium phosphate and calcium carbonate, which gives bone its unique hardness. Most of the calcium in our bodies is stored in the skeleton. The endocrine system controls the release of calcium from the bone when the level of _____ in the blood is decreased.

14-4 The chief characteristic of bone is its rigid nature, but it is important to remember that bone contains living cells and is richly supplied with blood vessels and nerves.

> ➤ **KEY** POINT <u>Bones may be classified as long, short, flat, or irregular.</u> Examples of long bones are those in the arm, leg, and thigh. Bones of the wrist are examples of short bones. Most of the bones of the skull are flat bones, and bones of the spine are classified as irregular bones. The general features of a long bone are shown in Figure 14-1. The drawing shows that some parts of bone are hard and compact (compact bone), whereas other parts are spongy (spongy bone).

compact

Which type of bony tissue do you suspect serves as protection and support, compact or spongy? _____

diaphysis (di-af′ə-sis)

14-5 Answer these questions as you look at Figure 14-1. The long shaft of the long bone is called the _____. This long shaft is thick, compact bone that surrounds yellow marrow in adults.

epiphysis (ə-pif′ə-sis)

At each end of the diaphysis, there is an expanded portion called the _____. The **epiphysis** is spongy bone that is covered by a thin layer of compact bone. The two ends are covered by articular cartilage (kahr′tĭ-ləj) to provide smooth surfaces for movement of the joints. Except in the areas where there is articular cartilage, the bone is covered with a tough membrane called **periosteum** (per″e-os′te-əm). Analyzing the word parts of peri/ost/eum will help you remember its meaning. The prefix peri- means around, oste(o) means _____,

bone

and -ium means membrane. (In writing periosteum, an "i" is omitted to facilitate pronunciation.)

Bone is richly supplied with blood vessels. Like other body tissues, bone requires oxygen and nutrients and produces wastes, the end products of metabolism.

14-6 Note that bone has four types of tissue: compact bone, spongy bone, yellow marrow, and periosteum. The **medullary cavity** contains the yellow marrow.

compact

The type of bone tissue that lies just beneath the periosteum is called _____ bone. It has a system of small canals (**haversian canals**) that run parallel to the bone's long axis and contain blood vessels (Figure 14-1, *B*). The canals are surrounded by concentric rings characteristic of mature bone.

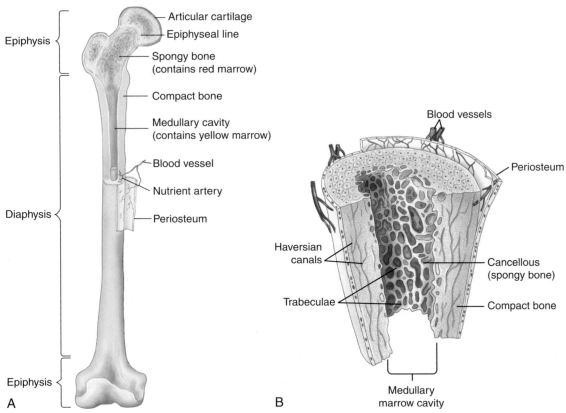

Figure 14-1 A typical long bone, partially sectioned. A, Major features of a long bone. Diaphysis is the long, main portion of a bone. Epiphyses are the knoblike ends of the bone. The outer part is compact, dense bone. The inner part is spongy and contains large spaces filled with bone marrow. **B,** Cross-section showing the haversian canals.

medullary
(med´u-lar˝e)

Spongy bone is lighter than compact bone and contains large spongy meshworks called **tra-beculae** (trə-bek´u-le). Spongy bone is found largely in the epiphyses (plural form of epiphysis) and inner portions of long bones and is filled with red and yellow marrow.

The _____ cavity contains yellow marrow. The periosteum is composed of fibrous tissue that covers the bone.

Learn the following word parts.

General Word Parts for Describing Bone

Combining Form	Meanings
blast(o), -blast	embryonic form
myel(o)	bone marrow or spinal cord
oste(o)	bone

embryonic

osteocyte
(os´te-o-sīt˝)

14-7 The combining form blast(o) and its corresponding suffix -blast mean embryonic or early form. An **osteo/blast** (os´te-o-blast˝) is an _____ bone cell. With growth, osteoblasts develop into mature bone cells. Use oste(o) to write a word that literally means a bone cell: _____. **Osteocytes** are mature bone cells that become embedded in the calcified intercellular substance of bone.

14-8 Calcium in bone is radiopaque; thus bones can block x-rays so that they do not reach image receptors. Bones are represented by white areas in an x-ray image (Figure 14-2). Unimpeded x-rays expose image receptors and cause a black or dark area in the image.

calcium

14-9 Calci/fication (kal˝sĭ-fi-ka´shən) is the process by which organic tissue becomes hardened by deposit of what substance in tissue? _____

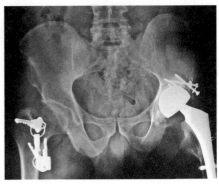

Figure 14-2 X-ray film of the pelvis. Keys were left in the pocket of a lightweight hospital robe during the examination, so radiography had to be repeated. Note also the metal fixation devices in the hip. Metal objects are radiopaque. Bones appear *white*, and soft tissue appears *gray*.

Normally calcium is deposited in bone in large amounts to give bone its hardness. Calcification in soft tissue is abnormal.

bone

14-10 Osteo/genesis (os″te-o-jen′ə-sis) or **ossification** (os″ĭ-fĭ-ka′shən) is the formation of bone substance. Human embryos contain no bone but do contain cartilage, a more flexible tissue that is shaped like bone. Osteo/genesis is the process whereby cartilage is used as a model to form what kind of tissue? _____

> ➤ **KEY** POINT <u>The Latin term for bone, *os* (plural, *ossa*), is often used in the naming of bones.</u> For example, os coccygis is the formal name for the coccyx, or the tailbone. *Os* and *ossa* are not word parts but instead are Latin terms that mean bone and are commonly used in naming them.

myel(o)

14-11 The combining form for bone marrow is _____. This combining form also means the spinal cord.
   The cells of red marrow are responsible for producing new blood cells. An embryonic bone marrow cell is called a _____.

myeloblast
(mi′ə-lo-blast)

   Myeloblasts mature into **myelocytes** (mi′ə-lo-sītz), which mature into leukocytes that are normally found in blood.

EXERCISE 1

Write a word in each blank to complete these sentences.

1. The soft tissue that fills the cavities of the bones is bone _____.

2. The long shaft of a long bone is called the diaphysis, and the expanded portions at the ends are called the

   _____.

3. Most of the bone is covered with a tough membrane called _____.

4. An osteoblast is an embryonic form of a/an _____ cell.

5. A term that means pertaining to the muscles and the skeleton is _____.

6. Osteogenesis is also called _____.

BONES OF THE SKELETON

skeleton

14-12 The human skeleton* is the bony framework of the body. **Skeletal** means pertaining to the _____. The skeletal system consists of the bones and the cartilages, ligaments, and tendons that are associated with the bones. Bones and muscles work together to enable us to bend our arms and legs, turn our heads, and perform other voluntary movements.

*Skeleton (Greek: a dried body or a mummy).

14-13 The adult human skeleton usually consists of 206 named bones. There are also a few others that vary in number from one individual to another, so they are not counted with the other 206 bones. The major bones are identified in Figure 14-3. Study the names of the bones and their locations.

Note that the skeleton is divided into the axial (ak′se-əl) skeleton and the appendicular (ap″en-dik′u-lər) skeleton. The division of the skeleton that forms the vertical axis of the body is the **axial skeleton.** The free appendages and their attachments are called the _____ **skeleton.**

appendicular

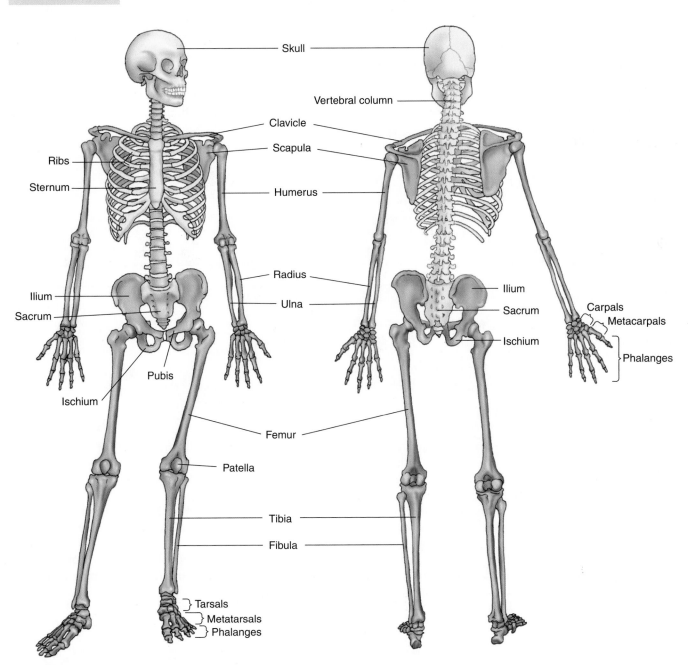

Figure 14-3 Anterior and posterior views of the human skeleton with major bones identified. The bones are grouped in two divisions: The axial skeleton forms the vertical axis of the body and is *shown here as bone colored.* The appendicular skeleton includes the free appendages and their attachments and is *shown in blue.*

EXERCISE 2

Write a word in each blank to complete these sentences.

1. The bony framework of the body is the _____.

2. A term that means pertaining to the skeleton is _____.

3. The division of the skeleton that forms the vertical axis of the body is the _____ skeleton.

4. Bones of the extremities and their attachments to the axial skeleton are called the _____ skeleton.

axial	**Axial Skeleton** **14-14** The skull, spinal column, sternum, and ribs make up the _____ skeleton. It consists of 80 major bones. These bones form the vertical axis to which the appendicular skeleton attaches. Learn the word parts associated with bones of the axial skeleton.

Word Parts: Bones of the Axial Skeleton

Combining Form	Bone	Common Name
cost(o)	costae	ribs
crani(o)	cranium	skull
rach(i), rachi(o), spin(o)	vertebral or spinal column	spine (backbone)
spondyl(o), vertebr(o)	vertebrae	bones of the spine
stern(o)	sternum	breastbone

Types of Vertebrae (Uppermost to Lowermost)

Combining Form	Meaning
cervic(o)	cervical
thorac(o)	thoracic
lumb(o)	lumbar
sacr(o)	sacral
coccyg(o)	coccygeal

skull **cranial** (kra′ne-əl)	**14-15** The **cranium** serves as protection for the brain and forms the framework of the face. The common name for the cranium is the _____. It is composed of three types of bones: cranial bones; facial* bones; and the six **auditory ossicles** (os´ĭ-kəlz), three tiny bones in each middle ear cavity (Figure 14-4). You learned that crani(o) means cranium or skull. The cranium is the major portion of the skull, that which encloses and protects the brain. Write a word that means pertaining to the skull: _____. The bones that make up the skull are listed in Table 14-1. The opening at the base of the skull through which the spinal cord passes is called the **foramen magnum** (fo-ra′mən mag′nəm).

*Facial (Latin: *facialis*, from *facies*, face).

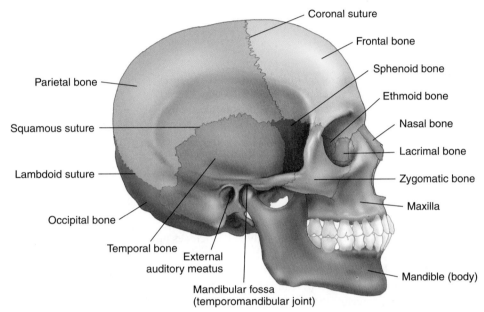

Figure 14-4 Major bones of the skull, lateral view. The cranium, that portion of the skull that encloses the brain, is composed of eight cranial bones (parietal, temporal, frontal, occipital, ethmoid, and sphenoid.) Sutures are immovable fibrous joints between many of the cranial bones. The 14 facial bones (not all are shown) form the basic framework and shape of the face. The auditory ossicles (not shown) are three tiny bones in each middle ear cavity. The external auditory meatus is the external opening of the ear.

TABLE 14-1	Named Bones of the Skull			
Cranial Bones		**Facial Bones**		**Auditory Ossicles**
Parietal (2)	Occipital (1)	Maxilla (2)	Palatine (2)	Malleus (2)
Temporal (2)	Ethmoid (1)	Zygomatic (2)	Inferior nasal concha (2)	Incus (2)
Frontal (1)	Sphenoid (1)	Mandible (1)	Lacrimal (2)	Stapes (2)
		Nasal (2)	Vomer (1)	

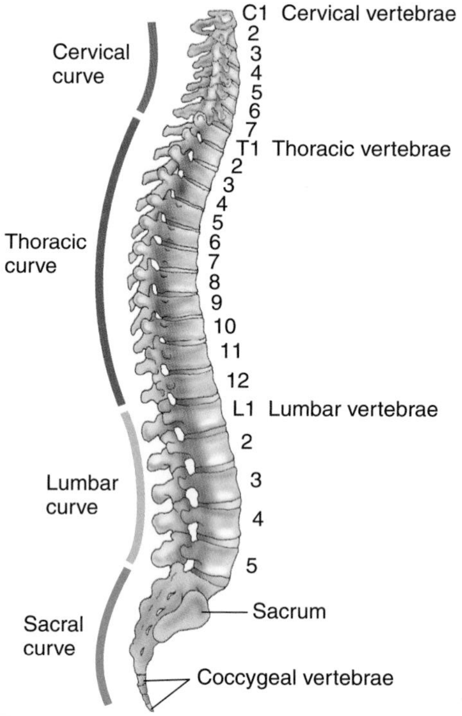

Figure 14-5 **The vertebral column with normal curvatures noted.** The vertebrae are numbered from above downward. There are seven cervical vertebrae in the neck region, 12 thoracic vertebrae behind the chest cavity, five lumbar vertebrae supporting the lower back, five sacral vertebrae fused into one bone called the sacrum, and four coccygeal vertebrae fused into one bone called the coccyx.

spine

14-16 The vertebral or spinal column is attached at the base of the skull. The **vertebral column** is commonly called the backbone or the _____, and it extends from the base of the skull to the pelvis. It encloses and protects the spinal cord, supports the head, and serves as a place of attachment for the ribs and muscles of the back.

spinal (spī′nəl)

The combining forms rach(i), rachi(o), and spin(o) mean spine. Combine spin(o) and -al to write a word that means pertaining to the spine: _____. Most medical terms pertaining to the spine use rach(i) and rachi(o). Rachi(o) is more commonly used than rach(i).

vertebrae

14-17 The vertebral column is composed of 26 **vertebrae.** Vertebrae (vur′tə-bre) is the plural form of **vertebra** (vur′tə-brə). **Inter/vertebral** (in″tər-vur′tə-brəl) means between two adjoining _____. Cushions of cartilage between adjoining vertebrae are called **intervertebral disks.** These layers of cartilage absorb shock.

neck

The vertebrae are named and numbered from the top downward (Figure 14-5). The combining form cervic(o) means neck. There are seven **cervical** (sur′vĭ-kəl) **vertebrae** (C1 through C7) located in the region called the _____.

chest

14-18 Thorac/ic refers to the _____. The 12 **thoracic vertebrae** (T1 through T12) are part of the posterior wall of the chest.

back

The combining form lumb(o) means the lower back. The five **lumb/ar** (lum′bahr, lum′bər) **vertebrae** (L1 through L5) are just below the thoracic vertebrae. In what part of the body are lumbar vertebrae located? lower _____

lumbar

Thoraco/lumbar (thor″ə-ko-lum′bər) means pertaining to two particular types of vertebrae. To what types of vertebrae does thoracolumbar refer? thoracic and _____

sacral (sa´krəl)

14-19 Use sacr(o) to write words about the sacrum, the triangular bone below the lumbar vertebrae. In adults, five vertebrae fuse to form the **sacrum.** Which vertebrae are fused into one bone, the sacrum? _____ **vertebrae**

coccygeal
(kok-sij´e-əl)

14-20 The combining form coccyg(o) means coccyx, or the tailbone. In adults the **coccyx** (kok´siks) is the bone at the base of the vertebral column. It is formed by four fused vertebrae. Which vertebrae fuse to form the coccyx? _____ **vertebrae**

breastbone

sternum

14-21 Locate the elongated flattened sternum (stur´nəm) in Figure 14-3. The common name of the **sternum** is the _____.
    The combining form that means sternum is stern(o). **Stern/al** (ster´nəl) pertains to the _____. **Intra/sternal** means within the sternum.
    The prefix infra- means situated below. **Infrasternal** (in˝frə-stur´nəl) means beneath the sternum. If infra/sternal means beneath the sternum, form a new word using retro- that means situated or occurring behind the breastbone: _____.

retrosternal
(ret˝ro-stur´nəl)
substernal
(səb-stur´nəl)

    Supra/sternal (soo˝prə-ster´nəl) means above the sternum. Using the prefix sub-, write the word that means below the sternum: _____.

14-22 The sternum is one of the bones that make up the thoracic cage, which protects the heart, lungs, and great vessels and also plays a role in breathing. **Thoracic** means pertaining to the

thorax (chest)

_____.
    Attached to the sternum are the ribs, which support the chest wall and protect the lungs and heart. See the thoracic cage in Figure 14-6 and note the 12 pairs of ribs, which are numbered from the top rib, beginning with 1. Note that the first seven ribs on each side join directly with the sternum by a strip of cartilage and are called _____ ribs.

true

    Also note the **xiphoid** (zif´oid, zi´foid) **process,** the smallest and lowermost part of the sternum, which is often used as a point of reference when examining the chest.

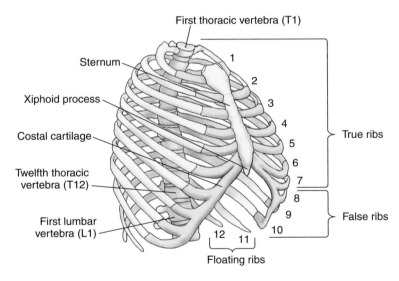

First thoracic vertebra (T1)

Sternum

Xiphoid process

Costal cartilage

Twelfth thoracic
vertebra (T12)

First lumbar
vertebra (L1)

1
2
3
4
5
6
7
8
9
10
12 11

True ribs

False ribs

Floating ribs

Figure 14-6 The thoracic cage. The ribs exist in pairs, 12 on each side of the chest, and are numbered from the top rib, beginning with *1*. The upper seven pairs join directly with the sternum by a strip of cartilage and are called *true ribs*. The remaining five pairs are referred to as *false ribs* because they do not attach directly to the sternum. The last two pairs of false ribs, called *floating ribs*, are attached only on the posterior aspect.

supracostal
(soo″prə-kos′təl)
ribs

sternum

sternum

14-23 The combining form cost(o) means ribs. Another term for a rib is **costa** (kos′tə), and the plural is costae (kos′te). **Cost/al** (kos′təl) means pertaining to the ribs. The location of **sub/cost/al** (səb-kos′təl) is below a rib. Write a term using supra- that means above or upon a rib: _____. **Infra/cost/al** (in″frə-kos′təl) means below a rib.

    Inter/costal (in″tər-kos′təl) is a term that means between the _____. Intercostal muscles lie between the ribs and draw adjacent ribs together to increase the volume of the thorax in breathing.

14-24 Sterno/cost/al (stur″no-kos′təl) pertains to the _____ and the ribs.

    Both vertebr(o) and spondyl(o) are combining forms that mean vertebrae. **Vertebro/costal** (vur″tə-bro-kos′təl) and **costo/vertebral** (kos″to-vur′tə-brəl) both mean pertaining to a vertebra and a rib.

14-25 Two other terms, **vertebrosternal** (vur″tə-bro-stur′nəl) and **sternovertebral** (stər″no-vər′tə-brəl), can also be reversed in this way. These terms mean pertaining to the vertebrae and the _____.

EXERCISE 3

Write a word in each blank to complete these sentences.

1. The axial skeleton is composed of the skull, the spinal column, the _____, and the ribs.
2. The combining form crani(o) means the _____ or the skull.
3. The combining form that means rib is _____.
4. The combining forms rach(i) and rachi(o) mean _____.
5. The combining form that means the breastbone is _____.
6. The spine is composed of 26 bones that are called _____.
7. The uppermost vertebrae are located within the neck and are called _____ vertebrae.
8. The coccyx is formed by four fused _____ vertebrae.

EXERCISE 4

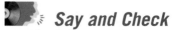 ***Build It!*** *Use the following word parts to build terms. (Some word parts will be used more than once.)*

infra-, inter-, supra-, cost(o), crani/o, lumb(o), stern(o), thorac(o), vertebr(o), -al, -ar

1. pertaining to the chest and the lower back   _____/_____/_____
2. pertaining to the skull   _____/_____
3. pertaining to above a rib   _____/_____/_____
4. pertaining to beneath the breastbone   _____/_____/_____
5. between two adjoining spinal bones   _____/_____/_____

Say and Check

Say aloud the terms you wrote for Exercise 4. Use the Companion CD to check your pronunciations.

Appendicular Skeleton

14-26 Bones of the extremities, the shoulder girdle, and the pelvic girdle comprise the appendicular skeleton. In other words, the appendicular skeleton includes the bones of the limbs and their attachments to the axial skeleton. The **shoulder girdle** includes the clavicle and the scapula, and the **pelvic girdle** includes the bones of the pelvis.

The major division of the skeleton that attaches to the axial skeleton is called the

appendicular

_____ skeleton.

Learn the following word parts for the names of the bones of the appendicular skeleton.

Word Parts: Bones of the Appendicular Skeleton

Combining Form	Bone	Common Name	Bones of the Lower Extremities		
clavicul(o)	clavicle	collarbone	**Combining Form**	**Bone**	**Common Name**
scapul(o)	scapula	shoulder blade	calcane(o)	calcaneus	heel bone
			femor(o)	femur	thigh bone
Bones of the Pelvic Girdle*			fibul(o)	fibula	calf bone
ili(o)	ilium		patell(o)	patella	kneecap
ischi(o)	ischium		phalang(o)	phalanx	toe
pub(o)	pubis			(plural,	
				phalanges)	
Bones of the Upper Extremities			tars(o)	tarsus	ankle
carp(o)	carpus	wrist		(sometimes,	
humer(o)	humerus	upper arm bone		edge of eyelid)	
phalang(o)	phalanx (plural,	finger	tibi(o)	tibia	shin bone
	phalanges)				
radi(o)	radius or	bone of the			
	(radiant energy)	forearm			
uln(o)	ulna	bone of the			
		forearm			

*These bones fuse to form the pelvic bone.

EXERCISE 5

Write a combining form for each of the following bones of the appendicular skeleton.

1. ankle _____

2. calf bone _____

3. collarbone _____

4. fingers or toes _____

5. heel bone _____

6. kneecap _____

7. shinbone _____

8. shoulder blade _____

9. thighbone _____

10. upper arm bone _____

11. wrist _____

collarbone

14-27 Locate the clavicle (klav´ĭ-kəl) in Figure 14-3. The **clavicle** is also known as the _____. **Infra/clavicul/ar** (in″frə-klə-vik´u-lər) means below the clavicle.

The clavicles are long, curved horizontal bones that attach to the sternum and either the left or right scapula. The **scapula** (skap´u-lə) is a large triangular bone that is commonly called the shoulder blade. **Infra/scapul/ar** (in″frə-skap´u-lər) means below the _____.

scapula

forearm

14-28 Each scapula is joined to the upper arm bone, the **humerus** (hu´mər-əs), by muscles and tendons. The **ulna** (ul´nə) and the **radius** (ra´de-əs) are bones of the _____.

carpals (kahr´pəlz)

14-29 The wrist is composed of eight carpal bones, also called _____. Bones of the hand also include **meta/carpals** (meta-, next) and **phalanges** (fə-lan´jēz), bones of the fingers.

clavicle
ribs

14-30 Many of the 126 bones that make up the appendicular skeleton are small and are found in the hands and feet, but several of the remaining bones in this part of the skeleton are the longest bones in the body. Bones of the appendicular skeleton are designed for movement.

Studying the individual bones of the appendicular skeleton, the combining form clavicul(o) means the clavicle. **Sterno/clavicul/ar** (stur″no-klə-vik′u-lər) pertains to the sternum and the _____. **Costo/clavicul/ar** (kos″to-klə-vik′u-lər) means pertaining to or involving the _____ and the clavicle.

14-31 The combining form scapul(o) means scapula (shoulder blade). **Scapul/ar** (skap′u-lər) means pertaining to the scapula. Write a term that means between the two shoulder blades: _____.

interscapular
(in″tər-skap′u-lər)

Scapulo/clavicul/ar (skap″u-lo-klə-vik′u-lər) means pertaining to the scapula and the clavicle. The clavicles and the two scapulae form the shoulder girdle, the connection between the arms and the axial skeleton.

14-32 Both the clavicle and the upper arm bone are attached to the scapula. The upper arm bone is the humerus and has the combining form humer(o). **Humer/al** (hu′mər-əl) pertains to the _____.

humerus

Humero/scapul/ar (hu″mər-o-skap′u-lər) means pertaining to the humerus and the _____.

scapula

14-33 The bones of the forearm, the portion of the arm between the elbow and the wrist, are the ulna and the _____, and their combining forms are uln(o) and radi(o), respectively. Also remember that radi(o) will sometimes refer to radiant energy, as you learned earlier. Use a combining form with radial to write a word that means pertaining to both the ulna and the radius: _____.

radius

ulnoradial
(ul″no-ra′de-əl)

14-34 Use another combining form with radial to write a word that means pertaining to the humerus and the radius: _____.

Humeroulnar (hu″mər-o-ul′nər) means pertaining to the humerus and the ulna.

humeroradial
(hu″mər-o-ra′de-əl)

14-35 The combining form carp(o) means the **carpus,** or wrist. Observe in Figure 14-7 that the wrist consists of eight small bones, arranged in two transverse rows. **Carp/al** (kahr′pəl) pertains to the _____. Bones of the wrist are called carpals. Therefore carpals is a word that means the same as carp/al bones.

carpus

14-36 The metacarpals (met″ə-kahr′pəlz) connect the wrist bones (carpals) to the phalanges. You learned that meta- is a prefix that means a change or next, as in a series. The meta/carpals lie _____ to the carpals. The five metacarpals constitute the palm. The proximal ends of the metacarpals join with the distal row of what type of bones? _____

next

carpal

14-37 The distal ends of the metacarpals join with the phalanges (fə-lan′jēz). The combining form phalang(o) means phalanges. The phalanges are bones of the _____, as well as bones of the toes. **Carpo/phalang/eal** (kahr″po-fə-lan′je-əl) pertains to the carpus and the _____—in this case, the fingers.

fingers

phalanges

See Figure 14-7 to observe that there are three phalanges in each finger (a proximal, middle, and distal phalanx) but not in the thumb.

14-38 The pelvic girdle consists of two hipbones. Each of these bones consists of three separate bones in the newborn, but eventually the three fuse to form one bone. Names of the three bones are the ilium, the ischium, and the _____. Their combining forms are ili(o), ischi(o), and pub(o), respectively. The **ilium** (il′e-əm) is the largest of the three bones. The **ischium** (is′ke-əm) is the posterior part of the pelvic girdle, and the **pubis** (pu′bis) is the anterior part of the pelvic girdle. **Ili/ac** (il′e-ak), **ischi/al** (is′ke-əl), and **pub/ic** (pu′bik) mean pertaining to the ilium, the _____, and the pubis, respectively.

pubis

ischium

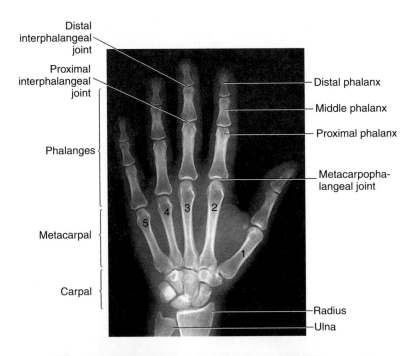

Distal interphalangeal joint
Proximal interphalangeal joint
Phalanges
Metacarpal
Carpal

Distal phalanx
Middle phalanx
Proximal phalanx
Metacarpophalangeal joint

5 4 3 2
1

Radius
Ulna

Figure 14-7 Radiograph of the human hand, postero-anterior view. The ulna and radius, as well as the bones of the hand, are identified. Eight small carpal bones make up the wrist. The palm of the hand contains five metacarpal bones, which are numbered *1* to *5* starting on the thumb side. There are three phalanges in each finger (a proximal, middle, and distal phalanx) except the thumb, which has two. The sesamoid bone is a small round bone embedded in the tendon that provides added strength for the thumb.

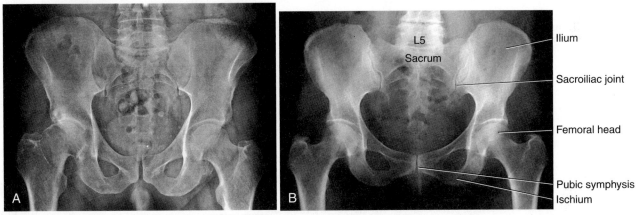

L5
Sacrum

Ilium
Sacroiliac joint
Femoral head
Pubic symphysis
Ischium

A

B

Figure 14-8 Radiographs comparing the male pelvis with that of the female, anterior views. A, Male pelvis. Bones of the male are generally larger and heavier. The pelvic outlet, the space surrounded by the lower pelvic bones, is heart shaped. **B,** Female pelvis. The pelvic outlet is larger and more oval than that of the male. The size and shape of the female pelvis varies and is important in childbirth. L5 is the fifth lumbar vertebra. The pubic symphysis is the joint where the two pubic bones are joined.

14-39 Locate these three bones that are fused to form each of the hipbones. The hipbones unite with the sacrum and coccyx to form the pelvis (Figure 14-8). Also compare the male pelvis with the female pelvis.

ilium	**Ilio/pubic** (il″e-o-pu′bik) pertains to the _____ and the pubis.
ischium	**Ischio/pubic** (is″ke-o-pu′bik) means pertaining to the _____ and the pubis.
	Ischio/coccyg/eal (is″ke-o-kok-sij′e-əl) is pertaining to the ischium and the
coccyx	_____.

14-40 Sub/pubic (səb-pu′bik) means a location _____ the pubis.
Supra/pubic (soo″prə-pu′bik) means above the pubis.

beneath

The hairs growing over the pubic region are called **pubes** (pu′bēz). This term is also used to denote the pubic region. The pubic region or the hairs that grow in this region are called the

pubes

_____.

The **pubic symphysis** is the **inter/pubic** (in″tər-pu′bik) joint where the two pubic bones meet.

14-41 The lower extremities, like the two upper extremities, are composed of sixty bones. The **femur** (fem′ər), or the thigh bone, is the longest and heaviest bone in the body (Figure 14-9). The combining form femor(o) means femur. **Femor/al** pertains to the _____.

femur

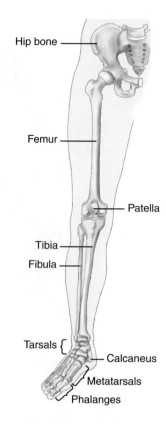

Figure 14-9 Right lower extremity, anterior view. The lower extremity consists of the bones of the thigh, leg, foot, and patella (kneecap). The lower leg has two bones, the tibia and the fibula. The foot is composed of the ankle, instep, and five toes. The ankle has seven bones, the calcaneus (heel bone) being the largest. The instep has five metatarsals, numbered 1 through 5 starting on the medial side. There are three phalanges in each of the toes, except in the great (or big) toe, which has only two.

femur
pubis
 	
ischiofemoral
(is″ke-o-fem′o-rəl)
 	
patella
 	
below
	Ilio/femor/al (il″e-o-fem′or-əl) means pertaining to the ilium and the _____.
	     Pubo/femor/al (pu″bo-fem′ə-rəl) means pertaining to the _____ and the femur. Use pubofemoral as a model to write a word that means pertaining to the ischium and the femur: _____.
	
	14-42 The patella (pə-tel′ə), or kneecap, is anterior to the knee joint. The combining form patell(o) means patella. **Patello/femor/al** (pə-tel″o-fem′ə-rəl) pertains to the _____ and the femur.
	     Infra/patell/ar (in″frə-pə-tel′ər) means _____ the patella.
	
	14-43 The lower leg is composed of two bones, the tibia and the fibula. The tibia, or shinbone, is the larger of the two bones. The combining form tibi(o) means tibia; the combining form fibul(o) means fibula.

fibula	**Fibul/ar** (fib′u-lər) means pertaining to the _____.
	14-44 The foot is composed of the ankle, instep, and toes. The ankle, or **tarsus,** consists of a group of seven short bones that resemble the bones of the wrist but are larger. The combining form tars(o) means the tarsus, or sometimes the edge of the eyelid. This is because a second meaning of tarsus is a curved plate of dense white fibrous tissue forming the supporting structure of the eyelid. It is not always obvious, when looking at a word containing tars(o), which meaning is intended. Words used in the following frames refer to the ankle, but one should be aware that a second meaning of tarsus is the edge of the eyelid.
tarsus (or ankle) **tarsals** (tahr′səlz)	**14-45 Tars/al** (tahr′səl) means pertaining to the _____. The ankle is composed of seven tarsal bones called the _____. One of the tarsal bones is the **calcaneus,** or heel bone. Bones of the feet are **metatarsals.** Like bones of the fingers, those of the toes are called phalanges. **14-46** The combining form calcane(o) refers to the calcaneus. **Calcane/al** (kal-ka′ne-əl) pertains to the calcaneus.

calcaneus	**Calcaneo/plantar** (kal-ka″ne-o-plan′tər) pertains to the _____ and the sole. **Plantar** is a word that means concerning the sole.
tibia	**Calcaneo/tibial** (kal-ka″ne-o-tib′e-əl) means pertaining to the calcaneus and the _____. **Calcaneo/fibular** (kal-ka″ne-o-fib′u-lər) means pertaining to the calcaneus and the fibula.
distal	**14-47** The bones between the tarsus and the toes are the metatarsals (met″ə-tahr′səlz). Which end of the metatarsals joins with the toes? _____
phalang(o)	**14-48** Bones of the toes are phalanges. Finger bones are also called phalanges. What is the combining form for phalanges? _____ There are two bones in the great toe and three in each of the lesser toes.
carpus (wrist)	**Carpo/ped/al** (kahr″po-ped′əl) pertains to the _____ and the foot. A carpopedal spasm, for example, is involuntary contraction of the muscles of the hands and feet.

EXERCISE 6

1. List three bones that fuse to form the pelvic bone: _____

2. Write the names of the two bones of the forearm: _____

EXERCISE 7

Word Analysis. *Break these words into their component parts by placing a slash between the word parts. Write the meaning of each term.*

1. ischiococcygeal   _____

2. humeroscapular   _____

3. infrapatellar   _____

4. ulnoradial   _____

5. metacarpal   _____

EXERCISE 8

Build It! *Use the following word parts to build terms.*

calcane(o), carp(o), clavicul(o), femor(o), ili(o), ischi(o), phalang(o), pub(o), scapul(o), tibi(o), -al, -ar, -eal, -ic

1. pertaining to the shoulder blade and the collarbone   _____/_____/_____

2. pertaining to the wrist and fingers   _____/_____/_____

3. pertaining to the ischium and the pubis   _____/_____/_____

4. pertaining to the ilium and the thigh bone   _____/_____/_____

5. pertaining to the calcaneus and the tibia   _____/_____/_____

Say and Check

Say aloud the terms from Exercises 7 and 8. Use the Companion CD to check your pronunciations.

JOINTS, TENDONS, AND LIGAMENTS

	14-49 Connective tissues, characterized by an abundance of intercellular material with relatively few cells, support and bind other body tissue and parts. Bone is the most rigid of all the connective tissues. The joints, tendons, and ligaments are also connective tissues. Tissue that supports
connective	and binds other body tissue and parts is called _____ tissue. Learn the following word parts for the joints, tendons, and ligaments.

Word Parts: Joints and Tendons

Combining Form	Meaning	Combining Form	Meaning
arthr(o), articul(o)	joint; articulation	synov(o), synovi(o)	synovial membrane
burs(o)	bursa	ten(o), tend(o), tendin(o)	tendon
chondr(o)	cartilage		

> ➤ **KEY** POINT A joint, or **articulation** (ahr-tik″u-la´shən), is a place of union between two or more bones. You are familiar with many joints—for example, the ankle, wrist, and knee. Joints are classified according to their structure and the amount of movement they allow. Joints are immovable, slightly movable, and freely movable. Table 14-2 shows examples of the three types.

joint

14-50 Two combining forms that mean joint are articul(o) and arthr(o). Most terms use arthr(o), but **articul/ar** (ahr-tik´u-lər) means pertaining to a _____.

14-51 Most joints in the adult body are freely movable joints, also called **synovial** (sĭ-no´ve-əl) **joints.** The combining forms synov(o) and synovi(o) mean synovial joint. The knee is an example of a synovial joint. The **tibio/femoral** (tib″e-o-fem´ə-rəl) or knee joint is the largest joint of the body.

Articular cartilage covers the ends of the opposing bones in a synovial joint, and they are separated by a space called the joint cavity that is filled with synovial fluid for lubrication (Figure 14-10). Synovial fluid is also called synovia (sĭ-no´ve-ə).

The articular cartilage provides protection and support for the joint. Some joints also have pads and cushions that help stabilize the joint and act as shock absorbers. **Bursae** (bur´se) are fluid-filled sacs that help reduce friction. The combining form burs(o) means a bursa. Note the location of the bursa in Figure 14-10. Bursae are commonly located between the skin and underlying bone or between tendons and ligaments.

tendons
ligaments

14-52 **Tendons** are bands of strong, fibrous tissue that attach the muscles to the bones (Figure 14-11). **Ligaments** connect bones or cartilage and serve to support and strengthen joints. What type of connective tissue attaches the muscles to the bones? _____
What type of connective tissue connects bones or cartilage? _____

14-53 The **temporomandibular** (tem″pə-ro-man-dib´u-lər) **joint** is one of a pair of joints connecting the mandible of the jaw to the temporal bone of the skull. It is abbreviated TMJ.

chondral
(kon´drəl)

14-54 Embryos contain a great deal of translucent, elastic tissue that, for the most part, is transformed into bone as the embryo matures. This elastic tissue is **cartilage.** Not all cartilage becomes bone, as evidenced by cartilage found in several parts of the adult body, such as the nose and ear. The combining form chondr(o) means cartilage. Use -al to write a term that means pertaining to cartilage: _____. **Chondr/oid** (kon´droid) means resembling cartilage.

vertebrae

14-55 **Vertebro/chondral** (vur″tə-bro-kon´drəl) means pertaining to the _____ and the adjacent cartilage.

TABLE 14-2   Types of Movement in Joints

Type of Movement	Examples
Immovable: Bones come in close contact and are separated by only a thin layer of fibrous connective tissue	Sutures in the skull
Slightly movable: Bones are connected by cartilage and joint, which allows slight movement only	Symphysis pubis, joints that connect the ribs to the sternum
Freely movable: Ends of the opposing bones are covered with articular cartilage and separated by a space called the joint cavity; these joints are sometimes called synovial joints	Shoulder, wrist, knee, elbow

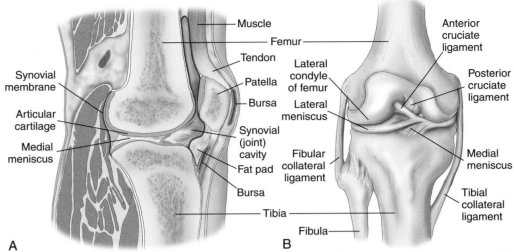

Figure 14-10 The knee joint. A, Lateral view, sagittal section. The hinged joint at the knee is a synovial joint. The ends of the opposing bones are covered by articular cartilage. The synovial membrane secretes synovial fluid into the joint cavity for lubrication. Menisci and bursae are special structures that act as protective cushions. **B,** Anterior view. Twelve ligaments, flexible bands of fibrous tissue, bind the structures of the knee to provide strength. Note how the anterior and posterior cruciate ligaments cross each other, a characteristic from which their name is derived (Latin: *crux*, cross, and *ligare*, to bind).

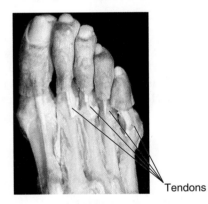

Figure 14-11 Tendons. Strong and flexible bands of dense fibrous connective tissue attach muscles to bones.

Chondro/costal (kon″dro-kos´təl) pertains to what structures and their associated cartilage? _____

ribs

14-56 Perichondrium (per″ĭ-kon´dre-əm) is the membrane around the surface of cartilage. **Peri/chondrial** (per″ĭ-kon´dre-əl) means pertaining to or composed of perichondrium, the

cartilage   membrane around the _____, or concerning the perichondrium.

EXERCISE 9

Write a word in each blank to complete these sentences.

1. Tissue that supports and binds other body tissue and parts is _____ tissue.

2. Another name for a joint is a/an _____.

3. Freely movable joints are filled with a fluid for lubrication and are called _____ joints.

4. Articular cartilage provides protection and support for the _____.

5. Fluid-filled sacs that help reduce friction in a joint are called _____.

6. Tissues that attach muscles to bones are _____.

7. Connective tissue that connects bones or cartilages and supports and strengthens joints is called a/an

_____.

8. The membrane around the surface of cartilage is called the _____.

MUSCLES

bone

14-57 Muscle is a type of tissue that is composed of fibers or cells that are able to contract, causing movement of body parts and organs. Before a skeletal muscle contracts, it receives an impulse from a nerve cell. The muscle exerts force on tendons, which in turn pull on bones, producing movement. You learned in the previous section that tendons attach a muscle to a _____.

Hyper/tonicity of muscle is abnormally increased muscle tone or strength. **Hypo/tonicity** is diminished tone or tension in any body structure, such as in paralysis.

Word Parts: Muscle

Combining Form	Meaning
fasci(o)	fascia
muscul(o), my(o)*	muscle

*My(o) (Greek: *myos,* of muscle).

muscle
embryonic

14-58 You know that my(o) and muscul(o) mean muscle. **Muscul/ar** means pertaining to _____.

A **myo/blast** (mi′o-blast) is an _____ cell that develops into muscle fiber.

> ➤ **KEY** POINT There are three types of muscle tissue in the body: skeletal, visceral, and cardiac. **Skeletal muscle,** with the primary function of movement of the body and its parts, is voluntarily controlled by the nervous system. **Visceral muscle,** located in the walls of organs and blood vessels, is involuntary. **Cardiac muscle** is only located in the heart.

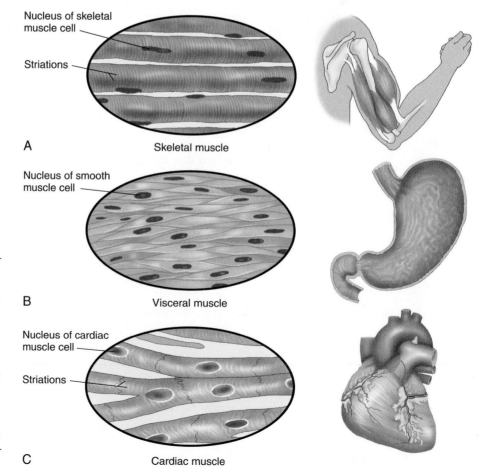

Figure 14-12 **Types of muscle. A,** Skeletal muscle cells (fibers) are long and cylindrical with alternating light and dark bands that give the cell a striated appearance. Skeletal muscles are also known as voluntary muscles because we have conscious control over them. **B,** Visceral muscle cells are elongated, spindle-shaped, and involuntary. Visceral muscle is also called smooth muscle because it lacks striations. **C,** Cardiac muscle cells are cylindrical and are striated but are shorter than skeletal muscle cells and are involuntary. These cells branch and interconnect.

Nucleus of skeletal muscle cell

Striations

A — Skeletal muscle

Nucleus of smooth muscle cell

B — Visceral muscle

Nucleus of cardiac muscle cell

Striations

C — Cardiac muscle

not

heart

In/voluntary means it is _____ voluntary, or not under our conscious control. (Visceral muscle is controlled by the autonomic nervous system described in Chapter 15.) The combining form viscer(o) means viscera, the internal organs enclosed within a body cavity, including the abdominal, thoracic, pelvic, and endocrine organs.

Cardiac muscle, **myocardium,** is also involuntary. Myo/cardium is _____ muscle. Characteristics of the three types of muscle tissues are shown in Figure 14-12.

14-59 Skeletal muscle makes up more than 600 muscles that are attached to and control the movement of the bones of the skeleton. The major muscles are shown in Figure 14-13.

Most skeletal muscles have names that describe some feature of the muscle, sometimes with several features combined in one name. Muscle features such as size, shape, direction of fibers,

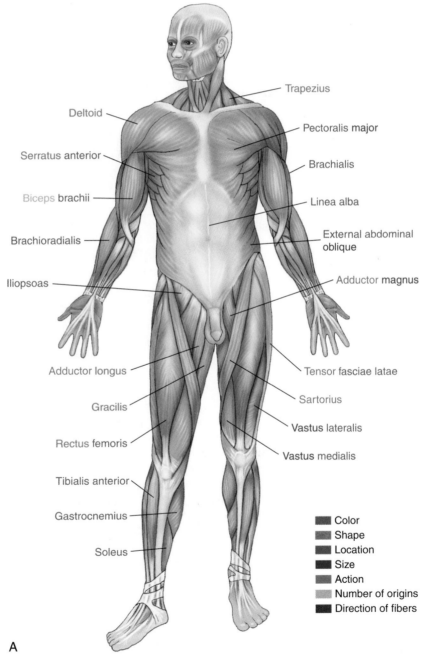

A

Figure 14-13 Major skeletal muscles of the body. A, Anterior view. Muscle features such as size, shape, direction of fibers, location, number of attachments, origin, and action are often used in naming muscles. This is demonstrated by the use of color-coding of the names on the anterior view.

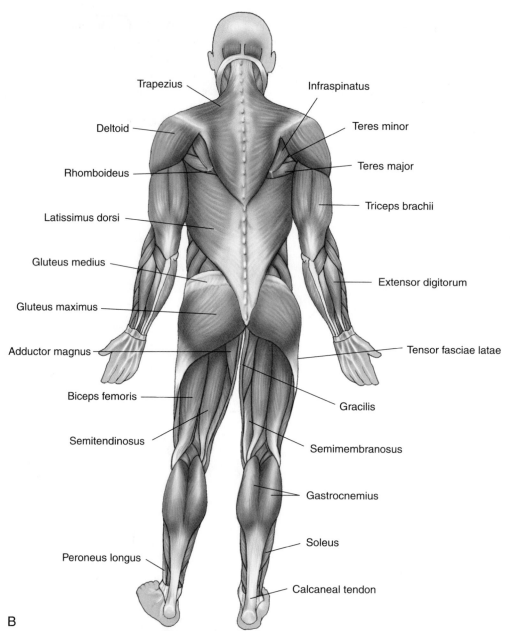

Trapezius

Infraspinatus

Deltoid

Teres minor

Rhomboideus

Teres major

Latissimus dorsi

Triceps brachii

Gluteus medius

Gluteus maximus

Extensor digitorum

Adductor magnus

Tensor fasciae latae

Biceps femoris

Gracilis

Semitendinosus

Semimembranosus

Gastrocnemius

Soleus

Peroneus longus

Calcaneal tendon

B

Figure 14-13 cont'd B, Posterior view.

location and number of attachments, origin, and action are often used in naming muscles. The name pectoralis major tells us it is a large muscle of the _____; major indicates the large size of the muscle. The names of the muscles in the anterior view have been color coded to indicate the origin of their names. For practice, color code as many muscles shown in the posterior view as you can, using terms you have learned together with a medical dictionary.

chest

14-60 A fibrous membrane called **fascia** (fash´e-ə) covers, supports, and separates muscles. The combining form for fascia is fasci(o). **Fascial** means pertaining to a _____.

fascia

Most skeletal muscles are attached to bones by tendons that span joints. When the muscle contracts, one bone moves relative to the other bone, and muscles sometimes work in groups to perform a particular movement. Muscles are arranged in antagonistic pairs. This means that when one muscle of the pair is contracted, the other is relaxed. For example, the biceps brachii muscle on the anterior arm bends the forearm at the elbow. The triceps brachii muscle on the posterior arm straightens the forearm at the elbow. When the former muscle contracts, the other is _____.

relaxed

14-61 There are several commonly used terms to describe different types of movement brought about by muscular activity (Figure 14-14). Use the information to write the answers in the following blanks.

The movement that straightens a limb is called _____. The movement that is opposite and means to bend a limb is **flexion** (flek´shən). The muscles responsible for these movements are called **extensors** and **flexors,** respectively.

14-62 Abduct/ion (ab-duk´shən) is the drawing away from the midline of the body, and the responsible muscles are called **abductors** (ab-duk´torz). The prefix ab- means away from. Abductors make movement possible away from the midline of the body.

The prefix ad- means toward. If ab/duction is the drawing away from the midline of the body, **ad/duction** (ad-duk´shən) is drawing _____ the midline.

The muscles responsible for adduction are called **adductors** (ă-duk´torz).

14-63 Rotation is the movement of a bone around its own axis, and the muscle that is responsible for rotation is called a **rotator.**

extension
(ek-sten´shən)

toward

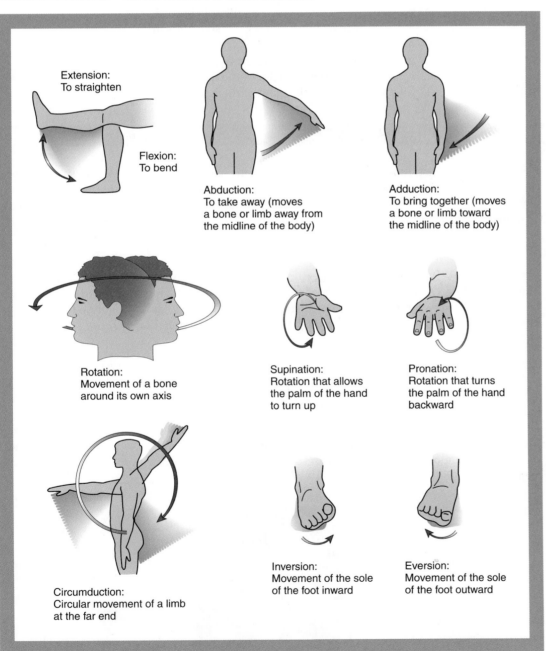

Extension:
To straighten

Flexion:
To bend

Abduction:
To take away (moves
a bone or limb away from
the midline of the body)

Adduction:
To bring together (moves
a bone or limb toward
the midline of the body)

Rotation:
Movement of a bone
around its own axis

Supination:
Rotation that allows
the palm of the hand
to turn up

Pronation:
Rotation that turns
the palm of the hand
backward

Circumduction:
Circular movement of a limb
at the far end

Inversion:
Movement of the sole
of the foot inward

Eversion:
Movement of the sole
of the foot outward

Figure 14-14 Types of muscular actions.

supination (soo″pī-na′shən)	The rotation that allows the palm of the hand to turn up is called _____.
pronation (pro-na′shən)	The rotation that turns the palm of the hand backward is called _____.
circumduction (sər″kəm-duk′shən)	**14-64** A circular movement of a limb at the far end is _____.
inversion (in-vər′zhən)	Movement of the sole of the foot inward is _____, and the opposite movement is **eversion** (e-vur′zhən).

EXERCISE 10

Match the types of body movements in 1 through 5 with their meanings (A through I). Not all selections will be used.

_____ 1. adduction

_____ 2. circumduction

_____ 3. eversion

_____ 4. flexion

_____ 5. supination

A. circular movement of a limb at the far end
B. drawing toward the midline of the body
C. movement of a bone around an axis
D. movement that allows turning the sole inward
E. movement that allows turning the sole outward
F. movement that bends a limb
G. movement that straightens a limb
H. rotation that turns the palm of the hand up
I. rotation that turns the palm of the hand down

DIAGNOSTIC TESTS AND PROCEDURES

14-65 Initial examination for musculoskeletal problems may include testing for range of motion (ROM), muscle strength, and reflexes. Range of motion is the maximum amount of movement that a healthy joint is capable of, and it is measured in degrees of a circle (Figure 14-15). Range-of-motion exercises are used to increase muscle strength and joint mobility. ROM means range

motion

of _____.

> ➤ **KEY** POINT <u>Range of motion is measured as either active ROM or passive ROM.</u> Active range of motion (AROM) is the range of movement through which a patient can actively, without assistance, move a joint by the adjacent muscles. Passive range of motion (PROM) is the maximum range of movement through which the examiner can safely move a person's joint.

Muscle strength can be graded by asking the patient to apply resistance to the force exerted by the examiner (for example, the examiner tries to pull the bent arm down while the patient tries to raise it).

Reflex action is the immediate and involuntary functioning or movement of an organ or body part in response to a particular stimulus. The **reflex hammer** is a mallet with a rubber head that is used to tap tendons, nerves, or muscles to test reflex reactions (see Figure 15-11). This instru-

hammer

ment for testing reflex reactions is called a reflex _____.

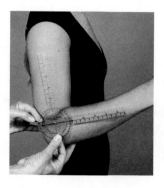 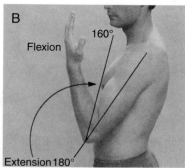

Figure 14-15 Range of motion and its measurement.
A, A goniometer is used to measure the angles of the range of motion. **B,** Demonstration of the normal range of motion of the elbow joint.

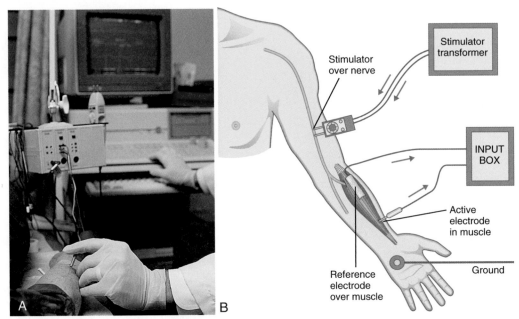

Figure 14-16 Electromyography. A, Patient and technician are shown with electromyographic equipment. Normal muscle at rest shows no electrical activity. Needle electrodes are inserted into the muscle to record skeletal muscle activity when the muscle contracts. **B,** Schematic drawing of electromyography, showing the stimulator transformer and the active electrode that has been placed in the muscle to detect skeletal muscle activity.

electrical

14-66 Electro/myo/graphy (e-lek″tro-mi-og´rə-fe), EMG, is used to record the response of a muscle to _____ stimulation (Figure 14-16). This is particularly useful in studying nerve damage and certain other disorders. The resulting record is called an **electromyogram** (e-lek″tro-mi´o-gram).

14-67 Diagnostic studies of the bones and connective tissues include radiologic studies, bone scans, laboratory tests, and a few invasive procedures. Standard x-rays provide information about the joints and bone density or congenital deformities or fractures. Bone density testing, also called **bone densito/metry** (den″sĭ-tom´ə-tre), is any one of several methods of

measures

determining bone mass with a machine that _____ how well the rays penetrate the bone. This is helpful in diagnosing osteoporosis and determining the effectiveness of therapy.

tomography

14-68 Bone tumors may be discovered during a routine radiologic examination. Computed tomography (CT), magnetic resonance imaging (MRI), bone scans, and biopsy are used to distinguish between benign and malignant tumors. Computed _____ produces an image of a cross-section of tissue. Magnetic resonance imaging is used to view soft tissue (for example, to visualize a cartilage tear). A **bone scan** is often useful in demonstrating malignant bone tumors, which appear as areas of increased uptake of radioactive material.

marrow

14-69 A bone marrow examination may include biopsy of the bone, as well as aspiration of bone marrow for microscopic study. These studies may be performed for other reasons, such as hemato/logic (hem″ə-to-loj´ik) evaluation. Bone marrow studies are used to diagnose leukemia, identify tumors or other disorders of the bone marrow, and determine the extent of myelosuppression. **Myelo/suppression** (mi″ə-lo-sə-pres´ən) is inhibition of the bone _____.
  The posterior iliac crest is generally the preferred site for **bone marrow aspiration** (Figure 14-17). In adults the anterior iliac crest or the sternum may also be used.

14-70 A **lumbar puncture,** commonly called a spinal tap, is performed for various therapeutic and diagnostic procedures. Diagnostic purposes include obtaining cerebrospinal fluid, measuring its pressure, or injecting substances for radiographic studies of the nervous system. Therapeutic indications include removing blood or pus, injecting drugs, and introducing an anesthetic for spinal anesthesia (Figure 14-18).

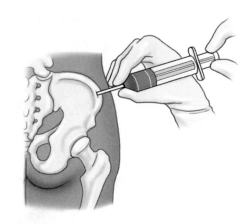

Figure 14-17 **Bone marrow aspiration from the posterior iliac crest.**

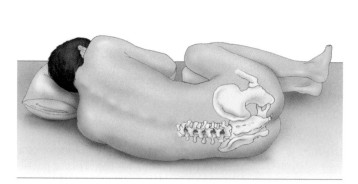

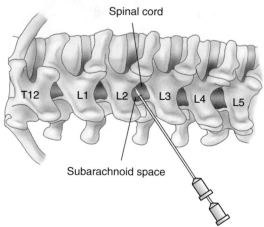

Spinal cord

T12 L1 L2 L3 L4 L5

Subarachnoid space

Figure 14-18 **Lumbar puncture.** The patient is generally positioned in the flexed lateral (fetal) position. The needle is inserted between the second and third or the third and fourth lumbar vertebrae. Cerebrospinal fluid can be removed or its pressure can be measured, and drugs can be introduced as done for spinal anesthesia.

vertebrae

The lumbar puncture is so named because the needle is inserted between two _____, usually the second and third or the third and fourth lumbar vertebrae (L2-3 or L3-4).

joint
within

14-71 Arthro/graphy (ahr-throg´rə-fe) is radiographic visualization of the inside of a _____. This is usually done by an intraarticular injection of a radiopaque substance. Both **intraarticular** and intra-articular mean _____ the joint.

The radiographic record produced after introduction of opaque contrast material into a joint is an **arthrogram** (ahr´thro-gram).

arthroscopy
(ahr-thros´kə-pe)

14-72 An **arthro/scope** (ahr´thro-skōp) is a fiberoptic instrument used for direct visualization of the interior of a joint. The process is called _____.

This procedure permits biopsy of cartilage or damaged synovial membrane, diagnosis of a torn cartilage, and, in some instances, removal of loose bodies in the joint space (Figure 14-19).

puncture

14-73 Arthro/centesis (ahr˝thro-sen-te´sis) is surgical _____ of a joint with a needle. This is performed to obtain samples of synovial fluid for diagnostic purposes, to remove excess fluid from joints to relieve pain, or to instill medications.

14-74 Table 14-3 lists several important laboratory tests that are used to assess musculoskeletal disorders. Use the material in the table to complete the next several blanks. In an **anti/nuclear antibody** (an˝te-, an˝ti-noo´kle-ər an´tĭ-bod˝e) (ANA) **test,** serum is tested for

antibodies

_____ that react with nuclear material. The ANA test is used primarily to diagnose systemic lupus erythematosus (described in Arthritis and Connective Tis-

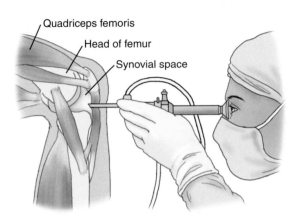

Figure 14-19 Arthroscopy of the knee. The examination of the interior of a joint is performed by inserting a specially designed endoscope through a small incision. This procedure also permits biopsy of cartilage or damaged synovial membrane, diagnosis of a torn meniscus, and in some instances, removal of loose bodies in the joint space.

TABLE 14-3	Abnormal Findings in Laboratory Testing for Musculoskeletal Disorders
Gland	**Principal Action**
Antinuclear antibody (ANA)	Serum is tested for antinuclear antibodies. Findings are positive in most patients with systemic lupus erythematosus, sometimes positive with scleroderma or rheumatoid arthritis.
Erythrocyte sedimentation rate (ESR)	Blood test shows elevated levels with any inflammatory process, especially rheumatoid arthritis and osteomyelitis.
Rheumatoid factor (RF) test	Blood test is positive in most patients with rheumatoid arthritis; sometimes there are lower levels in other connective tissue diseases.
Serum calcium	Decreased in osteomalacia; increased in some bone tumors.
Serum creatine phosphokinase (CPK)	Elevated levels are found in skeletal muscle disorders and myocardial infarction (death of heart muscle).
Serum phosphorus	Decreased in osteomalacia; increased in certain bone tumors.
Serum uric acid	Elevated levels are usually found in patients with gout.
Urine calcium	Sometimes detected in metastatic bone disease.

sue Diseases, later in this chapter), although a positive result may indicate other autoimmune diseases, such as rheumatoid arthritis or other connective tissue diseases.

erythrocyte

14-75 ESR means _____ **sedimentation rate.** This is the rate at which red blood cells (erythrocytes) settle out in a tube of blood that has been treated to prevent clotting. Elevated levels are found in any inflammatory process, especially rheumatoid arthritis.

rheumatoid

14-76 RF means the _____ **factor.** The result of this test is positive in most patients with rheumatoid arthritis.

decreased

14-77 The levels of serum calcium and serum phosphorus are _____ in osteomalacia (os″te-o-mə-la′shə), a disorder characterized by excessive loss of calcium from the bone.

creatine

14-78 CPK means _____ **phosphokinase.** Increased serum levels of CPK are found in skeletal muscle disorders and myocardial infarction (death of a portion of cardiac muscle, commonly called a heart attack).

gout (gout)

14-79 Elevated levels of serum uric acid are usually found in patients with a condition called _____, a disease associated with an inborn error of uric acid metabolism that can result in painful swelling of joints.

calcium

14-80 Calci/uria (kal″se-u′re-ə) means _____ in the urine. Although calcium may be present in normal urine in minute amounts, it is not readily detectable. (Urinary excretion of calcium is affected by several things, including diet.) **Hyper/calciuria** (hi″pər-kal″se-u′re-ə) is often seen in metastatic bone disease, in which there is rapid bone destruction.

EXERCISE 11

Write a word in each blank to complete these sentences.

1. BDT means _____ density testing.

2. EMG is the abbreviation for _____.

3. ROM means range of _____.

4. ESR means _____ sedimentation rate.

5. RF means _____ factor.

6. Arthrography is radiographic visualization of the inside of a/an _____.

7. A fiberoptic instrument that is used for direct visualization of the inside of a joint is a/an _____.

8. Surgical puncture of a joint is _____.

EXERCISE 12

Build It! *Use the following word parts to build terms. (Some word parts will be used more than once.)*

intra-, articul(o), arthr(o), calc(i), electr(o), my(o), oste(o), -ar, -gram, -graphy, -malacia, -uria

1. radiographic visualization inside a joint   _____/_____

2. calcium in the urine   _____/_____

3. pertaining to within a joint   _____/_____/_____

4. the record produced by electrical stimulation of a muscle

       _____/_____/_____

5. condition of softening of bone   _____/_____

Say and Check

Say aloud the terms you wrote for Exercise 12. Use the Companion CD to check your pronunciations.

PATHOLOGIES

connective	**14-81** Although injury is a primary cause of problems of the musculoskeletal system, the bones, muscles, and associated tissue are subject to various pathologies, including infections, metabolic disturbances, congenital disorders, and connective tissue diseases. You learned earlier that bone, cartilage, ligaments, and tendons are called _____ tissue because they support and bind other tissues.

Word Parts: Musculoskeletal Disorders

Combining Form	Meanings	Suffixes	Meanings
ankyl(o)	stiff	-asthenia	weakness
scler(o)	hard	-sarcoma	malignant tumor from
troph(o)	nutrition		connective tissue

STRESS AND TRAUMA INJURIES

14-82 Common musculoskeletal injuries include simple muscle strains, sprains, dislocations, and fractures. A **strain** is damage, usually muscular, that results from excessive physical effort.

A **sprain** is a traumatic injury to the tendons, muscles, or ligaments around a joint, characterized by pain, swelling, and discoloration of the skin over the joint. Radiography is often needed to rule out fractures. Strains and sprains are common traumatic injuries that cause much discomfort and can interfere with normal activities.

If a muscle in the arm is very sore but shows no swelling or discoloration of the skin after many hours playing games at the computer, is this more likely to be a strain or a sprain?

strain

pain

14-83 My/algia (mi-al′jə) is muscular _____. Another word that means the same as myalgia is **myodynia** (mi″o-din′e-ə).

A muscle cramp is a painful, involuntary muscle spasm, often caused by inflammation of the muscle, but it can be a symptom of electrolyte imbalance. An example of the latter is **tetany** (tet′ə-ne), a condition characterized by cramps, convulsions, twitching of the muscles, and sharp flexion of the wrists and ankle joints. It is caused by an imbalance in calcium metabolism.

14-84 A break in a bone is called a **fracture.**

> ➤ **KEY** POINT Fractures are classified as complete or incomplete and simple vs. compound. They are classified as complete fractures, with the break across the entire width of the bone so it is divided into two sections, or incomplete fractures. They are also described by the extent of associated soft tissue damage as simple or compound. The bone protrudes through the skin in a **compound fracture,** also called an **open fracture.** If a bone is fractured but does not protrude through the skin, it is called a **simple** or **closed fracture** (Figure 14-20).

compound
(or open)

Which type of fracture is a broken bone that causes an external wound? _____
An incomplete fracture in which the bone is bent and fractured on one side only, as in Figure 14-20, is called a **greenstick fracture** and is seen principally in children, whose bones are still pliant.

14-85 Figure 14-21 illustrates four types of fractures. In an **impacted fracture,** one bone fragment is firmly driven into the fractured end of another fragment.

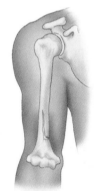
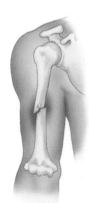
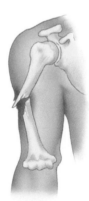

Incomplete, simple (closed)　　Complete, simple (closed)　　Compound (open)

Figure 14-20 Classification and description of the severity of fractures. Fractures are classified as either complete or incomplete and are described as either open or closed.

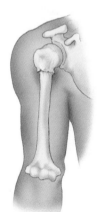
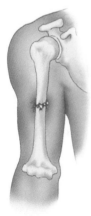
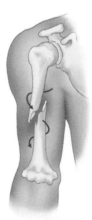
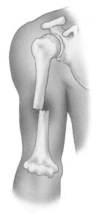

Impacted　　Comminuted　　Displaced spiral　　Displaced transverse

Figure 14-21 Common types of fractures. The spiral and transverse fractures are also displaced. The ends of broken bones in displaced fractures often pierce the surrounding skin, resulting in open fractures; however, these two examples are closed fractures.

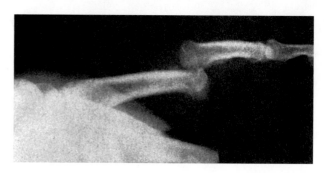

Figure 14-22 Radiograph demonstrating an interphalangeal dislocation of the finger.

spiral	Notice the many fragments of bone present in the **comminuted** (kom´ĭ-noŏt´əd) **fracture.** In which type of fracture is the bone twisted apart? _____ **fracture.** The bone is also displaced in the example. Displacement of a bone from a joint is also called a **dislocation** (Figure 14-22). Dislocations and fractures are usually evident on x-ray images of the affected bones.
across	The example of a **transverse fracture,** one in which the break is at right angles to the axis of the bone, also shows displacement. It will be helpful to remember that trans- in transverse means _____. Fractures are classified by the bone involved, the part of that bone, and the nature of the break, such as a compression fracture of the L4 vertebra. A **compression fracture** is a bone break caused by excessive vertical force. Pieces of the bone tend to move out in horizontal directions, and the affected bone collapses. The spinal cord is sometimes damaged in compression fractures of the vertebrae.
atrophy	**14-86** Treatments for dislocations and fractures are included later in this chapter, but immobilization of fractures by use of a cast is common. Muscle shrinks when a limb is immobilized for a long period. The term **atrophy** (at´rə-fe) means a decrease in size of an organ or tissue. This type of atrophy is called disuse _____. Atrophy is noticeable in these cases because the limb has decreased in size.
wrist	**14-87 Carpal tunnel syndrome** (CTS) is an example of trauma that results from prolonged, repetitive movements. CTS is a condition in which the median nerve in the wrist becomes compressed, causing pain and discomfort. Excessive hand exercise, a potential occupational hazard, can lead to a chronic condition of CTS. Carpal in its name will help you remember that CTS is a condition of the _____. Surgery to relieve the pressure on the nerve may be necessary.
rotation	**14-88** Rotator cuff injury may occur as a result of repetitive motions, injury, or the degenerative processes of aging. The **rotator cuff** is a structure of muscles and tendons that stabilizes and allows range of motion in the shoulder joint and, as the name implies, _____ of the humerus.
bursitis (bər-si´tis)	**14-89** Inflammation of a bursa is called _____. This condition can result from repetitive motion, as well as trauma, infection, or other disorders of the musculoskeletal system.
tendon	Both **tendin/itis** (ten″dĭ-ni´tis) and **tendon/itis** (ten″də-ni´tis) mean inflammation of a _____, but tendinitis is the preferred spelling. Bursitis and tendinitis can be related to overuse, repetitive motion, or irritation; symptoms usually disappear with rest.
pain	**14-90** Tenodynia (ten″o-din´e-ə) may be caused by tendinitis. **Teno/dynia** means _____ in a tendon and is the same as **tenalgia** (te-nal´jə).
synovitis (sin″o-vi´tis)	Using synov(o), write a word that means inflammation of a synovial joint: _____.
	14-91 Common symptoms of persons with musculoskeletal disorders include pain, weakness, deformity, limitation of movement, stiffness, and **joint crepitus** (krep´ĭ-təs), the crackling sound produced when a bone rubs against another bone or roughened cartilage.

spine	Both **rachio/dynia** (ra″ke-o-din′e-ə) and **rachialgia** (ra″ke-al′jə) mean a painful condition of the _____. **Spondyl/algia** (spon″dĭ-lal′jə) is pain in a vertebra.

spine

ischialgia (is″ke-al′jə)
ischium
sternum
pain

Sacro/dynia (sa″kro-din′e-ə) is pain of the sacrum. Using a different suffix, write another word that means pain in the ischium: _____. **Ischio/dynia** (is″ke-o-din′e-ə) is also pain in the _____.

Stern/algia (stər-nal′jə) is pain in the _____.
Tibi/algia (tib″e-al′jə) is _____ of the tibia.

calcaneitis
(kal-ka″ne-i′tis)

14-92 Calcaneo/dynia (kal-ka″ne-o-din′e-ə) is a painful heel. Write a word that means inflammation of the heel bone: _____.

chondralgia
(kon-dral′jə)
bone

14-93 The knee is subject to many injuries, particularly tearing of the cartilage. **Chondr/itis** (kon-dri′tis), inflammation of the cartilage, can cause **chondro/dynia** (kon″dro-din′e-ə), pain of the cartilage. Another term that means painful cartilage, _____, uses a different suffix.

Osteo/chondr/itis (os″te-o-kon-dri′tis) is inflammation of cartilage and _____.

cartilage
chondropathy
(kon-drop′ə-the)

14-94 Arthro/chondr/itis (ahr″thro-kon-dri′tis) is inflammation of an articular _____.

Write a word that means any disease of a cartilage: _____.

14-95 An abnormal condition characterized by facial pain and by mandibular dysfunction, apparently caused by a defective or dislocated temporomandibular joint (TMJ), is called TMJ pain dysfunction syndrome or is sometimes shortened to TMJ disorder.

temporomandibular

Some indications of this disorder are clicking of the joint when the jaw moves, limitation of jaw movement, and temporomandibular dislocation. TMJ is an abbreviation for the _____ joint.

14-96 Low back pain that radiates down the buttock and below the knee, resulting from pressure on spinal nerve roots, is the most common symptom of a **herniated disk,** rupture of an intervertebral disk, the tough fibrous cushion between two vertebral bodies. This condition can result either from repeated stress or injury to the spine, or from natural degeneration with aging.

herniated

This is also called a slipped disk, but a more appropriate name is a _____ disk (Figure 14-23).

14-97 Feet absorb considerable shock while running and walking, activities that can bring about a variety of disorders, particularly when structural weaknesses and other problems exist or improperly fitted shoes are worn.

tarsus

Tarso/ptosis (tahr″sop-to′sis) is prolapse of the _____.
This is commonly called flatfoot.

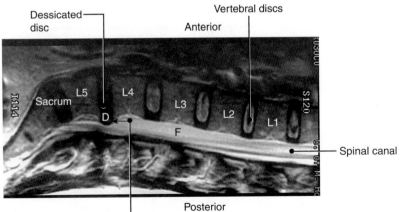

Figure 14-23 A lumbar MRI scan of a herniated disk.

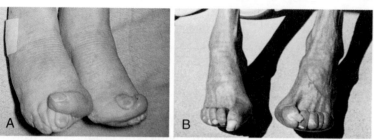

Figure 14-24 Deformities of the feet. A, Hallux valgus. The great toe rides over the second toe in this example. **B,** Hammertoe. The toes are permanently flexed. Hallux valgus is also present.

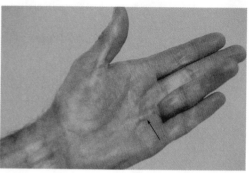

Figure 14-25 Dupuytren contracture. This painless progressive shortening, thickening, and fibrosis of the subcutaneous tissue of the palm causes the fourth and fifth fingers to bend into the palm and resist extension.

hallux

Hallux means the great toe. **Hallux valgus** (hal´əks val´gəs) is a deformity of the foot, sometimes called a bunion. The great toe deviates laterally at the **metatarso/phalang/eal** (MTP) **joint** (Figure 14-24, *A*). The medically correct name for bunion is _____ valgus.

A **hammertoe** is a toe that is permanently flexed at the midphalangeal joint, producing a clawlike appearance. This common abnormality often occurs simultaneously with hallux valgus (Figure 14-24, *B*). Hammertoe may be present in more than one digit, but the second toe is most often affected. **Corns** (hard masses of epithelial cells overlying a bony prominence) may develop on the dorsal side, and **calluses** (thickening of the outer layers of the skin at points of friction or pressure) may appear on the plantar surface.

tumor

14-98 In **Morton neur/oma** (no͞o-ro´mə) a small, painful _____ grows in a digital nerve of the foot. Surgical removal of the neuroma is generally indicated if the pain persists and interferes with walking.

Tarsal tunnel syndrome is the ankle version of the carpal tunnel syndrome. Treatment is similar to that for carpal tunnel syndrome.

14-99 The cause is not known for some musculoskeletal disorders, such as **Dupuytren contracture**, a thickening and tightening of the palmar fascia, causing the fourth or fifth finger to bend into the palm and resist extension (Figure 14-25).

EXERCISE 13

Word Analysis. *Break these words into their component parts by placing a slash between the word parts. Write the meaning of each term.*

1. myodynia _____

2. spondylalgia _____

3. arthrochondritis _____

4. calcaneodynia _____

5. atrophy _____

INFECTIONS

bone

14-100 Oste/itis (os˝te-i´tis) is inflammation of a _____. It may be caused by infection, degeneration, or trauma. Osteitis results in **oste/algia** (os˝te-al´jə),

pain

also called **osteo/dynia** (os˝te-o-din´e-ə), which means bone _____.

Osteo/mye/litis (os˝te-o-mi˝ə-li´tis) is an infection of the bone and bone marrow caused by infectious microorganisms that are introduced by trauma or surgery, by extension from a nearby infection, or via the bloodstream. Staphylococci are common causes of osteomyelitis.

14-101 Sometimes it is difficult to know if myel(o) in a word refers to bone marrow or the spinal cord, and in some words it can refer to either. For example, **myel/itis** (mi″ə-li′tis) means inflammation of either the bone _____ or the spinal cord.

marrow

14-102 Cellul/itis (sel″u-li′tis) is an acute, spreading, swollen, pus-forming inflammation of the deep subcutaneous tissues. It may be associated with abscess formation. If the muscle is also involved, it is called **myocellulitis** (mi″o-sel″u-li′tis).

You learned earlier that cellul(o) means small cell, but that may not be helpful in remembering this term. Write the term that means an acute, pus-forming inflammation of the tissues and muscle: _____.

myocellulitis

TUMORS AND MALIGNANCIES

14-103 The cause of bone tumors is largely unknown, unless cancer originates in other tissues and metastasizes to the bone. Bone tumors are either benign or malignant. Benign bone tumors are often asymptomatic.

> ➤ **KEY** POINT <u>There are many types of benign bone tumors.</u> Benign tumors arise from several types of tissue. The major classifications include chondrogenic tumors, osteogenic tumors, and fibrogenic tumors.

cartilage

Chondro/genic tumors develop in the _____. A **chondr/oma** (kon-dro′mə) is a benign tumor or tumor-like growth of mature cartilage. An **osteo/chondr/oma** (os″te-o-kon-dro′mə), composed of bone and cartilage, is the most common benign bone tumor.

bone

Osteo/genic (os″te-o-jen′ik) tumors arise in the _____. These are usually benign, but one type, giant cell tumor of the bone, sometimes metastasizes.

Fibro/genic tumors are derived from fibrous tissue.

14-104 Malignant bone tumors may be primary (originating in the bone) or secondary (originating in other tissue and metastasizing to the bone).

> ➤ **KEY** POINT <u>Terms using the word part -sarcoma name or describe malignant tumors.</u> There may be rare instances of misnomers. **Osteo/sarcoma** (os″te-o-sahr-ko′mə) is the most common type of primary malignant bone tumor. In addition to osteosarcoma, other primary bone tumors include these cancers:
> - **chondrosarcoma** (kon″dro-sahr-ko′mə)
> - **fibrosarcoma** (fi″bro-sahr-ko′mə)
> - Ewing sarcoma

malignant

cartilage

Words ending in sarcoma generally describe tumors that are _____.

A chondro/sarcoma is derived from _____, spreads to the bone, and destroys it.

fibrous

A fibro/sarcoma arises from _____ tissues. **Ewing sarcoma** is an aggressive bone tumor.

14-105 Metastatic bone cancer occurs far more often than primary bone cancer. That is because certain types of cancer metastasize frequently to the bone, much more often than other types of primary cancer. Primary cancers of the breast, prostate, kidney, thyroid, and lung are sometimes called bone-seeking cancers because they frequently metastasize to _____ tissue, especially bone marrow.

bone

marrow

14-106 Multiple myel/oma (mi″ə-lo′mə) is a malignant neoplasm of the bone _____ that disrupts and destroys bone marrow function. Both multiple myeloma and leukemia are white blood cell cancers, with proliferation of certain types of cells and limited production of normal red blood cells, white blood cells, and platelets.

14-107 Leukemia is a broad term given to a group of malignant diseases that are characterized by replacement of bone marrow with proliferating immature leukocytes and abnormal numbers of immature leukocytes in the blood circulation. Leukemia is classified according to the predominant type of proliferating leukocytes. It is classified as either acute or chronic. Leuk/emia received its name from the large number of _____ blood cells in the circulation.

Environmental and genetic factors are believed to be involved in the development of leukemia, but the exact mechanism is generally unknown. Certain chemicals and drugs as well as ionizing radiation exposure (for example, the atomic bomb at Hiroshima or the Chernobyl nuclear accident) increase the risk for development of leukemia. The damage to genes that control cell growth changes cells from a normal to a malignant state.

Classification of the type of leukemia is complex, but the disease is classified according to the predominant proliferating cells. **Lympho/cyt/ic** or **lympho/blast/ic** and **myelo/cyt/ic** or **myelo/gen/ous** leukemias are broad classifications, and several subtypes exist. Lympho/blasts are immature cells that develop into _____. The immature cells in myelogenous leukemias are granulocytes.

Acute leukemia has a sudden onset. Chronic leukemia develops slowly, and signs and symptoms similar to those of acute leukemia may not appear for years. Diagnosis is made by blood tests and bone marrow biopsies. Acute myelocytic leukemia is often abbreviated AML. CML means _____ myelogenous leukemia. ALL and CLL mean acute lymphocytic and chronic lymphocytic leukemia, respectively.

Margin answers: white, lymphocytes, chronic

EXERCISE 14

■■ **Build It!** *Use the following word parts to build terms. (Some word parts will be used more than once.)*

cellul(o), chondr(o), leuk(o), myel(o), my(o), oste(o), -emia, -itis, -oma, -sarcoma

1. inflammation of the bone _____/_____

2. malignant tumor derived from cartilage _____/_____

3. inflammation of the bone and bone marrow _____/_____/_____

4. inflammation of muscle and deep subcutaneous tissues _____/_____/_____

5. blood condition with many immature white blood cells _____/_____

🔊 **Say and Check**

Say aloud the terms you wrote for Exercise 14. Use the Companion CD to check your pronunciations.

METABOLIC DISTURBANCES

14-108 There is a delicate balance between bone destruction and bone formation. Excessive formation can lead to abnormal hardness and unusual heaviness of bone, called **osteo/sclerosis** (os″te-o-sklə-ro′sis).

Despite its density, osteosclerotic bone is brittle and subject to fracture. Literal interpretation of osteosclerotic is pertaining to bone that is _____.

Softening and destruction of bone is called **osteo/lysis** (os″te-ol′ĭ-sis). **Paget disease** (named for Sir James Paget, an English surgeon) is a skeletal disease in which osteolysis is usually evident. Osteo/lysis is _____ of bone.

14-109 Vitamin D aids in the absorption of calcium from the intestinal tract. A deficiency of vitamin D results in insufficient calcium absorption and **calci/penia** (kal″sĭ-pe′ne-ə), a deficiency of _____ in the body.

Margin answers: hard, destruction, calcium

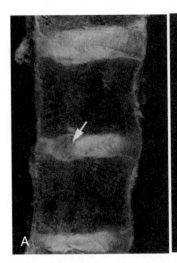
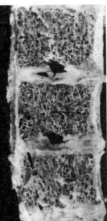
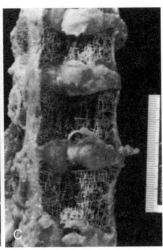

Figure 14-26 Normal versus osteoporotic vertebral bodies. A, Normal vertebral bodies. **B,** Vertebrae showing moderate osteoporosis. **C,** Vertebrae showing severe osteoporosis. The vertebral bodies are sectioned to show internal structure. *A* shows well-formed, normal vertebrae and disks. The *white arrow* points to a small focus of degeneration. In *B* the overall shape of the vertebrae is preserved, but osteoporosis is already well developed. The disks show severe degeneration *(black arrows).* Note in *C,* severe osteoporosis, how the vertebrae have been compressed by the bulging disks.

Remember that de- means down or from. **De/calci/fication** (de-kal″sĭ-fĭ-ka′shən) is loss of calcium from bone or teeth.

14-110 Osteo/penia (os″te-o-pe′ne-ə) is not a disease but a condition that is common to metabolic bone disease. **Osteopenia** is a reduced bone mass, usually the result of synthesis not compensating for the rate of destruction of bone. Write this term that means a reduced bone mass:

osteopenia _____.

14-111 Osteo/porosis (os″te-o-pə-ro′sis) is a metabolic disease in which reduction in the amount of bone mass leads to subsequent fractures. It occurs most commonly in postmenopausal women, sedentary individuals, and patients on long-term steroid therapy. The bones appear thin and fragile, and fractures are common (Figure 14-26). This metabolic bone disease in which there is a reduction in bone mass and increased porosity is called _____.

osteoporosis

It may cause pain, especially in the lower back, and loss of height; spinal deformities are common. Figure 14-27 shows the effect of the disease on height and shape of the spine with advancing years.

14-112 Translated literally, **osteo/malacia** (os″te-o-mə-la′shə) means abnormal

softening _____ of bone. It is a reversible metabolic disease in which there is a defect in the mineralization of bone, resulting from inadequate phosphorus and cal-

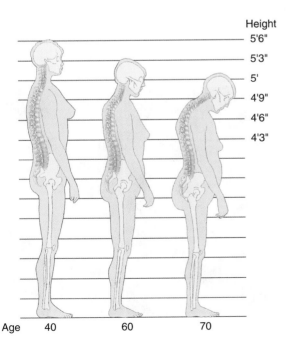

Height
— 5'6"
— 5'3"
— 5'
— 4'9"
— 4'6"
— 4'3"

Age   40   60   70

Figure 14-27 Osteoporotic changes in the curvature of the spine. The spine appears normal at age 40 and shows osteoporotic changes at age 60 and 70. These changes bring about a loss of as much as 6 to 9 inches in height, and the so-called dowager's hump in the upper thoracic vertebrae.

cium. The deficiency may be caused by a diet lacking phosphorus and calcium or vitamin D, which is necessary for bone formation. Other causes include malabsorption or a lack of exposure to sunlight, which is necessary for the body to synthesize vitamin D. Osteomalacia is the adult equivalent of rickets in children.

Insufficient calcium for bone mineralization during the growing years causes **rickets** (rik´əts). Skeletal deformities of rickets are much more severe than those of osteomalacia in adults. In children, the disorder takes the form of _____.

In adults, the disorder is called _____.

14-113 Osteitis deformans (os″te-i´tis de-for´manz), also called Paget disease, is a disorder characterized by excessive bone destruction and unorganized bone repair. The disease was thought to be an infectious inflammatory process and was named osteitis deformans. The other name for osteitis deformans is _____ disease.

> rickets
> osteomalacia
>
> Paget

CONGENITAL DEFECTS

14-114 The skeletal system is affected by several developmental defects, including malformations of the spine. **Spina bifida** (spi´nə bif-ə-də, bi´fə-də) is a congenital abnormality characterized by defective closure of the bones of the spine. It can be so extensive that it allows herniation of the spinal cord, or it might be evident only on radiologic examination. Remember that the prefix bi- in bi/fida means _____.

A **cranio/cele** (kra´ne-o-sēl″) is a hernial protrusion of the brain through a defect in the _____. This is the same as an **encephalocele**.

14-115 Literal translation of **rachi/schisis** (ra-kis´kĭ-sis) is split _____. This is congenital **fissure** (split) of one or more vertebrae.

14-116 Sterno/schisis (stern[o], sternum + -schisis, split) means _____ sternum. In sternoschisis (stər-nos´kĭ-sis), there is congenital fissure of the sternum. The suffix -schisis means split.*

14-117 Scoliosis (sko″le-o´sis) is lateral curvature of the spine, a fairly common abnormality of childhood, especially in females. Write this term that means lateral curvature of the spine: _____. Causes include congenital malformations of the spine, poliomyelitis, spastic paralysis, and unequal leg lengths.

Lordosis (lor-do´sis) is an abnormal anterior concavity of the lumbar spine as viewed from the side. **Kyphosis** (ki-fo´sis) refers to an abnormal convexity in the curvature of the thoracic spine as viewed from the side. Compare these abnormal curvatures of the spine (Figure 14-28).

> two
>
> skull
>
> spine
>
> split
>
> scoliosis

---

*-Schisis (Greek: *schizein*, split).

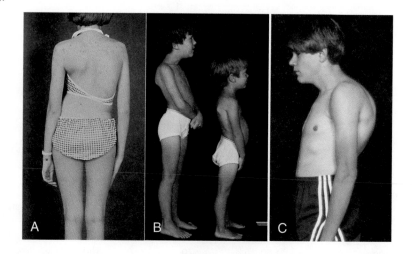

Figure 14-28 Three abnormal curvatures of the spine. A, Scoliosis, lateral curvature of the spine. **B,** Lordosis, abnormal anterior concavity of the lumbar spine. **C,** Severe kyphosis of the thoracic spine.

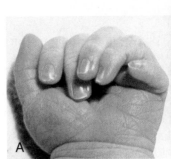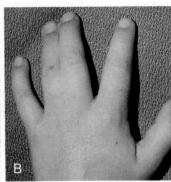

Figure 14-29 **Comparison of the fingers in polydactyly and syndactyly. A,** Polydactyly. Note the presence of six fingers. **B,** Syndactyly. Note the webbing of the third and fourth phalanges.

muscular	**14-118** The suffix -trophy means nutrition. **Dystrophy** is any abnormal condition caused by defective nutrition, often entailing a developmental change in muscles. 　**Muscular dystrophy** is a group of inherited diseases that are characterized by weakness and atrophy of muscle without involvement of the nervous system. In all forms of muscular dystrophy, there is progressive disability and loss of strength. The name of this disease, the cause of which is unknown but appears to be an inborn error of metabolism, is _____ dystrophy.
many	**14-119** An **anomaly*** (ə-nom′ə-le) is a deviation from what is regarded as normal, especially as a result of congenital defects. Each hand and foot normally has five digits. **Poly/dactyl/ism** (pol″e-dak′təl-iz-əm) or **poly/dactyly** (pol″e-dak′tə-le) is the presence of _____ digits on the hands or feet. In either of these terms, it is understood that the number of digits is greater than the expected number of five.
syndactyly	**Syndactyly** (sin-dak′tə-le) is a congenital anomaly of the hand or foot, marked by persistence of the webbing between adjacent digits, so they are more or less completely attached. It can be so severe that there is complete union of the digits and fusion of the bones. Write this term that means a congenital anomaly marked by webbing between adjacent digits: _____. This is also called **syndactylism** (sin-dak′tə-liz-əm). Compare polydactyly and syndactyly in Figure 14-29.

*Anomaly (Greek: *anomalos,* irregular).

EXERCISE 15

Word Analysis. *Break these words into their component parts by placing a slash between the word parts. Write the meaning of each term.*

1. craniocele _____

2. syndactylism _____

3. osteosclerosis _____

4. osteopenia _____

5. rachischisis _____

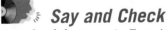 **Say and Check**

Say aloud the terms in Exercise 15. Use the Companion CD to check your pronunciations.

ARTHRITIS AND CONNECTIVE TISSUE DISEASES

joints

14-120 Arthr/itis is any inflammatory condition of the _____, characterized by pain, heat, swelling, redness, and limitation of movement. Write a word

arthropathy
(ahr-throp′ə-the)

that means any disease of the joints: _____. An **osteo/arthro/pathy** (os″te-o-ahr-throp′ə-the) is a disease of the bones and joints.

14-121 Arthr/algia (ahr-thral′jə) means pain in a joint. Write another word that means pain in a

arthrodynia
(ahr″thro-din′e-ə)

joint, using a different suffix: _____.

Many forms of arthritis are accompanied by pain and stiffness in adjacent parts. **Spondyl/arthritis** (spon″dəl-ahr-thri′tis) is accompanied by **dors/algia** (dor-sal′jə), pain in the

hardening

back. **Arthro/scler/osis** (ahr″thro-sklə-ro′sis) is _____ of the joints.

14-122 Osteo/arthritis (os″te-o-ahr-thri′tis), also called **degenerative joint disease** (DJD), is a form of arthritis in which one or many joints undergo degenerative changes, particularly loss of articular cartilage (Figure 14-30). This is the most common type of arthritis and is often classified as a connective tissue disease. **Connective tissue diseases** are a group of acquired disorders that cause immunologic and inflammatory changes in small blood vessels and connective tissue.

Hips, knees, the vertebral column, and the hands are primarily affected because they are used most often and bear the stress of body weight. DJD is characterized by progressive deterioration

cartilage

and loss of articular _____.

Possible causes of DJD include the wear-and-tear effects of aging, genetics, mechanical stress (abuse or overuse of certain joints), and certain metabolic diseases such as diabetes mellitus. Routine x-rays are usually helpful in confirming the diagnosis. CT and MRI may be used to determine the extent of vertebral involvement.

14-123 Rheumatoid arthritis (RA) is the second most commonly occurring connective tissue disease. It is also the most destructive to joints. It is a chronic, progressive, systemic inflammatory process that affects primarily synovial joints.

RA affects females more often than males, and people with a family history of RA two or three times more often than the rest of the population. It is believed to be an **autoimmune disease**—that is, one that is characterized by an alteration of the immune system, resulting in the production of antibodies against the body's own cells. You have learned that the combining form aut(o) means self. An alteration in the immune system resulting in the production of antibodies

autoimmune

against the body's own cells is called an _____ disease.

Fever and fatigue are common findings in rheumatoid arthritis. As the disease worsens, the joints become progressively inflamed and painful. Joint deformity is common (Figure 14-31).

14-124 Lupus erythematosus (loo′pəs er″ə-them″ə-to′sis), systemic scleroderma (sklēr″o-dur′mə), and Sjögren (shər′gren) syndrome are also autoimmune diseases that involve connective tissue. **Lupus erythematosus** (LE) is named for the characteristic butterfly rash that appears

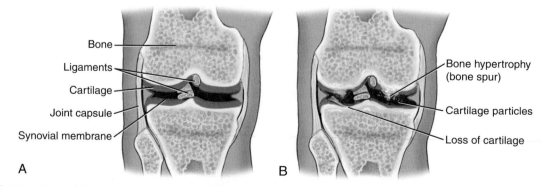

A

B

Bone
Ligaments
Cartilage
Joint capsule
Synovial membrane

Bone hypertrophy
(bone spur)
Cartilage particles
Loss of cartilage

Figure 14-30 Joint changes that occur in degenerative joint disease involving the knee. A, Normal knee joint. **B,** Bone hypertrophy and loss of cartilage in DJD of the knee.

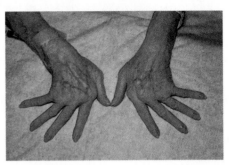

Figure 14-31 Hand deformities characteristic of chronic rheumatoid arthritis. There is marked deformity of the metacarpophalangeal joints, causing deviation of the fingers to the ulnar side of the hand.

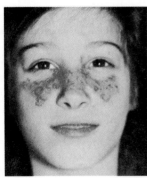

Figure 14-32 The characteristic "butterfly" rash of systemic lupus erythematosus. The word *lupus* is the Latin term for wolf. The rash is usually red, and thus the term *erythematosus*, a Latin word meaning reddened, was added in naming this disease.

across the bridge of the nose in some cases (Figure 14-32). There are two classifications of lupus: **cutaneous** or **discoid** lupus erythematosus (DLE) and **systemic lupus erythematosus** (SLE). The discoid type affects only the skin. The systemic type can cause major body organs and systems to fail and is potentially fatal. Prolonged exposure to sunlight and other forms of ultraviolet lighting aggravates the skin rash. The name of this autoimmune disease is _____ erythematosus.

> lupus

14-125 **Systemic scleroderma,** also called **systemic sclerosis** (sklə-ro´sis), is another connective tissue disease. Translated literally, sclero/derma means hardening of the _____. Associated with a high mortality rate, systemic sclerosis is characterized by inflammation, fibrosis, and sclerosis of the skin and vital organs. The cause is unknown, but autoimmunity is suspected.

> skin

14-126 **Sjögren syndrome** is an immunologic disorder characterized by deficient fluid production, which leads to dry eyes, dry mouth, and dryness of other mucous membranes. This disorder primarily affects women over 40 years of age.

14-127 **Gout** is a systemic disease associated with an inborn error of uric acid metabolism. Urate crystals deposit in the joints, myocardium, kidneys, and ears, causing inflammation. The disease can cause painful swelling of a joint, accompanied by chills and fever. Males are affected more often than females, and diet and medication are critical in the management of this disease called _____.

> gout

14-128 The literal interpretation of **polyarthritis** (pol″e-ahr-thri´tis) is inflammation of _____ joints; however, this term means inflammation of more than one joint. The inflammation either may migrate from one joint to the other, or several joints may be affected by inflammation simultaneously.

> many

14-129 **Spondylo/arthro/pathy** (spon″də-lo-ahr-throp´ə-the) is a term that means any one of a group of inflammatory disorders that affect the joints and spine.

14-130 The combining form ankyl(o) means stiff. **Ankylosing spondylitis** causes inflammation and stiffening of the _____. **Ankylosis** (ang″kə-lo´sis) means stiffening of a joint.

> spine

14-131 **Lyme disease** is an infection caused by the bite of an infected deer tick. Symptoms in the early stages of the disease are a circular rash, ill feeling, fever, headache, and muscle and joint aches. Prompt antibiotic treatment is effective. Without treatment, a small percentage of infected persons will develop arthritis as well as heart and neurologic problems. This disease, called _____ disease, is named for the place where it was originally described, Lyme, Connecticut.

> Lyme

*Discoid (Greek: *diskos,* flat plate).

MUSCULAR DISORDERS

many

myopathy
(mi-op′ə-the)
muscle

fatigue

muscles

joints

softening

myasthenia

muscle

muscle

14-132 Polymyositis (pol″e-mi″o-si′tis) is an inflammatory myo/pathy that involves _____ muscles, which leads to atrophy of the muscle. Weight loss, fatigue, and gradual weakness of the muscles are characteristic. A disease of the muscles is called a _____.

14-133 Myo/fascial (mi″o-fash′e-əl) pertains to a _____ and its fascia. Myofascial pain syndrome is pain in one region of the body, often diagnosed by palpation of a "trigger point" that causes pain and twitching of a muscle some distance away from the point of palpation. Myo/fascial means pertaining to a muscle and its fascia.

14-134 Chronic fatigue syndrome is a disorder characterized by disabling fatigue accompanied by a variety of associated complaints, including muscle pain, joint pain, and headache. This disabling disorder that is named for its chief symptom is called chronic _____ syndrome.

14-135 Poly/my/algia (pol″e-mi-al′jə) means pain of many _____. **Polymyalgia rheumatica** (roo-mat′ik-ə) is a chronic, inflammatory disease that primarily affects the arteries in muscles. The major symptoms are stiffness, weakness, and aching, most commonly in the shoulder or pelvic girdle.

14-136 Fibro/my/algia (fi″bro-mi-al′jə), also called **fibromyalgia syndrome,** is characterized by widespread non/articular pain of the torso, extremities, and the face. It may be attributable to deep sleep deprivation. **Non/articular** means that the _____ are not involved in this chronic disorder.

14-137 Atrophy of muscle tissue occurs as one ages, but the rate is slowed by exercise. Therapeutic exercise that increases muscle strength and tone is helpful with balance in walking and provides support for the joints as one ages.
   Myo/lysis (mi-ol′ĭ-sis) means disintegration or degeneration of muscle, and **myo/malacia** (mi″o-mə-la′shə) is abnormal _____ of muscular tissue.

14-138 My/asthenia (mi″əs-the′ne-ə) is a term specifically applied to muscle weakness. The suffix -asthenia means weakness. Write this new word that means muscle weakness: _____.
   Myasthenia gravis is a disease of unknown cause, characterized by fatigue and muscle weakness resulting from a defect in the conduction of nerve impulses. It may either be restricted to one muscle group or become generalized. The disorder may affect any muscles of the body but especially those of the eyes, face, lips, tongue, neck, and throat.

14-139 A **myo/cele** (mi′o-sēl) is herniation of a _____ through its ruptured sheath.

14-140 Myo/fibr/osis (mi″o-fi-bro′sis) is a condition in which _____ tissue is replaced by fibrous tissue.

EXERCISE 16

Match the terms in the left column (1 through 6) with their meanings in the right column (A through I). Not all choices will be used.

_____ 1. comminuted fracture

_____ 2. compound fracture

_____ 3. dislocation

_____ 4. greenstick fracture

_____ 5. sprain

_____ 6. strain

A. bone is shattered, producing numerous fragments
B. broken bone is at right angle to the axis of the bone
C. broken bone protrudes through the skin
D. displacement of a bone from a joint
E. incomplete fracture in which the bone is fractured on one side only
F. muscular damage that results from excessive physical effort
G. one bone fragment is firmly driven into another fragment
H. painful, involuntary muscle spasm
I. injury to the tendons, muscles, or ligaments around a joint

EXERCISE 17

Write a word in each blank space to complete these sentences.

1. A condition in which the median nerve in the wrist becomes compressed, causing pain, is

   _____ tunnel syndrome.

2. Inflammation of a bursa is _____.

3. Inflammation of an articular cartilage is _____.

4. TMJ disorder is a dysfunction of the _____ joint.

5. Another name for flatfoot is _____.

6. An osteosarcoma is a malignant bone _____.

7. A metabolic disease in which there is a defect in the mineralization of bone, resulting from inadequate phosphorus

   and calcium, is _____.

8. A congenital abnormality characterized by defective closure of the spine is called spina _____.

9. Degenerative joint disease is also called _____.

10. A disease of the nervous system that is characterized by fatigue and muscle weakness is called

    _____ gravis.

EXERCISE 18

Build It! *Use the following word parts to build terms. (Some word parts will be used more than once.)*

poly-, ankyl(o), arthr(o), fibr(o), my(o), scler(o), spondyl(o), -algia , -derma, -osis, -pathy

1. hardening of the skin   _____/_____

2. condition of stiffening of a joint   _____/_____

3. condition where muscle is replaced by fibrous tissue

   _____/_____/_____

4. pain in many muscles   _____/_____/_____

5. disorder affecting the joints and spine   _____/_____/_____

Say and Check

Say aloud the terms you wrote for Exercise 18. Use the Companion CD to check your pronunciations.

SURGICAL AND THERAPEUTIC INTERVENTIONS

reduction

14-141 Orthopedics (or″tho-pe´diks) is the branch of medicine that specializes in the prevention and correction of disorders of the musculoskeletal system. Orthopedic surgeons, also called **orthopedists,** restore fractures to their normal positions by **reduction,** pulling the broken fragments into alignment. Pulling a fracture (fx) into alignment is called _____.

A fracture is usually restored to its normal position by manipulation without surgery. This is called **closed reduction.**

> ➤ **KEY** POINT <u>Management of a closed reduction usually involves immobilization with a splint, bandage, cast, or traction.</u> A **splint** immobilizes, restrains, or supports the injured part (for example, the finger) until healing occurs (Figure 14-33). A **cast** is a stiffer, more solid dressing form with plaster of Paris or other material. **Traction** is the use of a pulling force to a part of the body to produce alignment and rest, while decreasing muscle spasm and correcting or preventing deformity.

14-142 If a fracture must be exposed by surgery before the broken ends can be aligned, it is an **open reduction.** The fracture shown in Figure 14-34 was corrected by surgery that included **internal fixation** to stabilize the alignment. Internal fixation uses pins, rods, plates, screws, and/or other materials to immobilize the fracture. After healing, the fixation devices may be either removed or left in place.

External fixation may be used in both open and closed reductions. This method uses metal pins attached to a compression device outside the skin surface (Figure 14-35).

After a bone is broken, the body begins the healing process to repair the injury. Electrical bone stimulation, bone grafting, and ultrasound treatment may be used when healing is slow or does not occur.

14-143 Persons with osteoporosis are predisposed to fractures. Calcium therapy, vitamin D, and osteo/porotics (os″te-o-pə-rot´ikz) are used to treat osteoporosis. Estrogen therapy, begun soon after the start of menopause, may help in the prevention and maintenance of osteoporosis, but there is no agreement on its value versus its risks. **Osteoporotics** are medications that are used

osteoporosis

to treat _____. Read more about hormone replacement therapy (HRT) for women at high risk for osteoporosis in Chapter 12.

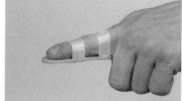

Figure 14-33 Finger splint. This type of orthopedic rigid device made of plastic or wood immobilizes, restrains, and supports the finger.

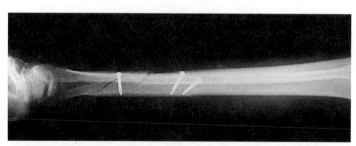

Figure 14-34 Internal fixation following a leg fracture. A lateral view of a lower leg break after reduction and internal fixation using screws.

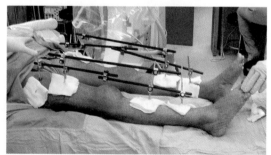

Figure 14-35 External fixation of a fracture. The fractured bone is held together by pins that are attached to a compression device. The pins are removed when the fracture is healed.

osteotome (os′te-o-tōm″) bone	**14-144** Excision of a bone (or a portion of it) is **oste/ectomy** (os″te-ek′tə-me). (One "e" is often dropped, and this is written **ostectomy** [os-tek′tə-me].) _____ is the name of the instrument used to cut bone. **Osteo/plasty** (os′te-o-plas″te) means surgical repair of a _____.
skull	**14-145 Cranio/plasty** (kra′ne-o-plas″te) is plastic surgery, or surgical repair, of the _____. **Crani/ectomy** (kra″ne-ek′tə-me) means excision of a segment of the skull. Incision into the cranium is **cranio/tomy** (kra″ne-ot′ə-me). Write the name of the instrument used in performing craniotomy: _____.

craniotome
(kra′ne-o-tōm″)
sternotomy
(stər-not′ə-me)
	14-146 Incision of the sternum is _____. This is a common incision used in open-heart surgery.
	    Excision of a rib is **costectomy** (kos-tek′tə-me), and excision of a vertebra is **vertebrectomy** (ver″tə-brek′tə-me).
	    Write a word that means excision of the coccyx: _____.

coccygectomy (kok″sĭ-jek′tə-me)	**14-147 Carp/ectomy** (kahr-pek′tə-me) is excision of one or more of the bones of the wrist. Write a word that means excision of a bone of a finger or toe: _____.
phalangectomy (fal″ən-jek′tə-me)	**14-148** Tendons may become damaged when a person suffers a deep wound. **Tendo/plasty** (ten′do-plas″te) is surgical repair of a _____. **Teno/tomy** (tə-not′ə-me) is _____ of a tendon.
tendon incision	Write a word using ten(o) and -rrhaphy that means union of a divided tendon by a suture (suture of a tendon): _____.

tenorrhaphy
(tə-nor′ə-fe)
bursectomy
(bər-sek′tə-me)
muscle
	14-149 Write a word that means excision of a bursa: _____.
	    Myo/plasty (mi′o-plas″te) is surgical repair of muscle. **Teno/myo/plasty** (ten″o-mi′o-plas″te) is surgical repair of a tendon and _____.
	    Myorrhaphy (mi-or′ə-fe) means suture of a torn or cut muscle.
	    Learn the two suffixes in the box below that are used to write surgical terms pertaining to the musculoskeletal system.

Word Parts: Orthopedics

Suffix	Meaning
-clasia	break
-desis	binding; fusion

binding or fusion	**14-150** Analyze spondylo/syn/desis: spondyl(o) means vertebra; syn- means joined (or together); and -desis means _____. **Spondylosyndesis** (spon″də-lo-sin-de′sis) is spinal fusion. It is fixation of an unstable segment of the spine, generally accomplished by surgical fusion with a bone graft or a synthetic device.
	14-151 Muscle relaxants are prescribed to relieve muscle spasms, such as the spasms that accompany a herniated disk. If bed rest and other clinical measures do not alleviate the problem, a **lamin/ectomy** (lam″ĭ-nek′tə-me) may be indicated. This is surgical removal of the bony posterior arch of a vertebra to permit surgical access to the disk so that the herniated material can be removed. Write this term that means the surgical removal of the bony arch of a vertebra:
laminectomy	_____. Complete excision of an intervertebral disk is a **disk/ectomy** (dis-kek′tə-me).
vertebroplasty	**14-152** Vertebral fractures can sometimes be repaired by **vertebro/plasty** (vur′tə-bro-plas″te). In this procedure, a plastic-like substance is injected on each side of the fractured vertebra to hold the fragments in position while the bone heals. The name of the procedure used to assist the healing of a fractured vertebra is called _____.

excision

bunion

arthrotomy
(ahr-throt′ə-me)
repair

chondroplasty
(kon′dro-plas″te)

arthrocentesis
(ahr″thro-sen-te′sis)
arthrodesis
(ahr″thro-de′sis)

joint

arthrolysis
(ahr-throl′ə-sis)

inflammation

14-153 A partial **fasciectomy** (fas″e-ek′tə-me) is generally performed to relieve Dupuytren contracture when function becomes impaired. A partial fasci/ectomy is _____ of fascia.

14-154 Numerous surgeries are performed to straighten the toes, remove bunions, and correct various deformities of the feet. A **bunion/ectomy** (bun″yən-ek′tə-me) is excision of a _____. Surgical repair to straighten the great toe can be done at the same time. Surgery may be performed to correct the alignment in hammertoe also.

14-155 Write a word that means incision of a joint, using arthr(o) and the suffix that means incision: _____. **Arthr/ectomy** (ahr-threk′tə-me) is excision of a joint.

14-156 **Arthro/plasty** (ahr′thro-plas″te) is surgical _____ of a joint. When other measures are inadequate to provide pain control for degenerative joint disease, surgery may be indicated, often total joint replacement (TJR).
   Replacement of hips, knees, elbows, wrists, shoulders, and joints of the fingers and toes has become common. Total knee replacement is the surgical insertion of a hinged device to relieve pain and restore motion to a knee that is severely affected by arthritis or injury.

14-157 Surgical repair of damaged cartilage is _____. This may be necessary if the cartilage becomes torn or displaced.
   Chondrectomy (kon-drek′tə-me) means surgical removal of cartilage.

14-158 Sometimes, excessive fluid accumulates in a synovial joint after injury and must be extracted with a needle. Write a word that means surgical puncture of a joint: _____.
   The suffix -desis means binding or fusion. Use this suffix with arthr(o) to form a word that literally means fusion of a joint: _____.
   Arthrodesis is a surgical procedure that is used to immobilize a joint. It is artificial ankylosis. Fusing the bones together stabilizes painful joints that have become unable to bear weight. Thus a stiff but stable and painless joint results.

14-159 **Arthro/clasia** (ahr″thro-kla′zhə) is artificial breaking of an ankylosed _____ to provide movement. Arthroclasia is a surgical procedure that is used to break adhesions of an ankylosed joint. Another term that means operative loosening of adhesions in an ankylosed joint is formed by combining the word part for joint and the suffix that means dissolving or destruction. Use these word parts to write the new term: _____.

14-160 Many drugs are available to treat different forms of arthritis and other connective tissue diseases. **Antiinflammatories** (an″te-in-flam′ə-to″rēz) are generally used to reduce inflammation and pain, especially drugs classified as **nonsteroidal antiinflammatory drugs** (NSAIDs). These drugs primarily reduce _____ that leads to pain. Ibuprofen is an example of an NSAID. Aspirin, a salicylate, is also used to reduce pain and inflammation.
   COX-2 inhibitors (for example, Celebrex) are also commonly used to reduce the inflammation of arthritis. These drugs are less likely to cause stomach distress and ulcers. (See the Pharmacology Section on the Companion CD for more information.)
   Anti/arthritics (an″te-ahr-thrit′ikz) are various forms of therapy that relieve the symptoms of arthritis.
   DMARDs, **disease-modifying antirheumatic drugs,** may actually modify the course of inflammatory conditions, such as rheumatoid arthritis, slowing progression of the disease. They tend to be slower acting than NSAIDs and may be prescribed with antiinflammatories.

14-161 Hematologists and oncologists treat persons with cancer or leukemia. The mode of treatment differs for different types of leukemia, but aggressive chemotherapy is common. A major side effect of chemotherapy is severe bone marrow suppression, so a combination of chemother-

myelosuppressive
(mi´ə-lo-sə-pres´iv)

apy, antibiotics to prevent infection, and blood transfusions to replace red cells and platelets is often given. Write a word that is an adjective that means inhibiting bone marrow activity: _____. (Drugs that inhibit bone marrow are called myelosuppressive agents or simply myelosuppressives.)

14-162 Bone marrow transplantation (BMT) is used to stimulate the production of normal blood cells. The patient's bone marrow is first destroyed with radiation and chemotherapy. Healthy bone marrow cells (stem cells) are transfused into the patient's blood; they migrate to the spongy bone and multiply into cancer-free bone marrow cells. (Cord blood, collected immediately after birth, is rich in stem cells and may be an alternative to **bone marrow transplants.**) In **autologous transplants,** clients receive their own stem cells (which were collected before chemotherapy was begun).

bone

14-163 Bone cancers are treated with a combination of drugs and surgery. Excision of the tumor tissue is common in benign bone tumors. Oste/ectomy is excision of a _____.
The treatment of primary bone tumors is surgical, often combined with chemotherapy and radiation. Pain can be intense in malignant bone tumors, so controlling pain is an important part of a patient's care.

EXERCISE 19

Match the surgical terms in the left columns with their meanings in the right column.

_____ 1. closed reduction
_____ 2. internal fixation
_____ 3. open reduction
_____ 4. osteectomy
_____ 5. osteoplast

A. excision of a bone
B. exposing a broken bone by surgery and aligning it
C. pulling a broken bone into alignment without surgery
D. surgery that uses pins or other materials to immobilize a broken bone
E. surgical repair of a bone

EXERCISE 20

Write terms for the following meanings.

1. breaking an ankylosed joint _____
2. excision of a rib _____
3. incision of a joint _____
4. inhibiting bone marrow activity _____
5. medications that reduce inflammation _____
6. spinal fusion _____
7. surgical puncture of a synovial joint _____
8. surgical removal of cartilage _____
9. surgical repair of the skull _____
10. suture of a torn or cut muscle _____

EXERCISE 21

Word Analysis. *Break these words into their component parts by placing a slash between the word parts. Then write the meaning of each term.*

1. craniotomy _____
2. myorrhaphy _____
3. tenomyoplasty _____
4. spondylosyndesis _____
5. fasciectomy _____

CHAPTER ABBREVIATIONS*

ALL	acute lymphocytic leukemia	**ESR**	erythrocyte sedimentation rate
AML	acute myelogenous leukemia	**fx**	fracture
ANA	antinuclear antibody	**L1, L2, etc.**	first, second, etc., lumbar vertebrae
AROM	active range of motion	**LE**	lupus erythematosus
BMT	bone marrow transplant	**MTP**	metatarsophalangeal
C1, C2, etc.	first, second, etc., cervical vertebrae	**NSAID**	nonsteroidal antiinflammatory drug
CLL	chronic lymphocytic leukemia	**PROM**	passive range of motion
CML	chronic myelogenous leukemia	**RA**	rheumatoid arthritis
CPK	creatine phosphokinase	**RF**	rheumatoid factor
CTS	carpal tunnel syndrome	**ROM**	range of motion
DJD	degenerative joint disease	**SLE**	systemic lupus erythematosus
DLE	discoid lupus erythematosus	**T1, T2, etc.**	first, second, etc., thoracic vertebrae
DMARD	disease-modifying antirheumatic drug	**TJR**	total joint replacement
EMG	electromyography	**TMJ**	temporomandibular joint

*Many of these abbreviations share their meanings with other terms.

▶ CHAPTER 14 REVIEW

Basic Understanding

Labeling

I. *Label the diagram with the combining forms for the bones that are indicated. For example, number 1 is clavicul(o).*

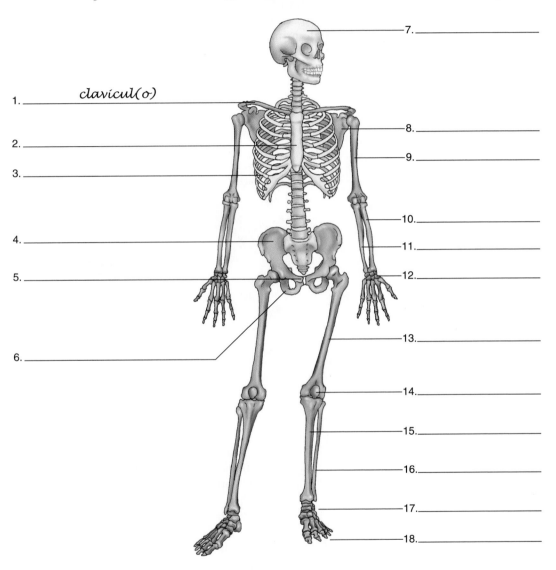

1. _____ clavicul(o)

2. _____

3. _____

4. _____

5. _____

6. _____

7. _____

8. _____

9. _____

10. _____

11. _____

12. _____

13. _____

14. _____

15. _____

16. _____

17. _____

18. _____

Matching

II. *Match the following anatomic structures with their descriptions.*

_____ 1. bone   _____ 5. ligament

_____ 2. bursa   _____ 6. synovial membrane

_____ 3. cartilage   _____ 7. tendon

_____ 4. joint

A. connects bones or cartilages
B. fluid-filled sac that helps reduce friction
C. fluid-secreting tissue lining the joint
D. place of union between two or more bones
E. provides protection and support for a joint
F. strong, fibrous tissue that attaches muscles to bones
G. the most rigid connective tissue

III. *Match the types of body movements in 1 through 10 with their meanings (A through J).*

_____ 1. abduction   _____ 6. flexion

_____ 2. adduction   _____ 7. inversion

_____ 3. circumduction   _____ 8. pronation

_____ 4. eversion   _____ 9. rotation

_____ 5. extension   _____10. supination

A. circular movement of a limb at the far end
B. movement of a bone around an axis
C. movement of the sole of the foot inward
D. movement of the sole of the foot outward
E. rotation that allows the palm of the hand to turn up
F. rotation that turns the palm of the hand backward (down)
G. to bend
H. to bring together
I. to straighten
J. to take away

Photo Match

IV. *Label the figures with the types of fractures in A through D.*
   A. comminuted; B. impacted; C. spiral; D. transverse

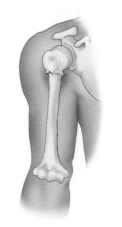 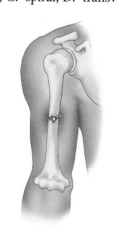 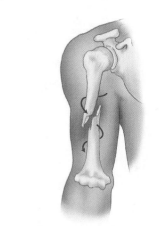 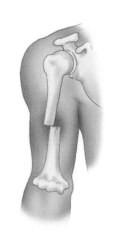

1. _____   2. _____   3. _____   4. _____

V. *Match the bones in 1 through 10 with their common names (A through J).*

_____ 1. carpal   _____ 6. pelvis

_____ 2. clavicle   _____ 7. phalanges

_____ 3. coccyx   _____ 8. scapula

_____ 4. femur   _____ 9. sternum

_____ 5. patella   _____ 10. tarsal

A. ankle bone
B. bones of the fingers and toes
C. breastbone
D. collarbone
E. hip bone
F. kneecap
G. shoulderblade
H. tailbone
I. thigh bone
J. wrist bone

VI. *Label the types of vertebrae that are indicated in the illustration.*

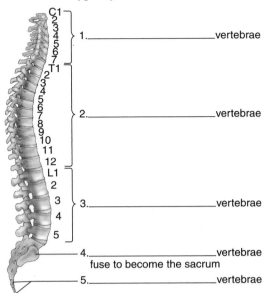

1._____vertebrae

2._____vertebrae

3._____vertebrae

4._____vertebrae
fuse to become the sacrum

5._____vertebrae

Listing

VII. *List five functions of the skeletal system.*

1. _____

2. _____

3. _____

4. _____

5. _____

VIII. *List the three major types of muscle, and describe their functions.*

1. _____

2. _____

3. _____

Photo ID

IX. *Use word parts to build terms to label these illustrations.*

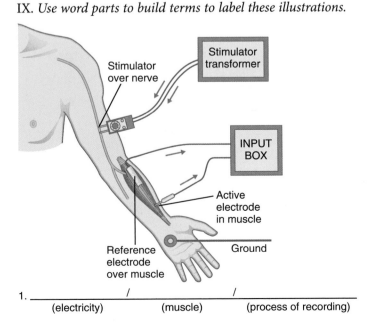

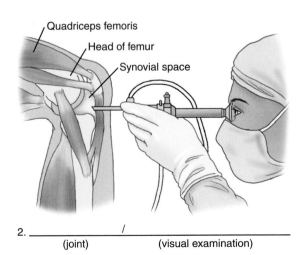

1. _____ / _____ / _____
  (electricity)   (muscle)   (process of recording)

2. _____ / _____
    (joint)   (visual examination)

Word Analysis

X. *Divide these words into their component parts, then define each term.*

1. carpophalangeal _____

2. chondrosarcoma _____

3. osteolysis _____

4. osteoarthropathy _____

5. scapuloclavicular _____

Multiple Choice

XI. *Circle the correct answers in the following multiple choice questions.*

1. Which term means congenital fissure of the breastbone? (costectomy, rachischisis, spondylosyndesis, sternoschisis)

2. Which term means pertaining to two bones of the forearm?
   (carpopedal, carpophalangeal, humeroulnar, ulnoradial)

3. Which term means any disease of the joints? (arthropathy, bursopathy, chondropathy, osteopathy)

4. Which of the following is the record produced in a procedure that records the response of a muscle to electrical stimulation? (arthrocentesis, electromyogram, myograph, range-of-motion reading)

5. Which of the following means loss of calcium from bone? (calcification, calciuria, decalcification, osteogenesis)

6. What is the term for the presence of extra fingers or toes?
   (carpopedal disease, Paget disease, phalangitis, polydactylism)

7. What is the name of the soft tissue that fills the cavity of a bone? (bone marrow, diaphysis, epiphysis, periosteum)

8. Which term means the process of using a fiberoptic instrument to view the interior of a joint?
   (arthrogram, arthrography, arthroscope, arthroscopy)

9. Which of the following pathologies means flatfoot?
   (Dupuytren contracture, hallux valgus, tarsal tunnel syndrome, tarsoptosis)

10. Which term means a reversible metabolic disease in which there is a defect in the bone resulting from inadequate phosphorus and calcium? (osteitis deformans, osteolysis, osteomalacia, osteoporosis)

Writing Terms

XII. *Write a term for each of the following meanings.*

1. aligning a broken bone _____

2. between the ribs _____

3. degenerative joint disease _____

4. excision of the tailbone _____

5. herniation of a muscle _____

6. inflammation of a bone _____

7. lateral curvature of the spine _____

8. pertaining to muscle and fascia _____

9. pertaining to the joints _____

10. surgical puncture of a joint _____

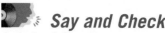 ## Say and Check

Say aloud the terms you wrote for Exercise XII. Use the Companion CD to check your pronunciations.

Greater Comprehension

Health Care Reports

XIII. *Answer the questions after reading the following preoperative history and physical.*

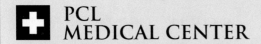 **PCL MEDICAL CENTER**

7700 Lexicon Way
St. Louis, MO 63146

Phone (555) 437-0000 • Fax (555) 437-0001

PREOPERATIVE HISTORY AND PHYSICAL

Patient Name: Thomas Shaw   **ID No**: 014-0001   **Date of Exam**: Feb 11, ----
ATTENDING PHYSICIAN: John T. Riley, M.D.   **Date of Surgery:** Feb 12, ----
HPI: 40-year-old man who fell yesterday, injuring left leg. Radiologic findings show comminuted proximal left femur fracture. Admitted for surgical repair of fracture.
ROS: A 12-point ROS is negative except for edema, left thigh. Sensation intact in left foot. Able to move left ankle and toes.
MEDICATIONS: insulin, Neurontin, Effexor, Paxil
ALLERGIES: penicillin, which causes hives and swelling of the tongue
PAST MEDICAL HISTORY: Insulin-dependent diabetes mellitus, neuropathy, herniated disk, arthralgias, depression
PAST SURGICAL HISTORY: SP laminectomy, right knee, and arthroscopy in the past
FAMILY HISTORY: Diabetes mellitus in his father; osteoporosis in his mother
SOCIAL HISTORY: Divorced, lives alone, does not smoke, drinks 2 six-packs weekly
DIAGNOSIS/PLAN: Patient with comminuted proximal left femur fracture, admitted for surgical repair in the AM. Need CBC, chem-18, HgA$_{1c}$, consult with anesthesia team

Michael Rawlings, MD
Michael Rawlings, MD

D: Feb 11, ----
T: Feb 11, ----

---

1. Describe the meaning of a comminuted proximal left femur fracture. _____

   _____

2. Describe the two procedures mentioned in the patient's surgical history. _____

   _____

3. What is meant by a herniated disk? _____

   _____

4. What is meant by the term arthralgias? _____

   _____

5. Describe the mother's medical history. _____

   _____

XIV. *Read the following report and define the terms that are indicated.*

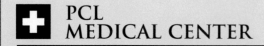

PCL MEDICAL CENTER

7700 Lexicon Way
St. Louis, MO 63146

Phone (555) 437-0000 • Fax (555) 437-0001

DISCHARGE SUMMARY

Patient Name: Martha Watkins   **ID No**: 014-0002   **DOB**: Oct 6, ----
DATE ADMITTED: 1/31/----   **Date Discharged:** 2/5/----   **Sex:** Female
FINAL DIAGNOSES
1. Osteoarthritis of the right knee
2. Rheumatoid arthritis
3. Degenerative joint disease, left knee
COMPLICATIONS: Postoperative deep vein thrombosis, right lower extremity
PRINCIPAL TREATMENT RENDERED: Right total knee arthroplasty, posterior stabilized, cemented.
DISCHARGE INSTRUCTIONS: Up ad lib with full weight-bearing to right lower extremity. Ambulate with wheeled walker.
Home health for physical and occupational therapy 3× weekly, and nursing visits to monitor incision and medication. Patient
to change dry dressing to incision daily. Regular diet.
MEDICATION: Coumadin 5 mg daily; Arthrotec for pain, 1 tablet 3× daily with food.
DISPOSITION: Patient to follow up with Dr. Withers for staple removal in 10 days. She is to call the Coumadin Clinic for an
appointment

John Robert Withers, MD

John Robert Withers, MD

JRW:pai
D: Feb 5, ----
T: Feb 7, ----

Define:

1. osteoarthritis _____

2. rheumatoid arthritis _____

3. degenerative joint disease, left knee _____

4. arthroplasty _____

5. right lower extremity _____

6. ad lib _____

XV. Read the following orthopedic clinic note, and answer the questions that follow the report.

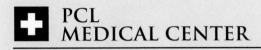 **PCL**
MEDICAL CENTER

7700 Lexicon Way
St. Louis, MO 63146

Phone (555) 437-0000 • Fax (555) 437-0001

ORTHOPEDIC CLINIC NOTE

Patient Name: Joseph A. Bluhm   ID No.: 014-0003   Date: Mar 9, ----

HISTORY: MSgt Bluhm visits today in follow-up for his L2 compression fracture. Again, he has a history of having been injured in Iraq, at which time he fell 15 to 20 feet from a guard tower. We have talked to him in the past regarding different options, conservative versus operative, and he has continued to be undecided about the best course of
therapy. He does report that he can now stay somewhat active with his pain. He is taking only one Aleve a day for his discomfort.

PHYSICAL EXAMINATION: Patient continues to have slight prominence on the right side with some mild tenderness to palpation. He does have a normal neurologic exam with 5/5 strength throughout. Normal sensation in bilateral lower extremities. Patient denies radicular symptoms.

X-RAY DATA: Radiographic data, including CT and MRI of the spine, were again reviewed. These were from March of last year. He also has plain films, which were repeated today, and they show no significant change. He does have a significant compression deformity of the L2 vertebral body, both in the anterior compression on the lateral view and right-sided compression on the AP or coronal view. Looking again at the MRI changes, patient also has L3, L4,
L4-5, and L5-SI grade I retrolisthesis.

IMPRESSION: Patient has an L2 compression fracture, multilevel lumbar spondylosis, and back pain.

PLAN: At this time the patient would like to decide whether or not he wants surgical management. We discussed with him the length of recovery and the risks versus benefits, and he is going to think about this at home. He will get back to us if he decides to have surgery. If he does decide to have surgery, we will need to repeat an MRI. We would also like to get a diskogram of his lumbar segments to see what component of pain that is, as well as to determine fusion levels. Again, he will contact us depending on his decision.

Michael Rawlings, MD

Michael Rawlings, MD

MR:pai
D: Mar 10, ----
T: Mar 12, ----

Answer these questions.

1. What is a compression fracture, and where is L2? _____

   _____

2. What is meant by "Normal sensation in bilateral lower extremities"? _____

   _____

3. What does multilevel lumbar spondylosis mean? _____

   _____

4. Break the term "diskogram" into its component parts, and write its meaning: _____

   _____

5. What is meant by the term "fusion"? _____

   _____

Spelling

XVI. *Circle all misspelled terms and write their correct spelling.*

adductor   anomaly   femural   fissure   ileofemoral

Interpreting Abbreviations

XVII. *Write the meanings of these abbreviations.*

1. ANA _____

2. DJD _____

3. EMG _____

4. ROM _____

5. SLE _____

Pronunciation

XVIII. *The pronunciation is shown for several medical words. Indicate which syllable has the primary accent by marking it with an ´.*

1. arthroclasia (ahr thro kla zhə)

2. chondrosarcoma (kon dro sahr ko mə)

3. lumbar (lum bahr)

4. myasthenia (mi əs the ne ə)

5. sternocostal (stər no kos təl)

Say and Check

Say aloud the five terms in Exercise XVIII. Use the Companion CD to check your pronunciations. In addition, be prepared to pronounce aloud these terms in class:

arthropathy	chondrogenic	fissure	myelogenous leukemia
autologous transplant	chondroma	foramen magnum	osteochondroma
bone marrow aspiration	cranial	hypertonicity	polydactyly
bone marrow transplant	Dupuytren contracture	interpubic	systemic scleroderma
calcaneitis	fibromyalgia syndrome	intrasternal	thoracolumbar

Categorizing Terms

XIX. *Classify the terms in the left columns (1 through 10) by selecting A, B, C, D, or E.*

_____ 1. antiarthritics

_____ 2. atrophy

_____ 3. bone densitometry

_____ 4. calcaneofibular

_____ 5. epiphysis

_____ 6. fibromyalgia

_____ 7. infrapatellar

_____ 8. reflex hammer

_____ 9. vertebroplasty

_____ 10. xiphoid process

A. anatomy
B. diagnostic test or procedure
C. pathology
D. surgery
E. therapy

Challenge

XX. *Break the following words apart, then write the meaning of each term.*

1. bursopathy _____

2. musculotendinous _____

3. osteochondral _____

4. suprapatellar _____

5. tenosynovitis _____

(Check your answers with the solutions in Appendix VI.)

PRONUNCIATION LIST

Use the Companion CD to review the terms that have been presented. Look closely at the spelling of each term as it is pronounced and be sure you know the meaning of each term.

abduction
abductor
adduction
adductor
ankylosing spondylitis
ankylosis
anomaly
antiarthritic
antiinflammatory
antinuclear antibody test
appendicular skeleton
arthralgia
arthrectomy
arthritis
arthrocentesis
arthrochondritis
arthroclasia
arthrodesis
arthrodynia
arthrogram
arthrography
arthrolysis
arthropathy
arthroplasty
arthrosclerosis
arthroscope
arthroscopy
arthrotomy
articular
articulation
atrophy
auditory ossicle
autoimmune disease
autologous transplant
axial skeleton
bone densitometry
bone marrow
bone marrow aspiration
bone marrow transplant
bone scan
bunionectomy
bursa
bursectomy
bursitis
calcaneal
calcaneitis
calcaneodynia
calcaneofibular
calcaneoplantar
calcaneotibial
calcaneus

calcification
calcipenia
calciuria
callus
cardiac muscle
carpal
carpal tunnel syndrome
carpals
carpectomy
carpopedal
carpophalangeal
carpus
cartilage
cast
cellulitis
cervical vertebrae
chondral
chondralgia
chondrectomy
chondritis
chondrocostal
chondrodynia
chondrogenic
chondroid
chondroma
chondropathy
chondroplasty
chondrosarcoma
chronic fatigue syndrome
circumduction
clavicle
closed fracture
closed reduction
coccygeal vertebrae
coccygectomy
coccyx
comminuted fracture
compound fracture
compression fracture
connective tissue
connective tissue disease
corns
costa
costal
costectomy
costoclavicular
costovertebral
COX-2 inhibitors
cranial
craniectomy
craniocele

cranioplasty
craniotome
craniotomy
cranium
creatine phosphokinase
cutaneous lupus
    erythematosus
decalcification
degenerative joint disease
diaphysis
discoid lupus
    erythematosus
disease-modifying
    antirheumatic drugs
diskectomy
dislocation
dorsalgia
Dupuytren contracture
dystrophy
electromyogram
electromyography
encephalocele
epiphysis
erythrocyte sedimentation
    rate
eversion
Ewing sarcoma
extension
extensor
external fixation
fascia
fascial
fasciectomy
femoral
femur
fibrogenic tumors
fibromyalgia
fibromyalgia syndrome
fibrosarcoma
fibula
fibular
fissure
flexion
flexor
foramen magnum
fracture
gout
greenstick fracture
hallux valgus
hammertoe
haversian canals

herniated disk
humeral
humeroradial
humeroscapular
humeroulnar
humerus
hypercalciuria
hypertonicity
hypotonicity
iliac
iliofemoral
iliopubic
ilium
impacted fracture
infraclavicular
infracostal
infrapatellar
infrascapular
infrasternal
intercostal
internal fixation
interpubic
interscapular
intervertebral
intervertebral disk
intraarticular
intrasternal
inversion
ischial
ischialgia
ischiococcygeal
ischiodynia
ischiofemoral
ischiopubic
ischium
joint crepitus
kyphosis
laminectomy
leukemia
ligament
lordosis
lumbar puncture
lumbar vertebrae
lupus erythematosus
Lyme disease
lymphoblastic leukemia
lymphocytic leukemia
medullary cavity
metacarpals
metatarsals
metatarsophalangeal joint

Morton neuroma
multiple myeloma
muscle relaxants
muscular
muscular dystrophy
musculoskeletal
myalgia
myasthenia
myasthenia gravis
myelitis
myeloblast
myelocyte
myelocytic leukemia
myelogenous leukemia
myelosuppression
myelosuppressive
myoblast
myocardium
myocele
myocellulitis
myodynia
myofascial
myofibrosis
myolysis
myomalacia
myopathy
myoplasty
myorrhaphy
nonarticular
nonsteroidal
    antiinflammatory
    drugs
open fracture
open reduction
orthopedics
orthopedist
ossification
ostealgia
ostectomy
osteectomy
osteitis
osteitis deformans
osteoarthritis
osteoarthropathy
osteoblast

osteochondritis
osteochondroma
osteocyte
osteodynia
osteogenesis
osteogenic
osteolysis
osteomalacia
osteomyelitis
osteopenia
osteoplasty
osteoporosis
osteoporotics
osteosarcoma
osteosclerosis
osteotome
Paget disease
patella
patellofemoral
pelvic girdle
perichondrial
perichondrium
periosteum
phalangectomy
phalanges
plantar
polyarthritis
polydactylism
polydactyly
polymyalgia
polymyalgia rheumatica
polymyositis
pronation
pubes
pubic
pubic symphysis
pubis
pubofemoral
rachialgia
rachiodynia
rachischisis
radius
reduction
reflex hammer
retrosternal

rheumatoid arthritis
rheumatoid factor
rickets
rotation
rotator
rotator cuff
sacral vertebrae
sacrodynia
sacrum
scapula
scapular
scapuloclavicular
scoliosis
shoulder girdle
simple fracture
Sjögren syndrome
skeletal
skeletal muscle
spina bifida
spinal
spiral fracture
splint
spondylalgia
spondylarthritis
spondylarthropathy
spondylosyndesis
sprain
sternal
sternalgia
sternoclavicular
sternocostal
sternoschisis
sternotomy
sternovertebral
sternum
strain
subcostal
subpubic
substernal
supination
supracostal
suprapubic
suprasternal
syndactylism
syndactyly

synovial joint
synovitis
systemic lupus
    erythematosus
systemic scleroderma
systemic sclerosis
tarsal
tarsal tunnel syndrome
tarsals
tarsoptosis
tarsus
temporomandibular
    joint
tenalgia
tendinitis
tendon
tendonitis
tendoplasty
tenodynia
tenomyoplasty
tenorrhaphy
tenotomy
tetany
thoracic
thoracic vertebrae
thoracolumbar
tibia
tibialgia
tibiofemoral
trabeculae
traction
transverse fracture
ulna
ulnoradial
vertebra
vertebrae
vertebral column
vertebrectomy
vertebrochondral
vertebrocostal
vertebroplasty
vertebrosternal
visceral muscle
xiphoid process

Español ENHANCING SPANISH COMMUNICATION

English	Spanish (pronunciation)
ankle	tobillo (to-BEEL-lyo)
back	espalda (es-PAHL-dah)
bones	huesos (oo-AY-sos)
calcium	calcio (CAHL-se-o)
cartilage	cartílago (car-TEE-lah-go)
cheek	mejilla (may-HEEL-lyah)
chew, to	masticar (mas-te-CAR)
collarbone	clavícula (clah-VEE-coo-lah)
cranium	cráneo (CRAH-nay-o)
elbow	codo (CO-do)
extremity	extremidad (ex-tray-me-DAHD)
forearm	antebrazo (an-tay-BRAH-so)
fracture	fractura (frac-TOO-rah)
heel	talón (tah-LON)
jaw	mandíbula (man-DEE-boo-lah)
joint	articulacíon (ar-te-coo-lah-se-ON), coyuntura (co-yoon-TOO-rah)
knee	rodilla (ro-DEEL-lyah)
kneecap	rótula (RO-too-lah)
ligament	ligamento (le-gah-MEN-to)
movement	movimiento (mo-ve-me-EN-to)
neck	cuello (coo-EL-lyo)
phalanges	falanges (fah-LAHN-hays)
phosphorus	fósforo (FOS-fo-ro)
reduction	reducción (ray-dooc-se-ON)
sacrum	hueso sacro (oo-AY-so SAH-cro)
shoulder	hombro (OM-bro)
shoulder blade	espaldilla (es-pal-DEEL-lyah)
skeleton	esqueleto (es-kay-LAY-to)
spinal column	columna vertebral (co-LOOM-nah ver-tay-BRAHL)
spine	espinazo (es-pe-NAH-so)
spiral	espiral (es-pe-RAHL)
sprain, to	torcer (tor-SERR)
sternum	esternón (es-ter-NON)
stiff	tieso (te-AY-so)
support	sustento (sus-TEN-to)
tear	lágrima de los ojos (LAH-gre-mah day los O-hos)
temple	sien (se-AYN)
tendon	tendón (ten-DON)
thumb	pulgar (pool-GAR)
toe	dedo del pie (DAY-do del pe-AY)
vertebral column	columna vertebral (co-LOOM-nah ver-tay-BRAHL)
weakness	debilidad (day-be-le-DAHD)

Nervous System and Psychologic Disorders

15

FUNCTION FIRST

The nervous system is the body's control center and communications network. It stimulates movement, senses changes both within and outside the body, and provides us with thought, learning, and memory. With the help of the hormonal system, the nervous system maintains homeostasis, a dynamic equilibrium of the internal environment of the body.

ANATOMY AND PHYSIOLOGY

nerve

15-1 The nervous system is the network of structures that activates, coordinates, and controls all functions of the body. The terms **nervous** (nur´vəs) and **neur/al** (noor´əl) mean pertaining to a _____ or the nerves, but the nervous system includes the brain and spinal cord as well as the nerves.

15-2 The nervous system is the body's most organized and complex system. It affects both psychologic and physiologic functions. In addition to being the center of thinking and judgment, the nervous system influences other body systems. For example, damage to the spinal nerves that supply nerve impulses to the diaphragm may result in respiratory arrest.

sensory

The various activities of the nervous system can be grouped as sensory, integrative, and motor functions. Sensory receptors detect changes that occur inside and outside the body. For example, receptors monitor changes in external conditions such as light or room temperature. They also monitor changes within the body, such as changes in body temperature and blood pressure. The gathering of this type of information is the _____ function of the nervous system.

15-3 Integrative functions create sensations, produce thoughts and memory, and make decisions based on sensory input. The nervous system responds to sensory input and integration by sending signals to muscles or glands and causing an effect. Responding and causing an effect in muscles or glands is the motor function of the nervous system.

motor

The activities of the nervous system include sensory receptors that detect change, integrative functions that produce thoughts and memory and help us make decisions, and _____ functions that enable us to respond to a stimulus.

ORGANIZATION OF THE NERVOUS SYSTEM

central
peripheral

15-4 The two principal divisions of the nervous system are the **central nervous system** (CNS) and the **peripheral** (pə-rif´ər-əl) **nervous system** (PNS). CNS is an abbreviation for _____ nervous system.

PNS means _____ nervous system.

brain

15-5 Looking at Figure 15-1, you see that the CNS is composed of the _____ and the spinal cord. This part of the system is the control center.

The second division of the nervous system is the PNS, the various nerves and nerve masses that connect the brain and the spinal cord with receptors, muscles, and glands. Observing the diagram, you see that the PNS is divided into a sensory or **afferent** (af´ər-ənt) system and a motor or **efferent** (ef´ər-ənt) system. Which system conveys information from the CNS to muscles and glands? _____

efferent

nerve

15-6 The nervous system is composed of two types of cells: neurons (noor´onz) and neuroglia (noo-rog´le-ə). Both types of cells that comprise nervous tissue are named using neur(o), which means _____.

Neurons conduct impulses either to or from the central nervous system. **Neuroglia, or glia**[*] **cells,** provide special support and protection. If a neuron is destroyed, it cannot replace itself. On

---

[*]Glia (Greek: *glia*, glue).

Nervous system

Central nervous system (CNS)	Peripheral nervous system (PNS)

Central nervous system (CNS)

Brain

Receives and integrates data. Regulates body activities.

Spinal cord

Carries information to and from brain. Provides reflexes.

Peripheral nervous system (PNS)

Kidney   Adrenal gland

Sensory (afferent)

Conveys information from receptors to CNS

Motor (efferent)

Conveys information from CNS to muscles and glands

Figure 15-1 Major divisions of the nervous system.

the other hand, neuroglia are far more numerous and, because they can reproduce, are the only source of primary malignant brain tumors, those originating in the brain.

Learn the following word parts.

Word Parts: Cells of the Nervous System

Combining Form	Meaning
dendr(o)	tree
gli(o)	neuroglia or a sticky substance
nerv(o), neur(o)	nerve

15-7 The neuron, or nerve cell, is the basic unit of the nervous system. Neurons carry out the function of the nervous system by conducting nerve impulses. Each neuron has a cell body, a single **axon** (ak´son), and one or more **dendrites** (den´drīts) (Figure 15-2).

The axon and dendrites are cytoplasmic projections, or processes, that project from the cell body. They are sometimes called nerve fibers. An axon carries impulses away from the cell body. Dendrites transmit impulses to the cell body. Which type of cytoplasmic projection carries a

axon

nervous impulse away from the cell body? _____

The combining form dendr(o) means tree. Which type of cytoplasmic projection has numer-

dendrite

ous branches? _____

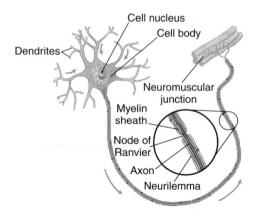

Cell nucleus

Cell body

Dendrites

Neuromuscular junction

Myelin sheath

Node of Ranvier

Axon

Neurilemma

Figure 15-2 Structure of a typical neuron. The basic parts of a neuron are the cell body, a single axon, and several dendrites. *Arrows* indicate the direction that an impulse travels to or from the cell body. The axon is surrounded by a segmented myelin sheath with neurilemma that forms a tight covering over each segment. The unmyelinated regions between the myelin segments are called the nodes of Ranvier. A myelinated nerve fiber is capable of conducting an impulse many times faster than if it were not myelinated.

gray

15-8 Many axons are surrounded by a white lipid covering called a **myelin sheath.** The myelinated axons appear whitish and are called white matter. Those that are not myelinated appear grayish and are called _____ matter.

In a myelinated fiber, the nerve impulse "jumps" from one **node of Ranvier** (see Figure 15-2) to the next and results in a faster rate of conduction than in an unmyelinated nerve fiber. If the myelin sheath becomes damaged, as it does in diseases such as multiple sclerosis, conduction of the impulse is impaired.

The region of communication between one neuron and another is called the **synapse** (sin´aps). An axon terminates in several short branches that together form a **synaptic bulb.** The synaptic bulb releases a neurotransmitter that either inhibits or enhances a nervous impulse. A

nervous

neuro/transmitter is a chemical that transmits a _____ impulse that either inhibits or enhances a reaction.

15-9 Some of the best known neurotransmitters are **acetylcholine** (ACh) (as˝ə-təl-, as˝ə-tēl-ko´lēn), **epinephrine** (ep˝ĭ-nef´rin), **dopamine** (do´pə-mēn), **serotonin** (ser˝o-to´nin), and **endorphins** (en-dor´finz, en´dor-finz). To prevent prolonged reactions, a neurotransmitter is quickly inactivated by an enzyme.

Disorders involving neurotransmitters have been implicated in the origin of various psychological disorders. The substances released at the synapse that either enhance or inhibit a nervous

neurotransmitters

impulse are called _____.

nerves

15-10 Neuro/muscul/ar (noor˝o-mus´ku-lər) means concerning both _____ and muscles.

> ➤ **KEY** POINT A neuro/muscular junction is the area of contact between a neuron and adjoining skeletal muscle. When a nerve impulse reaches the neuromuscular junction, acetylcholine is released, which leads to contraction of the muscle. Acetylcholine acts rapidly on muscle tissue, and most of it is then promptly inactivated by an enzyme, **acetylcholinester/ase** (as˝ə-təl-, as˝ə-tēl-ko˝lĭ-nes´tə-rās).

enzyme

The latter ends in the suffix -ase, meaning _____, which should help you distinguish between these two terms.

Certain drugs can block transmission of impulses to the skeletal muscle. The transmission is blocked at the neuromuscular junction.

15-11 Conduction of nervous impulses is often described as a **reflex arc.** A reflex is an automatic, involuntary response to some change, either inside or outside the body. Reflexes help maintain homeostasis by making constant adjustments to our blood pressure, breathing rate, and pulse. A common reflex is that of quickly removing your hand from a hot object.

A **deep tendon reflex** (DTR) is one way of assessing the reflex arc. For example, a sharp tap on the tendon just below the kneecap normally causes extension of the leg at the knee. This is called the **patellar** (pə-tel´ər) **response** or knee jerk response. A normal response indicates an intact reflex arc between the nervous system and the muscles that are involved in the response. Other areas are also assessed for reflex activities. An automatic, involuntary response to some

reflex

change, either inside or outside the body, is called a _____.

15-12 The reflex arc involves two types of neurons: a sensory neuron and a motor neuron. **Sensory neurons** transmit nerve impulses toward the spinal cord and the brain. **Motor neurons** transmit nerve impulses from the brain and the spinal cord (Figure 15-3).

motor

Note that the _____ neuron causes the muscle to contract.

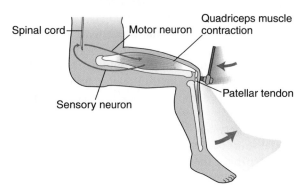

Figure 15-3 Conceptual drawing of the reflex arc. A receptor detects the stimulus, the tap on the patellar tendon with the reflex hammer. The sensory neuron transmits the nerve impulse to the spinal cord. The motor neuron conducts a nervous impulse that causes the quadriceps muscle to contract. Extension of the leg at the knee, also called knee jerk, is the normal patellar response.

EXERCISE 1

1. List four functions of the nervous system:

   _____.

2. The various activities of the nervous system can be grouped as detecting changes, producing thoughts and making decisions, and causing an effect in muscles or glands. What are the names of these three activities?

   _____, _____, and _____ functions

3. Name the two principal divisions of the nervous system: _____ and _____.

4. Name the two types of cells of the nervous system: _____ and _____.

5. Name the two types of cytoplasmic projections of a basic nerve cell: _____ and _____.

CENTRAL NERVOUS SYSTEM

brain

15-13 The central nervous system consists of the _____ and spinal cord. The brain, a soft mass of tissue weighing approximately 1360 grams (3 pounds) in the average adult, receives thousands of bits of information and integrates all the data to determine the appropriate response. The brain is surrounded by the **cranium** (kra′ne-əm) (skull), and the spinal cord is protected by the vertebrae. In addition to the skull and vertebrae, the brain and spinal cord are protected by three membranes called **meninges** (mə-nin′jēz) and circulating **cerebrospinal fluid.** The singular form of meninges is meninx (me′ninks).

Learn the following word parts.

Word Parts: Central Nervous System

Combining Form	Meaning	Combining Form	Meaning
cerebell(o)	cerebellum	mening(i), mening(o)	meninges
cerebr(o), encephal(o)	brain (cerebr[o] sometimes means cerebrum)	arachn(o)	spider or arachnoid (a meningeal membrane)
myel(o)	spinal cord (sometimes, bone marrow)		

15-14 The meninges (singular, meninx) enclose the brain and the spinal cord (Figure 15-4).

> ➤ **KEY** POINT <u>Remember the three layers that make up the meninges.</u> The tough outer layer, the **dura mater*** (doo′rə ma′tər), lies just inside the cranial bones and lines the vertebral canal. The middle layer is the **arachnoid** (ə-rak′noid), a thin layer with numerous threadlike strands that attach it to the innermost layer. The combining form arachn(o) means either the arachnoid membrane or spider. The innermost layer, the **pia mater**† (pi′ə ma′tər, pe′ə mah′tər), is thin and delicate and is tightly attached to the surface of the brain and spinal cord.

*Dura mater (Latin: *durus,* hard; *mater,* mother).
†Pia mater (Latin: *pia,* tender; *mater,* mother).

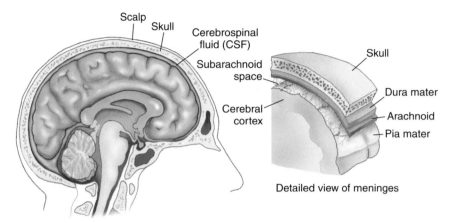

Scalp
Skull
Cerebrospinal fluid (CSF)
Subarachnoid space
Cerebral cortex
Skull
Dura mater
Arachnoid
Pia mater

Detailed view of meninges

Figure 15-4 The brain and its protective coverings, the meninges. The tough outer membrane, the dura mater, lies just inside the skull. The threadlike strands of the middle layer, the arachnoid, resemble a cobweb. The pia mater is the innermost meningeal layer and is so tightly bound to the brain that it cannot be removed without damaging the surface.

dura pia	The outer layer is the _____ mater. The middle layer is the arachnoid, and the innermost layer is the _____ mater.
meninges	**15-15** The combining form mening(o) means the _____. **Meningeal** (mə-nin′je-əl) means pertaining to the meninges.
below (or beneath)	**15-16 Sub/dural** (səb-doo′rəl) means _____ the dura mater, so it refers to the area between the dura mater and the arachnoid. The potential space between these two membranes is the **subdural space.**
	15-17 The **cerebrum** is the largest and uppermost portion of the brain, and the combining form cerebr(o) means either the cerebrum or the brain in general. It is concerned with interpretation of impulses and all voluntary muscle activities. It is the center of higher mental faculties.
cerebrum cranium	**Cerebr/al** (sə-re′brəl, ser′ə-brəl) means pertaining to the _____. **Craniocerebral** (kra″ne-o-ser′ə-brəl) means pertaining to the _____ and the cerebrum.
	15-18 The brain is that part of the CNS contained within the skull. A longitudinal fissure almost completely divides it into two **cerebral hemispheres** (hemi- means half). The surface of each hemisphere is covered with a convoluted layer of gray matter called the **cerebral cortex.** Division of the cortex into lobes provides useful reference points (Figure 15-5).
frontal	The lobe that is located near the front of the cerebrum is the _____ lobe.
temporal (tem′pə-rəl)	The regions of the head in front of the ears are known as the temples. The parts of the cerebrum that are located in the areas of the temples are called the _____ lobes.
occipital	Occipital (ok-sip′ĭ-təl) is an adjective that means concerning the back part of the head. The lobe that is located at the back part of the head, just behind the temporal lobe, is the _____ **lobe.**
parietal (pə-ri′ə-təl)	Another lobe, just above the occipital lobe, is the _____ lobe. The lobe deep within the brain is the **insula** (in′sə-lə).

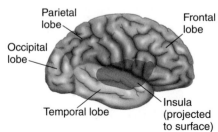

Parietal lobe
Frontal lobe
Occipital lobe
Insula (projected to surface)
Temporal lobe

Figure 15-5 Lateral view of the cerebrum. The surface of the cerebrum is marked by convolutions. The pia mater closely follows the convolutions and goes deep into the grooves (sulci). Each cerebral hemisphere is divided into five lobes: the frontal lobe, the parietal lobe, the occipital lobe, the temporal lobe, and an insula that is covered by parts of the other lobes.

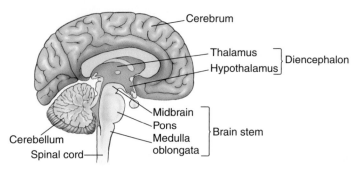

Figure 15-6 Midsagittal view of the principal structures of the brain. The brainstem consists of the midbrain, the pons, and the medulla. Its lower end is a continuation of the spinal cord. The diencephalon is above the brainstem and consists of the thalamus and the hypothalamus. The cerebrum is about seven eighths of the total weight of the brain and spreads over the diencephalon. The cerebellum is inferior to the cerebrum.

Note that different lobes are associated with different functions. The frontal lobes are associated with personality, behavior, emotion, and intellectual functions. The temporal lobes are associated with hearing and smell, the occipital lobes are associated with vision, and the parietal lobes are associated with language and the general function of sensation.

15-19 The brain consists of several parts: the cerebrum, diencephalon (di″ən-sef′ə-lon), brain stem, and cerebellum (ser″ə-bel′əm) (Figure 15-6). The **cerebellum** lies just under the cerebrum, the largest portion of the brain. The **thalamus** and **hypothalamus** are parts of the

diencephalon
_____ .

   The **midbrain, pons,** and **medulla** are parts of the **brain** _____ .

stem
The medulla (mə-dul′ə) is continuous with the spinal cord at an opening in the bone called the **foramen*** **magnum** (fo-ra′mən mag′nəm).

15-20 The **spinal cord** is a cylindric structure located in the canal of the vertebral column. Thirty-one pairs of spinal nerves arise from the spinal cord and are named and numbered according to the region and level of the spinal cord from which they emerge (Figure 15-7).

*Foramina (Latin: hole).

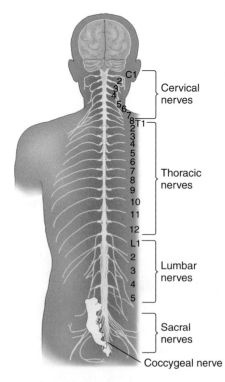

Figure 15-7 The spinal cord and nerves emerging from it. The spinal cord, about 44 cm (16 to 18 inches) long, extends from the medulla to the second lumbar vertebra. It ends as the cauda equina (meaning horse's tail), a group of nerves that arise from the lower portion of the cord and hang like wisps of coarse hair. There are 31 pairs of spinal nerves: 8 cervical, 12 thoracic, 5 lumbar, 5 sacral, and 1 coccygeal. The sciatic nerve, actually two nerves bound together by a common sheath of connective tissue, is often considered to be the largest nerve in the body. It supplies the entire musculature of the leg and foot. Irritation or injury to this nerve causes pain, often from the thigh down its branches into the toes. Neuralgia along the course of the sciatic nerve is called sciatica.

sciatic

The **sciatic** (si-at´ik) **nerve** is actually two nerves bound together by a common sheath of connective tissue but is collectively called the sciatic nerve. It is often considered to be the largest nerve in the body, arising from spinal nerves on either side, and is called the _____ nerve.

within

15-21 A word that means within the spinal canal is **intra/thecal** (in″trə-the´kəl), which means _____ a sheath (or the spinal canal). An intrathecal injection, for example, is an injection into a particular place in the spinal canal for diffusion of a material throughout the spinal fluid.

brain

15-22 In addition to the protection offered by the meninges, cerebrospinal fluid (CSF) surrounds and cushions the spinal cord and brain. **Cerebro/spinal** means pertaining to the _____ and the spinal cord.

ventricles

Cerebrospinal fluid is formed in the ventricles, four cavities in the brain. The fluid circulates through the ventricles, the subarachnoid space, and the central canal of the spinal cord. Cavities in the brain that produce CSF are called **cerebral** _____.

cerebellum

15-23 The combining form cerebell(o) means cerebellum. **Cerebell/ar** (ser″ə-bel´ər) pertains to the _____.

EXERCISE 2

Write words in the blanks to complete the following:

1. The CNS consists of the _____ and _____ _____.

2. List the three types of meninges: _____, _____, and _____.

EXERCISE 3

Word Analysis. *Break these words into their component parts by placing a slash between the word parts. Write the meaning of each term.*

1. cerebrospinal _____

2. craniocerebral _____

3. meningeal _____

4. neuromuscular _____

5. subdural _____

Say and Check

Say aloud the terms in Exercise 3. Use the Companion CD to check your pronunciations.

PERIPHERAL NERVOUS SYSTEM AND THE SENSE ORGANS

15-24 The peripheral nervous system is that portion of the nervous system that is outside the central nervous system.

> ➤ **KEY** POINT The PNS forms the communication network between the central nervous system and the rest of the body. The PNS consists of the nerves that branch out from the brain and spinal cord which communicate with the rest of the body. It is further divided into the **sensory** (afferent) and **motor** (efferent) **systems**. Special sense organs have receptors that detect sensations, and then sensory neurons transmit the information to the CNS. Motor neurons carry impulses that initiate muscle contraction.

central

Peripheral means located away from the center. The PNS is located away from the nervous system control center, the CNS or the _____ nervous system.

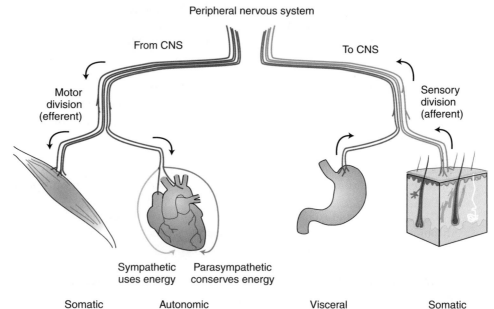

Figure 15-8 **Schematic drawing of the divisions of the peripheral nervous system.** The motor (efferent) division is subdivided into the somatic and autonomic systems. The sensory (afferent) division is subdivided into the visceral and somatic systems.

sensory

15-25 Receptors are sensory nerve endings that respond to various kinds of stimulation. The awareness that results from the stimulation is what we know as sensation. The major senses are sight, hearing, smell, taste, and touch. Receptors are _____ nerve endings.

Touch is subdivided into several sensations that we receive through the skin: touch, pressure, pain, heat, and cold. The skin contains numerous sense receptors for these sensations. Hair has no receptors, but the movement of hair can be detected by receptors near the hair follicle (see Chapter 16 for more information). The skin and many tissues have pain receptors.

The PNS consists of nerves that connect with **somatic** (so-mat´ik) tissues (skin and muscles that are involved in conscious activities) and also nerves that link the CNS to **autonomic** (aw″tə-nom´ik) tissues (the visceral organs, such as the stomach and heart, which function without conscious effort). These further divisions of the PNS are illustrated in Figure 15-8.

The autonomic system regulates and coordinates visceral activities without our conscious effort. This helps maintain a stable internal environment. The autonomic system has two divisions, the sympathetic and parasympathetic nervous systems.

autonomic

15-26 Sympathetic (sim″pə-thet´ik) and **parasympathetic** (par″ə-sim″pə-thet´ik) systems are divisions of the _____ nervous system. In general, impulses transmitted by the nerve fibers of one division stimulate an organ, whereas impulses from the other division either decrease or halt organ activity.

Activation of the sympathetic division causes a series of physiologic responses called the fight-or-flight response. These responses increase the heart and breathing rates and prepare the body for fighting off danger. When danger is past, which system would counteract these responses? _____ system

parasympathetic

15-27 Sympathetic and parasympathetic nerve fibers, like other axons of the nervous system, release neurotransmitters and are classified on the basis of the substance produced. **Cholinergic** (ko″lin-ər´jik) fibers release acetylcholine. **Adrenergic** (ad″ren-ur´jik) fibers release epinephrine. (Epinephrine is also called **adrenaline;** hence the term adren/ergic.)

acetylcholine
epinephrine

Cholinergic fibers release _____.
Adrenergic fibers release _____.

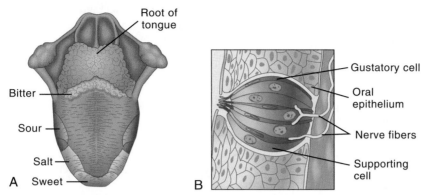

Figure 15-9 Taste buds and the taste regions of the tongue. **A,** Taste regions of the tongue. In addition to the four basic taste sensations (sweet, sour, bitter, and salty), there are combined perceptions plus the input from olfactory receptors. **B,** Drawing of an individual taste bud. Each taste bud rests in a pocket. Many taste buds are distributed over the tongue and the roof of the mouth.

15-28 Special sense organs—the eyes, ears, skin, mouth, and nose—have receptors that enable us to see, hear, feel, taste, and smell. The receptors that detect changes in our environment can be grouped into five types: chemoreceptors (ke″mo-re-sep´tərz), mechanoreceptors (mek″ə-no-re-sep´tərz), photoreceptors (fo″to-re-sep´tərz), thermoreceptors (thur″mo-re-sep´tərz), and nociceptors (no″sĭ-sep´tərz). Review the combining forms used to name the receptors below.

Word Parts: Types of Receptors

Combining Form	Meaning	Combining Form	Meaning
chem(o)	chemical	phot(o)	light
mechan(o)	mechanical	therm(o)	heat
noc(i)	cause harm, injury, or pain		

chemical

Chemo/receptors are nerve endings in the nose and tongue that are adapted for excitation by what type of substances? _____

chemoreceptors

Taste buds contain chemoreceptors for sweet, sour, bitter, and salty tastes (Figure 15-9). Receptors that are stimulated by chemical stimuli are called _____.

15-29 **Mechano/receptors** that are sensitive to mechanical changes in touch or pressure are widely distributed in the skin. Mechanoreceptors for hearing are located within the ear.

light

The eyes contain **photoreceptors** that detect _____.

Thermoreceptors are located immediately under the skin and are widely distributed throughout the body. Thermo/receptors detect changes in temperature, sensing both cold and

heat

_____, as the name implies.

The sense of pain is initiated by special receptors, **nociceptors,** that are widely distributed throughout the skin and the internal organs.

15-30 The sense organs contain the receptors that help us detect changes in our environment.

The eyes are the paired organs of sight. Having earlier learned the meaning of ophthalm(o) and ocul(o), both **ophthalm/ic** and **ocul/ar** mean pertaining to the _____,

eye

because ocul(o) and ophthalm(o) mean eye.

Intra/ocul/ar (in″trə-ok´u-lər), **inter/ocul/ar** (in″tər-ok´u-lər), and **extra/ocul/ar** (eks″trə-

outside

ok´u-lər) mean within, between, and _____ the eye, respectively.

15-31 The structures of the eye and ear are shown in Figure 15-10, A. Although it is probably not necessary to memorize the structures that make up these two sense organs, it is important to recognize names associated with them.

Eyelids open and close the eye and keep foreign objects from entering the eye. The eyelids, as well as the anterior portion of the sclera, are lined with a mucous membrane called **conjunctiva** (kən-jənk´ti-və).

15-32 The eyeball, or globe, is composed of three layers (Figure 15-10, *B*). The tough outer layer is composed of the **sclera** (the white, opaque membrane covering most of the eyeball) and the transparent **cornea** (the convex, transparent structure at the front of the eyeball that helps focus light rays entering the eye). The combining form kerat(o) means the cornea, but it also means hard, like horn.

The lens of the eye is located posterior to the pupil and is responsible for focusing the light rays so they form a perfect image on the retina. The **iris** is the pigmented portion that accounts for blue, brown, gray, green, and combinations of these colors in eyes. The **retina,** the innermost layer of the eye, contains photoreceptors (rods and cones) that receive images of external objects. The retina is continuous with the **optic nerve,** which carries the nervous impulse to the cerebrum and enables vision. Examine the appearance of the optic nerve and retina in Figure 15-10, *C*.

Learn the following word parts.

Word Parts: Eye and Ear

Combining Form	Meaning	Combining Form	Meaning
ir(o), irid(o)	iris	audi(o)	hearing
kerat(o)	cornea; hard, horny	ot(o)	ear
ocul(o), ophthalm(o)	eye		
dacry(o), lacrim(o)	tear		
opt(o), optic(o)	vision		

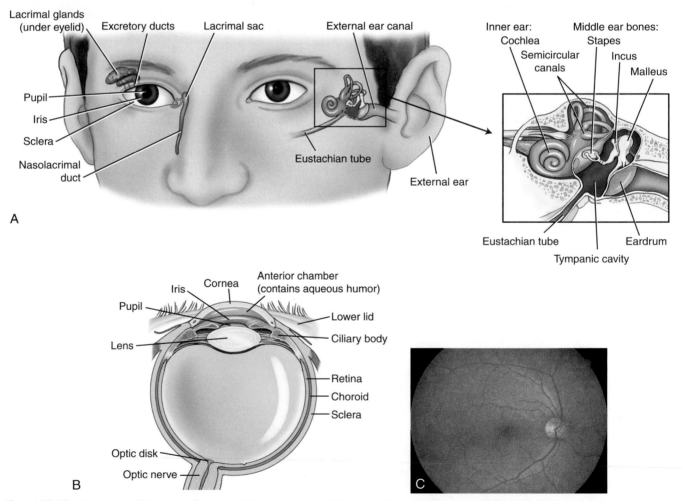

Figure 15-10 Structures of the ear and eye. A, Major structures of the eye and ear. **B,** Structures of the eyeball. **C,** Ophthalmoscopic view of the interior of the eye. A normal retina and optic nerve are shown. The normal retina and blood vessel walls are mainly transparent. Note that the branching points of the blood vessels "point" toward the optic nerve.

crying

15-33 The combining forms dacry(o) and lacrim(o) mean tear, as in crying. The **lacrim/al gland** produces fluid (tears) that keeps the eye moist. (Refer again to Figure 15-10.) If more lacrimal (lak´rĭ-məl) fluid is produced than can be removed, we say that the person is _____. (This is also called **tearing.**)
 Lacrim/ation (lak″rĭ-ma´shən) refers to crying, the production and discharge of tears.

lacrimal

15-34 Tears produced by the _____ gland wash over the eyeball and are drained through small openings in the inner corner of the eye. Tears pass through these openings into small ducts that lead to the **lacrimal sac.** From here they pass into the large **nasolacrimal duct** (na″zo-lak´rĭ-məl dukt) that ends in the nasal cavity. Naso/lacrimal pertains

nose

to the _____ and the lacrimal apparatus.
 Another name for the lacrimal sac is **dacryo/cyst** (dak´re-o-sist″).

15-35 The ears have receptors that detect touch, pain, heat, and cold, but the mechanoreceptors that enable us to hear usually come to mind when we think of the ear as a sense organ. We depend on our ears not only for hearing but also for the sense of equilibrium, both functions of mechanoreceptors.
 Anatomically, the ear is divided into the external ear, middle ear, and inner ear. (Refer

external

again to Figure 15-10.) The part of the ear that is visible is the _____ ear. With the function of collecting sound waves and directing them into the ear, the outer (external) ear ends at the **tympanic membrane** (eardrum).
 The middle ear is an air-filled cavity and has three tiny bones. When the eardrum vibrates, these bones transmit the vibrations to fluids in the inner ear. The inner ear contains the cochlea (kok´le-ə) and the semicircular canals. The **cochlea** contains receptors that enable us to hear. The **semicircular canals** enable us to maintain a sense of balance.

hearing

15-36 Audi/ble pertains to _____. **Audio/logy** is the science of hearing, particularly the study of impaired hearing that cannot be improved by medication or surgery. An **audiologist** (aw″de-ol´ə-jist) is a person skilled in audiology.

15-37 The nose is responsible for the sense of smell, and this sense is intricately linked with chemoreceptors in the tongue that enable us to experience different tastes of food and other substances.
 The term **olfaction** (ol-fak´shən) means the sense of smell, and **olfactory** (ol-fak´tə-re)

smell

means pertaining to the sense of _____. **Anosmia**[*] (an-oz´me-ə) is loss or impairment of the sense of smell, and **hyperosmia** (hi″pər-oz´me-ə) is an abnormally increased sensitivity to odors.

---

[*]Anosmia (Greek: *a,* without; *osme,* smell).

EXERCISE 4

Write words in the blanks to complete these sentences.

1. The peripheral nervous system is divided into the afferent or _____ system and the motor system.

2. The organs that have receptors that detect sensations are called _____ organs.

3. Cholinergic nerve fibers release _____.

4. Adrenergic nerve fibers release _____.

5. Nerve endings that are stimulated by chemical stimuli are called _____.

6. Nerve endings that detect light are called _____.

7. Nerve endings that detect changes in temperature are called _____.

8. Nerve endings that detect pain are called _____.

9. The _____ gland produces tears.

10. Hyperosmia means an abnormally increased sensitivity to _____.

EXERCISE 5

 Build It! *Use the following word parts to build terms. (Some word parts will be used more than once.)*

inter-, audi(o), dacry(o), lacrim(o), nas(o), ocul(o), somat(o), -al, -ar, -cyst, -ic, -logy

1. the study of hearing   _____/_____

2. pertaining to between the eyes   _____/_____/_____

3. pertaining to the nose and the tear apparatus   _____/_____/_____

4. lacrimal sac   _____/_____

5. pertaining to the body   _____/_____

Say and Check

Say aloud the terms you wrote for Exercise 5. Use the Companion CD to check your pronunciations.

DIAGNOSTIC TESTS AND PROCEDURES

15-38 A change in the level of consciousness may be the first indication of a decline in central nervous system function.

> ➤ **KEY** POINT <u>Levels of consciousness are cognitive function involving arousal mechanisms of the brain.</u> The levels of consciousness include alert wakefulness (normal); response to stimuli, although it may be slow; drowsiness; **stupor** (patient is vaguely aware of the environment); and **coma** (patient does not appear to be aware of the environment).

The various stages of response of the mind to stimuli are called the levels of _____.

consciousness

Memory, another means of assessing neurologic function, is classified as long-term, recent, and immediate memory. Loss of memory is often an early sign of neurologic problems.

15-39 Deep tendon reflex (DTR) and superficial reflex are used to assess neurologic and muscular damage. A deep tendon reflex, a brisk contraction of a muscle in response to a sharp tap by a finger or rubber hammer on a tendon, is often helpful in diagnosing stroke (Figure 15-11). A **superficial reflex** is evaluated by stimulation of the skin, such as stroking the sole of the foot to evaluate the response.

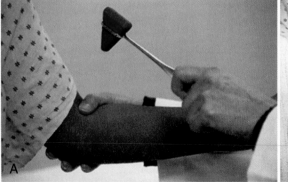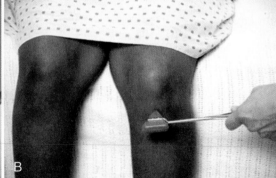

Figure 15-11 Tendon reflex, brisk contraction of a skeletal muscle in response to a sharp tap with a reflex hammer on a tendon.
A, Biceps reflex. The examiner elicits the biceps reflex by placing the thumb over the biceps tendon and striking the thumb with a hammer.
B, Patellar reflex. This reflex is elicited by striking the patellar tendon just below the kneecap. The normal response is extension of the leg.

tendon

The two types of reflex that are easily tested are the deep _____ reflex and the superficial reflex.

15-40 Certain illnesses may require chemical analysis and microscopic examination of the cerebrospinal fluid. Only a few cells are normally present, and a large number of leukocytes may indicate infection. Bacterial and fungal cultures of the CSF are done if indicated.

Cerebrospinal fluid is obtained by spinal puncture (usually a lumbar puncture); this is performed both for diagnostic purposes and sometimes to introduce substances into the spinal canal.

lumbar

The **lumbar puncture** is the introduction of a hollow needle into the subarachnoid space of the _____ part of the spinal canal (see Figure 14-18). It is performed not only for diagnostic purposes but also for the injection of an anesthetic solution for spinal anesthesia or contrast media for imaging procedures.

15-41 You are probably familiar with the term electrocardiography, which means the process of recording the electrical activity of the heart. **Electro/encephalo/graphy** (e-lek″tro-ən-sef″ə-log′rə-fe) is the process of recording the electrical activity of the _____.

brain
instrument

An **electroencephalograph** (e-lek″tro-ən-sef′ə-lo-graf″) is the _____ used in electroencephalography.

Electrodes are attached to various areas of the patient's head using a special gel (Figure 15-12). During neurosurgery, the electrodes can be applied directly to the brain. Electroencephalography is used to diagnose several disorders, including seizures, lesions, and impaired consciousness.

15-42 Although the legal definition of brain death varies from state to state, it is generally defined as an irreversible form of unconsciousness characterized by a complete loss of brain function while the heart continues to beat. A diagnosis of brain death may require a demonstration that electrical activity of the brain is absent. An **electro/encephalo/gram** (e-lek″tro-en-sef′ə-lo-

record

gram″), abbreviated EEG, is the _____ produced by the electrical activity of the brain.

15-43 A number of radiographic examinations are available to assess the nervous system. Plain x-ray studies of the skull and spine are often helpful in diagnosing fractures, abnormal curvatures, or other bony abnormalities.

Computed tomography (CT) and MRI are used to assess structural changes of the brain and spinal cord. CT is particularly helpful in detecting intracranial bleeding, lesions, and cerebral edema (see Figure 3-10).

brain

Echo/encephalo/graphy uses ultrasonic waves beamed through the head to record structural aspects of the _____. The record produced is an **echo/encephalo/gram** (ek″o-en-sef′ə-lə-gram″).

15-44 **Positron emission tomography** is a computerized nuclear medicine technique that uses radioactive substances to assess the function of various body structures, particularly the brain.

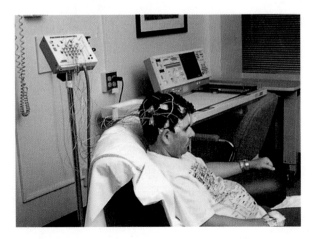

Figure 15-12 Electroencephalography. Electrodes are attached to various areas of the patient's head. The patient generally remains quiet with closed eyes during the procedure. In certain cases prescribed activities may be requested. The test is used to diagnose epilepsy, brain stem disorders, lesions, and impaired consciousness.

> ▶ **KEY** POINT The PET equipment constructs color-coded images that indicate the intensity of metabolic activity. The patient either inhales or is injected with radioactive material. The positrons of the injected material are absorbed by body cells and the equipment constructs color-coded images of the gamma rays that result. The radioactivity used in PET is short lived, so that patients are exposed to only small amounts of radiation.

function

An important advantage of positron emission tomography is that it assesses
_____, whereas most radiographic imaging studies of the brain assess structure.

brain

15-45 Encephalo/graphy (en-sef″ə-log′rə-fe) is radiography of the _____.
It is accomplished by withdrawal and replacement of the cerebrospinal fluid by a gas. Because of the risks involved, it is generally used only when results of CT and MRI are not definitive.

myelography
(mi″ə-log′rə-fe)
myelogram
(mi′ə-lo-gram)
brain

15-46 Write a word that means radiography of the spinal cord (after injection of a contrast medium): _____.
    Myelography can be useful in studying spinal lesions, spinal injuries, or disk disease. It is often supplemented by CT. The record produced in myelography is a _____.

15-47 Cerebral angio/graphy is used to visualize the blood vessels of the _____ after injection of a radiopaque contrast medium. Although it is not used as often as less invasive tests, such as CT, it can be used to diagnose abnormalities of blood vessels, such as an **aneurysm** (an′u-riz″əm), a ballooning out of the wall of a vessel (Figure 15-13).

15-48 Brain scans are used to assess aneurysms as well as to locate abscesses, tumors, or hematomas. In this diagnostic test a radioisotope that is selective for certain types of abnormal brain tissue is injected intravenously. Imaging with a gamma camera demonstrates the area of accumulation of the radioisotope.

radioisotope

    In a brain scan, imaging is accomplished using a _____.

ophthalmoscope
(of-thal′mə-skōp)
instrument

15-49 You learned earlier that **ophthalmo/scopy** (of″thəl-mos′kə-pe) is visual examination of the eye (see Figure 3-4). The instrument is an _____.

    An **ophthalmo/meter** (of″thəl-mom′ə-ter) is an _____ for measuring the eye.

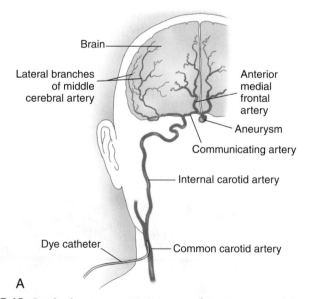

Brain
Lateral branches of middle cerebral artery
Anterior medial frontal artery
Aneurysm
Communicating artery
Internal carotid artery
Dye catheter
Common carotid artery

A

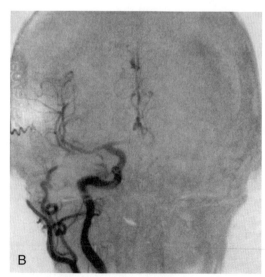

B

Figure 15-13 Cerebral aneurysm. A, Diagram of an aneurysm and the major cerebral arteries visible in cerebral angiography. **B,** A cerebral angiogram. Cerebral angiography is used to study intracranial circulation and is especially helpful in visualizing aneurysms and vascular occlusions. A contrast medium is used that outlines the vessels of the brain.

TABLE 15-1	Decibel Intensity and Safe Exposure Time for Common Sounds	
Sound	**Decibel Intensity (dB)**	**Safe Exposure Time***
Threshold of hearing	0	
Whispering	20	
Average residence or office	40	
Conversational speech	60	
Car traffic	70	>8 hr
Motorcycle	90	8 hr
Chain saw	100	2 hr
Rock concert, front row	120	3 min
Jet engine	140	Immediate danger
Rocket launching pad	180	Immediate danger

From Ignatavicius DD, Workman ML: *Medical-surgical nursing: critical thinking for collaborative care*, ed 5, St Louis, 2006, Saunders.
*For every 5-dB increase in intensity, the safe exposure time is cut in half.

otoscope (o′to-skōp)

15-50 The ear is examined in **oto/scopy** (o-tos′kə-pe) (see Figure 3-3). The instrument used in otoscopy is an _____.

hearing

15-51 An **audio/meter** (aw″de-om′ə-tər) is an electronic device for measuring _____. The record produced is an **audiogram** (aw′de-o-gram″). Hearing is tested by using tones from very low to very high frequencies at various decibels (dB) of intensity. The lowest intensity at which a young, normal ear can detect sound (about 51% of the time) is 0 dB. Conversational speech is around 60 dB, and sounds at that decibel intensity are not harmful. Exposure to loud noises, even for a short time, can damage the cochlear hair cells and result in hearing loss. Looking at Table 15-1, what is considered a safe exposure time if

3

you are sitting in the front row at a rock concert? _____ minutes

15-52 Sleep studies are not invasive and are used to diagnose **sleep apnea** (ap′ne-ə), a sleep disorder characterized by short periods in which respiration is absent. These tests are performed in a sleep laboratory where the patient is monitored electronically while sleeping.
    Tests that consist of electronic monitoring of a sleeping person to diagnose sleep apnea are

sleep

called _____ studies.

EXERCISE 6

Match diagnostic procedures in the left columns with their descriptions in the right column.

_____ 1. brain scan   _____ 4. echoencephalography   A. brisk muscular contraction in response to stimuli

_____ 2. cerebral angiography   _____ 5. myelography   B. imaging of the brain using radioisotopes

_____ 3. deep tendon reflex   C. radiography of the spinal cord
                                                                D. use of ultrasound to study brain structure
                                                                E. visualization of blood vessels of the brain

EXERCISE 7

Word Analysis. *Break these words into their component parts by placing a slash between the word parts. Write the meaning of each term.*

1. ophthalmometer   _____

2. electroencephalograph   _____

3. audiogram   _____

4. ophthalmoscopy   _____

5. encephalography   _____

Say and Check

Say aloud the terms in Exercise 7. Use the Companion CD to check your pronunciations.

PATHOLOGIES

15-53 The nervous system is a complicated body system, and many of its functions are not well understood, particularly in the realm of psychologic disorders. Disturbances of the central nervous system vary from acute to chronic, short term to long term, and minor to life-threatening. Pathologies include trauma, congenital disorders, infections, tumors, degenerative disorders, diseases of the sense organs, and psychologic disturbances.

Some disorders of the nervous system do not fit into the categories presented here. For example, the learning disorder **dyslexia** (dis-lek′se-ə) is an impairment of the ability to read, spell, and write words; it results from a variety of pathologic conditions, some of which are associated with the nervous system. The prefix dys- means _____, and *lexis* is a Greek term meaning word. Dyslexic persons often reverse letters and words, cannot adequately distinguish the letter sequences in written words, and have difficulty determining right from left. The exact cause of dyslexia is not known, but it is unrelated to intelligence.

difficult

Learn the meanings of the following word parts.

Additional Word Parts: Nervous System Pathologies

Combining Form	Meaning		Suffixes	Meaning
pseud(o)	false		-asthenia	weakness
			-esthesia	sensitivity to pain
			-lexia	words, phrases

15-54 Pain, which is caused by stimulation of the sensory nerve endings, is the most common symptom for which patients seek medical advice. You have learned that -algia means _____.

pain

Algesia (al-je′ze-ə) is a word that refers to sensitivity to pain and is also used as a suffix. **Hyper/algesia** (hi″pər-al-je′ze-ə) is _____ sensitivity to pain.

increased

Literal interpretation of **hyp/algesia** (hi″pal-je′ze-ə) or **hypo/algesia** (hi″po-al-je′ze-ə) is _____ sensitivity to pain. Either term means a decrease in sensation in response to stimulation of the sensory nerves.

decreased

Paresthesia (par″es-the′zhə) is a subjective sensation, experienced as numbness, tingling, or a "pins and needles" feeling, often in the absence of an external stimulus.

Pseud/esthesia (sōōd″es-the′zhə) is an imaginary or false sensation. The prefix pseudo- means false. Pseud/esthesia is a sensation occurring in the absence of the appropriate stimulus, and its cause is not well understood. (Pseudesthesia is also called **pseudoesthesia**. Two spellings are accepted for many terms in which pseud[o] is joined to a combining form that begins with a vowel.)

Pseudesthesia can occur in a lost arm or leg after amputation. This imaginary or false sensation is termed _____.

pseudesthesia

neuralgia
(nōō-ral′jə)

15-55 Using -algia, write a word that means pain of a nerve: _____.

Poly/neur/algia (pol″e-nōō-ral′jə) is a type of neuralgia that affects many nerves simultaneously.

> ► KEY POINT <u>A **poly/neuro/pathy** (pol″e-nōō-rop′ə-the) is a condition in which many peripheral nerves are affected.</u> **Poly/neur/itis** (pol″e-nōō-ri′tis) is an example of a polyneuropathy. Polyneuritis means inflammation of many nerves (simultaneously). Damage to cranial or peripheral nerves can lead to various neuropathies that may be evidenced by tingling, burning, or decreased sensitivity in an extremity.

15-56 Sciatica (si-at´ĭ-kə) is inflammation of the sciatic nerve, usually marked by pain and tenderness along the course of the nerve through the thigh and leg. This may arise from problems in the lower back as a result of a herniated intervertebral disk or arthritis and is accompanied by lower back pain (LBP). Write this term that means inflammation of the sciatic nerve:

sciatica

_____.

HEADACHES

headache

15-57 A headache, pain in the head from any cause, is a symptom. Most headaches do not indicate serious disease. **Cephal/algia** (sef″ə-lal´jə), often shortened to **ceph/algia** (sə-fal´jə), is a synonym for _____.

The most common types of headaches are pain related to the eyes, ears, teeth, and paranasal structures (for example, a sinus headache). Other kinds of headaches include tension headaches (muscle contraction headaches), cluster headaches, and migraine headaches (Figure 15-14).

15-58 Tension headaches result from the long-sustained contraction of skeletal muscles around the scalp, face, neck, and upper back. This is the primary source of many headaches associated with excessive emotional tension, anxiety, and depression. Also called muscle contraction head-

tension

aches, _____ headaches result from long-sustained contraction of skeletal muscles of the head and upper back.

15-59 Cluster headaches are characterized by intense unilateral pain. Uni/lateral means occur-

side

ring on one _____ only. They are very painful, occur in clusters, and fortunately do not last long.

15-60 A **migraine headache** is a vascular disorder characterized by recurrent throbbing headaches, often accompanied by loss of appetite, photophobia, and nausea with or without vomiting. Photophobia is sensitivity of the eyes to light. Translated literally, **photo/phobia** means an ab-

light

normal fear of _____. This term also means a morbid fear of light with an irrational need to avoid light places.

Migraine headaches occur more often in females than in males and sometimes begin in childhood. The classic migraine begins with depression, irritability, restlessness, and perhaps loss of appetite. There may also be transient neurologic disturbances, including visual problems (flashes of light, distorted or double vision, seeing spots), dizziness, and nausea. The headache increases in severity until it becomes intense and may last a few hours or up to several days if not treated.

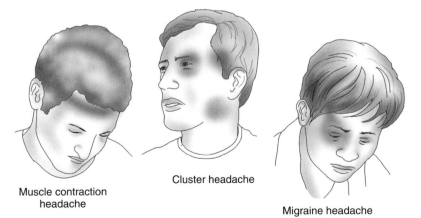

Muscle contraction
headache

Cluster headache

Migraine headache

Figure 15-14 Three types of headaches. Shaded areas show regions of most intense pain.

EXERCISE 8

Build It! *Use the following word parts to build terms. (Some word parts will be used more than once.)*

dys-, hyper-, poly-, cephal(o), neur(o), phot(o), -algia, -algesia, -itis, -lexia, -phobia

1. headache   _____/_____

2. sensitivity to or fear of light   _____/_____

3. inflammation of many nerves   _____/_____/_____

4. increased sensitivity to pain   _____/_____

5. condition of difficulty with reading   _____/_____

Say and Check

Say aloud the terms you wrote for Exercise 8. Use the Companion CD to check your pronunciations.

TRAUMA	

15-61 Craniocerebral trauma is commonly called head trauma or head injury. It is a traumatic insult to the brain caused by an external physical force that may produce a diminished or altered state of consciousness. It may result in impairment of cognitive abilities (perception, reasoning, judgment, and memory) or physical functions and may be temporary or permanent. Skull fractures, gunshot wounds, and knife injuries are examples of open head traumas. Blunt trauma as seen in motor vehicle accidents can lead to **concussions** (kən-kush´ənz), **contusions** (bruises), or tearing of the brain.

An abnormal condition in which language function is absent or disordered because of an injury to certain areas of the cerebral cortex can result in **a/phasia** (ə-fa´zhə) or **dys/phasia** (disfa´zhə). Literal translation of a/phasia is absence of _____.

speech

Difficult, poorly articulated speech, usually caused by damage to a central or peripheral motor nerve, is called **dys/arthria*** (dis-ahr´thre-ə).

15-62 Consciousness is responsiveness of the mind to the impressions made by the senses. A **cerebral concussion** usually causes loss of consciousness. A concussion is an injury resulting from impact with an object. A blow to the head can cause a cerebral _____.

concussion

A person who is responsive to impressions made by the senses is said to be conscious. A person who is **semi/conscious** (sem˝e-kon´shəs) is only partially aware of his or her surroundings.

A **coma** is a profound unconsciousness from which the patient cannot be aroused. Using semiconscious as a model, write a word that means a partial or mild coma from which the patient can be aroused: _____.

semicoma
(sem˝e-ko´mə)

15-63 The **Glasgow Coma Scale** is a standardized system for assessing the degree of conscious impairment in the critically ill (especially those with head injuries) and for predicting the duration and ultimate outcome of coma. The system involves determination of the degree of eye opening, verbal response, and motor response. Each of the three determinants is assessed numerically by the best response, and the numbers can be used to determine improvement, stability, or deterioration of a person's level of consciousness (Table 15-2). This standardized system for assessing the degree of conscious impairment is called the Glasgow _____ Scale.

Coma

The sum of the numeric values can be used as an objective measurement. A sum of 15 of the three numeric values generally indicates no impairment, 3 is compatible with brain death, and 7 is usually accepted as a state of coma.

15-64 Head injuries can also result in a spinal cord injury (SCI). An **encephalo/myelo/pathy** (en-sef˝ə-lo-mi˝əl-op´ə-the) is any disease involving the _____ and the spinal cord.

brain

---

*Dysarthria (dys-, difficult + Greek: *arthroun,* to articulate).

TABLE 15-2 Glasgow Coma Scale Scoring

Eyes Open		Best Motor Response	
4	Spontaneously	6	Obeys a command ("Hold out three fingers.")
3	On request	5	Localizes a painful stimulus
2	To pain stimuli (supraorbital or digital)	4	Withdraws in response to pain
1	No opening	3	Flexes either arm
		2	Extends arm to painful stimulus
Best Verbal Response		1	No response
5	Oriented to time, place, person		
4	Engages in conversation, confused in content		
3	Words spoken but conversation not sustained		
2	Groans evoked by pain		
1	No response		

From *Mosby's medical dictionary,* ed 7, St Louis, 2006, Mosby.

Forceful injuries to the vertebral column can damage the spinal cord and lead to neurologic problems. Injuries to the vertebral column that can result in damage to the spinal cord include excessive rotation, hyperextension, hyperflexion, and vertical compression (Figure 15-15).

15-65 Three types of **hemat/omas** associated with head injuries are shown in Figure 15-16. You learned earlier that a hematoma is a collection of blood in the tissues of the skin or in an organ.

Because epi- means above or on, epi/dural means situated on or outside the dura mater. Accumulation of blood in the epidural space is an _____

epidural
(ep″ĭ-doo´rəl)

hematoma. This hematoma compresses the dura mater and thus compresses the brain.

Accumulation of blood between the dura mater and the arachnoid is called a **subdural hematoma.** The acute form is often the result of a tear in the arachnoid associated with a head injury.

within

Note that bleeding occurs _____ the brain in an **intra/cerebral** (in″trə-ser´ə-brəl) **hematoma.** Fortunately this type of hematoma is less common than a subdural or epidural hematoma. Intracerebral hematomas have a high mortality rate because of the damage they cause to brain tissue.

15-66 **Cerebro/vascular** (ser″ə-bro-vas´ku-lər) **accident** (CVA) is also called stroke or stroke syndrome.

> ➤ **KEY** POINT Normal blood supply to the brain has been disrupted in CVA. CVA results in insufficient oxygen to brain tissue, caused by hemorrhage, occlusion (closing), or constriction of the blood vessels that normally supply oxygen to the brain.

A **cerebral aneurysm** (sə-re´brəl, ser´ə-brəl an´u-rizm) is an abnormal, localized dilation of a cerebral artery. The aneurysm may rupture to produce a **cerebral hemorrhage. Hemorrhagic strokes** are caused by the rupture of a cerebral artery.

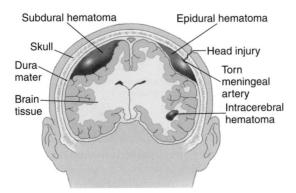

Figure 15-16 **Three types of hematomas associated with head injuries: subdural hematoma, epidural hematoma, and intracerebral hematoma.**

brain

artery

stroke (CVA)

Embolic strokes are caused by a **cerebral embolus** (em´bo-ləs), a plug of matter (usually a blood clot) brought by the blood to the _____. A cerebral embolus is one cause of a CVA.

Thrombotic strokes are caused by plaque deposits that build up on the interior of a cerebral _____. Both embolic and thrombotic strokes are commonly preceded by warning signs, such as a **transient ischemic attack** (TIA), caused by a brief interruption in cerebral blood flow. The term ischemic pertains to deficient blood circulation (in this case, in the brain). TIA symptoms often include disturbance of normal vision, dizziness, weakness, and numbness. A transient ischemic attack is important because it may be a warning sign of an impending _____. The types of stroke are shown in Figure 15-17.

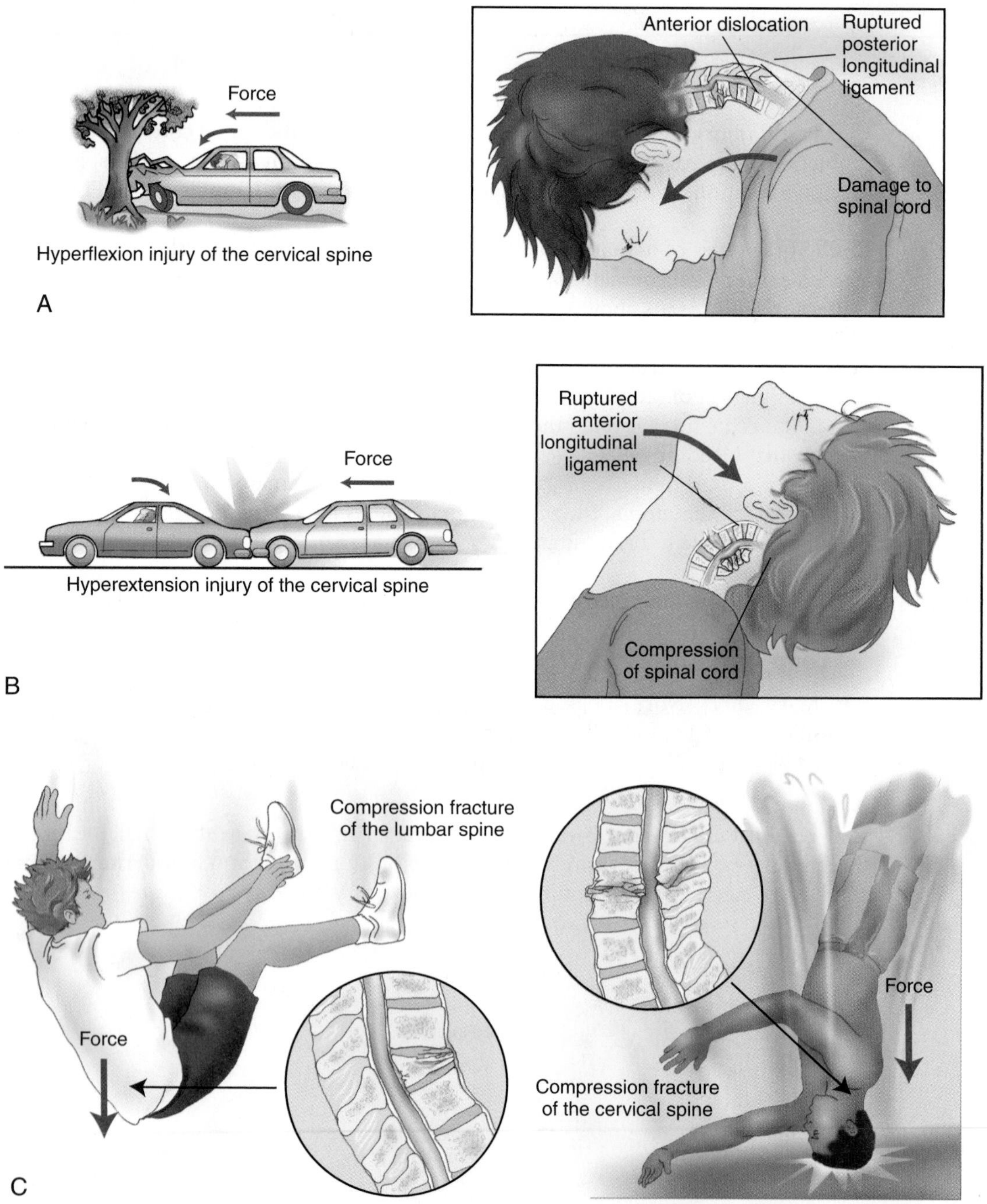

Force

Hyperflexion injury of the cervical spine

A

Anterior dislocation

Ruptured posterior longitudinal ligament

Damage to spinal cord

Force

Hyperextension injury of the cervical spine

B

Ruptured anterior longitudinal ligament

Compression of spinal cord

Compression fracture of the lumbar spine

Force

Force

Compression fracture of the cervical spine

C

Figure 15-15 Closed spinal cord injuries. Fractures and dislocations to the vertebral column can result in injury to the spinal cord. These types of vertebral injuries occur most often at points where a relatively mobile portion of the spine meets a relatively fixed segment. **A,** Hyperflexion of the cervical vertebrae. **B,** Hyperextension of the cervical vertebrae. **C,** Vertical compression of the cervical spine and the lumbar spine.

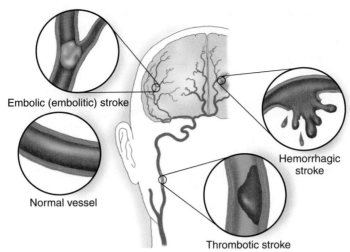

Figure 15-17 Types of stroke. A cerebrovascular accident, commonly referred to as a stroke, is a disruption in the normal blood supply to the brain. An embolic stroke is caused by an embolus or a group of emboli that breaks off from one area of the body, often the heart, and travels to the cerebral arteries. Thrombotic strokes are caused by plaque deposits that build up on the interior of a cerebral artery, gradually occluding it. Hemorrhagic strokes are caused by rupture of a cerebral arterial wall.

disease	**15-67** The peripheral nerves are subject to many types of trauma. A **peripheral neuropathy** (noo-rop´ə-the) is any _____ of the peripheral nerves. Those of the extremities are commonly affected. An example is wristdrop, in which nerve damage results in the hand remaining in a flexed position at the wrist, and it cannot be extended. Write the term that means wristdrop by combining carp(o) and -ptosis: _____.
carpoptosis (kahr˝pop-to´sis)	

EXERCISE 9

Match terms in the left columns with their meanings in the right column.

_____ 1. encephalomyelopathy   _____ 4. neurosclerosis

_____ 2. hypalgesia   _____ 5. polyneuritis

_____ 3. hyperalgesia   _____ 6. pseudesthesia

A. any disease involving the brain and spinal cord
B. decreased response to stimulation of the sensory nerves
C. hardening of nervous tissue
D. imaginary or false sensation
E. increased sensitivity to pain
F. inflammation of many nerves simultaneously

PARALYSIS

paralysis	**15-68 Paralysis** is the loss of muscle function, loss of sensation, or both and is a sign of an underlying problem. Paralysis may be caused by trauma, disease, or poisoning. Injury to different areas of the spinal cord results in different types of paralysis. Remembering that -plegia means paralysis, in **hemi/plegia** (hem˝e-ple´jə) there is _____ of one half of the body (only one side).
	Paralysis of both sides of the body is **di/plegia** (di-ple´je-ə). In diplegia there is paralysis of similar parts on both sides of the body.
four	**Quadri/plegia** (kwod˝rĭ-ple´jə) is paralysis of all _____ extremities.
paralysis	**15-69** In **para/plegia** (par˝ə-ple´jə), the upper limbs are not affected. Para/plegia is _____ of the lower portion of the body and both legs. The prefix para- means near, beside, or abnormal. Some interpretation is needed in the term paraplegia.
	Mono/plegia (mon˝o-ple´jə) is paralysis of one limb.

facial

15-70 Facial paralysis, or **Bell palsy,** is a neuropathy that drastically affects the body image. The cause is unknown; the onset is acute and is characterized by a drawing sensation with paralysis of all facial muscles on the affected side. Bell palsy is acute paralysis of a cranial nerve affecting one side of the face, also called _____ paralysis.

CONGENITAL DISORDERS

meninges
meninges

15-71 Congenital defects of the nervous system may be obvious at birth and may vary from minor to severe. An abnormal protrusion near the spine may be a meningocele (mə-ning´go-sēl″) or meningo/myelo/cele (mə-ning″go-mi´ə-lo-sēl″). A **meningo/cele** is hernial protrusion of _____ through a defect in the skull or vertebral column (Figure 15-18).

A **meningo/myelo/cele** is hernial protrusion of parts of the _____ and spinal cord through a defect in the vertebral column. Both these congenital defects are generally repaired by surgery, but either defect may result in residual motor and sensory deficits.

palsy

15-72 **Cerebral palsy** (pawl´ze) is a motor function disorder caused by a permanent, nonprogressive brain defect present at birth or occurring shortly thereafter. It may result in spastic paralysis in various forms, seizures, and varying degrees of impaired speech, vision, and hearing. It is often associated with asphyxia during birth. This congenital defect is called cerebral _____.

Huntington

15-73 Huntington disease, also called **Huntington chorea** (kə-re´ə), is a hereditary disorder that affects both genders equally. Symptoms begin between 30 and 50 years of age. The two main signs and symptoms are progressive mental status changes leading to dementia and rapid, jerky movements in the trunk, facial muscles, and extremities. Neurotransmitters have been implicated in the symptoms of this inherited disorder called _____ disease.

anotia
(an-o´shə)

15-74 One developmental defect that is not life-threatening but life-altering is absence of one or both ears. Combine an- + ot(o) + -ia to write a word that means absence of the ear: _____.

Anotia is absence of one or both external ears. It is generally accompanied by lack of an internal ear also. Cosmetic reconstructive surgery, generally performed while the child is still young, does not, of course, correct the deafness.

INFECTIONS

brain

15-75 Infections of the CNS include encephalomyelitis (en-sef″ə-lo-mi″ə-li´tis), meningitis (men″in-ji´tis), and encephalitis (en-sef″ə-li´tis). **Encephalomyelitis** is inflammation of the _____ and spinal cord.

meninges

15-76 **Mening/itis** is inflammation of the _____ of the brain and the spinal cord. Although other infectious organisms can invade the nervous system, bacterial or viral organisms are most often responsible for meningitis.

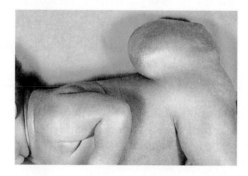

Figure 15-18 Meningocele. The spinal meninges have formed a hernial cyst that is filled with cerebrospinal fluid and is protruding through a defect in the vertebral column.

15-77 Encephal/itis is inflammation of the brain tissue. It is most often caused by a virus, usually having gained access to the bloodstream from a viral infection elsewhere in the body.

brain

Encephalo/meningitis (en-sef″ə-lo-men″in-ji´tis) is inflammation of the _____ and its coverings.

15-78 If the inflammation is confined to the cerebellum, this condition (inflammation of the cerebellum) is _____.

cerebellitis
(ser′ə-bel-i´tis)

You learned in another chapter that the combining form ventricul(o) means ventricle. The word part can refer to a ventricle in either the brain or the heart. Ventricul/itis (ven-trik″u-li´tis)

ventricle

is inflammation of a _____. Although it is not obvious, **ventriculitis** refers especially to inflammation of a ventricle of the brain.

15-79 Four other diseases caused by infectious microorganisms that have a devastating effect on the central nervous system are tetanus (tet´ə-nəs), botulism (boch´ə-liz-əm), poliomyelitis (po″le-o-mi″ə-li´tis), and rabies (ra´bēz, ra´be-ēz).

Tetanus, also known as lockjaw, is caused by a bacterium and is easily preventable through immunization. The infection is commonly transmitted through a wound contaminated with the bacteria. The bacterial toxin attacks the nervous system and results in muscle rigidity and spasms. Taking its name from the "locked jaw" rigidity that results, this disease is known as

tetanus

_____.

15-80 Botulism is caused by a type of bacteria that is toxic to nervous tissue and causes paralysis of both voluntary and involuntary motor activity. Most cases are caused by eating improperly canned foods. Symptoms usually appear 12 to 36 hours after eating contaminated food in this

botulism

neurotoxic disease, called _____.

15-81 Poliomyelitis is an acute viral disease that attacks the gray matter of the spinal cord and parts of the brain. It can be asymptomatic, mild, or paralytic. This disease is rarely seen in North America because it can be prevented by immunization. It is informally called polio.[*]

15-82 Rabies is an acute, often fatal, disease of the central nervous system transmitted to humans by infected animals. After introduction of the virus into the human body, often by an animal bite, the virus travels along nerve pathways to the brain and later to other organs. Without medical intervention and possibly the use of vaccine, coma and death are likely.

A nontechnical term for rabies that is obsolete is **hydrophobia** (hi″dro-fo´be-ə). This name was given after observation that rabid animals avoid water. Infected animals avoid water because paralysis prevents them from being able to swallow. Hydrophobia is an obsolete term for

rabies

_____.

[*]Polio (Greek: _polios_, gray).

EXERCISE 10

Word Analysis. _Break these words into their component parts by placing a slash between the word parts. Write the meaning of each term._

1. encephalomeningitis _____

2. hemiplegia _____

3. meningomyelocele _____

4. ventriculitis _____

5. hydrophobia _____

Say and Check

Say aloud the terms in Exercise 10. Use the Companion CD to check your pronunciations.

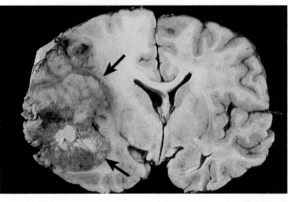

Figure 15-19 A primary brain tumor. This autopsy specimen of the brain shows a large tumor *(arrows)*. This patient had multiple distant metastases in the lung and spine.

TUMORS

neuroglia

15-83 Primary brain tumors arise within the brain structures and rarely spread outside the brain. Glia cells are the only source of primary malignant brain tumors. The tumors are called gliomas (gli-o′məz). A **gli/oma,** a primary tumor of the brain, is composed of which type of nerve cell? _____

A **meningi/oma** (mə-nin″je-o′mə) is a tumor of the meninges that grows slowly and may invade the skull. Tumors within the skull can invade and compress brain tissue, which generally leads to increased intracranial pressure (ICP), headaches, and many neurologic problems, such as a **neuro/genic** (noor″o-jen′ik) **bladder,** a dysfunction of the urinary bladder caused by a lesion (a tumor) of the nervous system. Normal control of urination and emptying of the bladder is usually absent.

within

15-84 You know that crani(o) means the cranium, or skull, therefore **intra/cranial** means _____ the skull. Brain tumors can become quite large, occupying considerable intracranial space, as shown in Figure 15-19.

water; head

15-85 Disorders such as brain tumors that interfere with the flow of CSF cause fluid accumulation in the skull, called hydrocephalus (hi″dro-sef′ə-ləs). Translated literally, hydro/cephalus means _____ in the _____. **Hydrocephalus** is a pathologic condition characterized by an abnormal accumulation of CSF within the skull and is usually accompanied by increased intracranial pressure. When this happens in an infant, before the cranial bones fuse, the cranium enlarges (see Figure 7-3). In an older child or adult, the pressure damages the soft brain tissue.

tumor

15-86 A **neur/oma** (noo-ro′mə) is a benign _____ composed chiefly of neurons and nerve fibers. Although they are benign, they can be painful (for example, a Morton neuroma that occurs in the foot) or can compress brain tissue (for example, an acoustic neuroma).

SEIZURE DISORDERS

seizure

15-87 A **seizure** is an abnormal, sudden, excessive discharge of electrical activity within the brain. Seizures are also known as **convulsions.** This abnormal activity is assessed in electroencephalography. A seizure may be recurrent, as in a seizure disorder, or transient and acute, as after a concussion. A concussion is damage to the brain caused by a violent jarring or shaking.
Remember that the suffix -lepsy means _____. **Epilepsy** (ep′ĭ-lep″se) is a group of chronic neurologic disorders characterized by recurrent episodes of convulsive seizures, sensory disturbances, loss of consciousness, or all of these.

15-88 Narcolepsy (nahr′ko-lep″se) is uncontrollable, brief episodes of sleep and uses the combining form narc(o), which means stupor. In narcolepsy the person cannot prevent a sudden attack of sleep while performing daytime activities. Its cause is unknown, and no pathologic lesions are found in the brain. The person may experience momentary loss of muscle tone. Visual or auditory hallucinations often occur at the onset of sleep. Stimulant drugs are often prescribed to prevent the sudden attacks of sleep at inappropriate times. The name of this disorder is

_____.

narcolepsy

DEGENERATIVE DISORDERS

15-89 Degenerative disorders are those in which there is deterioration of structure or function of tissue. Included in this section are neurologic disorders that affect motor ability or nerve transmission (Parkinson disease, multiple sclerosis, amyotrophic lateral sclerosis [a-mi″o-tro′fik lat′ər-əl sklə-ro′sis], myasthenia gravis [mi″əs-the′ne-ə gră′vis]) and involve mental deterioration (dementia, Alzheimer [awltz′hi-mər] disease).

    Parkinson disease is a slowly progressing, debilitating, neurologic disease that affects motor ability. It is characterized by muscle rigidity, bradykinesia (brad″e-kĭ-ne′zhə), and tremor (trem′ər, tre′mər). The suffix -kinesia means movement. **Brady/kinesia** means _____ movement, or slowness of all voluntary movement or speech. **Tremor** is rhythmic, purposeless, quivering involuntary movement. A characteristic posture and masklike facial expression are often seen.

    Parkinson disease occurs most often in people over 50 years of age and results from widespread degeneration of a part of the brain that produces dopamine. The cause is not known.

slow

15-90 **Multiple sclerosis** (MS) is a progressive degenerative disease that affects the myelin sheath and conduction pathways of the central nervous system.

> ➤ **KEY** POINT <u>In multiple sclerosis, the myelin sheath deteriorates and is replaced by scar tissue that interferes with normal transmission of the nerve impulse</u>. One of the earliest signs is paresthesia, abnormal sensations in the extremities or on one side of the face. The disease is characterized by periods of remission and exacerbation (flare). Disability increases as the disease progresses and the periods of exacerbation become more frequent.

    In multiple sclerosis, the myelin sheath deteriorates and is replaced by scar tissue that interferes with normal transmission of the nerve impulse. This disease that is named for the multiple areas of sclerotic tissue that replace the myelin sheath is multiple _____.

sclerosis

15-91 **Amyotrophic lateral sclerosis** (ALS) is also called Lou Gehrig disease. It is characterized by atrophy (wasting) of the hands, forearms, and legs. The disease results in paralysis and death. The cause of the disease is unknown. Analyzing the parts of a/myo/trophic, a- means without, my(o) means _____, and -trophic means nutrition.

    This rare degenerative disease of the motor neurons, characterized by weakness and atrophy of the muscles, is ALS, which means _____ lateral sclerosis.

muscle

amyotrophic

15-92 **My/asthenia gravis,** meaning grave muscle weakness, is a chronic neuromuscular disease characterized by muscular weakness and fatigue. The suffix -asthenia means weakness, so my/asthenia means weakness of the _____.

    This degenerative condition results from a defect in the conduction of nerve impulses at the neuromuscular junction. Characterized by chronic fatigue and muscle weakness, it is called _____ gravis.

muscle

myasthenia

15-93 **Dementia** (də-men′shə) is a progressive mental disorder of the brain.

> ➤ **KEY** POINT <u>There are many causes of dementia.</u> Conditions that cause the decline may be treatable or partially reversible. Dementia is characterized by confusion, disorientation, deterioration of memory and intellectual abilities, and personality disintegration. Dementia occurs most often in older adults. Dementia caused by drug intoxication, insulin shock, hydrocephalus, or certain other causes may be reversed by treating the underlying cause. Organic forms of dementia, such as Alzheimer disease, are generally considered incurable.

Alzheimer

Alzheimer disease is chronic, progressive mental deterioration that is sometimes called dementia, Alzheimer type. This accounts for more than half of the persons with dementia who are older than 65 years of age. It is less common in people in their 40s and 50s. Although the exact cause is not known, both chemical and structural changes occur in the brain. The disease is characterized by confusion, memory failure, disorientation, inability to carry out purposeful activities, and speech and gait disturbances. It involves irreversible loss of memory. The patient becomes increasingly mentally impaired, severe physical deterioration takes place, and death occurs. This type of dementia is called _____ disease.

EXERCISE 11

Build It! *Use the following word parts to build terms. (Some word parts will be used more than once.)*

a-, brady-, intra-, crani(o), gli(o), my(o), narc(o), troph(o), -al, -ic, -kinesia, -lepsy, -oma

1. slow movement _____/_____

2. uncontrollable brief episodes of sleep (or stupor) _____/_____

3. pertaining to the area within the skull _____/_____/_____

4. tumor of glial cells _____/_____

5. pertaining to a lack of muscle nutrition _____/_____/_____/_____

Say and Check

Say aloud the terms you wrote for Exercise 11. Use the Companion CD to check your pronunciations.

EYE AND EAR DISORDERS

15-94 We depend on the sense organs to detect sensations. Disorders of the eyes and ears can interfere with this ability; hence the inclusion of the eyes and ears in this chapter. The more common problems of the eyes and ears are injury and infection. The eyes are protected by the bony orbit, but more than a million eye injuries occur each year by blunt objects, by penetration of the eyeball, or by chemicals.

15-95 Blephar/optosis (blef″ə-rop-to′sis, blef″ə-ro-to′sis), also called **ptosis** (to′sis), is an abnormal condition in which one or both upper eyelids droop (Figure 4-4). It may be congenital or acquired as a result of weakness of the muscle (as in aging) or paralysis of the nerve.

eyelid

Blephar/itis (blef″ə-ri′tis) is inflammation of the _____ and is characterized by swelling and redness. Its causes include allergies, irritants, and infection. Crying can cause **blephar/edema** (blef″ər-ĭ-de′mə), swelling of the eyelid, and transient blephar/itis, but the crusts of dried mucus on the lids that are characteristic of true blepharitis are absent.

Blepharitis may be accompanied by **conjunctivitis** (kən-junk″tĭ-vi′tis), inflammation of the conjunctiva. Write this term that means inflammation of the conjunctiva:

conjunctivitis

_____.

15-96 A **hordeolum** (hor-de′o-ləm), also called sty or stye, is an infection of a sebaceous gland in the lid margin. It usually affects only one eye at a time (see Figure 7-9).

keratitis
(ker″ə-ti′tis)

Iritis (i-ri′tis) is inflammation of the iris.

Write a term that means inflammation of the cornea: _____.

Treatment of keratitis is important to avoid corneal scarring or perforation.

Dry eyes are caused by a variety of conditions and disorders caused by decreased tear secretion or increased evaporation of moisture from the eye, as in an extremely dry or windy environment.

Inflammation of the external eye is a common condition because the eye is sensitive to many external irritants, including cosmetics, dust, and fumes. In addition, microorganisms can cause infection.

softening	**15-97** Several terms are used to describe various eye conditions, such as **ophthalmo/malacia** (of-thal″mo-mə-la′shə), which is abnormal _____ of the eyeball. **Ophthalmo/plegia** (of-thal″mo-ple′jə) means paralysis of the eye.
hemorrhage	**Ophthalmo/rrhagia** (of-thal″mo-ra′jə) is _____ from the eye.
pain	**Ophthalm/algia** (of″thəl-mal′jə) means _____ in the eye. This can lead to excessive lacrimation.
cataract	**15-98** A **cataract** (kat′ə-rakt) is an abnormal progressive condition of the lens of the eye, characterized by loss of transparency. Write the name of this abnormal opacity of the lens of the eye, being careful with its spelling: _____.
	15-99 Glaucoma (glaw-, glou-ko′mə) is an abnormal condition of increased pressure within the eye. Prolonged pressure can damage the retina and optic nerve. Several drugs are available, and even laser surgery is used to relieve the increased pressure.
retina	**15-100** Any disease of the retina is a **retino/pathy** (ret″ĭ-nop′ə-the). A **detached retina** is separation of the retina from the back of the eye (Figure 15-20). Although it can be caused by severe trauma, most cases are associated with internal changes within the eye. Retinal detachment requires surgical treatment to avoid deterioration that can lead to blindness in the affected eye. This disorder is called detached _____.
	Macular degeneration is a progressive deterioration of the macula lutea of the retina, an oval yellow spot at the optical center of the retina; this can result in severe visual acuity problems.
calculus	**15-101** Concretions (calculi) can form in the lacrimal passages. A **dacryo/lith** (dak′re-o-lith″) is a lacrimal _____ or a tear stone. **Dacryo/lith/iasis** (dak″re-o-lĭ-thi′ə-sis) is the presence of lacrimal calculi.
lacrimal	**15-102 Dacryo/cyst/itis** (dak″re-o-sis-ti′tis) is inflammation of the _____ sac. **Dacryo/sinus/itis** (dak″re-o-si″nəs-i′tis) is inflammation of the lacrimal sac and the sinus.
vision	**15-103 Dipl/opia** (dĭ-plo′pe-ə) means double _____.
	Three common irregularities in vision are explained in Figure 15-21. These are refractive disorders, because light rays are not focused appropriately on the retina.
myopia (mi-o′pe-ə)	Another name for nearsightedness is _____. Farsightedness is the same as **hyperopia** (hi″pər-o′pe-ə). Uneven focusing of the image, resulting from distortion of the curvature of the lens or cornea, is **astigmatism** (ə-stig′mə-tiz-əm).
	Presby/opia* (pres″be-o′pe-ə) is hyperopia and impairment of vision due to advancing years or to old age.

*Presbyopia (Greek: *presbys,* old man; *-opia,* vision).

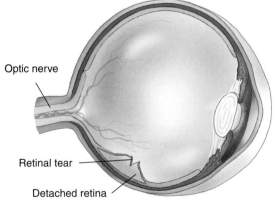

Figure 15-20 Retinal detachment. The onset of separation of the retina from the back of the eye is usually sudden and painless. The person may experience bright flashes of light or floating dark spots in the affected eye. Sometimes there is loss of visual field, as though a curtain is being pulled over part of the visual field. Retinal detachments are usually visible using ophthalmoscopy.

Optic nerve

Retinal tear

Detached retina

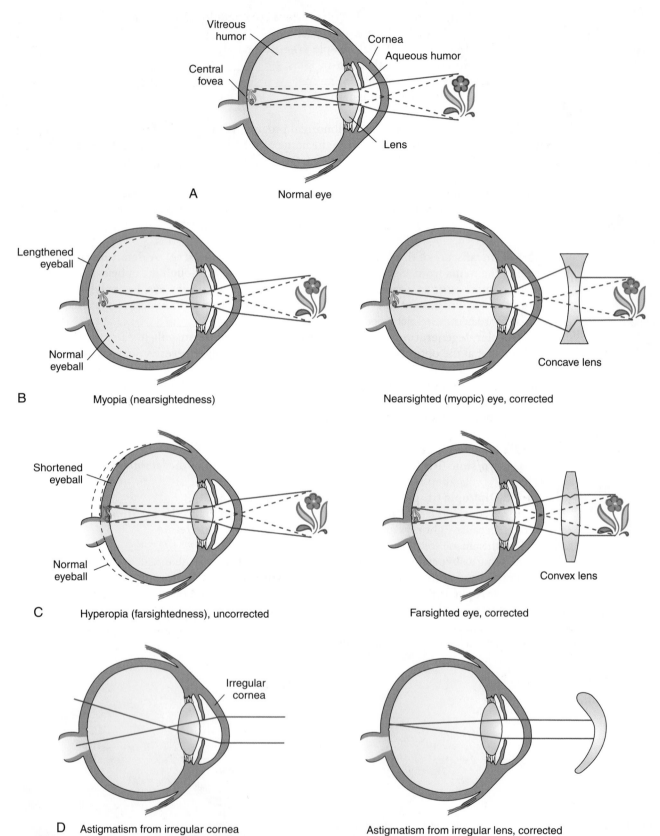

Figure 15-21 Normal and abnormal refraction in the eyeball. A, In the normal eye, a clear image is formed when light rays from an object are bent properly and converge on the center of the retina. **B,** In myopia (nearsightedness), the image is focused in front of the retina and is corrected by use of a concave lens. **C,** In hyperopia (farsightedness), the image is focused behind the retina and is corrected using a convex lens. **D,** In astigmatism, the curvature of the cornea or lens is uneven and results in the image being focused at two different points on the retina. A cylindrical lens is used to correct astigmatism.

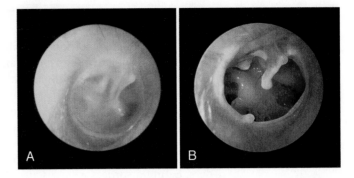

Figure 15-22 Comparison of the appearance of a normal eardrum and a perforated eardrum. A, Otoscopic view of a normal intact eardrum. **B,** Otoscopic view of a perforated eardrum.

15-104 Ear trauma can occur from a blow by a blunt object. The eardrum can be damaged by extended exposure to loud noises, penetrating injury, rupture, or perforation by shock waves from an explosion, deep sea diving, trauma, or acute middle ear infections. A perforated eardrum can be seen during an otoscopic examination (Figure 15-22).

otitis (o-ti´tis)

15-105 Write a word that means inflammation of the ear: _____.
Otitis may produce **ot/algia** (o-tal´je-ə), pain in the ear, which is also called earache.

inflammation

Otitis media (o-ti´tis me´de-ə) is _____ of the middle ear. The middle ear is separated from the external ear by the eardrum. **Mastoid/itis** (mas˝toid-i´tis) is an infection of one of the mastoid bones, usually an extension of a middle ear infection. It is difficult to treat and can result in hearing loss. Antibiotic therapy is aimed at treating middle-ear infections before they progress to mastoiditis.

otorrhea
(o˝to-re´ə)

15-106 A discharge from the ear may accompany otitis. Write a word that means discharge from the ear: _____. Otorrhea may contain blood, pus, or even spinal fluid. Ear infections are just one cause of otorrhea.

hardening

15-107 Oto/sclerosis (o˝to-sklə-ro´sis) means _____ of the ear. This condition is caused by formation of spongy bone around structures of the middle and inner ear, and it leads to hearing impairment.

tinnitus

15-108 Tinnitus[*] (tin´ĭ-təs, tĭ-ni´-təs), noise in the ears, is one of the most common complaints of persons with ear or hearing disorders. The noise includes ringing, buzzing, roaring, or clicking. It may be a sign of something as simple as accumulation of earwax or **cerumen**[†] (sə-roo´mən) or as serious as **Meniere** (mĕ-nyār´) **disease.** The latter is a chronic disease of the inner ear with recurrent episodes of hearing loss, tinnitus, and vertigo (vur´tĭ-go). **Vertigo** is also called dizziness. Ringing in the ears is called _____.

[*]Tinnitus (Latin: *tinnire,* to tinkle). [†]Cerumen (Latin: *cera,* wax).

EXERCISE 12

Word Analysis. *Break these words into their component parts by placing a slash between the word parts. Write the meaning of each term.*

1. blepharedema _____

2. ophthalmorrhagia _____

3. keratitis _____

4. retinopathy _____

5. dacryolithiasis _____

Say and Check

Say aloud the terms in Exercise 12. Use the Companion CD to check your pronunciations.

PSYCHOLOGIC DISORDERS

psychiatry	**15-109** Psychologic disorders are unlike most diseases or disorders that confront health professionals because there often is no change in the body structure and sometimes not even detectable changes in chemistry, thus making the abnormalities difficult to demonstrate and treat in the usual sense. A psychologist is one who is trained in methods of psychologic analysis, therapy, and research. You learned in Chapter 2 that the medical specialty that deals with the diagnosis, treatment, and prevention of mental illness is _____. Several disorders are discussed in this section, including mental retardation, mental deterioration, anxiety disorders, phobias, obsessions and compulsions, schizophrenia, and mood disorders. Eating disorders were discussed in Chapter 10, The Digestive System. Learn the meanings of the following combining forms related to psychology.

Additional Word Parts: Psychology

Combining Form	Meaning	Combining Form	Meaning
ment(o), psych(o)	mind	pyr(o)	fire
phren(o)	mind or diaphragm	schist(o), schiz(o)	split

mind	**15-110** Only a few psychologic disorders have observable pathologic conditions of the brain. Some examples of observable pathologic conditions are mental retardation, dementia, and Alzheimer disease. (The two latter disorders were discussed earlier in this chapter.) **Mental retardation** is a disorder characterized by subaverage general intelligence with deficits or impairments in the ability to learn and to adapt socially. Mental retardation is abnormally low intellectual functioning of the _____ or deficient intellectual development.
autism	**15-111** Signs of psychologic disorders can appear in a very young child. Such is the case with mental retardation, autism (aw´tiz-əm), and attention deficit disorder. **Autism** is characterized by withdrawal and impaired development in social interaction and communication. Write the name of this disorder that may be characterized by extreme withdrawal: _____. **Attention deficit disorder** and **attention deficit hyperactivity disorder** are abbreviated ADD and ADHD, respectively. These are characterized by short attention span, poor concentration, and, in ADHD, hyperactivity. Hyperactivity is also called **hyper/kinesia**. Translated literally,
movement	hyper/kinesia or **hyper/kinesis** is above normal _____.
exaggerated	**15-112** Most persons experience occasional feelings of sadness or discouragement resulting from personal loss or tragedy; however, **clinical depression** is an abnormal emotional state characterized by exaggerated feelings of sadness, despair, discouragement, emptiness, and hopelessness. Milder forms of this type of depression are sometimes called neurotic depression. It is important to remember that the feelings of sadness and hopelessness are _____ in clinical depression.
	15-113 **Neur/osis** is the former name for a category of mental disorders in which the symptoms are distressing to the person, reality testing is intact, behavior does not violate gross social norms, and there is no apparent organic cause.

> ➤ KEY POINT Many disorders that were formerly classified as neuroses are now classified as disorders or combinations of disorders. These include anxiety disorders, dissociative disorders, mood disorders, sexual disorders, and somatoform disorders.

mind	**15-114** **Anxiety disorders** are characterized by anticipation of impending danger and dread, the source of which is largely unknown or unrecognized. An anxiety attack is an acute, psychobiologic reaction that usually includes several of the following: restlessness, tension, tachycardia, and breathing difficulty. A **psycho/biological response** involves both the _____ and the physical body.

15-115 An **obsessive-compulsive disorder** (OCD) is an anxiety disorder characterized by recurrent and persistent thoughts, ideas, and feelings of obsessions or compulsions sufficiently severe to cause distress, consume considerable time, or interfere with the person's occupational, social, or interpersonal functioning. An **obsession** is a persistent thought or idea that occupies the mind and cannot be erased by logic or reasoning. A **compulsion** is an irresistible, repetitive impulse to act contrary to one's ordinary standards. An obsessive-compulsive disorder is a pattern of persistent behaviors that involve compulsion to act on an _____.

obsession

15-116 **Phobias** are obsessive, irrational, and intense fears of an object, an activity, or a physical situation. The suffix -phobia means abnormal _____. Phobias range from abnormal fear of public places, **agoraphobia** (ag″ə-rə-fo´be-ə), to abnormal fear of animals, **zoophobia** (zo″o-fo´be-ə), and even include an abnormal fear of acquiring a phobia, **phobophobia** (fo″bo-fo´be-ə).
    Write a word that means an irrational fear of heights by using the combining form for extremity and -phobia: _____.

fear

acrophobia
(ak´ro-fo´be-ə)
fear

    Claustro/phobia (klaws″tro-fo´be-ə) is a morbid _____ of closed places. (A claustrum is a barrier.)
    An abnormal fear of fire is **pyro/phobia** (pi″ro-fo´be-ə).

15-117 **Posttraumatic stress disorder** is characterized by an acute emotional response _____ a traumatic event or situation involving severe environmental stress, such as a physical assault or military combat.

after

15-118 A panic disorder or **panic attack** is an episode of acute anxiety that occurs unpredictably with feelings of intense apprehension or terror, accompanied by dyspnea (difficult breathing), dizziness, sweating, trembling, and chest pain.
    When these signs and symptoms occur unpredictably with feelings of extreme apprehension, the disorder is called a _____ attack.

panic

15-119 Emotional conflicts are so repressed in a **dissociative disorder** that a separation or split in the personality occurs, resulting in an altered state of consciousness or a confusion in identity. Existence within a person of two or more separate identities is an example of a _____ disorder. Symptoms may include amnesia, and in this case the loss of memory is generally caused by severe emotional trauma.

dissociative

15-120 A **mood disorder** is a variety of conditions characterized by a disturbance in mood as the main feature. In severe cases they may be a sign of depressive disorder or may be symptomatic of a bipolar disorder. Conditions characterized by a disturbance in mood are called _____ disorders.

mood

15-121 A **mania** is an unstable emotional state that includes excessive excitement, elation, ideas, and psychomotor activities. In an extreme manic episode a delusion of grandeur may occur. The suffix -mania is used to write terms pertaining to excessive preoccupation. **Megalo/mania** (meg″ə-lo-ma´ne-ə) is an abnormal mental state in which one believes oneself to be a person of great importance, power, fame, or wealth. You learned earlier that -mania means excessive preoccupation; therefore the literal translation of megalo/mania is excessive _____ with greatness.
    A **bipolar disorder** is a major mental disorder characterized by the occurrence of manic episodes, major depressive episodes, or mixed moods. The term bipolar in the name indicates that the disorder has two distinct aspects. Megalomania may occur in an extreme manic episode of bipolar disorder.

preoccupation

15-122 The combining form pyr(o) means fire. **Pyro/mania** (pi″ro-ma´ne-ə) is excessive preoccupation with _____. A **pyro/maniac** has an obsessive preoccupation with fires. The combining form pyr(o) means fire. Pyro/mania is a compulsion to set fires or watch fires.

fire

Klepto/mania[*] (klep″to-ma′ne-ə) is characterized by an abnormal, uncontrollable, and recurrent urge to steal.

15-123 Sexual disorders are those caused at least in part by psychologic factors. Such a disorder, characterized by a decrease or disturbance in sexual desire that is not the result of a general medical condition, is called a sexual dysfunction. Sexual perversion or deviation, in which the sexual instinct is expressed in ways that are biologically undesirable, socially prohibited, or socially unacceptable, is termed **para/phil/ia** (par″ə-fil′e-ə). Sexual dysfunctions and paraphilia are classified as _____ disorders.

sexual

15-124 Somatoform (so-mat′o-form) **disorders** are any of a group of disorders, characterized by symptoms suggesting physical illness or disease, for which there are no demonstrable organic causes or physiologic dysfunctions. Somato/form is derived from somat(o), meaning body, and -form, which is a suffix for shape.

Hypo/chondr/iasis (hi″po-kon-dri′ə-sis) or hypochondria is a chronic abnormal concern about the health of the body. It is characterized by extreme anxiety, depression, and an unrealistic interpretation of physical symptoms as indications of a serious illness or disease despite medical evidence to the contrary. Hypochondriasis is classified as a _____ disorder.

somatoform

15-125 The suffix -asthenia means weakness. **Neur/asthenia** (noor″əs-the′ne-ə) is a nervous disorder characterized by _____ and sometimes nervous exhaustion. It is often associated with a depressed state and is believed by some to be psychosomatic. You learned in Chapter 6 that **psychosomatic** disorders are emotional states that influence the physical body's functioning.

weakness

Pseudo/mania (soo″do-ma′ne-ə) is a false or pretended mental disorder. **Pseudo/plegia** (soo″do-ple′-jə) is hysterical paralysis. There is loss of muscle power without real paralysis.

15-126 A psychotic disorder, or **psychosis,** is any major mental disorder characterized by a gross impairment in reality testing. The latter is an ego function that enables one to differentiate between external reality and any inner imaginative world and to behave in a manner that exhibits an awareness of accepted norms. Impairment of reality testing is indicative of a disturbance that may lead to psychosis.

> ➤ **KEY** POINT <u>**Schizo/phrenia** (skiz″o-fre′ne-ə, skit″so-fre′ne-ə) is any of a large group of psychotic disorders.</u> Schizophrenia is characterized by gross distortion of reality, hallucinations, disturbances of language and communication, and disorganized or catatonic behavior (psychologically induced immobility with muscular rigidity that is interrupted by agitation).

Notice the two pronunciations of the term schizophrenia. The combining form schiz(o) means _____. Translated literally, schizophrenia means split mind and relates to the splitting off of a part of the psyche, which may dominate the psychic life of the patient even though it may express behavior contrary to the original personality. The concept of multiple personalities, two or more distinct subpersonalities, is not necessarily a characteristic of schizophrenia.

split

15-127 A number of personality disorders exist with which you may already be familiar. These include antisocial behavior, paranoia, and others. **Anti/social behavior** is acting _____ the rights of others.

Paranoia (par″ə-noi′ah) is characterized by persistent delusions of persecution, mistrust, and combativeness.

against

15-128 Additional information about psychologic disorders can be found in the *Diagnostic and Statistical Manual of Mental Disorders* (DSM), published by the American Psychiatric Association. It is based on the International Classification of Disease and uses diagnostic codes, which are fundamental to medical record keeping, greatly facilitating data record keeping and retrieving. DSM means _____ *and Statistical Manual of Mental Disorders.*

Diagnostic

---

[*]Kleptomania (Greek: *kleptein,* to steal; *mania,* madness).

EXERCISE 13

Build It! *Use the following word parts to build terms. (Some word parts will be used more than once.)*

hyper-, neur(o), pseudo-, psych(o), pyr(o), -asthenia, -kinesia, -mania, -osis, -phobia

1. false or pretended mental disorder   _____/_____

2. major mental disorder   _____/_____

3. nervous disorder characterized by muscular weakness   _____/_____

4. abnormal fear of fire   _____/_____

5. excessive movement   _____/_____

Say and Check

Say aloud the terms you wrote for Exercise 13. Use the Companion CD to check your pronunciations.

SURGICAL AND THERAPEUTIC INTERVENTIONS

skull (cranium)

15-129 Cranial surgery may be needed for brain tumors, trauma, brain abscesses, or vascular abnormalities. The individual's need determines the particular type of surgery. Selected cranial surgical procedures are presented in Table 15-3.

    In reading Table 15-3, you see that a **burr hole** is a hole drilled into the _____. It is particularly used to drain an abscess.

15-130 Any surgical opening into the skull is a **craniotomy** (kra″ne-ot′ə-me).

> ➤ **KEY** POINT <u>Craniotomies are performed to gain access to the brain, relieve intracranial pressure, or control bleeding inside the skull.</u> Surgical removal of a portion of the skull in order to perform surgery on the brain is a **craniectomy** (kra″ne-ek′tə-me). This type of surgery may be necessary to repair the brain or its vessels, remove a brain tumor, or repair an aneurysm.

excision

    An **aneurysm/ectomy** (an″u-riz-mek′tə-me) is _____ of an aneurysm.

repair

    Cranio/plasty (kra′ne-o-plas″te) is surgical _____ of the skull after surgery or injury to the skull.

    Use cerebr(o) to write a word that means incision of the brain:

cerebrotomy
(ser″ə-brot′ə-me)

_____.

TABLE 15-3   Types of Cranial Surgery

Type	Description
Burr hole	Opening into the cranium with a drill; used to remove localized fluid and blood beneath the dura
Craniotomy	Opening into the cranium with removal of a bone flap, and opening of the dura to remove a lesion, repair a damaged area, drain blood, or relieve increased ICP
Craniectomy	Excision into the cranium to cut away a bone flap
Cranioplasty	Repair of a cranial defect resulting from trauma, malformation, or previous surgical procedure; artificial material used to replace damaged or lost bone
Stereotaxis	Precision localization of a specific area of the brain using a frame or a frameless system based on three-dimensional coordinates; procedure is used for biopsy, radiosurgery, or dissection
Shunt procedures	Alternate pathway to redirect cerebrospinal fluid from one area to another using a tube or implanted device; for example, a ventriculoperitoneal shunt

Modified from Lewis SM, Heitemper MM, Dirksen SR: *Medical-surgical nursing: assessment and management of clinical problems,* St Louis, 2004, Mosby.

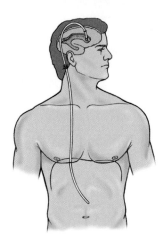

Figure 15-23 Ventriculoperitoneal shunt. This type of shunt consists of plastic tubing between a cerebral ventricle and the peritoneum for the draining of excess cerebrospinal fluid from the brain in hydrocephalus.

15-131 Shunts are used to redirect cerebrospinal fluid from one area to another using a tube or an implanted device. A **ventriculo/peritone/al shunt** creates a passageway between a cerebral _____ and the peritoneum for the draining of CSF from the brain in hydrocephalus (Figure 15-23).

ventricle

15-132 Stereotaxis (ster″e-o-tak′sis) uses a system of three-dimensional coordinates to locate a site to be operated on or irradiated. In **stereotactic surgery** the surgeon is assisted by a computer-guided apparatus that is used to target a specific area of the brain.

Stereotactic radiosurgery involves closed-skull destruction of a target (for example, a tumor) using ionizing radiation. The patient's head is held in a stereotactic frame (Figure 15-24, *A*). In a **gamma knife procedure,** a high dose of radiation is delivered to precisely targeted tumor tissue. In naming this procedure, "knife" was used because controlled destructive radiation replaces the surgical knife (Figure 15-24, *B*).

In combination with stereotactic procedures, surgical lasers are also used to destroy tumors.

destruction

15-133 Neuro/lysis (noo-rol′ĭ-sis) is _____ of nerves. Neurolysis has several meanings, but all of them have to do with nervous tissue. The word is used to mean release of a nerve sheath by cutting it longitudinally, loosening of adhesions surrounding a nerve, or disintegration of nerve tissue.

Write a word that means surgical repair of a nerve: _____.
Neuro/rrhaphy (noo-ror′ə-fe) specifically means suture of a nerve.

neuroplasty
(noo′o-plas″te)

15-134 Neuro/tripsy (noor″o-trip′se) is surgical crushing of a nerve.
Write a term that means excision of a nerve: _____.

neurectomy
(noo-rek′to-me)

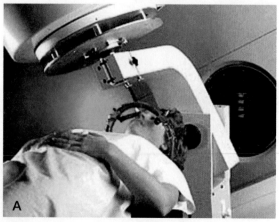

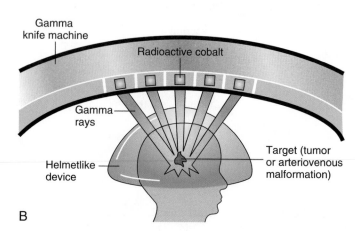

Figure 15-24 Gamma knife treatment assisted by stereotaxis. A, The stereotactic frame holds the head in a fixed position. **B,** In a gamma knife treatment, beams are intense only at the targeted area.

15-135 Pain management may be for a short time (for example, after surgery) or longer (chronic pain) and may include both drug therapy and nondrug treatments. **An/algesic** (an″əl-je′zik) means relieving pain or not being _____ to pain. Agents that relieve pain without causing loss of consciousness are also called analgesics. Three well-known analgesics that are used for mild to moderate pain are aspirin, ibuprofen, and acetaminophen.

    Opioid analgesics act on the CNS, are more often used for severe pain, and may alter the patient's perception, producing tolerance or dependency. Some examples are codeine and morphine.

15-136 Nerve blocks are used to reduce pain by temporarily or permanently blocking transmission of _____ impulses. **Nerve block anesthesia** is produced by injecting an anesthetic along the course of a nerve to inhibit the conduction of impulses to and from the area supplied by the nerve.

    Sympathectomy (sim″pə-thek′tə-me) is a surgical procedure in which one or more sympathetic nerves are severed. This surgery has special uses, including alleviation of pain.

15-137 **Epidural anesthesia** is injection of an anesthetic into the epidural space, which contains spinal fluid and spinal nerves. Epidurals, most commonly performed in the lumbar area, can be tailored to numb an area of the body from the lower extremities to the upper abdomen. They are often used in labor and childbirth. Epidural injections, containing various combinations of cortisone and anesthetics, are used by pain specialists to alleviate chronic pain of the lower back.

15-138 **Trans/cutane/ous electrical nerve stimulation** (TENS) is a method of pain control by the application of electric impulses to the nerve endings (Figure 15-25). Pain signals to the brain are blocked by electrical impulses generated by a stimulator that is attached to electrodes placed on the skin. Literal translation of transcutaneous is across or performed through the

_____.

15-139 In addition to analgesics and anesthetics, many drugs, including hypnotics, anticonvulsants, and antipyretics, act on the central nervous system.

    Hypnotics* are drugs often used as sedatives to produce a calming effect. Functional activity, irritability, and excitement are decreased by sedatives.

    Anti/convulsants act _____ convulsion, **anti/pyretics** are used to decrease fever, and antiparkinsonian drugs are used to treat Parkinson disease.

15-140 Both anti- and contra- mean against. A **contra/indication** (kon″trə-in″dĭ-ka′shən) is any condition that renders a particular treatment improper or undesirable. Contra- means

_____.

15-141 If a cerebral embolus is caused by a blood clot, a **thrombo/lytic** (throm″bo-lit′ik) may be used. **Thrombolytics** _____ blood clots.

---

*Hypnotics (Greek: *hypnos,* sleep).

Margin terms: sensitive · nerve · skin · against · against · dissolve

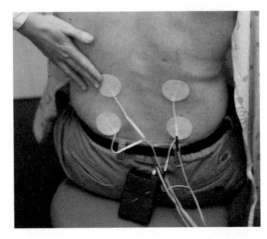

Figure 15-25 Transcutaneous electric nerve stimulation (TENS). The TENS unit is being used in this example to control low back pain. Electrodes are placed on the skin and attached to a stimulator by flexible wires. The electric impulses block transmission of pain signals to the brain. TENS is nonaddictive and has no known side effects, but it is contraindicated in patients with artificial cardiac pacemakers.

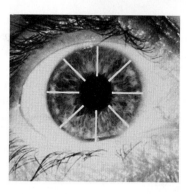

Figure 15-26 Radial keratotomy. Incisions are made in the cornea from the outer edge toward the center in spokelike fashion to flatten the cornea and thus correct myopia.

eyelid

15-142 A **blepharo/plasty** (blef´ə-ro-plas˝te) is just one of many types of eye surgery. Blepharo-plasty is the use of plastic surgery to restore or repair the _____. If vision is adversely affected by sagging of the eyelids, it can be corrected by plastic surgery. If appearance is the primary concern, this procedure can be done for cosmetic reasons. Write the name of this surgery: _____.

blepharoplasty

15-143 Cataracts are usually treated with removal of the cataract. To prevent the need for a special contact lens or glasses, an **intraocular lens** (IOL) is sometimes surgically implanted when the cataract is removed. An intra/ocular lens is implanted _____ the eye.

within

   Corneal grafting may be necessary to improve vision in cases of corneal scarring or perforation. The cornea was one of the first organs transplanted; rejection of the transplanted tissue is uncommon.

15-144 Corrective glasses or contact lenses can often correct uncomplicated problems with vision, such as nearsightedness and farsightedness. **Radial keratotomy** (ker˝ə-tot´ə-me) often reduces or eliminates the need for further correction in many persons with myopia, hyperopia, and astigmatism (Figure 15-26). Kerato/tomy is incision of the _____. The **excimer laser** is used in this type of corneal surgery and causes minimal damage to adjacent cells.

cornea

15-145 Dacryocyst/itis usually responds to systemic administration of antibiotics but rarely may require a **dacryo/cysto/rhino/stomy** (dak˝re-o-sis˝to-ri-nos´tə-me), surgical creation of a passageway between the lacrimal sac and the _____.

nose

   Dacryo/cysto/tomy (dak˝re-o-sis-tot´ə-me) means incision of the lacrimal sac.

15-146 A **vago/tomy** (va-got´ə-me) is severing of various branches of the vagus nerve and is done to reduce the amount of acid secreted in the stomach. This is done to prevent the recurrence of an ulcer. Write this term that means severing of the vagus nerve:

vagotomy

_____.

mind

15-147 **Psycho/analysis** (si˝ko-ə-nal´ĭ-sis) is a method of diagnosing and treating disorders of the _____. This is accomplished by ascertaining and studying the facts of the patient's mental condition.

   Psycho/therapy (si˝ko-ther´ə-pe) is treatment of disorders of the mind by psychologic means rather than by physical means.

➤ KEY POINT <u>**Psycho/pharmacology** (si˝ko-fahr˝mə-kol´ə-je) is the study of the action of drugs on functions of the mind.</u> **Anti/depressants** are medications that prevent or relieve depression. **Anti/anxiety drugs** are used to relieve feelings of anxiety. **Anti/psychotics** are medications that are used to treat the symptoms of severe psychiatric disorders. **Tranquilizers** are prescribed to calm anxious or agitated persons, ideally without decreasing their consciousness. **Narcotic drugs** produce stupor or sleep.

EXERCISE 14

Word Analysis. *Break these words into their component parts by placing a slash between the word parts. Write the meaning of each term.*

1. neurolysis _____

2. keratotomy _____

3. dacryocystorhinostomy _____

4. vagotomy _____

5. transcutaneous _____

EXERCISE 15

Match terms in the left columns with descriptions in the right column.

_____ 1. analgesics _____ 4. shunt

_____ 2. epidural _____ 5. TENS

_____ 3. neurotripsy

A. application of electric impulses to the nerve endings
B. injection of anesthesia to produce numbness in the lower part of the body
C. act on CNS to relieve pain without causing loss of consciousness
D. redirect fluids from one area to another
E. surgical crushing of a nerve

EXERCISE 16

Write a term for each of the following.

1. agents used to dissolve blood clots _____

2. excision of an aneurysm _____

3. surgical removal of a portion of the skull _____

4. suture of a nerve _____

5. surgical repair of the eyelid _____

Say and Check

Say aloud the terms you wrote for Exercise 16. Use the Companion CD to check your pronunciations.

CHAPTER ABBREVIATIONS*

ACh	abbreviation for acetylcholine	**EEG**	electroencephalogram
ADD	attention deficit disorder	**ICP**	intracranial pressure
ADHD	attention deficit hyperactivity disorder	**IOL**	intraocular lens
ALS	amyotrophic lateral sclerosis	**LBP**	lower back pain
CNS	central nervous system	**MS**	multiple sclerosis
CSF	cerebrospinal fluid	**OCD**	obsessive-compulsive disorder
CVA	cerebrovascular accident, costovertebral angle	**PNS**	peripheral nervous system
dB	decibel	**SCI**	spinal cord injury
DSM	*Diagnostic and Statistical Manual of Mental Disorders*	**TENS**	transcutaneous electrical nerve stimulation
DTR	deep tendon reflex	**TIA**	transient ischemic attack

*Many of these abbreviations share their meanings with other terms.

▶ CHAPTER 15 REVIEW

Basic Understanding

Labeling

I. *Label the drawing of the meninges with arachnoid, dura mater, and pia mater.*

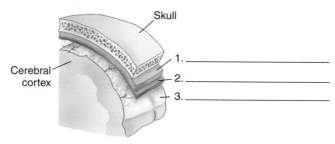

Detailed view of meninges

II. *Label the following structures in the drawing: brain stem, cerebellum, cerebrum, diencephalon, and spinal cord.*

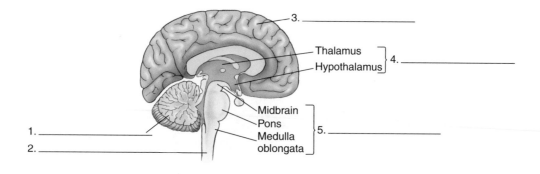

Photo ID
III. *Use the word parts to write terms to label the illustrations.*

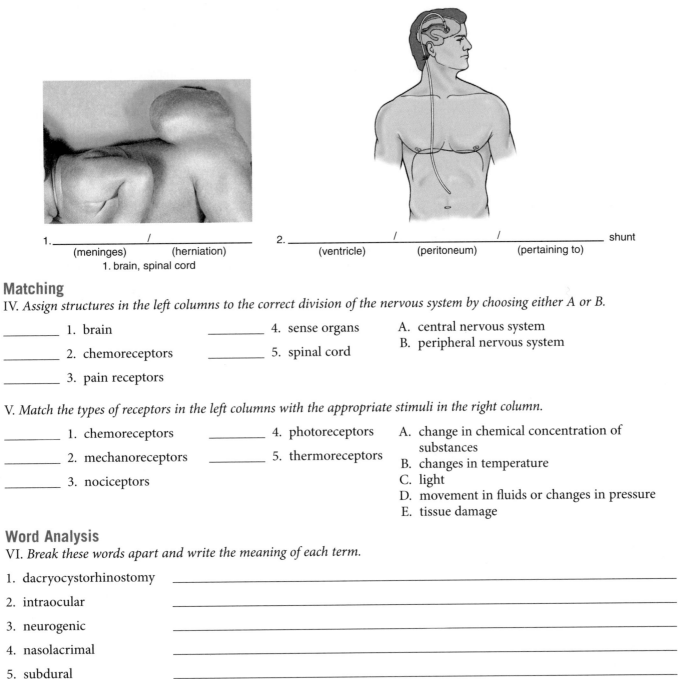

1._____/_____
    (meninges)   (herniation)
       1. brain, spinal cord

2. _____/_____/_____ shunt
    (ventricle)   (peritoneum)   (pertaining to)

Matching
IV. *Assign structures in the left columns to the correct division of the nervous system by choosing either A or B.*

_____ 1. brain   _____ 4. sense organs   A. central nervous system
                                                           B. peripheral nervous system

_____ 2. chemoreceptors   _____ 5. spinal cord

_____ 3. pain receptors

V. *Match the types of receptors in the left columns with the appropriate stimuli in the right column.*

_____ 1. chemoreceptors   _____ 4. photoreceptors   A. change in chemical concentration of
                                                              substances

_____ 2. mechanoreceptors _____ 5. thermoreceptors   B. changes in temperature
                                                              C. light

_____ 3. nociceptors   D. movement in fluids or changes in pressure
                                                               E. tissue damage

Word Analysis
VI. *Break these words apart and write the meaning of each term.*

1. dacryocystorhinostomy _____

2. intraocular   _____

3. neurogenic   _____

4. nasolacrimal   _____

5. subdural   _____

Multiple Choice
VII. *Circle the correct answer for each of the following.*

1. Which of the following structures is the outermost meningeal membrane? (arachnoid, cochlea, dura mater, pia mater)

2. Which of the following is chronic, progressive mental deterioration that involves irreversible loss of memory, disorientation, and speech and gait disturbances?
(Alzheimer disease, Lou Gehrig disease, Meniere syndrome, multiple sclerosis)

3. Which term means paralysis of the lower portion of the body and both legs?
(diplegia, hemiplegia, paraplegia, quadriplegia)

4. Which of the following is the correct name for a stroke?
(cerebrovascular accident, craniocerebral trauma, monoplegia, polyneuropathy)

5. Which of the following is the record produced in radiography of the spinal cord after injection of a contrast medium? (encephalogram, encephalography, myelogram, myelography)

6. Which term means a morbid fear of closed places? (acrophobia, agoraphobia, claustrophobia, zoophobia)

7. Which of the following means hernial protrusion of the meninges through a defect in the vertebral column? (meningitis, meningocele, myelocele, myelomalacia)

8. What is the term for any condition that renders a particular treatment improper or undesirable? (anotia, anticonvulsant, antipyretic, contraindication)

9. Which term means incision of the lacrimal sac? (cholecystotomy, cystolithectomy, dacryocystotomy, dacryolithiasis)

10. What does algesia mean? (oversensitivity to pain, pain, sensitivity to pain, undersensitivity to pain)

Fill in the Blanks

VIII. *Write the appropriate word in each blank.*

Three membranes collectively known as (1) _____ cover the brain and spinal cord.

The largest and uppermost portion of the brain is the (2) _____. A fluid called (3) _____ fluid surrounds and cushions the brain and spinal cord. The nervous system is composed of two types of cells. The basic unit of the nervous system is called a (4) _____. The other type of cell that serves as support is a (5) _____ cell.

A cytoplasmic projection that carries impulses away from the cell body of the neuron is called an (6) _____.

Another type of cytoplasmic process that carries an impulse to the cell body is a (7) _____.

Writing Terms

IX. *Write one term for each of the following meanings.*

1. absence of one or both ears _____

2. hardening and ossification of the ear _____

3. inflammation of the brain and spinal cord _____

4. inflammation of the cornea _____

5. nearsightedness _____

6. partially aware of one's surroundings _____

7. radiography of the spinal cord _____

8. recording the electrical activity of the brain _____

9. presence of lacrimal calculi _____

10. uncontrollable, brief episodes of sleep _____

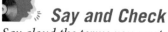 **Say and Check**

Say aloud the terms you wrote for Exercise IX. Use the Companion CD to check your pronunciations.

Greater Comprehension

Health Care Reports

X. *Read the following health care report. Then answer the questions that follow the report.*

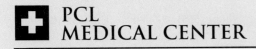

PCL MEDICAL CENTER

7700 Lexicon Way
St. Louis, MO 63146

Phone (555) 437-0000 • Fax (555) 437-0001

NEUROLOGIC CONSULTATION

Patient Name: Emma Lang   **ID No**: 015-0001   **DOB**: Dec 4, ----
PCP: Mollie E. Turner, MD, Family Physician
CHIEF COMPLAINT: Multiple sclerosis
HISTORY OF PRESENT ILLNESS: This 52-year-old black woman has a diagnosis of multiple sclerosis made 10 years ago via MRI scan. Family has noted progressive confusion over the last 3 to 4 months, especially in the morning, as well as dysphagia. She frequently chokes on liquids, has difficulty understanding speech, has weakness in both arms and legs with severe spasticity. She seldom speaks. She is catheterized 3× to 4× daily owing to urinary retention.
ALLERGIES: NKDA
MEDICATIONS: See chart for extensive list of meds.
PHYSICAL EXAMINATION: General: Is pleasant, carries out simple commands. HEENT: Normocephalic, atraumatic. Caries evident with possible gingivitis. TMs clear. CV & Lungs: Unremarkable. GI: Some esophageal stricture. Neuromuscular exam: Disoriented to time, place, and person. Muscle power is decreased in both arms. Tone is increased in right leg. There are no signs of vertigo or tinnitus. Genitourinary: Incontinent of urine.
FAMILY HISTORY: Parents deceased. No children, lives with sister and her family.
IMPRESSION/PLAN: Progressive neurologic disorder with dementia, ophthalmoplegia, diplopia, dysarthria, neurogenic bladder, dysphasia, and dysphagia. Will be admitted for multiple testing. Patient has obvious caries and possible gingivitis; to be scheduled for a stat dental checkup before admission to hospital. Consults with ophthalmology, GU, GI to be set up.

Match terms in the left columns with their meanings in the right column.

_____ 1. diplopia

_____ 2. dysphasia

_____ 3. ophthalmoplegia

_____ 4. tinnitus

_____ 5. vertigo

A. difficulty in language function
B. dizziness
C. double vision
D. paralysis of the eyes
E. ringing in the ears

Circle one answer for each of the following questions.

6. Multiple sclerosis is classified as which type of pathology? (congenital, degenerative, infectious, traumatic)

7. Which of the following is a progressive mental disorder characterized by confusion, disorientation, and personality disintegration? (dementia, dysphasia, multiple sclerosis, neurogenic bladder)

8. Which term in the report means difficult and poorly articulated speech? (Alzheimer, depression, dysarthria, paranoia)

XI. *Read the following report and define the terms that are underlined.*

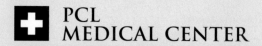

PCL
MEDICAL CENTER

7700 Lexicon Way
St. Louis, MO 63146

Phone (555) 437-0000 • Fax (555) 437-0001

REHABILITATION CONSULTATION

Patient Name: Richard Yu   **ID No.:** 015-0002   **Date of Exam:** Apr 16, ----
Referring Physician: Mollie E. Turner, MD, Family Practice
HISTORY OF PRESENT ILLNESS: This 69-year-old, left-handed Asian man is seen for management of ambulatory dys-function secondary to <u>Parkinson disease</u>. He has a history of diplopia secondary to <u>meningioma</u>. He was diagnosed with <u>peripheral neuropathy</u>. He is able to ambulate with a wheeled walker with standby assist. Requires moderate assist for transfers. Has a persistent problem with diplopia. No apparent problem with focal weakness.
PHYSICAL EXAM: HEENT: Left <u>ptosis</u> with extraocular movements. Flat affect. Mild decrease in left corneal reflex. Neck, Lungs, Heart, Extremities: Consistent with exam done 6 months ago. Neuromuscular exam: Decreased muscle mass and moderate <u>bradykinesia.</u> Resting tremor, right upper extremity. Bilateral arm strength decreased. Bilateral lower extremity strength is good. Babinski sign negative bilaterally. No report of vertigo. Good gag response bilaterally. A&O ×2. Exhibits short-term memory loss, short attention span. Has trouble maintaining balance without his walker.
IMPRESSION: Parkinson disease, ambulatory dysfunction, peripheral neuropathy
PLAN: Mr. Yu would benefit from a rehabilitation program that offers intensive physical therapy to maintain range of mo-tion, build strength and balance, and optimize his mobility. Occupational therapy will optimize strength, dexterity, and self-care skills. Speech therapy will optimize communication skills, swallowing, and speech. He can begin next week. Thank you for allowing me to share in this gentleman's care.

Vanessa Gale, RPT
Vanessa Gale, RPT
Physical Therapy

VG:pai
D: Apr 17, ----
T: Apr 17, ----

Define:

1. Parkinson disease: _____

2. meningioma: _____

3. peripheral neuropathy: _____

4. ptosis: _____

5. bradykinesia: _____

XII. Read the following Death Summary and write definitions of the terms that are underlined.

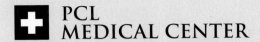

PCL MEDICAL CENTER

7700 Lexicon Way
St. Louis, MO 63146

Phone (555) 437-0000 • Fax (555) 437-0001

DEATH SUMMARY

Date of Admission: Jul 10, ----   **Date of Death:** Jul 10, ----
Patient Name: Henry Stein   **ID No.:** 015-0004   **Sex:** Male
INTRODUCTION: This patient, approximately 30 years old, was brought to the Emergency Room at 1602 hours in extremely unstable condition after he sustained a gunshot wound through-and-through the brain.
HISTORY OF PRESENT ILLNESS: This was reportedly a self-inflicted gunshot wound, <u>bihemispheric</u>, involving both of the ventricular systems. He was resuscitated after CT scan, resuscitated in the ICU. Vital signs initially improved,
but it was clear he was developing <u>coagulopathy</u>. We did have the neurosurgeons available for consideration of <u>ICP monitor</u>, but with his clinical and radiographic examination findings, the patient would have had no meaningful survival whatsoever. The neurosurgeon and I elected to go with an ICP monitor placement, which was accomplished in the Intensive Care Unit by Dr. Reid. (See separate dictation.) No family members were available at the time.
HOSPITAL COURSE: Patient's ICPs were extremely elevated. He became persistently more and more coagulopathic. He developed <u>sympathetic dysfunction</u>, causing wild variations in his vital signs. Andrea Nicole Stein, the patient's wife, arrived at the hospital; being the next of kin, she elected to discontinue this futile care. I agreed that this patient had an unsurvivable brain injury and bihemispheric gunshot wound.
At that point we withdrew care, and the patient succumbed shortly thereafter.

Linda Weaver, MD

Linda Weaver, MD
Trauma Team

LW:pai
D: Jul 10, ----
T: Jul 10, ----

Define the following terms.

1. bihemispheric _____

2. coagulopathy _____

3. ICP monitor _____

4. sympathetic dysfunction _____

Spelling
XIII. *Circle all misspelled terms and write their correct spelling.*

acetylcoline   Alzheimer   cerebrul   iritis   ophthalmoscopy

Interpreting Abbreviations
XIV. *Write the meanings of the following abbreviations.*

1. ADHD _____

2. ALS _____

3. CSF _____

4. DTR _____

5. SCI _____

Pronunciation

XV. Pronunciation is shown for several terms. Mark the primary accent in each term with an ´.

1. arachnoid (ə rak noid)

2. cerebrotomy (ser ə brot ə me)

3. efferent (ef ər ənt)

4. glioma (gli o mə)

5. kleptomania (klep to ma ne ə)

 Say and Check

Say aloud the five terms in Exercise XV. Use the Companion CD to check your pronunciations. In addition, be prepared to pronounce aloud these terms in class:

adrenergic	carpoptosis	encephalomyelopathy	hyperosmia
agoraphobia	cataract	excimer laser	Meniere disease
amyotrophic lateral sclerosis	cerebral aneurysm	foramen magnum	myasthenia gravis
antianxiety drugs	cholinergic	hordeolum	neuroglia
botulism	dacryocystotomy	hyperkinesia	stereotactic radiosurgery

Categorizing Terms

XVI. Classify the terms in the left column by selecting A, B, C, D, or E.

_____ 1. arachnoid

_____ 2. audiometer

_____ 3. botulism

_____ 4. carpoptosis

_____ 5. cerebral angiography

_____ 6. cochlea

_____ 7. myelogram

_____ 8. opioid analgesics

_____ 9. sciatica

_____ 10. sympathectomy

A. anatomy
B. diagnostic test or procedure
C. pathology
D. surgery
E. therapy

Challenge

XVII. Divide these words into their component parts and write the meaning of each term.

audiometric _____

cardiophobia _____

cerebrocerebellar _____

encephalomalacia _____

meningoencephalomyelitis _____

(Check your answers with the solutions in Appendix VI.)

 PRONUNCIATION LIST

Use the Companion CD to review the terms that have been presented. Look closely at the spelling of each term as it is pronounced and be sure you know the meaning of each term.

acetylcholine	amyotrophic lateral	antidepressant	attention deficit
acetylcholinesterase	sclerosis	antipsychotic	hyperactivity disorder
acrophobia	analgesic	antipyretic	audible
adrenaline	aneurysm	antisocial behavior	audiogram
adrenergic	aneurysmectomy	anxiety disorders	audiologist
afferent	anosmia	aphasia	audiology
agoraphobia	anotia	arachnoid	audiometer
algesia	antianxiety drugs	astigmatism	autism
Alzheimer disease	anticonvulsant	attention deficit disorder	autonomic

axon
Bell palsy
bipolar disorder
blepharedema
blepharitis
blepharoplasty
blepharoptosis
botulism
bradykinesia
brain scan
brain stem
burr hole
carpoptosis
cataract
central nervous system
cephalalgia
cephalgia
cerebellar
cerebellitis
cerebellum
cerebral
cerebral aneurysm
cerebral angiography
cerebral concussion
cerebral cortex
cerebral embolus
cerebral hemisphere
cerebral hemorrhage
cerebral palsy
cerebral ventricle
cerebrospinal
cerebrospinal fluid
cerebrotomy
cerebrovascular accident
cerebrum
cerumen
chemoreceptor
cholinergic
claustrophobia
clinical depression
cluster headache
cochlea
coma
compulsion
concussion
conjunctiva
conjunctivitis
contraindication
contusion
convulsion
cornea
corneal grafting
craniectomy
craniocerebral
cranioplasty
craniotomy
cranium

dacryocyst
dacryocystitis
dacryocystorhinostomy
dacryocystotomy
dacryolith
dacryolithiasis
dacryosinusitis
deep tendon reflex
dementia
dendrite
detached retina
diencephalon
diplegia
diplopia
dissociative disorders
dopamine
dura mater
dysarthria
dyslexia
dysphasia
echoencephalogram
echoencephalography
efferent
electroencephalogram
electroencephalograph
electroencephalography
embolic stroke
encephalitis
encephalography
encephalomeningitis
encephalomyelitis
encephalomyelopathy
endorphin
epidural anesthesia
epidural hematoma
epilepsy
epinephrine
excimer laser
extraocular
foramen magnum
frontal lobe
gamma knife procedure
Glasgow Coma Scale
glaucoma
glia cell
glioma
hematoma
hemiplegia
hemorrhagic stroke
hordeolum
Huntington chorea
hydrocephalus
hydrophobia
hypalgesia
hyperalgesia
hyperkinesia
hyperkinesis

hyperopia
hyperosmia
hypnotic
hypoalgesia
hypochondriasis
hypothalamus
insula
interocular
intracerebral hematoma
intracranial
intraocular
intraocular lens
intrathecal
iris
iritis
keratitis
kleptomania
lacrimal gland
lacrimal sac
lacrimation
lumbar puncture
macular degeneration
mania
mastoiditis
mechanoreceptor
medulla
megalomania
Meniere disease
meningeal
meninges
meningioma
meningitis
meningocele
meningomyelocele
mental retardation
midbrain
migraine headache
monoplegia
mood disorders
motor neuron
motor system
multiple sclerosis
myasthenia gravis
myelin sheath
myelogram
myelography
myopia
narcolepsy
narcotic drugs
nasolacrimal duct
nerve block anesthesia
nervous
neural
neuralgia
neurasthenia
neurectomy
neurogenic bladder

neuroglia
neurolysis
neuroma
neuromuscular
neuron
neuroplasty
neurorrhaphy
neurosis
neurotransmitter
neurotripsy
nociceptors
node of Ranvier
obsession
obsessive-compulsive
    disorder
occipital lobe
ocular
olfaction
olfactory
ophthalmalgia
ophthalmic
ophthalmomalacia
ophthalmometer
ophthalmoplegia
ophthalmorrhagia
ophthalmoscope
ophthalmoscopy
opioid analgesics
optic nerve
otalgia
otitis
otitis media
otorrhea
otosclerosis
otoscope
otoscopy
panic attack
paralysis
paranoia
paraphilia
paraplegia
parasympathetic
paresthesia
parietal lobe
Parkinson disease
patellar response
peripheral
peripheral nervous system
peripheral neuropathy
phobia
phobophobia
photophobia
photoreceptor
pia mater
poliomyelitis
polyneuralgia
polyneuritis

polyneuropathy
pons
positron emission
  tomography
posttraumatic stress
  disorder
presbyopia
pseudesthesia
pseudoesthesia
pseudomania
pseudoplegia
psychoanalysis
psychobiological response
psychopharmacology
psychosis
psychosomatic
psychotherapy
ptosis
pyromania
pyromaniac

pyrophobia
quadriplegia
rabies
radial keratotomy
receptor
reflex arc
retina
retinopathy
schizophrenia
sciatic nerve
sciatica
sclera
seizure
semicircular canals
semicoma
semiconscious
sensory neuron
sensory system
serotonin
sexual disorders

shunt
sleep apnea
somatic
somatoform disorders
spinal cord
stereotactic radiosurgery
stereotactic surgery
stereotaxis
stupor
subdural
subdural hematoma
subdural space
superficial reflex
sympathectomy
sympathetic
synapse
synaptic bulb
tearing
temporal lobe
tension headache

tetanus
thalamus
thermoreceptor
thrombolytic
thrombotic stroke
tinnitus
tranquilizers
transcutaneous electrical
  nerve stimulation
transient ischemic attack
tremor
tympanic membrane
vagotomy
ventriculitis
ventriculoperitoneal shunt
vertigo
zoophobia

Español ENHANCING SPANISH COMMUNICATION

English	Spanish (pronunciation)
adrenaline	adrenalina (ah-dray-nah-LEE-nah)
anxiety	ansiedad (an-se-ay-DAHD)
concussion	concusión (con-coo-se-ON)
conscious	consciente (cons-se-EN-tay)
consciousness	conciencia (con-se-EN-se-ah)
convulsion	convulsión (con-vool-se-ON)
cry	lloro (YO-ro)
epilepsy	epilepsia (ay-pe-LEP-se-ah)
eyeball	globo del ojo (GLO-bo del O-ho)
eyebrow	ceja (SAY-hah)
eyelash	pestaña (pes-TAH-nyah)
fatigue	fatiga (fah-TEE-gah)
gray	gris (grees)
headache	dolor de cabeza (do-LOR day cah-BAY-sa)
light	luz (loos)
lobe	lóbulo (LO-boo-lo)
neck	cuello (coo-EL-lyo)
nervous	nervioso (ner-ve-O-so)
optic	óptico (OP-te-co)
painful	doloroso (do-lo-RO-so)
paralysis	parálisis (pah-RAH-le-sis)
seizure	ataque (ah-TAH-kay)
sensation	sensación (sen-sah-se-ON)
sleep	sueño (soo-AY-nyo)
spinal column	columna vertebral (co-LOOM-nah ver-tay-BRAHL)
stroke	ataque de apoplejía (ah-TAH-kay de ah-po-play-HEE-ah)
vision	visión (ve-se-ON)
white	blanco (BLAHN-co)

Integumentary System

16

LEARNING GOALS

Basic Understanding
In this chapter you will learn to do the following:
1. State the function of the integumentary system, and analyze associated terms.
2. Write the meaning of the word parts associated with the integumentary system, and use them to build and analyze terms.
3. Match the epidermis, dermis, and adipose tissue with their characteristics.
4. List the four accessory skin structures and describe their functions.
5. Write the names of the diagnostic tests and procedures for integumentary system assessment when given descriptions of the procedures, or match the procedures with their descriptions.
6. Match the names of integumentary system pathologies with their descriptions, or write the names of the pathologies when given their descriptions.
7. Match the different types of skin lesions with their descriptions.
8. Match the integumentary system terms for surgical and therapeutic interventions with their descriptions, or write the names of the interventions when given their descriptions.

Greater Comprehension
9. Use word parts from this chapter to determine the meanings of terms in a health care report.
10. Spell the terms accurately.
11. Pronounce the terms correctly.
12. Write the meaning of the abbreviations.
13. Categorize terms as anatomy, diagnostic test or procedure, pathology, surgery, or therapy.

MAJOR SECTIONS OF THIS CHAPTER:

❏ **ANATOMY AND PHYSIOLOGY**
   The Skin
   Accessory Skin Structures
❏ **DIAGNOSTIC TESTS AND PROCEDURES**

❏ **PATHOLOGIES**
   Dermatitis and Skin Infections
   Skin Lesions
   Injuries to the Skin
   Disorders of Accessory Skin Structures
❏ **SURGICAL AND THERAPEUTIC INTERVENTIONS**

FUNCTION FIRST

The skin (integument) is the external covering of the body and is the largest organ of the body. It acts as a barrier to disease-causing organisms, helps regulate the temperature of the body, provides information about the environment through receptors, helps eliminate waste through perspiration, and is involved in the synthesis of vitamin D.

ANATOMY AND PHYSIOLOGY
THE SKIN

integumentary

16-1 The term **integument** (in-teg′u-mənt) means a covering or skin. The **integumentary** (in-teg-u-men′tar-e) system is the skin and its glands, hair, nails, and other structures that are derived from it. Because it is on the outside of our bodies, we are more familiar with the skin than with any other organ. Write the name of this body system that includes the skin and other structures derived from it: _____ system

Modified skin continues into various parts of the body, for example, the mucous membrane that lines the mouth, the nose, the intestines, and other cavities or canals that open to the outside. The skin that is studied in this chapter is the body covering, the integument.

Learn the following word parts and their meanings.

Word Parts: Anatomy and Physiology of the Skin

Word Part	Meaning	Combining Form	Meaning
Word Parts Pertaining to Skin Layers		**Accessory Skin Structures and Substances**	
adip(o), lip(o)	fat	hidr(o)	sweat
cutane(o), derm(o), dermat(o)	skin	onych(o), ungu(o)	nail
kerat(o)	horny or cornea	pil(o), trich(o)	hair
-derm	skin or germ layer	seb(o)	sebum

above

16-2 The skin consists of two main parts: the epidermis (ep″ĭ-dur′mis) and the dermis (dur′mis) (Figure 16-1). Remembering that epi- means above or on, where is the epi/dermis located? _____ the dermis

hard

16-3 The **epidermis** consists of four or five layers. **Epidermal** (ep″i-dur′məl) means pertaining to or resembling epidermis. The palms and soles have the greatest number of layers. The outermost layer of epidermis consists of cells that are nonliving and are constantly being shed and replaced. These cells contain **keratin** (ker′ə-tin), a waterproofing protein that hardens over several days. Keratin is a **scleroprotein** (sklēr″o-pro′tēn). The combining form scler(o) means _____, which helps to describe the scaly, or horny, nature of keratin.

horny

16-4 The combining form kerat(o) means either horny or the cornea—the convex, transparent structure at the front of the eye. When kerat(o) is used in discussions regarding the skin, it means hard or horny.

Kerato/genesis (ker″ə-to-jen′ə-sis) is the formation of keratin, a _____ material.

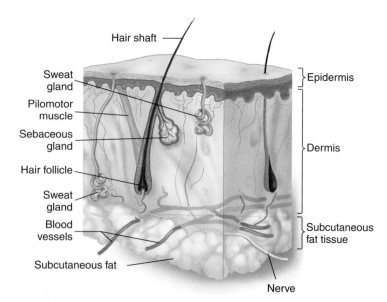

Hair shaft

Sweat gland

Pilomotor muscle

Sebaceous gland

Hair follicle

Sweat gland

Blood vessels

Subcutaneous fat

Nerve

Epidermis

Dermis

Subcutaneous fat tissue

Figure 16-1 The skin. The epidermis, the thin outer layer, is composed of four to five layers. Underneath the epidermis is the thicker dermis, composed of connective tissue containing lymphatics, nerves, blood vessels, hair follicles, sebaceous glands, and sweat glands. Beneath the dermis is a layer of subcutaneous adipose tissue.

16-5 The **dermis,** also called the **corium** (kor´e-əm), is the thicker layer of the skin. It is a noncellular connective tissue that is composed of collagen and elastic fibers that provide strength and flexibility. The dermis contains numerous blood vessels, nerves, and glands. Hair follicles also are embedded in this layer. Which layer of the skin is thicker, the epidermis or the dermis?

dermis

_____

The upper region of the dermis has many finger-like projections. The ridges marking the outermost layer of the skin are caused by the size and arrangement of these projections. The ridge patterns on the fingertips and thumbs (fingerprints) are different for each person.

16-6 Locate the subcutaneous (sub″ku-ta´ne-əs) **adipose** (ad´ĭ-pōs) tissue in Figure 16-1. Both derm(o) and cutane(o) mean skin. Dermal and cutaneous (ku-ta´ne-əs) mean pertaining to the skin. Sub/cutaneous means pertaining to _____ the skin.

below

The **subcutaneous adipose tissue** lies just under the dermis. It serves as a cushion against shock and insulates the body. The combining form adip(o) means fat. Adipose means pertaining

fat

to _____.

Both the dermis and the subcutaneous fat layer become thinner as a result of decreased blood flow that occurs with aging. Decreased tone and elasticity lead to wrinkles, and thin, transparent skin is more susceptible to injury.

16-7 Remembering that derm(a) and dermat(o) mean skin, a **dermato/logist** (dur″mə-tol´o-jist) is a physician who specializes in the skin. Which specialty is practiced by a dermatologist?

dermatology
(dər″mə-tol´o-je)

_____

16-8 The skin is derived from a tissue layer called **ectoderm** (ek´to-dərm) that forms during embryonic development. Sense receptors of the skin, as well as other parts of the nervous system, are also derived from ectoderm.

> ➤ **KEY** POINT <u>Three germ layers form during early stages of embryonic development</u>. Soon after fertilization, the fertilized egg undergoes cell division, producing a ball of cells that eventually differentiates into three distinct layers: **endoderm** (en´do-dərm), **mesoderm** (mez´o-, me″zo-dərm), and ectoderm. The suffix -derm means either skin or a germ layer. Here it is used to refer to a germ layer, a primary layer of cells of the developing embryo from which various organ systems develop.

ectoderm

Endo/derm, meso/derm, and ectoderm are the innermost, middle, and outermost germ layers, respectively. Skin is derived from which germ layer? _____

EXERCISE 1

Word Analysis. *Break these words into their component parts by placing a slash between the word parts. Then write the meaning of each term.*

1. keratogenesis _____

2. subcutaneous _____

3. ectoderm _____

4. dermatologist _____

5. endoderm _____

Say and Check

Say aloud the terms in Exercise 1. Use the Companion CD to check your pronunciations.

ACCESSORY SKIN STRUCTURES

trich(o)

16-9 The **accessory skin structures** include hair, nails, sebaceous (sə-ba´shəs) glands, and sweat glands. They are embedded in the dermis.

Hair protects the scalp from injury, eyebrows and eyelashes protect the eyes, and hair in the nostrils and external ear canals protects these structures from dust and insects. The differing distribution of hair in male and female individuals is controlled by hormones. At puberty, hair develops in the armpit and pubic regions and, in the male, on the face and other parts of the body. Two combining forms that mean hair are pil(o) and _____.

armpit

16-10 Remember that the combining form axill(o) means axilla (ak-sil´ə) or armpit. Hair develops in the axill/ary and pubic regions at puberty. Facial and chest hair also develop in males. The **axillary** (ak´sĭ-lar″e) region is the area of the _____.

epidermis

16-11 Observe the structure of a hair in Figure 16-2. The hair root is embedded in the dermis and is the portion of the hair below the surface. The shaft protrudes above the surface of the skin, or above what layer? _____

sebaceous

The **arrector pili** (ə-rek´tor pi´li) **muscles** contract under stresses of cold or fright, straighten the hair follicles, and raise the hairs, producing goose bumps or gooseflesh. Observing Figure 16-2, the names of the two glands that are directly connected with the hair follicle are the **apocrine** (ap´o-krin) **sweat gland** and the _____ gland.

seb(o)

16-12 Most **sebaceous glands** are structurally associated with hair follicles, but those of the eyelids, nipples, and genitalia are freestanding. Sebaceous glands are found in all areas of the body that have hair. **Sebum** (se´bəm), the oily material secreted by the sebaceous gland, keeps hair and skin soft and pliable and also inhibits growth of bacteria on the skin. Write the combining form that means sebum, the oily material for which sebaceous glands are named: _____.

sweat

16-13 Another type of gland found in the skin is a sweat* gland or **sudoriferous** (soo″do-rif´ər-əs) **gland.** Another name for a sudoriferous gland is a _____ gland. Sweat glands are found in most parts of the skin, being most numerous in the palms and soles.

Look again at Figure 16-2 and study the two types of sweat glands. Those that are associated with the hair follicles interact with bacteria on the skin to produce a characteristic body odor. Sweat glands that are not associated with hair follicles open to the surface of the skin through pores. When stimulated by temperature increases or emotional stress, these glands produce perspiration that evaporates on the skin surface and has a cooling effect.

---

*Sweat (Latin: *sudor*).

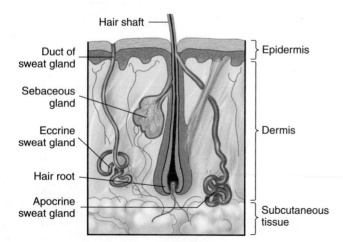

Figure 16-2 **The structure of hair and associated glands.** The hair shaft extends beyond the surface of the epidermis, and the root is the portion of the hair that is below the surface of the skin. Straight hair occurs when the hair shaft is round; wavy, if it is oval; curly or kinky, if it is flat. Hair can be cut without pain because it contains no nerves. The cuticle is the outermost covering and is the part that wears away at the tip of the shaft, resulting in split ends. Two types of glands (sebaceous glands and apocrine sweat glands) have ducts that open into hair follicles, and their secretions are transported to the skin surface. Stimulation of the eccrine sweat glands causes perspiration through ducts that open onto the surface of the skin. This is the single most important factor in the regulation of body temperature.

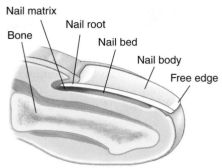

Nail matrix

Nail root

Bone

Nail bed

Nail body

Free edge

Figure 16-3 Structures of the nail. Each nail has a free edge, a nail body (the visible part), and a nail root, which is covered with skin. The nail bed is thickened to form the nail matrix, which is responsible for growth of the nail. The matrix is under the part of the nail body that appears as a whitish, crescent-shaped area called the lunula. Nails appear pinkish because of the rich supply of blood vessels in the underlying dermis.

16-14 Perspiration, or sweat, is the substance produced by the sweat glands. Sweat is a mixture of water, salt, and other waste products. Although elimination of waste is a function of the sweat glands, their principal function is to help regulate body temperature. As sweat evaporates on the skin surface, the skin is cooled and the body temperature is decreased. The principal function of sweat glands is to help regulate body _____.

temperature

water

16-15 Use hidr(o) to write terms pertaining to sweat. Do not confuse hidr(o) and hydr(o). The combining form hydr(o) means _____, whereas hidr(o) means sweat or perspiration.

16-16 Fingernails and toenails, modifications of the horny epidermal cells, are composed of keratin. (See the fingernail components in Figure 16-3. The cuticle is not shown in the illustration.)

Nails are thin plates of dead epidermis that contain a very hard type of keratin, which protects the fingers and toes and helps us pick up small objects. The nail matrix is responsible for growth of the nail and appears as a whitish, crescent-shaped area called the **lunula** (loo´nu-lə). Nails appear pink because of the rich supply of blood vessels in the underlying dermis.

Onycho/phagia (on″ĭ-ko-fa´jə) is the habit of nail biting. An **onycho/phag/ist** (on″ĭ-kof´ə-jist) habitually bites the _____.

nails

16-17 Another combining form, ungu(o), also means nail. It is used to write an adjective, **ungual** (ung´gwəl), which means pertaining to the _____.

nail

EXERCISE 2

Write the meaning of the following word parts.

1. adip(o) _____   6. onych(o) _____

2. axill(o) _____   7. pil(o) _____

3. cutane(o) _____   8. seb(o) _____

4. hidr(o) _____   9. trich(o) _____

5. kerat(o) _____   10. ungu(o) _____

11. Name the two layers of the skin: _____ and _____.

12. Name the germ layer from which the skin is derived: _____.

13. Write the name of the oily material secreted by sebaceous glands: _____.

14. Write another term for a sweat gland: _____.

15. Write an adjective that means pertaining to the nail: _____.

DIAGNOSTIC TESTS AND PROCEDURES

16-18 Diagnostic tests are generally performed when inspection of the skin is not sufficient to diagnose a suspected condition. A biopsy (bx) is performed to remove samples of lesions if malignancy is suspected. Laboratory cultures are performed to identify the cause of an infection, and skin tests are used to determine the existence of allergies.

Of the diagnostic tests just described, which term means the removal of a small piece of living tissue? _____

biopsy

16-19 A skin biopsy may involve removal of part of a lesion, either a punch biopsy or a shaved specimen. In a **punch biopsy** an instrument called a punch is used to remove a small amount of material (at least to the level of the dermis) for microscopic study (Figure 16-4). A **shaved specimen** is performed on superficial lesions, using a razor blade to obtain the specimen. Material may also be obtained by **curettage** (ku″rə-tahzh′), the scraping of material from a lesion using an instrument called a **curet** (ku-ret′) (Figure 16-5).

Write the name of the procedure that uses a curet to scrape material from a lesion for testing: _____.

curettage

16-20 Tissue or fluids (obtained by needle aspiration) can be examined microscopically, and bacterial and fungal cultures may be done in an effort to grow the causative organisms in an artificial culture medium to establish the cause of an infection. Special microscopic studies can demonstrate the presence of fungal or bacterial infections and the presence of certain parasites, such as lice. Fungal or bacterial infections are those caused by _____ or bacteria.

fungi

Some fungi are fluorescent when viewed with a Wood lamp, an ultraviolet (UV) light that is also called a black lamp (Figure 16-6).

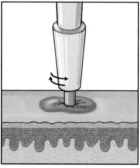
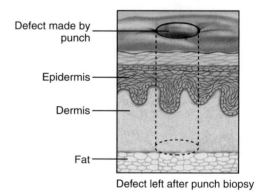

Insertion of biopsy tool

Defect made by punch

Epidermis

Dermis

Fat

Defect left after punch biopsy

Figure 16-4 Punch biopsy. With the use of a punch, living tissue is removed for microscopic examination.

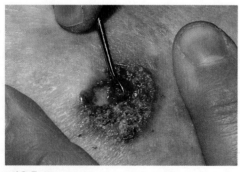

Figure 16-5 Curettage. A curet is used to scrape material from the surface of a wound. Curettage is performed to obtain tissue for either microscopic examination or culture or to clear unwanted material from areas of chronic infection.

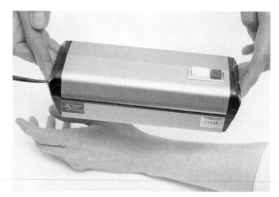

Figure 16-6 Wood lamp. This type of lamp is used to help diagnose certain bacterial and fungal infections. The light causes hairs infected with certain microorganisms to become fluorescent.

allergy

16-21 A skin test is one that is performed to determine the reaction of the body to a substance by observing the results of either injecting the substance or applying it to the skin. When it is done to determine if an allergy to a particular substance exists, it is called an allergy test.

A skin test called an _____ test is performed to detect allergic reactions.

16-22 A sweat test is specifically performed to diagnose **cystic fibrosis** (fi-bro´sis), a congenital disorder that causes abnormally thick secretions of mucus, particularly in the lungs. Increased levels of sodium and chloride are present in the sweat of individuals who have cystic fibrosis,

sweat

and _____ tests are used to diagnose the disorder.

EXERCISE 3

Write an answer in each blank in the following sentences.

1. The test in which a sample of living tissue is removed for diagnostic purposes is called a/an _____.

2. Fluids can be removed from a wound by _____ aspiration.

3. A/An _____ test is one that is done to determine the reaction to a substance by observing the results of either injecting the substance or applying it to the skin.

4. A/An _____ test demonstrates increased levels of sodium and chloride in cystic fibrosis.

PATHOLOGIES

away

16-23 An important characteristic of skin is its ability to communicate information to the trained observer. Normal skin has an even tone that is free of lesions, bruises, or signs of inflammation (pain, heat, redness, or swelling).

You learned that ex- means out, without, or away from. **Ex/foliation** (eks-fo″le-a´shən) is a falling _____ of tissue in scales or layers. **Induration** (in″du-ra´shən) is hardening of a tissue, especially the skin, and is usually caused by edema and inflammation.

Learn the following word parts and their meanings.

Word Parts: Skin Pathologies and Treatments

Combining Form	Meaning	Combining Form	Meaning
cry(o)	cold	rhytid(o)	wrinkle
erythemat(o)	erythema or redness	seps(o), sept(o)*	infection
follicul(o)	follicle	xer(o)	dry
heli(o)	sun	**Suffix**	
ichthy(o)	fish	-phoresis	transmission
necr(o)	dead or death		

*Sometimes sept(o) means septum.

pale

16-24 The skin is a reflection of the general health of a person. It can be excessively red in high blood pressure and other conditions involving dilation of the blood vessels. How might the skin appear in anemia? _____

Severe heart or lung disease may cause **cyanosis** (si″ə-no´sis), in which the skin would

bluish

appear _____. Unusually yellow skin suggests the presence of greater than the normal amount of bile pigment in the blood (**jaundice**).

16-25 A partial or total absence of pigment in the skin, hair, and eyes is called **albinism** (al´bĭ-niz-əm). Albinism is present at birth (see Figure 4-7). There is an absence of normal pigmentation caused by a defect in melanin precursors. In albinism, lack of pigmentation is implied

white

by albin(o), which means _____. Sometimes the skin and eyes appear pinkish. An **albin/o** (al-bi´no) is a person affected with albinism.

fish

16-26 Ichthy/osis (ik″the-o′sis) is a condition in which the skin is dry and scaly, resembling fish skin. The combining form ichthy(o) means fish. **Ichthy/oid** (ik′the-oid) means resembling a fish.

Some forms of ichthyosis, but not all, are hereditary. Ichthyosis is any of several generalized skin disorders marked by dryness and scaliness, resembling _____ skin.

xeroderma

16-27 A mild, nonhereditary form of ichthyosis is called **xero/derma** (zēr″o-der′mə). Xero/derma literally means dry skin. Write the name of this mild form of ichthyosis, characterized by roughness and dryness of the skin: _____.

xerosis (zēr-o′sis)

16-28 Using -osis, write a word that means any dry condition: _____. This word may refer to abnormal dryness, as of the eye, skin, or mouth; however, it is sometimes used to mean excessive dryness of the skin. Dry skin is vulnerable to scaling, thinning, and injury.

pediculosis

16-29 The skin can serve as a host to several parasitic diseases. **Pediculosis** (pə-dik″u-lo′sis) refers to infestation by human lice and is named for a genus of sucking lice, *Pediculus*. There are head lice, body lice, and pubic lice. Write the name of this disease that means infestation with lice: _____.

16-30 Skin changes may be related to specific skin diseases but also may reflect an underlying systemic disorder. **Discoid lupus erythematosus** (DLE) is a disease primarily of the skin. This chronic disorder is characterized by lesions that are covered with scales. The disorder was so named because of the reddish facial rash that appears in some patients, giving them a wolflike appearance (see Figure 14-32). The combining form erythemat(o) means erythema or redness. **Erythema** is redness (example, blushing) or inflammation of the skin (example, sunburn) or mucous membranes that is the result of dilation of the superficial capillaries. Write the name of the disorder that is believed to be a problem of autoimmunity: discoid lupus

erythematosus

_____.

hardened

16-31 Sclero/derma (sklēr″o-dur′mə) means hardening and thickening of the skin, a finding in various diseases. Literal translation of scleroderma is _____ skin. Systemic scleroderma is an autoimmune disorder of the connective tissue.

EXERCISE 4

Build It! *Use the following word parts to build terms. (Some word parts will be used more than once.)*

epi-, albin(o), cyan(o), derm(o), ichthy(o), xer(o), -al, -ism, -oid, -osis

1. lack of pigment in the skin, hair, and eyes   _____/_____

2. bluish discoloration   _____/_____

3. resembling a fish   _____/_____

4. pertaining to the outside layer of skin   _____/_____/_____

5. condition of dryness   _____/_____

Say and Check

Say aloud the terms you wrote for Exercise 4. Use the Companion CD to check your pronunciations.

DERMATITIS AND SKIN INFEC)TIONS

skin

16-32 Dermat/itis (der″mə-ti′tis) is an inflammatory condition of the _____. It may be acute or chronic and is a very general term that applies to any type of inflammation of the skin, including skin infections. A superficial dermatitis, inflammation on the surface of the skin, is called **eczema** (ek′zə-mə).

16-33 Contact dermatitis is a skin rash resulting from exposure to an irritant or antigen. Figure 4-2 shows the appearance of the skin of a person who is allergic to a necklace that contains nickel.

Sunburn is a type of dermatitis that results from overexposure to the sun. Remembering that phot(o) means light, the literal translation of photodermatitis (fo″to-dur″mə-ti′tis) is inflammation of the skin caused by _____. **Photodermatitis** is an abnormal skin reaction to light and is a common symptom of DLE.

light

16-34 Scabies (ska′bēz) is a contagious dermatitis caused by the itch mite and is transmitted by close contact. Write the name of this parasitic disease: _____.
The dermatitis results from irritation of the skin by the itch mite and is complicated by scratching caused by the intense itching.

scabies

16-35 Seborrheic (seb″o-re′ik) **dermatitis** is a chronic inflammatory condition of the _____ characterized by greasy scales and yellowish crusts. Dandruff is one type of seborrheic dermatitis. The cause is not known, but the sebaceous glands become overactive and the hair and scalp are excessively oily.

skin

16-36 Sebo/rrhea (seb″o-re′ə) means excessive production of sebum, the oily secretion of the sebaceous glands of the skin. The increased activity of the sebaceous glands at puberty may block the hair follicle and cause blackheads. Bacteria can infect the blocked follicle and result in a pus-filled pimple. Acne, a skin disease common where sebaceous glands are most numerous (face, chest, and upper back), is characterized by blackheads, whiteheads, pimples, nodules, and cysts (Figure 16-7). (See frame 16-42 for more information about nodules and cysts.) Acne is also called **acne vulgaris** (vəl-ga′ris). Pimples result from bacterial infection of blocked _____ glands.

sebaceous

16-37 Three words that mean the production of pus are **suppuration** (sup″u-ra′shən), **purulence** (pu′roo-ləns), and **pyogenesis** (pi″o-jen′ə-sis). Remember the meanings of suppuration and purulence, although they do not contain word parts that you necessarily recognize. Like _____, suppuration and purulence mean production of pus.
A **furuncle** (fu′rung-kəl), commonly called a boil, is a localized **suppurative** (sup′u-ra″tiv) infection that begins with infection of a hair follicle or sebaceous gland by pathogenic staphylococci.

pyogenesis

16-38 Skin infections are caused by specific types of bacteria, viruses, and fungi. A **verruca** (və-roo′kə) is a benign warty skin lesion (wart) with a rough surface caused by a common contagious virus (see Figure 16-8, *A*). The term for a wart is a _____.
Herpes simplex virus (HSV) infection is the most common viral infection of adult skin. Type 1 (HSV-1) causes the classic fever blisters. Another type of herpes virus, herpes zoster, causes shingles and occurs with reactivation of the herpes virus in individuals who have previously had chickenpox. The cause of fever blisters is an infection with the type 1 _____ simplex virus. HSV 1 is not to be confused with HSV 2, which causes genital herpes infections that are generally limited to the genital region.

verruca

herpes

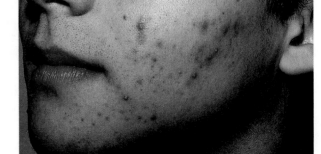

Figure 16-7 Acne vulgaris on the lower face. Acne is common where sebaceous glands are numerous (face, upper back, and chest).

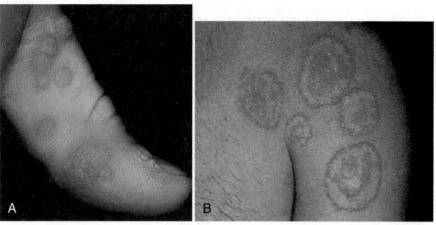

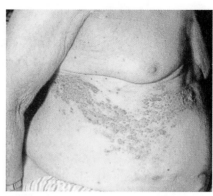

Figure 16-8 Two types of skin infections. A, A verruca, commonly called a wart, has a rough surface and is caused by a virus. **B,** Ringworm, a superficial fungal infection of the nonhairy skin of the body, is named for the circular lesions that are characteristic of the disease.

Figure 16-9 Herpes zoster. Also called shingles, this disease affects persons who have had chickenpox, and it is a reactivation of the dormant chickenpox virus. Note the pattern of the vesicles that follow the underlying route of nerves infected with the virus.

16-39 Herpes zoster, also called **shingles,** affects persons who have had chickenpox. It is an acute infection caused by reactivation of the dormant chickenpox virus. Herpes zoster is characterized by the development of painful vesicles that follow the underlying route of cranial or spinal nerves inflamed by the virus (Figure 16-9). It is a disease of immunosuppression and occurs most often and with greater severity in older persons. The lesions of herpes zoster are similar to those of herpes simplex (fever blisters), but they have a different distribution. The disease com-

zoster

monly called shingles is herpes _____.

A vaccination to prevent herpes zoster is available for persons who have had chickenpox. In addition, a vaccine for immunization against chickenpox is available for individuals 12 months of age or older.

16-40 A superficial fungal infection is called a **dermato/myc/osis** (dər″mə-to-mi-ko′sis) or **myco/dermat/itis** (mi″ko-der″mə-ti′tis). Either of these terms means a skin infection caused by

fungus

a _____. **Ringworm,** or **tinea** (tin′e-ə), is a group of dermatomycoses that can affect various parts of the body (see Figure 16-8, *B*).

Several skin infections caused by infectious microorganisms are presented in Table 16-1.

TABLE 16-1	Skin Eruptions Caused by Infectious Microorganisms	
Bacterial	**Fungal**	**Viral**
Erysipelas	Candidiasis	Herpes simplex type 1 fever blisters
Furuncles (boils) and carbuncles	Onychomycosis	Herpes zoster (shingles)
Impetigo	Tinea capitis (ringworm of scalp)	Rubella (German measles)
Leprosy	Tinea corporis (generalized)	Rubeola (measles)
Lyme disease	Tinea pedis (athlete's foot)	Varicella (chickenpox)
Meningococcemia		Verrucae (warts)
Paronychia (infection of marginal structures around nail)		
Scarlet fever		
Syphilis		

Consult a medical dictionary for explanations of the terms.

EXERCISE 5

Match the skin conditions in the left columns with their characteristics in the right column.

_____ 1. dermatitis   _____ 4. scleroderma

_____ 2. ichthyosis   _____ 5. seborrheic dermatitis

_____ 3. pediculosis   _____ 6. xeroderma

A. any inflammatory condition of the skin
B. autoimmune condition that often causes hard and thickened skin
C. greasy scales and yellowish crusts
D. infestation by human lice
E. dry, scaly skin
F. rough, dry skin

SKIN LESIONS

16-41 A skin **lesion** is any visible, local abnormality of the tissues of the skin, such as a sore, a rash, or a tumor. Most skin lesions are benign, but one type is among the most malignant of all kinds of cancer.

Trauma, such as cuts, punctures, or burns, exposes the underlying tissue to infection. Climate, hygiene, and general health also play a part. An **abscess** (ab´ses) is any pus-containing cavity that is surrounded by inflamed tissue and is characteristically caused by infection with staphylo/cocci (see Figure 4-12, *E* and *F*). Healing usually occurs when the abscess drains or is incised. Staphylococci, often abbreviated staph, are pyo/genic bacteria, which means they produce _____.

pus

16-42 Observe the two types of lesions shown in Figure 16-10. Both a **cyst** and a **nodule** cause a raised area of the overlying skin, but the cyst is filled with fluid or a semisolid material, whereas the _____ is solid and more than 1 cm wide and deep.

nodule (nod´ūl)

16-43 Examine the appearance of other types of lesions presented in Figure 16-11. The lesions are **primary lesions** because they are initial reactions to an underlying problem. A freckle is a nonraised, small dark spot on the skin, so it is called a _____.

macule (mak´ūl)

Both **papules** (pap´ūlz) and **plaques** (plaks) are elevated and circumscribed, but which type is less than 1 cm in diameter? _____. A small mole is a papule. Dandruff represents a type of plaque.

papule

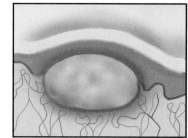
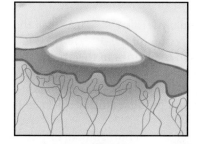

Figure 16-10 Schematic drawing of two types of lesions in cross section. Palpation by a physician will usually distinguish between a fluid-filled cyst and a solid nodule.

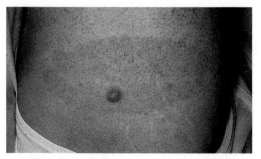
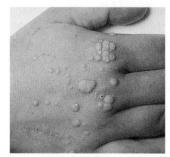
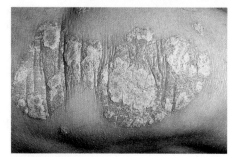

Macules: Nonraised, discolored spots less than 1 cm in diameter

Papules: Elevated lesion less than 1 cm in diameter

Plaques: Elevated and circumscribed patches more than 1 cm in diameter

Figure 16-11 Primary lesions of the skin. These initial reactions to an underlying problem alter one of the structural components of the skin.

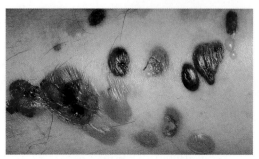

Bullae: Blisters greater than 1 cm and filled with clear fluid

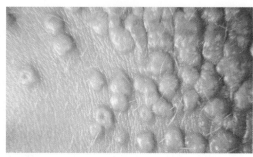

Vesicles: Blisters less than 1 cm and filled with clear fluid

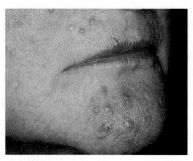

Pustules: Vesicles filled with cloudy fluid or pus

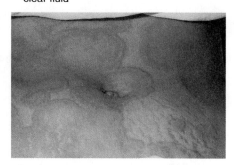

Wheals: Irregularly shaped, elevated lesions

Figure 16-11, cont'd Primary lesions of the skin.

pustules
bullae

urticaria

ulcers
fissures (fish′ərz)

petechiae

Vesicles (ves′ĭ-kəlz), **bullae** (bul′e), and **pustules** (pus′tūlz) are blister-like and contain fluid. Note that the singular form of bullae is bulla (bul′ə). The lesions of acne are filled with pus, so they are called _____.

Vesicles and bullae are differentiated by size. Which type of lesion is larger? _____

Urticaria (ur″tĭ-kar′e-ə) is an allergic skin eruption characterized by transient, elevated, irregularly shaped lesions that are called **wheals** (hwēlz, wēlz) (see Figure 16-11). Treatment includes antihistamines and removal of the stimulus or allergen. The name for this allergic skin reaction, also called hives, is _____.

16-44 Secondary lesions are changes in the appearance of the primary lesion and can occur with normal progression of the disease. See Figure 16-12 and use the accompanying information to write words in the blanks in this frame. **A/trophy** (at′rə-fe) of the skin is characterized by thinning with loss of skin markings. Stretch marks are an example of atrophy.

Deep, irregular erosions that extend into the dermis are called _____.

Athlete's foot produces linear cracks in the epidermis that are examples of _____.

16-45 Dried serum, sebum, blood, or pus on the skin surface produces a **crust.** Crusts frequently result from broken vesicles, bullae, or pustules.

Scales are dried fragments of sloughed epidermis. They appear dry and irregular in size and shape and are usually whitish. They are frequently seen in **psoriasis** (sə-ri′ə-sis), a common chronic skin disease characterized by circumscribed red patches covered by thick, dry, silvery scales (Figure 16-13, *A*).

Petechiae[*] (pə-te′ke-e) are tiny purple or red spots appearing on the skin as a result of tiny hemorrhages within the dermal or submucosal layers (see Figure 16-13, *B*). They are flush with the skin and range in size from pinpoint to pinhead size. Write the term for the spots that result from tiny hemorrhages in the skin: _____.

[*]Petechiae (Italian: *petecchie,* flea bite).

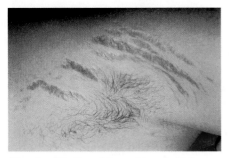

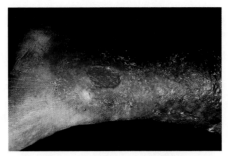

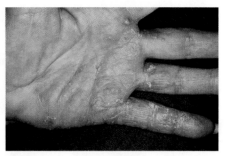

Atrophy: Wasting of the epidermis. Skin appears thin and transparent

Ulcer: Irregularly shaped erosions that extend into the dermis

Fissures: Deep linear splits through the epidermis into the dermis

Figure 16-12 Secondary lesions of the skin. The linear lines of atrophy, ulcerations, and fissures result from changes in the initial skin lesion.

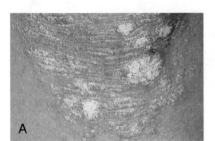

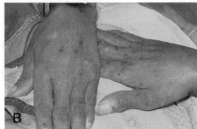

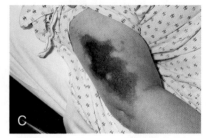

Figure 16-13 Common benign disorders of the skin. A, Psoriasis is characterized by circumscribed red patches covered by thick, dry silvery scales. **B,** Petechiae appear on the skin as a result of tiny hemorrhages beneath the surface. **C,** An ecchymosis is a hemorrhagic spot.

ecchymosis	An **ecchymosis** (ek″ĭ-mo´sis) is a hemorrhagic spot, larger than a petechia. It forms a nonelevated blue or purplish patch (see Figure 16-13, *C*). Write the term for this large hemorrhagic spot: _____.
nevus	**16-46** A new growth of tissue characterized by a disordered growth of cells is a tumor, also called a neoplasm. Several benign tumors have already been mentioned, for example, warts and moles. Another term for a mole is a **nevus** (ne´vəs); the plural is nevi (ne´vi). Write the term that means a mole: _____.
tumor	**16-47** The combining form lip(o) means fats. A **lip/oma** (lip-o´mə) is a common, benign _____ consisting of mature fat cells, usually removed by surgical excision. A **kerat/oma** (ker″ə-to´mə), also called a callus, is a flat, poorly defined mass, often on the sole over a bony prominence, and is caused by pressure. A **corn** is also caused by pressure or friction but, unlike a callus, is round or conical and usually painful.
lesion	**16-48 Kerat/osis** (ker″ə-to´sis) is a condition of the skin characterized by the formation of horny growths or excessive development of the epithelium. One type of keratosis, **sebo/rrhe/ic keratosis** (seb″o-re´ik ker″ə-to´sis), is a consequence of aging. The lesion of seborrheic keratosis is a common benign _____ that may occur anywhere on the body of an older person but it is more commonly found on the face, neck, upper trunk, and arms (Figure 16-14). Lesions such as this, with well-defined edges and definite boundaries, are described as circumscribed lesions because it would be possible to draw a circle around a lesion of this type.
actinic	**Actinic keratosis**[*] (ak-tin´ik ker″ə-to´sis) is a premalignant lesion that is common in people with chronically sun-damaged skin. Write the name of the type of keratosis that is considered a premalignant lesion: _____ keratosis. These premalignant lesions may progress to skin cancer if the lesions are not removed. They are usually treated, because this type of keratosis can progress to **squamous cell carcinoma.**

[*]Actinic (Greek: *aktis,* ray).

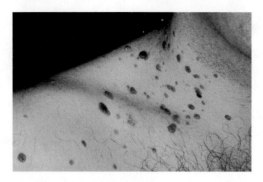

Figure 16-14 Seborrheic keratoses. Numerous seborrheic keratoses are present, some of which are deeply pigmented with melanin. The large lesions show the characteristic stuck-on appearance. Seborrheic keratoses are benign tumors that can be removed by curettage, cryotherapy, and application of caustic agents.

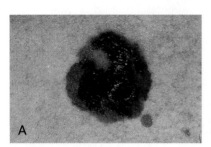
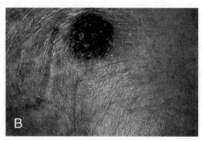
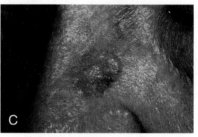

Figure 16-15 Three common types of skin cancer. A, Malignant melanoma. **B,** Squamous cell carcinoma. **C,** Basal cell carcinoma.

tumor

cancer
(or carcinoma)

Kaposi

16-49 Basal cell and squamous cell cancers are common types of skin cancer that are rarely invasive. In other words, they rarely spread to other organs. **Basal cell carcinoma** is a malignant epithelial cell tumor that begins as a papule and continues to enlarge. One type of skin cancer that is included in cancer statistics is malignant melanoma. Because about half of malignant melanomas (mel″ə-no′məz) arise from moles, nevi with irregular edges or variegated colors are usually surgically removed and examined microscopically to determine their cell type. Literal interpretation of melan/oma is a black _____.

A **malignant melanoma,** often shortened to melanoma, is a pigmented neoplasm that originates in the skin and is composed of **melano/cytes** (mel″ə-no-sītz, mə-lan′o-sītz). It is highly metastatic, one of the most aggressive of all skin cancers, and causes a high mortality rate in affected individuals. Figure 16-15 shows a melanoma with two other common types of skin cancer. Squamous cell carcinoma, basal cell carcinoma, and malignant melanoma are all types of skin _____.

16-50 Kaposi sarcoma (kah′po-she, kap′o-se sahr-ko′mə) is the most common malignancy associated with acquired immunodeficiency syndrome (AIDS). The lesions are small, purplish-brown papules that spread throughout the skin, the lymph nodes, and the internal organs. Other disorders associated with this lesion include diabetes and malignant lymphoma. The name of the lesion is _____ sarcoma (see Figure 13-17).

EXERCISE 6

Match skin lesions in the left columns with their characteristics in the right column.

_____ 1. bulla   _____ 4. macule

_____ 2. cyst   _____ 5. papule

_____ 3. fissure   _____ 6. pustule

A. blister, larger than 1 cm
B. crack in the skin
C. discolored spot, not elevated
D. fluid-filled sac containing pus
E. sac filled with clear fluid
F. solid elevation, less than 0.5 cm in diameter

INJURIES TO THE SKIN

16-51 A **wound** is a physical injury involving a break in the skin, usually caused by an act or accident other than a disease.

> ➤ **KEY** POINT <u>Intentional wounds are the result of planned invasive therapy or treatment, as in surgery.</u> The wound edges are clean, bleeding is controlled, the wound is usually made under sterile conditions, and the risk of infection is low. Unintentional wounds occur from unexpected trauma or forcible injury, as in scrapes, burns, or stabbing. This type of wound usually occurs in an unsterile environment, the edges are jagged, and bleeding may be uncontrolled. Because of the factors involved in unintentional wounds, the risk for infection is increased and there is often a longer healing time.

Surgery can be classified as which type of wound, intentional or unintentional?

intentional _____

16-52 The skin is subject to many injuries because it is exposed to the external environment. Trauma to the skin and underlying tissues requires healing to repair the defect, whether the wound was created by a surgical incision or an accident. A surgical wound generally heals faster and with less infection than accidental trauma because of its aseptic (free of infection) nature.

infected The combining forms seps(o) and sept(o) mean infection. **A/septic** means free of pathogenic organisms or _____ material.

> ➤ **KEY** POINT <u>Infection is just one of several things that slow the healing process.</u> Factors that slow the process of healing include the following:
> • infection, presence of foreign material, or necrotic tissue
> • movement (lack of immobilization) of the wound
> • poor blood circulation in the area of an abscess, or in the individual in general
> • decreased number of white blood cells in the blood
> • deficiency of antibodies in the blood
> • malnutrition in the individual

16-53 A pressure ulcer is a special type of injury to the skin that occurs almost exclusively in people with limited mobility. Also called bedsores or **decubitus ulcers** (de-ku´bĭ-təs ul´sərz), these sores occur as a result of mechanical trauma and lack of adequate blood circulation to the affected area. Once formed, they are slow to heal. Ulcerations that occur almost exclusively in pressure or persons with limited mobility are called _____ ulcers.
decubitus
A mark that is left by healing of a lesion where excess collagen was produced to replace the injured tissue is called a scar. Excessive overgrowth of unsightly scar tissue, called a **keloid** (ke´loid), occurs in some individuals, especially black individuals. Write the word that means keloid overgrowth of scar tissue: _____.

16-54 A **laceration** (las˝ər-a´shən) is a torn, jagged wound (Figure 16-16, *A*). A **puncture** is a wound made by piercing. Skin is scraped or rubbed away by friction in an **abrasion** (ə-bra´zhən). One type of injury, a **contusion** (kən-too´zhən), is caused by a blow to the body

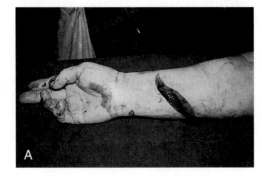
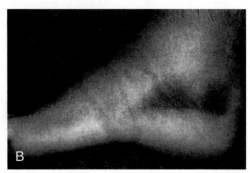

Figure 16-16 Two types of wounds. A, A laceration is a torn, jagged wound. **B,** A contusion is a bruise.

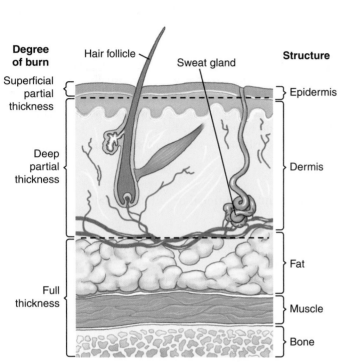

Type of Burn	Dermal Layers Involved	Appearance of the Skin
Partial-thickness:		
Superficial (1st degree)	Only the epidermis	Red; no immediate blisters, but may blister after 24 hours
Deep partial-thickness (2nd degree)	Extends into the dermis	Red and moist, blistered
Full-thickness:		
(3rd degree)	Throughout the dermis and epidermis, sometimes into subcutaneous fat layer	Hard, dry, and leathery; white, deep red, yellow, brown to black
Deep full-thickness (4th degree)	No skin layers remain; underlying bone and muscle are damaged	Wound is blackened and depressed; muscle and bone are exposed

Figure 16-17 Cross-section of skin indicating the degree of burn and structures involved.

that causes subcutaneous bleeding and does not disrupt the integrity of the skin. A contusion is called a bruise and is characterized by swelling, discoloration, and pain (Figure 16-16, *B*).

A torn, jagged wound is called a _____, whereas a wound that is made by piercing is called a puncture. *laceration*

When skin is scraped away by friction, it is called an _____. *abrasion*

16-55 Burns are tissue injuries resulting from excessive exposure to heat, electricity, chemicals, radiation, or gases, in which the extent of the injury is determined by the amount of exposure and the nature of the agent that causes the burn. The magnitude of the injury is based on the depth and extent of the total body surface area (TBSA) that is burned.

Burns are sometimes classified as first-, second-, third-, and fourth-degree injuries. The American Burn Association (ABA) advocates categorizing the burn injury according to the depth of tissue destruction as a **superficial** or **deep partial-thickness burn** or as a **full-thickness burn** (third or fourth degree). Study Figure 16-17 and read the descriptions of skin layer destruction and appearances of the burns.

In comparing superficial partial-thickness burns and full-thickness burns, _____-thickness burns destroy deeper layers of tissue. *full*

The superficial burn does not extend beyond which layer of skin? _____ *epidermis*

In a deep partial-thickness burn, damage does not extend beyond which layer of skin? _____ *dermis*

Muscle and bone are exposed in a _____ full-thickness burn. *deep*

Which type of burn is characterized by blisters? deep _____ thickness burn *partial*

16-56 Burned tissue usually represents various levels of damage. In addition to the burn depth, burn severity takes into consideration factors such as the size and location of the burn, mechanism of injury, duration and intensity of the burn, and the age and health of the individual. The very young as well as older persons are at greatest risk. The magnitude of the burn is determined by how much of the TBSA is affected. TBSA means total body _____ area. *surface*

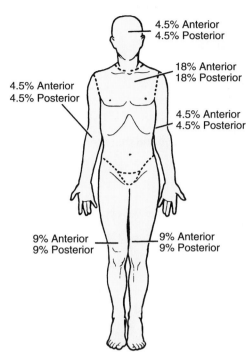

Figure 16-18 **The rule of nines for estimating burn percentage in an adult.** The rule of nines assigns 9% to the head and each arm, 18% to each leg and the anterior and posterior trunk, and 1% to the perineum. This formula can be used on adults whose weight is proportional to their height.

4.5% Anterior
4.5% Posterior

18% Anterior
18% Posterior

4.5% Anterior
4.5% Posterior

4.5% Anterior
4.5% Posterior

9% Anterior
9% Posterior

9% Anterior
9% Posterior

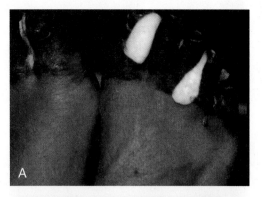

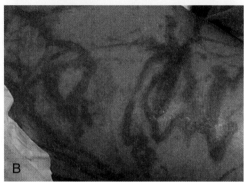

Figure 16-19 **Tissue necrosis. A,** Necrosis resulting from frostbite. **B,** Necrosis that resulted from contact with the stinging structures on the tentacles of a jellyfish.

> ➤ KEY POINT <u>The "rule of nines" calculates the size of a burn injury.</u> The **rule of nines** is a formula for estimating the percentage of adult body surface covered by burns (Figure 16-18) and is modified in infants and children because of the proportionately larger head size.

The rule of nines is relatively easy to remember and may be used for initial assessment of an adult burn patient; however, a more complicated system called the Lund-Browder system takes into account the patient's age.

Serious burn injuries can result in systemic disturbances, including fluid and protein losses, and abnormalities in many body systems. In addition, infection is a serious threat when the skin is destroyed and can no longer protect the underlying tissues from microorganisms. Another term for infection is **sepsis** (sep′sis).

16-57 **Frostbite** is damage to skin, tissues, and blood vessels as a result of prolonged exposure to cold (Figure 16-19, *A*). The extent of injury depends largely on the intensity and the duration of the exposure. Because injury is greater in **hypoxic tissue,** the individual's health affects the severity of injury. Hyp/oxia (hi-pok′se-ə) means a condition in which the amount of oxygen is

below

frostbite

_____ normal.

Damage to tissue as a result of exposure to cold is called _____.

16-58 **Necr/osis** (nə-kro′sis) is localized tissue death that occurs in response to disease or injury—in other words, death of areas of tissue or bone surrounded by healthy parts. When tissue is badly damaged, it becomes **necro/tic** (nə-krot′ik). The combining form necr(o) means dead or death. Necro/tic describes a characteristic of tissue that has been broken down. Necrotic

dead

tissue is _____ tissue.

Depending on the sensitivity of the person, the type of jellyfish, and the degree of contact, tissue necrosis can result from a jellyfish sting (Figure 16-19, *B*). But in most cases, limited contact with the tentacles of jellyfish causes only a tender, red welt on the skin.

EXERCISE 7

Write a word in each blank to complete these sentences.

1. A/An _____ is a cavity that contains pus.

2. A/An _____ is commonly called a boil.

3. Another name for a wart is a/an _____.

4. A mycodermatitis is a superficial _____ infection of the skin.

5. Tiny purple or red spots that result from tiny hemorrhages within the dermal or submucosal layers are called _____.

6. Another name for a mole is a/an _____.

7. A condition of the skin characterized by the formation of horny growths or excessive development of the horny growth is called a/an _____.

8. A common, benign tumor consisting of mature fat cells is called a/an _____.

9. The most common malignancy associated with AIDS is _____ sarcoma.

10. In a deep partial-thickness burn, damage does not extend beyond the layer of skin called the _____.

DISORDERS OF ACCESSORY SKIN STRUCTURES

trichopathy (trĭ-kop´ə-the)	**16-59** Pathologies also occur with the hair, nails, sebaceous glands, and sweat glands. Use trich(o) to write a term that means any disease of the hair: _____.
folliculitis	**16-60** Infections in intact skin often involve the hair follicles, where bacteria easily accumulate and grow well. **Follicul/itis** (fə-lik″u-li´tis) is a term that refers to superficial bacterial infection involving the hair follicles, and it uses the combining form follicul(o), which means follicle. Write the term that means inflammation of the hair follicles: _____. Without treatment, folliculitis can progress to **cellul/itis** (sel″u-li´tis), a localized bacterial invasion of subcutaneous tissue. Cellulitis can also occur independently of folliculitis and is characterized by pain, heat, swelling, and redness.
condition	**16-61** The literal translation of **trich/osis** (tri-ko´sis) is an abnormal _____ of the hair. Its extended meaning is any abnormal growth or development of hair.
alopecia	**16-62** Baldness is **alopecia** (al″o-pe´shə). Write this new word for baldness: _____. Alopecia prematura is baldness that occurs early in life (Figure 16-20).
onychopathy (on″ĭ-kop´ə-the) fungus	**16-63** Use onych(o) to write a term that means any disease of the nails: _____. **Onych/osis** (on″ĭ-ko´sis) is atrophy or other unhealthy condition of the nails, often caused by a fungal infection. **Onycho/myc/osis** (on″ĭ-ko-mi-ko´sis) is a condition of the nails resulting from a _____ (Figure 16-21). **Onychomalacia** (on″ĭ-ko-mə-la´shə) is abnormal softening of the nails.
sweat	**16-64** **Hidr/aden/itis** (hi″drad-ə-ni´tis) is inflammation of a _____ gland. (Hidr[o] loses the "o" when joined with aden[o].) A chronic form of hidradenitis is caused by closure of the pores with secondary bacterial infection of apocrine sweat glands, chiefly in the axillary and anogenital areas. It is characterized by the development of a tender red abscess that enlarges and eventually breaks through the skin or forms a cyst.

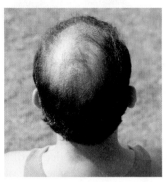

Figure 16-20 Alopecia prematura. This man is in his early thirties and is experiencing premature baldness.

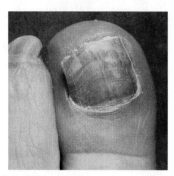

Figure 16-21 Onychomycosis. This is a fungal condition of the nails. Note the discoloration of the nail and the redness around the nail, indicating inflammation.

transmission	**16-65 Dia/phoresis** (di″ə-fə-re′sis) means excessive sweating. The suffix -phoresis means transmission. Translated literally, dia/phoresis means _____ through, so you will need to remember that diaphoresis means excessive sweating (or perspiration). Perspiration is only one means of ridding the body of excess heat. The level of heat produced within the body and lost from the body surface is regulated and controlled by the brain.
below	**16-66** Prolonged exposure to cold temperatures can lead to **hypo/therm/ia** (hi″po-thur′me-ə), a condition in which the body temperature is _____ normal. Literal translation of hypothermia is a condition of less than normal heat.
hyperthermia (hi″pər-thur′me-ə)	**16-67** Using hypothermia as a model, write a word that means a greatly increased body temperature: _____.
	16-68 In a healthy person, internal body temperature is maintained within a narrow range by the brain, resulting in a balance between generation and conservation of heat.
	➤ **KEY** POINT <u>Understand the difference between pyrexia and hyperthermia.</u> **Pyrexia** (pi-rek′se-ə), or fever, is an increased body temperature that is mediated by an increase in the heat regulatory set point. In contrast, hyperthermia overrides or bypasses normal heat regulation. Heat stroke and sunstroke are examples of hyperthermia. These conditions are caused by prolonged exposure to excessive heat or the sun and may be life-threatening. **Thermo/plegia** (thər″mo-ple′jə) is another name for heatstroke or sunstroke.
paralysis	Translated literally, thermoplegia means heat _____.

EXERCISE 8

Word Analysis. *Break these words into their component parts by placing a slash between the word parts. Write the meaning of each term.*

1. hidradenitis   _____

2. trichopathy   _____

3. photodermatitis   _____

4. hypothermia   _____

5. folliculitis   _____

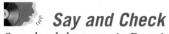 *Say and Check*

Say aloud the terms in Exercise 8. Use the Companion CD to check your pronunciations.

SURGICAL AND THERAPEUTIC INTERVENTIONS

16-69 Most surgical procedures involving the skin are for the purposes of repairing or treating damaged skin, removing lesions, or penetrating the skin to perform diagnostic or surgical procedures.

Wound irrigation is the flushing of an open wound using a medicated solution, water, sterile saline (a salt solution, usually an isotonic solution of sodium chloride), or an antimicrobial liquid preparation. **Anti/microbial** means pertaining to a substance that acts

against

_____ microorganisms, either killing or inhibiting their growth.

This type of irrigation is done to cleanse and remove debris and excessive drainage (Figure 16-22). The wound is irrigated and the rinsing solution is aspirated and discarded until the returning solution is clear. After irrigation is completed, the area is dried and some type of dressing is applied.

16-70 Wound management depends on the type and characteristics of the wound. Some types of wounds are left uncovered; others require coverings ranging from medicated transparent sprays to sterile dressings.

Superficial wounds often heal without **suturing** (soo´chər-ing). Deep wounds with gaping edges or wounds located over joints where movement opens the cut edges are generally stapled or sutured to stop the bleeding, hold the tissues together, and enhance the healing process. Adhesive sprays are used for closing certain wounds, but deep wounds generally require

suturing

_____.

16-71 Negative-pressure wound therapy (vacuum-assisted closure [VAC]) uses suction and controlled negative pressure (vacuum) to remove drainage and speed wound healing. The VAC system pulls infectious materials and other fluids from the wound via tubing. Wounds suitable for this type of therapy include acute or traumatic wounds, chronic ulcerated wounds, or surgical wounds that have dehisced. You probably remember from an earlier chapter that **dehiscence** (de-his´əns) is the rupture of a wound closure or the separation of a surgical incision, typically

closure

an abdominal incision. VAC means vacuum-assisted _____.

16-72 A skin graft is transplantation of skin to cover areas where skin has been lost through a burn or other trauma, or to replace diseased skin that has been removed. If the graft is from the patient's own body, it is called an **autograft** (aw´to-graft), for which the literal translation is

self

_____ graft.

An **allograft** (al´o-graft) is a graft of tissue between two genetically different individuals of the same species.

16-73 A **skin flap** is a special type of skin graft that involves moving a section of skin to a nearby area without cutting off the end of the transplanted tissue. This is done to leave some of the blood circulation intact.

skin

A **derma/tome** is used to cut thin slices of _____ for grafting.

16-74 Severe burns of the arms or legs can require **amputation** (am˝pu-ta´shən), the surgical removal of a limb or part of the body. All depths of burns except superficial partial-thickness burns may involve skin grafting.

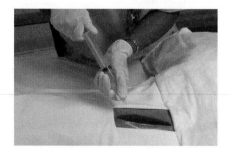

Figure 16-22 Wound irrigation. Flushing of an open wound to cleanse and remove debris and excessive drainage.

tissue	**Histo/compatibility** (his″to-kəm-pat″ĭ-bil´ĭ-te) is necessary for a successful transplant of any organ or tissue. Histo/compatibility means that the transplanted _____ is capable of surviving without ill effects. If the tissue is not compatible, this is called **in/compatibility.**

16-75 Remembering that top(o) means place, **topical** (top´ĭ-kəl) **medications** are placed directly on the skin. **Topical antimicrobial** (an″te-, an″ti-mi-kro´be-əl) **agents** and dressings are applied to injured or burned tissue to prevent infection, and aseptic procedures are followed. A/septic

without

means _____ infection.

16-76 Escharo/tomy (es″kə-rot´ə-me) is a surgical incision into necrotic tissue resulting from a severe burn; it is done to relieve pressure that results from severe swelling.

Débridement (da-brēd-maw´) is the removal of foreign material and dead or damaged tissue, especially from a wound. To **débride** (da-brēd´) is to remove by dissection. Write this word that means the removal of foreign material or damaged tissue by excision:

débridement

_____.

onychectomy
(on″ĭ-kek´tə-me)

16-77 Use onych(o) to write a word that means removal (excision) of the nail:

_____. (Declawing of an animal is also called onychectomy.)

16-78 Boils or other deep suppurative wounds may require incision and drainage (I&D) to relieve pressure and speed healing.

> ➤ **KEY** POINT The treatment of lesions depends on the type of lesion. **Anti/septics** help to clean a wound and inhibit the growth of microorganisms, **antibiotics** are used to treat infections, and **antipruritics** (an″te-, an″ti-proo-rit´iks) relieve or prevent itching.

Write the term that means medications that are used to relieve itching:

antipruritics

_____.

16-79 Topical medications may be found in many forms: aerosols, ointments, liquids, or creams. An **aero/sol** (ār´o-sol) medication is a liquid that is vaporized and propelled into the

air

_____ by gas under pressure within the container.

An **ointment** (abbreviated ung) is a medicated, fatty, soft substance for external application to

topical
feeling

the body. In other words, an ointment is for what type of use? _____

Topical an/esthetics are applied to produce a lack of _____.

16-80 Wart treatments include salicylic acid and **electrodesiccation** (e-lek″tro-des″ĭ-ka´shən). In

electricity

electro/desiccation, tissue is destroyed by burning with _____.

Warts may also be destroyed by **cryo/therapy** (kri″o-ther´ə-pe), a technique of exposing tissues to extreme cold to produce well-defined areas of cell destruction.

16-81 Plastic surgery is the replacement or restoration of parts of the body and is performed to correct a structural or cosmetic defect. Increased expenditures on cosmetics, surgery, and other treatments to improve our appearance attest to how we value our physical appearance.

A reconstructive technique in plastic surgery uses **collagen injections** to enhance the lips or "plump" sagging facial skin. The collagen injections are replacement of the lost collagen and elastic

dermis

from which layer of the skin? _____ This is sometimes used with injections of Botox (botulinum toxin), a potent bacterial toxin that relaxes facial wrinkles. (Botox is also used to relax the muscles involved in spasms of the eyelid or other spastic ailments.)

16-82 A combining form that means wrinkle or wrinkles is rhytid(o). **Rhytido/plasty** (rit´ĭ-do-plas″te) means face-lift. Literal translation of rhytido/plasty means surgical repair for

wrinkles

_____. Skin of the face is tightened, wrinkles are removed, and the skin is made to appear firm and smooth.

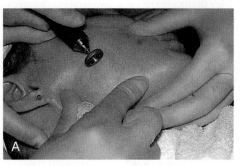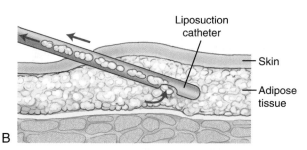

Figure 16-23 Two cosmetic surgical procedures. A, Dermabrasion, a treatment to remove superficial scars. **B,** Liposuction, also called suction lipectomy, removes adipose tissue with a suction pump device.

dermabrasion

16-83 Derm/abrasion (dur″mə-bra′zhən) is a treatment for removing superficial scars on the skin (Figure 16-23, *A*). This physical "sanding of the skin" is called _____. This procedure is also used to remove tattoos.

Alternatives to dermabrasion are chemical peels or laser destruction of the outermost epidermal layers. Chemical peels use a strong chemical solution to reduce wrinkles, blemishes, and sun-damaged areas of the skin. The top layers peel away, and new, smoother skin layers replace the old ones.

16-84 It may seem natural to think of excision of a lipoma as lip/ectomy (lĭ-pek′tə-me); however, this is incorrect. **Lipectomy** originally meant excision of a mass of subcutaneous fat tissue, as from the abdominal wall. The term has been extended to mean removal of fat from the neck, legs, arms, belly, and elsewhere by placing a narrow tube under the skin and applying a vacuum. The suction pulls the fat loose. This suction lipectomy is called **liposuction** (lip″o-suk′shən).

fat

Lipo/suction removes adipose tissue with a suction pump device, and it is used primarily as cosmetic surgery to remove or reduce localized areas of _____ (Figure 16-23, *B*).

16-85 Lipo/lysis (lĭ′pol′ə-sis) is the breakdown or destruction of fat. Injection lipolysis and laser lipolysis are alternatives to liposuction. Injection lipolysis is a procedure that involves injection of a combination of substances, including enzymes, into fat pockets, and the dissolved fat is eliminated by the body. Laser lipolysis eliminates fat by using a laser rather than by injecting substances.

EXERCISE 9

Match the terms in the surgical list in the left columns with their descriptions on the right.

_____ 1. allograft   _____ 5. liposuction
_____ 2. autograft   _____ 6. onychectomy
_____ 3. débridement   _____ 7. rhytidoplasty
_____ 4. escharotomy

A. cutting away of dead or damaged tissue in a wound
B. excision of the nail
C. face-lift
D. surgery to remove excess fat
E. surgical incision to relieve pressure after a severe burn
F. tissue graft between two genetically different individuals
G. tissue graft whereby one's tissue is transplanted to another site of one's body

destruction

16-86 Electro/lysis (e″lek-trol′ə-sis) is sometimes used to destroy the hair follicles when hair is growing in an undesirable place. By its word parts, you know that electro/lysis is _____ of a substance by passing electrical current through it. Most electrolysis is done for aesthetic reasons, for example, getting rid of facial hair.

16-87 The most popular aesthetic plastic surgery for male individuals is hair transplantation. Grafts or plugs of skin containing hair follicles are transplanted from some part of the body to the head. An oral medication is effective in restoring hair in certain types of hair loss but must be taken the remainder of one's life to prevent hair loss. You learned earlier of different types of

skin grafts. Which type of graft is transplantation of hair from one part of the body to
another? _____

autograft

16-88 Treatment of acne includes the use of topical and oral antibiotics. Topical antibiotics are
applied directly to the _____. Topical and oral retinoids
(ret´ĭ-noidz) are also used. **Retinoids** are compounds that are structurally related to substances
that exhibit vitamin A activity, such as retinal and retinol. Retinoids increase the sloughing of
epithelial cells and cause extrusion of blackheads.

skin

16-89 Several physical treatments are available for various skin conditions. Ultraviolet (UV) light
therapy is a common physical treatment in psoriasis and other skin conditions (see Figure 5-4).
UV radiation, one of the types of energy that is included in sunlight, is more readily accessible
and easier to control than exposure to the sun.
    Helio/therapy (he˝le-o-ther´ə-pe) is _____ of disease by
exposing the body to sunlight. The combining form heli(o) means the sun.

treatment

16-90 Certain wounds require the use of **heat hydro/therapy.** By its name, you know that heat
hydrotherapy makes use of warm _____.

water

16-91 The remaining types of physical therapy have to do with treatments for muscle pain, reduction of tissue swelling, or increasing circulation. The skin is involved in many cases, however,
because the treatment is delivered through the skin.
    Ultrasound is used therapeutically as a penetrating deep-heating agent for soft tissue. Ultra-
sound uses high-frequency _____ waves.
    Another method of generating heat in soft tissue is **diathermy** (di´ə-thur˝me). Both dia-
thermy and ultrasound are used to increase circulation to an inflamed area. Dia/therm/y means
passing high-frequency current through tissue to generate _____
in a particular part of the body.

sound

heat

16-92 Various types of stimulation to the skin and subcutaneous tissue offer pain relief.
Trans/cutaneous electrical nerve stimulation (TENS) is one of these methods (see Figure 15-25).
Trans/cutaneous means that the electrical current is delivered across (or through) the
_____. Electrodes are placed over the painful sites, and small
amounts of electrical current are delivered to painful areas.

skin

16-93 Transdermal drug delivery is a method of applying a drug to unbroken skin. The drug
is absorbed through the skin and then enters the circulatory system. It is used particularly for
estrogen, nicotine, and scopolamine (to prevent motion sickness). Not all medications can
be administered in this way. Administration of a drug through unbroken skin is called
_____ drug delivery.

transdermal

EXERCISE 10

Match the types of therapy with their characteristics.

_____ 1. diathermy

_____ 2. heat hydrotherapy

_____ 3. heliotherapy

_____ 4. TENS

_____ 5. transdermal drug delivery

A. administers a drug through unbroken skin
B. delivers electric current through the skin to painful areas
C. exposes the body to the sun
D. uses high-frequency current to generate heat for healing
E. uses warm water

CHAPTER ABBREVIATIONS*

ABA	American Burn Association	**I&D**	incision and drainage
AIDS	acquired immunodeficiency syndrome	**staph**	*Staphylococcus*
Bx, bx	biopsy	**TBSA**	total body surface area
DLE	discoid lupus erythematosus	**TENS**	transcutaneous electrical nerve stimulation
HSV	herpes simplex virus	**ung**	ointment
HSV 1	herpes simplex virus type 1	**UV**	ultraviolet
HSV 2	herpes simplex virus type 2	**VAC**	vacuum-assisted closure

*Many of these abbreviations share their meanings with other terms.

▶ CHAPTER 16 REVIEW

Basic Understanding

Labeling

I. *Label the degree of burn (1 to 3) and the structures (4 to 6) in the following illustration of the skin and underlying structures.*

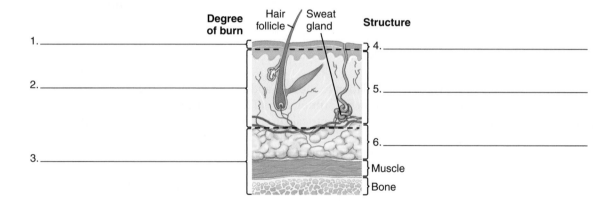

Listing

II. *List five functions of the skin.*

1. _____

2. _____

3. _____

4. _____

5. _____

III. *List the accessory skin structures and describe their functions.*

1. _____

2. _____

3. _____

4. _____

Matching

IV. *Match skin lesions in the left columns with their characteristics in the right column.*

_____ 1. bulla

_____ 2. cyst

_____ 3. fissure

_____ 4. macule

_____ 5. papule

_____ 6. pustule

_____ 7. scar

_____ 8. vesicle

A. blister, larger than 1 cm

B. blister, smaller than 1 cm

C. cracklike lesion of the skin

D. discolored spot, not elevated

E. excess collagen production after injury

F. fluid-filled sac containing pus

G. sac filled with clear fluid

H. solid elevation, less than 0.5 cm in diameter

Photo ID

V. *Use word parts to build words to label the illustrations.*

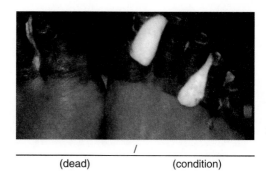

_____ / _____
(dead)   (condition)

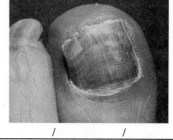

_____ / _____ / _____
(nail) (fungus) (condition)

Word Analysis

VI. *Divide these words into their component parts, and write the meaning of each term.*

1. electrolysis _____

2. ichthyosis _____

3. keratogenesis _____

4. melanocyte _____

5. scleroderma _____

Multiple Choice

VII. *Circle the correct answer for each multiple choice question.*

1. Which test determines an individual's reaction to a substance by observing the results after injecting the substance or applying it to the skin? (needle aspiration, punch biopsy, skin culture, skin test)

2. Which of the following destroys tissue using very cold temperatures? (cryotherapy, electrodesiccation, heliotherapy, ultrasound)

3. Which of the following means removal of foreign material and dead or contaminated tissue from an infected or traumatic lesion until surrounding healthy tissue is exposed? (débridement, necrosis, pyemia, rhytidectomy)

4. Which term means pertaining to the armpit? (adipose, alopecia, apocrine, axillary)

5. Which of the following is an inflammatory skin disease that begins on the scalp but may involve other areas, particularly the eyebrows? (acne vulgaris, basal cell carcinoma, seborrheic dermatitis, verruca)

6. Which of the following is a test that is used to diagnose cystic fibrosis? (shaved specimen, skin biopsy, sebum analysis, sweat test)

7. Which term means a disease characterized by chronic hardening and thickening of the skin? (ecchymosis, Kaposi sarcoma, keratosis, scleroderma)

8. Which of the following is a common name for decubitus ulcer? (bedsore, keratoma, mole, wart)

9. In describing a burn by "thickness," which type of burn is characterized by blisters?
(deep partial-thickness, deep full-thickness, full-thickness, superficial partial-thickness)

10. Which term means the death of areas of tissue or bone surrounded by healthy parts?
(atrophy, erosion, fissure, necrosis)

Fill In the Blanks
VIII. *Complete the sentences by writing a term in each blank space.*

1. Cells of the epidermis contain _____, which is a scleroprotein.

2. The corium is another name for the layer of skin called the _____.

3. An oily material secreted by the sebaceous glands is called _____.

4. Sweat glands, also called _____ glands, produce perspiration.

5. Diaphoresis means excessive _____.

Writing Terms
IX. *Write words for the following.*

1. a boil _____

2. a contagious dermatitis caused by the itch mite _____

3. a torn, jagged wound _____

4. absence of pigment in the skin, hair, and nails _____

5. another name for a bruise _____

6. any disease of the nails _____

7. baldness _____

8. condition in which the skin is dry and scaly _____

9. heatstroke or sunstroke _____

10. superficial infection involving hair follicles _____

Say and Check
Say aloud the terms you wrote for Exercise IX. Use the Companion CD to check your pronunciations.

Greater Comprehension

Health Care Reports

X. *Read the following operative report and, using your critical thinking skills, answer the questions that follow the report.*

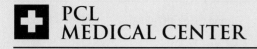

PCL
MEDICAL CENTER

7700 Lexicon Way
St. Louis, MO 63146

Phone (555) 437-0000 • Fax (555) 437-0001

OPERATION REPORT

Patient Name: Ames M. Weaver   **ID No.:** 016-0003   **Date of Surgery:** Jul 11, ----
Surgeon: Mark Bonneville, MD   **Anesthesia:** General endotracheal by Dr. Reid
PREOPERATIVE DIAGNOSIS: Improvised explosive device (IED) soft-tissue wounds, right lower extremity
POSTOPERATIVE DIAGNOSIS: Improvised explosive device (IED) soft-tissue wounds, right lower extremity
MATERIAL FORWARDED TO THE LABORATORY: Cultures were taken from his small proximal wound for microbiology
OPERATIONS PERFORMED
1. Irrigation and debridement   2. Wound VAC, right thigh wounds
Estimated blood loss: Minimal
Preop antibiotics: Ancef 2 grams
Complications: None
Tourniquet time: None
PREOPERATIVE HISTORY: Patient is a 24-year-old active duty airman assigned to Air Force Special Forces in Iraq. On 3 July, he sustained wounds from an IED and was initially treated with tourniquet, then had débridements in Iraq, then in Landstuhl. He was brought to PCL Clinic 9 July where he underwent irrigation and débridement by the General Surgery team. He was immediately transferred to my service when Dr. Janskin had to go TDY out of the country.

Past Medical History, negative. Past Surgical History: Childhood tonsillectomy. Allergies, none. Medications, just what he has been given at PCL.

I discussed all the risks of repeat surgery and our recommendations with the patient. He is a Senior Airman in the Air Force. I also discussed with him the need to consider stopping tobacco use. He indicated his understanding of all the many risks of surgery. He also understood the recommendations for repeated irrigation and débridement. Patient gave informed consent.

DESCRIPTION OF OPERATION: The patient was identified in the preoperative area, and his operative site was signed. He was brought to the operating room where a final time-out was called. He then underwent satisfactory endotracheal anesthesia. He was placed in the left lateral decubitus position. His large lateral thigh wound required minimal débridement. His other, smaller wounds also required minimal débridement. Copious irrigation was carried out.

The wound VAC was placed in his large lateral thigh wound with vessel loops. In addition, his distal thigh wound, which was the largest of the three smaller wounds, had a wound VAC placed. A bridge was placed on top of plastic, not on top of skin. His other two wounds were temporarily closed with plans to reopen and repeat I&D them. Cultures were taken from his small proximal wound.

The patient was extubated and taken to recovery room in good condition.

1. What is meant by débridement? _____

_____

2. What is meant by irrigation as described in the operation? _____

_____

3. Explain wound VAC. _____

_____

4. What does the abbreviation I&D mean? _____

XI. *Write the meanings of the underlined terms in the following H&P exam.*

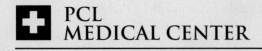

PCL MEDICAL CENTER

7700 Lexicon Way
St. Louis, MO 63146

Phone (555) 437-0000 • Fax (555) 437-0001

HISTORY & PHYSICAL EXAM

Patient Name: Rodney Masters   **ID No.:** 016-0002   **DOB:** Sept 28, ----
Admitted: 8/15/——   **Sex:** Male   **PCP:** Carlos Ayala, MD
CHIEF COMPLAINT: Warmth, edema, <u>erythema</u> from right knee to calf; febrile with <u>induration</u>
HISTORY: 39-year-old white man who scratched an area of probable <u>folliculitis</u> on his right lower extremity 3 days before admission. Patient had been water skiing in the river 2 days before that. He noticed discomfort within 12 hours after coming home from the river.
PAST HISTORY: Insulin-dependent diabetes mellitus for 2 years. Has frequent bacterial skin infections, very slow to heal. Has had no major surgeries.
FAMILY HISTORY: Mother is age 60 with <u>discoid lupus erythematosus</u>. Father, age 73, with history of <u>eczema</u>. Patient is married with 3 children, all L&W.
PHYSICAL EXAMINATION: Temp 100.8°F, otherwise VS are WNL. Exam limited to RLE, which is red and inflamed. Slight amount of serous drainage from lesion. Pitting edema is present.
LABORATORY TESTS: WBCs 12.0. Wound culture showed light growth of MRSA.
DIAGNOSIS: <u>Cellulitis</u>, right lower extremity
PLAN: IV antibiotic treatment. Dr. Ayala will follow for diabetes management.

Define:

1. erythema _____

2. induration _____

3. folliculitis _____

4. discoid lupus erythematosus _____

5. eczema _____

6. cellulitis _____

XII. *After reading the following Consult, match the descriptions (1 to 7) to the terms or phrases (A to G).*

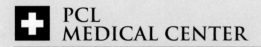

PCL MEDICAL CENTER

7700 Lexicon Way
St. Louis, MO 63146

Phone 555.437.0000 • Fax 555.437.0001

PLASTIC SURGERY CONSULTATION

Patient Name: Michael Turner   **ID No.:** 016-0001   **Date of Exam:** Feb 4, ----
REASON FOR CONSULTATION: Hypertrophic scarring and keloid formation, left upper extremity and neck
HISTORY OF PRESENT ILLNESS: 34-year-old black man who suffered 25% TBSA full- and partial-thickness flame burns to bilateral upper extremities and neck after tripping and falling into a campfire 4 months ago. Patient was treated with Silvadene dressing changes and split-thickness skin grafts to the bilateral upper extremities and neck with right and left thighs

as donor sites. Donor sites were treated with a single layer of petrolatum gauze and have healed well. Right upper extremity graft site has healed without sepsis or excessive scarring. Left upper extremity and neck show hypertrophic scarring and keloid formation despite his wearing elastic pressure bandage.

PAST MEDICAL HISTORY: Unremarkable except for onychomycosis of the toenails

FAMILY HISTORY: Mother, age 68, with melanoma. Father, age 70, with HTN and seborrheic dermatitis.

ALLERGIES: Neomycin ointment

MEDICATIONS: See chart for list of pain meds.

IMPRESSION: Keloid formation, left upper extremity and neck

PLAN: Surgery to correct keloid formation, left upper extremity and neck

_____ 1. an overgrowth of collagenous scar tissue

_____ 2. areas of skin removed from one site and transplanted to another site

_____ 3. fungal condition of the nails

_____ 4. infection

_____ 5. malignant skin cancer

_____ 6. pertaining to an increase in size

_____ 7. the classification of the type of burn

A. hypertrophic
B. keloid formation
C. melanoma
D. onychomycosis
E. sepsis
F. split-thickness skin grafts
G. 25% TBSA (total body surface area) full- and partial-thickness

Spelling

XIII. *Circle each misspelled term in this list and write the correct spelling.*

abrasion   aerosol   ektoderm   hydradenitis   onykectomy

Interpreting Abbreviations

XIV. *Write the meaning of each abbreviation.*

1. ABA _____

2. DLE _____

3. HSV-1 _____

4. TBSA _____

5. ung _____

Pronunciation

XV. *Pronunciation is shown for several medical terms. Indicate the primary accent in each term by marking it with an ´.*

1. cellulitis (sel u li tis)

2. dermabrasion (dər mə bra shən)

3. ichthyosis (ik the o sis)

4. urticaria (ur tĭ kar e ə)

5. xeroderma (zēr o der mə)

 Say and Check

Say aloud the five terms in Exercise XV. Use the Companion CD to check your pronunciations. In addition, be prepared to pronounce aloud these terms in class:

actinic keratosis	escharatomy	onychopathy	suppurative
antipruritic	hidradenitis	pediculosis	ungual
arrector pili muscle	ichthyoid	purulence	verruca
atrophy	lipectomy	rhytidoplasty	wheal
eczema	mycodermatitis	seborrheic dermatitis	xerosis

Categorizing Terms

XVI. *Classify the terms in the left columns by selecting A, B, C, D, or E.*

_____ 1. diathermy

_____ 2. eczema

_____ 3. escharotomy

_____ 4. liposuction

_____ 5. pediculosis

_____ 6. rhytidectomy

_____ 7. shaved specimen

_____ 8. skin flap

_____ 9. ungual

_____ 10. xerosis

A. anatomy
B. diagnostic test or procedure
C. pathology
D. surgery
E. therapy

Challenge

XVII. *Determine the meanings of these words by dividing them into their component parts, then define each term.*

1. anhidrosis _____

2. dermatographia _____

3. hyperkeratosis _____

4. onychodystrophy _____

5. trichophagia _____

(Check your answers with the solutions in Appendix VI.)

 PRONUNCIATION LIST

Use the Companion CD to review the terms that have been presented. Look closely at the spelling of each term as it is pronounced and be sure you know the meaning of each term.

abrasion
abscess
accessory skin structures
acne vulgaris
actinic keratosis
adipose
aerosol
albinism
albino
allograft
alopecia
amputation
antibiotic
antimicrobial
antipruritic
antiseptic
apocrine sweat gland
arrector pili muscle
aseptic
atrophy
autograft
axillary
basal cell carcinoma
bulla
burn
cellulitis
collagen injection

contact dermatitis
contusion
corium
corn
crust
cryotherapy
curet
curettage
cutaneous
cyanosis
cyst
cystic fibrosis
débride
débridement
decubitus ulcer
deep partial-thickness burn
dehiscence
dermabrasion
dermatitis
dermatologist
dermatology
dermatome
dermatomycosis
dermis
diaphoresis
diathermy

discoid lupus
    erythematosus
ecchymosis
ectoderm
eczema
electrodessication
electrolysis
endoderm
epidermal
epidermis
erythema
escharotomy
exfoliation
fissure
folliculitis
frostbite
full-thickness burn
furuncle
heat hydrotherapy
heliotherapy
herpes simplex virus
herpes zoster
hidradenitis
histocompatibility
hyperthermia
hypothermia
hypoxic tissue

ichthyoid
ichthyosis
incompatibility
induration
integument
integumentary
jaundice
Kaposi sarcoma
keloid
keratin
keratogenesis
keratoma
keratosis
laceration
lesion
lipectomy
lipolysis
lipoma
liposuction
lunula
macule
malignant melanoma
melanocyte
mesoderm
mycodermatitis
necrosis
necrotic

nevus
nodule
ointment
onychectomy
onychomalacia
onychomycosis
onychopathy
onychophagia
onychophagist
onychosis
papule
pediculosis
perspiration
petechia
photodermatitis
plaque
primary lesions
psoriasis

punch biopsy
puncture
purulence
pustule
pyogenesis
pyrexia
retinoid
rhytidoplasty
ringworm
rule of nines
scabies
scales
scleroderma
scleroprotein
sebaceous gland
seborrhea
seborrheic dermatitis
seborrheic keratosis

sebum
secondary lesions
sepsis
shaved specimen
shingles
skin flap
squamous cell carcinoma
subcutaneous adipose
    tissue
sudoriferous gland
superficial partial-thickness
    burn
suppuration
suppurative
suturing
thermoplegia
tinea
topical anesthetic

topical antimicrobial agent
topical medication
transcutaneous electrical
    nerve stimulation
transdermal drug delivery
trichopathy
trichosis
ulcer
ungual
urticaria
verruca
vesicle
wheal
wound
wound irrigation
xeroderma
xerosis

Español ENHANCING SPANISH COMMUNICATION

English	Spanish (pronunciation)
allergy	alergia (ah-LEHR-he-ah)
burn	quemadura (kay-mah-DOO-rah)
dermatology	dermatología (der-mah-to-lo-HEE-ah)
eyebrow	ceja (SAY-hah)
eyelash	pestaña (pes-TAH-nyah)
gland	glándula (GLAN-doo-lah)
hair	pelo (PAY-lo)
hives	roncha (RON-chah)
injury	daño (DAH-nyo)
nails	uñas (OO-nyahs)
perspiration	sudor (soo-DOR)
skin	piel (pe-EL)
ulcer	ulcera (OOL-say-rah)
wound	lesión (lay-se-ON)

Endocrine System

17

LEARNING GOALS

Basic Understanding

In this chapter you will learn to do the following:

1. State the function of the endocrine system, and analyze associated terms.
2. Write the meaning of the word parts associated with the endocrine system, and use them to build and analyze terms.
3. Define homeostasis, and describe two ways in which the pituitary gland cooperates with the nervous system to maintain it.
4. Write the names of the other glands of the endocrine system, describe their functions, and define the terms associated with these structures.
5. Recognize the hormones associated with the major endocrine organs and their target organs or functions.
6. Write the names of the diagnostic tests and procedures used for assessment of the endocrine system when given descriptions of the procedures, or match the procedures with their descriptions.
7. Write the names of endocrine system pathologies when given their descriptions, or match the pathologies with their descriptions.
8. Match the terms for endocrine system surgical and therapeutic interventions with their descriptions, or write the names of the interventions when given their descriptions.

Greater Comprehension

9. Use word parts from this chapter to determine the meanings of terms to answer questions about the terms in a health care report.
10. Spell the terms accurately.
11. Pronounce the terms correctly.
12. Write the meanings of the abbreviations.
13. Categorize terms as anatomy, diagnostic test or procedure, pathology, surgery, or therapy.

MAJOR SECTIONS OF THIS CHAPTER:

❑ **ANATOMY AND PHYSIOLOGY**
  Hormones of the Neurohypophysis
  Hormones of the Adenohypophysis
  Other Endocrine Tissues
❑ **DIAGNOSTIC TESTS AND PROCEDURES**

❑ **PATHOLOGIES**
  Pituitary, Thyroid, and Parathyroid
    Disorders
  Adrenal, Pancreas, and Breast Disorders
❑ **SURGICAL AND THERAPEUTIC INTERVENTIONS**

FUNCTION FIRST

The endocrine system cooperates with the nervous system to regulate body activities. This is accomplished by endocrine hormones that affect various processes throughout the body, such as growth, metabolism, and secretions from other organs.

ANATOMY AND PHYSIOLOGY

17-1 The **endocrine** (en´do-krīn, en´do-krin) **system** and the nervous system work together to maintain homeostasis (ho″me-o-sta´sis). Homeostasis (home[o], sameness or constant + -stasis, stopping or controlling) is a relative constancy in the internal environment of the body.

The nervous system communicates with the endocrine system through nerve impulses. The endocrine system acts through chemical messengers called hormones. Working together, the nervous system and the endocrine system help maintain constancy in the body that is called

homeostasis

_____.

secrete

17-2 You have learned that the combining form crin(o) means to _____.
The endocrine (endo-, inside + -crine, to secrete) system is composed of the ductless glands and other structures that secrete hormones into the bloodstream. The ductless glands are **endocrine glands,** which secrete **hormones** (hor´mōnz), chemical substances, into the blood that are carried to another part of the body, where they exert specific physiologic effects. Write the name of the chemical secretions of endocrine glands:

hormones

_____.

17-3 A **gland** is an organ that has specialized cells that secrete or excrete substances that are not related to the gland's ordinary metabolism. There are many glands in the body.

> ➤ **KEY** POINT Glands are classified as either exocrine or endocrine glands. The prefix exo- means outside, and **exo/crine** (ek´so-krin) **glands** have ducts that enable them to empty secretions onto an external or an internal body surface. A sweat gland is an example of an exocrine gland. Endocrine glands (for example, the thyroid and pituitary glands) are ductless, so they secrete their hormones into the bloodstream. Compare endocrine and exocrine glands (Figure 17-1).

ducts

Unlike exocrine glands, endocrine glands have no _____,
so they secrete their hormones into the bloodstream.

17-4 Dysfunctions in hormone production fall into two categories: either a deficiency or an excess in secretion. A deficiency is called **hypo/secretion** (hi″po-se-kre´shən). Excess secretion is

hypersecretion
(hi″pər-se-kre´shən)

called _____.

The organ or structure toward which the effects of a hormone are primarily directed is called the **target organ.** If a hormone has a specific effect on the thyroid gland, then the thyroid is the target organ. If a hormone has a specific effect on the ovaries, then the ovary is the

target

_____ organ.

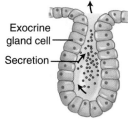

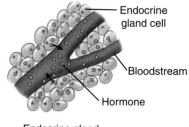

Exocrine gland cell

Secretion

Exocrine gland (has duct)

A

Endocrine gland cell

Bloodstream

Hormone

Endocrine gland (ductless)

B

Figure 17-1 Comparison of the structure of an exocrine gland vs. an endocrine gland. A, Exocrine glands, such as sweat glands, are simple glands that have a duct that enable them to empty secretions onto a body surface. **B,** Endocrine glands are ductless and produce and secrete hormones into the blood or lymph nodes.

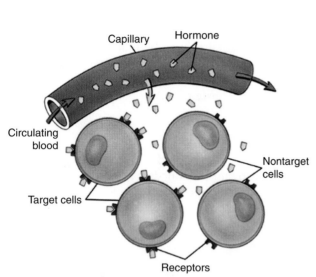

Figure 17-2 The target cell concept. The hormone recognizes the target tissue through receptors (the site that interacts with the hormone), so the hormones act only on cells that have receptors specific for that hormone. The shape of the receptor determines which hormone can react with it.

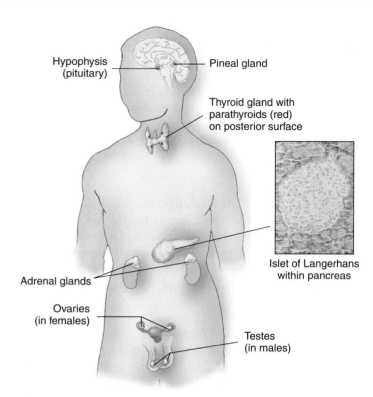

Figure 17-3 Location of major glands of the endocrine system.

---

hypophysis
(hi-pof′ə-sis)

17-5 The target cell concept explains how only certain cells of specific organs are affected by a specific hormone (Figure 17-2). Hormones are either proteins or steroids (ster′oidz). Most hormones in the human body are proteins, with the exception of the sex hormones and those from the adrenal cortex, which are **steroids** (a special group of lipids). Proteins are quickly inactivated in the digestive tract, so if there is a deficiency, these hormones are administered by injection. Sex hormones and other steroids can be taken orally.

17-6 The locations of the major glands of the endocrine system are shown in Figure 17-3. Note that the **pituitary** (pĭ-too′ĭ-tar″e) **gland** is also called the _____. This gland is a small, round structure about 1 cm (or ½ inch) in diameter that is attached by a stalk at the base of the brain.

kidneys

An **adrenal** (ə-dre′nəl) **gland** lies above each of the two kidneys. **Supra/renal** (soo″prə-re′nəl) means above the _____. Sometimes the adrenal glands are called the suprarenal glands.

The ovaries and testes are **gonads** (go′nads)—glands that provide ova and sperm, respectively.

17-7 Observing the endocrine glands that are labeled on the right side of Figure 17-3, the **pineal*** (pin′e-əl) **gland,** also called the pineal body, is shaped like a pine cone and is attached to the posterior part of the brain.

The **thyroid** (thi′roid), also called the thyroid gland, is located at the front of the neck. Note that it consists of bilateral lobes that are connected by a narrow strip of thyroid tissue. **Parathyroid** (par″ə-thi′roid) **glands** are located near the thyroid (as the name implies). They are actually embedded in its posterior surface.

The **pancreas** is an elongated structure that has digestive functions as well as endocrine functions. Clusters of cells within the pancreas that perform the endocrine function are shown in Figure 17-3. These clusters of cells in the pancreas are the _____ **of Langerhans** (lahng′ər-hahnz).

islets

---

*Pineal (Latin: pineus, *pine cone*).

Learn the meanings of the following terms.

Word Parts: Endocrine Anatomy and Physiology

Word Part	Meaning	Word Part	Meaning
Combining Forms Associated with Anatomy		**Word Parts Associated with Function**	
aden(o)	gland	andr(o)	male or masculine
adren(o), adrenal(o)	adrenal gland	calc(i)	calcium
cortic(o)	cortex	gigant(o)	large
gonad(o)	gonad	gluc(o)	glucose
mamm(o), mast(o)	breast	glyc(o), glycos(o)	sugar
pancreat(o)	pancreas	insulin(o)	insulin
parathyroid(o)	parathyroid glands	iod(o)	iodine
pituitar(o), hypophys(o)	pituitary gland	ket(o)	ketone
thyr(o), thyroid(o)	thyroid gland	lact(o)	milk
		trop(o)	to stimulate
		-crine	secrete
		-dipsia	thirst
		-physis	growth
		-tropic	stimulating
		-tropin	that which stimulates

17-8 Some hormones of the endocrine glands are released in response to the nervous system (i.e., the adrenal gland releases adrenaline in response to the sympathetic nervous system in stressful situations). In addition, the pituitary gland supplies hormones that act directly on cells or stimulate other glands that govern numerous vital processes. Because many endocrine glands respond to hormones produced by the pituitary gland, it is nicknamed "the **master gland**."

➤ **KEY** POINT <u>The pituitary gland has many names.</u> The pituitary gland is also called the pituitary, the hypophysis cerebri, or simply the hypophysis. The suffix -physis means growth. The pituitary is nicknamed the master gland.

under

The hypo/physis was so named because it grows _____ the cerebrum.

EXERCISE 1

1. Write the names of six major glands of the endocrine system: _____

_____

EXERCISE 2

Fill in the blanks in these sentences.

1. The endocrine system and the _____ system cooperate to maintain homeostasis.

2. The name of the master gland is the _____.

3. An organ that has specialized cells that secrete or excrete substances that are not related to its ordinary metabolism

   is called a/an _____.

4. Chemical substances that are produced in one part or organ and initiate or regulate the activity of an organ in

   another part are called _____.

nerve

neurohypophysis

gland

anterior

17-9 Examine the diagram of the pituitary and its target organs in Figure 17-4. The pituitary is divided structurally and functionally into an anterior lobe and a posterior lobe.

The posterior lobe of the pituitary is called the **neurohypophysis** (noor″o-hi-pof′ə-sis). The combining form neur(o) means _____. This lobe contains ends of neurons, the cell bodies of which are located in the **hypothalamus** (hi″po-thal′ə-məs), a portion of the lower part of the brain. The hormones of the neurohypophysis are stored in the axon endings and are released when a nerve impulse travels down the axon.

The portion of the pituitary that releases hormones when stimulated by nervous impulses from the hypothalamus is called the _____.

17-10 The anterior lobe of the pituitary is called the **adenohypophysis** (ad″ə-no-hi-pof′ĭ-sis). The word part aden(o) refers to a _____. This lobe is the glandular part of the hypophysis. The release of hormones from the adenohypophysis is controlled by regulating hormones produced by the hypothalamus.

17-11 Look again at Figure 17-4. Abbreviations such as ADH, STH, and MSH stand for pituitary hormones. The two hormones produced by the posterior lobe of the pituitary act directly on specific cells of the kidneys, the breasts, and the uterus.

The anterior lobe of the pituitary produces many hormones, several of which act on other endocrine glands, causing them also to secrete hormones. The green arrows in Figure 17-4 represent anterior pituitary hormones. Which lobe of the pituitary releases the greater number of hormones? _____ lobe

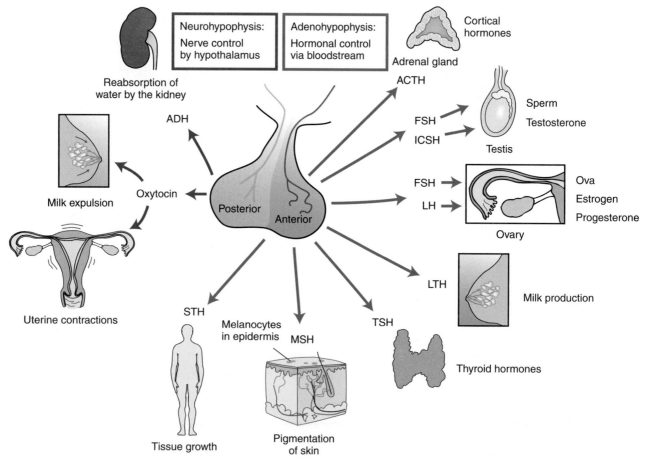

Figure 17-4 The pituitary, the master gland. The posterior pituitary lobe *(shown on the left)* is controlled by nervous stimulation by the hypothalamus and releases two hormones. In contrast, the anterior pituitary lobe is controlled by hypothalamic hormones brought by the blood stream and secretes many hormones.

EXERCISE 3

Word Analysis. *Break these words into their component parts by placing a slash between the word parts. Write the meaning of each term.*

1. adenohypophysis _____

2. neurohypophysis _____

3. hypothalamus _____

4. exocrine _____

5. homeostasis _____

Say and Check

Say aloud the terms in Exercise 3. Use the Companion CD to check your pronunciations.

HORMONES OF THE NEUROHYPOPHYSIS

17-12 The hypothalamus controls the neurohypophysis, the posterior lobe, by direct nervous stimulation.

> ➤ **KEY** POINT The hypothalamus synthesizes two hormones that are stored in the neurohypophysis. Antidiuretic (an″te-, an″ti-di″u-ret′tik) hormone and oxytocin (ok″se-to′sin) are synthesized in the hypothalamus and transported to the neurohypophysis for storage. On stimulation by the hypothalamus, the neurohypophysis releases them into the bloodstream.

against

Antidiuretic hormone (ADH) affects the volume of urine excreted. The prefix anti- means _____. **Diuretic** (di″u-ret′ik) means increasing urine excretion or the amount of urine. It also means an agent that promotes urine excretion. Anti/diuretic hormone acts against a diuretic. It acts in the kidneys to reabsorb water from the urine, producing concentrated urine. Absence of this hormone produces **diuresis** (di″u-re′sis), passage of large amounts of dilute urine.

17-13 Some common caffeinated drinks (tea, coffee, soda) and even water can act as diuretics. Physicians also prescribe diuretic drugs to rid the body of excess fluid in patients with edema.

increase

Diuretics (increase or decrease?) _____ urination. Anti/diuretic hormone causes a decrease in the amount of water lost in urination.

17-14 The second hormone, **oxytocin,** is released in large quantities just before a female gives birth. It causes uterine contractions, thus inducing childbirth. It also acts on the mammary glands to stimulate the release of milk. Write the name of the pituitary hormone that causes contraction

oxytocin

of the uterus and acts on the mammary glands: _____.

HORMONES OF THE ADENOHYPOPHYSIS

STH, MSH, LH, FSH, and TSH

17-15 The hypothalamus regulates the adenohypophysis, the anterior lobe, by producing regulatory and inhibitory hormones.

> ➤ **KEY** POINT Regulatory and inhibitory hormones stimulate or inhibit the adenohypophysis. Hypothalamic regulatory and inhibitory hormones act on the adenohypophysis to either stimulate or inhibit the secretion of its hormones. When the adenohypophysis secretes its hormones, they travel through the bloodstream and bring about changes in other organs, often another endocrine gland. Note that the control from the hypothalamus to the adenohypophysis is hormonal, whereas the control of the neurohypophysis—as mentioned above—is through nervous stimulation.

The adenohypophysis releases several hormones that regulate a large range of body activities. Look again at the target organs of these hormones (see Figure 17-4). Most of these pituitary secretions stimulate other glands, and many of their names contain trop(o), which means to stimulate or turn. **Tropic** (tro´pik) is an adjective that means to _____.

stimulate

17-16 Growth hormone (GH) is also called **somato/tropic hormone** (STH), or **somatotropin** (so´mə-to-tro˝pin). The suffix -tropin refers to that which stimulates. Somato/tropin is the hormone that _____ body growth.

stimulates

This hormone increases the rate of growth and maintains size once growth is attained. It is called GH or _____.

somatotropin

17-17 Melanocyte-stimulating hormone (MSH) from the pituitary stimulates melanocytes distributed throughout the epidermis. MSH promotes pigmentation and controls the amount of melanin produced by melanocytes. The name melanin (mel´ə-nin) implies the color _____. **Melanin** is a black or dark brown pigment that occurs naturally in the hair, skin, and parts of the eye.

black

17-18 The combining form gonad(o) means gonads (ovaries or testes).

> ➤ **KEY** POINT <u>Two important pituitary hormones have the gonads as target organs.</u> **Gonado/tropic** (go˝nə-do-tro´pik) **hormones** stimulate the ovaries of the female and the testes of the male. **Follicle-stimulating hormone** (FSH) and **luteinizing** (loo´te-in-i˝zing) **hormone** (LH) are produced by the adenohypophysis.

gonadotropin
(go˝nə-do-tro´pin)

Write a word that means a hormone that stimulates the gonads: _____.
FSH and LH are gonadotropins.

gonads

17-19 Gonad/al (go-nad´əl) means pertaining to the _____.
Gonadotropic (go˝nə-do-tro´pik) is an adjective that means stimulating the gonads. The first gonadotropic hormone, FSH, stimulates the ovaries to secrete estrogen and acts on the follicle (as its name implies). FSH stimulates production of sperm in the testes of male individuals.

LH stimulates ovulation and production of progesterone in the female ovary. LH often is called **interstitial cell–stimulating hormone** (ICSH) in male individuals because it promotes the growth of the interstitial cells of the testes and the secretion of testosterone.

17-20 The period of life at which reproduction becomes possible is **puberty** (pu´bər-te). It is recognized by maturation of the genitals and appearance of secondary sex characteristics. The onset of puberty is triggered by the hypothalamus and the anterior pituitary. FSH and LH act on the testes and ovaries (Figure 17-5). Male sex hormones are collectively called **androgens** (an´dro-jəns), with **testosterone** (tes-tos´tə-rōn) being the most abundant.

Figure 17-5 reinforces the concept that the main hormones secreted by the ovaries and testes are estrogen and _____, respectively. **Progesterone** (pro-jes´tə-rōn) is another important female hormone produced mainly by the ovaries (and by the placenta during pregnancy) and in minute amounts by the adrenal cortex.

testosterone

17-21 The combining form andr(o) means _____ or masculine. Testosterone is the most potent androgen and is produced in large quantities by the testes, making that produced by the adrenal glands insignificant in most cases. **Andro/genic** (an˝dro-jen´ik) means producing _____ characteristics or masculinization. In women, the masculinization effect of androgen secretion may become evident after menopause.

male

masculine

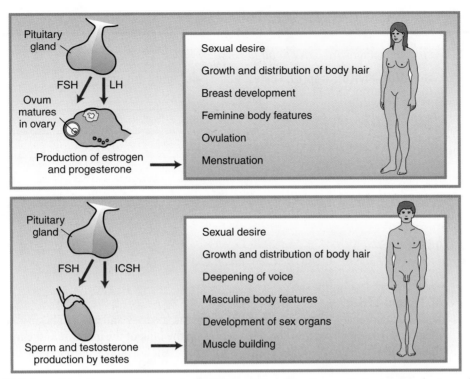

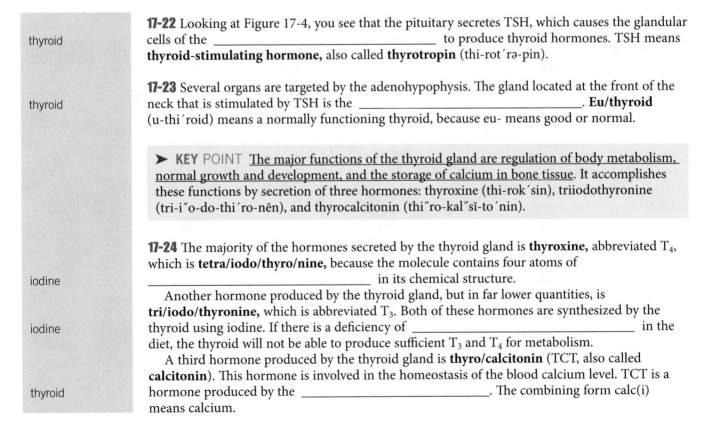

Figure 17-5 Secondary female and male sexual characteristics. The changes that occur at puberty are brought about by the hypothalamus and the anterior pituitary. Changes in the secretions of FSH and LH bring about changes in the ovaries and testes and the hormones they produce.

thyroid

17-22 Looking at Figure 17-4, you see that the pituitary secretes TSH, which causes the glandular cells of the _____ to produce thyroid hormones. TSH means **thyroid-stimulating hormone,** also called **thyrotropin** (thi-rot′rə-pin).

thyroid

17-23 Several organs are targeted by the adenohypophysis. The gland located at the front of the neck that is stimulated by TSH is the _____. **Eu/thyroid** (u-thi′roid) means a normally functioning thyroid, because eu- means good or normal.

> ➤ **KEY** POINT <u>The major functions of the thyroid gland are regulation of body metabolism, normal growth and development, and the storage of calcium in bone tissue.</u> It accomplishes these functions by secretion of three hormones: thyroxine (thi-rok′sin), triiodothyronine (tri-i″o-do-thi′ro-nēn), and thyrocalcitonin (thi″ro-kal″sĭ-to′nin).

iodine

17-24 The majority of the hormones secreted by the thyroid gland is **thyroxine,** abbreviated T_4, which is **tetra/iodo/thyro/nine,** because the molecule contains four atoms of _____ in its chemical structure.

iodine

Another hormone produced by the thyroid gland, but in far lower quantities, is **tri/iodo/thyronine,** which is abbreviated T_3. Both of these hormones are synthesized by the thyroid using iodine. If there is a deficiency of _____ in the diet, the thyroid will not be able to produce sufficient T_3 and T_4 for metabolism.

thyroid

A third hormone produced by the thyroid gland is **thyro/calcitonin** (TCT, also called **calcitonin**). This hormone is involved in the homeostasis of the blood calcium level. TCT is a hormone produced by the _____. The combining form calc(i) means calcium.

Build It! *Use the following word parts to build terms.*

eu-, andr(o), melan(o), somat(o), thyr(o), trop(o), -cyte, -genic, -ic, -oid, -tropin

1. that which stimulates body growth _____/_____

2. cell that produces melanin _____/_____

3. normal thyroid function _____/_____/_____

4. producing masculine characteristics _____/_____

5. to stimulate _____/_____

Say and Check

Say aloud the terms you wrote for Exercise 4. Use the Companion CD to check your pronunciations.

ACTH and LTH

17-25 Each adrenal (ə-dreʹnəl) gland has two parts, a cortex and a medulla, and each part has its own functions. The outer **cortex** (korʹteks) makes up the bulk of the gland, and the inner portion is called the **medulla** (mə-dulʹə). Table 17-1 lists the important hormones produced by the adrenal glands.

> ➤ **KEY** POINT The cortex and medulla of the adrenal gland are stimulated by different means, and they secrete different hormones. The hypothalamus influences both portions, but the medulla receives direct nervous stimulation. The cortex is stimulated by the **adrenocorticotropic** (ə-dreʺno-korʺtĭ-ko-troʹpik) **hormone** (ACTH) brought by the circulating blood.

TABLE 17-1	Hormones Secreted by the Adrenal Gland		
Gland	**Hormone**	**Target Tissue**	**Principal Action**
Adrenal cortex	Mineralocorticoids (main one is aldosterone)	Kidney	Increases water retention by changing sodium and potassium reabsorption in the kidney tubules
	Glucocorticoids (main ones are cortisol and cortisone)	Most body tissue	Increases blood glucose levels; inhibits inflammation and the immune response
	Androgens, estrogens	Most body tissue	Secreted in such small amounts that the effect is generally masked by ovarian and testicular hormones
Adrenal medulla	Epinephrine, norepinephrine	Heart and blood vessels, liver, adipose	Increases heart rate and blood pressure, increases blood flow and blood glucose level, helps the body cope with stress

17-26 Mineralocorticoids (minʺər-əl-o-korʹtĭ-koids), glucocorticoids (glooʺko-korʹtĭ-koids), androgens, and estrogens are secreted by the adrenal _____.
Mineralo/corticoids help maintain water balance in the body. As the name implies, **gluco/corticoids** increase blood _____, but they also inhibit inflammation. Individuals with severe inflammation, as in the joints, may receive injections of **cortisone** to relieve the pain and inflammation. Cortisone may also be included in topical creams and ointments to relieve skin inflammation. Androgens have masculinizing effects, and **estrogens** have feminizing effects.

cortex

glucose

17-27 ACTH is a hormone secreted by the adenohypophysis that stimulates the adrenal cortex. The combining forms adren(o) and adrenal(o) refer to the adrenal glands.
     Adreno/cortico/tropin (ə-dreʺno-korʺtĭ-ko-troʹpin) is another name for ACTH, the hormone that _____ the adrenal glands.
     The adrenal medulla secretes two hormones: epinephrine (epʺĭ-nefʹrin), also called **adrenaline** (ə-drenʹə-lin), and norepinephrine (noradrenaline). The medulla mostly secretes **epinephrine,**

stimulates

which stimulates the heart. **Norepinephrine** causes blood vessels to constrict. Together they prepare the body for strenuous activity and are sometimes called the fight-or-flight hormones.

17-28 Remembering the meaning of lact(o), the **lactogenic hormone** (LTH), also called **prolactin** (pro-lak′tin), is produced by the anterior pituitary and causes _____ production by the mammary glands.

milk

17-29 The **mammary** (mam′ər-e) **glands** are the two glands of the female breasts that secrete milk. The female breasts are accessory organs of the reproductive system. The breasts are located anterior to the chest muscles, and each breast contains 15 to 20 lobes of glandular tissue that radiate around the nipple. The milk-producing glands of the female are called the _____ glands.

mammary

Structural aspects of the breast are shown in Figure 17-6. The circular pigmented area of skin surrounding the nipple is the **areola** (ə-re′o-lə). **Lobule** (lob′ūl) means small lobe. The lobes are separated by connective and adipose (fatty) tissue. The amount of adipose tissue determines the size of the breasts but not the amount of milk that can be produced.

17-30 **Lacto/genic** means inducing the secretion of milk (lact[o] means milk).

> ➤ **KEY** POINT <u>Changes in the mammary glands prepare the breasts of a pregnant female for</u> <u>**lacto/genesis** (lak′to-jen′ə-sis), the production of milk.</u> The most important hormone that stimulates milk production is prolactin, also called LTH. The mammary glands secrete a cloudy fluid called **colostrum** (kə-los′trəm) the first few days after a female gives birth. Because of both high antibody and protein content, colostrum serves adequately as food for the infant until milk production begins 2 to 3 days after parturition.

17-31 Each breast lobule is drained by its own **lactiferous** (lak-tif′ər-əs) duct, which has a dilated portion called a sinus that serves as a reservoir for milk. The nipple, located near the center of the breast, contains the openings of the milk ducts.

Lactation (lak-ta′shən) is the secretion or ejecting of milk. Milk ejection is a normal reflex in a lactating woman and is elicited by tactile stimulation of the nipple (such as nursing by the infant). Impulses from the nipple to the hypothalamus stimulate the release of _____ by the pituitary gland, which brings about contractions that eject the milk from the breast (Figure 17-7). If a lactating mother stops nursing, milk production usually ceases within a few days.

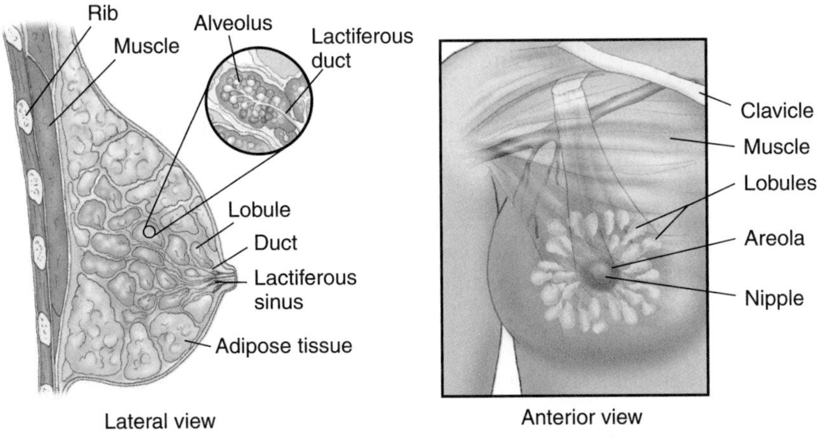

oxytocin

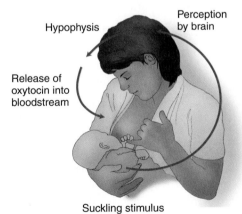

Figure 17-7 Interrelationships of hypothalamus, neurohypophysis, and breast. Suckling by the infant stimulates nerve endings at the nipple. Impulses are carried to the hypothalamus, which causes the neurohypophysis to secrete oxytocin into the blood stream. The oxytocin is carried to the breast, where it causes milk to be expressed into the ducts. Milk begins to flow within 30 seconds to 1 minute after a baby begins to suckle.

Figure 17-6 Structure of the adult female breast, lateral and anterior views. The breasts are mammary glands and function as part of both the endocrine and reproductive systems.

between

17-32 Several adjectives are used when describing locations near the breasts. Remembering that inter- means between, **inter/mammary** (in″tər-mam′ə-re) means situated _____ the breasts. **Retro/mammary** (ret″ro-mam′ər-e) means behind the mammary gland.

EXERCISE 5

Word Analysis. *Break these words into their component parts by placing a slash between the word parts. Write the meaning of each term.*

1. lactogenic   _____

2. adrenal   _____

3. retromammary   _____

4. lactation   _____

5. adrenocorticotropic   _____

Say and Check

Say aloud the terms in Exercise 5. Use the Companion CD to check your pronunciations.

OTHER ENDOCRINE TISSUES

17-33 In addition to the endocrine glands that have been studied in previous sections, the pineal gland, the pancreas, and the parathyroids are considered here with a few other organs that have hormonal activity.

The exact functions of the pineal gland have not been established, but there is evidence that it secretes the hormone **melatonin** (mel″ə-to′nin). The pineal gland usually begins to diminish around the age of 7 years. If degeneration does not occur, the production of melatonin remains high and puberty may be delayed in girls. This indicates that melatonin may inhibit the activities of the ovaries.

pineal

Melatonin is secreted by the _____ gland. In addition to a regulatory function in sexual development, effects of melatonin may influence the sleepiness-wakefulness cycle and mood and may cause a decrease in skin pigmentation.

17-34 Strict regulation of hormonal secretion is important to maintain homeostasis.

> ➤ **KEY** POINT The body uses three different methods to regulate hormones: direct nervous stimulation, secretion of hormones in response to other hormones, and a negative feedback mechanism.

The adrenal medulla is an example of the first method, direct nervous stimulation. The adrenal medulla secretes epinephrine and norepinephrine in response to stimulation by sympathetic nerves.

Tropic hormones cause secretion of other hormones. For example, thyrotropin (TSH) from the anterior pituitary gland causes the thyroid gland to secrete the _____ hormones.

thyroid

The interaction between two important pancreatic hormones and the concentration of glucose in the blood is an example of a negative feedback system. In negative feedback a gland is sensitive to the concentration of a substance that it regulates. Continue reading to see how this works.

17-35 The pancreas has an exocrine portion that secretes digestive enzymes that are carried through a duct to the duodenum and an endocrine portion that secretes hormones into the blood. The endocrine portion consists of many small cell groups called islets of Langerhans. These cells secrete two hormones that have a role in regulating blood glucose levels.

The two hormones secreted by the islets of Langerhans are **glucagon** (gloo´kə-gon) and **insulin** (in´sə-lin). The action of glucagon is to increase blood glucose levels. It is secreted in response to a low concentration of glucose in the blood. This mechanism prevents hypoglycemia (hi″po-gli-se´me-ə), a less than normal amount of _____ in the blood, from occurring between meals. Glucose, which the body uses for energy, is the type of sugar found in blood; therefore, **hypoglycemia** means less than a normal amount of blood glucose.

17-36 The action of insulin is opposite or antagonistic to that of glucagon. Insulin promotes the uptake and utilization of glucose for energy and is secreted in response to a high concentration of glucose in the blood. Because insulin opposes the action of glucagon, the action of insulin brings about a _____ in blood glucose levels.

Elevated glucose levels stimulate the secretion of insulin from the pancreas, and low levels of glucose decrease the secretion of insulin (Figure 17-8).

Insufficient insulin activity may be caused either by insufficient secretion or by insufficient or defective target cells, and leads to diabetes mellitus.

17-37 The parathyroid gland (any of four small structures attached to the dorsal surface of the thyroid) is an endocrine gland not directly controlled by the pituitary but closely linked with the thyroid gland.

> ➤ **KEY** POINT The thyroid gland regulates the parathyroid glands by negative feedback.
> Parathyroid glands secrete **parathyroid hormone** (PTH) or **parathormone** (para- is used here to mean near or beside). PTH increases the blood calcium level and its production and release is regulated by a negative feedback mechanism.

Negative feedback of PTH means that it is secreted in response to low levels of _____ in the blood.

PTH has the opposite effect, or is antagonistic, to calcitonin secreted by the _____ gland.

17-38 In addition to the endocrine glands you have studied, other organs that have some hormonal activity include the stomach, small intestines, thymus, heart, and placenta.

The lining of the stomach produces **gastrin** (gas´trin), which stimulates the production of hydrochloric acid, and the enzyme **pepsin** (pep´sin), each being a substance that is used in the digestion of food. The hormone gastrin (gastr[o] means stomach) is secreted in response to food in the stomach. Hormones secreted by the lining of the small intestine stimulate the pancreas and the gallbladder to produce substances that aid in digestion.

The **thymus** (thi´məs) is located near the middle of the chest cavity behind the breastbone. It produces **thymosin** (thi´mo-sin), which assists in the development of lymphocytes, blood cells that function in immunity. The thymus, usually largest at puberty, diminishes in size as an individual reaches adulthood. The hormone produced by the thymus is called _____.

Margin answers: sugar; decrease; calcium; thyroid; thymosin

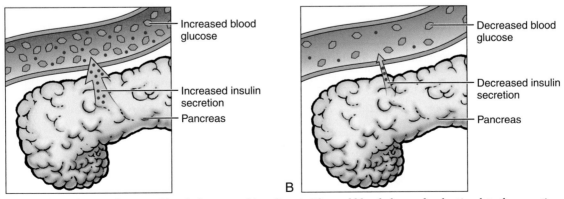

Figure 17-8 Feedback mechanism between blood glucose and insulin. A, Elevated blood glucose levels stimulate the secretion of insulin from the pancreas. **B,** As blood glucose levels decrease, the stimulus for insulin secretion also decreases.

Special cells in the atria, the upper chambers of the heart, produce a hormone, **atriopeptin** (a"tre-o-pep´tin), which increases the loss of sodium and water in urine.

The placenta of a pregnant female produces **human chorionic gonadotropin** (HCG), estrogen, and progesterone, which function to maintain the uterine lining during pregnancy.

17-39 The cells of most tissues throughout the body can produce prostaglandins (pros"tə-glan´dinz) when stimulated, particularly by injury. **Prostaglandins,** potent chemical regulators, are hormone-like substances that have a localized, immediate, and short-term effect on or near the cells where they are produced.

Prostaglandins have many effects, and the same substance sometimes has opposite effects on different tissues. Some of the effects include smooth muscle contraction, involvement in blood clotting, and many aspects of fever and pain. They are believed to be implicated in the symptoms of severe menstrual cramps, premenstrual syndrome, and premature labor. Write the name of these hormone-like substances: _____.

prostaglandins

The major endocrine glands and their secretions are summarized in Table 17-2.

TABLE 17-2 Major Endocrine Glands and Their Secretions

Gland	Primary Secretions
Pituitary gland, anterior lobe	ACTH, FSH, GH, ICSH, LH, LTH, MSH, and TSH
Pituitary gland, posterior lobe	ADH and oxytocin
Adrenal glands, cortex	Aldosterone, cortisol, and androgens
Adrenal glands, medulla	Epinephrine and norepinephrine
Gonads, ovaries	Estrogen, progesterone, and HCG
Gonads, testes	Testosterone
Pancreas (islets of Langerhans)	Insulin and glucagon
Parathyroid glands	PTH
Thyroid gland	Thyroxine, triiodothyronine, and calcitonin
Pineal gland	Melatonin and serotonin
Thymus	Thymosin

EXERCISE 6

Match the hormones in the left columns with the glands on the right that secrete them.

_____ 1. ACTH

_____ 2. antidiuretic hormone

_____ 3. epinephrine

_____ 4. follicle-stimulating hormone

_____ 5. growth hormone

_____ 6. insulin

_____ 7. luteinizing hormone

_____ 8. melanocyte-stimulating hormone

_____ 9. oxytocin

_____ 10. testosterone

_____ 11. thyrocalcitonin

_____ 12. thyrotropin

A. adrenals
B. gonads
C. pancreas
D. pituitary
E. thyroid

EXERCISE 7

Name the target organ for each of the following hormones.

1. ACTH _____

2. antidiuretic hormone _____

3. follicle-stimulating hormone _____

4. luteinizing hormone _____

5. prolactin _____

6. thyrotropin _____

DIAGNOSTIC TESTS AND PROCEDURES

17-40 Most endocrine glands are not accessible for examination in a routine physical examination; however, the thyroid gland and the male gonads are exceptions. The patient's neck can be observed for any unusual bulging over the thyroid area, and the gland can be palpated (Figure 17-9, *A*). Both enlargement and masses are abnormal findings and indicate additional testing is necessary.

palpation

Likewise, the testicles are examined visually for a difference in size and are palpated for masses. The method of using the hands or fingers to examine an organ is called

_____.

Physical indications of endocrine dysfunctions include unusually tall or short stature, coarsening of facial features, edema (accumulation of fluid in the interstitial tissues), hair loss, or excessive facial hair in female individuals.

increased

17-41 Hyper/thyroid/ism (hi″pər-thi′roid-iz-əm) is abnormally _____ activity of the thyroid. A classic finding associated with hyper/thyroid/ism is **ex/ophthal/mos** (ek″sof-thal′mos), that is, protrusion (bulging outward) of the eyeballs. Hyperthyroidism is not always the cause of exophthalmos, and further tests are required. The patient in Figure 17-9, *B* has exophthalmos and a **goiter** (goi′tər), an enlarged thyroid gland that is usually evident as a pronounced swelling in the neck. The metabolic processes of the body are accelerated as a result of the hypersecretion of thyroid hormones. Signs and symptoms include nervousness, fatigue, constant hunger, weight loss, heat intolerance, and palpitations (pounding or racing of the heart).

17-42 Laboratory testing includes blood tests and urine tests, depending on the symptoms. Pituitary studies include blood tests for levels of GH, gonadotropins, and other hormones secreted by the pituitary gland. The gonadotropins are FSH and _____ hormone.

luteinizing

MRI is useful in identifying tumors involving the pituitary or the hypothalamus.

17-43 There are a number of blood tests and radiologic tests to determine thyroid function. Blood studies include testing for TSH, thyroxine, and T_3.

Because the thyroid gland absorbs iodine from the blood to synthesize T_3 and T_4, radio/iodine can be used to study the gland. Radioiodine, ^{131}I, like all radionuclides (radioisotopes), gives off radiation. The **radioactive iodine uptake** (RAIU) **test** measures the ability of the thyroid gland to trap and retain the ^{131}I after oral ingestion. A radiation counter determines the amount of ^{131}I uptake by the thyroid gland. If a less than normal quantity of radioactive iodine is absorbed by the thyroid gland, which condition is expected, hypothyroidism or hyperthyroidism? _____

hypothyroidism

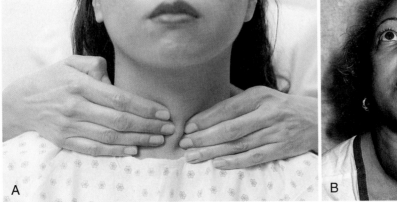
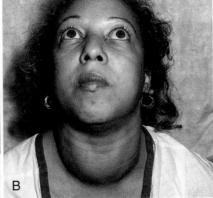

Figure 17-9 Physical examination of the thyroid gland. A, Using the hands to feel for thyroid enlargement or masses. **B,** Observing the patient for thyroid enlargement and exophthalmos, protrusion of the eyeballs. This patient shows both exophthalmos and a goiter, which is an enlarged thyroid gland evidenced by the swelling in the neck.

Thyroid scans consist of administration of a radiopharmaceutical, followed by passage of a scanner over the thyroid and creation of an image of the spatial distribution of the radionuclide.

17-44 Measurement of the levels of PTH, calcium, and phosphate in the blood helps to determine the functioning of the _____ gland.

parathyroid

Several hormones secreted by the adrenal glands can be measured in the blood and urine, as can the level of ACTH in the blood. Computed tomography, sometimes using contrast agents, can be used to detect tumors of the adrenal gland.

17-45 Blood tests to study pancreatic function include fasting blood sugar (FBS), **glycosylated hemoglobin** (HbA$_{1c}$), and **glucose tolerance** (GTT) **tests**. The FBS measures the glucose level in circulating blood. **Hyper/glyc/emia** is a greater than normal amount of glucose in the blood, and **hypo/glyc/emia** is a _____ than normal amount of glucose in the blood. HbA$_{1c}$ is an abbreviation for a type of hemoglobin, HbA$_{1c}$, and is also called glycosylated hemoglobin. HbA$_{1c}$ is more accurate than a fasting blood sugar, because A$_{1c}$ measures the degree of glucose control during the previous 3 months, rather than just 1 day.

less

A GTT test is a test of the body's ability to use carbohydrates by giving a standard dose of glucose to the patient and measuring the blood and urine for glucose levels at regular intervals.

17-46 Urine studies to evaluate pancreatic function include testing for glucose and ketones (ke′tōnz). Neither glucose nor ketone levels are detectable in normal urine specimens. Use glycos(o) and -uria to write a word that means the presence of sugar, especially glucose, in the urine: _____.

glycosuria
(gli″ko-su′re-ə)

Ketones are products of abnormal use of fat in the body (as in diabetes). Excessive production of ketones leads to their excretion in the urine. Combine ket(o) and -uria to write a word that means the presence of ketones in the urine: _____.

ketonuria
(ke′to-nu′re-ə)

Radiologic testing to identify pancreatic tumors or cysts usually includes computed tomography, with or without a contrast medium.

17-47 The breasts are part of several body systems, including the endocrine system. Self-examination of the breasts should be done periodically. A breast self-examination includes observing and palpating the breasts for changes that could indicate disease. Early diagnosis of breast cancer greatly improves the chance of survival.

Mammo/graphy (mə-mog′rə-fe) is a diagnostic procedure that uses x-rays to study the soft tissues of the breast. It is used as a screening test to detect various benign conditions and malignant tumors of the breast. The radiographic image produced in mammography is called a

mammogram
(mam′ə-gram)

_____.

Figure 17-10 is a mammogram showing carcinoma of the breast.

17-48 Breast masses are one of the most common disorders of the breast; and fortunately, most masses are benign.

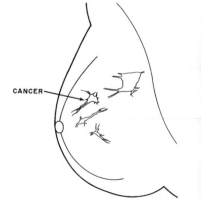
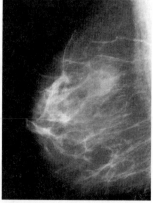

CANCER

Figure 17-10 Mammogram, including a drawing, of cancer of the breast. The *light areas* indicate carcinoma.

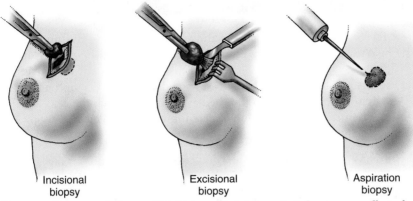

Incisional biopsy   Excisional biopsy   Aspiration biopsy

Figure 17-11 Breast biopsy techniques. If fluid is present, it is aspirated using a needle and syringe, and the material is examined histologically. If no fluid is aspirated, tissue is removed by incisional biopsy or excisional biopsy, the latter performed to remove all of the mass itself.

> ➤ **KEY** POINT Several diagnostic tools are available to evaluate a breast mass. In addition to mammography, any of several diagnostic tools may be indicated such as needle aspiration, incisional biopsy, or excisional biopsy (Figure 17-11). Needle aspiration, or **aspiration biopsy,** is the removal of fluid or tissue from the breast mass through a large-bore needle. An **incisional biopsy** is the surgical removal of tissue from the breast mass, and **excisional biopsy** removes the mass itself. The fluid or tissue removed in these procedures is examined histologically.

aspiration

When fluid or tissue is removed through a large-bore needle, this is called _____ biopsy.

EXERCISE 8

Match the test or abbreviation with the description of the diagnostic procedure.

_____ 1. blood test of fasting glucose level

_____ 2. examination with the hands or fingers

_____ 3. test of thyroid's ability to trap and retain iodine

_____ 4. test of hemoglobin attached to a glucose molecule

_____ 5. enlarged thyroid gland

A. goiter
B. RAIU
C. palpation
D. FBS
E. HbA$_{1c}$

EXERCISE 9

Build It! *Use the following word parts to build terms. (Some word parts will be used more than once.)*

hyper-, hypo-, glyc(o), glycos(o), keton(o), mamm(o), thyroid(o), -emia, -graphy, -ism, -uria

1. increased activity of the thyroid gland   _____/_____/_____

2. less than normal amount of glucose in the blood _____/_____/_____

3. presence of ketones in the urine   _____/_____

4. presence of sugar in the urine   _____/_____

5. radiographic examination of the breast   _____/_____

Say and Check

Say aloud the terms you wrote for Exercise 9. Use the Companion CD to check your pronunciations.

PATHOLOGIES

adenopathy
(ad″ə-nop′ə-the)

17-49 Too little or too much of a specific hormone leads to a dysfunction of the endocrine system. Write a term that has a literal translation of any disease of a gland: _____. This term means any disease of a gland, but remember that the term is sometimes used to mean any disease of the lymph nodes.

An **aden/oma** (ad″ə-no′mə) is a benign tumor in which the cells are clearly derived from glandular tissue. In contrast, **adeno/carcinoma** (ad″ə-no-kahr″sĭ-no′mə) means any of a large group of malignant tumors of the glands.

PITUITARY, THYROID, AND PARATHYROID DISORDERS

antidiuretic

thirst

decreased

somatotropin

17-50 Pituitary dysfunction can result in hypo/secretion or hyper/secretion of the pituitary hormones. Disorders of the posterior lobe of the pituitary are usually related to a deficiency or excess of ADH, which is the _____ hormone.

Diabetes insipidus (di″ə-be′tēz in-sip′ĭ-dəs) is a disorder associated with a deficiency of ADH or inability of the kidneys to respond to ADH. Do not confuse diabetes insipidus with **diabetes mellitus** (mel′lĕ-təs, mə-li′təs), the well-known type of diabetes that is associated with insufficient or improper use of insulin by the body. Diabetes insipidus has some of the characteristics of the other type of diabetes, poly/uria (pol″e-u′re-ə) and poly/dipsia (pol″e-dip′se-ə), but it is not associated with insulin deficiency. **Poly/uria** and **poly/dipsia** mean excessive urination and excessive _____, respectively.

Excessive release of ADH leads to an abnormal condition called the syndrome of inappropriate ADH secretion (SIADH) and usually develops in association with other diseases.

17-51 The effects and hormones of anterior pituitary disorders are excessive or deficient growth (somatotropin), metabolism (prolactin, STH, ACTH, and MSH), or sexual development (FSH and LH). Untreated endocrine dysfunctions during childhood generally have longer lasting and greater effects than those that occur after puberty. Because of better knowledge and improved testing, many endocrine dysfunctions in children are treated and long-lasting effects are avoided.

Hypo/pituitar/ism (hi″po-pĭ-too′ĭ-tə-riz″əm) is _____ activity of the pituitary gland. A person with hypopituitarism is deficient in one or more anterior pituitary hormones, with deficiencies of ACTH and TSH being the most life-threatening. This condition is a result of a congenital developmental defect, a tumor that destroys the pituitary or the hypothalamus, or lack of blood circulation to the pituitary.

17-52 Insufficient GH in childhood (Figure 17-12) leads to **dwarfism** (dworf′iz-əm). The adult dwarf may be no more than 3 to 4 feet tall. Pituitary dwarfism is caused by a deficiency of which hormone? _____

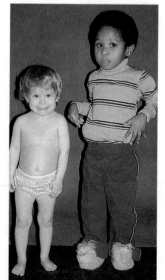

Figure 17-12 Childhood deficiency of growth hormone. Compare the normal 3-year-old boy with the short 3-year-old girl who exhibits the characteristic small stature and "Kewpie doll" appearance, suggesting a deficiency of growth hormone.

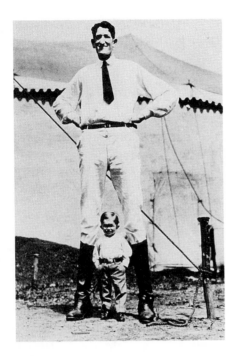

Figure 17-13 Gigantism and dwarfism, resulting from abnormal secretions of growth hormone. Hypersecretion of growth hormone during the early years results in gigantism. The person usually has normal body proportions and normal sexual development. The same hypersecretion in an adult causes acromegaly. Hyposecretion of growth hormone during the early years produces a dwarf unless the child is treated with injections of growth hormone.

pituitary

Pituitary insufficiency in childhood has more drastic effects than the same disorder in adults. Atrophy of the pituitary gland in an adult causes a state of ill health, malnutrition, and wasting known as **pituitary cachexia** (kə-kek´se-ə). Although **cachexia** may occur in many chronic diseases, pituitary cachexia is caused by hyposecretion of the _____ gland.

increased

17-53 Hyperpituitarism (hi˝pər-pĭ-too´ĭ-tə-riz˝əm) is _____ pituitary activity. A common cause of this overactivity is the presence of a benign tumor, especially a pituitary adenoma. Overproduction of GH during childhood leads to **gigantism** (ji-gan´tiz-əm, ji´gan-tiz-əm), and the person will become much taller than normal. Two opposite conditions, dwarfism and gigantism, are shown in Figure 17-13.

somatotropin

Pituitary gigantism is caused by hypersecretion of which hormone? _____

enlargement

17-54 Excess of GH in adults does not cause gigantism. Increased secretion of GH in adults causes **acromegaly** (ak˝ro-meg´ə-le). The name acro/megaly denotes a typical feature of the disease, _____ of the extremities. Bones of the feet, hands, cheeks, and jaws thicken in this disease because of oversecretion of GH (Figure 17-14).

Hyperpituitarism almost always involves excessive secretion of GH, but it may involve other pituitary hormones as well.

thyropathy
(thi-rop´ə-the)

17-55 Using thyr(o), write a word that means any disease of the thyroid gland: _____. Thyroid disorders include inflammation or enlargement of the thyroid and hypersecretion or hyposecretion of thyroid hormones.

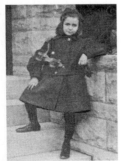 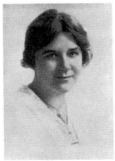 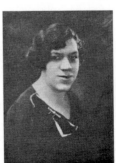 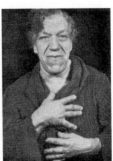

Figure 17-14 Progression of acromegaly. The patient is shown at age 9, age 16, age 33 with well-established acromegaly, and age 52 in the late stages of acromegaly.

inflammation

Thyroid/itis (thi″roid-i′tis) is _____ of the thyroid gland. Acute thyroiditis is generally the result of an infection, but there are different forms and causes of chronic thyroiditis.

excessive

17-56 Hyper/thyroid/ism is a condition caused by _____ secretion of two hormones of the thyroid gland. This increases the metabolic rate, which then causes an increased demand for food to support this metabolic activity.

The patient with hyperthyroidism becomes excitable and nervous, exhibiting moist skin, rapid pulse, increased metabolic rate, weight loss, and exophthalmos. In ex/ophthalmos, the

eyes

_____ protrude outward. (One "o" is dropped to prevent a double "o.")

17-57 The most common form of hyperthyroidism is **Graves disease**, believed to be an autoimmune disease. Three hallmarks of Graves disease are hyperthyroidism, exophthalmos, and goiter. The patient shown in Figure 17-9, *B* exhibits exophthalmos and goiter.

Goiter is a descriptive term that means an enlarged thyroid gland, usually evident as a pro-

neck

nounced swelling in the _____. It may be associated with hyperthyroidism, hypothyroidism, tumors, or thyroiditis.

17-58 **Thyro/toxic/osis** (thi″ro-tok″sĭ-ko′sis), also called thyroid storm, is a life-threatening event that is usually triggered by a major stressor, such as trauma or infection. Signs and symptoms result from a rapid increase in the metabolic rate and include fever, fast pulse, hypertension, gastrointestinal symptoms, agitation, and anxiety. A term for thyroid storm is

thyrotoxicosis

_____.

decreased

17-59 **Hypothyroidism** (hi″po-thi′roid-iz-əm) means _____ activity of the thyroid gland.

Hypothyroidism in childhood results in a condition called **cretinism** (kre′tin-iz-əm) and is caused by insufficient thyroxine. The condition is characterized by arrested physical and mental development (Figure 17-15).

17-60 **Myxedema** (mik″sə-de′mə) is caused by hyposecretion of thyroxine and T₃ during adulthood. The body retains water, and the resultant edema causes facial puffiness. This condition is caused by decreased secretion of the thyroid gland. Hormone therapy usually alleviates the symptoms.

17-61 **Hypo/parathyroid/ism** (hi″po-par″ə-thi′roid-iz-əm) is below normal functioning of the parathyroids. **Hyper/parathyroid/ism** (hi″pər-par″ə-thi′roid-iz-əm) means abnormally

increased

_____ activity of the parathyroids.

Hypoparathyroidism results in **hypocalcemia** (hi″po-kal-se′me-ə), which is a less than nor-

calcium

mal level of _____ in the blood. Early on, surgeons learned the importance of calcium when they inadvertently removed the parathyroids while removing the thyroid. Hypocalcemia occurred in the patients 1 to 2 days after the surgery.

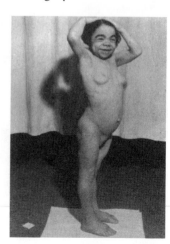

Figure 17-15 Cretinism. This 33-year-old untreated adult cretin exhibits characteristic features. She is only 44 inches tall, and has underdeveloped breasts, protruding abdomen, umbilical hernia, widened facial features, and scant axillary and pubic hair.

Hyperparathyroidism causes hypercalcemia. **Hyper/calc/emia** (hi″pər-kal-se′me-ə) is a greater than normal blood calcium level.

17-62 Pituitary hypogonadism (hi″po-go′nad-iz-əm) is caused by a decreased secretion of FSH or LH by the pituitary. **Hypo/gonad/ism** is decreased functional activity of the _____ and results in a deficiency in the hormones produced by the affected structures, ovaries or testes.

gonads

EXERCISE 10

Word Analysis. *Break these words into their component parts by placing a slash between the word parts. Write the meaning of each term.*

1. adenocarcinoma _____

2. polydipsia _____

3. hypopituitarism _____

4. hyperparathyroidism _____

5. hypocalcemia _____

Say and Check

Say aloud the terms in Exercise 10. Use the Companion CD to check your pronunciations.

ADRENAL, PANCREAS, AND BREAST DISORDERS

enlargement

adrenopathy
(ad″rən-op′ə-the)

adrenals

17-63 Adreno/megaly (ə-dre″no-meg′ə-le) is _____ of one or both adrenal glands. Using adren(o), write a word that means any disease of the adrenals: _____.

17-64 Hyper/adrenal/ism (hi″pər-ə-dre′nəl-iz-əm) is increased secretory activity of the _____. Hypersecretion of the adrenal cortex causes **Cushing syndrome,** which is characterized by increased blood glucose levels, edema resulting from imbalance of water in the body, and masculinization in female individuals.

Tumors that result in hypersecretion of androgens or estrogens before puberty usually have dramatic effects. This is called the **adrenogenital** (ə-dre″no-jen′ĭ-təl) **syndrome** or **adrenal virilism** (vir′ĭ-liz-əm). There is a rapid onset of puberty and sex drive in male individuals. In female individuals, the masculine distribution of body hair develops and the clitoris enlarges to look more like a penis.

17-65 Several dysfunctions of the gonadal hormones were discussed in Chapter 12. Hirsutism and gynecomastia are other disorders resulting from imbalances in estrogens and androgens.

Excessive growth and male distribution of body hair in the female is hirsutism* (hur′soot-iz-əm) (Figure 17-16, *A*). **Hirsutism,** however, means excessive growth of _____. It has several causes, including heredity, hormonal dysfunction, and medication. A decreased estrogen level or other hormonal dysfunction can result from abnormalities of the ovaries or adrenals.

Occasionally an adrenal tumor secretes excess estrogens. When this occurs, the male patient experiences development of gyneco/mast/ia (gi″-nə-, jin″ə-ko-mas′te-ə), which translated literally means a female breast condition (Figure 17-16, *B*). **Gynecomastia** means excessive growth of the male mammary glands.

Andro/pathy (an-drop′ə-the) means any disease peculiar to the male gender, such as gynecomastia. Write this word that means a disease seen only in males: _____.

hair

andropathy

*Hirsutism (Latin: *hirsutus,* shaggy).

Figure 17-16 Examples of estrogen and androgen imbalances. A, Hirsutism, excessive body hair in a masculine distribution pattern, can result from several causes, including heredity, hormonal dysfunction, and/or medication. **B,** Gynecomastia, a noninflammatory enlargement of both breasts in males, can be temporary and benign. The most common cause is a disturbance of the normal ratio of androgen to estrogen, and may occur as a side effect of drug therapy.

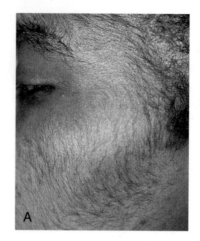
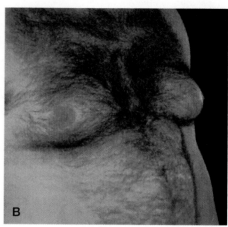

decreased

cortex

hyposecretion

pancreatitis
(pan″kre-ə-ti′tis)
insulin

greater

excessive

mellitus

17-66 Hypo/adrenal/ism (hi″po-ə-dre′nəl-iz-əm) is _____ adrenal activity. The loss of medullary activity does not cause as drastic an effect as the loss of adrenocortical activity. **Adreno/cortical** pertains to the adrenal _____.
   Hyposecretion of epinephrine produces no significant effect. Hypersecretion, usually from a tumor, puts the body in a prolonged or continual fight-or-flight mode.

17-67 Hyposecretion of the adrenal cortex in which all three classes of adrenal corticosteroids are reduced leads to **Addison disease.** This life-threatening condition is characterized by dehydration, low blood glucose levels, bronzing of the skin, and general ill health. Partial or complete failure of the adrenal glands can result from auto/immune processes, infection, tumors, or hemorrhage within the gland. Addison disease results from _____ of the adrenal cortex.

17-68 The pancreas is subject to inflammation and cancer, and both conditions can lead to insufficient secretion of insulin. Write a term that means inflammation of the pancreas: _____. This disorder, as well as pancreatic cancer, can result in a deficiency of insulin secretion by the pancreas. **Hypo/insulin/ism** (hi″po-in′su-lin-iz″əm) is a deficient secretion of _____ by the pancreas.

17-69 Diabetes mellitus (DM) is primarily a result of resistance to insulin or a deficiency or complete lack of insulin secretion by the insulin-producing cells of the pancreas. Without insulin, glucose builds up in the blood and hyperglycemia results. Hyper/glycem/ia means a _____ than normal level of glucose in the blood.
   Hyperglycemia causes serious fluid and electrolyte imbalances, ultimately resulting in the classic symptoms of diabetes: polyphagia, polyuria, and polydipsia. **Polyphagia** (pol″e-fa′jə) (poly, many + -phagia, eating) means excessive hunger and uncontrolled eating. Polyuria (-uria, urination) means _____ urination, and polydipsia (-dipsia, thirst) means excessive thirst.

17-70 When used alone, the term diabetes generally refers to diabetes mellitus, but one should be aware that the term diabetes means excessive excretion of urine, and diabetes insipidus, for example, is so named because of its classic symptoms, not because of its relationship to DM.
   Broad classifications of DM are type 1, type 2, gestational, and other types. **Type 1 diabetes mellitus** is genetically determined and results in absolute insulin deficiency. Individuals with this particular gene produce little or no insulin and are classified as having type 1 diabetes _____. This disease was previously called insulin-dependent diabetes mellitus (IDDM).

> ➤ **KEY** POINT <u>Chronic complications of DM include vascular diseases and neuro/pathy</u> <u>(noo-rop´ə-the)</u>. Vascular diseases include diseases of the heart and major vessels, as well as smaller vessels (e.g., **diabetic nephro/pathy** [nə-frop´ə-the], which is damage to the small vessels of the kidneys and is the leading cause of end-stage renal disease in the United States). **Diabetic retino/pathy,** another complication, is a disorder of the retinal blood vessels of the eye that can eventually lead to blindness. **Diabetic neuropathy** is nerve damage associated with DM. Foot complications are a common problem for the patient with diabetes, particularly the development of **peripheral vascular disease** (PVD), which can lead to amputation.

insulin

17-71 The specific genetic link and development of **type 2 diabetes mellitus** is unclear. Contributing causes may be genetic and environmental factors, as well as the aging process and obesity. It is characterized by insulin resistance, rather than insufficient _____ secretion. Type 2 DM was formerly called non–insulin-dependent diabetes (NIDDM), but this term was misleading, because some individuals with type 2 diabetes require insulin.

gestational

17-72 **Gestational diabetes mellitus** (GDM), first recognized during pregnancy, is carbohydrate intolerance, usually caused by a deficiency of insulin. It disappears after delivery of the infant, but in a significant number of cases, returns years later. This type of diabetes is called _____ diabetes mellitus.
   There are some other less common types of DM in addition to type 1, type 2, and gestational DM. An example is the type of DM associated with hyperthyroidism.

decreased

17-73 **Hyper/insulin/ism** (hi″pər-in´sə-lin-iz″əm) is excessive insulin in the body. Hyperinsulinism results in hypo/glyc/emia, a _____ amount of glucose in the blood.
   Hypo/glycemia is a less than normal amount of glucose in the blood. It is caused by administration of too much insulin, excessive secretion of insulin by the pancreas, or dietary deficiency. An individual with hypoglycemia usually experiences weakness, headache, hunger, visual disturbances, and anxiety. If untreated, hypoglycemia can lead to coma and death. Write the term that

hypoglycemia

means less than normal levels of glucose in the blood: _____.

17-74 The mammary glands are lactiferous glands in the female breasts that are the target organs of oxytocin and LTH. Many problems associated with the breast are not a result of hormones. However, hormones may be related to breast disorders, for example, inappropriate lactation (nipple discharge).
   Mamm/algia (mə-mal´jə), **masto/dynia** (mas″to-din´e-ə), and **mast/algia** (mas-tal´jə) mean

pain

breast _____.
   Frequently encountered breast disorders include fibrocystic (fi″bro-sis´tik) disease, breast cancer, and benign tumors.

17-75 **Fibro/cystic breast disease** is a disorder characterized by single or multiple benign cysts of the breast. The cysts must be considered potentially malignant until diagnostic tests indicate otherwise; thereafter, the breasts should be observed carefully for change. The cysts often occur as a result of cyclic breast changes that accompany the menstrual cycle. This disorder characterized

fibrocystic

by benign cysts of the breast is called _____ breast disease.

17-76 A number of breast tumors are benign and can be differentiated from cancerous tumors by mammography and biopsy. Excluding skin cancer, breast cancer has been the most common malignancy among women in the United States for years. The cause of breast cancer is still unknown, but early detection and improved treatment have contributed to a decrease in mortality rates. Breast cancer in female individuals is still a major cause of cancer death. Breast cancer in male individuals is rare.

	Breast cancer often begins as a small, painless lump; dimpled skin; or nipple retraction. As the cancer progresses, there may be nipple discharge, pain, and ulceration.
cancer	**Masto/carcinoma** (mas″tə-kahr″sĭ-no′mə) is a term that means breast _____.
breast	**17-77 Mast/itis** (mas-ti′tis) is an inflammatory condition of the _____ that occurs most frequently in lactating women. It is usually caused by bacterial infection. If mastitis is untreated, abscesses may form.

EXERCISE 11

Build It! *Use the following word parts to build terms. (Some word parts will be used more than once.)*

hyper-, adrenal(o), carcin(o), insulin(o), mast(o), pancreat(o), -dynia, -ism, -itis, -oma

1. inflammation of the pancreas _____/_____

2. pain in the breast _____/_____

3. cancer of the breast _____/_____/_____

4. increased secretory activity of the adrenals _____/_____/_____

5. excessive insulin in the body _____/_____/_____

Say and Check

Say aloud the terms you wrote for Exercise 11. Use the Companion CD to check your pronunciations.

EXERCISE 12

Match the pathologies in the left column with their characteristics in the right column.

_____ 1. acromegaly

_____ 2. Addison disease

_____ 3. Cushing syndrome

_____ 4. cretinism

_____ 5. diabetes mellitus

_____ 6. exophthalmos

_____ 7. gigantism

_____ 8. goiter

_____ 9. hypogonadism

_____ 10. myxedema

A. decreased functional activity of the ovaries or testes
B. enlarged thyroid gland
C. hypersecretion of the adrenal cortex
D. hypersecretion of GH in adults
E. hypersecretion of somatotropin during childhood
F. hyposecretion of the adrenal cortex
G. hyposecretion of thyroxine and T_3 during adulthood
H. hypothyroidism in childhood
I. insufficient secretion or resistance to insulin
J. outward protrusion of the eye

SURGICAL AND THERAPEUTIC INTERVENTIONS

	17-78 Because the most common cause of hypopituitarism is a pituitary tumor, treatment consists of surgery or radiation to remove the tumor, followed by administration of the deficient hormones.
	Certain types of pituitary tumors can cause overproduction of GH, and the treatment of choice is surgery to remove the tumor. Irradiation of the tumor and drugs may also be indicated. **Hypophysectomy** (hi-pof″ə-sek′tə-me) is surgical removal or destruction of the hypophysis (Figure 17-17). Hypophys/ectomy is removal or destruction of the _____.
hypophysis (pituitary)	Overproduction of a single tropic hormone (such as TSH) usually causes oversecretion by the target organ (e.g., overproduction of thyroxine and T_3). Drug therapy may be useful in suppressing the hormone production.

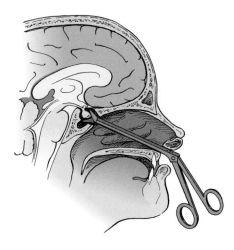

Figure 17-17 Hypophysectomy. Surgical removal of the pituitary gland may be performed to excise a pituitary tumor or to slow the growth and spread of endocrine-dependent malignant tumors. It is done only if other treatment fails to destroy all pituitary tissue.

excision

17-79 The treatment of hyperthyroidism is destruction of large amounts of the thyroid tissue by either surgery or radioactive materials or the use of **anti/thyroid drugs** to block the production of thyroid hormones. **Thyroid/ectomy** (thi″roid-ek′tə-me) is _____ of the thyroid.

adrenalectomy
(ə-dre″nəl-ek′to-me)

17-80 It may be necessary to surgically remove adrenal tumors that cause the adrenals to produce excess corticoids. Using adrenal(o), write a word that means excision of an adrenal gland: _____.

insulin

17-81 The goal of treatment of DM is to maintain a balance of the body's insulin and glucose. Type 1 diabetes is controlled by administration of insulin, proper diet, and exercise. Insulin is administered by injection on a regular basis, either sub/cutaneous injection or via an insulin pump. An **insulin pump** is a portable battery-operated instrument that delivers a measured amount of insulin through the abdominal wall. It can be programmed to deliver doses of insulin according to the body's needs (Figure 17-18). The individual with type 1 diabetes requires an outside source of _____ to sustain life.

Insulin is a **glucose-lowering agent**. Type 2 diabetes is controlled by diet, exercise, oral agents, and sometimes insulin. Oral agents are another means of lowering blood glucose.

Proper nutrition is important in gestational diabetes. Insulin is given if nutritional therapy is insufficient.

excessive

17-82 Treatment of hypoglycemia may consist of a glucose paste placed inside the cheek, administration of glucose (dextrose) such as that found in orange juice, or intravenously if the person is unconscious. Strict attention to diet is important for patients with hypoglycemia caused by _____ secretion of insulin.

mastopexy
(mas′to-pek-se)

17-83 Masto/ptosis (mas″top-to′sis, mas″to-to′sis) is sagging or prolapsed breasts. Write a word using mast(o) that means surgical fixation of the breasts: _____.

Mastopexy is performed to correct a pendulous breast. (This is also called breast lift.)

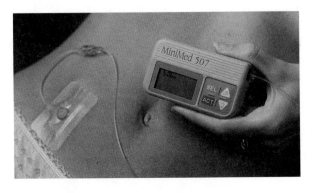

Figure 17-18 External insulin pump. This portable battery-operated instrument delivers a measured amount of insulin through the abdominal wall at preset intervals. It can be programmed to deliver varied amounts of insulin according to the body's needs at different times of the day.

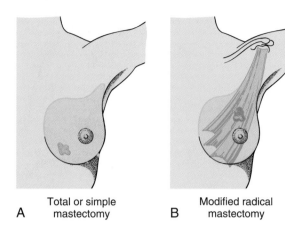

Total or simple mastectomy   A

Modified radical mastectomy   B

Figure 17-19 Simple vs. radical mastectomy. These are most commonly performed to remove a malignant tumor. **A,** In a simple mastectomy, only breast tissue is removed. **B,** In a radical mastectomy, axillary lymph nodes and some of the muscles of the chest are removed with the breast.

17-84 The extent and location of metastases determines the therapeutic strategy in breast cancer. For breast cancer with distant metastases, nonsurgical treatment (chemotherapy, hormone therapy, and sometimes radiation) may be prescribed. For women with breast cancer at a stage for which surgery is recommended, follow-up after the surgery with chemotherapy, radiation, hormone therapy, or targeted therapy may be prescribed.

Excision of the lump with removal of varying amounts of tissue is often the treatment of choice in breast cancer. The amount of extra tissue removed ranges from a small amount of surrounding healthy tissue to the entire breast. A **lumpectomy** (ləm-pek´tə-me) is surgical excision of a tumor that is known to be or suspected of being cancer. **Mast/ectomy** is removal of

breast

the _____. Only breast tissue is removed in a simple mastectomy, whereas axillary lymph nodes and muscles of the chest are removed in a radical mastectomy (Figure 17-19).

17-85 Breast reconstruction may begin during the original mastectomy or soon after surgical removal of the breast, using saline or silicone breast implants. **Mammo/plasty** (mam´o-plas˝te) is

breast

plastic surgery of the _____.

Mammoplasty, plastic reshaping of the breasts, can be done to reduce or lift large or sagging breasts and sometimes to enlarge small breasts. **Augmentation mammoplasty** is plastic surgery to increase the size of the female breast. **Reduction mammoplasty** is plastic surgery to

reduce

_____ the size of the breast.

EXERCISE 13

Write a term for each of the following:

1. excision of a lump in the breast   _____

2. excision of the thyroid   _____

3. plastic surgery of the breast   _____

4. removal of the adrenal gland   _____

5. surgical fixation of the breasts   _____

6. surgical removal of a breast   _____

CHAPTER ABBREVIATIONS*

ACTH	adrenocorticotropic hormone	LTH	lactogenic hormone
ADH	antidiuretic hormone	MSH	melanocyte-stimulating hormone
DM	diabetes mellitus	NIDDM	non–insulin-dependent diabetes mellitus
FBS	fasting blood sugar	PTH	parathormone (parathyroid hormone)
FSH	follicle-stimulating hormone	PVD	peripheral vascular disease
GDM	gestational diabetes mellitus	RAIU	radioactive iodine uptake
GH	growth hormone	SIADH	syndrome of inappropriate ADH secretion
GTT	glucose tolerance test		
HbA$_{1c}$	glycosylated hemoglobin	STH	somatotropic hormone
hCG or HCG	human chorionic gonadotropin	T$_3$	triiodothyronine
^{131}I	radioactive iodine	T$_4$	thyroxine
ICSH	interstitial cell stimulating hormone	TCT	thyrocalcitonin
IDDM	insulin-dependent diabetes mellitus	TSH	thyroid-stimulating hormone
LH	luteinizing hormone		

*Many of these abbreviations share their meanings with other terms.

▶ CHAPTER 17 REVIEW

Basic Understanding

Listing

I. *Write the names of the six major endocrine glands:* _____

_____

II. *Describe two ways in which the pituitary cooperates with the nervous system to maintain homeostasis.*

1. _____

2. _____

Matching

III. *Match each hormone with its target gland. (Some selections will be used more than once.)*

_____ 1. antidiuretic hormone   _____ 4. oxytocin   A. breasts
                                                                   B. gonads
_____ 2. follicle-stimulating hormone _____ 5. thyrotropin   C. kidneys
                                                                   D. thyroid gland
_____ 3. luteinizing hormone

IV. *Match each hormone with the gland(s) that secrete them.*

_____ 1. adrenocorticotropin   _____ 8. melanocyte-stimulating hormone   A. adrenals
                                                                                  B. gonads
_____ 2. antidiuretic hormone   _____ 9. oxytocin   C. pancreas
                                                                                  D. pituitary
_____ 3. epinephrine   _____ 10. testosterone   E. thyroid

_____ 4. follicle-stimulating hormone _____ 11. thyrocalcitonin

_____ 5. growth hormone   _____ 12. thyrotropin

_____ 6. insulin   _____ 13. thyroxine

_____ 7. luteinizing hormone

V. *Match these hormones with their principal action.*

_____ 1. calcitonin   _____ 5. melanocyte-stimulating hormone

_____ 2. epinephrine   _____ 6. mineralocorticoids

_____ 3. insulin   _____ 7. parathormone

_____ 4. glucocorticoids

A. has antidiuretic effect
B. decreases blood calcium level
C. decreases blood glucose level
D. increases blood calcium level
E. increases blood glucose level
F. increases heart rate and blood pressure
G. promotes pigmentation of skin and hair

Word Analysis

VI. *Break these words into their component parts, and define each term.*

1. adrenocortical   _____

2. endocrine   _____

3. hypercalcemia   _____

4. mastectomy   _____

5. somatotropin   _____

 Say and Check

Say aloud the terms in Exercise VI. Use the Companion CD to check your pronunciations.

Photo ID

VII. *Use word parts to build terms to label these illustrations.*

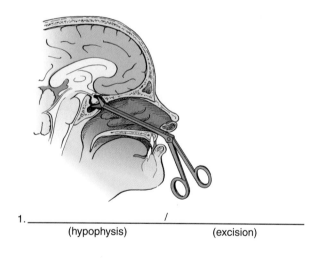

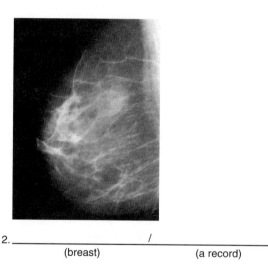

1. _____ / _____
      (hypophysis)   (excision)

2. _____ / _____
      (breast)   (a record)

Multiple Choice

VIII. *Circle the correct answer for each of the following questions.*

1. Which of the following is an exocrine gland? (adrenal gland, pituitary, sweat gland, thyroid)

2. Which of the following hormones produce masculine sex characteristics?
   (androgens, estrogens, prolactins, triiodothyronines)

3. What is the name of the diagnostic procedure that uses x-ray to study the breast?
   (mammogram, mammography, radioactive iodine uptake test, reduction mammoplasty)

4. Which of the following pathologies is associated with hypersecretion of the glucocorticoids?
   (Addison disease, Cushing syndrome, gigantism, thyrotoxicosis)

5. Which of the following is the expected result of increased secretion of growth hormone in adults?
   (acromegaly, cretinism, gigantism, gonadopathy)

6. Which of the following disorders is associated with a deficiency of ADH?
(cretinism, diabetes insipidus, hyperaldosteronism, pituitary dwarfism)

7. Which of the following disorders is caused by hyposecretion of thyroxine and T_3 during adulthood?
(cretinism, Graves disease, hypogonadism, myxedema)

8. The islets of Langerhans are structures in which of the following? (adrenal gland, kidney, pancreas, thyroid)

9. Which of the following tests is more accurate for determining the degree of blood glucose control?
(fasting blood sugar, glycosylated hemoglobin, radioactive iodine uptake, urinary ketones)

10. Which of the following terms means an enlarged thyroid gland?
(goiter, hyperadrenism, hyperthyroidism, hypothyroidism)

Writing Terms

IX. *Write a term for each of the following.*

1. adrenalin _____

2. decreased thyroid activity _____

3. excessive growth of hair _____

4. gland that produces either ova or sperm _____

5. increased level of blood glucose _____

6. lactogenic hormone _____

7. master gland _____

8. producing masculine characteristics _____

9. stability in the normal body state _____

10. sugar in the urine _____

 Say and Check

Say aloud the terms you wrote for Exercise IX. Use the Companion CD to check your pronunciations.

Greater Comprehension

Pronunciation

X. *The pronunciation of several medical terms is shown. Indicate the primary accented syllable by marking it with an ´.*

1. antidiuretic (an te, an tĭ di u ret ik)

2. gynecomastia (gi nə, jin ə ko mas te ə)

3. hypoadrenalism (hi po ə dre nəl iz əm)

4. mammoplasty (mam o plas te)

5. oxytocin (ok sĭ to sin)

 Say and Check

Say aloud the five terms in Exercise X. Use the Companion CD to check your pronunciations. In addition, be prepared to pronounce aloud these terms in class:

acromegaly	diabetes insipidus	hirsutism	mineralocorticoid
adenohypophysis	diabetic nephropathy	hypoparathyroidism	myxedema
adrenal virilism	euthyroid	hypophysis	tetraiodothyronine
cachexia	exophthalmos	lactiferous	thyropathy
colostrum	gynecomastia	mastoptosis	thyrotoxicosis

Health Care Reports

XI. *Read the Consultation and write the meaning of the underlined terms or abbreviations.*

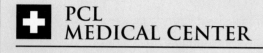

PCL MEDICAL CENTER

7700 Lexicon Way
St. Louis, MO 63146

Phone (555) 437-0000 • Fax (555) 437-0001

CONSULTATION

Patient Name: Wynona A. Harter   **ID No.:** 017-0002   **Date:** Jul 18, ----

CHIEF COMPLAINT: "I feel like my heart is racing, and my weight is falling off."

HISTORY: This 62-year-old woman is admitted with a fractured right hip following a mechanical fall. Orthopedics called us in consult to review the patient's <u>endocrinology</u> status owing to <u>palpitations</u>, hyperexcitability, weight loss, and <u>exophthalmos</u>.

PHYSICAL EXAM: <u>VS</u>: Pulse 120, <u>BP</u> 170/96, weight 160 pounds, down from 170 pounds 6 months ago. General: Appears anxious but is oriented ×3. <u>HEENT</u>: Eyes bulging, right greater than left. Oropharynx clear. Neck: <u>Goiter</u> present, protruding about 5 cm from the right neck. Heart: Rapid heartbeat, otherwise <u>WNL</u>. Musculoskeletal: Status post right hip replacement; has osteoporosis based on history and x-ray findings. Neurologic exam: Cranial nerves II through XII within normal limits. Psychiatric: Mood and affect pleasant but anxious.

DIAGNOSTIC DATA: I will order thyroid function tests and a full metabolic panel.

DIAGNOSES

1. Osteoporosis, status post right hip replacement following a mechanical fall
2. <u>Hyperthyroidism</u>

PLAN: Tapazole, 10 mg q. 8h. for now. Consider possible <u>thyroidectomy</u> after she has sufficiently recovered from her current procedure. Continue to follow with orthopedics. To be seen in my office after she has been discharged.

Thank you for allowing me to share in the care of this delightful patient. My full endocrinology report with recommendations will follow.

Daphnes Panagedes, MD

Daphnes Panagedes, MD, Endocrinologist

DP: pai
D: Jul 18, ----
T: Jul 18, ----

Define:

1. endocrinology   _____

2. palpitations   _____

3. exophthalmos   _____

4. VS   _____

5. BP   _____

6. HEENT   _____

7. goiter   _____

8. WNL   _____

9. hyperthyroidism   _____

10. thyroidectomy   _____

XII. *Read the History and Physical and answer the questions.*

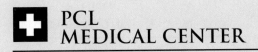

PCL
MEDICAL CENTER

7700 Lexicon Way
St. Louis, MO 63146

Phone (555) 437-0000 • Fax (555) 437-0001

ADMITTING HISTORY & PHYSICAL EXAM

Patient Name: Mary Ellen Sanders   **ID No.:** 017-0003   **Date:** Feb 9, ----

CHIEF COMPLAINT: "I feel tired all the time, I can't get enough to drink, also I seem to pee constantly."

HISTORY: 50-year-old woman with obesity and poorly healing skin wounds. Complains of fatigue, polydipsia, and polyuria. Has had frequent UTIs over the last couple of years. Was admitted to hospital for nonhealing leg ulcers.

MEDICAL/SURGICAL HISTORY: History of peripheral vascular disease, CA of right breast with mastectomy, and has hypercholesterolemia and hyperlipidemia.

FAMILY HISTORY: Mother, 75, with history of obesity, hypothyroidism, and fibrocystic breast disease. Father, 80, with history of hypertension, IDDM with retinopathy, neuropathy, and nephropathy.

LABORATORY TESTS: FBS 150, HbA$_{1c}$ 9%. Urinalysis with culture pending.

DIAGNOSIS: Diabetes mellitus type 2

PLAN: Weight loss with 1800-calorie diabetic diet; self-monitoring of blood sugar 4× a day; oral hypoglycemic medication; repeat HbA$_{1c}$ ×3 months. May order an antibiotic once culture results are known. Possible referral to Urology.

Daphnes Panagedes, MD

Daphnes Panagedes, MD
Endocrinology Consultants

DP: pai
D: Feb 9, ----
T: Feb 9, ----

---

1. Explain the complaints that the patient has had with her urinary tract. _____

   _____

2. Which term indicates that she had a cancerous breast removed? _____

3. Indicate the terms related to her levels of cholesterol and lipids, and explain their meanings. _____

   _____

4. Explain two things that the H&P tells us about her skin. _____

   _____

5. Define retinopathy, neuropathy, and nephropathy. _____

   _____

6. What part of the H&P reports the glycosylated hemoglobin? Explain its meaning. _____

   _____

XIII. Read the operative report and define the following terms.

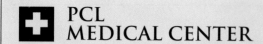

PCL MEDICAL CENTER

7700 Lexicon Way
St. Louis, MO 63146

Phone (555) 437-0000 • Fax (555) 437-0001

OPERATION REPORT

Patient Name: Gary Huffman   **ID No.:** 017-0004   **Date of Surgery:** Jun 13, ----
PREOPERATIVE DIAGNOSIS: Bilateral gynecomastia
POSTOPERATIVE DIAGNOSIS: Bilateral gynecomastia
SURGEON: Frank J. Wright, MD   **ASSISTANT:** Jane Stewart, MD
ANESTHETIST: Ron DeVittori, MD **ANESTHESIA:** General endotracheal via intubation and Marcaine infiltration
SPONGE COUNT VERIFIED: Correct at end of case
MATERIAL FORWARDED TO THE LABORATORY FOR EXAMINATION
1. Right breast tissue   2. Left breast tissue
OPERATION PERFORMED: Bilateral subcutaneous mastectomies
COMPLICATIONS: None
INDICATIONS: This 18-year-old Caucasian male patient, referred by Dr. Panagedes, has gynecomastia, which has been persistent for more than 1½ years and is affecting his social development and behavior. Desires surgical correction before leaving for college.
DESCRIPTION OF OPERATION
After discussion of risks, benefits, and alternatives, and after answering all questions, the patient signed informed consent and was taken to the operating room, sleep induced, intubated, and fully anesthetized. He was positioned squarely and symmetrically on the board with both arms out without hyperextension of the arms and with a pillow under the knees. Sterile prep with Betadine scrub and paint, sterile towels and drapes, was performed of the bilateral chest, shoulders, arms, and upper abdomen, and the patient was draped out.

An incision was made in a semicircle under each breast with a 5-mm extension to the right and left of the nipples. The incision was at the edge of the areola. Leaving an adequate depth of tissue behind the nipples to avoid nipple necrosis, the breasts were divided under the nipples; then the breast and fat pads surrounding the breasts were excised using electrocautery dissection on the right and left sides. Care was taken to avoid making the flap too thin. Good hemostasis was achieved. The pectoralis fascia was left intact; the axillary fat pad was left undisturbed.

Both wounds were irrigated with warm sterile saline solution. Good hemostasis was achieved. With the patient symmetric and midline marked, the breast tissue was examined with the skin flaps reapproximated.

Define:

1. gynecomastia   _____

2. bilateral mastectomies   _____

3. areola   _____

4. hemostasis   _____

5. axillary fat pad   _____

6. reapproximated   _____

Spelling

XIV. Circle each misspelled term in the following list and write its correct spelling.

adrenohypophysis   calcitonin   homostasis   neurohypophysis   tyrotropin

Interpreting Abbreviations

XV. *Write the meaning of these abbreviations.*

1. GDM _____

2. GH   _____

3. ICSH _____

4. ^{131}I   _____

5. TSH _____

Categorizing Terms

XVI. *Classify the terms in the left columns by selecting A, B, C, D, or E.*

_____ 1. acromegaly

_____ 2. dwarfism

_____ 3. glucose-lowering agent

_____ 4. hirsutism

_____ 5. hypogonadism

_____ 6. lobule

_____ 7. mammogram

_____ 8. mastectomy

_____ 9. radioactive iodine uptake

_____ 10. thyroiditis

A. anatomy
B. diagnostic test or procedure
C. pathology
D. surgery
E. therapy

Challenge

XVII. *Divide each of these terms into its component parts. Then write the meaning of each term.*

1. adrenalectomy   _____

2. endocrinopathy   _____

3. lactosuria   _____

4. pituitarism   _____

5. thyrogenic   _____

(Check your answers with the solutions in Appendix VI.)

 PRONUNCIATION LIST

Use the Companion CD to review the terms that have been presented. Look closely at the spelling of each term as it is pronounced and be sure you know the meaning of each term.

acromegaly	adrenopathy	Cushing syndrome	exophthalmos
Addison disease	androgen	diabetes insipidus	fibrocystic breast disease
adenocarcinoma	androgenic	diabetes mellitus	follicle-stimulating hormone
adenohypophysis	andropathy	diabetic nephropathy	gastrin
adenoma	antidiuretic hormone	diabetic neuropathy	gestational diabetes mellitus
adenopathy	antithyroid drugs	diabetic retinopathy	gigantism
adrenal gland	areola	diuresis	gland
adrenal virilism	aspiration biopsy	diuretic	glucagon
adrenalectomy	atriopeptin	dwarfism	glucocorticoid
adrenaline	augmentation mammoplasty	endocrine glands	glucose-lowering agent
adrenocortical	cachexia	endocrine system	glucose tolerance tests
adrenocorticotropic	calcitonin	epinephrine	glycosuria
hormone	colostrum	estrogen	glycosylated hemoglobin
adrenocorticotropin	cortex	euthyroid	goiter
adrenogenital syndrome	cortisone	excisional biopsy	gonad
adrenomegaly	cretinism	exocrine glands	gonadal

gonadotropic
gonadotropic hormones
gonadotropin
Graves disease
gynecomastia
hirsutism
hormone
human chorionic
    gonadotropin
hyperadrenalism
hypercalcemia
hyperglycemia
hyperinsulinism
hyperparathyroidism
hyperpituitarism
hypersecretion
hyperthyroidism
hypoadrenalism
hypocalcemia
hypoglycemia
hypogonadism
hypoinsulinism
hypoparathyroidism
hypophysectomy
hypophysis
hypopituitarism
hyposecretion
hypothalamus
hypothyroidism

incisional biopsy
insulin
insulin pump
intermammary
interstitial cell–stimulating
    hormone
islets of Langerhans
ketone
ketonuria
lactation
lactiferous
lactogenesis
lactogenic
lactogenic hormone
lobule
lumpectomy
luteinizing hormone
mammalgia
mammary gland
mammogram
mammography
mammoplasty
mastalgia
mastectomy
master gland
mastitis
mastocarcinoma
mastodynia
mastopexy

mastoptosis
medulla
melanin
melanocyte-stimulating
    hormone
melatonin
mineralocorticoid
myxedema
neurohypophysis
norepinephrine
oxytocin
pancreas
pancreatitis
parathormone
parathyroid glands
parathyroid hormone
pepsin
peripheral vascular disease
pineal gland
pituitary cachexia
pituitary gland
pituitary hypogonadism
polydipsia
polyphagia
polyuria
progesterone
prolactin
prostaglandin
puberty

radioactive iodine
    uptake test
reduction mammoplasty
retromammary
somatotropic hormone
somatotropin
steroid
suprarenal
target organ
testosterone
tetraiodothyronine
thymosin
thymus
thyrocalcitonin
thyroid
thyroid-stimulating
    hormone
thyroidectomy
thyroiditis
thyropathy
thyrotoxicosis
thyrotropin
thyroxine
triiodothyronine
tropic
type 1 diabetes mellitus
type 2 diabetes mellitus

Español ENHANCING SPANISH COMMUNICATION

English	Spanish (pronunciation)
adrenal	suprarenal (soo-prah-ray-NAHL)
adrenaline	adrenalina (ah-dray-nah-LEE-nah)
augmentation	aumento (ah-oo-MEN-to)
beard	barba (BAR-bah)
calcium	calcio (CAHL-se-o)
diabetes	diabetes (de-ah-BAY-tes)
dwarf	enano (ay-NAH-no)
giant	gigante (he-GAHN-tay)
glucose	glucosa (gloo-CO-sah)
goiter	papera (pah-PAY-rah)
growth	crecimiento (cray-se-me-EN-to)
hormone	hormona (or-MOH-nah)
insulin	insulina (in-soo-LEE-nah)
iodine	yodo (YO-do)
masculine	masculino (mas-coo-LEE-no)
nipple	pezón (pay-SON)
pancreas	páncreas (PAHN-cray-as)
pituitary	pituitario (pe-too-e-TAH-re-o)
synthesis	síntesis (SEEN-tay-sis)
thyroid	tiroides (te-RO-e-des)

Review of Chapters 1 Through 17

18

LEARNING GOALS

Basic Understanding

After completing Chapters 1 through 17, you will be able to do the following:

1. Match terms pertaining to anatomy, diagnostic tests or procedures, pathology, surgery, or therapy with their meanings or descriptions.
2. Write terms when presented with their definitions.

Greater Comprehension

3. Categorize terms as anatomy, diagnostic test or procedure, pathology, surgery, or therapy.

PREPARING FOR THE FINAL EXAMINATION

This chapter is included to help you test yourself on how well you remember the material. Work all questions in the review if you completed all chapters in the book. Questions are presented within chapter groups. If you did not complete all chapters in the book, do not work the questions relating to chapters that you did not cover.

It is better to do all questions in a set before checking the answers. When you find that you have answered incorrectly, prepare a study sheet of terms that you did not remember. When finished with this chapter, look through the earlier chapters and find the correct answer for all questions that you missed. Analyze the component parts of these items.

The review is a representative sample of chapter material but does not include every term. Before taking the test that your instructor prepares, refer to your study sheet several times and study the list of terms at the end of each chapter, being sure you remember the meaning of each term.

MAJOR SECTIONS OF THIS CHAPTER:

CHAPTERS ARE DESIGNATED IN EACH SECTION.

   I. Multiple Choice Questions
  II. Writing Terms
 III. Categorizing Terms

I. Multiple Choice Questions

Circle the correct answer for each of the following questions.

Chapter 2

1. Cynthia is pregnant. Which type of specialist should she see to care for her during her pregnancy, labor, and delivery? (gerontologist, obstetrician, orthopedist, otologist)

2. Which of the following physicians specializes in the diagnosis and treatment of newborns through the age of 28 days? (geriatrician, gynecologist, neonatologist, urologist)

3. Sally injures her arm while ice skating. The emergency room physician orders an x-ray examination. Which type of physician is a specialist in interpreting x-ray films? (gynecologist, ophthalmologist, plastic surgeon, radiologist)

4. What does the word neuron mean? (medical specialty that deals with the nervous system, nerve cell, neurosurgery, specialist in diseases of the nervous system)

5. Which physician is certified in the laboratory study of disease? (clinical pathologist, gastroenterologist, internist, surgical pathologist)

Chapter 3

6. Susie tells the doctor that she has a sore throat. Which term describes the sore throat? (diagnosis, prognosis, sign, symptom)

7. Mr. Jones has plastic surgery on his hand. What is the name of this procedure? (carpectomy, chiroplasty, ophthalmoplasty, otoplasty)

8. An elderly man is told he has an enlarged heart. Which term describes his condition? (cardiomegaly, carditis, coronary artery disease, megalomania)

9. Which term means a record of the electrical impulses of the heart? (electrocardiogram, electrocardiograph, electrocardiography, telecardiography)

10. Which diagnostic procedure produces an image of a detailed cross-section of tissue similar to what one would see if the organ were actually cut into sections? (computed tomography, contrast imaging, electrocardiography, nuclear medicine imaging)

Chapter 4

11. Johnny, a college student, sees the physician and is told that his appendix is inflamed. What is the name of his condition? (appendectomy, appendicitis, appendorrhexis, appendotomy)

12. Karen sustains a severe head injury in which there is herniation of the brain through an opening in the skull. What is the name of this pathology? (cerebritis, cerebrotomy, encephalocele, encephaloplasty)

13. Ken suffers an abnormal fear of heights. What type of pathology does he have? (dilatation, mania, phobia, ptosis)

14. Which of the following describes an unfavorable response to medical treatment? (autoimmune, contagious, iatrogenic, functional)

15. Which of the following are classified by their shape, such as cocci (spheric), bacilli (rod-shaped), spirilla (spiral), or vibrios (comma-shaped)? (viruses, fungi, protozoa, bacteria)

Chapter 5

16. Which term describes a structure that can be seen with the naked eye? (macroscopic, microscopic, ophthalmoscopic, ophthalmoscopy)

17. What does the prefix in antiperspirant mean? (against, before, effective, supporting)

18. What is the meaning of the prefix in quadruplets? (one, two, three, four)

19. In which type of injection is the needle placed in the muscular layer? (intradermal, intramuscular, intravenous, subcutaneous)

20. Which term means a set of symptoms that occur together and characterize a particular disease or condition? (dysphoria, symptomatic, syndrome, tachyphasia)

Chapter 6

21. A disease or condition that is determined by one's genes or a change in the number or structure of the chromosomes is a/an (genetic disorder, organelle, organism, tissue).

22. Pete is trying to explain a method of drawing imaginary lines to designate abdominal areas. Which term should he use to describe the areas when the abdomen is divided into four regions? (bilateral areas, nine regions, six regions, quadrants)

23. Dr. Ray explains in a radiology report that a fracture has occurred in the distal portion of the thigh bone. Distal means (farther from the origin, in the middle of the bone, nearer the origin, on the side of the bone).

24. Which plane divides the body into anterior and posterior portions? (frontal, midsagittal, sagittal, transverse)

25. Which of these terms means a muscular partition that separates the thoracic and abdominopelvic cavities? (diaphragm, paracentesis, peritoneum, pyrogen)

Chapter 7

26. Transportation of oxygen to body cells is a major function of (blood platelets, erythrocytes, leukocytes, thrombocytes).

27. A term that means having no tendency to repair itself or develop into new tissue is (analytic, anisocytosis, aplastic, hemolytic).

28. The surgical procedure whereby living organs are transferred from one part of the body to another or from one individual to another is (rejection, transmission, transplant, transreaction).

29. Interstitial fluid fills the spaces (around, between, inside, outside) most of the cells of the body.

30. A decrease in the number of blood platelets is called (hemophilia, leukemia, leukocytosis, thrombopenia).

Chapter 8

31. Charlie, a 60-year-old man, has just been diagnosed as having a coronary occlusion. He is most at risk for which of the following? (atrioventricular block, congenital heart disease, myocardial infarction, rheumatic fever)

32. Charlie is told that he has a form of arteriosclerosis in which yellowish plaque has accumulated on the walls of the arteries. What is the name of this form of arteriosclerosis? (aortostenosis, atherosclerosis, cardiomyopathy, coarctation)

33. Jim developed a blood clot in a coronary artery. What is Jim's condition called? (hypotension, coronary artery bypass, coronary thrombosis, fibrillation)

34. Baby Seth is born with cyanosis and a heart murmur. Which congenital heart disease does the neonatologist think is most likely? (atrial septal defect, atrioventricular block, megalocardia, pericarditis)

35. Ten-year-old Zack had a sore throat for several days before he developed painful joints and a fever. Which disease does the physician suspect that can cause damage to the heart valves? (defibrillator, pericardium, lymphoma, rheumatic fever)

Chapter 9

36. Mrs. Smith's doctor tells her that she has pneumonia. What is another name for her diagnosis? (congestive heart disease, pneumonitis, pulmonary edema, pulmonary insufficiency)

37. Which term means coughing up and spitting out sputum? (expectorate, expiration, exhalation, extrapleural)

38. What is the serous membrane that lines the walls of the thoracic cavity? (parietal pleura, rhinorrhea, silicosis, visceral pleura)

39. Which of the following expand the air passages? (antitussives, antihistamines, antineoplastics, bronchodilators)

40. Mrs. Sema has difficulty breathing except when sitting in an upright position. What is the term for her condition? (anoxia, hypocapnia, inspiration, orthopnea)

Chapter 10

41. Cal Jones has radiography of the gallbladder. What is the name of this diagnostic test?
    (barium enema, barium meal, cholecystography, esophagogastroscopy)

42. Tests show that Cal has a gallstone in the common bile duct. Which of the following is a noninvasive conservative procedure to alleviate Cal's problem?
    (cholecystostomy, choledochostomy, choledochojejunostomy, extracorporeal shock wave lithotripsy)

43. Linda M., a 16-year-old girl, is diagnosed as having self-induced starvation. Which of the following is the name of the disorder associated with Linda's problem? (anorexia nervosa, aphagia, malaise, polyphagia)

44. Unless there is intervention for Linda's self-induced starvation, which condition will result?
    (adipsia, atresia, emaciation, volvulus)

45. A 70-year-old man is diagnosed with cancer of the colon. Which term indicates a surgical intervention for this condition? (colectomy, colonoscope, colonic irrigation, colonic stasis)

Chapter 11

46. Which of the following terms means making radiographic images of the urinary system after the urine has been rendered opaque by a contrast medium?
    (cystoscopy, cystoureteroscopy, intravenous urography, nephrotomography)

47. Which of the following is indicated if the blood urea nitrogen is elevated?
    (pyelostomy, pyuria, renal clearance, renal failure)

48. Which term means pertaining to the urinary bladder and a ureter?
    (cystourethral, extracystic, urethrovaginal, vesicoureteral)

49. Which term means excretion of an abnormally large quantity of urine? (anuria, dysuria, oliguria, polyuria)

50. Which of the following is *not* a type of urinary tract catheterization?
    (endoscopy tube, nephrostomy tube, suprapubic tube, urethral tube)

Chapter 12

51. Which term means difficult or painful menstruation? (amenorrhea, dysmenorrhea, metrorrhagia, menorrhea)

52. Which term means absence of living sperm? (azoospermia, oligospermia, testalgia, orchiepididymitis)

53. Which term means surgical fixation of a prolapsed uterus? (cervicectomy, hysterectomy, hysteropexy, leiomyomectomy)

54. Which term means a condition in which tissue that contains typical endometrial elements is present outside the uterus? (endometriosis, endometritis, hysteropathy, salpingopathy)

55. Which term means absence of a testis? (anorchidism, aspermia, oligospermia, orchidectomy)

Chapter 13

56. Which term means abnormal or difficult labor? (abortion, dystocia, eclampsia, stillbirth)

57. Which of the following is a genetic disorder in which the fetus has an extra chromosome?
    (Down syndrome, erythroblastosis fetalis, hemolytic anemia, implantation)

58. Which term means the same as pregnancy? (embryonic, gestation, ovulation, parturition)

59. Which of the following is the normal presentation of the fetus during labor?
    (breech, cephalic, shoulder, transverse)

60. Which of the following is the common name for condyloma acuminatum?
    (genital herpes, genital warts, moniliasis, venereal ulcer)

Chapter 14

61. Which term means congenital fissure of the breastbone? (costectomy, rachischisis, spondylosyndesis, sternoschisis)

62. Which term means pertaining to two bones of the forearm?
    (carpopedal, carpophalangeal, humeroulnar, ulnoradial)

63. Which term means any disease of the joints? (arthropathy, bursopathy, chondropathy, osteopathy)

64. Which of the following is the record produced in a procedure that records the response of a muscle to electrical stimulation? (arthrocentesis, electromyogram, myograph, range-of-motion reading)

65. What is the term for the presence of extra fingers or toes? (carpopedal disease, Paget disease, phalangitis, polydactylism)

Chapter 15

66. Which part of the nervous system contains the brain and spinal cord? (peripheral nervous system, autonomic nervous system, central nervous system, thalamus)

67. Which term means paralysis of the lower portion of the body and both legs? (diplegia, hemiplegia, paraplegia, quadriplegia)

68. Which of the following means hernial protrusion of the meninges through a defect in the vertebral column? (meningitis, meningocele, myelocele, myelomalacia)

69. Which term means incision of the lacrimal sac? (cholecystotomy, cystolithectomy, dacryocystotomy, dacryolithiasis)

70. Which of the following is chronic, progressive mental deterioration that involves irreversible loss of memory, disorientation, and speech and gait disturbances? (Alzheimer disease, Lou Gehrig disease, Meniere syndrome, multiple sclerosis)

Chapter 16

71. Which of the following means removal of foreign material and dead or contaminated tissue from an infected or traumatic lesion until surrounding healthy tissue is exposed? (débridement, necrosis, pyemia, rhytidectomy)

72. Which of the following is an inflammatory skin disease that begins on the scalp but may involve other areas, particularly the eyebrows? (acne vulgaris, basal cell carcinoma, seborrheic dermatitis, verruca)

73. Which term means a disease characterized by chronic hardening and thickening of the skin? (ecchymosis, Kaposi sarcoma, keratosis, scleroderma)

74. In describing a burn by "thickness," which type of burn is characterized by blisters immediately after the injury? (deep partial-thickness, deep full-thickness, full-thickness, superficial partial-thickness)

75. Which term means the death of areas of tissue or bone surrounded by healthy parts? (atrophy, erosion, fissure, necrosis)

Chapter 17

76. The islets of Langerhans are structures in which of the following? (adrenal, kidney, pancreas, thyroid)

77. Which of the following terms means an enlarged thyroid gland? (goiter, hyperadenism, hyperthyroidism, hypothyroidism)

78. What is the name of the diagnostic procedure that uses x-rays to study the breast? (mammogram, mammography, radioactive iodine uptake test, reduction mammoplasty)

79. Which of the following disorders is associated with a deficiency of ADH? (cretinism, diabetes insipidus, hyperaldosteronism, pituitary dwarfism)

80. Which of the following pathologies is associated with hypersecretion of the glucocorticoids? (Addison disease, Cushing syndrome, gigantism, thyrotoxicosis)

II. Writing Terms

Write one word for each of the following clues.

Chapter 2

1. having a severe and relatively short duration   _____

2. method of prioritizing patients according to their needs   _____

3. pertaining to the heart   _____

4. study of the characteristics, causes, and effects of disease _____

5. specialist in internal medicine _____

Chapter 3
6. excision of the colon _____

7. incision of the eye _____

8. instrument used in encephalotomy _____

9. suture of a vessel _____

10. swelling of the eyelid _____

Chapter 4
11. a substance that causes hemolysis _____

12. a substance that produces cancer _____

13. any disease of the eye _____

14. inflammation of a bone _____

15. pertaining to the nose _____

Chapter 5
16. having no symptoms _____

17. abnormally slow speech _____

18. within cells _____

19. behind the nose _____

20. double vision _____

Chapter 6
21. affecting only one side _____

22. lying flat on the back _____

23. inflammation of the umbilicus _____

24. pertaining to the abdomen and pelvis _____

25. a record of electrical impulses of the brain _____

Chapter 7
26. any erythrocyte of irregular shape _____

27. below normal sodium in the blood _____

28. dissolving of a thrombus _____

29. neutral-staining granulocyte _____

30. production of blood _____

Chapter 8
31. absence of a heartbeat _____

32. agents that cause dilation of blood vessels _____

33. increased blood pressure _____

34. increased pulse _____

35. inflammation of a lymphatic vessel _____

Chapter 9

36. softening of the wind pipe _____

37. difficult or weak voice _____

38. presence of nasal calculi _____

39. pertaining to the air sacs of the lung _____

40. radiographic examination of the larynx _____

Chapter 10

41. any disease of the stomach _____

42. enzyme that breaks down starch _____

43. excessive vomiting _____

44. excision of the gallbladder _____

45. inflammation of the liver _____

Chapter 11

46. inflammation of the renal glomeruli _____

47. inflammation of the renal pelvis _____

48. pus in the urine _____

49. radiography of the urinary bladder _____

50. surgical crushing of a stone _____

Chapter 12

51. incision of the vas deferens _____

52. inflammation of the cervix uteri _____

53. inflammation of the vulva and vagina _____

54. insufficient sperm in the semen _____

55. surgical fixation of a fallopian tube _____

Chapter 13

56. a woman who has produced many viable offspring _____

57. attachment of a fertilized ovum to the endometrium _____

58. deliberate rupture of the fetal membranes to induce labor _____

59. incision made to enlarge the vaginal opening for delivery _____

60. painless sore of syphilis _____

Chapter 14

61. degenerative joint disease _____

62. excision of the tailbone _____

63. herniation of a muscle _____

64. inflammation of a bone _____

65. lateral curvature of the spine _____

Chapter 15

66. radiography of the spinal cord _____

67. process of recording the electrical activity of the brain _____

68. abnormal loss of transparency of the lens of the eye _____

69. inflammation of the brain and spinal cord _____

70. abnormal fear of public places _____

Chapter 16

71. another name for a bruise _____

72. any disease of the nails _____

73. superficial infection involving hair follicles _____

74. absence of pigment in the skin, hair, and nails _____

75. a torn, jagged wound _____

Chapter 17

76. master gland _____

77. producing masculine characteristics _____

78. decreased thyroid activity _____

79. gland that produces either ova or sperm _____

80. sugar in the urine _____

III. Categorizing Terms

Classify each term by writing A (anatomy), D (diagnostic test or procedure), P (pathology), S (surgery), or T (therapy).

Chapter 2

1. anesthetic ointment _____

2. gastric _____

3. neurosurgery _____

4. ophthalmic _____

5. carcinoma _____

Chapter 3

6. adenectomy _____

7. rhinoplasty _____

8. endoscopy _____

9. analgesics _____

10. edema _____

Chapter 4

11. metastasis _____

12. blepharal _____

13. dermatitis _____

14. jaundice _____

15. cephalometry _____

Chapter 5

16. subcutaneous _____

17. microtia _____

18. postnasal _____

19. suprarenal _____

20. tachyphasia _____

Chapter 6

21. acrocyanosis _____

22. antipyretic _____

23. aplasia _____

24. febrile _____

25. thoracotomy _____

Chapter 7

26. anticoagulant _____

27. dyscrasias _____

28. leukocyte _____

29. allograft _____

30. staphylococcemia _____

Chapter 8

31. aneurysm _____

32. angiostomy _____

33. arteriography _____

34. thymus _____

35. lymphedema _____

Chapter 9

36. acidosis _____

37. bronchogram _____

38. coryza _____

39. glottis _____

40. hydrothorax _____

Chapter 10

41. diverticulectomy _____

42. gastroscopy _____

43. gingiva _____

44. glossorrhaphy _____

45. pancreatography _____

Chapter 11

46. dysuria _____

47. hydronephrosis _____

48. lithotrite _____

49. nephrectomy _____

50. renal _____

Chapter 12

51. candidiasis _____

52. hysteroscopy _____

53. colporrhaphy _____

54. hydrocele _____

55. scrotal _____

Chapter 13

56. eclampsia _____

57. spermatoblast _____

58. endometrium _____

59. pelvimetry _____

60. fetoscope _____

Chapter 14

61. arthrocentesis _____

62. calcaneofibular _____

63. chondrectomy _____

64. dystrophy _____

65. myelosuppressives _____

Chapter 15

66. cerebellum _____

67. echoencephalography _____

68. hydrocephalus _____

69. neurasthenia _____

70. vagotomy _____

Chapter 16

71. dermatomycosis _____

72. liposuction _____

73. rhytidoplasty _____

74. trichopathy _____

75. ungual _____

Chapter 17

76. adrenalectomy _____

77. exophthalmos _____

78. mastectomy _____

79. myxedema _____

80. parathyroids _____

Appendix I: Medical Abbreviations

A&O	alert and oriented	CDC	Centers for Disease Control and Prevention
a.c.	before meals (*ante cibum*)	CHF	congestive heart failure
ABA	American Burn Association	CK (CPK)	creatine kinase (formerly called creatine phosphokinase)
ABG	arterial blood gas		
ACh	acetylcholine	CLL	chronic lymphocytic leukemia
ACS	American Cancer Society	cm	centimeter
ACTH	adrenocorticotropic hormone	CML	chronic myelogenous leukemia
ad lib.	freely as needed, at pleasure (*ad libitum*)	CMV	cytomegalovirus
		CNS	central nervous system
ADD	attention deficit disorder	CO$_2$	carbon dioxide
ADH	antidiuretic hormone	COLD	chronic obstructive lung disease
ADHD	attention deficit hyperactivity disorder	COPD	chronic obstructive pulmonary disease
ADL	activities of daily living	CPAP	continuous positive airway pressure
AHF	antihemophilic factor	CPD	cephalopelvic disproportion
AI	aortic insufficiency	CPK	creatine phosphokinase
AIDS	acquired immunodeficiency syndrome	CPR	cardiopulmonary resuscitation
		CRF	chronic renal failure
ALL	acute lymphoblastic leukemia	CS, C-section	cesarean section
ALS	amyotrophic lateral sclerosis	CSF	cerebrospinal fluid
ALT	alanine aminotransferase	CSR	Cheyne-Stokes respiration
AML	acute myelogenous leukemia	CT, CAT	computed tomography, computerized axial tomography, or computed axial tomography
ANA	antinuclear antibody		
AP	anteroposterior		
aq.	water (*aqua*)		
ARDS	acute or adult respiratory distress syndrome	CTS	carpal tunnel syndrome
		CVA	cerebrovascular accident, costovertebral angle
ARF	acute renal failure		
AROM	active range of motion	Cx	cervix
ASHD	arteriosclerotic heart disease	D&C	dilation and curettage
AST	aspartate aminotransferase (enzyme increased after myocardial infarction)	dB	decibel
		DFA	direct fluorescent antibody
		DIC	disseminated intravascular coagulation
AV, A-V	atrioventricular	DJD	degenerative joint disease
AVB	atrioventricular block	dL	deciliter
baso	basophil	DLE	discoid lupus erythematosus
BBT	basal body temperature	DM	diabetes mellitus
b.i.d.	twice a day (*bis in die*)	DMARD	disease-modifying antirheumatic drugs
BMI	body mass index	DNA	deoxyribonucleic acid
BMT	bone marrow transplant	DOB	date of birth
BP	blood pressure	DSA	digital subtraction angiography
BPH	benign prostatic hyperplasia	DSM	*Diagnostic and Statistical Manual of Mental Disorders*
BUN	blood urea nitrogen		
Bx, bx	biopsy	DTR	deep tendon reflex
C	Celsius, centigrade	Dx	diagnosis
C1, C2, etc.	cervical vertebrae	ECG, EKG	electrocardiogram
CC	chief complaint	ECMO	extracorporeal membrane oxygenation
C&S	culture and sensitivity	ED	emergency department
CABG	coronary artery bypass graft	EDD	expected delivery date
CAD	coronary artery disease	EEG	electroencephalogram
CAL	chronic airflow limitation	EFM	electronic fetal monitor
CBC, cbc	complete blood cell count		

EGD	esophagogastroduodenoscopy	IBS	irritable bowel syndrome
EIA	enzyme immunoassay	ICP	intracranial pressure
ELISA	enzyme-linked immunosorbent assay	ICSH	interstitial cell–stimulating hormone
EMG	electromyography	IDDM	insulin-dependent diabetes mellitus
ENT	ear, nose, and throat	IED	improvised explosive device
eos	eosinophil	IFA	immunofluorescent assay
ESR	erythrocyte sedimentation rate	INR	International Normalized Ratio
ESWL	extracorporeal shock wave lithotripsy	IOL	intraocular lens
F	Fahrenheit	IP	inpatient
FBS	fasting blood sugar	IUD	intrauterine device
FEMA	Federal Emergency Management Agency	IV	intravenous
		IVF	in vitro fertilization
FH	family history	IVP	intravenous pyelogram
FHR	fetal heart rate	kg	kilogram
FSH	follicle-stimulating hormone	KUB	kidneys, ureters, and bladder
fx	fracture	L	liter
g	gram	L&W	living and well
G	gravida (pregnant)	L1, L2, etc.	lumbar vertebrae
GC	gonococcus	LA	left atrium
GDM	gestational diabetes mellitus	LBP	lower back pain
GERD	gastroesophageal reflux disease	LDH	lactate dehydrogenase (enzyme increased after myocardial infarction)
GFR	glomerular filtration rate		
GH	growth hormone	LDL	low-density lipoprotein
GI	gastrointestinal	LE	lupus erythematosus
GP	general practitioner	LFT	liver function tests
GTT	glucose tolerance test	LH	luteinizing hormone
GU	genitourinary	LLQ	left lower quadrant
GYN, Gyn, gyn	gynecology	LMP	last menstrual period
h	hour (hora)	LPF	low-power field
H&P	history and physical	LPN	licensed practical nurse
HAV	hepatitis A virus	LTH	lactogenic hormone
HbA$_{1c}$	glycosylated hemoglobin	LUQ	left upper quadrant
Hb, Hgb	hemoglobin	LV	left ventricle
HBV	hepatitis B virus	LVN	licensed vocational nurse
HCG, hCG	human chorionic gonadotropin	lymph	lymphocyte
HCT, Hct	hematocrit	mcg	microgram
HCV	hepatitis C virus	MD	doctor of medicine
HDL	high-density lipoprotein	mg	milligram
HDV	hepatitis D virus	MI	myocardial infarction
HEENT	head, eye, ear, nose, and throat	MIDCAB	minimally invasive direct coronary artery bypass
HEV	hepatitis E virus		
HIPAA	Health Insurance Portability and Accountability Act	min	minute
		mL	milliliter
HIV	human immunodeficiency virus	mm Hg	millimeters of mercury
HPF	high-power field	mono	monocyte
HPI	history of present illness	MRI	magnetic resonance imaging
HPV	human papillomavirus	MS	multiple sclerosis
HRT	hormone replacement therapy	MSH	melanocyte-stimulating hormone
HSV	herpes simplex virus	MRSA	methicillin-resistant *Staphylococcus aureus*
HSV-1	herpes simplex virus type 1		
HSV-2	herpes simplex virus type 2	MTP	metatarsophalangeal
HTN	hypertension	MVP	mitral valve prolapse
hx, Hx	history	neut	neutrophil
^{131}I	radioactive iodine	NIDDM	non–insulin-dependent diabetes mellitus
I&D	incision and drainage	NIH	National Institutes of Health
I&O	intake and output	NPO	nothing by mouth (*nil per os*)
IBD	inflammatory bowel disease	NSAID	nonsteroidal antiinflammatory drug

O₂	oxygen
OB	obstetrics
OCD	obsessive-compulsive disorder
OD	overdose; right eye (*oculus dexter*)
OP	outpatient
OPCAB	off-pump coronary artery bypass
OR	operating room
OTC	over-the-counter drug
P	pulse
PA	physician assistant or posteroanterior
Pap	Papanicolaou smear, stain, or test
PAT	paroxysmal atrial tachycardia
PCI	percutaneous coronary intervention
PDA	patent ductus arteriosus
PE	physical examination
PET	positron emission tomography
PFT	pulmonary function test
pH	potential hydrogen or potential of hydrogen; hydrogen ion concentration
PID	pelvic inflammatory disease
PMH	past medical history
PMN	polymorphonuclear
PMS	premenstrual syndrome
PNS	peripheral nervous system
p.o.	orally (*per os*)
p.r.n.	as the occasion arises, as needed (*pro re nata*)
PROM	passive range of motion
PSA	prostate-specific antigen
Pt	patient
PT	prothrombin time
PTCA	percutaneous transluminal coronary angioplasty
PTH	parathormone (parathyroid hormone)
PTT	partial thromboplastin time
PVC	premature ventricular contraction
PVD	peripheral vascular disease
q.	every
q.i.d.	four times a day (*quater in die*)
R	respirations
RA	right atrium or rheumatoid arthritis
RAIU	radioactive iodine uptake
RBC	red blood cell, red blood cell count
RDA	recommended dietary allowance
RDS	respiratory distress syndrome
RF	rheumatoid factor
Rh	rhesus factor in blood
RLQ	right lower quadrant
RN	registered nurse
ROM	range of motion
ROS	review of systems
RPFT	registered pulmonary function therapist
RPR	rapid plasma reagin or rapid plasma reagin test (for syphilis)
RUQ	right upper quadrant
RV	right ventricle
Rx	prescription
SA	sinoatrial
SARS	severe acute respiratory syndrome
SCI	spinal cord injury
SGOT	serum glutamic-oxaloacetic transaminase
SGPT	serum glutamic-pyruvic transaminase
SIADH	syndrome of inappropriate ADH secretion
SIDS	sudden infant death syndrome
SLE	systemic lupus erythematosus
SOB	shortness of breath
SSN	social security number
staph	*Staphylococcus*
stat.	immediately (*statim*)
STD	sexually transmitted disease
STH	somatotropic hormone
strep	streptococci
T	temperature
Tl, T2, etc.	thoracic vertebrae
T₃	triiodothyronine
T₄	thyroxine
TAH	total abdominal hysterectomy
TB	tuberculosis
TBSA	total body surface area
TCT	thyrocalcitonin
TENS	transcutaneous electrical nerve stimulation
TFT	thyroid function test
TIA	transient ischemic attack
t.i.d.	three times a day (*ter in die*)
TJR	total joint replacement
TMJ	temporomandibular joint
TPN	total parenteral nutrition
TSH	thyroid-stimulating hormone
TSS	toxic shock syndrome
TTO	transtracheal oxygen
TUMT	transurethral microwave thermotherapy
TUNA	transurethral needle ablation
TUR	transurethral resection
TURP	transurethral resection of the prostate
Tx	treatment
UA, U/A	urinalysis
UGI	upper gastrointestinal series or upper GI
ung	ointment
URI	upper respiratory infection
UTI	urinary tract infection
UV	ultraviolet
VAC	vacuum-assisted closure
VC	vital capacity
VCUG	voiding cystourethrogram
VD	venereal disease
VDRL	Venereal Disease Research Laboratories
VS, v.s.	vital signs
WBC	white blood cell, white blood cell count
WD, WN	well developed, well nourished
WMD	weapons of mass destruction
WNL	within normal limits

Appendix II: Enhancing Spanish Communication

Appendix II is divided into three sections:
- A. English-Spanish Translation of Selected Terms
- B. Spanish-English Translation of Selected Terms
- C. Communication Quick Reference for Spanish-Speaking Clients

A. English-Spanish Translation of Selected Terms

ENGLISH	SPANISH (PRONUNCIATION)	ENGLISH	SPANISH (PRONUNCIATION)
abdomen	abdomen (ab-DOH-men), vientre (ve-EN-tray)	blood sample	muestra de sangre (moo-AYS-trah de SAHN-gray)
acidity	acidez (ah-se-DES)	blue	azul (ah-SOOL)
acute	agudo (ah-GOO-do)	body	cuerpo (coo-ERR-po)
adrenal	suprarenal (soo-prah-ray-NAHL)	bone	hueso (oo-AY-so)
adrenaline	adrenalina (ah-dray-nah-LEE-nah)	brain	cerebro (say-RAY-bro)
aged	envejecido (en-vay-hay-SEE-do)	breast	seno (SAY-no)
allergy	alergia (ah-LEHR-he-ah)	breasts	senos (SAY-nos)
anatomy	anatomía (ah-nah-to-MEE-ah)	breathe	alentar (ah-len-TAR), respirar (res-pe-RAR)
anemia	anemia (ah-NAY-me-ah)		
anesthesia	anestesia (ah-nes-TAY-se-ah)	breathing	respiración (res-pe-rah-se-ON)
anesthetic	anestésico (ah-nes-TAY-se-co)	burn	quemadura (kay-mah-DOO-rah)
ankle	tobillo (to-BEEL-lyo)	calcium	calcio (CAHL-se-o)
antibiotic	antibiótico (an-te-be-O-te-co)	calculus	cálculo (CAHL-coo-lo)
anxiety	ansiedad (an-se-ay-DAHD)	cancer	cáncer (KAHN-ser)
appendix	apéndice (ah-PEN-de-say)	capillary	capilar (cah-pe-LAR)
appetite	apetito (ah-pay-TEE-to)	cartilage	cartílago (car-TEE-lah-go)
arm	brazo (BRAH-so)	catheter	catéter (cah-TAY-ter)
armpit	sobaco (so-BAH-co)	cheek	mejilla (may-HEEL-lyah)
artery	arteria (ar-TAY-re-ah)	chest	pecho (PAY-cho)
asphyxia	asfixia (as-FEEC-se-ah)	chew, to	masticar (mas-te-CAR)
aspirate	aspirar (as-pe-RAR)	child	niña (NEE-nya), niño (NEE-nyo)
asthma	asma (AHS-mah)	childbirth	parto (PAR-to)
augmentation	aumento (ah-oo-MEN-to)	cholesterol	cholesterol (co-les-tay-ROL)
bacilli	bacilos (bah-SEE-los)	chronic	crónico (CRO-ne-co)
back	espalda (es-PAHL-dah)	circumcision	circumcisión (ser-coon-se-se-ON)
beard	barba (BAR-bah)	clot	coágulo (co-AH-goo-lo)
belch	eructo (ay-ROOK-to)	collarbone	clavicula (clah-VEE-coo-lah)
belly	barriga (bar-REE-gah)	conception	concepción (con-sep-se-ON)
benign	benigno (bay-NEEG-no)	concussion	concusión (con-coo-se-ON)
biopsy	biopsia (be-OP-see-ah)	condom	condón (con-DON)
birth	nacimiento (nah-se-me-EN-to)	conscious	consciente (cons-se-EN-tay)
black	negro (NAY-gro)	consciousness	conciencia (con-se-EN-se-ah)
bladder	vejiga (vah-HEE-gah)	constipation	estreñimiento (es-tray-nye-me-EN-to)
blood	sangre (SAHN-gray)		
blood pressure	presión sanguínea (pray-se-ON san-GEE-nay-ah)	contraception	contracepción (con-trah-cep-se-ON)

608

ENGLISH	SPANISH (PRONUNCIATION)
convulsion	convulsión (con-vool-se-ON)
cough	tos (tos)
cranium	cráneo (CRAH-nay-o)
cream	crema (CRAY-mah)
cry	lloro (YO-ro)
defecate	evacuar (ay-vah-coo-AR)
dentist	dentista (den-TEES-tah)
dermatology	dermatología (der-mah-to-lo-HEE-ah)
destruction	destrucción (des-trooc-se-ON)
diabetes	diabetes (de-ah-BAY-tes)
diagnosis	diagnóstico (de-ag-NOS-te-co)
diagnostic	diagnóstico (de-ag-NOS-te-co)
dialysis	diálisis (de-AH-le-sis)
diaphragm	diafragma (de-ah-FRAHG-mah)
diarrhea	diarrea (de-ar-RAY-ah)
digestion	digestión (de-hes-te-ON)
dilatation, dilation	dilatación (de-lah-tah-se-ON)
disease	enfermedad (en-fer-may-DAHD)
dizziness	vértigo (VERR-te-go)
dwarf	enano (AY-nah-no)
ear	oreja (o-RAY-hah)
edema	hidropesía (e-dro-pay-SEE-ah)
elbow	codo (CO-do)
electricity	electricidad (ay-lec-tre-se-DAHD)
enlargement	aumento (ah-oo-MEN-to)
enzyme	enzima (en-SEE-mah)
epilepsy	epilepsia (ay-pe-LEP-se-ah)
erect, straight	derecho (day-RAY-cho)
erection	erección (ay-rec-se-ON)
esophagus	esófago (ay-SO-fah-go)
excretion	excreción (ex-cray-se-ON)
extremity	extremidad (ex-tray-me-DAHD)
eye	ojo (O-ho)
eyeball	globo del ojo (GLO-bo del O-ho)
eyebrow	ceja (SAY-hah)
eyelash	pestaña (pes-TAH-nyah)
eyelid	párpado (PAR-pah-do)
face	cara (CAH-rah)
fainting	languidez (lan-gee-DES), desmayo (des-MAH-yo)
fatigue	fatiga (fah-TEE-gah)
fear	miedo (me-AY-do)
feces	excremento (ex-cray-MEN-to)
feminine	femenina (fay-may-NEE-na)
fetus	feto (FAY-to)
fever	fiebre (fe-AY-bray)
fiber	fibra (FEE-brah)
finger	dedo (DAY-do)
fingerprint	impresión digital (im-pray-se-ON de-he-TAHL)
fire	fuego (foo-AY-go)
fluid	fluido (floo-EE-do)
foam	espuma (es-POO-mah)
foot (pl., feet)	pie (PE-ay), pies (PE-ays)
forearm	antebrazo (an-tay-BRAH-so)

ENGLISH	SPANISH (PRONUNCIATION)
fracture	fractura (frac-TOO-rah)
gallbladder	vesícula biliar (vay-SEE-coo-la be-le-AR)
gallstone	cálculo biliar (CAHL-coo-lo be-le-AR)
giant	gigante (he-GAHN-tay)
gland	glándula (GLAN-doo-lah)
glucose	glucosa (gloo-CO-sah)
goiter	papera (pah-PAY-rah)
gray	gris (grees)
green	verde (VERR-day)
growth	crecimiento (cray-se-me-EN-to)
gum, gingiva	encía (en-SEE-ah)
gynecology	ginecología (he-nay-co-lo-HEE-ah)
hair	pelo (PAY-lo)
hand	mano (MAH-no)
head	cabeza (cah-BAY-sah)
headache	dolor de cabeza (do-LOR day cah-BAY-sa)
heart	corazón (co-rah-SON)
heat	calor (cah-LOR)
heel	talón (tah-LON)
hemorrhage	hemorragia (ay-mor-RAH-he-ah)
hernia	hernia (AYR-ne-ah), quebradura (kay-brah-DOO-rah)
high blood pressure	hipertensión, presión alta (e-per-ten-se-ON, pray-se-ON AHL-tah)
hip	cadera (cah-DAY-rah)
hives	roncha (RON-chah)
hormone	hormona (or-MOH-nah)
hunger	hambre (AHM-bray)
hypodermic	hipodérmico (e-po-DER-me-co)
imperfect	imperfecto (im-per-FEC-to)
impotency	impotencia (im-po-TEN-se-ah)
inflammation	inflamación (in-flah-mah-se-ON)
influenza	gripe (GREE-pay)
injection	inyección (in-yec-se-ON)
injury	daño (DAH-nyo)
instrument	instrumento (ins-troo-MEN-to)
insulin	insulina (in-soo-LEE-nah)
intercourse, sexual	cópula (CO-poo-lah)
intestine	intestino (in-tes-TEE-no)
iodine	yodo (YO-do)
jaw	mandíbula (man-DEE-boo-lah)
joint	articulación (ar-te-coo-lah-se-ON), coyuntura (co-yoon-TOO-rah)
kidney	riñon (ree-NYOHN)
knee	rodilla (ro-DEEL-lyah)
kneecap	rótula (RO-too-lah)
laxative	purgante (poor-GAHN-tay)
leg	pierna (pe-ERR-nah)
leukemia	leucemia (lay-oo-SAY-me-ah)
life	vida (VEE-dah)
ligament	ligamento (le-gah-MEN-to)
light	luz (loos)

ENGLISH	SPANISH (PRONUNCIATION)
lips	labios (LAH-be-os)
liver	hígado (EE-ga-do)
lobe	lóbulo (LO-boo-lo)
lung	pulmón (pool-MON)
lymph	linfa (LEEN-fa)
lymphatic	linfático (lin-FAH-te-co)
malignant	maligno (mah-LEEG-no)
masculine	masculino (mas-coo-LEE-no)
membrane	membrana (mem-BRAH-nah)
menopause	menopausia (may-no-PAH-oo-se-ah)
menstruation	menstruación (mens-troo-ah-se-ON)
microscope	microscopio (me-cros-CO-pe-o)
milk	leche (LAY-chay)
mind	mente (MEN-te)
mouth	boca (BO-cah)
movement	movimiento (mo-ve-me-EN-to)
mucus	moco (MO-co)
murmur	murmullo (moor-MOOL-lyo)
muscle	músculo (MOOS-coo-lo)
nails	uñas (OO-nyahs)
narcotic	narcótico (nar-CO-te-co)
narrow	estrecho (es-TRAY-cho)
navel	ombligo (om-BLEE-go)
neck	cuello (coo-EL-lyo)
nerve	nervio (NERR-ve-o)
nervous	nervioso (ner-ve-O-so)
neurology	neurología (nay-oo-ro-lo-HEE-ah)
newborn	recién nacida (ray-se-EN nah-SEE-dah)
nipple	pezón (pay-SON)
nose	nariz (nah-REES)
nostril	orificio de la nariz (or-e-FEE-se-o day lah nah-REES)
nutrition	nutrición (noo-tre-se-ON)
obstruction	obstrucción (obs-trooc-se-ON)
optic	óptico (OP-te-co)
optician	óptico (OP-te-co)
orange (color)	anaranjado (ah-nah-ran-HAH-do), naranjado (nah-ran-HAH-do)
orthodontist	ortodóntico (or-to-DON-te-co)
ovarian	ovárico (o-VAH-re-co)
ovary	ovario (o-VAH-re-o)
oxygen	oxígeno (ok-SEE-hay-no)
pain	dolor (do-LOR)
painful	doloroso (do-lo-RO-so)
palm	palma (PAHL-mah)
pancreas	páncreas (PAHN-cray-as)
paralysis	parálisis (pah-RAH-le-sis)
parasite	parásito (pah-RAH-se-to)
parturition	parto (PAR-to)
pathology	patología (pah-to-lo-HEE-ah)
penis	pene (PAY-nay)
perspiration	sudor (soo-DOR)
phalanges	falanges (fah-LAHN-hays)

ENGLISH	SPANISH (PRONUNCIATION)
phosphorus	fósforo (FOS-fo-ro)
physical examination	examen físico (ek-SAH-men FEE-se-co)
pink	rosa (RO-sah)
pituitary	pituitario (pe-too-e-TAH-re-o)
pneumonia	neumonía (nay-oo-mo-NEE-ah), pulmonía (pool-mo-NEE-ah)
pregnancy	embarazo (em-bah-RAH-so)
pregnant	embarazada (em-bah-rah-SAH-dah)
prolapse	prolapso (pro-LAHP-so)
prostate	próstata (PROS-ta-tah)
prostatic	prostático (pros-TAH-te-co)
prostatitis	prostatitis (pros-ta-TEE-tis)
protection	protección (pro-tec-se-ON)
psychiatry	psiquiatría (se-ke-ah-TREE-ah)
psychology	psicología (se-co-lo-HEE-ah)
pulse	pulso (POOL-so)
radiation	radiación (rah-de-ah-se-ON)
rectum	recto (REK-to)
red	rojo (ROH-ho)
redness	rojo (RO-ho)
reduction	reducción (ray-dooc-se-ON)
renal artery	arteria renal (ar-TAY-re-ah ray-NAHL)
renal calculus	cálculo renal (CAHL-coo-lo ray-NAHL)
reproduction	reproducción (ray-pro-dooc-se-ON)
respiration	respiración (res-pe-rah-se-ON)
rhythm	ritmo (REET-mo)
rhythm method	método de ritmo (MAY-to-do day REET-mo)
rib	costilla (cos-TEEL-lyah)
ringing	zumbido (zoom-BEE-do)
rupture	ruptura (roop-TOO-rah)
sacrum	hueso sacro (oo-AY-so SAH-cro)
saliva	saliva (sah-LEE-vah)
same	mismo (MEES-mo)
seizure	ataque (ah-TAH-kay)
sensation	sensación (sen-sah-se-ON)
sexual	sexual (sex-soo-AHL)
shoulder	hombro (OM-bro)
shoulder blade	espaldilla (es-pal-DEEL-lyah)
skeleton	esqueleto (es-kay-LAY-to)
skin	piel (pe-EL)
skull	cráneo (CRAH-nay-o)
sleep	sueño (soo-AY-nyo)
sole	planta (PLAHN-tah)
sound	sonido (so-NEE-do)
spasm	espasmo (es-PAHS-mo)
speech	habla (AH-blah), lenguaje (len-goo-AH-hay)
spinal column	columna vertebral (co-LOOM-nah ver-tay-BRAHL)
spine	espinazo (es-pe-NAH-so)

ENGLISH	SPANISH (PRONUNCIATION)	ENGLISH	SPANISH (PRONUNCIATION)
spiral	espiral (es-pe-RAHL)	tonsil	tonsila (ton-SEE-lah), amígdala (ah-MEEG-dah-lah)
spleen	bazo (BAH-so)		
sprain, to	torcer (tor-SERR)	tooth (pl., teeth)	diente (de-AYN-tay)
starch	almidón (al-me-DON)	trachea	tráquea (TRAH-kay-ah)
sterile	estéril (es-TAY-reel)	transfusion	transfusión (trans-foo-se-ON)
sternum	esternón (es-ter-NON)	trauma	daño (DAH-nyo), herida (ay-REE-dah)
stiff	tieso (te-AY-so)		
stomach	estómago (es-TOH-mah-go)	treatment	tratamiento (trah-tah-me-EN-to)
stone	cálculo (CAHL-coo-lo)	ulcer	ulcera (OOL-say-rah)
stroke	ataque de apoplejía (ah-TAH-kay de ah-po-play-HEE-ah)	urea	urea (oo-RAY-ah)
		urinalysis	urinálisis (oo-re-NAH-le-sis)
sugar	azúcar (ah-SOO-car)	urinary	urinario (oo-re-NAH-re-o)
support	sustento (sus-TEN-to)	urinary bladder	vejiga (vay-HEE-gah)
surgeon	cirujano(a) (se-roo-HAH-no) (na)	urinary system	sistema urinario (sis-TAY-mah oo-re-NAH-re-o)
surgery	cirugía (se-roo-HEE-ah)		
suture	sutura (soo-TOO-rah)	urinate	orinar (o-re-NAR)
swallow	tragar (trah-GAR)	urination	urinación (oo-re-nah-se-ON)
sweat	sudor (soo-DOR)	urine	orina (o-REE-nah)
swelling	hinchar (in-CHAR)	urology	urología (oo-ro-lo-HEE-ah)
symptom	síntoma (SEEN-to-mah)	uterus	útero (OO-tay-ro)
synthesis	síntesis (SEEN-tay-sis)	vagina	vagina (vah-HEE-nah)
tear	lágrima de los ojos (LAH-gre-mah day los O-hos)	varicose veins	venas varicosas (VAY-nahs vah-re-CO-sas)
teeth (sing., tooth)	dientes (de-AYN-tays)	vein	vena (VAY-nah)
temperature	temperatura (tem-pay-rah-TOO-rah)	vertebral column	columna vertebral (co-LOOM-nah ver-tay-BRAHL)
temple	sien (se-AN)	vessel	vaso (VAH-so)
tendon	tendón (ten-DON)	vision	visión (ve-se-ON)
testicle	testículo (tes-TEE-coo-lo)	voice	voz (vos)
tests	pruebas (proo-AY-bahs)	voiding	urinar (oo-re-NAR)
therapy	tratamiento (trah-tah-me-EN-to)	vomiting	vómito (VO-me-to)
thigh	muslo (MOOS-lo)	water	agua (AH-goo-ah)
thirst	sed (sayd)	weakness	debilidad (day-be-le-DAHD)
throat	garganta (gar-GAHN-tah)	white	blanco (BLAHN-co)
thumb	pulgar (pool-GAR)	wound	lesión (lay-se-ON)
thyroid	tiroides (te-RO-e-des)	wrist	muñeca (moo-NYAY-cah)
toe	dedo del pie (DAY-do del PE-ay)	x-ray	radiografía (rah-de-o-grah-FEE-ah)
tongue	lengua (LEN-goo-ah)	yellow	amarillo (ah-mah-REEL-lyo)

B. Spanish-English Translation of Selected Terms

SPANISH	ENGLISH	SPANISH	ENGLISH
acidez	acidity	cirujano(a)	surgeon
adrenalina	adrenaline	clavícula	collarbone
agua	water	coágulo	clot
agudo	acute	codo	elbow
alentar	breathe	colesterol	cholesterol
alergia	allergy	columna vertebral	spinal column, vertebral column
almidón	starch	concepción	conception
amarillo	yellow	conciencia	consciousness
amígdala	tonsil	concusión	concussion
anaranjado	orange-colored	condón	condom
anatomía	anatomy	consciente	conscious
anemia	anemia	contracepción	contraception
anestesia	anesthesia	convulsión	convulsion
anestésico	anesthetic	cópula	sexual intercourse
ansiedad	anxiety	corazón	heart
antebrazo	forearm	costilla	rib
antibiótico	antibiotic	coyuntura	joint
apéndice	appendix	cráneo	cranium, skull
apetito	appetite	crecimiento	growth
arteria	artery	crema	cream
arteria renal	renal artery	crónico	chronic
articulación	joint	cuello	neck
asfixia	asphyxia	cuerpo	body
asma	asthma	daño	trauma, injury
aspirar	aspirate	debilidad	weakness
ataque	seizure	dedo	finger
ataque de apoplejía	stroke	dedo del pie	toe
aumento	augmentation, enlargement	dentista	dentist
azúcar	sugar	derecho	erect, straight
azul	blue	dermatología	dermatology
bacilos	bacilli	desmayo	fainting
barba	beard	destrucción	destruction
barriga	belly	diabetes	diabetes
bazo	spleen	diafragma	diaphragm
benigno	benign	diagnóstico	diagnostic
biopsia	biopsy	diálisis	dialysis
blanco	white	diarrea	diarrhea
boca	mouth	diente, dientes	tooth (pl., teeth)
brazo	arm	digestión	digestion
cabeza	head	dilatación	dilation, dilatation
cadera	hip	dolor	pain
calcio	calcium	dolor de cabeza	headache
cálculo	calculus, stone	doloroso	painful
cálculo biliar	gallstone	electricidad	electricity
cálculo renal	renal calculus	embarazada	pregnant
calor	heat	embarazo	pregnancy
cáncer	cancer	enano	dwarf
capilar	capillary	encía	gum, gingiva
cara	face	enfermedad	disease
cartílago	cartilage	envejecido	aged
catéter	catheter	enzima	enzyme
ceja	eyebrow	epilepsia	epilepsy
cerebro	brain	erección	erection
circuncisión	circumcision	eructo	belch
cirugía	surgery	esófago	esophagus

SPANISH	ENGLISH
espalda	back
espaldilla	shoulderblade
espasmo	spasm
espinazo	spine
espiral	spiral
espuma	foam
esqueleto	skeleton
estéril	sterile
esternón	sternum
estómago	stomach
estrecho	narrow
estreñimiento	constipation
evacuar	defecate
examen físico	physical examination
excreción	excretion
excremento	feces
extremidad	extremity
falanges	phalanges
fatiga	fatigue
femenina	feminine
feto	fetus
fibra	fiber
fiebre	fever
fluido	fluid
fósforo	phosphorus
fractura	fracture
fuego	fire
garganta	throat
gigante	giant
ginecología	gynecology
glándula	gland
globo del ojo	eyeball
glucosa	glucose
gripe	influenza
gris	gray
habla	speech
hambre	hunger
hemorragia	hemorrhage
herida	trauma, injury
hernia	hernia
hidropesía	edema
hígado	liver
hinchar	swelling, to swell
hipertensión	high blood pressure
hipodérmico	hypodermic
hombro	shoulder
hormona	hormone
hueso	bone
hueso sacro	sacrum
imperfecto	imperfect
impotencia	impotency
impresión digital	fingerprint
inflamación	inflammation
instrumento	instrument
insulina	insulin
intestino	intestine
inyección	injection

SPANISH	ENGLISH
labios	lips
lágrima do los ojos	tears
languidez	fainting
leche	milk
lengua	tongue
lenguaje	speech
lesión	wound
leucemia	leukemia
ligamento	ligament
linfa	lymph
linfático	lymphatic
lloro	cry
lóbulo	lobe
luz	light
maligno	malignant
mandíbula	jaw
mano	hand
masculino	masculine
masticar	to chew
mejilla	cheek
membrana	membrane
menopausia	menopause
menstruación	menstruation
mente	mind
método de ritmo	rhythm method
microscopio	microscope
miedo	fear
mismo	same
moco	mucus
movimiento	movement
muestra de sangre	blood sample
muñeca	wrist
murmullo	murmur
músculo	muscle
muslo	thigh
nacimiento	birth
naranjado	orange-colored
narcótico	narcotic
nariz	nose
negro	black
nervio	nerve
nervioso	nervous
neumonía	pneumonia
neurología	neurology
niño(a)	child
nutrición	nutrition
obstrucción	obstruction
ojo	eye
ombligo	navel
óptico	optician, optic
oreja	ear
orificio de la nariz	nostril
orina	urine
orinar	urinate
ortodóntico	orthodontist
ovárico	ovarian
ovario	ovary

SPANISH	ENGLISH
oxígeno	oxygen
palma	palm
páncreas	pancreas
papera	goiter
parálisis	paralysis
parásito	parasite
parpado	eyelid
parto	childbirth, parturition
patología	pathology
pecho	chest
pelo	hair
pene	penis
pestaña	eyelash
pezón	nipple
pie (pl., pies)	foot (pl., feet)
piel	skin
pierna	leg
pituitario	pituitary
planta	sole
presión alta	high blood pressure
presión sanguínea	blood pressure
prolapso	prolapse
próstata	prostate
prostático	prostatic
prostatitis	prostatitis
protección	protection
pruebas	tests
psicología	psychology
psiquiatría	psychiatry
pulgar	thumb
pulmón	lung
pulmonía	pneumonia
pulso	pulse
purgante	laxative
quebradura	hernia
quemadura	burn
radiación	radiation
radiografía	x-ray examination
recién nacida	newborn
recto	rectum
reducción	reduction
reproducción	reproduction
respiración	breathing, respiration
respirar	breathe
riñón	kidney
ritmo	rhythm
rodilla	knee
rojo	red
roncha	hives
rosa	pink
rótula	kneecap
ruptura	rupture
saliva	saliva
sangre	blood

SPANISH	ENGLISH
sanguínea	blood pressure
sed	thirst
seno(s)	breast(s)
sensación	sensation
sexual	sexual
sien	temple
síntesis	synthesis
síntoma	symptom
sistema urinario	urinary system
sobaco	armpit
sonido	sound
sudor	sweat, perspiration
sueño	sleep
suprarenal	adrenal
sustento	support
sutura	suture
talón	heel
temperatura	temperature
tendón	tendon
testículo	testicle
tieso	stiff
tiroides	thyroid
tobillo	ankle
tonsila	tonsil
torcer	to sprain
tos	cough
tragar	swallow
transfusión	transfusion
tráquea	trachea
tratamiento	treatment, therapy
ulcera	ulcer
uñas	nails
urea	urea
urinación	urination
urinálisis	urinalysis
urinar	voiding
urinario	urinary
urología	urology
útero	uterus
vagina	vagina
vaso	vessel
vejiga	urinary bladder
vena	vein
venas varicosas	varicose veins
verde	green
vértigo	dizziness
vesícula biliar	gallbladder
vida	life
vientre	abdomen
visión	vision
vómito	vomiting
voz	voice
yodo	iodine
zumbido	ringing

C. Communication Quick Reference for Spanish-Speaking Clients

The Body • El Cuerpo (el coo-ERR-po)

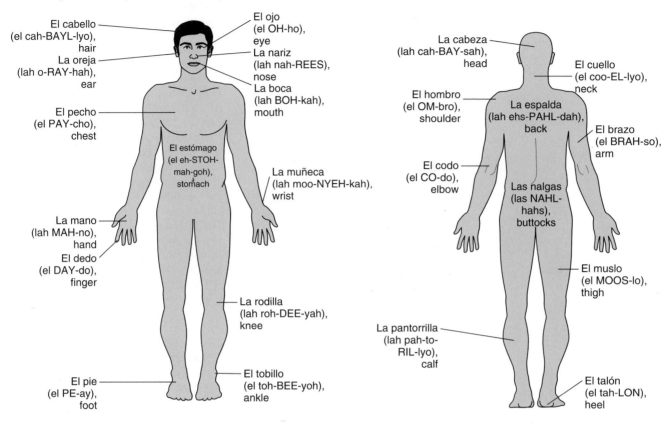

El cabello (el cah-BAYL-lyo), hair
La oreja (lah o-RAY-hah), ear
El pecho (el PAY-cho), chest
El estómago (el eh-STOH-mah-goh), stomach
La mano (lah MAH-no), hand
El dedo (el DAY-do), finger
El pie (el PE-ay), foot

El ojo (el OH-ho), eye
La nariz (lah nah-REES), nose
La boca (lah BOH-kah), mouth
La muñeca (lah moo-NYEH-kah), wrist
La rodilla (lah roh-DEE-yah), knee
El tobillo (el toh-BEE-yoh), ankle

La cabeza (lah cah-BAY-sah), head
El hombro (el OM-bro), shoulder
El codo (el CO-do), elbow
La pantorrilla (lah pah-to-RIL-lyo), calf

El cuello (el coo-EL-lyo), neck
La espalda (lah ehs-PAHL-dah), back
El brazo (el BRAH-so), arm
Las nalgas (las NAHL-hahs), buttocks
El muslo (el MOOS-lo), thigh
El talón (el tah-LON), heel

Common Instructions to be Used with the Body Parts

Move the, Mueva *(mooh-EH-bah)*   Touch the, Toque *(TOH-keh)*   Point to the, Señale *(seh-NYAH-leh)*

More Parts of the Body

Armpit, la axila *(lah ac-SEE-la)*
Breasts, los senos *(lohs SAY-nohs)*
Collarbone, la clavicula *(lah clah-VEE-coo-lah)*
Diaphragm, el diafragma *(el de-ah-FRAHG-mah)*

Forearm, el antebrazo *(el an-tay-BRAH-so)*
Groin, la ingle *(lah EEN-glay)*
Hip, la cadera *(lah cah-DAY-rah)*
Kneecap, la rótula *(lah RO-too-lah)*
Nail, la uña *(lah OON-yah)*
Pelvis, la pelvis *(lah PEL-ves)*

Rectum, el recto *(el REK-to)*
Rib, la costilla *(lah cos-TEEL-lyah)*
Spine, el espinazo *(el es-pe-NAH-so)*
Throat, la garganta *(lah gar-GAHN-tah)*
Tongue, le lengua *(lah LEN-goo-ah)*

Organs

Appendix, el apéndice *(el ah-PEN-de-say)*
Bladder, la vejiga *(lah vah-HEE-gah)*
Brain, el cerebro *(el seh-RAY-bro)*
Colon, el colon *(el KOH-lohn)*
Esophagus, el esófago *(el ay-SOH-fah-go)*
Gallbladder, la vesícula biliar *(lah vay-SEE-coo-la be-le-AHR)*

Genitals, los genitales *(los hay-ne-TAHL-as)*
Heart, el corazón *(el co-rah-SON)*
Kidney, el riñón *(el ree-NYOHN)*
Large intestine, el intestino grueso *(el in-tes-TEE-no groo-AY-so)*
Liver, el hígado *(el EE-gah-doh)*
Lungs, los pulmones *(los pool-MON-ays)*
Pancreas, el páncreas *(el PAHN-cray-as)*

Small intestine, el intestino delgado *(el in-tes-TEE-no del-GAH-do)*
Spleen, el bazo *(el BAH-so)*
Thyroid gland, la tiroides *(lah te-RO-e-des)*
Tonsils, las amígdalas *(las ah-MEEG-dah-lahs)*
Uterus, el útero *(el OO-tay-ro)*

Essential Phrases

Good…
    morning.
    afternoon.
    night.
Hello.
How are you?
Good (Fine).

Buenos(as)…
    días.
    tardes.
    noches.
Hola.
¿Cómo está?
Bien.

BWEH-nohs(nahs)…
    DEE-ahs.
    TAHR-days.
    NO-chays.
OH-lah.
¿Ko-mo ays-TAH?
Be-IN.

Essential Phrases—cont'd

Bad, Better, Worse.	Mal, Mejor, Peor.	*Mahl, May-HOR, Pay-ORE.*
The same.	Igual.	*E-goo-AHL.*
Do you speak English?	¿Habla inglés?	*¿AH-blah een-GLAYS?*
I don't understand.	No comprendo.	*No kom-PREHN-do.*
Excuse me.	Discúlpeme.	*Dis-COOL-pah-may.*
Please speak slowly.	Por favor, hable más lento.	*Por fah-VOHR, AH-blay MAHS LEHN-toh.*
Are you in pain?	¿Está adolorido(a)	*¿Ay-TAH ah-do-lo-REE-do(da)?*
Yes, No.	Sí, No.	*SEE, Noh.*
Tell me where it hurts.	Digame donde le duele.	*DEE-gah-me DOHN-day lay DWAY-lay.*
Here, There.	Aquí, Ahi.	*Ah-KEE, Ah-EE.*
Are you allergic to any medication?	¿Es usted alérgico(a) a alguna medicación?	*¿Ays oos-TAYD ah-LEHR-he-ko(ka) ah ahl-GOO-na may-de-cah-se-ON?*
I'm here to help you.	Estoy aquí para ayudarle.	*Ays-TOY ah-KEE pah-rah ah-yoo-DAHR-lay.*
Calm down.	Cálmese.	*KAHL-may-say.*
Please.	Por favor.	*Por fah-VOHR.*
Thank you.	Gracias.	*GRAH-syahs.*
You're welcome.	De nada.	*Day NAH-dah.*
May I?	¿Puedo?	*¿PWEH-do?*
Who, What, When, Where?	¿Quién, Qué, Cuándo, Dónde?	*¿Kyahn, Kay, KWAHN-do, DOHN-day?*
Zero, One, Two, Three, Four	Cero, Uno, Dos, Tres, Cuatro	*SAY-ro, OO-no, dos, trays, KWAH-tro*
Five, Six, Seven, Eight, Nine, Ten	Cinco, Seis, Siete, Ocho, Nueve, Diez	*SEEN-ko, says, se-AY-tay, OH-cho, noo-AY-vay, de-AZ*

Description of Pain

Is your pain…	Tiene un dolor…	*Tee-AY-nay oon do-LOR…*
burning?	¿quemante?	*¿kay-MANH-tay?*
constant?	¿constante?	*¿kohn-STAHN-tay?*
dull?	¿sordo?	*¿SOHR-do?*
intermittent?	¿intermitente?	*¿in-ter-mee-TEN-teh?*
mild?	¿moderado?	*¿moh-deh-RAH-doh?*
severe?	¿muy fuerte?	*¿MOO-ee foo-ERR-tay?*
sharp?	¿agudo?	*¿ah-GOO-do?*
throbbing?	¿pulsante?	*¿pool-SAHN-tay?*
worse?	¿peor?	*¿pay-ORE?*

Preliminary Examination

My name is _____, and I am your nurse.	Me llamo _____, y soy su enfermera(o).	*May YAH-mo _____, E SO-e soo en-fer-MAY-rah(ro).*
I'm going to…	Le voy a…	*Lay voy ah…*
take your vital signs.	tomar los signos vitales.	*to-MAHR los SEEG-nos vee-TAH-lays.*
weigh you.	pesarle.	*pay-SAHR-lay*
take your blood pressure.	tomar la presion.	*to-MAR la pray-SYON.*
Extend your arm and relax.	Extienda su brazo y descánselo.	*Eks-TAHN-da soo BRAH-so e days-KAHN-say-lo.*
I'm going to take your…	Le voy a tomar…	*Lay voy ah to-MAR*
pulse.	el pulso.	*el POOL-so.*
temperature.	su temperatura.	*soo tem-pay-rah-TOO-rah.*
I'm going to count your respirations.	Voy a contar sus respiraciones.	*Voy ah kon-TAR soos res-pe-rah-se-ON-as.*

Obtaining a Blood Sample

I need to draw a blood sample.	Necesito tomar una muestra de la sangre.	*Nay-say-SEE-to to-MAR OO-nah moo-AYS-trah day lah SAHN-gray.*
Please give me your arm.	Por favor, déme el brazo.	*Por fah-VOHR, DAY-MAY el BRAH-so.*
It may cause a little discomfort.	Le puede causar alguna molestia.	*Lay PWAY-day kaw-SAR ahl-GOO-nah mo-LAYS-tah.*
I am going to put a tourniquet around your arm.	Le voy a poner una liga alrededor del brazo.	*Lay VO-e ah po-NAR OO-nah LEE-gah ahl-ray-day-DOR del BRAH-so.*
I am going to draw blood from this vein.	Voy a sacar la sangre de esta vena.	*Voy ah sah-KAR la SAHN-gray day ES-tah VAY-nah.*

Appendix III: Genetics

The advances in the study of genetics are as dramatic as any in the field of medicine. Medical genetics involves studies of inherited diseases, mapping of disease genes, analyses of the molecular mechanism by which genes cause disease, and the diagnosis and treatment of genetic diseases.

The advances in medical genetics are so rapid that no selection or description of terms remains constant for long. Accordingly, this listing of terms is basic and intended only to stimulate further study in this exciting field.

Terms Related to the Number of Chromosomes in a Cell

aneuploid (an´u-ploid): Indicates that there is not (an-) a normal (eu-) set (ploid) of chromosomes.

autosomes (aw´to-sōmz): The 22 pairs of chromosomes that are homologs, meaning the pairs are the same (homo). These are the nongender, nonsex chromosomes.

clone (klōn): Genetically identical cells or organisms derived asexually from a single common ancestor.

diploid (dip´loid): Cell with two (di-) sets (ploid) of chromosomes. A normal somatic cell of the human body has two sets of chromosomes, or a total of 46, one set of 23 from each parent.

dispermy (di´spər-me): Indicates that an egg has been fertilized by two (di-) sperm and has received a set of chromosomes from both sperm (2 × 23) and a set from the egg (23), for a total of 69 chromosomes.

euploid (u´ploid): Cell that contains a normal number of chromosomes in its nucleus. The term means normal (eu) set (ploid), or 46 chromosomes in each cell in humans.

haploid (hap´loid): Cell with a single (hap) set (loid) of chromosomes, or 23 chromosomes. A sperm has a single set because it is intended to gain another set when it joins an egg, which is also haploid.

karyotype (kar´e-o-tīp): The symbolic representation, using numbers, letters, and other symbols, of the chromosomal content of an individual, tissue, or cell line.

monosomy (mon´o-so″me): Absence of one (mono-) chromosome of an otherwise diploid cell. In humans, the person has one full set (23) and one set of 22 (23 minus 1), for a total of 45 chromosomes; this is commonly known as having a missing chromosome.

polyploidy (pol´e-ploi″de): Term describing a cell that contains at least one complete set (ploid) of extra (poly) chromosomes, for a total of 69 (3 × 23) or more. Occurs in some animals (not viable humans) and some plants.

tetraploidy (tet´rə-ploi-de): Cell that contains four (tetra-) sets (ploid) of 23 chromosomes, for a total of 92 (4 × 23) chromosomes. Does not occur in viable humans.

triploidy (trip´loi-de): Cell that contains three (tri-) sets (ploid) of chromosomes. In humans, the presence of 23 chromosomes for a total of 69 (3 × 23) chromosomes, a frequent finding in abortuses.

trisomy (tri´so-me): Indicates that there is one extra chromosome (somy) in addition to the usual diploid; the person has two sets of chromosomes (2 × 23) plus one extra, for a total of 3 (tri-) units, or 47 chromosomes.

Terms Related to the Structure and Function of Genes and Chromosomes

allele (ə-lēl´): Any of several forms of a gene, usually arising through mutation, that are responsible for hereditary variation. Allele means "of one another," indicating the hereditary linkage. The term is short for allelomorph, which loosely translated means "the change of one another." *Note:* Different versions of the same allele are said to be allelic, meaning they are related but not the same.

bases (bā´ses) (A, C, G, T): Four nitrogenous substances (bases) that make up part of the DNA molecule: adenine (A), cytosine (C), guanine (G), and thymine (T). Combinations of these four bases specify amino acid sequences that form proteins.

chromosome (kro´mo-sōm): Dark-colored (chrom[o]) body (some, soma) formed just before a cell divides that carries the genetic information for the cell. It is made up of chromatin, a substance that gives the nucleus of a cell a granular or colored (chrom) appearance.

codon (ko´don): A set of three different bases that specifies an amino acid, which is a building block of protein (this is a very simple explanation of a complex interaction).

cytogenics, cytogenetics (si-to-jen´iks, si-to-jə-net´iks): Study of chromosomes and their abnormalities; a combination of the study of cytology and genetics.

DNA and RNA: Deoxyribonucleic acid (de-ok″se-ri-bo-noo-kle´ik as´id) and ribonucleic acid (ri″bo-noo-kle´ik as´id); the materials that make up a gene. DNA is the double-helix or twisted ladder shape molecule; the double helix has come to be the symbol of genetic studies.

dominant allele and recessive allele (dom´ĭ-nənt ə-lēl; re-ses´iv ə-lēl): A dominant allele is one that masks, or dominates, another, and a recessive allele is one that is dominated by the other. Some mutations are manifested when only one gene of an allelic pair carries the mutation and others only when both genes of an allelic pair carry the mutation. A mutation is a permanent, inheritable change in a gene. Some alleles are codominant, meaning that they are both expressed when they occur together; for example, blood type AB in the ABO blood typing system.

exon and intron (ek´son, in´tron): Portion of a gene that is located near the end (ex-) of the chromosome, thus its name, exon; intron describes the DNA sequence found between (in-) two exons.

flow cytometry (flo si-tom´ə-tre): Process in which the chromosomes in the cell (cyto[o]) are counted and measured (-metry). Because chromosome sequence is important, the sequence is also measured.

gene (jēn): One of the segments that make up a chromosome and carry the inheritance of characteristics and diseases. The term means stock, from which we inherit; the root word gen also means born or produced.

gene therapy (jēn ther´ə-pe): Insertion of normal genes into a cell to correct a disease (this is a simple definition of a complex process).

genome (je´nōm): Complete set of genes in the chromosomes of each cell of a particular organism.

genotype (je´no-tīp): The entire genetic constitution of an individual, or an individual's allelic, or genetic, makeup at a particular location on a chromosome.

germline gene therapy (jerm´līn jēn ther´ə-pe): Therapy that alters all the cells of the body, including the germ line, which means that these changes can be inherited. (See somatic.)

Human Genome Project: An international research effort to map and sequence the entire genetic makeup of humans, and to analyze, store, and make available the information obtained.

linkage analysis (lingk´əj ə-nal´ĭ-sis): Describes the determination of the order and distance between genes in genetic mapping.

locus (lo´kəs): The position of alleles on a chromosome. The location of alleles is important because they pair with other alleles according to location.

mutation (mu-ta´shən): A permanent, transmissible change in the genetic material, usually in a single gene; can also mean gross alteration in chromosomal structure.

phenotype (fe´no-tīp): The observable appearance (pheno) of characteristics of an individual (type) as a result of the interaction of genes and the environment.

pleiotropy (pli-ot´rə-pe): Describes genes that have multiple (pleio), seemingly unrelated effects. The suffix -tropy means turns, so an association of new symptoms at every turn (-tropy) is a way to learn this term. An example is Marfan syndrome, with long limbs, narrow face, detached lens, and scoliosis.

polygenic (pol-e-jen´ik): Trait caused by the combined effects of many (poly) genes (genic).

RNA, ribonucleic acid (ri˝bo-noo-kle´ik as´id): Found in both the nucleus and cytoplasm of cells; plays several roles in the translation of the genetic code and the assembly of proteins.

ROI: Abbreviation for region of interest; a part of the chromosome that is being studied.

sex chromosomes (seks kro´mo-sōms): Gender-, or sex-, specific chromosomes. A male is made up of a Y chromosome from the father and an X from the mother (XY). A female is made up of an X from the father and an X from the mother (XX). The mother produces only X chromosomes. The father can produce sperm containing X or Y chromosomes; therefore the father determines the gender of the child.

somatic cell gene therapy (so-mat´ik sel jēn ther´ə-pe): Therapy that alters only the body cells; the changes are not passed on to the next generation (see germ line).

Terms Related To Types of Genetic Diseases

chromosome disorder (kro´mo-sōm dis-or´dər): Disease in which entire chromosomes, or large segments of them, are missing, duplicated, or otherwise altered. An example is Down syndrome (also known as trisomy 21).

genomic imprinting (im-print´ing): Rare situation in which genetic defects cause a different disease when inherited from the mother than when inherited from the father. The genetic marking (imprint) is different depending on which parent contributed the gene. Examples are Prader-Willi syndrome, which is inherited from the father, and Angelman syndrome, which is inherited from the mother; the genetic defect is thought to be the same in both syndromes.

mitochondrial disorders (mi-to-kon´dre-əl dis-or´dərs): Disorders associated with alterations in the chromosomes in the mitochondria of the cell; these are very rare disorders. An example is MELAS syndrome (mitochondrial [M] encephalopathy [E], lactic [L] acidosis [A], and strokelike [S] episodes).

multifactorial disorders (mul˝te-fak-tor´e-əl dis-or´dərs): Genetic diseases that are caused by more than one (multi-) factor, such as multiple genetic disorders and environmental causes. Examples are cleft lip and cleft palate and diabetes.

single-gene disorders (sing´gəl jēn dis-or´dərs): Disorders in which a single gene is altered; these conditions are sometimes referred to as mendelian disorders, named for Gregor Johann Mendel (1822-1884), an Austrian monk, who is considered the father of genetics. Mendel's experiments on garden peas and the resultant knowledge transferred to human genetics is an example of the importance of genetics in both humans and plants. Examples of single-gene disorders are cystic fibrosis, hemophilia A, sickle cell disease, and Marfan syndrome.

Appendix IV: Conversion Tables

Weight Equivalents

1 lb	= 453.6 g = 0.4536 kg = 16 oz
1 oz	= 38.35 g
1 kg	= 1000 g = 2.2046 lb
1 g	= 1000 mg
1 mg	= 1000 mcg = 0.001 g
1 mcg	= 0.001 mg = 0.000001 g

1 mcg/g or 1 mg/kg is the same as parts per million (ppm).
g, gram; kg, kilogram; lb, pound; mcg, microgram; mg, milligram; oz, ounce.

Conversion Factors*

1 mg	= 1/65 gr	1/60
1 g	= 15.43 gr	15
1 kg	= 2.20 lb	Avoirdupois
	= 2.68 lb	Troy
1 gr	= 0.065 g	60 mg
1 dr	= 27.34 gr g	Avoirdupois
1 oz	= 31.1 g	30+
1 mL	= 16.23 min	16
1 L	= 1.06 qt	1+
	= 33.80 fl oz	34
1 min	= 0.062 mL	0.06
1 fl dr	= 3.7 mL	4
1 fl oz	= 29.57 mL	30
1 pt	= 473.2 mL	500
1 qt	= 946.4 mL	1000

*Commonly used approximate values
dr, dram; fl dr, fluid dram; fl oz, fluid ounce; g, gram; gr, grain; kg, kilogram; L, liter; min, minum; mL, milliliter; pt, pint; qt, quart.

Temperature Conversion

Degrees Celsius to degrees Fahrenheit: (°C) $\frac{9}{5}$ + 32
Degrees Fahrenheit to degrees Celsius: (°F − 32) $\frac{5}{9}$

Weight-Unit Conversion Factors

Units Given	Units Wanted	For Conversion Multiply by
lb	g	453.6
lb	kg	0.4536
oz	g	28.35
kg	lb	2.2046
kg	mg	1,000,000
kg	g	1,000
g	mg	1,000
g	mcg	1,000,000
mg	mcg	1,000
mg/g	mg/lb	453.6
mg/kg	mg/lb	0.4536
mcg/kg	mcg/lb	0.4536
kcal/kg	kcal/lb	0.4536
kcal/lb	kcal/kg	2.2046
ppm	mcg/g	1
ppm	mg/kg	1
ppm	mg/lb	0.4536
mg/kg	%	0.0001
ppm	%	0.0001
mg/g	%	0.1
g/kg	%	0.1

g, gram; kcal, kilocalorie; kg, kilogram; lb, pound; mcg, microgram; mg, milligram; oz, ounce; ppm, parts per million.

Volume Equivalents

Household	Metric
1 drop (gt)	= 0.06 milliliter (mL)
15 drops (gtt)	= 1 mL (1 cc)
1 teaspoon (tsp)	= 5 mL
1 tablespoon (tbs)	= 15 mL
2 tablespoons	= 30 mL
1 ounce (oz)	= 30 mL
1 teacup	= 180 mL (6 oz)
1 glass	= 240 mL (8 oz)
1 measuring cup	= 240 mL (0.5 pint)
2 measuring cups	= 500 mL (1 pint)

Appendix V: Word Parts

This appendix has two parts.
   A. Alphabetized Word Parts and Meanings
   B. English Words and Corresponding Word Parts

A. Alphabetized Word Parts and Meanings

WORD PART	MEANING
a-	no, not, without
ab-	away from
abdomin(o)	abdomen
-able	capable of, able to
-ac	pertaining to
acid(o)	acid
acr(o)	extremities (arms and legs)
ad-	toward
aden(o)	gland
adenoid(o)	adenoids
adip(o)	fat
adren(o), adrenal(o)	adrenal gland
aer(o)	air or gas
-al	pertaining to
alb(o), albin(o)	white
albumin(o)	albumin
algesi(o)	sensitivity to pain
-algia	pain
alkal(o)	alkaline, basic
alveol(o)	alveoli, air sac
amni(o)	amnion
amyl(o)	starch
an-	no, not, without
ana-	upward, excessive, again
an(o)	anus
andr(o)	male or masculine
aneurysm(o)	aneurysm
angi(o)	vessel
ankyl(o)	stiff
-ant	that which causes
ante-	before in time or in place
anter(o)	anterior or front
anthrac(o)	coal
anti-	against
aort(o)	aorta
append(o), appendic(o)	appendix
arachn(o)	spider or arachnoid membrane
arter(o), arteri(o)	artery
arteriol(o)	arteriole
arthr(o), articul(o)	joint; articulation
-ary	pertaining to

WORD PART	MEANING
-ase	enzyme
-asthenia	weakness
-ate	to cause an action or the result of an action
atel(o)	imperfect or incomplete
ather(o)	yellowish, fatty plaque
-ation	process
atri(o)	atrium
audi(o)	hearing
aut(o)	self
axill(o)	axilla (armpit)
bacter(i), bacteri(o)	bacteria
balan(o)	glans penis
bi-	two
bi(o)	life or living
bil(i)	bile or gall
blast(o), -blast	immature, embryonic form
blephar(o)	eyelid
brady-	slow
bronch(o), bronchi(o)	bronchi
bronchiol(o)	bronchioles
bucc(o)	cheek
burs(o)	bursa
calc(i)	calcium
calcane(o)	calcaneus (heel bone)
cancer(o)	cancer
-capnia	carbon dioxide
carcin(o)	cancer
cardi(o)	heart
carp(o)	carpus (wrist)
caud(o)	tail or toward the tail
cec(o)	cecum
-cele	hernia
cellul(o)	little cell or compartment
-centesis	surgical puncture to aspirate or remove fluid
centi-	one hundred or one hundredth
cephal(o)	head
cerebell(o)	cerebellum
cerebr(o)	brain, cerebrum
cervic(o)	neck; cervix uteri

WORD PART	MEANING
cheil(o)	lip
chem(o)	chemical
chir(o)	hand
chlor(o)	green
chol(e)	bile
cholecyst(o)	gallbladder
choledoch(o)	common bile duct
chondr(o)	cartilage
chori(o)	chorion
chrom(o)	color
-cidal	killing
circum-	around
-clasia	break
clavicul(o)	clavicle (collarbone)
coagul(o)	coagulation
coccyg(o)	coccyx (tail bone)
col(o), colon(o)	colon or large intestine
colp(o)	vagina
coni(o)	dust
contra-	against
coron(o)	crown
cost(o)	costae (ribs)
crani(o)	cranium (skull)
crin(o)	to secrete
-crine	secrete
cry(o)	cold
crypt(o)	hidden
cutane(o)	skin
cyan(o)	blue
-cyesis	pregnancy
cyst(o)	bladder, cyst, fluid-filled sac
cyt(o), -cyte	cell
dacry(o), lacrim(o)	tear
dactyl(o)	finger or toe (digit)
de-	down, from, or reversing
dendr(o)	tree
dent(i), dent(o)	tooth
derm(a), derm(o), dermat(o)	skin
-derm	skin or germ layer
-desis	binding, fusion
di-	two
dia-	through
diplo-	double
-dipsia	thirst
dist(o)	distant, far
diverticul(o)	diverticula
dors(o)	dorsal, back
duoden(o)	duodenum
-dynia	pain
dys-	bad, difficult
-eal	pertaining to
ech(o)	sound
-ectasia, ectasis	dilatation (dilation, enlargement) or stretching of a structure or part
ecto-	out, without, away from

WORD PART	MEANING
-ectomy	excision (surgical removal or cutting out)
-edema	swelling
electr(o)	electricity
embol(o)	embolus
-emesis	vomiting
-emia	condition of the blood
en-, end-, endo-	inside
encephal(o)	brain
endocardi(o)	endocardium
enter(o)	small intestine; intestines
epi-	above, on
epididym(o)	epididymis
epiglott(o)	epiglottis
-er	one who
erythemat(o)	erythema or redness
erythr(o)	red
esophag(o)	esophagus
esthesi(o)	feeling or sensation
-esthesia	sensitivity to pain
eu-	good, normal
-eum	membrane
ex-, exo-, extra-	out, without, away from
fasci(o)	fascia
femor(o)	femur
fet(o)	fetus
fibr(o)	fiber or fibrous
fibrin(o)	fibrin
fibul(o)	fibula
fluor(o)	emitting or reflecting light
follicul(o)	follicle
fung(i)	fungus
gastr(o)	stomach
gen(o)	beginning, origin
-genesis	producing or forming
-genic	produced by or in
genit(o)	organs of reproduction
ger(a), ger(o), geront(o)	elderly
gigant(o)	large
gingiv(o)	gums
gli(o)	neuroglia or a sticky substance
glomerul(o)	glomerulus
gloss(o), lingu(o)	tongue
gluc(o)	glucose
glyc(o), glycos(o)	sugar
gon(o)	genitals or reproduction
gonad(o)	gonad
-gram	a record
-graph	instrument for recording
-graphy	process of recording
-gravida	pregnant female
gynec(o)	female
heli(o)	sun
hem(a), hem(o), hemat(o)	blood
hemi-	half, partly
hemoglobin(o)	hemoglobin
hepat(o)	liver

WORD PART	MEANING	WORD PART	MEANING
herni(o)	hernia	lith(o), -lith	stone; calculus
hidr(o)	perspiration, sweat	lob(o)	lobe
hist(o)	tissue	log(o)	knowledge, words
home(o)	sameness, constant	-logic, -logical	pertaining to
humer(o)	humerus (upper arm bone)	-logist	one who studies; specialist
hydr(o)	water	-logy	study or science of
hyper-	excessive, more than normal	lumb(o)	lower back
hypo-	beneath or below normal	lymph(o)	lymph, lymphatics
hypophys(o)	pituitary gland (hypophysis)	lymphaden(o)	lymph node
hyster(o)	uterus	lymphangi(o)	lymph vessel
-ia-, -iasis	condition	lymphat(o)	lymphatics
-iac	one who suffers	lys(o)	destruction, dissolving
iatr(o)	physician or treatment	-lysin	that which destroys
-iatrician	practitioner	-lysis	process of loosening, freeing, or destroying
-iatrics, -iatry	medical profession or treatment	-lytic	capable of destroying
-ible	able to, capable of	macro-	large or great
-ic	pertaining to	mal-	bad
ichthy(o)	fish	malac(o)	soft, softening
idi(o)	individual	-malacia	soft; abnormal softening
ile(o)	ileum	mamm(o)	breast
ili(o)	ilium	mandibul(o)	mandible
immun(o)	immune	-mania	excessive preoccupation
in-	not or inside (in)	-maniac	one who shows excessive preoccupation
infer(o)	lowermost or below	mast(o)	breast
infra-	beneath, under	maxill(o)	maxilla
insulin(o)	insulin	mechan(o)	mechanical
inter-	between	medi(o), medio-	middle
intestin(o)	intestines	mediastin(o)	mediastinum
intra-	within	mega-, megalo-	large, enlarged, or great
iod(o)	iodine	-megaly	enlargement
ipsi-	same	melan(o)	black
ir(o), irid(o)	iris	men(o)	month
is(o)	equal	mening(i), mening(o)	meninges
ischi(o)	ischium	ment(o)	mind
-ism	condition or theory	meso-	middle
-ist	one who	meta-	change; next, as in a series
-itis	inflammation	metr(o)	measure; uterine tissue
-ium	membrane	-meter	instrument used to measure
-ive	pertaining to	-metry	process of measuring
jejun(o)	jejunum	micro-	small
kal(i)	potassium	mid-	middle
kary(o)	nucleus	milli-	one thousandth
kerat(o)	cornea; hard, horny	mono-	one
ket(o), keton(o)	ketone bodies	morph(o)	shape; form
kinesi(o)	movement	muc(o)	mucus
-kinesia, -kinesis	movement, motion	multi-	many
lacrim(o)	tear	muscul(o), my(o)	muscle
lact(o)	milk	myc(o)	fungus
lapar(o)	abdominal wall	myel(o)	bone marrow or spinal cord
laryng(o)	larynx	my(o)	muscle
later(o)	side	myocardi(o)	myocardium
leps(o), -lepsy	seizure	narc(o)	stupor
leuk(o); occasionally leuc(o)	white	nas(o)	nose
-lexia	words, phrases	nat(o)	birth
lingu(o)	tongue	natr(o)	sodium
lip(o)	fat, lipid		

WORD PART	MEANING
ne(o)	new
necr(o)	death
nephr(o)	kidney
nerv(o), neur(o)	nerve
noc(i)	cause harm, injury, or pain
noct(i)	night
norm(o)	normal
nos(o)	disease
nucle(o)	nucleus
nulli-	none
nyct(o)	night
o(o)	ovum
obstetr(o)	midwife
ocul(o)	eye
odont(o)	teeth
-oid	resembling
-ole	small
olig(o)	few, scanty
-oma	tumor
omphal(o)	umbilicus (navel)
onc(o)	tumor
onych(o)	nail
oophor(o)	ovary
ophthalm(o)	eye
-opia, opt(o), optic(o)	vision
or(o)	mouth
orchi(o), orchid(o)	testis
-orexia	appetite
orth(o)	straight
-ose	sugar
-osis	condition (often an abnormal condition; sometimes, an increase), disease
oste(o)	bone
ot(o)	ear
-ous	pertaining to or characterized by
ovari(o)	ovary
ox(i)	oxygen
palat(o)	palate
pan-	all
pancreat(o)	pancreas
para-	near, beside, or abnormal
par(o)	bearing offspring
-para	woman who has given birth
parathyroid(o)	parathyroid gland
patell(o)	patella
path(o), -pathy	disease
ped(o)	child (sometimes, foot)
pelv(i)	pelvis
pen(o)	penis
-penia	deficiency
-pepsia	digestion
per-	through or by
peri-	around
pericardi(o)	pericardium
perine(o)	perineum

WORD PART	MEANING
peritone(o)	peritoneum
pex(o), -pexy	surgical fixation
phag(o)	eat, ingest
-phagia, -phagic, -phagy	eating, swallowing
phalang(o)	phalanx (bones of fingers or toes)
pharmac(o), pharmaceut(i)	drugs or medicine
pharyng(o)	pharynx
phas(o), -phasia	speech
phil(o)	attraction
phleb(o)	vein
-phobia	abnormal fear
phon(o)	voice
-phoresis	transmission
phot(o)	light
phren(o)	mind or diaphragm
-phylaxis	protection
-physis	growth
pil(o)	hair
pituitar(o)	pituitary gland
plas(o), -plasia	formation, development
plast(o)	repair
-plasty	surgical repair
pleg(o), -plegia	paralysis
pleur(o)	pleura
-pnea	breathing
pneum(o)	lungs or air
pneumon(o)	lungs
pod(o)	foot
-poiesis	production
-poietin	that which causes production
poikil(o)	irregular
poly-	many
post-	after, behind
poster(o)	back, behind
pre-	before in time or in place
primi-	first
pro-	for, favoring, supporting
proct(o)	anus, rectum
prostat(o)	prostate
prote(o), protein(o)	protein
proxim(o)	near
pseudo-	false
psych(o)	mind
-ptosis	prolapse (sagging or drooping)
-ptysis	spitting
pub(o)	pubis
pulm(o), pulmon(o)	lung
py(o)	pus
pyel(o)	renal pelvis
pylor(o)	pylorus
pyr(o)	fire
quad-, quadri-	four
rach(i), rachi(o)	vertebral or spinal column, spine (backbone)

WORD PART	MEANING
radi(o)	radiant energy (sometimes, radius)
rect(o)	rectum
ren(o)	kidney
retro-	behind, backward
rheumat(o)	rheumatism
rhin(o)	nose
rhythm(o), rrhythm(o)	rhythm
rhytid(o)	wrinkle
-rrhage, -rrhagia	excessive bleeding or hemorrhage
-rrhaphy	suture (uniting a wound by stitches)
-rrhea	flow or discharge
-rrhexis	rupture
sacr(o)	sacrum
salping(o)	fallopian or uterine tube or auditory tube
-sarcoma	malignant tumor from connective tissue
scapul(o)	scapula (shoulder blade)
schis(o), schiz(o), schist(o), -schisis	split, cleft
scler(o)	hard
-sclerosis	hardening
scop(o)	to examine, to view
-scope	instrument used for viewing
-scopy	visual examination with a lighted instrument
scrot(o)	scrotum
seb(o)	sebum
semi-	half, partly
semin(o)	semen
seps(o)	infection
sept(i), sept(o)	infection; septum
sial(o)	saliva; salivary glands
sialaden(o)	salivary glands
sigmoid(o)	sigmoid colon
sin(o), sinus(o)	sinus
som(a), somat(o)	body
son(o)	sound
-spasm	twitching, cramp
sperm(o), spermat(o)	spermatozoa
spher(o)	round
spin(o)	spine
spir(o)	to breathe (sometimes, spiral)
splen(o)	spleen
spondyl(o)	vertebrae
-stalsis	contraction
staphyl(o)	grapelike cluster; uvula
-stasis	stopping, controlling
-stenosis	narrowing; stricture
stern(o)	sternum (breastbone)
steth(o)	chest
stomat(o)	mouth
-stomy	formation of an opening

WORD PART	MEANING
strept(o)	twisted
sub-	beneath, under
super-	above, beyond, excessive
super(o), supra-	above, beyond
sym-, syn-	joined, together
synov(o), synovi(o)	synovial membrane
tachy-	fast
tars(o)	ankle (sometimes, edge of eyelid)
tel(e)	distant, far
ten(o), tend(o), tendin(o)	tendon
test(o), testicul(o)	testicle
tetra-	four
therapeut(o), -therapy	treatment
therm(o)	heat
thorac(o)	thorax (chest)
thromb(o)	thrombus; clot
thym(o)	thymus
thyr(o), thyroid(o)	thyroid gland
tibi(o)	tibia
-tic	pertaining to
tom(o)	to cut
-tome	an instrument used for cutting
-tomy	incision (cutting into tissue)
tonsill(o)	tonsil
top(o)	place or position
tox(o), toxic(o)	poison
trache(o)	trachea
trans-	across
tri-	three
trich(o)	hair
-tripsy	surgical crushing
trop(o)	to stimulate
-tropic	stimulating
-tropin	that which stimulates
troph(o), -trophic, -trophy	nutrition
uln(o)	ulna (a bone of the forearm)
ultra-	excessive
umbilic(o)	umbilicus
ungu(o)	nail
uni-	one
ur(o)	urinary tract, urine
ureter(o)	ureter
urethr(o)	urethra
-uria	urine or urination
urin(o)	urine
uter(o)	uterus
vag(o)	vagus nerve
vagin(o)	vagina
valv(o), valvul(o)	valve
varic(o)	twisted and swollen
vas(o)	vessel; ductus deferens
vascul(o)	vessel
ven(i), ven(o)	vein

WORD PART	MEANING	WORD PART	MEANING
ventr(o)	belly	viscer(o)	viscera
ventricul(o)	ventricle	vulv(o)	vulva
venul(o)	venule	xanth(o)	yellow
vertebr(o)	vertebra	xer(o)	dry
vesic(o)	bladder or blister	-y	state or condition
vir(o), virus(o)	virus		

B. English Words and Corresponding Word Parts

MEANING	WORD PART	MEANING	WORD PART
abdomen	abdomin(o)	basic	alkal(o)
abdominal wall	lapar(o)	bearing offspring	par(o)
able to	-able, -ible	before	ante-, pre-, pro-
abnormal	para-	beginning	gen(o), -genic, -genesis,
abnormal softening	-malacia		-genous
above	epi-, super-, super(o), supra-	behind	poster(o), post-, retr(o)
acid	acid(o)	belly side	ventr(o)
across	trans-	below normal	hypo-
adenoids	adenoid(o)	below or beneath	hypo-, infer(o), infra-, sub-
adrenaline	adrenalin(o)	beside	para-
adrenals	adren(o), adrenal(o)	between	inter-
after	post-	beyond	super-, super(o), supra-
again	ana-	bile	bil(i), chol(e)
against	anti-, contra-	binding	-desis
aged	ger(a), ger(o), geront(o)	birth	nat(o)
air	aer(o), pneum(o)	birth (give birth)	par(o)
air sac	alveol(o)	woman who has	-para
albumin	albumin(o)	given birth	
alkaline	alkal(o)	black	melan(o)
all	pan-	bladder	cyst(o), vesic(o)
alveolus	alveol(o)	bleeding, excessive	-rrhage, -rrhagia
amnion	amni(o)	blister	vesic(o)
aneurysm	aneurysm(o)	blood	hem(a), hem(o), hemat(o),
ankle bone	tars(o)		-emia
anterior	anter(o)	blue	cyan(o)
anus	an(o)	body	som(a), somat(o)
anus and rectum	proct(o)	bone	oste(o)
aorta	aort(o)	bone marrow	myel(o)
appendix	append(o), appendic(o)	brain	cerebr(o), encephal(o)
appetite	-orexia	break	-clasia
arachnoid	arachn(o)	breast	mamm(o), mast(o)
armpit	axill(o)	breast bone	stern(o)
arms and legs	acr(o)	breathe, breathing	-pnea, spir(o)
around	circum-, peri-	bronchi	bronch(o), bronchi(o)
arteriole	arteriol(o)	bronchiole	bronchiol(o)
artery	arter(o), arteri(o)	bursa	burs(o)
articulation	arthr(o), articul(o)	by	per-
atrium	atri(o)	calcaneus	calcane(o)
attraction	phil(o)	calcium	calc(i)
away from	ab-, ecto-, ex-, exo-, extra-	calculus	lith(o), -lith
axilla	axill(o)	cancer	cancer(o), carcin(o)
back	dors(o), poster(o)	capable of	-able, -ible
backward	retr(o)	carbon dioxide	-capnia
bacteria	bacter(i), bacteri(o)	carpus	carp(o)
bad	dys-, mal-	cartilage	chondr(o)

MEANING	WORD PART
(to) cause an action or the result of an action	-ate
cause harm, injury, or pain	noc(i)
(that which) causes	-ant
cecum	cec(o)
cell	cyt(o), -cyte
cell, little	cellul(o)
cerebellum	cerebell(o)
cerebrum	cerebr(o)
cervix uteri	cervic(o)
change	meta-
characterized by	-ous
cheek	bucc(o)
chemical	chem(o)
chest	steth(o), thorac(o)
child	ped(o)
chorion	chori(o)
clavicle	clavicul(o)
cleft	-schisis, schis(o), schist(o), schiz(o)
clot (thrombus)	thromb(o)
cluster	staphyl(o)
coagulation	coagul(o)
coal	anthrac(o)
coccyx	coccyg(o)
cold	cry(o)
collarbone	clavicul(o)
colon	col(o), colon(o)
color	chrom(o)
common bile duct	choledoch(o)
compartment	cellul(o)
condition	-ia, -iasis, -ism, -osis, -y
condition of the blood	-emia
constant	home(o)
contraction	-stalsis
controlling	-stasis
cornea	kerat(o)
costae	cost(o)
cramp	-spasm
cranium	crani(o)
crown	coron(o)
cut (to cut)	tom(o)
incision or cutting	-tomy
instrument used to cut	-tome
cyst	cyst(o)
death	necr(o)
decreased or deficient	-penia
destruction	lys(o)
that which destroys	-lysin
process of destroying	-lysis
capable of destroying	-lytic
development	plas(o), -plasia
diaphragm	phren(o)
difficult	dys-

MEANING	WORD PART
digestion	-pepsia
digit	dactyl(o)
dilation	-ectasia, -ectasis
discharge	-rrhea
disease	nos(o), path(o), -osis, -pathy
dissolving	lys(o)
distant	dist(o), tel(e)
diverticula	diverticul(o)
dorsal	dors(o)
double	dipl(o)
down	de-
drooping	-ptosis
drugs	pharmac(o), pharmaceut(i)
dry	xer(o)
ductus deferens (vas deferens)	vas(o)
duodenum	duoden(o)
dust	coni(o)
ear	ot(o)
eat	phag(o)
eating	-phagia, -phagic, -phagy
edge of eyelid	tars(o)
egg (ovum)	o(o)
elderly	ger(a), ger(o), geront(o)
electricity	electr(o)
embolus	embol(o)
embryonic form	-blast, blast(o)
emitting or reflecting light	fluor(o)
endocardium	endocardi(o)
enlargement	-megaly
enzyme	-ase
epididymis	epididym(o)
epiglottis	epiglott(o)
equal	is(o)
erythema	erythemat(o)
esophagus	esophag(o)
examine	scop(o)
instrument used	-scope
process of examining	-scopy
excessive	ana-, hyper-, super-, ultra-
excessive preoccupation	-mania
excision	-ectomy
extremities	acr(o)
eye	ocul(o), ophthalm(o)
eyelid	blephar(o)
fallopian tube	salping(o)
false	pseudo-
far	dist(o), tel(e)
fascia	fasci(o)
fast	tachy-
fat	adip(o), lip(o)
favoring	pro-
fear (abnormal)	-phobia
feeling	esthesi(o), -esthesia

MEANING	WORD PART
female	gynec(o)
femur	femor(o)
fetus	fet(o)
few	olig(o)
fiber, fibrous	fibr(o)
fibrin	fibrin(o)
fibula	fibul(o)
fingers or toes	dactyl(o)
fire	pyr(o)
first	primi-
fish	ichthy(o)
flow	-rrhea
follicle	follicul(o)
foot	ped(o), pod(o)
for	pro-
form	morph(o)
forming	-genesis
formation	plas(o), -plasia
formation of an opening	-stomy
four	quad-, quadri-, tetra-
from	de-
front	anter(o)
fungus	fung(i), myc(o)
fusion	-desis
gall	bil(i), chol(e)
gallbladder	cholecyst(o)
gas	aer(o)
genitals	genit(o), gon(o)
germ layer	-derm
gland	aden(o)
glans penis	balan(o)
glomerulus	glomerul(o)
glucose	gluc(o)
gonads (ovaries and testes)	gonad(o)
good	eu-
green	chlor(o)
growth	-physis
gums	gingiv(o)
hair	pil(o), trich(o)
half	hemi-, semi-
hand	chir(o)
hard	kerat(o), scler(o)
hardening	scler(o), -sclerosis
head	cephal(o)
hearing	audi(o)
heart	cardi(o)
heat	therm(o)
heel bone	calcane(o)
hemoglobin	hemoglobin(o)
hemorrhage	-rrhage, -rrhagia
hernia	-cele, herni(o)
hidden	crypt(o)
horny	kerat(o)
humerus	humer(o)

MEANING	WORD PART
hypophysis	hypophys(o), pituitar(o)
ileum	ile(o)
ilium	ili(o)
immature form	blast(o), -blast
immune	immun(o)
imperfect	atel(o)
incision	tom(o), -tomy
instrument used	-tome
incomplete	atel(o)
increase	-osis
individual	idio-
infection	seps(o), sept(i), sept(o)
inferior	infer(o)
inflammation	-itis
ingest	phag(o)
inside	en-, end-, endo-, in-
insulin	insulin(o)
intestine	enter(o), intestin(o)
iodine	iod(o)
iris	ir(o), irid(o)
irregular	poikil(o)
irrigation	-clysis
ischium	ischi(o)
jejunum	jejun(o)
joined together	syn-, sym-
joint	arthr(o), articul(o)
ketone bodies	ket(o), keton(o)
kidney	nephr(o), ren(o)
killing	-cidal
kneecap	patell(o)
knowledge	log(o)
large	gigant(o), macr(o), megal(o), mega-, -megaly
large intestine	col(o), colon(o)
larynx	laryng(o)
life	bi(o)
light	phot(o)
lip	cheil(o)
lipid	lip(o)
liver	hepat(o)
living	bi(o)
lobe	lob(o)
location	top(o)
lower back	lumb(o)
lowermost	infer(o)
lung	pneum(o), pneumon(o), pulm(o), pulmon(o)
lymph	lymph(o)
lymph node	lymphaden(o)
lymph vessel	lymphangi(o)
lymphatics	lymph(o), lymphat(o)
male	andr(o)
mandible	mandibul(o)
many	multi-, poly-
masculine	andr(o)
maxilla	maxill(o)

MEANING	WORD PART
measure	metr(o)
instrument used	-meter
process	-metry
mechanical	mechan(o)
mediastinum	mediastin(o)
medicine	-iatrics, -iatry, pharmac(o), pharmaceut(i)
membrane	-eum, -ium
meninges	mening(i), mening(o)
middle	mid-, medi(o), meso-
midwife	obstetr(o)
milk	lact(o)
mind	ment(o), phren(o), psych(o)
month	men(o)
more than normal	hyper-
mouth	or(o), stomat(o)
movement	kinesi(o), -kinesia
mucus	muc(o)
muscle	muscul(o), my(o)
myocardium	myocardi(o)
nail	onych(o), ungu(o)
narrowing	-stenosis
nature	physi(o)
near	para-, proxim(o)
neck	cervic(o)
nerve	neur(o), nerv(o)
neuroglia	gli(o)
new	neo-
new opening	-stomy
next (as in a series)	meta-
night	noct(i), nyct(o)
no	a-, an-
none	nulli-
normal	norm(o), eu-
nose	nas(o), rhin(o)
not	a-, an-, in-
nucleus	kary(o), nucle(o)
nutrition	-trophic, troph(o), -trophy
old	ger(a), ger(o), geront(o)
on	epi-
one	uni-, mon(o)
one hundred, one-hundredth	centi-
one-thousandth	milli-
one who	-er, -ist
one who studies	-logist
one who suffers	-iac
one with excessive preoccupation	-maniac
organs of reproduction	genit(o), gon(o)
origin	gen(o), -gen, -genic, -genesis, -genous
out	ecto-, ex-, exo-, extra-
outside	ecto-, exo-, extra-
outward	exo-
ovary	oophor(o)

MEANING	WORD PART
ovum (egg)	o(o)
oxygen	ox(i)
pain	-algia, -dynia
palate	palat(o)
pancreas	pancreat(o)
paralysis	pleg(o), -plegia
parathyroid gland	parathyroid(o)
partly	semi-
patella (kneecap)	patell(o)
pelvis	pelv(i)
penis	pen(o)
pericardium	pericardi(o)
perineum	perine(o)
peritoneum	peritone(o)
perspiration	hidr(o)
pertaining to	-ac, -al, -ary, -eal, -ic, -ive, -logic, -logical, -ous, -tic
phalanges	phalang(o)
pharynx	pharyng(o)
phrases	-lexia
physician or treatment	iatr(o)
pituitary gland	hypophys(o), pituitar (o)
place (position)	top(o)
pleura	pleur(o)
poison	tox(o), toxic(o)
potassium	kal(i)
practitioner	-iatrician
pregnancy	-cyesis
pregnant female	-gravida
preoccupation (excessive)	-mania
process	-ation
production	-poiesis
that which causes	-poietin
produced by or in	-genic
producing	-genesis
prolapse	-ptosis
prostate gland	prostat(o)
protection	-phylaxis
protein	prote(o), protein(o)
pubis	pub(o)
pus	py(o)
pylorus	pylor(o)
radiant energy	radi(o)
radius	radi(o)
(to) record	gram(o)
record (the record)	-gram
recording instrument	-graph
recording process	-graphy
rectum	rect(o)
red, redness	erythr(o), erythemat(o)
removal	-ectomy
renal pelvis	pyel(o)
repair	plast(o)
reproduction	gon(o)
resembling	-oid

MEANING	WORD PART
reversing	de-
rheumatism	rheumat(o)
rhythm	rhythm(o), rrhythm(o)
ribs	cost(o)
round	spher(o)
rupture	-rrhexis
sac, fluid-filled	cyst(o)
sacrum	sacr(o)
sag	-ptosis
saliva	sial(o)
salivary gland	sial(o), sialaden(o)
same	ipsi-
sameness	home(o)
scanty	olig(o)
scapula (shoulder blade)	scapul(o)
scrotum	scrot(o)
sebum	seb(o)
secrete	crin(o), -crine
seizure	-lepsy, leps(o)
self	aut(o)
semen	semin(o)
sensation	esthesi(o)
sensitivity to pain	algesi(o), -esthesia
septum	sept(o)
shape	morph(o)
shoulder blade	scapul(o)
side	later(o)
sigmoid colon	sigmoid(o)
single	mon(o)
sinus	sin(o), sinus(o)
situated above	super(o), super-, supra-
situated below	infer(o), infra-
skin	cutane(o), derm(a), dermat(o), -derm
skull	crani(o)
slow	brady-
small	micr(o), -ole
small intestine	enter(o)
sodium	natr(o)
soft, softening	-malacia
sound	ech(o), son(o)
specialist	-logist
speech	phas(o), -phasia
sperm, spermatozoa	spermat(o), sperm(o)
spider	arachn(o)
spinal cord	myel(o)
spine	rach(i), rachi(o), spondyl(o), spin(o)
spitting	-ptysis
spleen	splen(o)
split	schis(o), schist(o), schiz(o), -schisis
starch	amyl(o)
state	-y
sternum (breast bone)	stern(o)
sticky substance	gli(o)

MEANING	WORD PART
stiff	ankyl(o)
stimulate	trop(o), -tropic
that which stimulates	-tropin
stomach	gastr(o)
stone	lith(o), -lith
stopping	-stasis
straight	orth(o)
stretching	-ectasia, -ectasis
stricture	-stenosis
study or science of	-logy
stupor	narc(o)
sugar	glyc(o), glycos(o), -ose
sun	heli(o)
supporting	pro-
surgical crushing	-tripsy
surgical fixation	pex(o), -pexy
surgical puncture	-centesis
surgical repair	-plasty
suture	-rrhaphy
swallowing	-phagia, -phagic, -phagy
sweat	hidr(o)
swelling	-edema
symptom	sympt(o)
synovial membrane	synov(o), synovi(o)
tail	caud(o)
tail bone	coccyg(o)
tarsals (ankle bones)	tars(o)
tear (crying)	dacry(o), lacrim(o)
teeth	dent(i), dent(o), odont(o)
tendon	ten(o), tend(o), tendin(o)
testis, testicle	orchi(o), orchid(o), test(o)
theory	-ism
thirst	dips(o), -dipsia
three	tri-
throat	pharyng(o)
thrombus	thromb(o)
through	dia-, per-, trans-
thymus	thym(o)
thyroid gland	thyr(o), thryoid(o)
tibia	tibi(o)
tissue	hist(o)
toe	dactyl(o)
together	sym-, syn-
tongue	gloss(o), lingu(o)
tonsil	tonsill(o)
toward	ad-
trachea	trache(o)
transmission	-phoresis
treatment	iatr(o), -iatry, therapeut(o), -therapy
tree	dendr(o)
tumor	onc(o), -oma
tumor, malignant from connective tissue	-sarcoma
turn	trop(o)

MEANING	WORD PART
twice	di-
twisted	strept(o)
twisted and swollen	varic(o)
twitching	-spasm
two	bi-, di-
ulna	uln(o)
umbilicus	omphal(o), umbilic(o)
under	infra-, sub-
upon	epi-
upper arm bone	humer(o)
uppermost	super(o)
ureter	ureter(o)
urethra	urethr(o)
urinary tract	ur(o)
urination	-uria
urine	ur(o), -uria, urin(o)
uterine tissue	metr(o)
uterine tube	salping(o)
uterus	hyster(o), uter(o)
uvula	staphyl(o)
vagina	colp(o), vagin(o)
vagus nerve	vag(o)
valve	valv(o), valvul(o)
varicose vein	varic(o)
vein	phleb(o), ven(o), ven(i)
ventral	ventr(o)
ventricle	ventricul(o)

MEANING	WORD PART
venule	venul(o)
vertebra	spondyl(o), vertebr(o)
vertebral column	rach(i), rachi(o), spondyl(o), spin(o)
vessel	angi(o), vas(o), vascul(o)
view	scop(o)
instrument used	-scope
process of viewing	-scopy
virus	vir(o), virus(o)
viscera	viscer(o)
vision	opt(o), optic(o)
voice	phon(o)
vomiting	-emesis
vulva	vulv(o)
water	hydr(o)
weakness	-asthenia
white	alb(o), albin(o), leuk(o), leuc(o)
windpipe	trache(o)
within	intra-
without	a-, an-, ecto-, ex-, exo-, extra
words	-lexia, log(o)
wrinkle	rhytid(o)
wrist bone	carp(o)
yellow	xanth(o)
yellow, fatty plaque	ather(o)

Appendix VI: Solutions to Review Exercises

Exercise 1
1. frame
2. answer
3. write
4. check

Exercise 2
1. CF
2. CF
3. WR
4. CF
5. WR
6. WR
7. CF
8. WR
9. WR

Exercise 3
1. P
2. S
3. P
4. S
5. CF
6. S
7. P
8. CF
9. S

Exercise 4
1. P
2. S
3. S
4. S
5. P
6. S
7. P
8. P
9. P

Exercise 5
1. tonsillitis
2. uremia
3. cardioaortitis
4. urogenital
5. enteritis
6. enterocyst

Exercise 6
1. periappendicitis
2. unilateral
3. antiseptic
4. anemia

Exercise 7
1. CF
2. CF

3. S
4. CF
5. P
6. P
7. S
8. P
9. P
10. CF

Exercise 8
1. acidosis
2. acromegaly
3. antiemesis
4. bronchoscopy
5. dysphagia
6. hypothyroidism
7. leukocytosis
8. malabsorption
9. myometrium
10. thrombophlebitis

Exercise 9
1. A
2. A
3. B
4. B
5. A
6. A

7. B
8. A

Exercise 10
1. six
2. se
3. hi
4. i in hi, e in se, e in me

Exercise 11
1. capsules
2. cataracts
3. calculi
4. cortices
5. diagnoses
6. meninges
7. neuroses
8. protozoa
9. vertices
10. viruses
11. appendix
12. fungus
13. larynx
14. prognosis
15. sarcoma
16. spermatozoon
17. syndrome
18. thrombus

Chapter 1 Review

I.
1. A combining form is a word root with an attached vowel to which prefixes and suffixes can be added.
2. A prefix is placed before a word root to modify its meaning.
3. A suffix is attached to the end of a word or word part to modify its meaning.
4. A word root is the main body of a word.

II.
1. CF
2. CF
3. S
4. CF
5. S
6. P
7. P
8. S
9. S
10. CF

III.
1. hypodermic
2. leukemia
3. melanoid
4. myocardial
5. thrombosis

IV.
1. atria
2. bullae
3. bursa
4. cervix
5. enchondroma
6. ganglia

7. index
8. microvilli
9. septa
10. syndromes

V.
cancer, ophthalmoplasty

VI.
1. ad; pos; ad, i
2. ar; ar, o; sol
3. kor; son; kor, ti
4. lak; tos, lak
5. nef; ro, skop; nef

Chapter 2

Exercise 1
1. E
2. B
3. D
4. A
5. E
6. B
7. C
8. F

Exercise 2
1. to secrete
2. feeling or sensation
3. stomach
4. elderly
5. female
6. larynx
7. birth
8. new
9. straight
10. nose

Exercise 3
1. ped(o)
2. ot(o)
3. ophthalm(o)
4. ped(o)
5. cardi(o)

6. immun(o)
7. psych(o)
8. neur(o)
9. dermat(o)
10. ur(o)

Exercise 4
1. cardio/logist
2. endo/crino/logist
3. gyneco/logy
4. gastro/entero/logist
5. cardio/logy
6. onco/logist
7. an/esthesio/logy
8. neo/nato/logy

Exercise 5
1. oto/logist
2. immuno/logist
3. ortho/ped/ist
4. psych/iatry
5. neuro/surgery
6. uro/logist

Exercise 6
1. D
2. I
3. H

4. E
5. G
6. F
7. J
8. C
9. B
10. A

Exercise 7
1. cardiology
2. radiology
3. immunology
4. endocrinology
5. otolaryngology or rhinology
6. obstetrics
7. gastroenterology
8. urology
9. orthopedics
10. rheumatology

Exercise 8
1. pharmaco/logy
2. bio(hazards)
3. radio/logic
4. or/al
5. therapeut/ic
6. endo/crine

Exercise 9
1. chief complaint
2. diagnosis
3. family history
4. history and physical
5. history of present illness
6. history
7. outpatient
8. physical examination
9. past medical history
10. review of systems
11. treatment
12. vital signs

Exercise 10
1. inpatients
2. outpatients
3. HIPAA

Exercise 11
1. E
2. A
3. B
4. C
5. D

Chapter 2 Review

I.
1. cardi/ac: cardi(o) is CF: -ac is S
2. gyneco/logist: gynec(o) is CF; -logist is S
3. ophthalmo/logical: oph-thalm(o) is CF; -logical is S
4. patho/logy: path(o) is CF; -logy is S
5. psych/iatry: psych(o) is CF; -iatry is S

II.
1. life or living
2. secrete
3. tooth
4. inside
5. vision
6. vision
7. mouth
8. drugs or medicine
9. nose
10. urinary tract or urine

III.
(No particular order)
1. anatomy
2. diagnostic test or procedure
3. pathology

4. surgery
5. therapy

IV.
1. B
2. K
3. F
4. J
5. E
6. H
7. L
8. D
9. C
10. A
11. G
12. I

V.
1. A
2. D
3. B
4. C
5. E

VI.
1. dent/al: dent(o) means tooth; -al means pertaining to
2. gastr/ic: gastr(o) means

stomach; -ic means pertaining to
3. neuro/logy: neur(o) means nerve; -logy means the study of
4. onco/logy: onc(o) means tumor; -logy means study or science of
5. ot/ic: ot(o) means ear; -ic means pertaining to

VII.
1. cardiologist
2. obstetrician
3. anesthetist
4. neonatologist
5. gastroenterologist
6. radiologist
7. orthopedist
8. nerve cell
9. clinical pathologist
10. radiopaque

VIII.
1. internist
2. chronic
3. acute
4. triage

5. radiolucent
6. cardiac
7. pathology
8. neurosurgery
9. malignant
10. hormones

IX.
cardiac, psychiatry

X.
1. chief complaint
2. general practitioner
3. licensed vocational nurse
4. obstetrics
5. surgery (or operating room)

XI.
1. an es the ze ol´ə je
2. fə ren´zik
3. gas tro en tər ol´ə je
4. or tho pe´diks
5. ra de o loj´ik

Chapter 3

Exercise 1
1. E
2. B
3. G
4. H
5. F
6. C
7. D
8. A

Exercise 2
1. -penia
2. -rrhea
3. -oid
4. -rrhexis
5. -spasm

Exercise 3
1. ophthalmo/malacia
2. calci/penia
3. oto/rrhea
4. oto/dynia
5. cardio/megaly
6. ophthalmo/scopy

7. oste/oid
8. blepharo/spasm

Exercise 4
1. pulse
2. respiration
3. auscultation
4. percussion
5. palpation
6. ambulation

Exercise 5
1. contrast
2. tomography
3. radioactive
4. resonance
5. sound

Exercise 6
1. analgesic
2. anesthesia
3. neuromuscular
4. therapeutic
5. narcotic

6. radiation
7. thermotherapy
8. cryotherapy

Exercise 7
1. G
2. A
3. F
4. H
5. I
6. J
7. B
8. D
9. C
10. E

Exercise 8
1. neur/ectomy
2. neuro/lysis
3. amnio/centesis
4. oto/plasty
5. ophthalmo/plasty
6. neuro/tripsy

Exercise 9
1. loosening, freeing, destroying
2. eye
3. suture
4. ear
5. brain
6. surgical repair
7. vessel
8. gland
9. incision
10. eyelid

Exercise 10
1. colono/scopy
2. append/ectomy
3. encephalo/tomy
4. osteo/tome
5. mammo/plasty
6. blepharo/plasty
7. chiro/plasty
8. angio/rrhaphy

Chapter 3 Review

I.
1. E
2. A
3. D
4. F
5. G
6. H
7. B
8. C

II.
1. E
2. A
3. I
4. J
5. H
6. B
7. F
8. C
9. D
10. G

III.
1. amnio/centesis: amnion: surgical puncture
2. blepharo/plasty: eyelid; surgical repair
3. colo/scopy: colon; visual examination

4. echo/graphy: sound; process of recording
5. electro/cardio/graph: electricity; heart; instrument used to record
6. fluoro/scope: emitting or reflecting light; instrument used to view
7. oste/oid: bone; resembling
8. tomo/gram: to cut; a record

IV.
1. medications used to treat malignant neoplasms
2. treatment using chemical agents
3. treatment of disease with medicine
4. treatment of disease with heat

V.
1. palpation
2. percussion
3. auscultation

VI.
1. symptom
2. chiroplasty
3. stasis
4. cardiomegaly
5. electrocardiogram
6. tracheostomy
7. adenectomy
8. ophthalmomalacia
9. otodynia
10. computed tomography

VII.
1. hemorrhage
2. colectomy or colonectomy
3. ophthalmotomy
4. encephalotome
5. otoplasty
6. neurotripsy
7. colopexy
8. angiorrhaphy
9. blepharedema
10. otoscopy

VIII.
neurotripsy, ophthalmoplasty, symptom

IX.
1. computed tomography
2. computed tomography
3. electrocardiogram
4. electrocardiogram
5. magnetic resonance imaging

X.
1. ap en dek´ tə me
2. kal sĭ pe´ne ə
3. en sef ə lot´ə me
4. nŏŏ rol´ĭ sis
5. sə nog´rə fe

XI.
1. appendic/itis: inflammation of the appendix
2. chiro/spasm: cramping of the hand
3. encephal/itis: inflammation of the brain
4. rhino/plasty: surgical repair of the nose
5. tracheo/scopy: visual examination of the trachea

Chapter 4

Exercise 1
1. condition
2. inflammation
3. fear
4. prolapse
5. -mania
6. -oma
7. -pathy
8. -cele
9. -emia
10. -lith

Exercise 2
1. adeno/pathy: any disease of a gland
2. carcin/oma: a cancerous tumor (or cancer)
3. neur/osis: a nervous condition
4. ot/itis: inflammation of the ear

Exercise 3
1. dermat/itis
2. angi/oma
3. encephalo/cele
4. bacter/emia

Exercise 4
1. A
2. C
3. D
4. E
5. B
6. J
7. I
8. G
9. F
10. H

Exercise 5
1. blephar/al: pertaining to the eyelid
2. cerebr/al: pertaining to the brain

3. lact/ase: the enzyme that breaks down lactose
4. mamm/ary: pertaining to the breast
5. neur/al: pertaining to a nerve

Exercise 6
1. B
2. G
3. D
4. I
5. J
6. E
7. A
8. H
9. C
10. F

Exercise 7
1. C
2. E
3. H
4. A
5. B
6. I
7. G
8. J
9. D
10. F

Exercise 8
1. microscope
2. hemolysin
3. hemolytic
4. ophthalmopathy
5. carcinogen
6. cephalometry
7. phagocyte
8. epilepsy

Exercise 9
1. white
2. green
3. blue
4. red

5. white
6. black
7. yellow

Exercise 10
1. xanthoderma
2. cyanosis
3. erythrocyte
4. albinism

Exercise 11
1. E
2. C
3. B
4. G
5. F
6. A
7. D

Exercise 12
1. cephal
2. histo
3. bio
4. my
5. toxico
6. pod
7. nas
8. pyro

Exercise 13
1. C
2. A
3. B

Exercise 14
1. E
2. C
3. A
4. D
5. B
6. F

Exercise 15
(No particular order)
1. bacteria
2. fungi
3. viruses
4. protozoa

Exercise 16
1. B
2. D
3. F
4. C
5. E
6. A

Exercise 17
1. weapons
2. disease
3. bioterrorism
4. disseminated

Exercise 18
(No particular order)
1. Direct invasion of surrounding tissue
2. Invasion of the bloodstream, so the cancer cells may be carried to distant sites
3. Invasion of lymphatic vessels, so the cancer cells may be transported to implant in the lymph nodes or other distant sites
4. Spread of cancer cells throughout a body cavity

Exercise 19
1. heart
2. cancer
3. cervical

Chapter 4 Review

I.
1. F
2. D
3. C
4. B
5. E
6. H
7. A
8. G

II.
1. E
2. C
3. B

4. D
5. A
6. F

III.
1. dermatitis
2. jaundice
3. appendicitis
4. encephalocele
5. phobia
6. biopsy
7. otopathy
8. tissue
9. phagocyte

10. hemolyze
11. organic disease
12. nosocomial
13. heart disease
14. lung
15. breast
16. strep throat

IV.
(No particular order, one feature)
1. viruses: much smaller than bacteria; replicate only within a cell

2. bacteria: classified according to shape
3. fungi: absorb organic molecules from surroundings; may be parasitic
4. protozoa: only a few are pathogenic

V.
(No particular order)
1. cocci
2. bacilli
3. spirochetes and spirilla
4. vibrios

VI.
(No particular order)
1. Direct invasion of surrounding tissue
2. Invasion of the bloodstream, so the cancer cells may be carried to distant sites
3. Invasion of lymphatic vessels, so the cancer cells may be transported to implant in the lymph nodes or other distant sites
4. Spread of cancer cells throughout a body cavity

VII.
1. encephalocele
2. dermatitis
3. albinism
4. blepharoptosis

VIII.
1. erythrocyte
2. hemolysin
3. carcinogen
4. ophthalmopathy
5. pyromania
6. osteitis
7. myalgia
8. nasal
9. calculi
10. microscopy

IX.
cephalic, cerebral

X.
1. American Cancer Society
2. Federal Emergency Management Association
3. high power field
4. improvised explosive device
5. weapons of mass destruction

XI.
1. ad ə nop´ə the
2. aw´top se
3. sef ə lom´ə tre
4. he mo lit´ik
5. lak´tōs

XII.
1. blephar/itis: inflammation of the eyelid
2. leuko/cyte: white cell (white blood cell)
3. myo/cele: hernia of muscle
4. neuro/genic: originating in the nervous system
5. xanth/ous: yellowish

Chapter 5

Exercise 1
1. B
2. B
3. A
4. D
5. C
6. A

Exercise 2
1. half, partly
2. many
3. none
4. many
5. first

Exercise 3
1. centi-, one hundred
2. diplo-, double
3. hyper-, excessive or more than normal
4. hypo-, below
5. milli-, one-thousandth

Exercise 4
1. away from, toward
2. behind
3. inside

4. between
5. above
6. around
7. postdate
8. extracellular
9. same
10. across

Exercise 5
1. anesthesia
2. anhydrous
3. aplastic
4. atraumatic
5. asymptomatic

Exercise 6
1. inconsistent
2. inanimate
3. inattentive
4. incapable
5. invisible

Exercise 7
1. A
2. F
3. A
4. B

5. D
6. B
7. G
8. E
9. E
10. C

Exercise 8
1. tachy(phasia)
2. mal(aise)
3. pre(cancerous)
4. macro(scopic)
5. eu(phoria)
6. post(anesthetic)
7. micr(otia)
8. dys(lexia)
9. contra(ceptive)
10. brady(phasia)

Exercise 9
1. centimeter
2. deciliter
3. gram
4. kilogram
5. liter
6. microgram
7. milligram

8. milliliter
9. alert and oriented
10. blood pressure
11. chief complaint
12. date of birth
13. diagnosis
14. history
15. pulse
16. physical examination
17. respirations
18. range of motion
19. review of systems
20. temperature

Exercise 10
1. b.i.d.
2. h
3. IV
4. min
5. p.o.
6. p.r.n.
7. q.
8. t.i.d.
9. L&W
10. WD
11. WNL
12. HPI

Chapter 5 Review

I.
1. J
2. C
3. F
4. B
5. G
6. A
7. E
8. D
9. I
10. H

II.
1. A
2. I
3. C
4. G
5. E
6. D
7. D
8. C
9. B
10. B
11. K

III.
1. first
2. fast
3. difficult
4. beneath
5. macroscopic
6. against
7. half
8. two
9. intradermal
10. syndrome

IV.
1. extra
2. intra
3. inter

V.
1. macro/scop/ic: macro-, large; scop(o), to view; -ic, pertaining to
2. micr/ot/ia: micro-, small; ot(o), ear; -ia, condition
3. post/nas/al: post-, behind; nas(o), nose; -al, pertaining to

4. tachy/phas/ia: tachy-, fast; phas(o), speech; -ia, condition
5. trans/derm/al: trans-, across; derm(o), skin; -al, pertaining to

VI.
1. anesthesia
2. anhydrous
3. aplastic
4. asymptomatic
5. atraumatic

VII.
1. bradyphasia
2. postnasal
3. microtia

4. diplopia
5. contralateral
6. ultrasonic
7. ultraviolet
8. intercellular
9. semipermeable
10. fatigue

VIII.
addiction, ipsilateral, postanesthetic

IX.
1. alert and oriented
2. date of birth
3. intravenous
4. as needed
5. review of systems

X.
1. ab dukt′
2. kon trə sep′tiv
3. hi po dər′mik
4. sin′drōm
5. trans dur′məl

XI.
1. ad/duct: to draw toward (the median plane or the axial line of a limb)
2. exo/skeleton: a hard structure developed on the outside of the body

3. peri/appendicitis: inflammation of the tissue around the appendix
4. pre/nat/al: before birth
5. sym/bi/osis: the living together or close association of two (dissimilar) organisms

---

Chapter 6

Exercise 1
organelles, cells, tissues, organs

Exercise 2
(No particular order)
1. nucleus
2. cytoplasm
3. cell membrane

Exercise 3
1. cell
2. tissue
3. organ
4. connective
5. epithelial
6. muscle
7. nervous
8. somatic
9. stem
10. congenital

Exercise 4
1. nervous
2. epithelial
3. connective
4. muscle

Exercise 5
1. midsagittal
2. transverse
3. frontal or coronal
4. anterior
5. posterior
6. lateral

Exercise 6
1. front, anterior
2. tail or lower part of body, caudal (caudad)
3. head, cephalad
4. distant or far, distal
5. back side, dorsal
6. situated below, inferior
7. side, lateral
8. middle, medial, or median
9. behind (toward the back), posterior
10. near, proximal
11. uppermost, superior
12. belly, ventral

Exercise 7
1. supine
2. prone

Exercise 8
1. RUQ
2. RLQ
3. LUQ
4. LLQ

Exercise 9
1. cranial
2. spinal
3. thoracic
4. abdominal
5. pelvic

Exercise 10
1. thorac(o)
2. acr(o)
3. dactyl(o)
4. pelv(i)
5. spin(o)
6. crani(o)

Exercise 11
1. abdomino/centesis: abdomin(o), abdomen; -centesis, surgical puncture
2. acro/megaly or acro/megal/y: acr(o), extremities; -megaly, enlargement
3. chiro/plasty: chir(o), hand; -plasty, surgical repair

4. dactylo/graphy: dactyl(o), digit; -graphy, process of recording
5. dermato/plasty: dermat(o), skin; -plasty, surgical repair
6. periton/eum: peritone(o), peritoneum; -eum, membrane
7. pod/iatr/ist: pod(o), foot; -iatry, medical profession or treatment; -ist, one who
8. viscer/al: viscer(o), viscera; -al, pertaining to

Exercise 12
1. pyrogen
2. dysplasia
3. aplasia
4. hypoplasia
5. hyperplasia
6. anaplasia

Exercise 13
1. umbilicus
2. somatic
3. brain
4. omphalocele
5. somatopsychic
6. dehiscence
7. evisceration

Chapter 6 Review

I.
1. hyperplasia
2. hypertrophy

II.
1. B
2. H
3. C
4. I
5. F
6. A

7. G
8. D
9. E

III.
1. E
2. D
3. B
4. C
5. H
6. F

7. B
8. G
9. A
10. E

IV.
1. cells
2. tissues
3. organs
4. body systems

V.
1. tissue
2. four quadrants
3. mediolateral
4. farther from the origin
5. frontal
6. encephalitis
7. prone
8. dermatosis
9. umbilicus
10. diaphragm

VI.
1. suprathoracic
2. unilateral
3. supine
4. peritoneal
5. plantar
6. dermatitis
7. abdominopelvic
8. chirospasm
9. dysplasia
10. electroencephalogram

VII.
abdomen, acrocyanosis

VIII.
1. anteroposterior
2. deoxyribonucleic acid
3. left lower quadrant
4. right lower quadrant
5. right upper quadrant

IX.
1. bi lat´ər əl
2. sə fal´ik
3. om fal´ik
4. pos tər o soo pĕr´e ər
5. vis´ər əl

X.
1. cephalo/centesis: surgical puncture of the skull (implied meaning)
2. dactyl/edema: swelling of the fingers or toes

3. dorso/dynia: pain of the back
4. extra/peritone/al: occurring or located outside the peritoneal cavity (implied meaning)
5. thoraco/stomy: surgical opening into the chest wall performed to provide a place for a drainage tube (implied meaning)

Chapter 7

Exercise 1
1. intra(cellular)
2. extra(cellular)
3. inter(stitial)

Exercise 2
1. F
2. A
3. B
4. D
5. G
6. C
7. E
8. F

Exercise 3
1. homeo/stasis: a relative constancy of the body's internal environment
2. hydro/cephal/us: a condition characterized by abnormal accumulation of cerebrospinal fluid within the skull
3. hyper/kal/emia: greater than normal blood potassium levels
4. hyper/natr/emia: greater than normal blood sodium levels
5. hypo/calce/emia: deficiency of blood calcium

Exercise 4
1. excessive loss of water from body tissue
2. swelling caused by excessive accumulation of fluid in the body tissues
3. molecules that conduct an electrical charge
4. the regulation of water by the body
5. to redirect the flow of body fluid from one part of the body to another, or the device that is implanted to accomplish that purpose

Exercise 5
1. A
2. A
3. C
4. G
5. B
6. D
7. E
8. F

Exercise 6
1. F
2. C
3. B
4. G
5. A
6. E
7. D

Exercise 7
1. A
2. D
3. C
4. F
5. H
6. J
7. E
8. B
9. G
10. I

Exercise 8
1. hemato/log/ic: pertaining to hematology
2. hemato/poiesis: production of blood
3. hemato/poietic: pertaining to hematopoiesis

Exercise 9
1. anti/coagul/ant: a substance that prevents coagulation
2. coagul/ant: a substance that promotes coagulation
3. coagul/ate: to cause to clot or to become clotted
4. coagulo/pathy: any disorder of coagulation

Exercise 10
(No particular order)
1. erythrocyte, red (blood) cell
2. leukocyte, white (blood) cell
3. thrombocyte, blood platelet

Exercise 11
(No particular order)
1. basophil
2. eosinophil
3. neutrophil
4. lymphocyte
5. monocyte

Exercise 12
1. karyo/megaly: enlarged nucleus
2. poly/morpho/nucle/ar: having a nucleus that may appear to have several nuclei (literally, many-shaped nuclei)
3. nucle/oid: resembling a nucleus
4. nucleo/protein: a protein found in the nucleus

Exercise 13
1. thrombocyte
2. thrombus
3. clot
4. thrombolysis
5. hemolysis

6. leukemia
7. leukocytes (white blood cells)
8. thrombocytosis
9. anemia
10. fainting

Exercise 14
1. microcyte
2. macrocytosis
3. anisocytosis
4. spherocyte
5. poikilocyte
6. hyperchromia
7. hypochromia
8. hemoglobinopathy
9. aplastic
10. hemoglobin

Exercise 15
1. fibrinolysis
2. coagulation
3. hemostasis
4. fibrinolysin
5. fibrinogen

Exercise 16
1. agglutination
2. transfusion
3. autologous
4. homologous
5. clots (or coagulation)

Exercise 17
1. antigen
2. susceptible
3. nonspecific
4. specific
5. active
6. immunodeficiency

Chapter 7 Review

I.
1. A
2. C
3. B
4. C
5. B

II.
1. A
2. C
3. D
4. B

III.
1. T
2. T
3. F
4. F
5. T

IV.
1. thrombocyte
2. leukocyte (sometimes leuco-cyte)
3. erythrocyte

V.
1. cellul/ar: pertaining to or consisting of cells
2. coagul/ant: a substance that promotes coagulation
3. hemato/poiesis: production of blood
4. hypo/calc/emia: decreased blood calcium
5. necro/tic: pertaining to death of tissue in response to injury or disease

VI.
(Any five; no particular order)
1-5. natural barriers (unbroken skin), complement, interferon, phagocytes, inflammation, mucus, cilia, normal flora, urination, chemicals in human tears, and acids of the stomach, vagina, and skin

VII.
(No particular order)
1. cell-mediated immunity
2. antibody-mediated immunity

VIII.
1. potassium
2. coagulation
3. interstitial
4. thrombus
5. anticoagulant
6. wastes
7. homeostasis
8. differential
9. hemolysis
10. leukemia

IX.
1. fibrinogen
2. virulence
3. erythrocytes
4. aplastic
5. transplant
6. inside
7. cell-mediated immunity
8. inflammation
9. intracellular
10. thrombopenia

X.
1. poikilocyte
2. hyponatremia
3. immunity
4. thrombosis
5. thrombolysis
6. allograft
7. abscess
8. neutrophil
9. hematopoiesis
10. intracellular

XI.
1. decrease in the number of neutrophils in the blood
2. decrease in the number of blood platelets
3. a pigmented malignant tumor
4. a bursting open, splitting, or gaping of a wound

5. above the normal dosage needed for treatment
6. internal blood clot
7. deficiency in erythrocytes, hemoglobin, or both
8. twice a day
9. pertaining to hematology
10. lack of body's natural ability to ward off infectious disease(s)

XII.
1. pertaining to difficulty in breathing
2. paleness
3. feeling of general discomfort
4. pertaining to both sides
5. swelling caused by excess fluid in interstitial spaces
6. hemoglobin
7. hematocrit
8. decreased blood sodium
9. within normal limits
10. head is of normal size

XIII.
1. chief complaint
2. history of present illness
3. review of systems (of the body)
4. physical examination
5. transplantation from one individual to another of the same species
6. a stem cell from which all red and white blood cells develop; can replace bone marrow that has been destroyed by disease; can continue to produce mature blood cells
7. oriented to person, place, time, and future plans
8. occurring from time to time
9. (L) *pro re nata* or as needed
10. graft versus host disease

XIV.
1. A
2. E
3. B
4. F

XV.
fibrinolysis, polymorphonuclear, toxicity

XVI.
1. antihemophilic factor
2. complete blood cell count
3. hemoglobin
4. human immunodeficiency virus
5. prothrombin time (also physical therapy)

XVII.
1. ko ag u lop´ə the
2. ə rith ro poi´ə tin
3. al o jen´ik
4. nə krot´ik
5. pro fə lak´sis

XVIII.
1. B
2. E
3. A
4. C
5. D

XIX.
1. eosinophil/ia: an increase in the number of eosinophils in the blood
2. erythr/oid: pertaining to erythrocytes; reddish in color
3. hemoglobino/meter: instrument used to measure hemoglobin
4. leuko/poiesis: production and development of leukocytes
5. thromb/oid: clotlike, resembling a thrombus

Chapter 8

Exercise 1
1. artery
2. arteriole
3. capillary
4. venule
5. vein
6. superior and inferior venae cavae

Exercise 2
1. B
2. B
3. A
4. D
5. C
6. D
7. D
8. E

Exercise 3
1. myocardium
2. endocardium
3. pericardium
4. arteriovenous
5. endocardial
6. ventricular
7. septal
8. atrial

Exercise 4
1. E
2. D
3. B
4. A
5. C

Exercise 5
1. aorta
2. endocardium
3. mediastinum
4. myocardium
5. pericardium
6. valve

Exercise 6
1. venae cavae
2. atrium
3. right ventricle
4. lungs
5. left atrium
6. bicuspid (or mitral)
7. aorta
8. arterioles
9. capillaries
10. veins

Exercise 7
1. electrocardiograph
2. tachycardia
3. aortography
4. arteriogram or arteriograph
5. stethoscope

Exercise 8
1. hypertension
2. bradycardia
3. diastole
4. systolic
5. Holter
6. lipids
7. lipoproteins
8. echocardiography

Exercise 9
1. atriomegaly
2. cyanosis
3. dysrrhythmia
4. microcardia
5. anoxia

Exercise 10
1. cardiomegaly
2. fibrillation
3. asystole
4. infarct
5. ischemia
6. cardiovalvulitis

7. pericarditis
8. stenosis
9. endocarditis
10. shock

Exercise 11
1. angiostenosis
2. aneurysmal
3. lymphangioma
4. arteriosclerosis
5. angiocarditis

Exercise 12
1. aneurysm
2. coronary
3. occlusion
4. thrombosis
5. atherosclerosis
6. aortosclerosis
7. thrombophlebitis
8. stenosis

Exercise 13
1. pericardiocentesis
2. angiostomy
3. cardioplegia
4. phleboplasty
5. endarterectomy

Exercise 14
1. D
2. B
3. F
4. A
5. C
6. E

Exercise 15
1. A
2. D
3. C
4. B

Exercise 16
1. adenoid(o)
2. lymphaden(o)
3. lymphangi(o)
4. thym(o)
5. tonsill(o)

Exercise 17
1. lymphatic
2. lymph
3. veins
4. systemic
5. splenic
6. thymic
7. tonsillar

Exercise 18
1. lymphography
2. lymphadenography
3. biopsy

Exercise 19
1. D
2. B
3. A
4. E
5. C

Exercise 20
1. B
2. A
3. C
4. G
5. F
6. H

Exercise 21
1. thymic
2. lymphedema
3. splenorrhagia
4. tonsillectomy
5. lymphadenopathy

Chapter 8 Review

I.
1. lymphangi(o)
2. arter(o), arteri(o)
3. arteriol(o)
4. phlebo, ven(i), ven(o)
5. venul(o)

II.
1. tonsill(o)
2. lymphaden(o)
3. thym(o)
4. lymphangi(o)
5. splen(o)

III.
1. H
2. B
3. D

4. I
5. E
6. F
7. G
8. C
9. J
10. A

IV.
1. E
2. C
3. A
4. B
5. D

V.
(No particular order)
Maintains the internal fluid en-

vironment by returning proteins and tissue fluids to the blood; aids in the absorption of fats into the bloodstream; helps defend the body against microorganisms and disease

VI.
1. lymphangitis
2. atherosclerosis
3. arteriogram
4. lymphedema

VII.
1. adenoid/ectomy: excision of the adenoids
2. angio/graphy: radiographic

visualization of the blood vessels
3. an/ox/ia: lack of oxygen in body tissues
4. atrio/megaly: enlargement of an atrium of the heart
5. cardio/vascul/ar: pertaining to the heart and blood vessels
6. echo/cardio/graphy: process of recording the heart using ultrasonic waves
7. end/arter/ectomy: excision of plaque from the inner wall of an artery
8. hemo/pericard/ium: blood within the pericardium
9. phleb/ectomy: excision of a vein

10. thrombo/phleb/itis: inflammation of a vein accompanied by a blood clot

VIII.
1. myocardial infarction
2. atherosclerosis
3. coronary artery bypass
4. endocarditis
5. defibrillation
6. coronary thrombosis
7. atrial septal defect
8. rheumatic fever
9. peripheral artery disease
10. aneurysm

IX.
1. thymoma
2. aortosclerosis
3. asystole
4. vasodilator
5. hypertension
6. tachycardia
7. lymphangitis
8. angiostenosis
9. tonsillectomy
10. splenorrhaphy

X.
1. cerebrovascular accident: a stroke; an abnormal condition of occlusion or hemorrhage of a vessel in the brain that results in lack of oxygen to brain tissue
2. computed tomography: a radiographic procedure that produces images of

cross sections of brain tissue
3. No. Atrial fibrillation is a cardiac arrhythmia characterized by disorganized, rapid electrical activity in the atria.
4. No. Arrhythmia is a disordered pattern of the heartbeat.
5. Telemetry is an electronic transmission of data between distant points.
6. Right and left endarterectomies: surgical removal of the lining of the right and left carotid arteries.
7. hypertension
8. congestive heart failure
9. myocardial infarction
10. coronary artery disease
11. atherosclerotic heart disease

XI.
1. heart attack
2. high blood pressure
3. elevated level of cholesterol in the blood
4. listening for sounds within the body, most commonly using a stethoscope
5. electrocardiogram (also EKG)
6. passage of a catheter (flexible tube) through an artery or vein in the leg up into the heart for diagnostic purposes
7. diagnostic radiographic pro-

cedure; passing a catheter through the coronary arteries after a contrast medium has been infiltrated
8. severe constricting pain in the chest; can radiate to the shoulders, neck, jaw, and so on
9. pronounced "cabbage," this is the abbreviation for coronary artery bypass procedure

XII.
1. Emergency Medical Services
2. absence of heartbeat
3. cardiopulmonary resuscitation
4. pertaining to an increased pulse rate
5. the first number in a blood pressure reading, representing contraction of the ventricles
6. pertaining to an artery

XIII.
atherosclerosis, ischemia

XIV.
1. atrioventricular
2. coronary artery bypass graft
3. congestive heart failure
4. cardiopulmonary resuscitation
5. myocardial infarction

XV.
1. kahr de o mi op´ə the
2. lim fad ə nop´ə the

3. lim fog´rə fe
4. per ĭ kahr´de əl
5. vas o di la´shən

XVI.
1. B
2. C
3. D
4. C
5. C
6. C
7. B
8. D
9. E
10. A

XVII.
1. aneurysm/ectomy: surgical excision of an aneurysm
2. epi/cardi/al: pertaining to the outer membrane of the heart; pericardial
3. lymph/angi/ectasia: dilation of (smaller) lymphatic vessels
4. pericardio/stomy: creation of an opening into the pericardium, usually for drainage
5. vascul/itis: inflammation of the blood vessels

Chapter 9

Exercise 1
1. oropharynx
2. larynx
3. bronchi
4. alveoli

Exercise 2
1. in/spir/ation: process of breathing in
2. para/nas/al: near the nose
3. pharyng/eal: pertaining to the pharynx
4. pulmon/ary: pertaining to the lungs
5. retro/nas/al: behind the nose

Exercise 3
1. pharynx
2. septum
3. larynx
4. sinuses
5. epiglottis

Exercise 4
1. phrenic
2. bronchoalveolar
3. endotracheal
4. extrapleural
5. subpulmonary

Exercise 5
1. trachea
2. bronchioles
3. alveoli
4. apex
5. pleura

Exercise 6
1. D
2. B
3. C
4. A
5. E

Exercise 7
1. oximeter
2. spirometry

3. bronchography
4. laryngoscopy
5. pharyngoscope

Exercise 8
1. anoxia
2. hypocapnia
3. dyspnea
4. apnea
5. alkalosis

Exercise 9
1. oxygen
2. hyperpnea
3. hyperventilation
4. hypercapnia
5. acidemia

Exercise 10
1. brady/pnea: slow breathing
2. eu/pnea: normal rate of breathing
3. hyp/ox/emia: decreased blood oxygen

4. ortho/pnea: breathing is difficult except in an upright position
5. phreno/plegia: paralysis of the diaphragm
6. tachy/pnea: greater than normal number of breaths per minute

Exercise 11
1. rhinorrhea
2. dysphasia
3. sinusitis
4. pharyngodynia
5. aphasia

Exercise 12
1. B
2. D
3. C
4. A
5. E

Exercise 13
1. D
2. A
3. B
4. C

Exercise 14
1. aplasia
2. laryngotracheitis
3. bronchiolitis
4. bronchiectasis
5. bronchopulmonary

Exercise 15
1. G
2. E
3. A
4. D
5. F
6. B
7. C
8. H

Exercise 16
1. anthracosis
2. pneumoconiosis
3. atelectasis
4. hemoptysis

Exercise 17
1. emphysema
2. COPD (chronic obstructive pulmonary disease)
3. emphysema
4. cystic fibrosis

Exercise 18
1. laryngectomy
2. thoracocentesis
3. tracheoplasty
4. tracheotomy
5. pneumonectomy

Exercise 19
1. asphyxia or asphyxiation
2. resuscitation
3. ventilator
4. tracheostomy
5. obstructive
6. transtracheal
7. orotracheal
8. lung
9. thoracostomy
10. antitussive

Chapter 9 Review

I.
1. G
2. A
3. B
4. F
5. D
6. E
7. C

II.
1. A
2. G
3. D
4. B
5. C
6. E
7. F

III.
1. sin(o)
2. nas(o), rhin(o)
3. pharyng(o)
4. laryng(o)
5. trache(o)
6. bronch(o), bronchi(o)
7. phren(o)
8. alveol(o)
9. bronchiol(o)

IV.
nasal cavity 1; bronchi 5; larynx 3; pharynx 2; trachea 4; alveoli 7; bronchioles 6

V.
(No particular order)
1. provide oxygen and remove carbon dioxide
2. maintain acid-base balance
3. produce speech
4. facilitate smell
5. maintain body's heat and water balance

VI.
1. B
2. B
3. B

4. A
5. A
6. A
7. B

VII.
1. pneumothorax
2. hemothorax
3. bronchoscopy
4. thoracocentesis or thoracentesis

VIII.
1. normal (eupnea)
2. bradypnea
3. tachypnea
4. hyperpnea

IX.
1. pneumonitis
2. expectoration
3. apnea
4. exchanging CO_2 for O_2
5. parietal pleura
6. paroxysmal
7. orthopnea
8. alkalosis
9. spirometry
10. pulmonary edema

X.
1. thrombus
2. dysphonia
3. bronchoscopy
4. aspiration
5. pharyngitis
6. rhinolithiasis
7. alveolar
8. laryngography
9. rhinorrhagia
10. intranasal

XI.
1. chronic obstructive pulmonary disease
2. device used to produce a fine spray or mist

3. reduced respiration
4. subnormal levels of oxygen in arterial blood
5. contraction (spasm) of smooth muscle in the bronchi
6. dilatation (enlarging) of the bronchi, usually by prescription drugs
7. referring to a marked, episodic increase in symptoms
8. difficult, painful breathing
9. device for delivering oxygen through the nostrils
10. registered pulmonary function therapist

XII.
1. malaise
2. pleural effusion
3. wheezes
4. crackle
5. pneumothorax
6. bronchitis
7. COLD
8. pulmonary embolism
9. bronchodilator
10. expectorant

XIII.
1. without a known cause
2. a condition of abnormally high blood pressure within the pulmonary circulation
3. breathed in
4. pertaining to difficult breathing
5. coughing up or spitting up of blood from the respiratory tract
6. continuous positive airway pressure

XIV.
laryngography, pneumonitis

XV.
1. lar ing gop´ə the
2. pə ri´ə təl
3. fə rin´je əl
4. spi rom´ə tər
5. tra ke os´tə me

XVI.
1. arterial blood gas
2. extracorporeal membrane oxygenation
3. herpes simplex virus
4. severe acute respiratory syndrome
5. upper respiratory infection

XVII.
1. C
2. E
3. B
4. C
5. A
6. A
7. B
8. D
9. B
10. C

XVIII.
1. broncho/spiro/metry: the study of the ventilation of each lung separately
2. laryngo/stomy: surgical creation of an artificial opening into the larynx
3. pharyngo/plegia: paralysis of the muscles of the pharynx
4. pneumo/myc/osis: fungal disease of the lungs
5. sino/scopy: endoscopic examination of a paranasal sinus

Chapter 10

Exercise 1
1. starch
2. bile
3. sugar
4. milk
5. fats
6. protein
7. thirst
8. appetite
9. digestion
10. contraction

Exercise 2
1. H
2. I
3. J
4. G
5. B
6. F
7. E
8. D
9. C
10. A

Exercise 3
1. anus
2. gallbladder
3. common bile duct
4. large intestine; colon
5. duodenum
6. small intestine; intestines
7. stomach
8. liver
9. ileum
10. jejunum
11. mouth
12. pancreas
13. rectum
14. salivary gland
15. mouth

Exercise 4
1. enteritis
2. gastric
3. oropharyngeal
4. colonic
5. mucoid

Exercise 5
1. lingual
2. mandibular
3. periodontist
4. palatine
5. interdental

Exercise 6
1. oral
2. mandible
3. maxilla
4. palate
5. cheek
6. gingiva
7. tongue
8. tongue

9. pharynx
10. endodontium
11. periodontium
12. orthodontics
13. pedodontics
14. gerodontics
15. salivary
16. esophagus
17. sphincter
18. pyloric

Exercise 7
1. B
2. B
3. B
4. A
5. A
6. A
7. B

Exercise 8
1. duodenal
2. proctologist
3. retrocecal
4. ileal
5. pericolic

Exercise 9
1. choledochal
2. biliary
3. cholecystic
4. hepatic
5. pancreatic

Exercise 10
1. cholecystogastric
2. hepatolytic
3. hypoglycemia
4. hyperglycemia
5. extrahepatic

Exercise 11
1. coloscopy
2. sialolith
3. esophagogastroscopy
4. cholecystogram
5. fluoroscopy

Exercise 12
1. A
2. D
3. B
4. C
5. H
6. F
7. E
8. G

Exercise 13
1. anorexia
2. hyperemesis
3. eupepsia
4. exogenous
5. adipsia

Exercise 14
1. cheil/osis: splitting of the lips and angles of the mouth
2. gingiv/algia: painful gums
3. end/odont/itis: inflammation of the endodontium
4. glosso/pyr/osis: sensation of pain, burning, and stinging of the tongue
5. pyo/rrhea: inflammation of the gingiva and the periodontal ligament
6. stomato/myc/osis: disease of the mouth caused by a fungus

Exercise 15
1. gastralgia
2. gastropathy
3. gastroesophageal
4. esophagomalacia
5. esophagodynia, esophagalgia

Exercise 16
1. F
2. B
3. C
4. A
5. G
6. I
7. J
8. M
9. L
10. E
11. D
12. H
13. K

Exercise 17
1. enterostasis
2. appendicitis
3. gastroduodenitis
4. lipopenia

Exercise 18
1. gastroenteritis
2. dysentery
3. fistula
4. diverticulosis
5. fissure
6. irritable
7. hemorrhoids
8. impaction
9. intussusception
10. volvulus

Exercise 19
1. A
2. D
3. F
4. E
5. B
6. C
7. G
8. H

Exercise 20
1. hepatomegaly
2. cholestasis
3. hepatorenal
4. pancreatolysis
5. pancreatolith

Exercise 21
1. cheilo/rrhaphy: suture of the lip
2. cheilo/stomato/plasty: surgical repair of the lips and mouth
3. esophago/myo/tomy: incision into the esophageal muscle
4. esophago/stomy: new opening into the esophagus
5. gingiv/ectomy: excision of the gums
6. glosso/rrhaphy: suture of the tongue
7. jejuno/stomy: formation of a new opening into the jejunum
8. lip/ectomy: excision of subcutaneous fat
9. naso/gastr/ic: pertaining to the nose and stomach
10. stomato/plasty: surgical repair of the mouth

Exercise 22
1. pylorotomy
2. gastropexy
3. jejunoileostomy
4. vagotomy
5. gastroduodenostomy

Exercise 23
1. hemicolectomy
2. cecoileostomy
3. ileostomy
4. laparoenterostomy
5. diverticulectomy

Exercise 24
1. lithotripsy
2. pancreatotomy
3. pancreatolithectomy
4. hepatotomy
5. choledochostomy

Exercise 25
1. D
2. G
3. E
4. B
5. A
6. I
7. F
8. J
9. H
10. C

Chapter 10 Review

I.
1. pharyng(o)
2. sial(o), sialaden(o)
3. hepat(o)
4. cholecyst(o)
5. duoden(o)
6. or(o), stomat(o)
7. esophag(o)
8. gastr(o)
9. pancreat(o)
10. jejun(o)
11. ile(o)
12. col(o)
13. an(o)

II.
1. C
2. B
3. D
4. A

III.
1. D
2. C
3. I
4. A
5. E
6. G
7. J
8. H
9. B
10. F

IV.
1. C
2. B
3. H
4. G
5. F
6. A
7. J
8. D
9. E
10. I

V.
(No particular order)
1. carbohydrates: basic source of cell energy
2. fats: energy reserve, and help cushion and insulate vital organs
3. proteins: building material for development, growth, and maintenance of the body

VI.
(No particular order)
1. liver = hepat(o)
2. gallbladder = cholecyst(o)
3. pancreas = pancreat(o)
4. salivary glands = sial(o) or sialaden(o)

VII.
1. cholecystogram
2. cheilosis
3. biliary lithotripsy
4. gastroscopy

VIII.
1. ileo/cec/al: pertaining to the cecum and the ileum
2. choledocho/litho/tripsy: surgical crushing of a stone in the common bile duct
3. chole/stasis: interruption of the flow of bile
4. esophago/myo/tomy: incision (longitudinal) of the muscle of the esophagus to treat achalasia
5. gastro/duodeno/stomy: anastomosis of the stomach and duodenum
6. gingivo/stomat/itis: inflammation of the mouth and gums
7. glosso/plegia: paralysis of the tongue
8. naso/gastr/ic: pertaining to the nose and stomach
9. sialo/lith/iasis: presence of salivary stones
10. stomato/plasty: surgical repair of the mouth

IX.
1. gastroenterology
2. cholecystography
3. extracorporeal shock wave lithotripsy
4. anorexia nervosa
5. emaciation
6. colectomy
7. pyloric stenosis
8. ileocecal valve
9. hiatal hernia
10. lips and mouth
11. enterostasis
12. gastroscope
13. glucose
14. bulimia
15. gastroenterostomy

X.
1. adipsia
2. gastropathy
3. amylase
4. hyperemesis

5. cholecystectomy
6. vagotomy
7. gastritis
8. pharyngeal
9. dyspepsia
10. duodenoscopy

XI.
1. large intestine
2. abnormal new growth
3. gallbladder
4. abdominal wall
5. large intestine
6. abdomen
7. T
8. T
9. F
10. T
11. F
12. F

XII.
1. large intestine
2. chronic
3. diagnostic procedure
4. pus
5. colonic obstruction
6. chronic disease with ulceration of colon and rectum, rectal bleeding, pain, diarrhea; unknown cause
7. diagnostic procedure, examination of interior of a canal by means of an instrument
8. inflammation of the gastrointestinal tract
9. disease of unknown cause of upper GI tract with ulcers, fever, abdominal pain, cramping, diarrhea, weight loss
10. test (brand name) for occult (hidden) blood in the stool

XIII.
1. removal of approximately half of the colon
2. a bursting open or gaping along sutured lines
3. a method of filtration, separation of substances
4. surrounding the colon
5. the segment of large intestine that extends from the end of the ascending colon to the beginning of the descending colon
6. enlarged, stretched

7. to stop the flow of blood; the arrest of bleeding

XIV.
glossorrhaphy, nasogastric, varices

XV.
1. body mass index
2. gastrointestinal
3. hepatitis B virus
4. herpes simplex virus
5. total parenteral nutrition

XVI.
1. ko lə sis to gas′trik
2. ko led′ə kəl
3. dis′ən ter e
4. fis′tu lə
5. hem ə roid ek′tə me

XVII.
1. C
2. E
3. B
4. A
5. C
6. B
7. D
8. C
9. C
10. C

XVIII.
1. ceco/colo/stomy: surgical creation of an anastomosis between the cecum and the colon
2. esophago/gastr/ectomy: removal of the esophagus and stomach
3. hemi/gastr/ectomy: surgical removal of one half of the stomach
4. sialo/genous: producing saliva
5. sigmoido/sigmoido/stomy: surgical creation of an anastomosis of portions of the sigmoid colon

Chapter 11

Exercise 1
(No particular order)
1. kidneys
2. ureters
3. bladder
4. urethra

Exercise 2
1. urethral
2. urinary
3. interrenal
4. extracystic
5. vesicoureteral, cystoureteral, or ureterocystic

Exercise 3
1. pelvis
2. ureter
3. urethra
4. nephron
5. bladder
6. glomerulus
7. tubules
8. meatus

Exercise 4
1. proteinuria
2. glycosuria
3. urinometer
4. pyuria
5. ketonuria

Exercise 5
1. cysto/metro/graphy: a urologic procedure that measures the amount of pressure on the bladder
2. nephro/stomy: surgical formation of a new opening into the renal pelvis
3. cysto/meter: an instrument used to measure aspects of the bladder
4. electro/myo/graphy: electrical recording of muscular contraction

Exercise 6
1. urinalysis
2. urea
3. cystometrography
4. renography
5. nephrotomography

Exercise 7
1. nephromalacia
2. urethrorrhagia
3. nocturia
4. nephromegaly
5. nephrotoxic

Exercise 8
1. F
2. C
3. A
4. D
5. G
6. B
7. E
8. J
9. I
10. H

Exercise 9
1. urethrocystitis or cystourethritis
2. nephropathy
3. ureteropyelonephritis
4. ureterolithiasis
5. nephrosclerosis

Exercise 10
1. bilateral
2. uremia
3. nephromalacia
4. urethrorrhea
5. renovascular
6. cystitis
7. pyelonephritis
8. polycystic
9. glomerulonephritis
10. mellitus

11. hydronephrosis
12. hydroureter
13. cystocele
14. hyperplasia
15. nephrolithiasis
16. insipidus
17. stenosis
18. thrombosis
19. hypospadias
20. epispadias

Exercise 11
1. transureteroureterostomy
2. lithotripsy
3. cystectomy
4. nephroureterectomy
5. lithotomy

Exercise 12
1. nephrectomy
2. ureterostomy
3. infection
4. pyelolithotomy
5. anticoagulant therapy
6. transurethral resection

Chapter 11 Review

I.
1. ren(o), nephr(o)
2. ureter(o)
3. cyst(o)
4. urethr(o)

II.
1. E
2. D
3. A
4. C
5. B

III.
(1 through 3, in no particular order)
filtering the blood; maintaining proper balance of water, salts, and acids; excreting waste products

IV.
1. F
2. F
3. T
4. F
5. F

6. F
7. F
8. T

V.
1. an/ur/ic: pertaining to absence of urine production or a urinary output of less than 100 mL per day
2. litho/tomy: the surgical excision of a calculus
3. noct/uria: excessive urination at night
4. olig/uria: a diminished capacity to form and pass urine—less than 500 mL per day
5. trans/urethral: through or across the wall of the urethra

VI.
1. urinometer
2. nephrotomogram
3. nephrostomy
4. cystoscopy

VII.
1. glomerulus
2. pyelolithotomy
3. renal enlargement
4. lithotripsy
5. intravenous pyelography
6. renal failure
7. incontinence
8. polyuria
9. endoscopy tube
10. transurethral resection
11. uremia
12. excessive number of white cells
13. hydroureter
14. stenosis
15. pyelonephritis

VIII.
1. uropathy
2. interrenal
3. hematuria
4. urethrocele
5. glomerulonephritis
6. pyelitis
7. hemodialysis
8. extracystic

9. cystography
10. lithotripsy

IX.
1. glomerulus
2. proximal convoluted tube
3. Bowman capsule
4. distal convoluted tubule
5. collecting duct

X.
1. difficult or painful
2. inflammation of the bladder and kidney
3. prostate
4. kidney stones
5. stone in the ureter
6. examination of the ureter
7. benign prostatic hyperplasia
8. kidney, ureter, and bladder
9. intravenous
10. urinalysis

XI.
1. nighttime frequency
2. kidney stones
3. insulin
4. cystoscope
5. carcinoma (cancer)
6. urinary tract infection
7. transurethral resection of the prostate

XII.
1. a developmental defect in which the urethral orifice (opening) is too low, lying on the undersurface of the penis
2. narrowing of the urinary meatus

3. surgical repair of the urinary meatus

XIII.
hydronephrosis, gonorrhea

XIV.
1. acute renal failure
2. electromyography
3. blood urea nitrogen
4. extracorporeal shock wave lithotripsy
5. voiding cystourethrogram

XV.
1. di u re´sis
2. lith´o trip se

3. nef ro lĭ thi´ə sis
4. pi´ə lo gram
5. u re´tər o plast te

XVI.
1. B
2. E
3. A
4. C
5. E
6. D
7. C
8. B
9. A
10. C

XVII.
1. cysto/rrhagia: hemorrhage from the bladder
2. keton/emia: the presence of ketones in the blood
3. nephro/toxic: toxic or destructive to a kidney
4. perineo/cele: a hernia in the perineal area
5. uro/genit/al: pertaining to the urinary and reproductive systems; genitourinary

Chapter 12

Exercise 1
1. vagina
2. organs of reproduction
3. uterus
4. month
5. measure or uterine tissue
6. ovum
7. ovary
8. ovary
9. uterus
10. vagina
11. perine(o)
12. cervic(o)
13. salping(o)
14. vulv(o)

Exercise 2
1. A
2. D
3. B
4. E
5. C

Exercise 3
1. cervical
2. ovarian
3. intrauterine
4. perimetrium
5. myometrium
6. endometrium

Exercise 4
1. menstruation
2. climacteric
3. menarche
4. ovulation
5. estrogen

Exercise 5
1. speculum
2. cytology
3. dysplasia
4. gonadotropin
5. colposcopy

6. hysteroscopy
7. hysterosalpingography
8. laparoscopy

Exercise 6
1. E
2. B
3. D
4. A
5. C

Exercise 7
1. B
2. C
3. A
4. D

Exercise 8
1. premenstrual
2. ovulation
3. anovulation
4. ovarian
5. pelvic
6. prolapse
7. retroversion
8. leiomyoma
9. fistula
10. cystocele

Exercise 9
1. salpingo/cele: hernial protrusion of a fallopian (or uterine) tube
2. oophoro/pathy: any disease of an ovary
3. cervic/itis: inflammation of the cervix
4. colpo/dynia: pain of the vagina
5. endo/metr/itis: inflammation of the lining of the uterus (endometrium)

Exercise 10
1. hormone
2. vulvectomy
3. oophoropexy
4. hysterectomy
5. laparohysterectomy
6. salpingectomy
7. ligation
8. salpingostomy
9. curettage
10. cryotherapy or cryosurgery

Exercise 11
1. colporrhaphy
2. salpingopexy
3. oophorohysterectomy
4. hysteropexy
5. laparoscope

Exercise 12
1. epididymis
2. testicle
3. rectum
4. urethra
5. vessel, vas deferens

Exercise 13
1. penile
2. prostatic
3. scrotal
4. seminal
5. testicular

Exercise 14
1. spermatogenesis
2. testicle
3. seminiferous
4. testosterone
5. luteinizing

Exercise 15
1. C
2. A

3. B
4. D

Exercise 16
1. urology
2. torsion
3. oligospermia
4. cryptorchidism
5. epididymitis
6. hydrocele
7. varicocele
8. phimosis
9. balanitis
10. hyperplasia

Exercise 17
1. a/zoo/sperm/ia: condition of the absence of living sperm
2. orchid/algia: testicular pain
3. prostat/itis: inflammation of the prostate gland
4. an/orch/ism: condition of absence of the testis
5. hyper/trophy: enlargement in size

Exercise 18
1. A
2. G
3. D
4. E
5. C
6. F
7. B
8. H

Exercise 19
1. orchiotomy
2. vasostomy
3. transurethral
4. prostatectomy

Chapter 12 Review

I.
1. oophor(o)
2. salping(o)
3. hyster(o)
4. cervic(o)
5. colp(o)

II.
1. vas(o)
2. urethr(o)
3. pen(o)
4. prostat(o)
5. epididym(o)
6. orchi(o)
7. scrot(o)

III.
1. A
2. B
3. C

IV.
1. A
2. B
3. C
4. A
5. D
6. F
7. E

V.
1. hysterosalpingogram
2. vasectomy
3. cystocele
4. rectocele

VI.
1. hystero/scope: an endoscope used to visually examine the cervix and uterine cavity
2. salping/itis: inflammation of a uterine tube
3. oophor/ectomy: surgical removal of one or both ovaries
4. spermato/genesis: development or production of sperm
5. vaso/vaso/stomy: restoring the cut ends of the vas deferens

VII.
1. dysmenorrhea
2. speculum
3. laparoscopy
4. oophoritis
5. menarche
6. hysteropexy
7. leukorrhea
8. endometriosis
9. colpoplasty
10. anorchidism
11. sterility
12. prepuce
13. cryptorchidism
14. torsion
15. orchialgia

VIII.
1. ovarian
2. ovulation
3. estrogen
4. uterine
5. menstruation (or menses)

IX.
1. anteversion
2. retroversion
3. anteflexion
4. retroflexion

X.
1. hysterectomy
2. menorrhagia
3. salpingocele
4. vasotomy
5. cervicitis
6. vulvovaginitis
7. oligospermia
8. salpingopexy
9. colposcopy
10. prostatectomy

XI.
1. per ĭ me´tre əm
2. per ĭ ne´əm
3. pro jes´tə rōn
4. tes tik´u lər
5. sper mə to jen´ə sis

XII.
1. ovary
2. uterus
3. inner lining of the uterus
4. dilation and curettage
5. last menstrual period
6. gynecology
7. hematology/oncology

XIII.
1. implantation of a fertilized ovum outside the uterine cavity
2. removal of the uterus through the vagina
3. removal of an ovary and its fallopian tube
4. nonmalignant enlargement of the prostate
5. herniation of the urinary bladder through the vaginal wall
6. herniation of the rectum through the vaginal wall
7. loss of support that holds the vagina in place, allowing it to sag
8. surgical repair of the perineum
9. surgical fixation of the vagina

XIV.
1. the semen discharged in a single emission (ejaculate is also a verb but is used here as a noun)
2. pertaining to the testicle
3. pertaining to the penis

XV.
dysplasia, gynecology, salpingorrhaphy

XVI.
1. benign prostatic hyperplasia
2. follicle-stimulating hormone
3. human chorionic gonadotropin
4. Papanicolaou
5. transurethral needle ablation

XVII.
1. C
2. C
3. B
4. D
5. B
6. C
7. A
8. B
9. D
10. A

XVIII.
1. balano/plasty: plastic surgery of the glans penis
2. epididymo/orch/itis: inflammation of the epididymis and the testicle
3. gonad/al shield: a shield used to protect the gonads during a radiographic procedure
4. leio/myo/fibr/oma: a benign uterine leiomyoma with fibrous connective tissue
5. oo/sperm: a fertilized ovum; the cell resulting from the union of the sperm and ovum after fertilization

Chapter 13

Exercise 1
1. gonad
2. gamete
3. zygote
4. ovulation
5. conception
6. implantation
7. fetus
8. chorion
9. spermatoblast
10. progesterone

Exercise 2
1. nat(o)
2. par(o)
3. false
4. pregnancy
5. pregnant female
6. that which stimulates

Exercise 3
1. post/nat/al: pertaining to after birth

2. amnio/rrhexis: rupture of the amnion (inner fetal membrane)
3. primi/gravida: a female during her first pregnancy
4. quadri/para: a woman who has had four viable offspring
5. neo/nato/logist: a physician who specializes in the study of newborn infants

Exercise 4
1. pregnancy
2. pelvimetry
3. amniocentesis
4. chorionic
5. fetoscope

Exercise 5
1. E
2. A
3. C
4. D
5. B

Exercise 6
1. E
2. B

3. A
4. D
5. C

Exercise 7
1. vasectomy
2. ligation
3. fertilization
4. abortion
5. episiotomy

Exercise 8
1. laparotomy
2. amniorrhexis
3. erythroblastosis
4. laparorrhaphy

Exercise 9
1. A
2. B
3. C
4. D
5. E

Chapter 13 Review

I.
1. umbilical cord
2. chorion
3. amnion
4. placenta
5. amniotic fluid
6. uterus

II.
1. D
2. C
3. A
4. B
5. E

III.
1. E
2. D
3. A
4. B
5. C

IV.
1. endo/metr/ium: lining of the uterus
2. erythro/blast/osis: a condition of embryonic forms of erythrocytes
3. laparo/rrhaphy: suture of the abdominal wall
4. neo/nato/logy: a specialty that cares for newborns
5. protein/uria: protein in the urine

V.
1. sonogram
2. intrauterine
3. fetoscope

VI.
1. HCG
2. pelvimetry
3. dystocia

4. Down syndrome
5. gestation
6. cephalic
7. spermicide
8. para 1
9. genital warts
10. candidiasis

VII.
1. neonate
2. multipara
3. spermatoblast
4. implantation
5. amniotomy
6. episiotomy
7. chancre
8. amniochorial or amniochorionic
9. fetal
10. ovulation

VIII.
1. an abnormal pregnancy in which the embryo implants outside the uterine cavity; extrauterine pregnancy
2. a surgical incision into the peritoneal cavity to establish a diagnosis and perform laparoscopic surgery as needed
3. destruction or cutting away of adhesions
4. the uterine tubes
5. the arrest of bleeding, as during surgery

IX.
1. description as seen with the naked eye
2. location of biopsy, as on a clock
3. sample of tissue from cervix, neck of uterus
4. totally, entirely

5. location of biopsy, as on a clock
6. samples of tissue from within the cervix
7. description as seen under a microscope
8. abnormal cells covering surface of the cervix (within the epithelium)
9. normal tissue from within the cervix
10. diagnoses made while looking at specimens under a microscope
11. early stage of cancer; in situ = confined, without invasion
12. warty growth, usually sexually transmitted

X.
1. vaginal swab (collection of fluid from the vagina)
2. cocci in pairs that are located inside and outside a cell
3. gonorrhea
4. Neisseria gonorrhoeae
5. penicillin or another antibiotic if patient is allergic to penicillin

XI.
amniocentesis, contraceptive

XII.
1. acquired immunodeficiency syndrome
2. cephalopelvic disproportion
3. fetal heart rate
4. gonococcus
5. intrauterine device

XIII.
1. am´ne on
2. shang´kər
3. gam´ ēt
4. im u no də fish´ən se
5. se kən dip´ə rə

XIV.
1. D
2. E
3. E
4. A
5. D
6. B
7. C
8. D
9. C
10. C

XV.
1. amnio/in/fusion: introduction of a fluid into the uterus during labor
2. feto/scopy: directly observing the fetus in utero, using a fetoscope introduced through a small incision in the abdomen
3. gono/cocc/al pyo/myos/itis: inflammation of a muscle caused by infection with gonococci
4. o/o/cyte donation: a method of aspirating an oocyte from a fertile woman for incubation in the uterus of a woman who has female factor infertility
5. spermato/path/ia: pertaining to diseased sperm or their associated organs

Chapter 14

Exercise 1
1. marrow
2. epiphyses
3. periosteum
4. bone
5. musculoskeletal
6. ossification

Exercise 2
1. skeleton
2. skeletal
3. axial
4. appendicular

Exercise 3
1. sternum
2. cranium
3. cost(o)
4. spine
5. stern(o)
6. vertebrae
7. cervical
8. coccygeal

Exercise 4
1. thoracolumbar
2. cranial
3. supracostal
4. infrasternal
5. intervertebral

Exercise 5
1. tars(o)
2. fibul(o)
3. clavicul(o)
4. phalang(o)
5. calcane(o)
6. patell(o)
7. tibi(o)
8. scapul(o)
9. femor(o)
10. humer(o)
11. carp(o)

Exercise 6
1. (No particular order) ilium, ischium, and pubis
2. (No particular order) ulna and radius

Exercise 7
1. ischio/coccyg/eal: pertaining to the ischium (sit bone) and the coccyx (tail bone)
2. humero/scapul/ar: pertaining to the humerus (upper arm bone) and the scapula (shoulder blade)
3. infra/patell/ar: pertaining to below the patella (kneecap)
4. ulno/radi/al: pertaining to the radius and ulna (lateral and medial forearm bones)
5. meta/carp/al: pertaining to the bones of the palm

Exercise 8
1. scapuloclavicular
2. carpophalangeal
3. ischiopubic
4. iliofemoral
5. calcaneotibial

Exercise 9
1. connective
2. articulation
3. synovial
4. joint
5. bursae
6. tendons
7. ligament
8. perichondrium

Exercise 10
1. B
2. A
3. E
4. F
5. H

Exercise 11
1. bone
2. electromyography
3. motion
4. erythrocyte
5. rheumatoid
6. joint
7. arthroscope
8. arthrocentesis

Exercise 12
1. arthrography
2. calciuria
3. intraarticular
4. electromyogram
5. osteomalacia

Exercise 13
1. myo/dynia: pain in a muscle
2. spondyl/algia: pain in a vertebra
3. arthro/chondr/itis: inflammation of an articular cartilage
4. calcaneo/dynia: pain in the heel
5. a/trophy: decrease in size (wasting)

Exercise 14
1. osteitis
2. chondrosarcoma
3. osteomyelitis
4. myocellulitis
5. leukemia

Exercise 15
1. cranio/cele: hernial protrusion of the brain through a defect in the skull
2. syn/dactyl/ism: condition of fused digits
3. osteo/sclerosis: abnormal hardness of bone
4. osteo/penia: decreased bone mass
5. rachi/schisis: fissure (split) of one or more vertebrae

Exercise 16
1. A
2. C
3. D
4. E
5. I
6. F

Exercise 17
1. carpal
2. bursitis

3. arthritis
4. temporomandibular
5. tarsoptosis
6. tumor
7. osteomalacia
8. bifida
9. osteoarthritis
10. myasthenia

Exercise 18
1. scleroderma
2. ankylosis
3. myofibrosis
4. polymyalgia
5. spondylarthropathy

Exercise 19
1. C
2. D
3. B
4. A
5. E

Exercise 20
1. arthroclasia
2. costectomy
3. arthrotomy
4. myelosuppression
5. antiinflammatories
6. spondylodesis
7. arthrocentesis
8. chondrectomy
9. cranioplasty
10. myorrhaphy

Exercise 21
1. cranio/tomy: surgical incision into the skull
2. myo/rrhaphy: suture of a muscle
3. teno/myo/plasty: repair of a tendon and muscle
4. spondylo/syn/desis: spinal fusion
5. fasci/ectomy: excision of fascia

Chapter 14 Review

I.
1. clavicul(o)
2. stern(o)
3. cost(o)
4. ili(o)
5. pub(o)
6. ischi(o)
7. crani(o)
8. scapul(o)
9. humer(o)
10. radi(o)
11. uln(o)
12. carp(o)
13. femor(o)
14. patell(o)
15. tibi(o)
16. fibul(o)
17. tars(o)
18. phalang(o)

II.
1. G
2. B
3. E
4. D
5. A
6. C
7. F

III.
1. J
2. H
3. A
4. D
5. I
6. G
7. C
8. F
9. B
10. E

IV.
1. B
2. A
3. C
4. D

V.
1. J
2. D
3. H
4. I
5. F
6. E
7. B
8. G
9. C
10. A

VI.
1. cervical
2. thoracic
3. lumbar
4. sacral
5. coccygeal

VII.
(No particular order)
support for the body, protection of soft body parts, movement, blood cell formation, and storage

VIII.
(No particular order)
skeletal: control movement of bones; visceral: contraction of organs and blood vessels; cardiac: contraction of the heart

IX.
1. electromyography
2. arthroscopy

X.
1. carpo/phalang/eal: pertaining to the wrist and fingers
2. chondro/sarcoma: malignant tumor derived from cartilage

3. osteo/lysis: destruction of bone
4. osteo/arthro/pathy: any disease affecting bones and joints
5. scapulo/clavicul/ar: pertaining to the shoulder blade and collarbone

XI.
1. sternoschisis
2. ulnoradial
3. arthropathy
4. electromyogram
5. decalcification
6. polydactylism
7. bone marrow
8. arthroscopy
9. tarsoptosis
10. osteomalacia

XII.
1. reduction
2. intercostal
3. osteoarthritis
4. coccygectomy
5. myocele
6. osteitis
7. scoliosis
8. myofascial
9. articular
10. arthrocentesis

XIII.
1. fracture of the right thigh bone resulting in many bone fragments
2. laminectomy: surgical removal of the bony arches of one or more vertebrae; right knee arthroscopy: examination of the interior of the right knee with an arthroscope
3. rupture of the cartilage surrounding an intervertebral disk
4. painful conditions of the joints
5. osteoporosis: abnormal loss of bone density and deterio-

ration of the bone with increased fracture risk

XIV.
1. degenerative joint disease; degenerative changes in the joints
2. chronic, inflammatory, and sometimes deforming disease of the joints that has an autoimmune component
3. osteoarthritis (noninflammatory, degenerative arthritis) of the left knee
4. arthroplasty: an operation to restore the integrity and function of a joint, as much as is possible
5. right leg
6. ad libitum (L), freely, as desired

XV.
1. A compression fracture is breaking of a bone caused by excessive vertical force and causing loss of height of the vertebral body (often causing the bone to collapse). L2 designates the second lumbar vertebra.
2. The feeling in both legs is normal.
3. Degeneration or deficient development of the articulating part of the lumbar vertebrae. Because the lumbar spine vertebrae are numbered L1 through L5, multilevel indicates involvement of more than one of these vertebrae.
4. Disko/gram means a record of a vertebral disk. (This is accomplished by introduction of a radiopaque contrast medium into the center of the disk.)
5. joining or uniting

XVI.
femoral, iliofemoral

XVII.
1. antinuclear antibody
2. degenerative joint disease
3. electromyography
4. range of motion
5. systemic lupus erythematosus

XVIII.
1. ahr thro kla′zhə
2. kon dro sahr ko′mə
3. lum′bahr
4. mi əs the′ne ə
5. stər no kos′təl

XIX.
1. E
2. C
3. B
4. A
5. A
6. C
7. A
8. B
9. D
10. A

XX.
1. burso/pathy: any disease of a bursa
2. musculo/tendin/ous: pertaining to the muscle and the tendon
3. osteo/chondr/al: pertaining to bone and cartilage
4. supra/patell/ar: pertaining to a location above the kneecap
5. teno/synov/itis: inflammation of the tendon and synovial membrane (joint lining)

Chapter 15

Exercise 1
1. (No particular order) stimulates movement; senses changes both within and outside the body; provides us with thought, learning, and memory; maintains homeostasis with the help of the hormonal system
2. sensory, integrative, motor
3. (No particular order) central nervous system, peripheral nervous system

4. (No particular order) neurons, neuroglia
5. (No particular order) axons, dendrites

Exercise 2
1. brain, spinal cord
2. (No particular order) dura mater, arachnoid, pia mater

Exercise 3
1. cerebro/spin/al: pertaining to the

cerebrum and the spinal cord
2. cranio/cerebr/al: pertaining to the skull and the cerebrum
3. mening/eal: pertaining to the meninges
4. neuro/muscul/ar: pertaining to the nerves and muscles
5. sub/dural: beneath the dura mater

Exercise 4
1. sensory
2. sense
3. acetylcholine
4. epinephrine
5. chemoreceptors
6. photoreceptors
7. thermoreceptors
8. nociceptors
9. lacrimal
10. odors

Exercise 5
1. audiology
2. interocular
3. nasolacrimal
4. dacryocyst
5. somatic

Exercise 6
1. B
2. E
3. A
4. D
5. C

Exercise 7
1. ophthalmo/meter: instrument to measure the eye
2. electro/encephalo/graph: instrument to measure electrical activity of the brain
3. audio/gram: record produced from measuring hearing
4. ophthalmo/scopy: visual examination of the eye
5. encephalo/graphy: radiography of the brain

Exercise 8
1. cephalalgia
2. photophobia
3. polyneuritis
4. hyperalgesia
5. dyslexia

Exercise 9
1. A
2. B
3. E
4. C
5. F
6. D

Exercise 10
1. encephalo/mening/itis: inflammation of the meninges and brain
2. hemi/plegia: paralysis of half of the body (one side only)
3. meningo/myelo/cele: an abnormal protrusion of the meninges and spinal cord
4. ventricul/itis: inflammation of a ventricle of the brain
5. hydro/phobia: rabies; fear of water (literal translation)

Exercise 11
1. bradykinesia
2. narcolepsy
3. intracranial
4. glioma
5. amyotrophic

Exercise 12
1. blephar/edema: swelling of the eyelid
2. ophthalmo/rrhagia: hemorrhage from the eye
3. kerat/itis: inflammation of the cornea
4. retino/pathy: any disease of the retina
5. dacryo/lith/iasis: calculus in the tear duct

Exercise 13
1. pseudomania
2. psychosis
3. neurasthenia
4. pyrophobia
5. hyperkinesia

Exercise 14
1. neuro/lysis: release of a nerve sheath
2. kerato/tomy: incision into the cornea
3. dacryo/cysto/rhino/stomy: surgical creation of a passageway between the lacrimal sac and the nose
4. vago/tomy: severing branches of the vagus nerve
5. trans/cutane/ous: through the skin

Exercise 15
1. C
2. B
3. E
4. D
5. A

Exercise 16
1. thrombolytics
2. aneurysmectomy
3. craniectomy
4. neurorrhaphy
5. blepharoplasty

Chapter 15 Review

I.
1. dura mater
2. arachnoid
3. pia mater

II.
1. cerebellum
2. spinal cord
3. cerebrum
4. diencephalon
5. brain stem

III.
1. meningocele
2. ventriculoperitoneal

IV.
1. A
2. B
3. B
4. B
5. A

V.
1. A
2. D
3. E
4. C
5. B

VI.
1. dacryo/cysto/rhino/stomy: creating a new opening into the nose from the lacrimal sac

2. intra/ocul/ar: pertaining to structures or substances within the eyeball
3. neuro/genic: originating in the nervous system
4. naso/lacrim/al: pertaining to the nose and associated lacrimal ducts
5. sub/dur/al: pertaining to the area under the dura mater

VII.
1. dura mater
2. Alzheimer disease
3. paraplegia
4. cerebrovascular accident
5. myelogram
6. claustrophobia
7. meningocele
8. contraindication
9. dacryocystotomy
10. sensitivity to pain

VIII.
1. meninges
2. cerebrum
3. cerebrospinal
4. neuron
5. neuroglia
6. axon
7. dendrite

IX.
1. anotia
2. otosclerosis

3. encephalomyelitis
4. keratitis
5. myopia
6. semiconscious
7. myelography
8. electroencephalography
9. dacryolithiasis
10. narcolepsy

X.
1. C
2. A
3. D
4. E
5. B
6. degenerative
7. dementia
8. dysarthria

XI.
1. degenerating neurologic disorder characterized by resting tremors, masklike facial expression, shuffling gait, muscle rigidity, and weakness
2. benign, encapsulated tumor of the meninges
3. any disorder of the peripheral nervous system
4. sagging or prolapse of an organ
5. slowing of spontaneity and movement

XII.
1. hemisphere is a synonym for the cerebral hemisphere; bihemispheric would pertain to both sides of the cerebral hemisphere
2. disease affecting the ability of the blood to clot; this would lead to uncontrollable bleeding
3. device to monitor a patient's intracranial pressure
4. dysfunction of the sympathetic part of the nervous system (the autonomic division of the nervous system)

XIII.
acetylcholine, cerebral

XIV.
1. attention deficit hyperactivity disorder
2. amyotrophic lateral sclerosis
3. cerebrospinal fluid
4. deep tendon reflex
5. spinal cord injury

XV.
1. ə rak´noid
2. ser ə brot´ə me
3. ef´ər ənt
4. gli o´mə
5. klep to ma´ne ə

XVI.
1. A
2. B
3. C
4. C
5. B
6. A
7. B

8. E
9. C
10. D

XVII.
1. audio/metr/ic: pertaining to the measurement of hearing

2. cardio/phobia: abnormal fear of heart disease
3. cerebro/cerebell/ar: pertaining to the cerebrum and the cerebellum
4. encephalo/malacia: softening of the brain

5. meningo/encephalo/myel/itis: inflammation of the meninges, brain, and spinal cord

Chapter 16

Exercise 1
1. kerato/genesis: formation of keratin, a horny material
2. sub/cutane/ous: pertaining to beneath the skin
3. ecto/derm: outside (outermost) germ layer
4. dermato/logist: specialist in treatment of the skin
5. endo/derm: innermost germ layer

Exercise 2
1. fat
2. axilla (armpit)
3. skin
4. sweat
5. horny or cornea
6. nail
7. hair
8. sebum
9. hair
10. nail
11. dermis and epidermis
12. ectoderm

13. sebum
14. sudoriferous gland
15. ungual

Exercise 3
1. biopsy
2. needle
3. skin (or allergy)
4. sweat

Exercise 4
1. albinism
2. cyanosis
3. ichthyoid
4. epidermal
5. xerosis

Exercise 5
1. A
2. E
3. D
4. B
5. C
6. F

Exercise 6
1. A
2. E
3. B
4. C
5. F
6. D

Exercise 7
1. abscess
2. furuncle
3. verruca
4. fungal
5. petechiae
6. nevus
7. keratosis
8. lipoma
9. Kaposi
10. dermis

Exercise 8
1. hidr/aden/itis: inflammation of a sweat gland
2. tricho/pathy: any hair disease

3. photo/dermat/itis: inflammation of skin reacting to light
4. hypo/therm/ia: condition of lack of heat
5. follicul/itis: inflammation of the hair follicles

Exercise 9
1. F
2. G
3. A
4. E
5. D
6. B
7. C

Exercise 10
1. D
2. E
3. C
4. B
5. A

Chapter 16 Review

I.
1. superficial partial thickness (first degree)
2. deep partial thickness (second degree)
3. full thickness (third degree)
4. epidermis
5. dermis
6. subcutaneous fat

II.
(Any 5, no particular order)
external body covering; acts as a barrier to microorganisms; helps regulate body temperature; provides information about the environment; helps eliminate wastes; synthesizes vitamin D

III.
(No particular order)
hair protects the scalp, eyes, nostrils, and ears; nails protect the fingers and toes, and fingernails help us pick up small things; sebaceous glands produce sebum to keep hair and skin soft and inhibit bacterial growth; sweat glands eliminate waste and help regulate body temperature

IV.
1. A
2. G
3. C
4. D
5. H
6. F
7. E
8. B

V.
1. necrosis
2. onychomycosis

VI.
1. electro/lysis: destruction by electricity
2. ichthy/osis: a condition in which the skin is dry, resembling scales

3. kerato/genesis: the formation of horny tissue (keratin)
4. melano/cyte: a cell capable of producing melanin
5. sclero/derma: hardening and thickening of the skin

VII.
1. skin test
2. cryotherapy
3. débridement
4. axillary
5. seborrheic dermatitis
6. sweat test
7. scleroderma
8. bedsore
9. deep partial thickness
10. necrosis

VIII.
1. keratin
2. dermis
3. sebum
4. sudoriferous
5. sweating (perspiration)

IX.
1. furuncle
2. scabies
3. laceration
4. albinism
5. contusion
6. onychopathy
7. alopecia
8. ichthyosis
9. thermoplegia
10. folliculitis

X.
1. the removal of foreign material or dead and damaged tissue
2. abundant flushing of the open wound
3. VAC means vacuum-assisted closure. It is used to remove drainage and speed wound healing, using tubes and a pump to draw off fluids from the wound.
4. incision and drainage

XI.

1. redness of the skin that is the result of dilation and congestion of superficial capillaries
2. hardening of the tissue, usually caused by edema and inflammation
3. inflammation of hair follicles
4. a chronic disease, primarily of the skin, characterized by lesions that are covered with scales
5. a superficial dermatitis
6. a superficial bacterial infection involving the hair follicles

XII.

1. B
2. F

3. D
4. E
5. C
6. A
7. G

XIII.

ectoderm, hidradenitis, onychectomy

XIV.

1. American Burn Association
2. discoid lupus erythematosus
3. herpes simplex virus type 1
4. total body surface area
5. ointment

XV.

1. sel u li´tis
2. dər mə bra´shən

3. ik the o´sis
4. ur tĭ kar´e ə
5. zēr o der´mə

XVI.

1. E
2. C
3. D
4. D
5. C
6. D
7. B
8. D
9. A
10. C

XVII.

1. an/hidr/osis: inadequate (literal translation: lack of) perspiration

2. dermato/graph/ia: a skin condition characterized by wheals that develop from tracing on the skin with the fingernail or a blunted instrument
3. hyper/kerat/osis: overgrowth of the cornified epithelial layer of the skin
4. onycho/dys/trophy: a condition of malformed or discolored fingernails or toenails
5. tricho/phag/ia: the habit of eating hair

Chapter 17

Exercise 1

1. pituitary, adrenals, gonads, thyroid, pancreas, and pineal gland

Exercise 2

1. nervous
2. pituitary
3. gland
4. hormones

Exercise 3

1. adeno/hypo/physis: gland portion (anterior) of the hypophysis (growth below the brain) or pituitary gland
2. neuro/hypo/physis: nerve portion (posterior) of the hypophysis (growth below the brain) or pituitary gland
3. hypo/thalamus: portion of the lower part of the brain (beneath the thalamus)
4. exo/crine: to secrete outside; the glands with ducts—different from endocrine
5. homeo/stasis: controlling the sameness, maintaining a balance

Exercise 4

1. somatotropin
2. melanocyte
3. euthyroid
4. androgenic
5. tropic

Exercise 5

1. lacto/genic: inducing the secretion of milk
2. ad/ren/al: pertaining toward the kidney, the gland situated atop each kidney
3. retro/mamm/ary: pertaining to behind the breasts
4. lact/ation: (process of) milk production
5. adreno/cortico/tropic: stimulating the adrenal cortex

Exercise 6

1. D
2. D
3. A
4. D
5. D
6. C
7. D
8. D
9. D
10. B
11. E
12. D

Exercise 7

1. adrenals
2. kidneys
3. ovaries or testes
4. ovaries or testes
5. female breasts
6. thyroid

Exercise 8

1. D
2. C
3. B
4. E
5. A

Exercise 9

1. hyperthyroidism
2. hypoglycemia
3. ketonuria
4. glycosuria
5. mammography

Exercise 10

1. adeno/carcin/oma: malignant tumor of a gland
2. poly/dipsia: excessive thirst
3. hypo/pituitar/ism: decreased activity of the pituitary gland
4. hyper/parathyroid/ism: abnormally increased activity of the parathyroid glands
5. hypo/calc/emia: low level of calcium in the blood

Exercise 11

1. pancreatitis
2. mastodynia
3. mastocarcinoma
4. hyperadrenalism
5. hyperinsulism

Exercise 12

1. D
2. F
3. C
4. H
5. I
6. J
7. E
8. B
9. A
10. G

Exercise 13

1. lumpectomy
2. thyroidectomy
3. mammoplasty
4. adrenalectomy
5. mastopexy
6. mastectomy

Chapter 17 Review

I.
(No particular order)
pituitary, adrenals, gonads, pineal gland, thyroid, pancreas

II.
(No particular order)
nervous system stimulates endocrine glands by nerve impulses; endocrine glands release hormones

III.
1. C
2. B
3. B
4. A
5. D

IV.
1. D
2. D
3. A
4. D
5. D
6. C
7. D
8. D
9. D
10. B
11. E
12. D
13. E

V.
1. B
2. F
3. C
4. E
5. G
6. A
7. D

VI.
1. adreno/cortic/al: pertaining to the adrenal cortex (outer portion)
2. endo/crine: to secrete internally (into the blood or lymph)
3. hyper/calc/emia: greater than normal amounts of calcium in the blood
4. mast/ectomy: surgical excision of one or both breasts
5. somato/tropin: growth hormone; agent that influences body growth

VII.
1. hypophysectomy
2. mammogram

VIII.
1. sweat gland
2. androgens
3. mammography
4. Cushing syndrome
5. acromegaly
6. diabetes insipidus
7. myxedema
8. pancreas
9. glycosylated hemoglobin
10. goiter

IX.
1. epinephrine
2. hypothyroidism
3. hirsutism
4. gonad
5. hyperglycemia
6. prolactin
7. pituitary
8. androgenic (or masculinizing)
9. homeostasis
10. glycosuria

X.
1. an tĭ di u ret´ik
2. jin ə ko mas´te ə
3. hi po ə dre´nəl iz əm
4. mam´o plas te
5. ok sĭ to´sin

XI.
1. study and treatment of the endocrine system
2. irregular heartbeat with increase in frequency or force or both; can be felt by the patient
3. protrusion of one or both eyeballs; can be due to thyroid disease
4. vital signs
5. blood pressure
6. head, ears, eyes, nose, throat
7. chronic, benign enlargement of the thyroid gland
8. within normal limits
9. abnormality of thyroid gland to include increased thyroid hormone, weight loss, shakiness, and exophthalmos
10. excision of the thyroid gland (surgical)

XII.
1. polyuria (excessive urination) and chronic UTIs (urinary tract infections)
2. mastectomy
3. Both are high—she has hypercholesterolemia and hyperlipidemia.
4. Nonhealing leg ulcers and poorly healing skin wounds—both due to diabetes, which affects the blood vessels, causing slow healing.
5. retinopathy (diseased eyes), neuropathy (diseased nerves), and nephropathy (diseased kidneys)
6. HbA_{1c} 9%, the amount of hemoglobin A_{1c} in the blood, provides an accurate long-term index of the patient's average blood glucose level.

XIII.
1. excessive development of the male mammary glands, frequently secondary to increased estrogen levels; may occur in normal adolescents
2. excision of both breasts
3. the circular pigmented area around the nipple
4. the arrest of bleeding
5. the mass of fat cells in the area of the axilla

6. reapproximated: to approximate is to bring close together; to reapproximate is to bring close together again, as in suturing together the edges of the skin after surgery

XIV.
adenohypophysis, homeostasis, thyrotropin

XV.
1. gestational diabetes mellitus
2. growth hormone
3. interstitial cell hormone
4. radioactive iodine
5. thyroid-stimulating hormone

XVI.
1. C
2. C
3. E
4. C
5. C
6. A
7. B
8. D
9. B
10. C

XVII.
1. adrenal/ectomy: the total or partial excision of one or both adrenal glands
2. endo/crino/pathy: a disease involving an endocrine gland or a dysfunction that decreases its secretion or response to a hormone
3. lactos/uria: lactose in the urine, a condition that may occur in late pregnancy or during lactation
4. pituitar/ism: any condition caused by a failure or defect of the pituitary gland
5. thyro/genic: originating in the thyroid gland

Chapter 18

I.

1. obstetrician
2. neonatologist
3. radiologist
4. nerve cell
5. clinical pathologist
6. symptom
7. chiroplasty
8. cardiomegaly
9. electrocardiogram
10. computed tomography
11. appendicitis
12. encephalocele
13. phobia
14. iatrogenic
15. bacteria
16. macroscopic
17. against
18. four
19. intramuscular
20. syndrome
21. genetic disorder
22. quadrants
23. farther from the origin
24. frontal
25. diaphragm
26. erythrocytes
27. aplastic
28. transplant
29. between
30. thrombopenia
31. myocardial infarction
32. atherosclerosis
33. coronary thrombosis
34. atrial septal defect
35. rheumatic fever
36. pneumonitis
37. expectorate
38. parietal pleura
39. bronchodilators
40. orthopnea
41. cholecystography
42. extracorporeal shock wave lithotripsy
43. anorexia nervosa
44. emaciation
45. colectomy
46. intravenous urography
47. renal failure
48. vesicoureteral
49. polyuria
50. endoscopy tube
51. dysmenorrhea
52. azoospermia
53. hysteropexy
54. endometriosis
55. anorchidism
56. dystocia
57. Down syndrome
58. gestation
59. cephalic
60. genital warts
61. sternoschisis
62. ulnoradial
63. arthropathy
64. electromyogram
65. polydactylism
66. central nervous system
67. paraplegia
68. meningocele
69. dacryocystotomy
70. Alzheimer disease
71. débridement
72. seborrheic dermatitis
73. scleroderma
74. deep partial thickness
75. necrosis
76. pancreas
77. goiter
78. mammography
79. diabetes insipidus
80. Cushing syndrome

II.

1. acute
2. triage
3. cardiac (sometimes coronary)
4. pathology
5. internist
6. colectomy or colonectomy
7. ophthalmotomy
8. encephalotome
9. angiorrhaphy
10. blepharedema
11. hemolysin
12. carcinogen
13. ophthalmopathy
14. osteitis
15. nasal
16. asymptomatic
17. bradyphasia
18. intracellular
19. retronasal or postnasal
20. diplopia
21. unilateral
22. supine
23. omphalitis
24. abdominopelvic
25. electroencephalogram
26. poikilocyte
27. hyponatremia
28. thrombolysis
29. neutrophil
30. hematopoiesis
31. asystole
32. vasodilators
33. hypertension
34. tachycardia
35. lymphangitis
36. tracheomalacia
37. dysphonia
38. rhinolithiasis
39. alveolar
40. laryngography
41. gastropathy
42. amylase
43. hyperemesis
44. cholecystectomy
45. hepatitis
46. glomerulonephritis
47. pyelitis
48. pyuria
49. cystography
50. lithotripsy
51. vasotomy
52. cervicitis
53. vulvovaginitis
54. oligospermia
55. salpingopexy
56. multipara
57. implantation
58. amniotomy
59. episiotomy
60. chancre
61. osteoarthritis
62. coccygectomy
63. myocele
64. osteitis
65. scoliosis
66. myelography
67. electroencephalography
68. cataract
69. encephalomyelitis
70. agoraphobia
71. contusion
72. onychopathy
73. folliculitis
74. albinism
75. laceration
76. pituitary
77. androgenic (or masculinizing)
78. hypothyroidism
79. gonad
80. glycosuria

III.

1. T
2. A
3. S
4. A
5. P
6. S
7. S
8. D
9. T
10. P
11. P
12. A
13. P
14. P
15. D
16. A
17. P
18. A
19. A
20. P
21. P
22. T
23. P
24. P
25. S
26. T
27. P
28. A
29. S
30. P
31. P
32. S
33. D
34. A
35. P
36. P
37. D
38. P
39. A
40. P
41. S
42. D
43. A
44. S
45. D
46. P
47. P
48. S
49. S
50. A
51. P
52. D
53. S
54. P
55. A
56. P
57. A
58. A
59. D
60. D
61. S
62. A
63. S
64. P
65. T
66. A
67. D
68. P
69. P
70. S
71. P
72. S
73. S
74. P
75. A
76. S
77. P
78. S
79. P
80. A

Bibliography/Illustration Credits

Bibliography

American Cancer Society: *Ca—A Cancer Journal for Clinicians*, Vol 57, No 1, Atlanta, 2007, American Cancer Society.

Applegate EJ: *The anatomy and physiology learning system: textbook,* ed 3, Philadelphia, 2006, Saunders.

Bedolla M: *Essential Spanish for health care,* New York, 1997, Living Language.

BJC Health Care: *Weapons of mass destruction awareness training,* St Louis, 2002.

Bonewit K: *Clinical procedures for medical assistants,* ed 6, Philadelphia, 2004, Saunders.

Centers for Disease Control and Prevention, Atlanta, 2007, www.cdc.gov.

Destafano C, Federman FM: *Essentials of medical transcription: a modular approach,* ed 2, Philadelphia, 2004, Saunders.

Dorland's illustrated medical dictionary, ed 31, Philadelphia, 2007, Saunders.

Dunmore CW, Fleischer RM: *Medical terminology: exercises in etymology,* ed 3, Philadelphia, 2004, FA Davis.

Ignatavicius DD, Workman ML, Mishler MA: *Medical-surgical nursing: critical thinking for collaborative care,* ed 5, Philadelphia, 2006, Saunders.

Joyce EV, Villanueva ME: *Say it in Spanish: a guide for health care professionals,* Philadelphia, 1996, Saunders.

Lewis SM, Heitkemper MM, Dirksen SR: *Medical-surgical nursing: assessment and management of clinical problems,* ed 6, St Louis, 2004, Mosby.

Mosby's medical, nursing, and allied health dictionary, ed 7, St Louis, 2006, Mosby.

Seidel HM, Ball JW, Dains JE, Benedict GW: *Mosby's guide to physical examination,* ed 6, St Louis, 2006, Mosby.

Taber's cyclopedic medical dictionary, ed 20, Philadelphia, 2005, FA Davis.

Velasquez M: *Velasquez Spanish and English dictionary,* Clinton, NJ, 1985, New Win Publishing.

Illustration Credits

Note: All Exercise Figures also appear as numbered figures within the same chapter. Please check the listing of the numbered figures to obtain credit information for exercise figures.

Chapter 1
Figures 1-2 and 1-5 From Polaski AL, Tatro SE: *Luckmann's core principles and practice of medical-surgical nursing,* Philadelphia, 1996, Saunders.

Chapter 2
Figure 2-2 From Seidel HM, Ball JW, Dains JE, Benedict GW: *Mosby's guide to physical examination,* ed 4, St Louis, 1999, Mosby.

Figure 2-3 From Ballinger PW, Frank ED: *Merrill's atlas of radiographic positions and radiologic procedures,* vol 1, ed 9, St Louis, 1999, Mosby.

Figure 2-4 From Thibodeau GA, Patton KT: *Anatomy & physiology,* ed 6, St Louis, 2007, Mosby/Elsevier.

Figure 2-5 From Seidel HM, Ball JW, Dains JE, Benedict GW: *Mosby's guide to physical examination,* ed 5, St Louis, 2003, Mosby.

Figure 2-6 From Polaski AL, Tatro SE: *Luckmann's core principles and practice of medical-surgical nursing,* Philadelphia, 1996, Saunders.

Figure 2-7 From Zakus S: *Mosby's clinical skills for medical assistants,* ed 4, St Louis, 2001, Mosby.

Figure 2-8 From Gerdin J: *Health careers today,* ed 4 St Louis, 2007, Mosby.

Figure 2-9 From Ignatavicius MS, Workman ML: *Medical-surgical nursing: critical thinking for collaborative care,* ed 5, 2006, Philadelphia, Saunders.

Chapter 3
Figure 3-1 From Goldstein BJ, Goldstein AO: *Practical dermatology,* ed 2, St Louis, 1997, Mosby.

Figure 3-2, A From Bonewit-West K: *Clinical procedures for medical assistants,* ed 7, Philadelphia, 2008, Saunders.

Figure 3-3 From Zitelli BJ, Davis HW: *Atlas of pediatric physical diagnosis,* ed 5, St Louis, 2007, Mosby.

Figure 3-4 From Ignatavicius MS, Workman ML: *Medical-surgical nursing: critical thinking for collaborative care,* ed 5, Philadelphia, 2006, Saunders.

Figure 3-5 From Phipps WJ, Monahan FD, Sands JK, Marek JF, Neighbors M: *Medical-surgical nursing,* ed 8, St Louis, 2007, Mosby.

Figure 3-6 From Potter PA, Perry AG: *Fundamentals of nursing,* ed 3, St Louis, 1993, Mosby.

Figure 3-7 From Seidel HM, Ball JW, Dains JE, Benedict GW: *Mosby's guide to physical examination,* ed 6, St Louis, 2006, Mosby.

Figure 3-8, A and B From Seidel HM, Ball JW, Dains JE, Benedict GW: *Mosby's guide to physical examination,* ed 5, St Louis, 2003, Mosby.

Figure 3-8, C From Seidel HM, Ball JW, Dains JE, Benedict GW: *Mosby's guide to physical examination,* ed 6, St Louis, 2006, Mosby.

Figures 3-9 and 3-14 From Frank ED, Long BW, and Smith BJ: *Merrill's atlas of radiographic positioning and radiologic procedures,* ed 11, St Louis, 2007, Mosby.

Figures 3-10, A, and 3-12, C Courtesy Siemens.

Figure 3-10, B From Seeley RS, Stephens TD, Tate P: *Anatomy and physiology,* ed 3, St Louis, 1995, Mosby.

Figure 3-11 From Ballinger PW, Frank ED: *Merrill's atlas of radiographic positions and radiologic procedures,* ed 10, St Louis, 2003, Mosby.

Figure 3-12, A from Mourad LA: *Orthopedic disorders,* St Louis, 1991, Mosby; B Courtesy of Professor A. Jackson, Department of Diagnostic Radiology, University of Manchester.

Figure 3-13 From Curry RA, Tempkin BB: *Sonography: introduction to normal structure and function,* St Louis, 2004, Saunders.

Figure 3-15 From Gruber RP, Peck GC: *Rhinoplasty: state of the art,* St Louis, 1993, Mosby.

Chapter 4
Figure 4-1 From Zacarian SA: *Cryosurgery,* St Louis, 1985, Mosby.

Figure 4-2 From Weston WL, Lane AT, Morelli JG: *Color textbook of pediatric dermatology,* ed 4, St Louis, 2007, Mosby.

Figure 4-3 From Clark DA: *Atlas of neonatology,* Philadelphia, 2000, Saunders.

Figure 4-4 From Palay DA, Krachmer JH, eds: *Ophthalmology for the primary care physician,* St Louis, 1998, Mosby.

Figure 4-5 From Hoffbrand AV: *Color atlas of clinical hematology,* London, 1987, Mosby.

Figure 4-6 From Kumar V, Abbas AK, Fasto N, and Mitchell RN: *Robbins' Basic pathology,* ed 8, Philadelphia, 2007, Saunders.

Figure 4-7 and 4-14, A and B From Zitelli BJ, Davis HW: *Atlas of pediatric physical diagnosis,* ed 5, St. Louis, 2007, Mosby. A, also: Courtesy Ellen Wald, MD, University of Wisconsin Children's Hospital.

Figures 4-8 From Kamal A, Brockelhurst JC: *Color atlas of geriatric medicine,* ed 2, St Louis, 1991, Mosby.

Figure 4-9 From Emond RT, Welsby PD, and Rowland HA: *Colour atlas of infectious diseases,* ed 4, London, 2003, Mosby, Ltd.

Figure 4-10 From Callen JP, Greer KE, Paller AS, Swinyer LJ: *Color atlas of dermatology,* ed 2, Philadelphia, 2000, Saunders.

Figures 4-11, A, and 4-12, F From Murray PR, Rosenthal KS, Kobayashi GS, Pfaller MA: *Medical microbiology,* ed 3, St Louis, 1994, Mosby.

Figures 4-11, B and 4-12, B and D From Forbes BA, Sahm DF, Weissfeld AS: *Bailey & Scott's diagnostic microbiology,* ed 11, St Louis, 2002, Mosby.

Figure 4-13 From Atlas RM: *Principles of microbiology,* St Louis, 1995, Mosby.

Figure 4-15 From Cotran RS, Kumar V, Collins T: *Robbin's pathologic basis of disease,* ed 7, Philadelphia, 2004, Saunders.

Chapter 5

Figure 5-4 Courtesy Department of Dermatology, College of Medicine, Houston, TX.

Figure 5-5 From Sanders MJ: *Mosby's paramedic textbook,* ed 3, St Louis, 2005, Mosby.

Figure 5-6 From Herlihy B, Maebius NK: *The human body in health and illness,* ed 3, Philadelphia, 2007, Saunders.

Figure 5-8 From Moore KL, Persaud TVN: *The developing human: clinically oriented embryology,* ed 7, Philadelphia, 2003, Saunders.

Chapter 6

Figure 6-3 From Greer I, Cameron I, Kitchner H, Prentice A: *Mosby's color atlas and text of obstetrics and gynecology,* London, 2001, Mosby Ltd.

Figure 6-4, A and D From Herlihy B, Maebius NK: *The human body in health and illness,* ed 3, Philadelphia, 2007, Saunders.

Figure 6-6, B, C, and D From Kelley LL, Petersen CM: *Sectional anatomy for imaging professionals,* ed 2, St Louis, 2007, Mosby-Yearbook.

Figure 6-7 From Frank ED, Long BW, and Smith BJ: *Merrill's atlas of radiographic positioning and radiologic procedures,* vol 1, ed 11, St Louis, 2007, Mosby.

Figure 6-9, A From Thompson JM, Wilson SF: *Health assessment for nursing practice,* St Louis, 1996, Mosby; B from Jacob S: *Atlas of human anatomy,* Philadelphia, 2002, Churchill Livingstone.

Figure 6-12 From Lewis SM, Heitkemper MM, Dirksen SR, O'Brien PG, Bucher L: *Medical-surgical nursing: assessment and management of clinical problems,* ed 7, St Louis, 2007, Mosby.

Figure 6-14 From Barkauskas VH, Bauman LC, Darling-Fisher CS: *Health & physical assessment,* ed 3, St Louis, 2002, Mosby, Inc.

Figure 6-15 From Ignatavicius MS, Workman ML: *Medical-Surgical Nursing: critical thinking for collaboratorive care,* ed 5, Philadelphia, 2006, Saunders.

Figure 6-16 From Zitelli & Davis: *Atlas of pediatric physical diagnosis,* ed 4, Philadelphia, 2002, Mosby.

Chapter 7

Figures 7-6, 7-12, and 7-13 From Applegate EJ, Thomas P: *The anatomy and physiology learning system: textbook,* ed 2, Philadelphia, 2000, Saunders.

Figure 7-3 From Hart CA, Broadhead RL: *Color atlas of pediatric infectious diseases,* London, 1992, Mosby-Wolfe.

Figure 7-4 From *Dorland's illustrated medical dictionary,* ed 31, Philadelphia, 2007, Saunders.

Figure 7-5 From Dennis Kunkel Microscopy, Inc., 1994.

Figure 7-7, A, C, D, and E From Rodak BF: *Hematology, clinical principles and applications,* ed 3, Philadelphia, 2007, Saunders.

Figure 7-7, B From Carr JH, Rodak BF: *Clinical hematology atlas,* ed. 2, Philadelphia, 2004, Saunders.

Figure 7-8 From Conlon CP, Snydman DR: *Mosby's color atlas and text of infectious diseases,* 2000, Mosby Ltd.

Figure 7-9 From Kanski J, Nischal KK: *Ophthalmology: clinical signs and differential diagnosis,* 1999, Mosby International.

Figure 7-10 From Hayhoe FGJ, Flemans RJ: *Color atlas of hematological cytology,* ed 3, London, 1992, Mosby-Wolfe.

Figure 7-11, A and B From Male D, Brostoff J, Roth D, and Roitt I: *Immunology,* ed 7, 2006, Mosby.

Chapter 8

Figure 8-10 From Applegate EJ: *The anatomy and physiology learning system: textbook,* ed 2, Philadelphia, 2000, Saunders.

Figure 8-12 From Snopek AM: *Fundamentals of special radiographic procedures,* 5e, St Louis, 2006, Saunders.

Figure 8-13 From Frank ED, Long BW, Smith BJ: *Merrill's atlas of radiographic positioning and radiologic procedures,* vol 3, ed 11, St Louis, 2007, Mosby.

Figure 8-14 From Braunwald: *Heart disease: a textbook of cardiovascular medicine,* ed 6, Philadelphia, 2001, Saunders.

Figure 8-18 From Thibodeau GA and Patton KT: *Anatomy & physiology,* ed 6, St Louis, 2007, Mosby.

Figure 8-21, A From Lewis SM, Heitkemper MM, Dirksen SR, O'Brien PG, Bucher L: *Medical-surgical nursing: assessment and management of clinical problems,* ed 7, St Louis, 2007, Mosby.

Figure 8-22, A Courtesy Medtronic Physio-Control, Redmond, Washington.

Figure 8-27, A From Topol E: *Textbook of interventional cardiology,* 1990, Saunders.

Figure 8-29 From Drake R, Vogl W, Mitchell A: *Gray's anatomy for students,* 2005, Churchill-Livingstone.

Figure 8-30 From Seidel HM, Ball JW, Dains JE, Benedict GW: *Mosby's guide to physical examination,* ed 6, St Louis, 2006, Mosby.

Figure 8-31 From Behrman R, Kliegman R, Jenson HB: *Nelson's textbook of pediatrics,* ed 17, Philadelphia, 2004, Saunders.

Figure 8-32 From Stone DR, Gorbach SL: *Atlas of infectious diseases,* Philadelphia, 2000, Saunders.

Chapter 9

Figures 9-3 and 9-13 From Ignatavicius MS, Workman ML: *Medical-surgical nursing: critical thinking for collaborative care,* ed 5, Philadelphia, 2006, Saunders.

Figure 9-5 From Monahan FD, Neighbors M: *Medical-surgical nursing: foundations for clinical practice,* ed 2, Philadelphia, 1998, Saunders.

Figure 9-7 From Talbot LA, Myers-Marquardt M: *Pocket guide to critical care assessment,* ed 3, St Louis, 1997, Mosby.

Figure 9-8 From Wilson SF, Thompson JM: *Respiratory disorders,* St Louis, 1990, Mosby.

Figure 9-9 Courtesy of Ohmeda, Boulder, Colorado.

Figures 9-10 and 9-15, B From Seidel HM, Ball, JW, Dains JE, Benedict GW: *Mosby's guide to physical examination,* ed 6, St Louis, 2006, Mosby.

Figure 9-14 From Earis JE, Pearson MG: *Respiratory medicine,* London, 1995, Times Mirror International Publishers.

Figure 9-15, A From Lemmi FO, Lemmi CAE: *Physical assessment findings CD-ROM,* Philadelphia, 2000, Saunders.

Figure 9-16 From Wilson SF, Giddens JF: *Health assessment for nursing practice,* ed 2, St Louis, 2001, Mosby.

Figure 9-18 From Kumar V, Robbins SL, and Cotran RS: *Pathologic basis of disease,* ed 7, Philadelphia, 2005, Saunders.

Figure 9-23, A Courtesy Lifecare, Westminster, Colorado.

Figure 9-23, B Courtesy Spacelabs Medical, Redmond, Washington.

Figure 9-26 From Elkin MK, Perry AG, Potter PA: *Nursing interventions and clinical skills,* ed 4, St Louis, 2007, Mosby.

Figure 9-27 From Potter PA, Perry AG: *Fundamentals of nursing,* ed 7, St Louis, 2009, Mosby.

Chapter 10

Figure 10-10 From Carlson K, Eisenstat S: *Primary care of women,* 1995, Mosby.

Figure 10-12, C From Aspinall RJ, Taylor-Robinson SD: *Mosby's colour atlas and text of gastroenterology and liver disease,* London, 2002, Mosby, Ltd.

Figure 10-13 From Sapp JP, Eversole LR, Wysocki GW: *Contemporary oral and maxillofacial pathology,* ed 2, St Louis, 2004, Mosby.

Figure 10-14 From Lemmi FO, Lemmi CAE: *Physical assessment findings CD-ROM,* Philadelphia, 2000, Saunders.

Figure 10-15 From *Dorland's illustrated medical dictionary,* ed 31, Philadelphia, 2007, Saunders.

Figure 10-16 From Callen JP, Greer KE, Hood AF, et al: *Color atlas of dermatology,* Philadelphia, 1992, Saunders.

Figure 10-17 From Clark DA: *Atlas of neonatology,* 2000, Saunders.

Figure 10-20 From Damjanov I, Linder J: *Anderson's pathology,* ed 10, St Louis, 1996, Mosby.

Chapter 11

Figure 11-6, A From Zakus S: *Mosby's clinical skills for medical assistants,* 2001, Mosby.

Figure 11-6, B From Belchetz PE, Hammond P: *Mosby's color atlas and text of diabetes and endocrinology,* London, 2003, Mosby, Ltd.

Figure 11-7 From Brunzel NA: *Fundamentals of urine & body fluid analysis,* ed 2, St Louis, 2004, Saunders.

Figure 11-9 From Harkreader H, Hogan MA, Thobaben M: *Fundamentals of nursing,* ed 3, St Louis, 2007, Saunders.

Figure 11-10 From Bontrager KL, Lampignano J: *Textbook of radiographic positioning and related anatomy,* ed 6, St Louis, 2005, Mosby.

Figures 11-11 and 11-22, B From Lewis S, Heitkemper MM, Dirksen SR: *Medical-surgical nursing, assessment and management of clinical problems,* ed 6, St Louis, 2004, Mosby.

Figure 11-12 From Price S, Wilson L: *Pathophysiology: clinical concepts of disease processes,* ed 6, St Louis, 2003, Mosby.

Figure 11-15 Courtesy Department of Pathology, Duke University Medical Center, Durham, North Carolina.

Figure 11-16 From Kumar V, Abbas AK, Fauston N, Mitchell RN: *Robbins' basic pathology,* ed 8, Philadelphia, 2007, Saunders.

Figure 11-21, A and B From Zitelli BJ, Davis HW: *Atlas of pediatric physical diagnosis,* ed 5, St Louis, 2007, Mosby.

Figure 11-22, A From Ignatavicius MS, Workman ML: *Medical-surgical nursing: critical thinking for collaborative care,* ed 5, Philadelphia, 2006, Saunders.

Figure 11-24, A and B From Athanasoulis CA et al: *Interventional radiology,* Philadelphia, 1982, Saunders.

Figure 11-26 From Lewis S, Heitkemper MM, Dirksen SR, O'Brien PG, Bucher L: *Medical-surgical nursing, assessment and management of clinical problems,* ed 7, St Louis, 2007, Mosby.

Chapter 12

Figure 12-7 From Black JM, Hawks JH: *Medical-surgical nursing,* ed 7, 2005, Saunders.

Figure 12-8 From Greer I, Cameron I, Kitchner H, Prentice A: *Mosby's color atlas and text of obstetrics and gynecology,* 2001, Mosby Ltd.

Figure 12-10, A From Symonds EM, MacPherson MBA: *Color atlas of obstetrics and gynecology,* London, 1994, Mosby-Wolfe.

Figure 12-10, B Courtesy the Royal College of Obstetricians and Gynaecologists.

Figure 12-11 From Polaski AL, Tatro SE: *Luckmann's core principles and practice of medical-surgical nursing,* Philadelphia, 1996, Saunders.

Figure 12-17 From Ignatavicius MS, Workman ML: *Medical-surgical nursing: Critical thinking for collaborative care,* ed 5, Philadelphia, 2006, Saunders.

Figure 12-18 From Lewis S, Heitkemper MM, Dirksen, SR, O'Brien PG, Bucher L: *Medical-surgical nursing, assessment and management of clinical problems,* ed 7, St Louis, 2007, Mosby.

Figure 12-21, B Courtesy of Fisher Scientific Company.

Figure 12-23 Courtesy Dr. Ellen Wald, Children's Hospital of Pittsburgh.

Chapter 13

Figures 13-3 and 13-8 From Moore KL, Persaud TVN: *The developing human,* ed 8, Philadelphia, 2008, Saunders.

Figure 13-5, A From Curry RA, Tempkin BB: *Sonography: introduction to normal structure and function,* St Louis, 2004, Saunders.

Figure 13-6 From Bonewit-West K: *Clinical procedures for medical assistants,* ed 7, St Louis, 2008, Saunders.

Figure 13-9 From Seidel HM, Ball JW, Dains JE, Benedict GW: *Mosby's guide to physical examination,* ed 6, St Louis, 2006, Mosby.

Figure 13-11 From Zitelli BJ, Davis HW: *Atlas of pediatric physical diagnosis,* ed 5, St Louis, 2007, Mosby.

Figure 13-13 From Zakus S: *Mosby's clinical skills for medical assistants,* ed 4, St Louis, 2001, Mosby.

Figure 13-15, A From Morse S, Moreland A, Homes K, eds: *Atlas of sexually transmitted diseases and AIDS,* London, 1996, Mosby-Wolfe.

Figure 13-15, B From Forbes BA, Sahm DF, Weissfeld AS: *Bailey & Scott's diagnostic microbiology,* ed 10, St Louis, 1998, Mosby.

Figure 13-16 Courtesy Antoinette Hadd, MD, Indiana University School of Medicine, Indianapolis.

Figure 13-17 From Noble J, ed: *Textbook of primary care medicine,* ed 3, St Louis, 2001, Mosby.

Figures 13-18 and 13-19 Courtesy Glaxo SmithKline, Research Triangle Park, North Carolina.

Chapter 14

Figures 14-2, 14-7, 14-8, and 14-34 From Frank ED, Long BW, Smith BJ: *Merrill's atlas of radiographic positioning and radiologic procedures,* vol 1, ed 11, St Louis, 2007, Mosby.

Figure 14-11 From Thibodeau GA, Patton KT: *Anatomy & physiology,* ed 3, St Louis, 1996.

Figure 14-15, A From Barkauskas VH, Bauman LC, Darling-Fisher CS: *Health & physical assessment,* ed 3, St Louis, 2002, Mosby, Inc.

Figures 14-15, B and 14-25 From Seidel HM, Ball JW, Dains JE, Benedict GW: *Mosby's guide to physical examination,* ed 6, St Louis, 2006, Mosby.

Figure 14-16, A From Mourad LA: *Orthopedic disorders,* St Louis, 1991, Mosby.

Figure 14-16, B From Black JM, Hawks JH: *Medical-surgical nursing,* ed 7, St Louis, 2005, Saunders.

Figure 14-22 From Canale ST: *Operative orthopaedics,* ed 9, St Louis, 1998, Mosby.

Figure 14-23 From Ballinger PW, Frank ED: *Merrill's atlas of radiographic positions and radiologic procedures,* vol 1, ed 10, St Louis, 2003, Mosby.

Figure 14-24 From Kamal A, Brockelhurst JC: *Coloratlas of geriatric medicine,* ed 2, St Louis, 1991, Mosby.

Figure 14-26 From Walter JB: *An introduction to the principles of disease,* ed 2, Philadelphia, 1982, Saunders.

Figures 14-28, A and C, and 14-29, B from Zitelli BJ, Davis HW: *Atlas of pediatric physical diagnosis,* ed 5, St Louis, 2007, Mosby.

Figure 14-28, B from Zitelli BJ, Davis HW: *Atlas of pediatric physical diagnosis,* St Louis, 1997, Mosby.

Figure 14-29, A Courtesy Dr. Christine L. Williams, New York Medical College.

Figure 14-31 From Swartz MH: *Textbook of physical diagnosis: history and examination,* ed 2, Philadelphia, 1994, Saunders.

Figure 14-32 From Behrman R, Kliegman R, Jenson HB: *Nelson's textbook of pediatrics,* ed 17, Philadelphia, 2004, Saunders.

Figure 14-33 From Chapleau W: *Emergency first responder: making the difference,* St Louis, 2004, Mosby.

Figure 14-35 Courtesy Zimmer, Inc., Warsaw, Indiana.

Chapter 15

Figures 15-9, A and B From Thibodeau GA, Patton KT: *Anatomy & physiology,* ed 6, St Louis, 2007, Mosby.

Figure 15-10, C From Palay DA, Krachmer JH, editors: *Ophthalmology for the primary care physician,* ed 2, St Louis, 2005, Mosby.

Figure 15-11 From Lewis SM, Heitkemper MM, Dirksen SR, O'Brien PG, Bucher L: *Medical-surgical nursing: assessment and management of clinical problems,* ed 7, St Louis, 2007, Mosby.

Figure 15-12 From Chipps EM, Clanin NJ, Campbell VG: *Neurologic disorders,* St Louis, 1992, Mosby.

Figure 15-13 From Polaski AL, Tatro SE: *Luckmann's core principles and practice of medical-surgical nursing,* Philadelphia, 1996, Saunders.

Figure 15-18 From Zitelli BJ, Davis HW: *Atlas of pediatric physical diagnosis,* ed 3, St Louis, 1997, Mosby.

Figure 15-19 From Osborn AG: *Diagnostic neuroradiology,* St Louis, 1994, Mosby.

Figures 15-22, 15-24, B, and 15-25 From Ignatavicius DD, Workman ML: *Medical-surgical nursing: critical thinking for collaborative care*, ed 5, Philadelphia, 2006, Saunders.

Figure 15-23 From Monahan FD, Sands JK, Neighbors, M, Marek JF, Green CH: *Phipps' medical-surgical nursing: health and illness perspectives*, ed 8, St Louis, 2007, Mosby.

Figure 15-24, A Courtesy Department of Neurological Surgery, Vanderbilt University Medical Center, Nashville, Tennessee.

Figure 15-26 From Phipps WJ, Monahan FD, Sands JK, Marek JF, Neighbors M: *Medical-surgical nursing*, ed 6, St Louis, 2003, Mosby.

Chapter 16

Figure 16-4 From Monahan FD, Neighbors M: *Medical-surgical nursing: foundations for clinical practice*, ed 2, Philadelphia, 1998, Saunders.

Figures 16-5 and 16-8, A From Habif TP: *Clinical dermatology: a color atlas guide to diagnosis and therapy*, ed 3, St Louis, 1996, Mosby.

Figure 16-6 From Wilson SF, Giddens JF: *Health assessment for nursing practice*, ed 3, St Louis, 2005, Elsevier.

Figure 16-7 From Callen JP, Greer KE, Paller AS, Swinyer LJ: *Color atlas of dermatology*, ed 2, Philadelphia, 2000, Saunders.

Figures 16-8, B, and 16-13, A From Habif TP: *Clinical dermatology: a color atlas guide to diagnosis and therapy*, ed 4, St Louis, 2004, Elsevier.

Figures 16-10, 16-12, 16-13, C From Noble J, ed: *Textbook of primary care medicine*, St Louis, 1996, Mosby.

Figure 16-11 Courtesy Mary Braham, Abbott Northwestern Hospital.

Figures 16-13, B, and 16-18 From Ignatavicius DD, Workman ML: *Medical-surgical nursing: Critical thinking for collaborative care*, ed 5, Philadelphia, 2006, Saunders.

Figure 16-14 From Bork K, Brauninger W: *Skin diseases in clinical practice*, ed 2, 1999, Saunders.

Figure 16-15, A, B, and C From Habif TP: *Clinical dermatology: a color atlas guide to diagnosis and therapy*, ed 2, St Louis, 1985, Mosby.

Figure 16-16, A and B From Stoy WA: *Mosby's EMT-basic textbook*, St Louis, 1996, Mosby.

Figure 16-19, A and B From Auerbach PS: *Wilderness medicine: management of wilderness and environmental emergencies*, ed 5, 2007, Mosby/Elsevier.

Figure 16-20 From Ignatavicius MS, Workman ML, Mishler MA: *Medical-surgical nursing across the health care continuum*, ed 3, Philadelphia, 1999, Saunders.

Figure 16-21 From Conlon CP, Snydman DR: *Mosby's color atlas and text of infectious diseases*, 2000, Mosby Ltd.

Figure 16-22 From Harkreader H, Hogan MA, Thobaben M: *Fundamentals of nursing*, ed 3, St Louis, 2007, Saunders.

Figure 16-23, A From Fewkes JL, Cheney ML, Pollack SV: *Illustrated atlas of cutaneous surgery*, 1992, Gower.

Chapter 17

Figure 17-2 Modified from Thibodeau GA, Patton KT: *Anatomy & physiology*, ed 5, St Louis, 2003, Mosby.

Figure 17-3 Photomicrograph by Bodansky HJ: *Pocket picture guide to diabetes*, London, 1989, Gower Medical Publishing.

Figure 17-8 From Herlihy B: *The human body in health and illness*, ed 3, 2007, St. Louis, Saunders.

Figure 17-9, A From Thompson JM, Wilson SF: *Health assessment for nursing practice*, St Louis, 1996, Mosby.

Figure 17-9, B From Swartz MH: *Textbook of physical diagnosis*, ed 5, Philadelphia, 2006, Saunders.

Figure 17-10 From Svane G, Potchen EJ, Sierra A, Azavedo E: *Screening mammography, breast cancer diagnosis in asymptomatic women*, St Louis, 1993, Mosby.

Figure 17-11 From Ignatavicius MS, Workman ML: *Medical-surgical nursing: critical thinking for collaborative care*, ed 5, Philadelphia, 2006, Saunders.

Figure 17-12 From Zitelli BJ, Davis HW: *Atlas of pediatric physical diagnosis*, ed 5, St Louis, 2007, Mosby.

Figure 17-13 Courtesy Ewing Galloway.

Figure 17-14 From Mendeloff AI, Smith DE, eds: Acromegaly, diabetes, hypermetabolism, proteinuria and heart failure. *Clin Pathol Conf Am J Med* 20:133, 1956.

Figure 17-15 From Ignatavicius DD, Workman ML, Mishler MA: *Medical-surgical nursing across the health care continuum*, ed 3, Philadelphia, 1999, Saunders.

Figure 17-16, A From Hordinsky MK, Sawaya ME, Scher RK: *Atlas of hair and nails*, 2000, Churchill Livingstone.

Figure 17-16, B From Evans A et al: *Atlas of breast disease management*, Philadelphia, 1998, Saunders.

Figure 17-17 From Black JM, Hawks JH: *Medical-surgical nursing*, ed 7, 2005, Saunders.

Figure 17-18 From Monahan FD, Neighbors M: *Medical-surgical nursing: foundations for clinical practice*, ed 2, Philadelphia, 1998, Saunders.

Figure 17-19 From Beare PG, Myers JL: *Adult health nursing*, ed 3, 1998, Mosby.

Appendix II

Figure from Ignatavicius MS, Workman ML: *Medical-surgical nursing: critical thinking for collaborative care*, ed 5, Philadelphia, 2006, Saunders.

Index/Glossary

Note: Page numbers followed by the letter *f* refer to figures; those followed by the letter *t* refer to tables.

adrenalectomy (ə-dreˮnəl-ekˊtə-me) surgical removal of one or both adrenal glands. 585

adrenaline (ə-drenˊə-lin) epinephrine; a hormone produced by the adrenal glands. 492, 570

adrenergic (adˮren-urˊjik) sympathomimetic (activated by, characteristic of, or secreting epinephrine). 492

adrenocortical (ə-dreˮno-korˊtĭ-kəl) pertaining to or arising from the adrenal cortex. 582

adrenocorticotropic hormone (ə-dreˮno-korˮtĭ-ko-troˊpik) a hormone capable of stimulating the adrenal cortex. 570

adrenocorticotropin (ə-dreˮno-korˮtĭ-ko-troˊpin) adrenocorticotropic hormone (ACTH); the hormone secreted by the adenohypophysis that stimulates the adrenal cortex. 570

adrenomegaly (ə-dreˮno-megˊə-le) enlargement of one or both of the adrenal glands. 581

adrenopathy (adˮrən-opˊə-the) any disease of the adrenal glands. 581

aerobic (ār-oˊbik) having molecular oxygen present; growing, living, or occurring in the presence of molecular oxygen; requiring oxygen for respiration; designed to increase oxygen consumption by the body. 86

aerosol (ārˊo-sol) a suspension of fine particles in air or gas. 551

afebrile (a-febˊril) without fever. 130

afferent (afˊər-ənt) conducting or conveying toward a center. 485, 486f

agglutination (ə-glooˮtĭ-naˊshən) aggregation of suspended cells into clumps or masses; also the process of union in wound healing. 162, 162f

agoraphobia (agˮə-rə-foˊbe-ə) intense, irrational fear of open spaces, characterized by marked fear of being alone or of being in public places where escape would be difficult or help might be unavailable. 515

agranulocyte (a-granˊu-lo-sītˮ) nongranular leukocyte. 153

agranulocytosis (a-granˮu-lo-si-toˊsis) a condition involving greatly decreased numbers of granulocytes. 157, 157t

AIDS *see* acquired immunodeficiency syndrome.

albinism (alˊbĭ-niz-əm) congenital absence of pigment in the skin, hair, and eyes, caused by absence or defect of tyrosinase, an enzyme that catalyzes the oxidation of tyrosine, a precursor of melanin. 78, 79f, 537

albino (al-biˊno) a person affected with a congenital absence of normal pigmentation in the body caused by a defect in melanin precursors. 78, 537

albumin (al-buˊmin) a protein found in animal tissue and the major serum protein. 327

albuminuria (alˮbu-mĭ-nuˊre-ə) the presence of albumin in the urine. 328

algesia (al-jeˊze-ə) sensitivity to pain; hyperesthesia. 500

alimentary tract (alˊə-menˊtər-e trakt) the part of the digestive structures formed by the esophagus, stomach, and the intestines; digestive tract. 266, 270f

alimentation (alˮə-men-taˊshən) the act of giving or receiving nutriment. 267, 301

alkalemia (alˮkə-leˊme-ə) increased pH (abnormal increased alkaline condition) of the blood. 237

alkalosis (alˮkə-loˊsis) increased alkaline nature of body fluids caused by accumulation of base or loss of acid. 237

allergen (alˊər-jen) an antigenic substance capable of producing immediate-type hypersensitivity (allergy). 165

allergy (alˊər-je) a hypersensitive state acquired through exposure to a particular allergen. 165

allogeneic, allogenic (alˮo-jə-neˊik, alˮo-jenˊik) having cell types that are antigenically distinct; denoting individuals or tissues that are of the same species but antigenically distinct. 163

allograft (alˊo-graft) a graft of tissue between individuals of the same species but not of the same genotype. 163, 550

alopecia (alˮo-peˊshə) baldness; absence of hair from skin areas where it is normally present. 548, 549f

alveolar (al-veˊə-lər) pertaining to the alveoli. 230

alveolus (al-veˊə-ləs) a small, saclike dilatation. 230
  pulmonary a., one of a cluster of small outpocketings at the end of the bronchioles through which the exchange of carbon dioxide and oxygen takes place between alveolar air and capillary blood. 230

Alzheimer disease (awltzˊhi-mər dǐ-zēzˊ) a progressive degenerative disease of the brain of unknown cause and characterized by diffuse atrophy throughout the cerebral cortex with distinctive histopathologic changes; sometimes called primary degenerative dementia. 509, 510

ambulant, ambulatory (amˊbu-lənt, amˊbu-lə-torˮe) walking or able to walk; not confined to bed. 50

ambulation (amˮbu-laˊshən) the act of walking. 50

amenorrhea (ə-menˮo-reˊə) absence or abnormal stoppage of the menses. 370

amniocentesis (amˮne-o-sen-teˊsis) percutaneous transabdominal puncture of the amnion for the purpose of removing amniotic fluid. 57, 407, 408f

amniochorial, amniochorionic (amˮne-o-korˊe-əl, amˮne-o-korˮe-onˊik) relating to both amnion and chorion. 401

amnion (amˊne-on) the thin membrane that lines the chorion and contains the fetus and the amniotic fluid around it. 57, 400, 401f

amnionic (amˮne-onˊik) pertaining to or developing an amnion; amniotic. 400

amniorrhexis (amˮne-o-rekˊsis) rupture of the amnion. 405

amniotic (amˮne-otˊik) pertaining to or developing an amnion. 57, 400
  a. fluid, the liquid or albuminous fluid contained in the amnion. 57, 400, 401f

amniotomy (amˮne-otˊə-me) deliberate rupture of the fetal membranes to induce labor. 412

amputation (amˮpu-taˊshən) the removal of a limb or other appendage or outgrowth. 500

amylase (amˊə-lās) an enzyme that breaks down starch. 268

amylolysis (amˮə-lolˊə-sis) the breaking down of starch, or its conversion to sugar. 268

amyotrophic lateral sclerosis (ALS) (a-miˮo-troˊfik latˊər-əl sklə-roˊsis) a motor neuron disease marked by progressive muscular weakness and atrophy with spasticity and exaggerated reflexes, caused by degeneration of motor neurons of the spinal cord, medulla, and cortex; also called Lou Gehrig disease. 509

anaerobic (anˮə-roˊbik) thriving best without oxygen. 86

anal (aˊnəl) pertaining to the anus. 271
  a. canal, the terminal portion of the digestive tract. 271, 279f, 280

analgesic (anˮəl-jeˊzik) relieving pain; a medication that relieves pain. 56, 519

anaphylactic (anˮə-fə-lakˊtik) pertaining to anaphylaxis. 165

anaphylaxis (anˮə-fə-lakˊsis) a manifestation of immediate hypersensitivity in which exposure of a sensitized individual to a specific antigen or hapten results in urticaria, pruritus, and angioedema, followed by vascular collapse and shock and often accompanied by life-threatening respiratory distress; a general term originally applied to the situation in which exposure to a toxin resulted not in development of immunity (prophylaxis) but in hypersensitivity. 165

anaplasia (anˮə-plaˊzhə) a loss of differentiation of cells and of their orientation to one another and to their axial framework and blood vessels, a characteristic of tumor tissue. 131, 131t

anastomose (ə-nasˊtə-mōs) to create a connection between two formerly separate structures. 303, 303f

anastomosis (ə-nasˮtə-moˊsis) an opening created by surgical, traumatic, or pathologic means between two normally distinct organs or spaces; a communication between two vessels by collateral channels. 303
  gastrojejunal a., a surgical procedure in which the stomach is directly attached to the jejunum. 303

anatomic (anˮə-tomˊik) pertaining to anatomy or to the structure of the body. 118
  a. pathologist, a physician specializing in the study of the effects of disease on the structure of the body. 22
  a. pathology, the study of the effects of disease on the structure of the body.
  a. plane, points of reference by which imaginary dissecting lines are drawn through the body to describe locations. 22
  a. position, the position in which the body is erect, facing forward with the arms at the sides and the palms toward the front. 117, 118f

anatomy (ə-natˊə-me) the science of the structure of living organisms. 34, 117

androgen (anˊdro-jən) any substance that possesses masculinizing activities, such as the testicular hormone, testosterone. 568, 570t

androgenic (anˮdro-jenˊik) producing masculine characteristics. 568

andropathy (an-dropˊə-the) any disease peculiar to the male sex. 581

anemia (ə-neˊme-ə) a condition in which the blood is deficient in red blood cells, hemoglobin, or both. 155, 155t
  hemolytic a., any of a group of acute or chronic anemias characterized by shortened survival of mature erythrocytes and inability of bone marrow to compensate for the decreased life span. 160
  sickle cell a., a genetically caused defect of hemoglobin synthesis, occurring almost exclusively in black individuals, characterized by the presence of sickle-shaped erythrocytes in the blood and homozygosity for S hemoglobin. Signs and symptoms include arthralgia, acute abdominal pain, and leg ulcerations. 159

anesthesia (anˮes-theˊzhə) having no feeling or sensation. 56
  epidural a., regional anesthesia produced by injection into the epidural space. 519
  general a., a reversible state of unconsciousness produced by anesthetics. 56
  local a., anesthesia confined to one area of the body. 56

anesthesia—cont'd

nerve block a., a loss of sensation in a region of the body, produced by injecting a local anesthetic along the course of a nerve or nerves. 519

regional a., the production of insensibility of a part by interrupting sensory nerve conductivity from that region of the body. 56

anesthesiologist (an″əs-the″ze-ol′ə-jist) a physician who specializes in the administration of anesthetics during surgery. 22

anesthesiology (an″əs-the″ze-ol′ə-je) the branch of medicine that studies anesthesia and anesthetics. 22

anesthetic (an″əs-thet′ik) pertaining to or producing anesthesia; an agent that produces anesthesia. 22, 56

topical a., a local anesthetic applied directly to the area to be anesthetized. 551

anesthetist (ə-nes′thə-tist) a nurse or technician trained to administer anesthetics. 22

aneurysm (an′u-riz″əm) a sac formed by localized dilation of an artery or vein, or of the heart. 200, 201*f*, 498

aneurysmal (an″u-riz′məl) pertaining to or resembling an aneurysm. 200

aneurysmectomy (an″u-riz-mek′tə-me) surgical removal of the sac of an aneurysm. 517

angiectomy (an″je-ek′tə-me) removal or resection of a vessel. 206

angina pectoris (an-ji′nə, an′ji-nə pek′to-ris) severe pain and constriction about the heart caused by an insufficient supply of blood to the heart itself. 119, 196

angiocardiography (an″je-o-kahr″de-og′rə-fe) radiography of the heart and major vessels after injection of a radiopaque contrast medium into a blood vessel or one of the cardiac chambers. 193

angiocarditis (an″je-o-kahr-di′tis) inflammation of the heart and great blood vessels. 200

angiogram (an′je-o-gram″) a radiograph of blood vessels filled with a contrast medium. 193, 498*f*

angiography (an″je-og′rə-fe) radiographic visualization of vessels of the body. 193

digital subtraction a., radiographic visualization that provides computer-enhanced radiographic images of blood vessels filled with contrast material. 193

pulmonary a., the radiographic examination of the blood vessels of the lungs. 234

renal a., the process of producing a radiograph of the renal arteries. 333

angioma (an″je-o′mə) a tumor whose cells tend to form blood or lymph vessels. 70, 70*f*, 200

angioplasty (an′je-o-plas″te) surgical repair of the blood vessels. 61

balloon a., a method of dilating or opening an obstructed blood vessel by threading a small, balloon-tipped catheter into the vessel, inflating the balloon, and compressing arteriosclerotic lesions against the walls of the vessel. 205, 206*f*

excimer laser a., the opening of an occluded artery with laser energy delivered through a fiberoptic probe. 205

percutaneous transluminal coronary a., compression of fatty deposits of plaque in a coronary artery by an inflated balloon on the end of a catheter; balloon catheter dilation. 205

angiorrhaphy (an″je-or′ə-fe) suture of a vessel or vessels. 61

angiostenosis (an″je-o-stə-no′sis) narrowing of the caliber of a vessel. 200

angiostomy (an″je-os′tə-me) surgical formation of a new opening into a blood vessel. 206

angiotomy (an″je-ot′ə-me) incision or severing of a blood or lymph vessel. 206

anhydrous (an-hi′drəs) lacking water. 6, 104

anisocytosis (an-i″so-si-to′sis) a condition in which erythrocytes are not of equal size. 158, 159*f*

ankylosing spondylitis (ang″kə-lo′sing spon″də-li′tis) inflammation of the spine marked by stiffening of the spinal joints and ligaments, so that movement becomes increasingly painful and difficult. It is a form of rheumatoid arthritis that affects the spine, and affects the male sex almost exclusively. 465

ankylosis (ang″kə-lo′sis) immobility of a joint. 465

anomaly (ə-nom′ə-le) marked deviation from the normal standard, especially as a result of congenital defects. 463

anorchidism (an-or′kĭ-diz″əm) absence of testes. 385

anorchism (an-or′kiz-əm) congenital absence of the testis, either unilaterally or bilaterally. 385

anorexia (an″o-rek′se-ə) lack or loss of appetite for food. 286

a. nervosa, a mental disorder occurring predominantly in female individuals, having onset usually in adolescence, and characterized by refusal to maintain a normal minimal body weight; intense fear of becoming obese that is undiminished by weight loss; disturbance of body image resulting in a feeling of being fat even when extremely emaciated; and amenorrhea (in the female sex). 286

anorexiant (an″o-rek′se-ənt) causing anorexia or loss of appetite. 301

anosmia (an-oz′me-ə) absence of the sense of smell. 495

anotia (an-o′shə) congenital absence of one or both ears. 131, 506

anovulation (an″ov-u-la′shən) absence of ovulation. 371

anoxia (ə-nok′se-ə) a total lack of oxygen; often used interchangeably with *hypoxia* to mean a reduced supply of oxygen to the tissues. 196, 236

antacid (ant-as′id) 1. counteracting acidity; 2. a substance that counteracts or neutralizes acidity, usually of the stomach. 302

anteflexion (an-te-flek′shən) 1. forward curvature of an organ or part; 2. the forward curvature of the uterus. 373, 373*f*

antenatal (an″te-na′təl) occurring or formed before birth; prenatal. 406

antepartum (an″te-pahr′təm) in obstetrics, before the onset of labor, with reference to the mother. 406

anterior (an-tēr′e-ər) situated in front or in the forward part of an organism. 118, 120

anterolateral (an″tər-o-lat′ər-əl) situated anteriorly and to one side. 121

anteromedial (an″tər-o-me′de-əl) situated anteriorly and to the medial side. 120

anteroposterior (an″tər-o-pos-tēr′e-ər) from front to back of the body, such as the direction of a radiographic projection. 121, 121*f*

anterosuperior (an″tər-o-soo-pēr′e-ər) situated anteriorly and superiorly. 122

anteversion (an″te-vur′zhən) the forward tipping or tilting of an organ; displacement in which the uterus is tipped forward but is not bent at an angle. 373, 373*f*

anthracosis (an-thrə-ko′sis) a usually asymptomatic form of pneumoconiosis caused by deposition of coal dust in the lungs. 247

antianxiety (an″te-ang-zi′ə-te) reducing anxiety. 520

antiarrhythmic (an″te-ə-rith′mik) preventing or alleviating cardiac arrhythmia; an agent that prevents or alleviates arrhythmia. 207

antiarthritic (an″te-ahr-thrit′ik) an agent that alleviates arthritis; alleviating arthritis. 470

antiasthmatic (an″te-az-mat′ik) alleviating asthma; a drug that alleviates asthma. 254

antibiotic (an″te-, an″ti-bi-ot′ik) destructive of life; a chemical substance that inhibits the growth of or kills other microorganisms. 130, 551

a. sensitivity test, a laboratory method of determining the susceptibility of organisms to therapy with antibiotics. 329

antibody (an′ti-bod″e) an immunoglobulin that interacts only with the antigen that induced its synthesis or with an antigen closely related to it. 164, 165

anticancer (an″ti-kan′sər) against cancer; a drug used to treat cancer. 254

anticoagulant (an″te-, an″ti-ko-ag′u-lənt) preventing blood clotting; any substance that prevents blood clotting. 150

anticonvulsant (an″te-, an″ti-kən-vul′sənt) preventing or relieving convulsions; an agent that prevents or relieves convulsions. 519

antidepressant (an″te-, an″ti-de-pres′ənt) preventing or relieving depression; an agent that is used to treat the symptoms of depression. 520

antidiarrheal (an″te-, an″ti-di″ə-re′əl) counteracting diarrhea; an agent that is effective in combating diarrhea. 306

antidiuretic (an″te-, an″ti-di″u-ret′ik) suppressing the rate of urine formation; an agent that suppresses urine formation. 567

a. hormone, a hormone produced by the hypothalamus that decreases the amount of water lost in urination. 324, 567

antiemetic (an″te-ə-met′ik) preventing or alleviating nausea and vomiting; an agent that prevents or alleviates nausea and vomiting. 306

antifebrile (an″te-, an″ti-feb′ril) relieving or reducing fever; an agent that relieves or reduces fever. 130

antigen (an′ti-jən) any substance that is capable, under appropriate conditions, of inducing a specific immune response and of reacting with the products of that response. 164

prostate-specific a., a protein produced by the prostate that may be elevated in patients with cancer or other disease of the prostate. 383

antihistamine (an″te-, an″ti-his′tə-mēn) a drug that counteracts the action of histamine. 166, 255

antihypertensive (an″te-, an″ti-hi′pər-ten′siv) counteracting high blood pressure; an agent that reduces high blood pressure. 207

antiinfective (an″te-in-fek′tiv) capable of killing or preventing the multiplication of infectious agents; an agent that so acts. 130

antiinflammatory (an″te-in-flam′ə-tor″e) counteracting or suppressing inflammation; an agent that counteracts or suppresses the inflammatory process. 130

nonsteroidal a. drug, any of a group of drugs acting against fever, pain, and inflammation by inhibiting prostaglandin synthesis. 470

antilipidemic (an″ti-lip″ĭ-de′mik) promoting a reduction of lipid levels in the blood; an agent that reduces lipids in the blood. 207

antimicrobial (an″te-, an″ti-mi-kro′be-əl) killing microorganisms or suppressing their multiplication or growth; an agent that kills microorganisms or suppresses their multiplication or growth. 130, 550

antineoplastic (an″te-, an″ti-ne″o-plas′tik) inhibiting or preventing the development of neoplasms; checking the maturation and proliferation of malignant cells; an agent having such properties. 55, 167, 254

antinuclear antibody test (an″te-, an″ti-noo′kle-ər) a blood test used primarily to help diagnose systemic lupus erythematosus, although a positive result may also indicate other autoimmune diseases. 452, 453*t*

antiperspirant (an″te-, an″ti-pur′spər-ant) inhibiting or preventing perspiration; an agent that inhibits or prevents perspiration. 106

antipruritic (an″te-, an″ti-proo-rit′ik) relieving or preventing itching; an agent that relieves or prevents itching. 551

antipsychotic (an″te-, an″ti-si-kot′ik) drugs that are effective in the treatment of psychosis. 520

antipyretic (an″te-, an″ti-pi-ret′ik) relieving or reducing fever; an agent that relieves or reduces fever. 130, 519

antiseptic (an″tĭ-sep′tik) pertaining to asepsis; a substance that inhibits the growth and development of microorganisms without necessarily killing them. 86, 551

antispasmodic (an″te-, an″ti-spaz-mod′ik) relieving spasm, usually of smooth muscle; an agent that relieves muscle spasms. 349

antithyroid (an″te-thi′roid) counteracting the functioning of the thyroid. 585

antitussive (an″te-, an″ti-tus′iv) relieving or preventing cough; an agent that relieves or prevents cough. 255

anuria (an-u′re-ə) complete suppression of urinary secretion by the kidneys. 335

anuric (an-u′rik) pertaining to or characterized by lack of secretion of urine. 335

anus (a′nəs) the distal or terminal opening of the alimentary canal. 271, 279*f*, 280

aorta (a-or′tə) the main trunk from which the systemic arterial system proceeds. 185, 188*f*

abdominal a., continuation of the thoracic aorta. 187

arch of a., the continuation of the ascending aorta that gives rise to the descending aorta. 187, 188*f*, 189*f*

ascending a., the proximal portion of the aorta arising from the left ventricle, giving origin to the right and left coronary arteries before continuing as the arch of the aorta. 187, 188*f*, 189*f*

coarctation of the a., a localized malformation of the aorta that causes narrowing of the lumen of the vessel. 195

descending a., the continuation of the aorta from the arch of the aorta, in the thorax, to the point of its division into the common iliac arteries. 187, 189*f*

thoracic a., the proximal portion of the descending aorta. 187, 188*f*, 189*f*

aortic (a-or′tik) of or pertaining to the aorta. 187

a. insufficiency, aortic regurgitation. 200

a. regurgitation, blood flow from the aorta back into the left ventricle during diastole. 200

a. stenosis, a narrowing or stricture of the aortic valve. 200

aortitis (a″or-ti′tis) inflammation of the aorta. 8, 200

aortogram (a-or′to-gram) the radiographic record resulting from aortography. 193

aortography (a″or-tog′rə-fe) radiography of the aorta after the injection of an opaque medium. 193, 200

aortosclerosis (a-or″to-sklə-ro′sis) abnormal hardening of the aorta. 200

aphagia (ə-fa′jə) refusal or loss of the ability to swallow. 288

aphasia (ə-fa′zhə) defect or loss of the power of expression by speech, writing, or signs, or of comprehending spoken or written language, because of injury or disease of the brain. 241, 502

aphonia (a-fo′ne-ə) loss of voice. 241

apical (ap′ĭ-kəl) pertaining or located at the apex. 230

aplasia (ə-pla′zhə) lack of development of an organ or tissue. 131, 131*t*, 244

aplastic (a-plas′tik) pertaining to or characterized by aplasia. 160

apnea (ap′ne-ə) cessation of breathing. 236

sleep a., transient periods of cessation of breathing during sleep. 236, 499

appendectomy (ap″en-dek′tə-me) surgical removal of the vermiform appendix. 61, 305

appendicitis (ə-pen″dĭ-si′tis) inflammation of the vermiform appendix. 70, 294, 305

appendicular (ap″en-dik′u-lər) pertaining to the vermiform appendix; pertaining to an appendage. 279, 434

appendix (ə-pen′diks) a general term used to designate a supplementary, accessory, or dependent part attached to a main structure; also called appendage. It is frequently used alone to refer to the appendix vermiformis. 278*f*, 279

vermiform a., a wormlike appendage of the cecum. 279, 279*f*

approximate (ə-prok′sĭ-māt′) to bring close together. 59

arachnoid (ə-rak′noid) resembling a spider's web; the middle of the three meninges. 488

areola (ə-re′o-lə) a circular area of a different color, surrounding a central point. 571

arrhythmia (ə-rith′me-ə) any variation from the normal rhythm of the heartbeat. 195

arterial (ahr-tēr′e-əl) pertaining to an artery or to the arteries. 179

arteriogram (ahr-tēr′e-o-gram) a radiograph of an artery after injection of a radiopaque medium. 192, 192*f*

renal a., a radiographic record of the renal arteries. 333, 333*f*

arteriograph (ahr-tēr′e-o-graf) a film produced by arteriography. 192

arteriography (ahr-tēr-e-og′rə-fe) radiography of arteries after injection of radiopaque material into the bloodstream. 192

coronary a., radiography of the coronary arteries. 193

arteriole (ahr-tēr′e-ōl) a minute arterial branch, especially one just proximal to a capillary. 179, 180*f*

arteriopathy (ahr-tēr′e-op′ə-the) any arterial disease. 200

arteriosclerosis (ahr-tēr″e-o-sklə-ro′sis) a group of diseases characterized by thickening and loss of elasticity of arterial walls. 191, 199

arteriosclerotic (ahr-tēr″e-o-sklə-rot′ik) pertaining to or affected with arteriosclerosis. 199

a. heart disease, arteriosclerotic heart disease. 199

arteriovenous (ahr″tēr″e-o-ve′nəs) pertaining to or affecting an artery and vein; both arterial and venous. 180

arteritis (ahr″tə-ri′tis) inflammation of an artery. 200

artery (ahr′tə-re) a vessel through which the blood passes away from the heart to the various parts of the body. 179, 180*f*

coronary a., one of a pair of arteries that branch from the aorta, or their branches, which supply blood to the heart. 182, 183*f*

pulmonary a., either of the arteries supplying blood to the lungs. 181

renal a., one of two arteries that carries blood to the kidneys. 321, 321*f*

arthralgia (ahr-thral′jə) pain in a joint. 464

arthrectomy (ahr-threk′tə-me) the excision of a joint. 470

arthritis (ahr-thri′tis) inflammation of joints. 464

rheumatoid a., a chronic systemic disease primarily of the joints, marked by inflammatory changes in the synovial membranes and articular structures and by muscle atrophy and bone loss. In late stages, deformity and ankylosis develop. 464, 465*f*

arthrocentesis (ahr″thro-sen-te′sis) puncture and aspiration of a joint. 452, 470

arthrochondritis (ahr″thro-kon-dri′tis) inflammation of the cartilage of a joint. 457

arthroclasia (ahr″thro-kla′zhə) the surgical breaking down of an ankylosis to secure free movement. 470

arthrodesis (ahr″thro-de′sis) the surgical fixation of a joint. 470

arthrodynia (ahr″thro-din′e-ə) pain in a joint. 464

arthrogram (ahr′thro-gram) a radiographic record after introduction of opaque contrast material into a joint. 452

arthrography (ahr-throg′rə-fe) radiography of a joint after injection of opaque contrast material. 452

arthrolysis (ahr-throl′ə-sis) destruction of a joint; the operative loosening of adhesions in an ankylosed joint. 470

arthropathy (ahr-throp′ə-the) any joint disease. 464

arthroplasty (ahr′thro-plas″te) plastic surgery of a joint or joints. 470

arthrosclerosis (ahr″thro-sklə-ro′sis) hardening of the joints. 464

arthroscope (ahr′thro-skōp) an endoscope for examining the interior of a joint and for carrying out diagnostic and therapeutic procedures within the joint. 452

arthroscopy (ahr-thros′kə-pe) examination of the interior of a joint with an arthroscope. 452, 453*f*

arthrotomy (ahr-throt′ə-me) surgical incision of a joint. 470

articular (ahr-tik′u-lər) of or pertaining to a joint. 444

articulation (ahr-tik″u-la´shən) the place of union or junction between two or more bones of the skeleton; a joint; the enunciation of words and sentences. 444

asbestosis (as″bes-to´sis) a form of lung disease caused by inhaling fibers of asbestos. 248

ascites (ə-si´tēz) effusion and accumulation of serous fluid in the abdominal cavity. 128, 128f

aspermatogenesis (a-spur″mə-to-jen´ə-sis) absence of development of spermatozoa. 384

aspermia (ə-spur´me-ə) failure of formation or emission of semen. 384

asphyxia (as-fik´se-ə) pathologic changes caused by lack of oxygen in respired air. 237, 239

asphyxiation (as-fik″se-a´shən) the causing of or state of asphyxia; suffocation. 237

aspiration (as″pĭ-ra´shən) the removal of fluids or gases from a cavity by the application of suction; drawing in or out as by suction. 80

asthma (az´mə) a condition marked by recurrent attacks of paroxysmal dyspnea, with wheezing caused by spasmodic contraction of the bronchi. 245

astigmatism (ə-stig´mə-tiz-əm) unequal curvature of the refractive surfaces of the eye. 511, 512f

asymptomatic (a″simp-to-mat´ik) showing or causing no symptoms. 104

asystole (a-sis´to-le) cardiac arrest; absence of a heartbeat. 195

atelectasis (at″ə-lek´tə-sis) incomplete expansion of a lung or a portion of a lung; airlessness or collapse of a lung that had once been expanded. 248

atherectomy (ath″ər-ek´tə-me) the removal of atherosclerotic plaque from an artery. 205, 206f

atherosclerosis (ath″ər-o-sklə-ro´sis) a common form of arteriosclerosis in which deposits of yellowish plaques are formed within the arteries. 199, 199f

atraumatic (a″traw-mat´ik) not causing damage or injury. 104

atresia (ə-tre´zhə) congenital absence or closure of a normal body orifice or tubular organ. 291

atrial (a´tre-əl) pertaining to an atrium. 183
    a. fibrillation, a cardiac arrhythmia characterized by disorganized electrical activity in the atria. 196
    a. septal defect, a congenital heart defect in which there is an opening between the atria. 195

atriomegaly (a″tre-o-meg´ə-le) abnormal dilatation or enlargement of an atrium of the heart. 195

atriopeptin (a″tre-o-pep´tin) a hormone involved in the regulation of renal and cardiovascular homeostasis. 574

atrioseptoplasty (a″tre-o-sep´to-plas″te) plastic repair to correct an abnormal opening between the atria. 203

atrioventricular (a″tre-o-ven-trik´u-lər) pertaining to an atrium of the heart and to a ventricle. 183
    a. block, a disorder of cardiac impulse transmission that reflects prolonged, intermittent, or absent conduction of impulses between the atria and ventricles. 196
    a. node, specialized heart muscle fibers that receive impulses from the sinoatrial node and transmit them to the bundle of His. 186

atrium (a´tre-əm) a chamber; used in anatomy to designate a chamber affording entrance to another structure or organ. Usually used alone to designate an atrium of the heart. 183

atrophy (at´rə-fe) a wasting away; a diminution in the size of a cell, tissue, organ, or part. 456, 542, 543f

audible (aw´də-bəl) capable of being heard. 495

audiogram (aw´de-o-gram″) a record of the thresholds of hearing of an individual for various sound frequencies. 499

audiologist (aw″de-ol´ə-jist) a person skilled in audiology, including diagnostic testing and the rehabilitation of those whose impaired hearing cannot be improved by medical or surgical means. 495

audiology (aw″de-ol´ə-je) the science of hearing, particularly diagnostic testing and the study of impaired hearing that cannot be improved by medication or surgical therapy. 495

audiometer (aw″de-om´ə-tər) an electronic device that produces acoustic stimuli of known frequency and intensity for the measurement of hearing. 499

auditory (aw´dĭ-tor″e) pertaining to the sense of hearing. 229
    a. ossicle, one of the three small bones in the middle ear. 434, 435t
    a. tube, the narrow channel connecting the middle ear and the nasopharynx. Formerly called the eustachian tube. 229

auscultation (aws″kəl-ta´shən) the act of listening for sounds within the body, chiefly for ascertaining the condition of the lungs, heart, pleura, abdomen, and other organs, and for the detection of pregnancy. 50, 50f
    abdominal a., listening for abdominal sounds, especially those of the stomach and intestines. 283

autism (aw´tiz-əm) preoccupation with inner thoughts, daydreams, fantasies, delusions, and hallucinations; egocentric, subjective thinking lacking objectivity and connection with reality. 514

autograft (aw´to-graft) a graft of tissue derived from another site in or on the body of the organism receiving it. 550

autoimmune (aw″to-ĭ-mūn´) pertaining to autoimmunity, a condition characterized by a specific humoral or cell-mediated immune response against constituents of the body´s own tissues. 82
    a. disease, one of a large group of diseases characterized by altered function of the immune system. 164, 464

autologous (aw-tol´ə-gəs) related to self; originating within an organism itself. 163
    a. graft, the transfer of tissue from one site to another on the same body. 163
    a. transfusion, a procedure in which blood is removed from a donor and stored for a variable period before it is returned to the donor´s circulation. 163

autonomic (aw″tə-nom´ik) self-controlling; functionally independent. 492
    a. nervous system, the part of the nervous system related to involuntary body functions. 492

autopsy (aw´top-se) the postmortem examination of a body. 80

axilla (ak-sil´ə) the armpit. 534

axillary (ak´sĭ-lar″e) pertaining to the axilla. 49, 534
    a. nodes, lymph nodes located in the axilla. 72f, 209f, 210

axon (ak´son) the nerve process by which impulses travel away from the cell body of a neuron. 27f, 486, 486f

azoospermia (a-zo″ə-spur´me-ə) lack of live spermatozoa in the semen. 384

bacilli (bə-sil´i) rod-shaped bacteria. 84, 85f

bacteremia (bak″tər-e´me-ə) the presence of bacteria in the blood. 71, 154

bactericidal (bak-tēr″ĭ-si´dəl) capable of killing bacteria. 86

bacteriostatic (bak-tēr″e-o-stat´ik) inhibiting the growth or multiplication of bacteria; an agent that inhibits the growth or multiplication of bacteria. 86

bacterium (bak-tēr´e-əm) in general, any of the unicellular prokaryotic microorganisms that commonly multiply by cell division (fission) and the cell of which is typically contained within a cell wall. 84

balanitis (bal″ə-ni´tis) inflammation of the glans penis. 386

Bartholin gland (bahr´to-lin gland) one of two small mucous glands located one in each lateral wall of the vestibule of the vagina, near the vaginal opening. 360

basophil (ba´so-fil) a granular leukocyte that has cytoplasm that contains coarse bluish-black granules of variable size. 152, 152f, 153

benign (bə-nīn´) not malignant; not recurrent; favorable for recovery. 24

bicuspid (bi-kus´pid) having two cusps; a mitral valve; a premolar tooth. 185, 274
    b. valve, mitral valve. 184f, 185

bilateral (bi-lat´ər-əl) having two sides, or pertaining to both sides. 122
    b. nephromegaly, enlargement of both kidneys. 336

bile (bīl) a fluid secreted by the liver and poured into the small intestine. Important constituents are conjugated bile salts, cholesterol, phospholipid, bilirubin diglucuronide, and electrolytes. 268, 281

biliary (bil´e-ar-e) pertaining to bile, to bile ducts, or to the gallbladder. 282

biohazard (bi´o-haz″ərd) a potentially dangerous infectious agent such as may be found in a clinical microbiology laboratory or used in experimental studies on genetic recombination. 30

biology (bi-ol´ə-je) the science that deals with the phenomena of life and living organisms in general. 80

biopsy (bi´op-se) removal and examination, usually microscopic, of tissue from the living body. A biopsy is performed to establish a precise diagnosis. 80, 577
    aspiration b., removal of living tissue for microscopic examination by suction through a fine needle attached to a syringe. 577, 577f
    excisional b., removal of an abnormal mass for microscopic examination. 577, 577f
    incisional b., removal of tissue from an abnormal mass for microscopic examination. 577, 577f
    punch b., the removal of living tissue for microscopic examination by means of a punch. 536, 536f

bioterrorism (bi″o-ter´ər-izm) the use of pathogenic biological agents to cause terror in a population. 89

bladder (blad´ər) a membranous sac serving as a receptacle for a secretion, especially the urinary bladder, which serves as a reservoir for urine. 321, 321f
    neurogenic b., dysfunction of the urinary bladder caused by a lesion of the nervous system. 339

blepharal (blef´ə-ral) pertaining to the eyelid. 73

blepharedema (blef″ə-rĭ-de´mə) swelling of the eyelids. 45, 510

blepharitis (blef″ə-ri´tis) inflammation of the eyelids. 6, 510

blepharoplasty (blef″ə-ro-plas″te) plastic surgery of the eyelid. 60, 520

blepharospasm (blef″ə-ro-spaz″əm) spasm of the eyelid. 45

blocker (blok´ər) something that obstructs passage or activity. 207

> *beta b.,* a popular term for beta-adrenergic block agents often used to decrease blood pressure. 207

> *calcium channel b.,* a drug that inhibits the flow of calcium ions across the membranes of smooth muscle cells, used primarily in treating heart diseases marked by coronary artery spasms. 207

blood (blud) the fluid that circulates through the heart and blood vessels, carrying nutrients and oxygen to the body cells. 142, 145, 148

> *b. cells,* red and white corpuscles. 150, 151, 152*f*

> *b. pressure,* the pressure existing in the large arteries at the height of the pulse wave. 49, 190

> *b. urea nitrogen,* the amount of urea in the blood. 329*t*, 330

body system (bod´e sis´təm) several organs of the body that work together to accomplish a set of functions. 114, 116, 116*t*

bolus (bo´ləs) a rounded mass of food or a pharmaceutical preparation ready to swallow, or such a mass passing through the gastrointestinal tract. 269

bone (bōn) the rigid connective tissue constituting most of the skeleton of vertebrates. 430

> *b. densitometry,* determining blood mass by measuring radiation absorption by the skeleton. 451

> *b. marrow,* the soft material filling the cavities of bones. 430

botulism (boch´ə-liz-əm) a type of food poisoning caused by a neurotoxin produced by the growth of *Clostridium botulinum* in improperly canned or preserved foods. 86, 507

Bowman capsule (bo´mən kap´səl) part of the kidney that functions as a filter in the formation of urine. 324, 324*f*

bradycardia (brad″e-kahr´de-ə) slow heartbeat, as evidenced by slowing of the pulse rate to less than 60 beats per minute. 191

bradykinesia (brad″e-kĭ-ne´zhə) abnormal slowness of muscular movement. 509

bradyphasia (brad″ĭ-fa´zhə) slow speech. 106

bradypnea (brad″e-ne´ə) abnormal slowness of breathing. 239, 239*f*

brain (brān) that part of the central nervous system contained within the cranium, consisting of the cerebrum, cerebellum, pons, medulla oblongata, and midbrain. 488, 489*f*

> *b. stem,* the stemlike portion of the brain connecting the cerebral hemispheres with the spinal cord and constituting the pons, medulla oblongata, and mesencephalon. 490, 490*f*

breast (brest) the anterior aspect of the chest; mammary gland. 571, 571*f*

> *b. augmentation,* insertion of an implant behind the breast to increase its size. 61, 61*f*, 586

> *b. reduction,* surgical removal of excess breast and skin tissue. 586

bronchial (brong´ke-əl) pertaining to a bronchus. 230

> *b. examination,* the visual examination of the tracheobronchial tree using a bronchoscope. 233, 233*f*

bronchiectasis (brong″ke-ek´tə-sis) chronic dilatation of the bronchi. 44, 244

bronchiole (brong´ke-ōl) one of the fine divisions of the bronchial tree. 230

bronchiolectasis (brong″ke-o-lek´tə-sis) dilation of the bronchioles. 245

bronchiolitis (brong″ke-o-li´tis) inflammation of the bronchioles; bronchopneumonia. 245

bronchitis (brong-ki´tis) inflammation of the bronchi. 244

bronchoalveolar (brong″ko-al-ve´ə-lər) pertaining to a bronchus and alveoli. 230

bronchoconstriction (bron″ko-kən-strik´shən) the act or process of decreasing the caliber of a bronchus; bronchostenosis. 244

bronchodilator, (brong″ko-di´la-tər, -di-la´tər) stretching or expanding the air passages; an agent that causes dilation of the bronchi. 254

bronchogenic (brong-ko-jen´ik) originating in a bronchus. 244

bronchogram (brong´ko-gram) the record obtained by bronchography. 233

bronchography (brong-kog´rə-fe) radiography of the bronchial tree after injection of an opaque solution. 233

broncholithiasis (brong″ko-lĭ-thi´ə-sis) a condition in which calculi are present within the lumen of the tracheobronchial tree. 244

bronchopathy (brong-kop´ə-the) any disease of the bronchi. 244

bronchopneumonia (brong″ko-nŏŏ-mo´ne-ə) a name given to an inflammation of the lungs that usually begins in the terminal bronchioles. These become clogged with a mucopurulent exudate, forming consolidated patches in adjacent lobules. 245

bronchopulmonary (brong″ko-pool´mə-nar″e) pertaining to the lungs and their air passages; both bronchial and pulmonary. 244

bronchoscope (brong´ko-skōp) instrument for viewing the bronchi. 232

bronchoscopic (brong″ko-skop´ik) pertaining to either bronchoscopy or the bronchoscope. 233

bronchoscopy (brong-kos´kə-pe) examination of the bronchi through a bronchoscope. 233, 233*f*

bronchospasm (brong´ko-spaz″əm) spasmodic contraction of the smooth muscle of the bronchi, as occurs in asthma. 244

bronchus (brong´kəs) either of the two main branches of the trachea. 230

buccal (buk´ əl) pertaining to or directed toward the cheek. 273

> *b. cavity,* the vestibule of the mouth, specifically the area lying between the teeth and cheeks. 273

> *b. mucosa,* the mucous membrane lining the inside of the mouth. 290

bulbourethral glands (bul″bo-u-re´thrəl glands) Cowper´s glands; two small glands, one on each side of the prostate gland. They secrete a viscid fluid that forms part of the seminal fluid. 380

bulimia (bŏŏ-le´me-ə) an emotional disorder characterized by episodic binge eating, usually followed by purging behaviors. 286

bulla (bul´ə) a large vesicle, greater than 1 cm in circumference, containing fluid. 542

bunionectomy (bun″yən-ek´tə-me) excision of an abnormal prominence on the first metatarsal head. 470

burn (bərn) injury to tissues caused by contact with dry heat (fire), moist heat (steam or hot liquid), chemicals (corrosive substances), electricity (current or lightning), friction, or radiant and electromagnetic energy. 546, 546*f*

> *deep partial-thickness b.,* one in which damage extends through the epidermis into the dermis; second-degree burn. 546, 546*f*

> *full-thickness b.,* one in which the epidermis and dermis are destroyed and damage extends into the underlying tissue; third-degree burn. Burn is classified as fourth-degree burn if underlying bone and muscle are damaged. 546, 546*f*

> *superficial partial-thickness b.,* a burn in which damage is limited to the epidermis; first-degree burn. 546, 546*f*

burr hole (bər) a hole drilled in the skull. 517

bursa (bur´sə) a sac or saclike cavity filled with a viscid fluid and situated at places in the tissues at which friction would otherwise develop. 444, 445*f*

bursectomy (bər-sek´tə-me) excision of a bursa. 469

bursitis (bər-si´tis) inflammation of a bursa. 456

bypass (bi´pas) an auxiliary flow; a shunt. 203

> *coronary artery b.,* a section of saphenous vein or other material grafted between the aorta and a coronary artery distal to an obstructive lesion. 203, 204*f*

> *coronary artery b. graft,* use of a vessel from elsewhere in the patient´s body to provide an alternate route for the blood to circumvent an obstructed coronary artery. 203, 204*f*

cachexia (kə-kek´se-ə) general ill health and malnutrition. 579

> *pituitary c.,* generalized insufficiency of pituitary hormones. 579

calcaneal (kal-ka´ne-əl) pertaining to the calcaneum, or heel bone. 442

calcaneitis (kal-ka″ne-i´tis) inflammation of the heel bone. 457

calcaneodynia (kal-ka″ne-o-din´e-ə) pain in the heel. 457

calcaneofibular (kal-ka″ne-o-fib´u-lər) pertaining to the heel bone and the fibula. 443

calcaneoplantar (kal-ka″ne-o-plan´tər) pertaining to the heel bone and the sole. 443

calcaneotibial (kal-ka″ne-o-tib´e-əl) pertaining to the heel bone and the tibia. 443

calcaneus (kal-ka´ne-əs) the irregular quadrangular bone at the back of the tarsus. It is also called the heel bone or os calcis. 442, 442*f*

calcification (kal″sĭ-fĭ-ka´shən) process whereby tissue becomes hardened by a deposit of calcium salts. 431

calcipenia (kal″sĭ-pe´ne-ə) deficiency of calcium. 45, 460

calcitonin (kal″sĭ-to´nin) a hormone elaborated by the thyroid gland in response to hypercalcemia. 569

calciuria (kal″se-u´re-ə) calcium in the urine. 453

calculus (kal´ku-ləs) an abnormal concretion, occurring within the animal body, chiefly in hollow organs or their passages. 72

> *renal c.,* a stone occurring in the kidney. 340, 345*f*

callus (kal´əs) localized hyperplasia of the horny layer of the epidermis caused by pressure or friction. 458, 543

cancer (kan´sər) a neoplastic disease the natural course of which is fatal. Cancer cells, unlike benign tumor cells, exhibit the properties of invasion and metastasis and are highly anaplastic. Cancer includes the two broad categories of carcinoma and sarcoma, but in normal usage it is often used synonymously with carcinoma. 24, 24*t*, 89

candidiasis (kan″dĭ-di´ə-sis) infection with a fungus of the genus *Candida*, especially *Candida albicans*. It is usually a superficial infection of the moist cutaneous areas of the body. 288, 418*t*, 420

cannula (kan´u-lə) a tube for insertion into a duct or cavity. 47
  nasal c., a device for delivering oxygen by way of two small tubes inserted into the nares. 250, 251*f*

capillary (kap´ĭ-lar″e) one of the minute vessels connecting the arterioles and venules. Walls of capillaries act as a semipermeable membrane for exchange of various substances between the blood and tissue fluid. In a less common meaning, capillary also means pertaining to or resembling a hair (Latin: *capillaris*, hairlike). 179, 180*f*, 187*f*

carcinogen (kahr-sin´ə-jen) any substance that produces cancer. 76

carcinogenesis (kahr″sĭ-no-jen´ə-sis) the origin of cancer. 76, 76*t*

carcinoma (kahr″sĭ-no´mə) a malignant tumor; cancerous tumor. 24
  basal cell c., an epidermoid carcinoma common on the face in the elderly and having a low degree of malignancy. 544, 544*f*
  lymphatic c., malignancy of the lymphatic system, generally spread to the lymphatics by lymph from another part of the body. 213
  squamous cell c., carcinoma developed from squamous epithelium. 543, 544, 544*f*

cardiac (kahr´de-ak) pertaining to the heart. 21
  c. arrest, ceasing of heart activity. 21, 195
  c. arrhythmia, irregular heart action or irregular pulse. 195
  c. insufficiency, the inability of the heart to pump efficiently. 196
  c. muscle, special striated muscle of the myocardium. 182
  c. pacemaker, an electrical device that can substitute for a defective sino-atrial node and control the beating of the heart by a series of electrical discharges. 202, 203*f*
  c. region, the portion of the stomach that is immediately adjacent to and surrounding the esophageal orifice. 276
  c. tamponade, compression of the heart produced by the accumulation of fluid in the pericardial sac. 198

cardiologist (kahr″de-ol´ə-jist) a physician who is specially trained in the prevention, diagnosis, and treatment of heart disease. 21

cardiology (kahr″de-ol´ə-je) the study of the heart and its functions. 21

cardiomegaly (kahr″de-o-meg´ə-le) enlargement of the heart. 45, 196

cardiomyopathy (kahr″de-o-mi-op´ə-the) a general diagnostic term designating primary disease of the heart muscle itself. 197

cardioplegia (kahr″de-o-ple´jə) arrest of myocardial contraction, as may be induced in performance of surgery on the heart. 203

cardioplegic (kahr″de-o-plej´ik) pertaining to arrest of myocardial contraction. 203
  c. solutions, drugs that are used to stop myocardial contractions so that surgery can be performed on the heart. 203

cardiopulmonary (kahr″de-o-pool´mə-nar-e) pertaining to the heart and lungs. 202
  c. bypass, a procedure used in heart surgery in which the blood is diverted from the heart and lungs by means of a pump oxygenator and returned directly to the aorta. 203, 204*f*
  c. resuscitation, the reestablishing of heart and lung action as indicated for cardiac arrest or apparent sudden death. 202

cardiovalvulitis (kahr″de-o-val″vu-li´tis) inflammation of the valves of the heart. 197

cardiovascular (kahr″de-o-vas´ku-lər) pertaining to the heart and blood vessels. 145, 179

cardioversion (kahr´de-o-vur″zhən) the restoration of normal heart rhythm by electrical shock. 203

cardioverter (kahr´de-o-vur″tər) a device that delivers a direct-current shock to restore normal heart rhythm. 203, 204*f*

caries (kar´ēz, kar´e-ēz) decay or death of bone or teeth. 289

carpal (kahr´pəl) pertaining to the carpus, or wrist. 8, 439, 440
  c. tunnel syndrome, a complex of symptoms resulting from compression of the median nerve in the carpal tunnel. 456

carpals (kahr´pəls) the bones of the wrist. 439, 440, 441*f*

carpectomy (kahr-pek´tə-me) surgical removal of the wrist bones. 469

carpopedal (kahr″po-ped´əl) pertaining to the wrist and foot. 443

carpophalangeal (kahr″po-fə-lan´je-əl) pertaining to the wrist and bones of the fingers. 440

carpoptosis (kahr″pop-to´sis) wristdrop. 505

carpus (kahr´pəs) the wrist; the joint between the arm and the hand. 8, 440, 441*f*

cartilage (kahr´tĭ-ləj) fibrous connective tissue present in adults and forming most of the temporary skeleton in the embryo. 430, 444
  articular c., a thin layer of cartilage on the articular surface of bones in synovial joints. 430, 431*f*, 444

cast (kast) a solid reproduction of an enclosed space such as a hollow organ; a rigid dressing, molded to the body while pliable, and hardening as it dries, to give firm support. 468

cataract (kat´ə-rakt) an opacity of the eye, or in the lens or capsule, that impairs vision or causes blindness. 511

catheter (kath´ə-tər) a flexible tube passed through body channels for withdrawal from or introduction of fluids into a body cavity. 47, 329
  Foley c., an indwelling catheter that has a balloon filled with air or liquid to train it in place in the bladder. 330, 330*f*
  indwelling c., a urethral catheter that is held in position in the urethra. 330

catheterization (kath″ə-tur-ĭ-za´shən) passage of a tubular, flexible instrument into a body channel or cavity for withdrawal or introduction of fluids into a body cavity. 47, 330
  cardiac c., passage of a long catheter through a vein in an arm, a leg, or the neck into the chambers of the heart. 193, 193*f*
  ureteral c., insertion of a catheter into the ureter. 331, 331*f*
  urethral c., insertion of a catheter through the urethra into the urinary bladder. 331, 331*f*, 332
  urinary c., passage of a catheter through the urethra into the bladder. 330

catheterize (kath´ə-ter-īz) to introduce a catheter within a body cavity. 47

catheterized urine specimen (kath´ə-ter-īzd) a sample of urine obtained from the bladder by catheterization. 329

caudad, caudal (kaw´dad, kaw´dəl) pertaining to a tail or tail-like appendage; denoting a position more toward the tail. 122

cauterization (kaw″tər-ĭ-za´shən) destruction of tissue with a hot or cold instrument, electric current, caustic substance, or other agent. 378

cauterize (kaw´tər-īz) to perform cauterization. 378

cecoileostomy (se″ko-il″e-os´tə-me) formation of a new opening between the cecum and the ileum. 305

cecum (se´kəm) the first part of the large intestine, extending from the ileum to the colon. 279, 279*f*

cellular (sel´u-lər) pertaining to or made up of cells. 142

cellulitis (sel″u-li´tis) an acute, spreading, edematous, suppurative inflammation of the deep subcutaneous tissue and sometimes muscle, which may be associated with abscess formation. 459, 548

Celsius (sel´se-əs) a temperature scale in which 0° is the freezing point of water and 100° is the boiling point of water at sea level. 98, 99*f*

centigrade (sen´tĭ-grād) consisting of or having steps or degrees. 98, 99*f*

centimeter (sen´tĭ-me″tər) a unit of length equal to one hundredth of a meter. 99

central nervous system (sen´trəl nur´vəs sis´təm) the control center of the body, composed of the brain and the spinal cord. 485, 486*f*, 488

cephalad (sef´ə-lad) referring to the head; toward the head. 122

cephalgia (sə-fal´jə) headache. 501

cephalic (sə-fal´ik) pertaining to the head or the head end of the body. 80, 123

cephalometer (sef″ə-lom´ə-tər) an instrument for measuring the head, or also for positioning the head in radiography. 5, 76

cephalometry (sef″ə-lom´ə-tre) measurement of the dimensions of the head. 23*f*, 76

cephalopelvic (sef″ə-lo-pel´vik) pertaining to the relationship of the fetal head to the maternal pelvis. 407
  c. disproportion, an unusually large fetal head in proportion to the maternal pelvis. 407

cerebellar (ser″ə-bel´ər) pertaining to the cerebellum, the part of the brain concerned with coordination of movements. 491

cerebellitis (ser″ə-bel-i´tis) inflammation of the cerebellum. 507

cerebellum (ser″ə-bel´əm) a large, dorsally projecting part of the hindbrain that is concerned with the coordination of movements. It consists of a median lobe and two lateral lobes. 490, 490*f*

cerebral (sə-re´brəl, ser´ə-brəl) pertaining to the cerebrum. 73, 489
  c. aneurysm, a thin sac filled with blood, formed by dilatation of the walls of an artery in the brain. 498*f*, 503
  c. angiography, radiography of the cerebral blood vessels. 498, 498*f*
  c. concussion, loss of consciousness as a result of a blow to the head. 502
  c. cortex, the convoluted layer of gray matter covering each cerebral hemisphere. 489, 489*f*
  c. embolus, a mass of undissolved matter present in a blood vessel in the brain and brought from another place, where it originated. 504
  c. hemisphere, either half of the cerebrum. 489
  c. hemorrhage, the rupture of a blood vessel, usually an artery, within the brain. 503

colon—cont'd

descending c., the portion of the colon on the left side of the abdomen that extends from the transverse colon to the sigmoid colon. 279, 279f

sigmoid c., the S-shaped part of the colon. 279, 279f

transverse c., the part of the colon that runs transversely across the upper part of the abdomen. 279, 279f

colonoscope (ko-lon´o-skōp) a flexible endoscope that permits visual examination of the colon; coloscope. 60, 285

colonoscopy (ko˝lən-os´kə-pe) examination by means of the colonoscope. 60, 285, 285f

colopexy (ko´lo-pek˝se) surgical fixation or suspension of the colon. 60

colorectal (ko˝lo-rek´təl) pertaining to or affecting the colon and rectum. 280

colorrhaphy (ko-lor´ə-fe) suture of the colon. 60

coloscope (kol´o-skōp) colonoscope. 60

coloscopy (ko-los´ko-pe) examination of the colon by means of an elongated flexible endoscope; same as colonoscopy. 60, 285

colostomy (kə-los´tə-me) surgical formation of a new opening from the large intestine to the surface of the body. 304, 305f

colostrum (kə-los´trəm) the thin, milky fluid secreted by the mammary gland the first few days before or after birth. 571

colpectomy (kol-pek´tə-me) excision of the vagina. 376

colpitis (kol-pi´tis) inflammation of the vagina; vaginitis. 370

colpocystitis (kol˝po-sis-ti´tis) inflammation of the vagina and of the bladder. 362

colpodynia (kol˝po-din´e-ə) vaginal pain. 374

colpohysterectomy (kol˝po-his˝tər-ek´tə-me) surgical removal of the uterus by way of the vagina. 377

colpoplasty (kol´po-plas˝te) plastic surgery of the vagina. 376

colporrhagia (kol˝po-ra´jə) vaginal hemorrhage. 374

colporrhaphy (kol-por´ə-fe) suture of the vagina. 376

colposcope (kol´po-skōp) an instrument for examining the vagina and cervix. 368, 368f

colposcopy (kol-pos´ko-pe) examination of the vagina and cervix using a colposcope. 368, 368f

coma (ko´mə) a profound unconsciousness from which the patient cannot be aroused. 502

complement (kom´plə-mənt) proteins in the blood that play a vital role in the body's immune defenses. 164, 165f

compulsion (kom-pul´shən) a persistent and irresistible impulse; a compulsive act or ritual. 515

computed tomography (kom-pu´tid to-mog´rə-fe) a special noninvasive roentgenographic technique that involves reconstruction of the body in cross-section from x-ray transmission measurements through the patient. Also called computerized axial tomography or computed axial tomography, CT, CAT. 52, 52f, 192

conception (kən-sep´shən) the onset of pregnancy, marked by implantation of the blastocyst in the endometrium. 400

concussion (kən-kush´ən) an injury resulting from impact with an object; loss of function associated with a blow or fall. 502, 508

cerebral c., loss of consciousness caused by a blow to the head. 502

condom (kon´dəm) a cover for the penis, worn during coitus to prevent impregnation or infection. 413, 413t

condyloma acuminatum (kon˝də-lo´mə ə-ku˝mĭ-nāt´um) a papilloma usually occurring on the mucous membrane or skin of the external genitals or in the perianal region, caused by an infectious virus; venereal wart. 418t, 419

congenital (kən-jen´ĭ-təl) present at or existing from the time of birth. 78, 116

c. heart disease, any structural or functional abnormality or defect of the heart or great vessels present at birth. 195

congestive (kən-jes´tiv) pertaining to or associated with abnormal accumulation of blood or fluid in a part. 197

c. heart failure, a condition characterized by weakness, breathlessness, and edema in lower portions of the body resulting from venous stasis and reduced outflow of blood. 197, 247

conjunctiva (kən-jənk´tĭ-və, kən-jənk-ti´və) the thin membrane lining the eyelids and covering the exposed whites of the eyes. 493

conjunctivitis (kən-junk˝tĭ-vi´tis) inflammation of the conjunctiva, the membrane that lines the eyelids and covers the exposed surface of the sclera. 510

contagious (kən-ta´jəs) capable of being transmitted from one individual to another. 82

contraception (kon˝trə-sep´shən) prevention of conception or impregnation. 412

contraceptive (kon˝trə-sep´tiv) anything used to diminish likelihood of or to prevent impregnation. 106, 375, 412

oral c., a hormonal compound taken orally that blocks ovulation. 412

contraindication (kon˝trə-in˝dĭ-ka´shən) any condition that renders some particular line of treatment improper or undesirable. 519

contralateral (kon˝trə-lat´ər-əl) associated with a particular part on an opposite side. 102

contusion (kən-too´zhən) a bruise; an injury of a part without a break in the skin. 545, 545f, 546

convulsion (kən-vul´shən) a violent involuntary contraction or series of contractions of the involuntary muscles; seizure. 508

copulation (kop˝u-la´shən) sexual union between male and female; coitus. 380

corium (kor´e-əm) alternative for dermis. 533

corn (korn) a hardening and thickening of the skin of the toes, caused by pressure. 458, 543

cornea (kor´ne-ə) the transparent structure forming the anterior part of the fibrous tunic of the eye. 494, 494f

coronary (kor´ə-nar˝e) encircling in the manner of a crown. This term is applied to vessels and ligaments, but especially to the heart's arteries. 182

c. arteriography, radiographic examination of the coronary arteries. 193

c. artery bypass, open heart surgery in which a prosthesis or a section of a blood vessel is grafted onto one of the coronary arteries. 203, 204f

c. artery bypass graft, a section of vein or other conduit grafted between the aorta and a coronary artery distal to an obstruction. 203, 204f

c. artery disease (CAD), myocardial damage caused by insufficient blood supply; also called coronary heart disease (CHD). 199

c. occlusion, complete obstruction of an artery of the heart, usually from progressive atherosclerosis. 199

c. thrombosis, development of an obstructive thrombus in a coronary artery. 199

coronavirus (kə-ro´nə-vi˝rəs) any virus belonging to the family Coronaviridae, which causes respiratory disease and possibly gastroenteritis in humans. 242

corpus luteum (kor´pəs loo´te-um) a yellow mass in the ovary formed by an ovarian follicle that has matured and discharged its ovum. 364

corpuscle (kor´pəs-əl) any small mass or body. 150

cortex (kor´teks) the outer layer of an organ. 570

adrenal c., the outer portion of the adrenal, which makes up the bulk of the gland. 570, 570t

cerebral c., the convoluted layer of gray matter covering each cerebral hemisphere. 489, 489f

cortisone (kor´tĭ-sōn) a natural glucocorticoid secreted by the adrenal cortex. 570

coryza (ko-ri´zə) an acute condition of the nasal mucous membrane, with a profuse discharge from the nostrils. 240

costa (kos´tə) rib. 438

costal (kos´təl) pertaining to the ribs. 438

costectomy (kos-tek´tə-me) removal of a rib. 469

costoclavicular (kos˝to-klə-vik´u-lər) pertaining to the ribs and collarbone. 440

costovertebral (kos˝to-vur´tə-brəl) pertaining to the ribs and vertebrae. 438

COX-2 inhibitors (koks) a group of nonsteroidal antiinflammatory drugs (NSAIDs) that have fewer gastrointestinal side effects than other NSAIDs. 470

crackle (krak´əl) an abnormal nonmusical sound heard on auscultation, primarily during inhalation. 235, 235f

cranial (kra´ne-əl) pertaining to the cranium or skull. 127, 434

c. cavity, the space within the skull that contains the brain. 126

craniectomy (kra˝ne-ek´tə-me) excision of a segment of the skull. 469, 517, 517t

craniocele (kra´ne-o-sēl˝) protrusion of the brain through a defect in the skull. 462

craniocerebral (kra˝ne-o-ser´ə-brəl) pertaining to the cranium and the cerebrum. 489

cranioplasty (kra´ne-o-plas˝te) plastic surgery of the skull. 469, 517, 517t

craniotome (kra´ne-o-tōm˝) an instrument used in craniotomy. 469

craniotomy (kra˝ne-ot´ə-me) cutting into the skull. 469, 517, 517t

cranium (kra´ne-əm) the skull; the skeleton of the head. 434, 435f

creatine kinase test (kre´ə-tin ki´nās) a blood test used to detect damage to the cardiac muscle. Also called creatine phosphokinase. 191

creatinine (kre-at´ĭ-nin) a substance formed from the metabolism of creatine. 327, 329

c. clearance, the rate at which creatinine is cleared from the blood by the kidneys. 330, 331

cretinism (kre´tin-iz-əm) a condition caused by congenital lack of thyroid secretion, marked by arrested physical and mental development. 580, 580*f*

croup (kro͞op) a condition resulting from acute obstruction of the upper airway caused by allergy, foreign body, infection, or new growth, occurring chiefly in infants and children, and characterized by resonant barking cough and hoarseness. 242

crust (krust) an outer layer of solid matter formed by the drying of a secretion. 542

cryosurgery (kri″o-sur´jər-e) destruction of tissue by application of extreme cold. 378

cryotherapy (kri″o-ther´ə-pe) treatment of tissue using cold temperatures. 55, 378, 420

cryptorchidism (krip-tor´kĭ-diz″əm) a developmental defect in which the testes remain in the abdominal cavity; undescended testes. 385, 385*f*

curet (ku-ret´) a spoon-shaped instrument for removing material from a surface. 378, 536, 536*f*

curettage (ku″rə-tahzh´) scraping of a cavity for removal of a growth or other material; curettement. 536, 536*f*

    dilation and c., surgical scraping of the uterus with a curette to remove contents of uterus after incomplete abortion, to obtain specimens for diagnosis, or to remove polyps. 378

Cushing syndrome (koosh´ing sin´drōm) a group of signs and symptoms associated with hypersecretion of the glucocorticoids by the adrenal cortex. 581

cuspid (kus´pid) having one point; a canine tooth. 274

    c. valve, a flap of tissue that controls the blood flow between an atrium and ventricle of the heart. 185

cutaneous (ku-ta´ne-əs) pertaining to the skin. 4, 533

cyanosis (si″ə-no´sis) blueness of the skin and mucous membranes. 78, 79*f*, 195, 537

cyst (sist) any sac that contains a fluid, either normal or abnormal, and is lined by epithelium. 541, 541*f*

cystectomy (sis-tek´tə-me) excision of a cyst; excision or resection of the urinary bladder. 344

cystic (sis´tik) pertaining to a cyst; pertaining to the urinary bladder or to the gallbladder. 322

    c. fibrosis, an inherited disease of exocrine glands that affects the pancreas, the respiratory system, and the sweat glands. 248, 537

cystitis (sis-ti´tis) inflammation of the bladder. 338

cystocele (sis´to-sēl) herniation of the urinary bladder into the vagina. 340, 341*f*, 374, 374*f*

cystography (sis-tog´rə-fe) roentgenography of the bladder after injection of the organ with an opaque solution. 333

cystolith (sis´to-lith) a calculus within the bladder. 340

cystolithotomy (sis″to-lĭ-thot´ə-me) the removal of a calculus by incision of the bladder. 347

cystometer (sis-tom´ə-ter) an instrument for measuring the neuromuscular mechanism of the bladder. 332

cystometrography (sis″to-mə-trog´rə-fe) the graphic recording of the pressure exerted at varying degrees of filling of the urinary bladder. 332

cystoplasty (sis´to-plas″te) plastic surgery of the bladder. 347

cystoscope (sis´to-skōp″) an instrument used for visual examination of the bladder. 334, 334*f*

cystoscopy (sis-tos´kə-pe) visual examination of the urinary tract with an instrument inserted through the urethra. 334, 334*f*

cystostomy (sis-tos´tə-me) formation of an opening into the urinary bladder. 348

cystotomy (sis-tot´ə-me) incision of the bladder. 348

cystourethritis (sis″to-u″re-thri´tis) inflammation of the bladder and urethra. 338

cystourethrography (sis″to-u″rə-throg´rə-fe) x-ray examination of the urinary bladder and the urethra. 333

cytology (si-tol´ə-je) study of cells. 366

cytotoxic (si´to-tok″sik) pertaining to or exhibiting a deleterious effect on cells. 80

cytotoxicity (si″to-tok-sis´ĭ-te) having a deleterious effect on cells. 167

cytotoxin (si´to-tok″sin) a toxin or antibody that has specific toxic action on cells of special organs. 167

dacryocyst (dak´re-o-sist″) the lacrimal sac; tear sac. 495

dacryocystitis (dak″re-o-sis-ti´tis) inflammation of the lacrimal sac. 511, 520

dacryocystorhinostomy (dak″re-o-sis″to-ri-nos´tə-me) surgical creation of a communication between the nasal cavity and the lacrimal sac. 520

dacryocystotomy (dak″re-o-sis-tot´ə-me) incision of the lacrimal sac. 520

dacryolith (dak´re-o-lith) a stone in the lacrimal sac or duct. 511

dacryolithiasis (dak″re-o-lĭ-thi´ə-sis) formation of tear stones. 511

dacryosinusitis (dak″re-o-si″nəs-i´tis) inflammation of the lacrimal duct and the ethmoidal sinus. 511

dactylitis (dak″tə-li´tis) inflammation of a finger or toe. 129

dactylogram (dak-til´o-gram) a fingerprint taken for purposes of identification. 129

dactylography (dak″tə-log´rə-fe) the study of fingerprints. 129

dactylospasm (dak´tə-lo-spaz″əm) cramping or twitching of the fingers or toes. 129

débride (da-brēd´) to remove foreign material and contaminated or devitalized tissue by sharp dissection. 551

débridement (da-brēd-maw´) the removal of foreign material and necrotized or contaminated tissue from or adjacent to an infected or traumatic lesion until surrounding healthy tissue is exposed. 551

decalcification (de-kal″sĭ-fĭ-ka´shən) the loss of calcium from bone. 461

decongestant (de″kən-jes´tənt) tending to reduce congestion or swelling; an agent that reduces congestion or swelling. 254

defecate (def´ə-kāt) to evacuate feces from the rectum. 295

defecation (def″ə-ka´shən) the evacuation of fecal material from the rectum. 280

defibrillation (de-fib″rĭ-la´shən) termination of fibrillation, usually by electroshock. 195

defibrillator (de-fib″rĭ-la´tər) an apparatus used to stop fibrillation by application of brief electroshock to the heart, directly or through electrodes placed on the chest wall. 195

degenerative joint disease (de-jen´ər-ə-tiv joint dĭ-zēz´) a chronic disease involving the joints, especially those bearing weight, characterized by destruction of articular cartilage, overgrowth of bone with lipping and spur formation, and impaired function; osteoarthritis. 464, 464*f*

dehiscence (de-his´əns) a splitting open. 134, 134*f*, 550

dehydration (de″hi-dra´shən) removal of water from a substance; the condition that results from excessive loss of body water. 143, 294

dementia (də-men´shə) loss of intellectual function caused by organic brain disease. 509

dendrite (den´drīt) one of the threadlike extensions of a neuron´s cytoplasm. 27*f*, 486, 486*f*

dental (den´təl) pertaining to the teeth. 273

dentalgia (den-tal´jə) toothache. 289

dentilingual (den″tĭ-ling´wəl) pertaining to the teeth and tongue. 273

dentist (den´tist) a person who has received a degree in dentistry and is authorized to practice dentistry. 274, 275

dentistry (den´tis-tre) the branch of the healing arts concerned with the teeth, oral cavity, and associated structures, including prevention, diagnosis, and treatment of disease and restoration of defective or missing tissue; the creation of restorations, crowns, and bridges; surgical procedures performed in and about the oral cavity; the practice of the dental profession collectively. 31, 274

denture (den´chər) a complement of teeth, either natural or artificial; ordinarily used to designate artificial replacement for the natural teeth. 273

dermabrasion (dur″mə-bra´zhən) a surgical procedure that uses an abrasive disk or other mechanical method to plane the skin. 552, 552*f*

dermal (dur´məl) pertaining to the skin. 533

dermatitis (dur″mə-ti´tis) inflammation of the skin. 70*f*, 71, 538

    contact d., acute or chronic dermatitis caused by materials or substances coming in contact with the skin. 70*f*, 538

dermatologic, dermatological (dur″mə-to-loj´ik, dur″mə-to-loj´ĭ-kəl) pertaining to dermatology; of or affecting the skin. 21

dermatologist (dur″mə-tol´o-jist) a specialist in skin diseases. 533

dermatology (dur″mə-tol´ə-je) the study of the skin and skin diseases. 21, 533

dermatome (dur´mə-tōm) an instrument for cutting thin skin slices for skin grafts; the area of skin supplied with afferent nerve fibers by a single posterior spinal root. 550

dermatomycosis (dur″mə-to-mi-ko´sis) a superficial infection of the skin or its appendages by fungi. 540

dermatoplasty (dur´mə-to-plas″te) plastic surgery of the skin; operative replacement of destroyed or lost skin. 129

dermatosis (dur″mə-to´sis) any skin condition not characterized by inflammation. 129

dermis (dur´mis) the layer of skin that lies under the epidermis. 102, 532, 532*f*, 533

diabetes insipidus (di´ə-be´tēz in-sip´ĭ-dəs) a metabolic disease characterized by polyuria and polydipsia. It is caused by inadequate secretion or release of antidiuretic hormone (ADH), or inability of the kidney tubules to respond to ADH. 341, 578, 582

diabetes mellitus (di″ə-be′tēz mel′lĕ-təs, mə-li′tis) a disorder of carbohydrate metabolism characterized by hyperglycemia and glycosuria, resulting from inadequate production or use of insulin. 282, 306, 339, 582

 type 1 d. m., diabetes mellitus caused by an autoimmune process; persons with this type of diabetes mellitus are dependent on insulin to prevent ketosis. 339, 582, 585

 type 2 d.m., type of diabetes mellitus in which affected persons are non–insulin-dependent. 339, 583, 585

diabetic (di″ə-bet′ik) pertaining to or affected with diabetes; a person with diabetes. 583

 d. nephropathy, a disease process of the kidneys associated with diabetes mellitus. 339, 583

 d. neuropathy, a disease process associated with diabetes mellitus and characterized by sensory or motor disturbances, or both, in the peripheral nervous system. 583

 d. retinopathy, a disorder of retinal blood vessels associated with diabetes mellitus. 583

diagnosis (di″əg-no′sis) the art of distinguishing one disease from another; determination of the nature of a cause of disease. 34, 44

diagnostic (di″əg-nos′tik) pertaining to diagnosis. 34, 44

dialysis (di-al′ə-sis) the diffusion and ultrafiltration of blood across a semipermeable membrane to remove toxic materials and maintain proper balance of fluid and blood electrolytes, and so forth, in cases of improper kidney function; hemodialysis. 336, 343

 peritoneal d., dialysis in which the lining of the peritoneal cavity is used as the dialysis membrane. 343, 344*f*

diaphoresis (di″ə-fə-re′sis) sweating or perspiration, especially profuse perspiration. 549

diaphragm (di′ə-fram) the muscular partition that separates the chest and abdominal cavities and serves as the major inspiratory muscle; a contraceptive device of rubber or soft plastic material placed over the cervix before intercourse. 126, 127*f,* 226*f,* 231, 231*f,* 413

diaphragma (di″ə-frag′mə) diaphragm. 231

diaphragmatic (di″ə-frag-mat′ik) pertaining to or of the nature of a diaphragm. 231

diaphysis (di-af′ə-sis) the elongated, cylindric portion (shaft) of a long bone. 430, 431*f*

diastole (di-as′to-le) the relaxation or the period of relaxation of the heart, especially of the ventricles. 190, 190*f*

diastolic (di″ə-stol′ik) pertaining to diastole. 190

diathermy (di′ə-thur″me) a treatment in which heat is passed through body tissues. 553

diencephalon (di″ən-sef′ə-lon) the portion of the brain that consists of the hypothalamus and thalamus. 490, 490*f*

dietetics (di″ə-tet′iks) the science or study and regulation of the diet. 31

differential white cell count (dif″ər-en′shəl) an examination and enumeration of the distribution of leukocytes in a stained blood smear. 153

digestion (di-jes′chən) the process or act of converting food into chemical substances that can be absorbed and assimilated; the subjection of a body to prolonged heat and moisture, so as to disintegrate and soften it. 266

digit (dij′it) a finger or toe. 129, 130

digoxin (dĭ-jok′sin) a cardiac drug obtained from the leaves of *Digitalis lanata.* 207

dilatation (dil″ə-ta′shən) the condition of being dilated or stretched beyond normal dimensions. 44, 405

dilation and curettage (di-la′shən and ku″rə-tahzh′) (D&C) a surgical procedure that expands the opening into the uterus so that the surface of the uterine wall can be scraped. 378

diphtheria (dif-thēr′e-ə) an acute infectious disease caused by toxigenic strains of *Corynebacterium diphtheriae.* 242

diplegia (di-ple′je-ə) paralysis affecting like parts on both sides of the body. 505

diplococci (dip″lo-kok′si) a pair of spheric bacteria, resulting from incomplete separation after cell division; plural of diplococcus. 85*f,* 86

diplopia (dĭ-plo′pe-ə) the perception of two images of a single object. 99, 511

disease (dĭ-zēz′) any deviation from or interruption of the normal structure or function of any part, organ, or system of the body that is manifested by a characteristic set of symptoms and signs. 81

 communicable d., any disease transmitted by a person or animal to another, directly or indirectly, or by vectors. 82

 Graves d., a multisystem autoimmune disorder characterized by pronounced hyperthyroidism. 580

 idiopathic d., a disease that develops without an apparent or known cause. 82

disease—cont'd

 peripheral vascular d., any abnormal condition that affects the blood vessels and lymphatic vessels, except those that supply the heart. 200

diskectomy (dis-kek′tə-me) excision of an intervertebral disk. 469

dislocation (dis″lo-ka′shən) displacement of a bone from a joint. 456, 456*f*

disorder (dis-or′dər) a derangement or abnormality of function; a morbid physical or mental state. 81

 bipolar d., a major mental disorder characterized by episodes of mania, depression, or mixed mood. 515

 dissociative d., a disorder in which emotional conflicts are so repressed that a split in the personality occurs. 515

 genetic d., any abnormality resulting from heredity. 115, 115*t*

 iatrogenic d., an unfavorable response to medical treatment. 82

 mood d., a variety of conditions characterized by a disturbance in mood as the main feature. 515

 obsessive compulsive d., an anxiety disorder characterized by recurrent and persistent thoughts, ideas, and feelings of obsessions or compulsions. 515

 post-traumatic stress d., a psychiatric disorder characterized by an acute emotional response to a traumatic event or situation. 515

 sexual d., any disorder involving sexual functioning, desire, or performance. 516

 somatoform d., any of a group of disorders characterized by symptoms suggesting physical illness or disease, for which there are no demonstrable organic causes or physiologic dysfunctions. 516

disseminated (dĭ-sem′ĭ-nāt″əd) scattered; distributed over a considerable area. 89, 157

distension (dis-ten′shən) the state of being distended or enlarged. 128, 340

distal (dis′təl) far or distant from the origin or point of attachment. 122

diuresis (di″u-re′sis) increased urination. 348, 567

diuretic (di″u-ret′ik) increasing urination or an agent that increases urination. 207, 348, 567

diverticulectomy (di″vər-tik″u-lek′tə-me) excision of a diverticulum. 305

diverticulitis (di″vər-tik″u-li′tis) inflammation of a diverticulum, especially related to colonic diverticula. 295, 295*f*

diverticulosis (di″vər-tik″u-lo′sis) the presence of diverticula in the absence of inflammation. 295, 295*f*

diverticulum (di″vər-tik′u-ləm) a circumscribed pouch of variable size occurring normally or created by herniation of the lining through a defect in the muscular coat of a tubular organ. 295

dopamine (do′pə-mēn) an intermediate product in the synthesis of norepinephrine that acts as a neurotransmitter in the central nervous system. It also acts on peripheral receptors, for example, in blood vessels. 487

dorsal (dor′səl) pertaining to the back; denoting a position more toward the back surface than some other object of reference. 121

 d. cavity, the body cavity located near the posterior surface of the body. It is further divided into the cranial cavity and the vertebral canal. 126, 126*f*

dorsalgia (dor-sal′jə) pain in the back. 464

dorsocephalad (dor″so-sef′ə-lad) toward the back of the head. 122

dorsolateral (dor″so-lat′ər-əl) pertaining to the back and the side. 121

dorsoventral (dor″so-ven′trəl) pertaining to the back and belly surfaces; passing from the back to the belly surface. 121

Down syndrome (doun sin′drōm) a chromosome disorder characterized by a small flattened skull, short, flat-bridge nose, epicanthal fold, short phalanges, widened spaces between the first and second digits of hands and feet, and moderate to severe mental retardation. Also called trisomy 21 and nondisjunction; formerly called mongolism. 410, 410*f*

duct (dukt) a passage with well-defined walls. 270*f*

 ejaculatory d., the passage formed by the junction of the duct of the seminal vesicles and ductus deferens through which semen enters the urethra. 380, 380*f*

ductus (duk′təs) a general term for a passage with well-defined walls; a duct. 270*f*

 d. deferens, the excretory duct of the testis; vas deferens. 380, 381*f*

duodenal (doo″o-de′nəl, doo-od′ə-nəl) pertaining to the duodenum. 278

duodenitis (doo-od″ə-ni′tis) inflammation of the duodenum. 295

duodenoscope (doo″o-de′no-skōp) an endoscope for examination of the duodenum. 285

duodenoscopy (doo″o-də-nos′kə-pe) endoscopic examination of the duodenum. 285

duodenostomy (doo″o-də-nos′tə-me) formation of a new opening into the duodenum. 395

duodenotomy (doo″o-də-not′ə-me) incision into the duodenum. 395

duodenum (doo″o-de′nəm, doo-od′ə-nəm) the part of the small intestine that connects with the stomach. 270, 276f, 277, 278, 278f

Dupuytren contracture (du-pwe-trah′ kən-trak′chər) contracture of the palmar fascia causing the ring and little fingers to bend into the palm so that they cannot be extended. 458, 458f

dura mater (doo′rə ma′tər) the outermost and toughest of the three membranes of the brain and spinal cord. 488, 489f

dwarfism (dworf′iz-əm) a disease in which the person is much smaller than the normal size of humans. The condition is caused by insufficient growth hormone in childhood. 578, 578f

dysarthria (dis-ahr′thre-ə) a speech disorder consisting of imperfect articulation caused by loss of muscular control after damage to the nervous system. 502

dyscrasia (dis-kra′zhə) an abnormal state or condition. 161

dysentery (dis′ən-ter″e) any of a number of disorders marked by inflammation of the intestine, especially the large intestine, with abdominal pain and frequent stools. 294

dyslexia (dis-lek′se-ə) inability to read, spell, and write words, despite the ability to see and recognize letters. 106, 500

dysmenorrhea (dis-men″ə-re′ə) painful menstruation. 370, 375

dyspepsia (dis-pep′se-ə) poor digestion. 288

dysphagia (dis-fa′je-ə) difficulty in swallowing. 287

dysphasia (dis-fa′zhə) speech impairment. 241, 507

dysphonia (dis-fo′ne-ə) difficulty in speaking or weak voice. 241

dysphoria (dis-for′e-ə) disquiet, restlessness, or malaise. 106

dysplasia (dis-pla′zhə) abnormality of development; in pathology, alteration in size, shape, and organization of adult cells. 131, 367

dyspnea (disp-ne′ə) difficult breathing. 6, 156, 236

dyspneic (disp-ne′ik) referring to or characterized by difficult breathing. 236

dysrhythmia (dis-rith′me-ə) disturbance of rhythm. 195

dystocia (dis-to′shə) abnormal or difficult labor. 410

dystrophic (dis-tro′fik) pertaining to or characterized by dystrophy. 76

dystrophy (dis′trə-fe) faulty nutrition. 76, 463

dysuria (dis-u′re-ə) difficult or painful urination. 335

ecchymosis (ek′ĭ-mo′sis) a small hemorrhagic spot, larger than a petechia, in the skin or mucous membrane forming a nonelevated, rounded or irregular, blue or purplish patch. 543, 543f

echocardiogram (ek″o-kahr′de-o-gram″) the record produced by echocardiography. 192, 192f

echocardiography (ek″o-kahr″de-og′rə-fe) recording of the heart walls or internal structures of the heart and neighboring tissue by the echo obtained from beams of ultrasonic waves directed through the chest wall. 192, 192f

  Doppler e., an echocardiographic technique that records the flow of red blood cells through the cardiovascular system by means of Doppler ultrasonography. 192

echography (ə-kog′rə-fe) a diagnostic aid in which ultrasonic waves are directed at the tissues. A record is made of the sound waves reflected back through the tissues to differentiate structures. 52

  Doppler e., a technique in which ultrasonography is used to evaluate the direction and pattern of blood flow within the heart. 192

eclampsia (ə-klamp′se-ə) convulsions occurring in a pregnant woman with hypertension, proteinuria, and/or edema. 409

ectoderm (ek′to-dərm) in embryology, the outermost layer of cells in the blastoderm. 533

ectopic (ek-top′ik) out of the usual place. 372, 409

  e. pregnancy, the implantation of a fertilized egg in any place other than the uterus. 372, 409

eczema (ek′zə-mə) a dermatitis occurring as a reaction to many endogenous and exogenous agents, characterized in the acute stage by erythema, edema associated with a serous exudate oozing and vesiculation, and crusting and scaling. 538

edema (ə-de′mə) an abnormal accumulation of fluid in intercellular spaces in the tissues. 45, 142, 143

  pulmonary e., abnormal diffuse, extravascular accumulation of fluid in the pulmonary tissues. 247

effacement (ə-fās′mənt) the taking up or obliteration of the cervix in labor in which it is so changed that only the thin external os remains. 405

efferent (ef′ər-ənt) conveying away from a center. 491, 492f

effusion (ə-fu′zhən) the escape of fluid into a part or tissue; an effused material. 198

  pleural e., presence of liquid in the pleural space. 245, 246f

ejaculation (e-jak″u-la′shən) a sudden act of expulsion, as of the semen. 330

electrocardiogram (e-lek″tro-kahr′de-o-gram″) a tracing produced by the electrical impulses of the heart. 45, 191, 191f

electrocardiograph (e-lek″tro-kahr′de-o-graf″) an instrument used to record the electrical current produced by the heart contractions. 46, 191

electrocardiography (e-lek″tro-kahr″de-og′rə-fe) recording the electrical currents of the heart muscle. 46, 46f

electrodesiccation (e-lek″tro-des″ĭ-ka′shən) dehydration of tissue by the use of a high-frequency electric current. 551

electroencephalogram (e-lek″tro-en-sef′ə-lo-gram″) a record produced by the electrical impulses of the brain. 132, 497

electroencephalograph (e-lek″tro-ən-sef′ə-lo-graf″) a machine used to record the electrical impulses of the brain. 132, 497

electroencephalography (e-lek″tro-ən-sef″ə-log′rə-fe) the recording of the electrical currents of the brain by means of electrodes applied to the scalp or to the surface of the brain or placed within the substance of the brain. 132, 497, 497f

electrolysis (e″lek-trol′ə-sis) destruction by passage of a galvanic electrical current, as in removal of excessive hair from the body. 552

electrolyte (e-lek′tro-lit) a substance that dissociates into ions when fused or in solution and thus becomes capable of conducting electricity. 144

electromyogram (e-lek″tro-mi′o-gram) the record obtained by electromyography. 451

electromyography (e-lek″tro-mi-og′rə-fe) the recording and study of the intrinsic electrical properties of skeletal muscle. 332, 451, 451f

electrophoresis (e-lek″tro-fə-re′sis) the separation of ionic solutes in a liquid under the influence of an applied electric field. 160

  hemoglobin e., identification of different types of hemoglobin based on their differing electrophoretic mobilities. 160

electrophysiologic studies (e-lek″tro-fiz″ĭ-o-loj′ik stud′ēz) evaluations of the mechanisms of production of electrical phenomena and the use of electrode catheters to study the effects of electricity on tissue, such as study of the heart rhythm. 193

elephantiasis (el″ə-fən-ti′ə-sis) a disease caused by a parasitic infestation and characterized by inflammation and obstruction of the lymphatics and increased size of nearby tissue. 45, 45f

elimination (e-lim″ĭ-na′shən) the act of expulsion or of extrusion, especially of expulsion from the body; omission or exclusion, as in an elimination diet. 267

emaciation (e-ma″she-a′shən) excessive leanness; a wasted condition of the body. 286

embolectomy (em″bə-lek′tə-me) surgical removal of an embolus from a blood vessel where it has lodged. 207

embolism (em′bə-liz-əm) the sudden blocking of a vessel by a clot or foreign material brought to its site of lodgment by the bloodstream. 154

embolus (em′bo-ləs) a clot or other plug brought by the bloodstream and forced into a smaller vessel where it lodges, thus obstructing circulation. 154, 247f, 504

embryo (em′bre-o) derivatives of the fertilized ovum that eventually become the offspring. 400, 400f

emesis (em′ə-sis) vomiting; an act of vomiting. 45, 287

emphysema (em″fə-se′mə) an accumulation of air in tissues or organs; pulmonary disease characterized by destruction of many of the alveolar walls. 248

empyema (em″pi-e′mə) accumulation of pus in a cavity of the body. If used without a descriptive qualifier, it refers to thoracic empyema. 245

encephalitis (en-sef″ə-li′tis) inflammation of the brain. 132, 507

encephalocele (en-sef′ə-lo-sēl″) hernia of part of the brain and meninges through a skull defect. 71, 71f, 462

encephalography (en-sef″ə-log′rə-fe) radiography of the brain. 498

encephalomeningitis (en-sef″ə-lo-men″in-ji′tis) inflammation of the brain and its membranes. 507

encephalomyelopathy (en-sef″ə-lo-mi″əl-op′ə-the) a disease involving the brain and spinal cord. 502

encephalopathy (en-sef″ə-lop′ə-the) any disease of the brain. 132

encephalotome (en-sef′ə-lə-tōm) an instrument for incision of the brain. 61

encephalotomy (en-sef″ə-lot′ə-me) incision of the brain. 61

endarterectomy (end-ahr″tər-ek′tə-me) excision of the atheromatous inner wall of an artery. 205

  carotid e., surgical excision of atheromatous segments of the inner walls of a carotid artery. 206

endocardial (en″do-kahr′de-əl) pertaining to the endocardium; situated or occurring within the heart. 183

endocarditis (en″do-kahr-di′tis) inflammation of the inner lining of the heart. 198

endocardium (en″do-kahr′de-um) the membrane lining the inner surface of the heart. 183

endocrine (en´do-krīn, en´do-krin) secreting internally; applied to organs that secrete hormones into the bloodstream. 22, 563, 563*f*
  e. system, the network of ductless glands and other structures that elaborate and secrete hormones into the bloodstream. 562, 563
endocrinologist (en˝do-krĭ-nol´ə-jist) a physician who treats diseases arising from disordered internal secretions. 22
endocrinology (en˝do-krĭ-nol´ə-je) the science that studies the endocrine glands and the hormones they produce. 22
endoderm (en´do-dərm) the innermost of the three primary germ layers of the embryo. 533
endodontics (en˝do-don´tiks) the branch of dentistry concerned with the cause, prevention, diagnosis, and treatment of conditions that affect the tooth pulp, root, and periapical tissues. 274
endodontist (en˝do-don´tist) a dentist who specializes in prevention and treatment of conditions that affect the tooth pulp, root, and periapical tissues. 274
endodontitis (en˝do-don-ti´tis) inflammation of the dental pulp. 289
endodontium (en˝do-don´she-əm) dental pulp. 274, 289
endogastric (en˝do-gas´trik) pertaining to the interior of the stomach. 277
endometrial (en˝do-me´tre-əl) pertaining to the endometrium. 363
  e. biopsy, a microscopic examination of a sample of endometrial tissue. 366, 366*f*
endometriosis (en˝do-me˝tre-o´sis) ectopic endometrium located in various places, usually in the pelvic cavity. 373, 374*f*
endometritis (en˝do-me-tri´tis) inflammation of the lining of the uterus. 373
endometrium (en˝do-me´tre-əm) the membrane that lines the cavity of the uterus. 363
endorphin (en-dor´fin, en´dor-fin) any of three amino acid residues that bind to opioid receptors in the brain and have potent analgesic activity. 487
endoscope (en´do-skōp) an instrument for the examination of the interior of a hollow viscus. 47, 47*f*
endoscopic sphincterotomy (en˝do-skop´ik sfingk˝tər-ot´ə-me) incision of a constricting sphincter through an endoscope. 307
endoscopy (en-dos´kə-pe) visual inspection of any cavity of the body by means of an endoscope. 47
endotracheal (en˝do-tra´ke-əl) within the trachea. 230
  e. intubation, a procedure in which a tube is placed through the nose or mouth into the trachea to establish an airway. 250, 251*f*
enteral, enteric (en´tər-əl, en-ter´ik) pertaining to the small intestine. 271
enteritis (en˝tər-i´tis) inflammation of the intestine, especially the small intestine. 271
enterostasis (en˝tər-o-sta´sis) the stopping of food in its passage through the intestine. 296
enuresis (en˝u-re´sis) involuntary discharge of urine after the age at which urinary control should have been achieved; often used with specific reference to involuntary discharge of urine occurring during sleep at night (bedwetting). 336
enzyme (en´zīm) a protein molecule that catalyzes chemical reactions of other substances without itself being destroyed or altered. 74
eosinophil (e˝o-sin´o-fil) a granular leukocyte with a nucleus that usually has two lobes and cytoplasm containing coarse, round granules that are readily stained by eosin. 152*f*, 153
epicardium (ep˝ĭ-kahr´de-um) the layer of serous pericardium on the surface of the heart. 182, 183*f*
epidemic (ep˝ĭ-dem´ik) occurring suddenly in numbers clearly in excess of normal expectancy. 28
epidemiologist (ep˝ĭ-de˝me-ol´ə-jist) a specialist in epidemiology. 28
epidemiology (ep˝ĭ-de˝me-ol´ə-je) the study of the relationships of factors determining the frequency and distribution of diseases in the human community; the field of medicine dealing with the determination of causes of localized outbreaks of infection or other disease of recognized cause. 28
epidermal (ep˝ĭ-dur´məl) pertaining to or resembling epidermis. 532
epidermis (ep˝ĭ-dur´mis) the outermost, nonvascular layer in the skin. 532, 532*f*
epididymis (ep˝ĭ-did´ə-mis) the elongated cordlike structure along the posterior border of the testis that provides for storage, transit, and maturation of spermatozoa and is continuous with the ductus deferens. 380, 381*f*
epididymitis (ep˝ĭ-did˝ə-mi´tis) inflammation of the epididymis. 385
epigastric region (ep˝ĭ-gas´trik) the area of the upper middle region of the abdomen. 125, 125*f*
epiglottiditis (ep˝ĭ-glot˝ĭ-di´tis) inflammation of the epiglottis. 229, 242
epiglottis (ep˝ĭ-glot´is) the lidlike structure composed of cartilage that covers the larynx during swallowing. 229
epilepsy (ep´ĭ-lep˝se) a recurrent disorder of cerebral function characterized by sudden, brief attacks of altered consciousness, motor activity, or sensory phenomena. 76, 508

epinephrine (ep˝ĭ-nef´rin) a hormone secreted by the adrenal medulla. It is a potent stimulator of the sympathetic nervous system and a powerful vasopressor, increasing blood pressure and cardiac output. 487, 492, 570
epiphysis (ə-pif´ə-sis) either end of a long bone. 430, 431*f*
episiotomy (ə-pēz˝e-ot´o-me) surgical incision into the perineum and vagina to prevent traumatic tearing during delivery. 412
epispadias (ep˝ĭ-spa´de-əs) a developmental anomaly consisting of absence of the upper wall of the urethra. 342, 342*f*
epistaxis (ep˝ĭ-stak´sis) hemorrhage from the nose; nosebleed. 240
epithelial (ep˝ĭ-the´le-əl) pertaining to or composed of epithelium. 116, 116*f*
erectile dysfunction (ə-rek´tĭl dis-funk´shən) inability of the male individual to achieve or maintain an erection. 385
erection (ə-rek´shən) the condition of being made rigid and elevated, especially that of the penis. 385
eructation (ə-rək-ta´shən) the casting up of wind from the stomach through the mouth; belching. 288
erythema (er˝ə-the´mə) redness of the skin produced by congestion of the capillaries. 538
erythroblast (ə-rith´ro-blast) embryonic form of a red blood cell. 160, 411
erythroblastosis fetalis (ə-rith˝ro-blas-to´sis fĕ-tă´ləs) a type of hemolytic anemia of the fetus or newborn infant, caused by the transplacental transmission of maternally formed antibody. 160, 410
erythrocyte (ə-rith´ro-sīt) a red blood cell. Mature form is a nonnucleated, biconcave disk. 79, 150, 158
  e. count, enumeration of the number of red blood cells in a blood sample. 151
  e. sedimentation rate, the rate at which red blood cells settle out in a tube of unclotted blood, expressed in millimeters per hour. 453, 453*t*
erythrocytic (ə-rith´ro-sit˝ik) pertaining to, characterized by, or of the nature of red blood cells. 151
erythrocytopenia (ə-rith˝ro-si˝to-pe´ne-ə) a deficiency in the number of red blood cells; anemia. 155
erythrocytosis (ə-rith˝ro-si-to´sis) an increase in the number of red blood cells. 157
erythropenia (ə-rith˝ro-pe´ne-ə) a deficiency in the number of red blood cells. 155
erythropoiesis (ə-rith˝ro-poi-e´sis) the production of red blood cells. 151
erythropoietin (ə-rith˝ro-poi´ə-tin) a hormone chiefly secreted by the kidney in the adult that acts on stem cells of the bone marrow to stimulate red blood cell production. 151, 322
escharotomy (es˝kə-rot´ə-me) surgical incision of the constricting, damaged tissue of a burned area. 551
esophageal (ə-sof˝ə-je´əl) pertaining to the esophagus. 276
  e. atresia, an abnormal esophagus that ends in a blind pouch or narrows to a thin cord and does not provide a continuous passage to the stomach. 291
esophagectomy (ə-sof˝ə-jek´tə-me) excision of all or part of the esophagus. 300
esophagitis (ə-sof˝ə-ji´tis) inflammation of the esophagus. 291
esophagoduodenostomy (ə-sof˝ə-go-doo˝o-de-nos´tə-me) surgical anastomosis between the esophagus and the duodenum. 304
esophagodynia (ə-sof˝ə-go-din´e-ə) pain in the esophagus. 291
esophagogastroduodenoscopy (ə-sof˝ə-go-gas˝tro-doo˝od-ə-nos´kə-pe) endoscopic examination of the esophagus, stomach, and duodenum. 284, 284*f*
esophagogastroplasty (ə-sof˝ə-go-gas´tro-plas˝te) plastic surgery of the esophagus and stomach. 302
esophagogastrostomy (ə-sof˝ə-go-gas-tros´tə-me) forming a new opening between the stomach and the esophagus. 302
esophagogram (ə-sof´ə-go-gram) a roentgenogram of the esophagus. 283
esophagojejunostomy (ə-sof˝ə-go-je˝joo-nos´tə-me) surgically creating a new opening between the esophagus and jejunum. 304
esophagomalacia (ə-sof˝ə-go-mə-la´shə) softening of the esophagus. 291
esophagomyotomy (ə-sof˝ə-go-mi-ot´ə-me) incision through the muscular coat of the esophagus. 300
esophagoscopy (ə-sof˝ə-gos´ko-pe) examining the esophagus using an endoscope. 284
esophagostomy (ə-sof˝ə-gos´tə-me) creation of an opening into the esophagus. 300
esophagram (ə-sof´ə-gram) a roentgenogram of the esophagus. 283
esophagus (ə-sof´ə-gəs) a muscular canal extending from the throat to the stomach. 266, 270

estrogen (es´trə-jen) the female sex hormones, including estradiol, and estrone; a generic term for estrus-producing compounds. Estrogens are responsible for female secondary sex characteristics. During the menstrual cycle, estrogens act on the female genitalia to produce a suitable environment for fertilization, implantation, and nutrition of the early embryo. 364

eupepsia (u-pep´se-ə) normal digestion. 268

euphoria (u-for´e-ə) an exaggerated feeling of physical and mental well-being. 106

eupnea (ūp-ne´ə) normal breathing. 239, 239f

eustachian tube (u-sta´ke-ən tōōb) the auditory tube, which extends from the middle ear to the pharynx. 229, 494f

euthyroid (u-thi´roid) normal thyroid function. 569

eversion (e-vur´zhən) a turning inside-out; a turning outward, as of the sole of the foot or the eyelid. 449f, 450

evisceration (e-vis˝ər-a´shən) removal of the viscera from the abdominal cavity; the protrusion of an internal organ through a wound or surgical incision. 134, 134f

Ewing sarcoma (u´ing sahr-ko´mə) a highly malignant, metastatic tumor of bone. 459

excimer laser (ek´sĭ-mər la´zər) a laser whose beam, in the ultraviolet spectrum, breaks chemical bonds instead of generating heat to destroy tissue. 205, 520

excision (ek-sizh´ən) removal, as of an organ, by cutting. 58

excretion (eks-kre´shən) the act, process, or function of excreting; material that is excreted. 146, 321

exfoliation (eks-fo˝le-a´shən) a falling off in scales or layers. 537

exhalation (eks˝hə-la´shən) expelling air from the lungs by breathing. 226

exophthalmos (ek˝sof-thal´mos) abnormal protrusion of the eyeball. 575, 575f

expectorate (ek-spek´tə-rāt) spitting or coughing up materials from the air passageways leading to the lungs. 249

expiration (ek˝spĭ-ra´shən) the act of expelling air from the lungs or breathing out; death. 226, 231f

expulsion (ek-spul´shən) the act of expelling. 405

extension (ek-sten´shən) the movement by which the ends of a jointed part are pulled away from each other; a movement that brings the members of a limb into or toward a straight condition. 449, 449f

extensor (ek-sten´sor) any muscle that extends a joint. 449

external fixation (ek-stur´nəl fik-sa´shən) a method of stabilizing fractures by pins drilled into the bony parts through the overlying skin and held in a fixed position by a rigid connector. 468, 468f

extracellular (eks˝trə-sel´u-lər) situated or occurring outside a cell. 102, 102f

extracorporeal (eks˝trə-kor-por´e-əl) situated or occurring outside the body. 203, 251, 346

  e. membrane oxygenator, a device that oxygenates a patient´s blood outside the body and returns the blood to the patient´s circulatory system. 251

extracystic (eks˝trə-sis´tik) outside a cyst or the bladder. 322

extrahepatic (eks˝trə-hə-pat´ik) situated or occurring outside the liver. 282

extraocular (eks˝trə-ok´u-lər) outside the eye. 493

extrapleural (eks˝trə-ploor´əl) outside the pleural cavity. 231

extrapulmonary (eks˝trə-pool´mo-nar˝e) not connected with the lungs. 231

extrauterine pregnancy (eks˝trə-u´tər-in) an ectopic pregnancy. 409

extremities (ek-strem´ĭ-tēs) the upper or lower limbs; hands or feet. 128, 442f

facial (fa´shəl) pertaining to or directed toward the face. 434

fallopian tube (fə-lo´pe-ən tōōb) the duct that extends laterally from the fundal end of the uterus and terminates near the ovary; uterine tube. 360

family practice (fam´ĭ-le prak´tis) the medical specialty concerned with the planning and provision of the comprehensive primary health care of all family members, regardless of age or sex, on a continuing basis. 19

fascia (fash´e-ə) a sheet or band of fibrous tissue that covers the muscles and various other organs of the body. 448

fascial (fash´e-əl) pertaining to or of the nature of a fascia. 448

fasciectomy (fas˝e-ek´tə-me) excision of fascia. 470

fatigue (fə-tēg´) a state of increased discomfort and decreased efficiency resulting from prolonged or excessive exertion; loss of capacity to respond to stimulation. 106

  chronic f. syndrome, a condition characterized by disabling fatigue, accompanied by many symptoms. 466

febrile (feb´ril) pertaining to or characterized by fever. 130

feces (fe´sēz) the excrement discharged from the intestines. 280

femoral (fem´or-əl) pertaining to the femur, the thigh bone. 441

femur (fe´mər) the thigh; the thigh bone. 34, 433f, 441

fertilization (fur´tĭ-lĭ-za´shən) rendering gametes fertile or capable of further development. 364

fertilization—cont'd

  in vitro f., a method of fertilizing human ova outside the body, then later injecting them into the uterus through the cervix. 415

fetal (fe´təl) of or pertaining to a fetus. 400

fetoscope (fe´to-skōp) a specially designed stethoscope for listening to the fetal heartbeat; an endoscope for viewing the fetus in utero. 408, 408f

fetus (fe´təs) the unborn offspring in the postembryonic period, after major structures have been outlined, in humans from 7 to 8 weeks after fertilization until birth. 400

fibrillation (fĭ-brĭ-la´shən) involuntary muscle contraction caused by spontaneous activation of single muscle cells or muscle fibers. 195

  ventricular f., cardiac arrhythmia marked by rapid, uncoordinated, and ineffective contraction of the ventricles. 195

fibrin (fi´brin) an insoluble protein that forms long threads that compose blood clots. 161

fibrinogen (fi-brin´o-jən) a protein in plasma that is essential for clotting of blood. 161

fibrinolysin (fi˝brĭ-nol´ə-sin) a substance that dissolves fibrin clots and also breaks down certain coagulation factors. 161

fibrinolysis (fi˝brĭ-nol´ə-sis) destruction of fibrin. 161

fibrocystic breast disease (fi˝bro-sis´tik) the presence of single or multiple benign cysts that are palpable in the breast. 583

fibromyalgia (fi˝bro-mi-al´jə) chronic pain in muscles and soft tissues surrounding joints. 466

fibrosarcoma (fi˝bro-sahr-ko´mə) a malignant tumor composed of cells and fibers that produce collagen. 459

fibrous (fi´brəs) composed of or containing fiber. 245, 322

fibula (fib´u-lə) the smaller of the two lower leg bones. 433f, 442, 442f

fibular (fib´u-lər) pertaining to the fibula, a bone in the lower leg. 442

fimbria (fim´bre-ə) any structure that resembles a fringe or border, such as the long fringelike extension of a uterine tube that lies close to the ovary. 360, 361f

fissure (fish´ər) a split; a cleft or groove. 294, 294f, 543f

fistula (fis´tu-lə) an abnormal communication between two internal organs, or from an internal organ to the body surface. 294

flexion (flek´shən) the act of bending; being bent. 449, 449f

flexor (flek´sor) any muscle that flexes a joint. 449

fluoroscope (floor´o-skōp) a device used in fluoroscopy for examining deep structures by means of x-rays. 52

fluoroscopy (floo-ros´kə-pe) examination by means of a fluoroscope, a device that allows both structural and functional visualization of internal structures. 52, 283

flutter (flut´ər) a rapid vibration or pulsation. 195

follicle (fol´ĭ-kəl) a sac or pouchlike depression or cavity. 364

  graafian f., a mature vesicular follicle of the ovary. 364

  f.-stimulating hormone (FSH), one of the gonadotropic hormones of the anterior pituitary that stimulates the growth and maturation of ovarian follicles, stimulates estrogen secretion, and promotes endometrial changes. This hormone also stimulates spermatogenesis in the male sex. 364, 365f

folliculitis (fə-lik˝u-li´tis) inflammation of a follicle or follicles; used ordinarily in reference to hair follicles but sometimes in relation to follicles of other kinds. 548

foramen magnum (fo-ra´mən mag´nəm) the opening in the occipital bone through which the spinal cord passes from the brain. 434, 490

fracture (frak´chər) a break or rupture in a bone; the breaking of a part, especially a bone. 455, 455f

  closed f., one that does not produce an open wound in the skin. 455

  comminuted f., one in which the bone is crushed or splintered. 456

  compound f., open fracture. 455

  compression f., a break in which bone surfaces are forced into each other. 456

  greenstick f., one in which only one side of a bone is broken. 455

  impacted f., one in which one fragment is firmly driven into the other. 455

  open f., one in which a wound through the overlying or adjacent soft tissues communicates with the site of the break. 455

  simple f., closed fracture. 455

  spiral f., a bone break that is spiral to the bone´s long axis. 456

  transverse f., one at right angles to the axis of the bone. 456

frequency (fre´kwən-se) the number of occurrences of a periodic or recurrent process per unit time. 335

friction rub (frik´shən) a dry grating sound heard with a stethoscope during auscultation. 235, 235f

glaucoma (glaw-, glou-ko´mə) a group of eye diseases characterized by an increase in intraocular pressure, which causes pathologic changes in the optic disk and typical defects in the field of vision. 511

glia cell (gli´ə) one of the cells that make up the supporting nerve of nervous tissue. 485

glioma (gli-o´mə) a tumor composed of tissue that represents neuroglia. The term is sometimes extended to include all the primary intrinsic neoplasms of the brain and spinal cord. 508

globin (glo´bin) a member of a group of proteins that make up the protein constituent of hemoglobin. 159

globulin (glob´u-lin) any member of a group of proteins, most of which are insoluble in water but soluble in saline solutions. 159

glomerular filtration rate (glo-mer´u-lər) a kidney function value that can be determined from the amount of filtrate formed by the glomeruli of the kidney. 325, 325f

glomerulonephritis (glo-mer´u-lo-nə-fri´tis) a type of nephritis in which there is inflammation of the glomeruli. 339

glomerulopathy (glo-mer″u-lop´ə-the) any disease of the renal glomeruli. 339

glomerulus (glo-mer´u-ləs) a small cluster, as of blood vessels or nerve fibers; often used alone to designate one of the renal glomeruli, which act as filters. 323

glossal (glos´əl) pertaining to the tongue. 273

glossectomy (glos-ek´tə-me) surgical removal of the tongue. 300

glossitis (glos-i´tis) inflammation of the tongue. 289

glossopathy (glos-op´ə-the) any disease of the tongue. 289

glossopharyngeal (glos″o-fə-rin´je-əl) pertaining to the tongue and the pharynx. 273

glossoplasty (glos´o-plas″te) plastic surgery of the tongue. 300

glossoplegia (glos″o-ple´jə) paralysis of the tongue. 289

glossopyrosis (glos″o-pi-ro´sis) pain, burning, itching, and stinging of the mucous membranes of the tongue without apparent lesions of the affected areas. 289

glossorrhaphy (glos-or´ə-fe) suture of the tongue. 300

glottis (glot´is) the vocal apparatus of the larynx. 229

glucagon (gloo´kə-gon) hormone secreted by the alpha cells of the islets of Langerhans in response to hypoglycemia, acetylcholine, some amino acids, and growth hormone. 282, 573

glucocorticoid (gloo″ko-kor´tĭ-koid) any of a group of steroids produced by the adrenal cortex. 570

glucose (gloo´kōs) a sugar found in certain foodstuffs, especially fruit, and normal blood; dextrose. 267
    g. lowering agent, a drug that lowers the blood glucose. 306, 585
    g. tolerance test, a test of the body´s ability to metabolize carbohydrates; involves administering a standard dose of glucose and measuring the blood and urine for glucose levels. 576

glycolysis (gli″kol´ə-sis) the enzymatic breakdown of glucose to simpler compounds. 267

glycosuria (gli″ko-su´re-ə) the presence of sugar in the urine. 327, 576

goiter (goi´tər) enlargement of the thyroid gland, causing a swelling in the front part of the neck. 575, 575f

gonad (go´nad) an organ that produces eggs or sperm; ovary or testis. 359, 379, 400, 564

gonadal (go-nad´əl) pertaining to the ovaries or the testes. 568

gonadotropic (go″nə-do-tro´pik) capable of stimulating the ovaries or the testes. 568
    g. hormone, a general term that means a hormone that stimulates the gonads and includes follicle-stimulating hormone and luteinizing hormone. 568

gonadotropin (go″nə-do-tro´pin) a substance that stimulates the gonads, especially the hormone secreted by the pituitary gland that stimulates the ovaries or testes. 367, 568
    human chorionic g., a hormone present in the urine and many body fluids of pregnant female individuals that forms the basis of testing for pregnancy. 367, 407, 574

gonococcus (gon″o-kok´əs) an organism of the species *Neisseria gonorrhoeae,* the cause of gonorrhea. 416

gonorrhea (gon″o-re´ə) infection caused by *Neisseria gonorrhoeae;* transmitted sexually in most cases but also by contact with infected exudates in neonatal children at birth, or by infants in households with infected inhabitants. It is characterized by discharge and painful urination in male individuals and often is asymptomatic in female individuals. 342, 416, 416f

gout (gout) hereditary metabolic disease that is a form of acute arthritis and is marked by inflammation of the joints. Gout is characterized by hyperuricemia and deposits of urates in and around joints. Any joint may be affected, but gout usually begins in the knee or foot. 453, 453t, 465

graafian follicle (grah´fe-ən fol´ĭ-kəl) development of the primary oocyte in the ovary to the stage where the ovum is fully developed. 364

granulocyte (gran´u-lo-sīt″) a leukocyte containing neutrophil, basophil, or eosinophil granules in its cytoplasm. 152, 153

gravid (grav´id) pregnant. 403

gravida (grav´ĭ-də) a pregnant woman. 403
    g. I, primigravida; during the first pregnancy. 403

gumma (gum´ə) a lesion in late stages of syphilis. 417

gynecologic (gi″nə-, jin″ə-kə-loj´ik) pertaining to female individuals, particularly to the female genitourinary system. 359

gynecologist (gi″nə-, jin″ə-kol´ə-jist) a physician who treats diseases of the female sex. 22

gynecology (gi″nə-, jin″ə-kol´ə-je) the branch of medicine that treats female diseases, especially those of the genital and urinary systems. 22, 359

gynecomastia (gi″nə-, jin″ə-ko-mas´te-ə) excessive development of the male mammary glands, sometimes even to the functional state. 581, 582f

halitosis (hal″ĭ-to´sis) offensive breath. 289

hallux valgus (hal´əks val´gəs) angulation of the great toe away from the midline of the body, or toward the other toes. 458, 458f

hammertoe (ham´ər-to) a toe with dorsal flexion of the first phalanx and plantar flexion of the second and third phalanges. 458, 458f

haversian canals (ha-vur´zhən kə-nalz´) the channels of compact bone that contain blood vessels, lymph vessels, and nerves. 430, 431f

headache (hed´āk) pain in the head. 501
    cluster h., a headache similar to migraine, recurring as often as two or three times a day over a period of weeks; then there may be absence of symptoms for weeks or months. 501, 501f
    migraine h., paroxysmal attacks of headache frequently unilateral, usually accompanied by disordered vision and gastrointestinal disturbances. 501, 501f
    tension h., a pain that affects the head as a result of overwork or emotional strain and involving tension in the muscles of the neck. 501, 501f

heart block (hahrt blok) impairment in conduction of an impulse in heart excitation. 195

heart flutter a type of irregular heart rhythm. 195

heat hydrotherapy the use of warm water in the treatment of disease. 553

Heimlich maneuver (hīm´lik) an emerging procedure for dislodging a bolus of food or other obstruction from the trachea to prevent asphyxiation. 249, 250f

heliotherapy (he″le-o-ther´ə-pe) treatment of disease by exposing the body to sunlight. 553

hemangioma (he-man″je-o´mə) an extremely common benign tumor, occurring most commonly in infancy and childhood, made up of newly formed blood vessels and resulting from malformation of angioblastic tissue of fetal life. 200

hematemesis (he″mə-tem´ə-sis) vomiting of blood. 287

hematochezia (he″mə-to, hem″ə-to-ke´zhə) presence of blood in the feces. 286

hematocrit (he-mat´o-krit) a tube with graduated markings used to determine the volume of packed red cells in a blood specimen by centrifugation; by extension, the measurement obtained using this procedure or the corresponding measurements produced by automated blood cell counters. 151

hematologic (he″mə-to-loj´ik) pertaining to the blood and the blood-forming tissues. 148

hematologist (he″mə-tol´ə-jist) a specialist in hematology. 148

hematology (he″mə-tol´ə-je) the study of blood and blood-forming tissues and their physiology and pathology. 148

hematoma (he″mə-to´mə) any localized collection of blood, usually clotted, in an organ, tissue, or space. 147, 503, 503f
    epidural h., accumulation of blood in the epidural space. 503, 503f
    intracerebral h., accumulation of blood within the brain tissue. 503, 503f
    subdural h., accumulation of blood in the subdural space. 503, 503f

hematopoiesis (he″mə-to, hem″ə-to-poi-e´sis) the formation and development of blood cells. 149

hematopoietic (he″mə-to, hem″ə-to-poi-et´ik) pertaining to or affecting hematopoiesis. 155

hematuria (he″mə-, hem″ə-tu´re-ə) the presence of blood in the urine. 328

hemicolectomy (hem″e-ko-lek´tə-me) excision of approximately half of the colon. 304

hemiplegia (hem″e-ple´jə) paralysis of one side of the body. 505

hemodialysis (he″mo-di-al´ə-sis) the process of diffusing blood through a semipermeable membrane for the purpose of removing toxic materials and maintaining acid-base balance in cases of impaired kidney function. 343, 344f

hemoglobin (he´mo-glo˝bin) the oxygen-carrying red pigment of red blood cells. 154, 160

glycosylated h., a hemoglobin A molecule in which the concentration represents the average blood glucose level over the previous several weeks. 576

hemoglobinopathy (he˝mo-glo˝bin-op´ə-the) a hematologic disorder caused by genetically determined abnormal hemoglobin. 160

hemolysin (he-mol´ə-sin) a substance that causes destruction of red blood cells. 76, 154

hemolysis (he-mol´ə-sis) destruction of red blood cells that results in the liberation of hemoglobin. 76, 154, 162

hemolytic (he˝mo-lit´ik) pertaining to, characterized by, or producing hemolysis. 76, 160

h. disease of the newborn, hemolytic erythroblastosis fetalis. 160, 410

hemolyze (he´mo-līz) to subject to or to undergo hemolysis. 76, 160

hemopericardium (he˝mo-per˝ĭ-kahr´de-əm) an effusion of blood within the pericardium. 198

hemophilia (he˝mo-fil´e-ə) a hereditary hemorrhagic disorder caused by deficiency of antihemophilic factor VIII or IX. 156

hemoptysis (he-mop´tĭ-sis) the spitting of blood or blood-stained sputum. 249

hemorrhoid (hem´ə-roid) a varicose dilation of a vein of the anal canal inside or just outside the rectum that causes pain, itching, and bleeding. 201, 294f

hemorrhoidectomy (hem˝ə-roid-ek´tə-me) excision of hemorrhoids. 305

hemostasis (he˝mo-sta´sis, he-mos´tə-sis) the checking of the flow of blood either by coagulation or surgical means; interruption of blood flow through any vessel or to any part of the body. 161, 162

hemothorax (he˝mo-thor´aks) a collection of blood in the chest cavity. 245, 246f

heparin (hep´ə-rin) a naturally occurring substance that acts in the body as an antithrombin factor to prevent intravascular clotting. Heparin sodium is used therapeutically as an anticoagulant. 207

hepatectomy (hep˝ə-tek´tə-me) excision of part of the liver. 306

hepatic (hə-pat´ik) pertaining to the liver. 281

h. lobectomy, excision of a lobe of the liver. 306

hepatitis (hep˝ə-ti´tis) inflammation of the liver. 162, 298, 421t

viral h., hepatitis caused by a viral infection, such as HAV, HBV, or HCV. 298, 420

hepatolytic (hep˝ə-to-lit´ik) destructive to the liver; hepatotoxic. 281

hepatoma (hep˝ə-to´mə) a tumor of the liver, especially hepatocellular carcinoma. 298

hepatomegaly (hep˝ə-to-meg´ə-le) enlargement of the liver. 298

hepatopathy (hep˝ə-top´ə-the) any disease of the liver. 298

hepatorenal syndrome (hep˝ə-to-re´nəl sin´drōm) functional renal failure, without pathologic renal changes, associated with cirrhosis and ascites or with obstructive jaundice. 298

hepatosplenomegaly (hep˝ə-to-sple˝no-meg´ə-le) enlargement of the liver and spleen. 298

hepatotomy (hep˝ə-tot´ə-me) surgical incision of the liver. 306

hepatotoxic (hep´ə-to-tok˝sik) toxic to liver cells. 281

hernia (hur´ne-ə) protrusion of an organ or part of it through an abnormal opening. 71

femoral h., hernia into the femoral canal. 133, 133f

hiatal h., protrusion of any structure through the esophageal hiatus of the diaphragm. 292, 292f

inguinal h., a hernia in which a loop of the intestine enters the inguinal canal. 133, 133f, 296, 296f

umbilical h., protrusion of part of the intestine at the umbilicus, the defect in the abdominal wall and protruding bowel being covered with skin and subcutaneous tissue. 133, 133f

herniated disk (hur´ne-āt˝əd disk) herniation of an intervertebral disk. 457

herniation (hur´ne-a´shən) abnormal protrusion of an organ or other body structure through a defect or natural opening in a covering, membrane, muscle, or bone. 71

hernioplasty (hur´ne-o-plas˝te) surgical repair of a hernia. 133

herpes (hur´pēz) a word that at one time was used to indicate any inflammatory skin disease marked by small vesicles in clusters and caused by a virus. Its use as a single word is imprecise but often refers to the condition of cold sores or fever blisters. 539

h. genitalis, herpetic blisters on the male or female genitalia. 418t, 419, 419f

h. simplex virus, herpes simplex virus 1 or herpes simplex virus 2. 241, 539

h. zoster, an acute infection caused by reactivation of the latent varicella zoster virus; shingles. 540, 540f

hesitancy (hez´ə-tən-se) tending to hold back or delay momentarily. In urinary hesitancy there is decrease in the force of the stream, often with difficulty in beginning the flow. 335

hidradenitis (hi˝drad-ə-ni´tis) inflammation of a sweat gland. 548

hilum (hi´ləm) anatomic nomenclature for a depression or pit at the part of an organ where vessels and nerves enter. 230, 323

hirsutism (hur´soot-iz-əm) abnormal hairiness, especially an adult male pattern of hair distribution in women. 581, 582f

histamine (his´tə-mēn) a substance present in the body that has known pharmacologic action when released from injured cells. Histamine can also be produced synthetically. 166

histocompatibility (his˝to-kəm-pat˝ĭ-bil´ĭ-te) the ability of donor tissue to survive after a transplant, rather than being rejected by the immune system of the patient who receives the tissue. 551

histologist (his-tol´ə-jist) one who studies tissue. 80

histology (his-tol´ə-je) study of the minute structure, composition, and function of tissues. 80

holistic (ho-lis´tik) considering a person as a functioning whole. 19, 19f

Holter monitor (hōl´tər mon´ĭ-tər) a type of ambulatory ECG monitor. 191

homeostasis (ho˝me-o-sta´sis) sameness or stability in the normal body state of an organism. 143, 267, 563

homologous (ho-mol´ə-gəs) corresponding in structure, position, origin, etc.; denoting individuals of the same species but antigenically distinct; pertaining to an antibody and the antigen that elicited its production. 163

h. graft, a tissue removed from a donor for transplantation to a recipient of the same species. 163

hordeolum (hor-de´o-ləm) a localized, purulent, inflammatory staphylococcal infection of one or more sebaceous glands. 510

hormone (hor´mōn) a chemical substance produced in the body that has a specific effect on the activity of certain cells or organs. 22, 563

interstitial cell–stimulating h., a hormone secreted by the pituitary gland that stimulates the production of testosterone by the interstitial cells of the testes. 568

lactogenic h., a hormone secreted by the pituitary gland that stimulates lactation in postpartum mammals. 571

melanocyte-stimulating h., a hormone secreted by the anterior pituitary gland that controls the intensity of pigmentation in pigmented cells. 568

parathyroid h., a hormone secreted by the parathyroid glands. 573

thyroid-stimulating h., a substance secreted by the pituitary gland that controls the release of thyroid hormone. 569

humeral (hu´mər-əl) pertaining to the humerus, the upper arm bone. 440

humeroradial (hu˝mər-o-ra´de-əl) pertaining to the humerus and radius. 440

humeroscapular (hu˝mər-o-skap´u-lər) pertaining to the upper arm bone and the shoulder blade. 440

humeroulnar (hu˝mər-o-ul´nər) pertaining to the humerus and ulna. 440

humerus (hu´mər-əs) the bone of the upper arm, extending from shoulder to elbow. 433f, 439

Huntington chorea (hun´ting-tən kə-re´ə) an autosomal dominant disease characterized by chronic, progressive, complex, jerky movements and mental deterioration terminating in dementia. 506

hydrocele (hi´dro-sēl) a circumscribed collection of fluid, especially pertaining to fluid collection in the scrotum. 385, 386f

hydrocelectomy (hi˝dro-se-lek´tə-me) excision of a hydrocele. 388

hydrocephalus (hi˝dro-sef´ə-ləs) a condition characterized by abnormal accumulation of cerebrospinal fluid within the skull, with enlargement of the head, atrophy of the brain, mental retardation, and convulsions; hydrocephaly. 144, 144f, 508

hydronephrosis (hi˝dro-nə-fro´sis) distention of the kidney with urine, as a result of obstruction of the ureter. 340, 340f

hydrophobia (hi˝dro-fo´be-ə) rabies, a viral disease transmitted to a human by the bite of an infected animal. 507

hydrothorax (hi˝dro-thor´aks) a collection of water fluid in the pleural cavity. 245

hydroureter (hi˝dro-u-re´tər) abnormal distention of the ureter caused by obstruction from any cause. 340, 340f

hydrous (hi´drəs) containing water. 104

hypalgesia (hi˝pal-je´ze-ə) decreased sensitivity to pain. 500

hyperacidity (hi˝pər-ə-sid´ĭ-te) an excessive amount of acid. 302

hyperactive (hi˝pər-ak´tiv) pertaining to or characterized by hyperactivity. 99

hyperadrenalism (hi˝pər-ə-dre´nəl-iz-əm) increased activity of the adrenal glands. 581

hyperalgesia (hi˝pər-al-je´ze-ə) abnormally increased sensitivity to pain. 500

hyperalimentation (hi″pər-al″ĭ-men-ta′shən) the intravenous infusion of a hypertonic solution that contains sufficient nutrients to sustain life. 301

hypercalcemia (hi″pər-kal-se′me-ə) an increased level of calcium in the blood. 144, 581

hypercalciuria (hi″pər-kal″se-u′re-ə) excessive calcium in the urine. 453

hypercapnia (hi″pər-kap′ne-ə) excessive carbon dioxide in the blood. 237

hyperchromic (hi″pər-kro′mik) highly or excessively stained or colored. 159

hyperemesis (hi″pər-em′ə-sis) excessive vomiting. 287

hyperemia (hi″pər-e′me-ə) excessive blood flow to a part of the body. 147

hyperglycemia (hi″pər-gli-se′me-ə) an increased amount of sugar in the blood. 282, 339, 576, 582

hyperinsulinism (hi″pər-in′sə-lin-iz″əm) excessive secretion of insulin by the pancreas, resulting in an increased level of insulin in the blood and hypoglycemia. 583

hyperkalemia (hi″pər-kə-le′me-ə) abnormally high concentration of potassium in the blood. 144

hyperkinesia, hyperkinesis (hi″pər-kĭ-ne′zhə, hi″pər-kĭ-ne′sis) abnormally increased muscular function or activity. 514

hypernatremia (hi″pər-nə-tre′me-ə) a greater than normal concentration of sodium in the blood. 144

hyperopia (hi″pər-o′pe-ə) an error of refraction in which rays of light entering the eye are brought to a focus behind the retina; also called farsightedness. 511, 512f

hyperosmia (hi″per-oz′me-ə) increased sensitivity of smell. 495

hyperoxemia (hi″pər-ok-se′me-ə) increased amount of oxygen in the blood. 250

hyperparathyroidism (hi″pər-par″ə-thi′roid-iz-əm) increased secretion of hormone by the parathyroids. 580

hyperpituitarism (hi″pər-pĭ-too′ĭ-tə-riz″əm) increased secretion by the pituitary gland. 579

hyperplasia (hi″pər-pla′zhə) abnormal increase in the number of normal cells in a tissue. 131, 131f, 386

  benign prostatic h., nonmalignant, noninflammatory enlargement of the prostate. 340, 341f, 386

hyperpnea (hi″pər-ne′ə, hi″pərp-ne′ə) an abnormal increase in depth and rate of respiration. 237, 239f

hyperpyrexia (hi″pər-pi-rek′se-ə) a highly increased body temperature of around 105° F or higher. 130

hyperpyrexial (hi″pər-pi-rek′se-əl) pertaining to an increased body temperature. 130

hypersecretion (hi″pər-se-kre′shən) excessive secretion. 578

hypersensitivity (hi″pər-sen″sĭ-tiv′ĭ-te) a state in which the body reacts with an exaggerated response to a foreign agent. 165

hypertension (hi″pər-ten′shən) increased blood pressure. 190

  renal h., hypertension resulting from renal artery stenosis or other kidney disorders. 341

hyperthermia (hi″pər-thur′me-ə) greatly increased body temperature. 549

hyperthyroidism (hi″pər-thi′roid-iz-əm) increased activity of the thyroid gland. 575, 580

hypertonicity (hi″pər-to-nis′ĭ-te) the state of being hypertonic. 446

hypertrophy (hi-pur′trə-fe) enlargement of an organ caused by an increase in the size of preexisting cells. 131, 131f

hyperventilation (hi″pər-ven″tĭ-la′shən) abnormally increased pulmonary ventilation, resulting in greater than normal loss of carbon dioxide, which if prolonged may lead to alkalosis. 237

hypnotic (hip-not′ik) inducing sleep; pertaining to or of the nature of hypnotism; a drug that acts to induce sleep. 519

hypoadrenalism (hi″po-ə-dre′nəl-iz-əm) decreased activity of the adrenal glands. 582

hypoalgesia (hi″po-al-je′ze-ə) decreased sensitivity to pain. 500

hypocalcemia (hi″po-kal-se′me-ə) decreased amount of calcium in the blood. 144, 580

hypocapnia (hi″po-kap′ne-ə) deficiency of carbon dioxide in the blood resulting from hyperventilation and eventually leading to alkalosis. 238

hypochondriac (hi″po-kon′dre-ak) pertaining to the hypochondrium; a person who has morbid anxiety about his or her health but has no attributable cause. 125

  h. region, that part of the upper abdomen on both sides of the epigastric region and beneath the cartilages of the lower ribs. 124, 125f

hypochondriasis (hi″po-kon-dri′ə-sis) a stomatoform disorder characterized by an interpretation of normal sensations as indications of serious problems. 516

hypochromia (hi″po-kro′me-ə) abnormal decrease in the hemoglobin content of the erythrocytes. 159

hypochromic (hi″po-kro′mik) pertaining to or marked by hypochromia. 159

hypodermic (hi″po-dur′mik) applied or administered beneath the skin. 102

hypogastric region (hi″po-gas′trik) the abdominal region below the umbilical region. 125, 125f

hypoglossal (hi″po-glos′əl) beneath the tongue. 273

hypoglycemia (hi″po-gli-se′me-ə) an abnormally low concentration of glucose in the blood. 282, 576, 583

hypogonadism (hi″po-go′nad-iz-əm) decreased functional activity of the gonads, with retardation of sexual development. 581

hypoinsulinism (hi″po-in′su-lin-iz″əm) deficient secretion of insulin by the pancreas. 582

hypokalemia (hi″po-kə-le′me-ə) abnormally low potassium concentration in the blood. 144

hyponatremia (hi″po-nə-tre′me-ə) deficiency of sodium in the blood. 144

hypoparathyroidism (hi″po-par″ə-thi′roid-iz-əm) decreased secretion of hormone by the parathyroids. 580

hypophysectomy (hi″pof-ə-sek′tə-me) surgical removal or destruction of the pituitary. 584

hypophysis (hi-pof′ə-sis) the pituitary gland. 564, 565

hypopituitarism (hi″po-pĭ-too′ĭ-tə-riz″əm) decreased activity of the pituitary gland. 578

hypoplasia (hi″po-pla′zhə) incomplete development or underdevelopment of an organ or tissue. 131

hypopnea (hi-pop′ne-ə) abnormal decrease in the depth and rate of breathing. 239

hyposecretion (hi″po-sə-kre′shən) diminished secretion as of a gland. 563, 578

hypospadias (hi″po-spa′de-əs) a developmental anomaly in which the urethra opens inferior to its usual location. 342, 342f

hypotension (hi″po-ten′shən) decreased blood pressure. 190

hypothalamus (hi″po-thal′ə-məs) the part of the brain most concerned with moderating behavior related to internal physiologic states. 566, 567

hypothermia (hi″po-thur′me-ə) low body temperature. 549

hypothyroidism (hi″po-thi′roid-iz-əm) decreased activity of the thyroid gland. 580

hypotonicity (hi″po-to-nis′ĭ-te) the state of being hypotonic. 446

hypoventilation (hi″po-ven″tĭ-la′shən) a state in which there is a reduced amount of air entering the pulmonary alveoli. 237

hypovolemia (hi″po-vo-le′me-ə) decreased volume of circulating blood in the body. 198

hypoxemia (hi″pok-se′me-ə) deficient oxygen in the blood. 239

hypoxia (hi-pok′se-ə) a condition of decreased oxygen. 236, 547

hysterectomy (his″tər-ek′tə-me) removal of the uterus. 376, 377

  abdominal h., a hysterectomy performed through an incision in the abdominal wall. 377

  vaginal h., a hysterectomy performed through the vagina. 377, 377f

hysteria (his-ter′e-ə) a now somewhat nebulous term formerly used in psychiatry for a dramatic attack involving intense emotional display. 71

hysteropathy (his″tə-rop′ə-the) any uterine disease or disorder. 372

hysteropexy (his′tər-o-pek″se) surgical fixation of the uterus. 378

hysteroptosis (his″tər-op-to′sis) falling or prolapse of the uterus. 372, 373f

hysterosalpingogram (his″tər-o-sal-ping″go-gram) the record produced by x-ray examination of the uterus and uterine tubes after the injection of opaque material. 368

hysterosalpingography (his″tər-o-sal″ping-gog′rə-fe) roentgenography of the uterus and uterine tubes after injection of opaque material. 368

hysteroscope (his′tər-o-skōp″) an endoscope used in direct visual examination of the uterus. 368

hysteroscopy (his″tər-os′kə-pe) inspection of the interior of the uterus with an endoscope. 368, 368f

ichthyoid (ik′the-oid) resembling a fish. 538

ichthyosis (ik″the-o′sis) any of several generalized skin disorders marked by dryness and scaliness, resembling fish skin. 538

ileac (il′e-ak) pertaining to the ileum; ileal. 279

ileal (il′e-əl) pertaining to the ileum; ileac. 279

ileitis (il″e-i′tis) inflammation of the ileum. 295

ileocecal (il″e-o-se′kəl) pertaining to the ileum and cecum. 279

ileostomy (il″e-os′tə-me) surgical creation of an opening into the ileum, usually by establishing a stoma on the abdominal wall. 304, 305f

ileum (il′e-əm) the distal portion of the small intestine, which extends from the jejunum to the cecum. 278, 278f, 279

iliac (il′e-ak) pertaining to the ilium, a bone of the pelvis. 440

iliofemoral (il″e-o-fem′or-əl) pertaining to the ilium and the femur. 442

iliopubic (il″e-o-pu′bik) pertaining to the ilium and the pubis, two bones of the pelvis. 441

ilium (il´e-əm) the lateral flaring portion of the hip bone. 433*f*, 440

immunity (ĭ-mu´nĭ-te) being immune; security against a particular disease; nonsusceptibility to the invasive or pathogenic effects of certain antigens. 164, 166*f*

    active i., immunity developing in response to antigenic stimulus. 166, 166*f*

    passive i., immunity acquired by transfer of antibody from an immune donor. 166, 166*f*

immunization (im˝u-nĭ-za´shən) the induction of immunity. 166

immunocompromised (im˝u-no-kom´prə-mīzd) having the immune response attenuated by administration of immunosuppressive drugs, by irradiation, by malnutrition, or by some disease processes. 167

immunodeficiency (im˝u-no-də-fish´ən-se) a deficiency in immune response. 167

immunoglobulin (im˝u-no-glob´u-lin) a protein of animal origin that has known antibody activity. 165

immunologist (im˝u-nol´ə-jist) a person who makes a special study of immunology. 25

immunology (im˝u-nol´ə-je) the branch of medical science concerned with the response of the organism to antigenic challenge, recognition of self from nonself, and all of the aspects of immune phenomena. 25

immunosuppressant, immunosuppressive (im˝u-no-sə-pres´ənt, im˝u-no-sə-pres´iv) pertaining to or inducing immunosuppression. 167

impaction (im-pak´shən) the condition of being firmly lodged or wedged. 296

    fecal i., a collection of puttylike or hardened feces in the rectum or sigmoid. 296

implantation (im˝plan-ta´shən) attachment of the fertilized egg to the epithelial lining of the uterus and its embedding in the compact layer of the endometrium. 400, 400*f*

incision (in-sizh´ən) a cut or wound produced by a sharp instrument; the act of cutting. 58

incisor (in-si´zər) any of the four anterior teeth in either jaw. 274

incompatibility (in˝kəm-pat˝i-bil´i-te) the unsuitability of one thing to another. 160, 163, 410

incontinence (in-kon´tĭ-nəns) inability to control excretory functions. 336

    urinary i., inability to control urination. 336, 348

induration (in˝du-ra´shən) the quality of being or becoming hard; an abnormally hard spot. 537

infarct (in´fahrkt) an area of necrosis in a tissue caused by local ischemia resulting from obstruction of circulation to the area. 196

infarction (in-fahrk´shən) the formation of a localized area of necrosis caused by insufficient blood supply, produced by an occlusion. 196

    myocardial i., death of an area of the heart muscle, occurring as a result of oxygen deprivation. 196

infectious (in-fek´shəs) capable of being transmitted; pertaining to a disease caused by a microorganism; producing infection. 82, 83*t*

    i. mononucleosis, an acute infectious disease that primarily affects lymphoid tissue. The cause of most cases of infectious mononucleosis is the Epstein-Barr virus. 154

inferior (in-fēr´e-ər) situated below or directed downward; in anatomy it is used in reference to the lower surface of a structure or to the lower of two or more similar structures. 122

inferomedian (in˝fər-o-me´de-ən) situated in the middle of the underside. 122, 130

infertility (in˝fər-til´i-te) diminished or absent capacity to produce offspring. 414

inflammation (in˝flə-ma´shən) a localized protective response elicited by injury or destruction of tissues. 128, 165*f*

influenza (in˝floo-en´zə) an acute viral infection involving the respiratory tract. 242, 294

infraclavicular (in˝frə-klə-vik´u-lər) below the collarbone. 439

infracostal (in˝frə-kos´təl) below a rib. 438

infrapatellar (in˝frə-pə-tel´ər) beneath the kneecap. 442

infrascapular (in˝frə-skap´u-lər) beneath the shoulderblade. 439

infrasternal (in˝frə-stur´nəl) beneath the breastbone. 437

ingest (in-jest´) taking food, medicine, etc., into the body by mouth. 76

ingestion (in-jes´chən) the act of taking food, medicines, etc., into the body by mouth. 266

inguinal (ing´gwĭ-nəl) pertaining to the groin. 126

    i. node, one of several lymph nodes located in the groin. 210

    i. regions, the abdominal area on both sides of the pubic area. 126, 126*f*

inhalation (in˝hə-la´shən) drawing air or other substances into the nasal or oral respiratory route; any drug administered by the respiratory route. 226

inhale (in-hāl) to take into the lungs by breathing. 104

injection (in-jek´shən) the forcing of a liquid into a part; a substance that is injected. 102

    intradermal i., placement of a small amount of a drug into the outer layers of the skin with a very fine gauge, short needle. 102, 103*f*

    intramuscular i., the deposition of medication into a muscular layer, usually in the anterior thigh, deltoid, or one of the buttocks. 102, 103*f*

    intravenous i., injection into a vein. 102, 103*f*

    subcutaneous i., injection of a small amount of medication below the skin layer into the subcutaneous tissue. 102, 103*f*

inspiration (in˝spĭ-ra´shən) the drawing of air into the lungs. 226, 231*f*

insula (in´sə-lə) a portion of the cerebral cortex. 489, 489*f*

insulin (in´sə-lin) a hormone secreted by the beta cells of the islets of Langerhans of the pancreas into the blood. 282, 573

integument (in-teg´u-mənt) a covering or investment. 532

integumentary (in-teg-u-men´tə-re) pertaining to, composed of, or serving as skin. 532

interalveolar (in˝tər-al-ve´o-lər) between the alveoli. 230

intercellular (in˝tər-sel´u-lər) situated between the cells of a structure. 102, 142

intercostal (in˝tər-kos´təl) between the ribs. 438

    i. muscles, the muscles that move the ribs when breathing. 438

interdental (in˝tər-den´təl) between the teeth. 273

interferon (in˝tər-fēr´on) any of a family of glycoproteins that exert nonspecific antiviral activity, have immunoregulatory functions, and can inhibit the growth of nonviral intracellular parasites. 164, 165*f*

intermammary (in˝tər-mam´ə-re) between the breasts. 572

internal os (os) the internal opening of the cervical canal. 409

internist (in-tur´nist) a specialist in internal medicine. 19

interocular (in˝tər-ok´u-lər) between the eyes. 493

interrenal (in˝tər-re´nəl) situated between the kidneys. 322

interscapular (in˝tər-skap´u lər) between the shoulder blades. 440

interstitial (in˝tər-stish´əl) pertaining to or situated between parts or in the interspaces of a tissue. 142

    i. cells of Leydig, cells in the testes that are responsible for the production of testosterone. 381, 381*f*

    i. fluid, tissue fluid or fluid occupying spaces between tissue cells. 142

intervertebral (in˝tər-vur´tə-brəl) between two contiguous vertebrae. 436

    i. disk, the layer of fibrocartilage between the bodies of adjoining vertebrae. 436

intestinal (in-tes´tĭ-nəl) pertaining to the intestine. 271

intraarticular (in˝trə-ahr-tik´u-lər) within a joint. 452

intracellular (in˝trə-sel´u-lər) within a cell. 102

intracranial (in˝trə-kra´ne-əl) within the skull. 508

intradermal (in˝trə-dur´məl) situated within the skin. 102

intramuscular (in˝trə-mus´ku-lər) situated in the muscle. 102

intraocular (in˝trə-ok´u-lər) situated within the eye. 493

    i. lens, a plastic lens inserted into the capsule of the lens after cataract surgery. 520

intrathecal (in˝trə-the´kəl) within a sheath or within the spinal canal. 491

intrauterine (in˝trə-u´tər-in) within the uterus. 160, 411

    i. device (IUD), a contraceptive device inserted into the uterine cavity. 412, 412*f*, 413*t*

intravenous (in˝trə-ve´nəs) situated within the vein. 102

    i. pyelography, roentgenography of the ureter and renal pelvis after intravenous injection of a radiopaque material. 333

    i. urography, radiography of the urinary tract after intravenous introduction of a radiopaque medium. 333, 333*f*

intubation (in˝too-ba´shən) insertion of a tube into a body canal or organ. 250

    endotracheal i., insertion of a tube into the trachea. 250, 251*f*

    nasotracheal i., insertion of a tube through the nose into the trachea to serve as an airway. 250, 251*f*

    orotracheal i., insertion of a tube through the mouth into the trachea to serve as an airway. 250, 251*f*

intussusception (in˝tə-sə-sep´shən) the prolapse of one part of the intestine into the lumen of an immediately joining part. 296*f*, 297

inversion (in-vur´zhən) a turning inward, inside-out, upside-down, or other reversal of the normal relation of a part. 449*f*, 450

in vitro (in ve´tro) in an artificial environment or within a test tube. 150

in vivo (in ve´vo) within the living body. 150

ipsilateral (ip˝sĭ-lat´ər-əl) situated on, pertaining to, or affecting the same side. 102

iris (i´ris) the circular pigmented membrane behind the cornea. 494, 494*f*

iritis (i-ri´tis) inflammation of the iris, usually marked by pain, congestion in the ciliary region, photophobia, contraction of the pupil, and discoloration of the iris. 510

ischemia (is-ke´me-ə) deficiency of blood from functional constriction or actual obstruction of a blood vessel. 196

ischial (is´ke-əl) pertaining to the ischium, a bone of the pelvis. 440

ischialgia (is˝ke-al´jə) pain in the ischium. 457

ischiococcygeal (is˝ke-o-kok-sij´e-əl) pertaining to the ischium and the coccyx (tailbone). 441

ischiodynia (is˝ke-o-din´e-ə) pain in the ischium. 457

ischiofemoral (is˝ke-o-fem´o-rəl) pertaining to the ischium and the femur. 442

ischiopubic (is˝ke-o-pu´bik) pertaining to the ischium and pubic region. 441

ischium (is´ke-əm) the inferior, dorsal portion of the hip bone. 443*f*, 440

islets of Langerhans (i´lətz of lahng´ər-hahnz) irregular microscopic structures scattered throughout the pancreas and constituting the endocrine portion. In humans they are composed of at least three types of cells that secrete insulin, glucagon, and somatostatin. 282, 564, 564*f*

isograft (i´so-graft) surgical transplantation of tissue from identical twins. 163

isotonic (i´so-ton´ik) equal tension; denoting a solution in which body cells can be placed without net flow of water across the cell's semipermeable membrane; denoting a solution that has the same tonicity as another solution with which it is compared. 158

jaundice (jawn´dis) yellowness of the skin, sclerae, and excretions because of increased bilirubin in the blood and deposition of bile pigments. 79, 79*f*, 298

jejunal (jə-joo´nəl) pertaining to the jejunum. 278

jejunoileostomy (jə-joo˝no-il˝e-os´tə-me) formation of a new opening between the jejunum and the ileum. 304

jejunostomy (jě˝joo-nos´tə-me) surgical creation of a permanent opening between the jejunum and the surface of the abdominal wall; also the opening it creates. 300

jejunotomy (jě˝joo-not´ə-me) surgical incision of the jejunum. 305

jejunum (jə-joo´nəm) that portion of the small intestine that extends from the duodenum to the ileum. 278, 278*f*

joint (joint) the site of junction or union between two or more bones. 444

   j. crepitus, a clicking sound often heard in movement of joints. 456

   metatarsophalangeal j., any of the joints between the metatarsals and the bones of the toes. 458

   synovial j., a general classification of joints that have a cavity between articulating bones and are freely movable. 444, 445*f*

   temporomandibular j., one of a pair of joints connecting the mandible of the jaw to the temporal bone of the skull. 444

Kaposi sarcoma (kah´po-shē, kap´o-sē sahr-ko´mə) a malignant neoplastic proliferation characterized by the development of bluish-red cutaneous nodules, usually on the lower extremities, that slowly increase in size and number and spread to more proximal sites. 167, 417, 419*f*

karyomegaly (kar˝e-o-meg´ə-le) abnormal enlargement of the cell nucleus. 153

Kegel exercises (keg´əl ek´sər-sī-zəs) exercises performed to strengthen the pubococcygeal muscle. 348

keloid (ke´loid) a sharply elevated, irregularly shaped, progressively enlarging scar resulting from formation of excessive amounts of collagen in the dermis during connective tissue repair. 545

keratin (ker´ə-tin) a protein that forms the epidermis, hair, and all horny tissue. 532

keratitis (ker˝ə-ti´tis) inflammation of the cornea. 510

keratogenesis (ker˝ə-to-jen´ə-sis) the formation of horny material. 532

keratoma (ker˝ə-to´mə) a horny tumor; a tumor composed of keratin. 543

keratosis (ker˝ə-to´sis) any horny growth; a condition of the skin characterized by the formation of horny growths or excessive development of the horny growth. 543

   seborrheic k., a common benign, noninvasive tumor of the skin characterized by soft, crumbly plaques, varying in pigmentation and occurring most often on the face, trunk, and extremities usually in middle life. 543, 544*f*

keratotomy (ker˝ə-tot´ə-me) surgical incision of the cornea. 520

   radial k., an operation in which a series of incisions is made in the cornea from its outer edge toward its center in spokelike fashion; done to flatten the cornea and thus to correct myopia. 520

ketoacidosis (ke˝to-as˝ĭ-do´sis) acidosis accompanied by the accumulation of ketone bodies (ketosis) in the body tissues and fluids. 328

ketone (ke´tōn) a compound that is a normal end product of lipid metabolism. 576

ketonuria (ke˝to-nu´re-ə) excretion of ketones in the urine. 328, 576

kidney (kid´ne) either of the two bean-shaped organs in the lumbar region that filter the blood, excreting the waste products in the form of urine and regulating the concentration of certain ions in the extracellular fluid. 321, 321*f*, 322

kidney—cont'd

   k. dialysis, removal of impurities or wastes from the blood of patients with renal failure or various toxic conditions. 343

   polycystic k., a heritable disorder marked by cysts scattered throughout both kidneys. 336, 387*f*

kleptomania (klep˝to-ma´ne-ə) an uncontrollable impulse to steal objects unnecessary for personal use or monetary value. 71, 516

kyphosis (ki-fo´sis) abnormally increased convexity in the curvature of the thoracic spine as viewed from the side; hunchback. 462, 462*f*

labia (la´be-ə) fleshy edges, usually designating the labia majora and labia minora. 360

   l. majora, a pair of elongated folds running downward and backward from the mons pubis in the female. 360, 360*f*

   l. minora, a small fold of skin located on each side between the labium majorus and the opening of the vagina. 360, 360*f*

labor (la´bər) the function of the female by which the product of conception is expelled from the uterus through the vagina to the outside world. 405, 406*f*

laceration (las˝ər-a´shən) the act of tearing; a torn, ragged wound. 545, 545*f*

lacrimal (lak´rĭ-məl) pertaining to the tears. 228, 495

   l. sac, upper dilated portion of the nasolacrimal duct. 495

lacrimation (la˝rĭ-ma´shən) secretion and discharge of tears; crying. 495

lactase (lak´tās) an enzyme that breaks down lactose. A deficiency of this enzyme may result in symptoms of lactose intolerance. 74

lactate dehydrogenase test (lak´tāt de-hi´dro-jən-ās) a blood test used to detect levels of LDH. Disease or injury to body tissues such as the heart and liver results in increased levels of LDH. 191

lactation (lak-ta´shən) the secretion of milk or the period of milk secretion. 571

lactiferous (lak-tif´ər-əs) producing or conveying milk. 571

   l. duct, tubular channel that conveys milk from the mammary gland. 571

   l. sinus, a dilated portion of a lactiferous duct that serves as a reservoir for milk. 571

lactogenesis (lak˝to-jen´ə-sis) the origin or formation of milk. 571

lactogenic (lak˝to-jen´ik) stimulating the production of milk. 571

   l. hormone, one of the gonadotropic hormones produced by the anterior pituitary; stimulates and maintains secretion of milk in postpartum mammals. 571

lactose (lak´tōs) the main sugar present in milk of mammals. 74, 268

   l. intolerance, a sensitivity disorder resulting in the inability to digest lactose from milk products. 74, 268

laminectomy (lam˝ĭ-nek´tə-me) excision of the posterior arch of a vertebra. 469

laparocholecystotomy (lap´ə-ro-ko˝lə-sis-tot´ə-me) removal of the gallbladder by incision of the abdominal wall. 307

laparoenterostomy (lap´ə-ro-en˝tər-os´tə-me) surgical creation of an artificial opening into the intestine through the abdominal wall. 304

laparohysterectomy (lap´ə-ro-his˝te-rek´tə-me) laparoscopic fixation of the uterus. 378

laparorrhaphy (lap´ə-ror´ə-fe) suture of the abdominal wall. 412

laparoscope (lap´ə-ro-skōp˝) an endoscope used for examining the peritoneal cavity. 368, 369*f*

laparoscopic (lap´ə-ro-skop´ik) pertaining to laparoscopy. 344

   l. cholecystectomy, removal of the gallbladder through small incisions in the abdominal wall. 307

   l. nephrectomy, removal of a kidney through several small incisions in the abdominal wall. 344

laparoscopy (lap´ə-ros´kə-pe) examination of the interior of the abdomen with a laparoscope. 368, 369*f*

laparotomy (lap´ə-rot´ə-me) surgical incision through the abdominal wall. 412

laryngalgia (lar˝in-gal´jə) pain in the larynx. 412

laryngeal (lə-rin´je-əl) pertaining to the larynx. 229

laryngectomy (lar˝in-jek´tə-me) excision of the larynx. 250

laryngitis (lar˝in-ji´tis) inflammation of the voice box. 241

laryngography (lar˝ing-gog´rə-fe) roentgenography of the larynx after instillation of a radiopaque substance. 232

laryngopathy (lar-ing-gop´ə-the) any disease of the larynx. 242

laryngopharyngeal (lə-ring˝go-fə-rin´je-əl) pertaining to the voice box and throat. 229

laryngopharynx (lə-ring˝go-far´ənks) that portion of the pharynx below the upper edge of the epiglottis, opening into the larynx and esophagus. 229

laryngoplegia (lə-ring˝go-ple´jə) paralysis of the voice box. 242

laryngoscope (lə-ring´gə-skōp) instrument used for examination of the larynx. 232

laryngoscopy (lar″ing-gos′kə-pe) examination of the larynx with a laryngoscope. 232

laryngospasm (lə-ring′go-spaz″əm) spasmodic closure of the larynx. 242

laryngotracheal (lə-ring″go-tra′ke-əl) pertaining to the larynx and the trachea. 244

laryngotracheitis (lə-ring″go-tra″ke-i′tis) inflammation of the larynx and the trachea. 244

laryngotracheobronchitis (lə-ring″go-tra″ke-o-brong-ki′tis) inflammation of the larynx, trachea, and bronchi. 244

larynx (lar′inks) the organ of voice; the air passage between the lower pharynx and the trachea. 24, 228, 229

lateral (lat′ər-əl) pertaining to a side; denoting a position farther from the median plane or midline of the body or of a structure. 118

lavage (lah-vahzh′) the irrigation or washing out of an organ; to wash out or irrigate. 302

laxative (lak′sə-tiv) mildly cathartic; an agent that acts to promote evacuation of the bowel; a cathartic or purgative. 306

leiomyoma (li″o-mi-o′mə) a benign tumor derived from smooth muscle, most commonly of the uterus; also called fibroid and fibroid tumor. 373

lesion (le′zhən) any pathologic or traumatic discontinuity of tissue or loss of function of a part. 133, 541
  primary l., a sore or wound that is the initial reaction to injury or disease. 541, 541*f*
  secondary l., changes in the appearance of a primary lesion resulting in a different-appearing lesion. 542, 543*f*

lethargy (leth′ər-je) a lowered level of consciousness marked by listlessness, drowsiness, and lack of feeling or emotion. 106

leukemia (loo-ke′me-ə) a disease of the blood-forming organs characterized by a marked increase in the number of leukocytes, including young forms of leukocytes not usually seen in circulating blood. 155, 156, 460
  lymphoblastic l., leukemia in which lymphoblasts are the predominant type of leukocyte. 460
  lymphocytic l., leukemia in which lymphocytes are the predominant type of leukocyte. 460
  myelocytic l., leukemia in which myelocytes are the predominant type of leukocyte. 460
  myelogenous l., leukemia in which polymorphonuclear leukocytes are the predominant type of leukocyte. 460

leukocyte (loo′ko-sīt) a white blood cell. 151, 152*f*
  l. count, enumeration of the number of white blood cells in a blood sample. 151

leukocytopenia (loo″ko-si″to-pe′ne-ə) a deficiency in the number of white blood cells. 155

leukocytosis (loo″ko-si-to′sis) a transient increase in the number of leukocytes in the blood. 156

leukopenia (loo″ko-pe′ne-ə) a deficiency in the number of leukocytes in the blood. 155

leukoplakia (loo″ko-pla′ke-ə) a white patch on a mucous membrane. 290, 290*f*

leukorrhea (loo″ko-re′ə) a white, viscid discharge from the vagina or uterine cavity. 373

ligament (lig′ə-mənt) a band of fibrous tissue that connects bones or cartilages and supports and strengthens joints. 444, 445*f*

lingual (ling′gwəl) pertaining to or near the tongue. 273

lipase (lip′ās, li′pās) an enzyme that breaks down fats. 268

lipectomy (lĭ-pek′tə-me) excision of a mass of subcutaneous adipose tissue. 302, 552
  suction-assisted l., removal of fat by placing a narrow tube under the skin and applying a vacuum. 552, 552*f*

lipid (lip′id) a fat. 191, 268

lipoid (lip′oid) resembling fat. 268

lipolysis (lĭ-pol′ə-sis) the dissolution of fat. 552

lipoma (lip-o′mə) a tumor composed of fatty tissue. 543

lipopenia (lip″o-pe′ne-ə) a deficiency of fats in the body. 297

lipoprotein (lip″o-, li″po-pro′tēn) any of the lipid-protein complexes in which lipids are transported in the blood. 191
  high-density l., a plasma protein that contains approximately 50% lipoprotein along with cholesterol, triglycerides, and phospholipid and is associated with decreased cardiac risk profiles. 191
  low-density l., a plasma protein containing relatively more cholesterol and triglycerides than protein. 191

liposuction (lip″o-suk′shən) surgical removal of localized fat deposits using high-pressure vacuum, applied by means of a subdermal cannula. 302, 552, 552*f*

lithotomy (lĭ-thot′ə-me) incision of a duct or organ for removal of a calculus. 346

lithotripsy (lith′o-trip″se) the crushing of a calculus within the urinary system or gallbladder, followed at once by the washing out of the fragments. 307, 307*f*, 346, 346*f*
  extracorporeal shock wave l., a procedure for treating gallstones and upper urinary tract stones. The patient is immersed in a large tub of water or placed in contact with a water cushion. A high-energy shock wave is focused on the stone, which disintegrates into particles small enough to be expelled. 306, 307, 346, 346*f*

lithotriptor (lith′o-trip″tər) an instrument for crushing calculi. 307

lithotrite (lith′o-trīt) an instrument for crushing a urinary calculus. 346

lobectomy (lo-bek′tə-me) excision of a lobe, as removal of a lobe of the lung, brain, or liver. 252
  hepatic l., excision of a lobe of the liver. 306

lobule (lob′ūl) a small lobe. 571

loop of Henle (loop əv hen′le) a long, U-shaped part of the renal tubule, extending through the medulla from the end of the proximal convoluted tubule to the beginning of the distal convoluted tubule. 324, 324*f*

lordosis (lor-do′sis) the anterior concavity in the curvature of the lumbar and cervical spine as viewed from the side. The term is used to refer to abnormally increased curvature (swayback) and to the normal curvature (normal lordosis). 462, 462*f*

lumbar (lum′bahr, lum′bər) pertaining to the lower back. 436
  l. puncture, the introduction of a hollow needle into the subarachnoid space of the lumbar part of the spinal canal. 451, 452, 452*f*, 497
  l. region, lateral abdominal region on each side of the umbilical region. 125, 125*f*

lumen (loo′mən) the cavity or channel within a tube. 199

lumpectomy (ləm-pek′tə-me) surgical excision of only the palpable lesion in carcinoma of the breast; surgical removal of a mass. 586

lunula (loo′nu-lə) a small crescent- or moon-shaped area. 535

lupus erythematosis (LE) (loo′pəs er″ə-them″ə-to′sis) a group of connective tissue disorders primarily affecting women, with a spectrum of clinical forms in which cutaneous disease may occur with or without systemic involvement. 464, 465*f*
  cutaneous l. e., a form of lupus erythematosus in which the skin may be the only organ involved, or it may precede the involvement of other systems. 465
  discoid l. e. (DLE), a chronic form of cutaneous lupus erythematosus in which the skin lesions mimic those of the systemic form but systemic signs are rare, although multisystem manifestations may develop after many years. 465
  systemic l. e., a chronic inflammatory, collagen disease affecting many systems of the body. 465, 465*f*

luteinizing hormone (loo′te-in-i″zing hor′mōn) a hormone secreted by the anterior lobe of the hypophysis that stimulates development of the corpus luteum. 364, 568

Lyme disease (līm dĭ-zēz′) a recurrent multisystemic disorder, beginning with a rash and followed by arthritis of the large joints, myalgia, malaise, and neurologic and cardiac manifestations. It is caused by the bacteria *Borrelia burgdorferi,* carried by the deer tick *Ixodes dammini.* 465

lymph (limf) a transparent fluid found in lymphatic vessels consisting of a liquid portion and cells that are mostly lymphocytes. 145, 208
  l. node, any of the small knots of lymphatic tissue found at intervals along the course of the lymphatic vessels. 208, 209*f*, 210

lymphadenectomy (lim-fad″ə-nek′tə-me) surgical excision of a lymph node or nodes. 214

lymphadenitis (lim-fad″ə-ni′tis) inflammation of a lymph node. 212, 212*f*

lymphadenopathy (lim-fad″ə-nop′ə-the) any disease of the lymph nodes. 213

lymphangiography (lim-fan″je-og′rə-fe) roentgenography of the lymphatic vessels after the injection of contrast medium. 211

lymphangioma (lim-fan″je-o′mə) a tumor composed of newly formed lymph channels. 200

lymphangitis (lim″fan-ji′tis) inflammation of a lymphatic vessel. 213, 213*f*

lymphatics (lim-fat′iks) a system of vessels that collects tissue fluids from all parts of the body and returns the fluids to the blood circulation; lymphatic system. 145, 208, 209*f*

lymphedema (lim″fə-de′mə) chronic edema of an extremity because of obstruction within the lymph vessels or the lymph nodes, resulting in accumulation of interstitial fluid. 212, 212*f*

lymphocyte (lim′fo-sīt) any of the mononuclear leukocytes found in the blood, lymph, and lymphoid tissues that are responsible for humoral and cellular immunity. 152, 152*f*

lymphogenous (lim-foj′ə-nəs) producing lymph; produced from lymph or in the lymphatics. 209

menopause (men´o-pawz) that period in a woman´s life when menstruation ceases. 364

menorrhagia (men″ə-ra´jə) abnormally profuse menstruation. 370

menorrhea (men″ə-re´ə) menstruation; too profuse menstruation. 370

menses (men´sēz) menstruation, the monthly flow of blood from the female genital tract. 366, 370

menstruation (men″stroo-a´shən) the cyclic, physiologic discharge through the vagina of blood and mucosal tissues from the nonpregnant uterus. 364

mental retardation (men´təl) abnormally low intellectual functioning. 514

mesenteric (mez″ən-ter´ik) pertaining to the mesentery, a fold of the peritoneum. 297

　m. occlusion, a binding or closing off of a segment of the intestine by the mesentery. 296f, 297

mesoderm (mez´o-, me´zo-dərm) in embryology, the middle layer of cells in the blastoderm. 533

mesothelioma (mez″o-, me″zo-the″le-o´mə) a tumor derived from mesothelial tissue. 248

mesothelium (mez″o-, me″zo-the´le-əm) the layer of flat cells forming the squamous epithelium that covers all true serous membranes in adults. 248

metabolism (mə-tab´ə-liz″əm) the sum of all the physical and chemical processes by which living organized substance is produced and maintained (anabolism), and also the transformation by which energy is made available for the uses of the organism (catabolism). 267

metacarpal (met″ə-kahr´pəl) pertaining to the metacarpus, the part of the hand between the wrist and fingers; one of the bones of the metacarpus. 439, 440

metastasis (mə-tas´tə-sis) a growth of pathogenic microorganisms or of abnormal cells distant from the site primarily involved by the morbid process. 89

metastasize (me-tas´tə-sīz) to form new foci of disease in a distant part by metastasis. 89

metatarsal (met″ə-tahr´səl) pertaining to the metatarsus; a bone of the metatarsus. 442, 442f

metritis (mə-tri´tis) inflammation of uterine tissue. 363

metrorrhagia (me″tro-ra´jə) uterine bleeding, usually of normal amount, occurring at completely irregular intervals, the period of flow sometimes being prolonged. 370

microbe (mi´krōb) a minute living organism, such as a bacterium, protozoan, or fungus. 130

microbiology (mi″kro-bi-ol´ə-je) the science that deals with the study of microorganisms. 83

microcardia (mi″kro-kahr´de-ə) smallness of the heart. 196

microcyte (mi´kro-sīt) an abnormally small erythrocyte, microns or less in diameter. 158, 159f

microcytosis (mi″kro-si-to´sis) an increase in the number of undersized red blood cells. 158

microorganism (mi″kro-or´gən-iz-əm) a minute living organism, usually microscopic; types include bacteria, rickettsiae, viruses, molds, yeasts, and protozoa. 83

microscope (mi´kro-skōp) an instrument for viewing small objects that must be magnified to be seen. 76

microscopic (mi″kro-skop´ik) of extremely small size and visible only by the aid of a microscope. 105

microscopy (mi-kros´kə-pe) viewing things with a microscope. 76, 88

microtia (mi-kro´shə) severe hypoplasia or aplasia of the pinna of the ear, with a blind or absent external auditory meatus. 105, 105f

micturition (mik″tu-rĭ´shən) urination. 325

midbrain (mid´brān″) the part of the brain that connects the pons and the cerebellum with the hemispheres of the cerebrum; mesencephalon. 490, 490f

midsagittal plane (mid-saj´ĭ-təl) the plane vertically dividing the body through the midline into right and left halves. 118, 119f

milligram (mil´ĭ-gram) one thousandth of a gram. 99

millimeter (mil´ĭ-me″tər) a unit of length; one thousandth of a meter. 99

mineralocorticoid (min″ər-əl-o-kor´tĭ-koid) any of the group of corticosteroids, principally aldosterone, predominantly involved in the regulation of electrolyte and water balance in the body. 570

mitral (mi´trəl) pertaining to the mitral or bicuspid valve; shaped like a miter. 185

　m. valve, a bicuspid valve situated between the left atrium and the left ventricle; bicuspid valve. 185, 184f

　m. valve prolapse, protrusion of one or both cusps of the mitral valve back into the left atrium during ventricular contraction. 197

mittelschmerz (mit´əl-shmertz) pain associated with ovulation, usually occurring in the middle of the menstrual cycle. 370

molar (mo´lər) a posterior tooth that is used for grinding food and acts as a major jaw support in the dental arch. 274, 274f

Monilia (mo-nil´e-ə) a genus of fungi. 420

moniliasis (mon-ĭ-li´ə-sis) candidiasis; any infection caused by a species of *Candida,* especially *Candida albicans.* 420

monoplegia (mon″o-ple´jə) paralysis of a limb. 505

mons (monz) a general term for an elevation, or eminence. 359

　m. pubis, the rounded fleshy prominence over the symphysis pubis. 359

mucoid (mu´koid) resembling mucus. 272

mucolytic (mu″ko-lit´ik) dissolving mucus; an agent that dissolves or destroys mucus. 255

mucosa (mu-ko´sə) mucous membrane. 272

mucous (mu´kəs) pertaining or relating to or resembling mucus; mucoid; covered with mucus; secreting, producing, or containing mucus. 146, 272

　m. colitis, irritable bowel syndrome. 295

mucus (mu´kəs) the free slime of the mucous membranes, composed of secretion of the glands, various salts, desquamated cells, and leukocytes. 79, 146, 272

multigravida (mul″tĭ-grav´ĭ-də) a female who has been pregnant more than once. 404

multipara (məl″tip´ə-rə) a female who has produced more than one viable offspring. 405

multiple myeloma (mul´tĭ-pəl mi″ə-lo´mə) a disseminated type of plasma cell dyscrasia characterized by multiple bone marrow tumors. 459

murmur (mur´mər) an auscultatory sound, particularly a periodic sound of short duration of cardiac or vascular origin. 195

　heart m., an abnormal sound heard on auscultation of the heart, caused by altered blood flow into a chamber or through a valve. 195, 197

muscle (mus´əl) an organ that produces movement of an animal by contraction. 116, 116f, 446, 446f

　arrector pili m., minute smooth muscle attached to the connective tissue sheath of the hair follicle, capable of causing the hair to stand erect. 534

　cardiac m., the muscle of the heart. 446, 446f

　m. relaxant, an agent that causes the muscles to relax. 469

　skeletal m., striated muscles that are attached to bones and bring about voluntary movement. 446, 446f

　visceral m., muscle that is associated chiefly with the hollow viscera. 446, 446f

muscular (mus´ku-lər) pertaining to or composing muscle; having a well-developed musculature. 81, 446

　m. dystrophy, a genetically determined myopathy characterized by atrophy and wasting away of muscles. 463

musculoskeletal (mus″ku-lo-skel´ə-təl) pertaining to or being composed of the skeleton and the muscles, as musculoskeletal system. 430

myalgia (mi-al´jə) pain in a muscle or muscles. 81, 455

myasthenia (mi″əs-the´ne-ə) muscle weakness. 466

　m. gravis, a disease characterized by muscle weakness, caused by a functional abnormality. 466, 509

mycodermatitis (mi″ko-der″mə-ti´tis) inflammation of the skin caused by a fungus. 540

myelin sheath (mi´ə-lin shēth) the sheath surrounding the axon of some (the myelinated) nerve cells. 486f, 487

myelinated (mi´ə-lĭ-nāt″əd) having a myelin sheath. 487

myelitis (mi″ə-li´tis) inflammation of the bone marrow; inflammation of the spinal cord. 459

myeloblast (mi´ə-lo-blast) embryonic form of blood cell found in the bone marrow. 432

myelocyte (mi´ə-lo-sīt) a cell found in the bone marrow. 432

myelogram (mi´ə-lo-gram) x-ray film of the spinal cord. 498

myelography (mi″ə-log´rə-fe) roentgenography of the spinal cord after injection of a contrast medium into the subarachnoid space. 498

myelosuppression (mi″ə-lo-sə-presh´ən) inhibition of bone marrow activity. 451

myelosuppressive (mi″ə-lo-sə-pres´iv) inhibiting bone marrow activity; an agent that inhibits bone marrow activity. 471

myoblast (mi´o-blast) embryonic cell that becomes a cell of the muscle fiber. 446

myocardial (mi″o-kahr´de-əl) pertaining to the muscular tissue of the heart. 182

　m. infarction, development of an infarct in the myocardium, usually the result of ischemia after occlusion of a coronary artery. 196, 197f

myocarditis (mi″o-kahr-di´tis) inflammation of the heart muscle. 198

myocardium (mi″o-kahr´de-əm) the middle and thickest layer of the heart wall, made up of cardiac muscle. 447

myocele (mi´o-sēl) hernia of the muscle. 446

myocellulitis (mi″o-sel″u-li´tis) inflammation of cellular tissue and muscle. 459

myodynia (mi″o-din´e-ə) pain in a muscle. 455

myofascial (mi″o-fash´e-əl) pertaining to or involving the fascia surrounding and associated with muscle tissue. 466

myofibrosis (mi″o-fi-bro´sis) replacement of muscle tissue by fibrous tissue. 466

myolysis (mi-ol´ĭ-sis) destruction of muscle tissue. 466

myomalacia (mi″o-mə-la´shə) morbid softening of muscle. 466

myometritis (mi″o-mə-tri´tis) inflammation of the myometrium, the muscular substance of the uterus. 373

myometrium (mi-o-me´tre-əm) the smooth muscle of the uterus. 363

myopathy (mi-op´ə-the) any disease of muscle. 466

myopia (mi-o´pe-ə) the error of refraction in which rays of light entering the eye are brought to a focus in front of the retina; also called nearsightedness. 511, 512f

myoplasty (mi´o-plas″te) surgical repair of a muscle. 469

myorrhaphy (mi-or´ə-fe) suture of divided muscle. 469

myxedema (mik″sə-de´mə) a condition resulting from hypothyroidism characterized by dry, waxy swelling of the skin. 580

narcolepsy (nahr´ko-lep″se) recurrent, uncontrollable brief episodes of sleep. 508

narcotic (nahr-kot´ik) pertaining to or producing narcosis, nonspecific and reversible depression of function of the central nervous system marked by stupor or insensibility produced by drugs; an agent that produces insensibility or stupor, applied especially to the opioids. 56, 520

nares (na´rēz) the nostrils, the external opening of the nose. 228

naris (na´ris) either of the external orifices of the nose. 228

nasal (na´zəl) pertaining to the nose. 80, 228

nasogastric (na″zo-gas´trik) pertaining to the nose and stomach. 291
   n. tube, any tube passed into the stomach through the nose. 291, 300, 301f

nasolacrimal (na″zo-lak´rĭ-məl) pertaining to the nose and lacrimal apparatus. 228, 495
   n. duct, a tubular passage that carries tears from the eye to the nose. 228

nasopharyngeal (na″zo-fə-rin´je-əl) pertaining to the nasopharynx. 229

nasopharyngitis (na´zo-far″in-ji´tis) inflammation of the nasopharynx. 241

nasopharynx (na″zo-far´inks) the upper part of the pharynx, continuous with the nasal passages. 229

nasoscope (na´zo-skōp) instrument for examining inside the nose. 232

nasotracheal (na″zo-tra´ke-əl) pertaining to the nose and trachea. 250

natal (na´təl) pertaining to birth. 402

nebulizer (neb´u-li″zər) a device for creating and throwing an aerosol spray. 254

necrosis (nə-kro´sis) death of tissue. 147, 547, 547f

necrotic (nə-krot´ik) pertaining to or characterized by necrosis. 147

neonatal (ne″o-na´təl) pertaining to a newborn child, usually designating the first weeks after birth. 406

neonate (ne´o-nāt) a newborn child. 406

neonatologist (ne″o-na-tol´ə-jist) a physician who specializes in care of the newborn. 23, 406

neonatology (ne″o-na-tol´ə-je) the branch of medicine dealing with treatment of the newborn infant. 23, 406

neoplasm (ne´o-plaz-əm) a new or abnormal growth either benign or malignant. 291

nephrectomy (nə-frek´tə-me) surgical excision of a kidney. 344

nephritis (nə-fri´tis) inflammation of the kidney. 336, 339

nephrolith (nef´ro-lith) a kidney stone. 340

nephrolithiasis (nef″ro-lĭ-thi´ə-sis) a condition marked by the presence of kidney stones. 340

nephrolithotomy (nef″ro-lĭ-thot´ə-me) removal of renal calculi by cutting into the kidney. 347

nephrolysis (nə-frol´ə-sis) destruction of kidney tissue; freeing of a kidney from adhesions. 336

nephromalacia (nef″ro-mə-la´shə) softening of the kidney. 336

nephromegaly (nef″ro-meg´ə-le) enlargement of the kidney. 336

nephron (nef´ron) the structural and functional unit of the kidney. 323, 324f

nephropathy (nə-frop´ə-the) any disease of the kidneys. 339
   obstructive n., a kidney disease caused by obstruction of the urinary tract. 339

nephropexy (nef´ro-pek″se) surgical fixation of a floating kidney. 348

nephroptosis (nef″rop-to´sis, nef″ro-to´sis) downward displacement of the kidney; floating kidney. 348

nephrosclerosis (nef″ro-sklə-ro´sis) hardening of the kidney caused by renovascular disease. 341

nephroscope (nef´ro-skōp) an instrument inserted into an incision in the renal pelvis for viewing the interior of the kidney. 334, 334f

nephroscopy (nə-fros´kə-pe) visualization of the kidney using a nephroscope. 334

nephrosonography (nef″ro-so-nog´rə-fe) ultrasonic scanning of the kidney. 333

nephrostomy (nə-fros´tə-me) the creation of a fistula leading directly into the renal pelvis. 345, 345f
   n. catheter, a tube inserted into the renal pelvis for direct drainage of the urine through a percutaneous opening. 332
   percutaneous n., placement of a catheter into the kidney through the skin, providing for diversion of the renal output, certain surgical procedures, including biopsies, and infusion of substances to dissolve calculi. 331, 331f

nephrotic syndrome (nə-frot´ik sin´drōm) a clinical classification that includes all diseases of the kidney characterized by chronic loss of protein in the urine and subsequent depletion of body protein. 339

nephrotomogram (nef″ro-to´mo-gram) a sectional radiograph of the kidney obtained by nephrotomography. 333, 333f

nephrotomography (nef″ro-to-mog´rə-fe) radiologic visualization of the kidney by tomography after intravenous introduction of contrast medium. 333

nephrotoxic (nef´ro-tok″sik) destructive to kidney cells. 336

nephroureterectomy (nef″ro-u-re″tər-ek´tə-me) excision of a kidney and all or part of the ureter. 344

neural (noor´əl) pertaining to a nerve or the nerves. 73, 485

neuralgia (noo-ral´jə) pain of a nerve. 500

neurasthenia (noor″əs-the´ne-ə) a nervous condition characterized by chronic weakness, easy fatigability, and sometimes exhaustion. 516

neurectomy (noo-rek´tə-me) excision of a part of a nerve. 57, 518

neuritis (noo-ri´tis) inflammation of a nerve. 70

neuroglia (noo-rog´le-ə) the supporting structure of nervous tissue. 485

neurohypophysis (noor″o-hi-pof´ə-sis) the posterior lobe of the pituitary gland. 566

neurologic (noor″o-loj´ik) pertaining to neurology or the nervous system. 76

neurologist (noo-rol´ə-jist) a specialist in the treatment of nervous diseases. 26

neurology (noo-rol´ə-je) the branch of medicine that deals with the study of the nervous system. 26

neurolysis (noo-rol´ĭ-sis) release of a nerve sheath by cutting it longitudinally; operative breaking up of perineural adhesions; relief of tension on a nerve; exhaustion of nervous energy; destruction of nerve tissue. 57, 518

neuroma (noo-ro´mə) a tumor made up of nerve cells and nerve fibers. 508
   Morton n., a neuroma resulting from compression of a branch of the plantar nerve by the metatarsal heads. 458

neuromuscular (noor″o-mus´ku-lər) pertaining to the nerves and muscles. 56, 487
   n. blocking agent, a drug used to stop muscle contraction. 56

neuron (noor´on) any of the conducting cells of the nervous system. 26, 27f, 117f, 485, 486, 486f
   motor n., one of various efferent nerve cells that transmit impulses from either the brain or spinal cord. 487
   sensory n., an afferent nerve cell conveying sensory impulses. 487

neuroplasty (noor´o-plas″te) plastic repair of a nerve. 518

neurorrhaphy (noo-ror´ə-fe) suturing of a cut nerve. 518

neurosis (noo-ro´sis) former name for a category of mental disorders characterized by anxiety and avoidance behavior. In general, the term refers to disorders in which the symptoms are distressing to the person, behavior does not violate gross social norms, and there is no apparent organic cause. 71, 514

neurosurgeon (noor″o-sur´jən) a surgeon who specializes in work on the nervous system. 26

neurosurgery (noor´o-sur´jər-e) surgery of the nervous system. 26

neurosyphilis (noor″o-sif´ĭ-lis) the central nervous system manifestations of syphilis. 417

neurotransmitter (noor″o-trans´mit-ər) any of a group of substances that are released on excitation from the axon terminal of a neuron and travel across the synaptic cleft either to excite or to inhibit the target cell. 487

neutrophil (noo´tro-fil) a granular leukocyte having a nucleus with three to five lobes and cytoplasm containing fine inconspicuous granules. 152, 152f

nevus (ne´vəs) any congenital lesion of the skin; a birthmark. 543

nitroglycerin (ni´tro-glis´ər-in) a drug used chiefly in the prophylaxis and treatment of angina pectoris, administered sublingually. 207

nociceptor (no″sĭ-sep′tər) a receptor for pain caused by injury to body tissues. 493

nocturia (nok-tu′re-ə) excessive urination at night. 336

node (nōd) a small mass of tissue as a swelling, knot, or protuberance, either normal or abnormal. 72f, 186, 210, 210f

    n. of Ranvier, one of several constrictions in the myelin sheath of a nerve fiber. 486f, 487

nodule (nod′ūl) a small node that is solid and can be detected by touch. 541, 541f

nonarticular (non″ahr-tik′u-lər) not associated with a joint. 466

noninflammatory (non″in-flam′ə-tor″e) not characterized by inflammation. 293, 295

norepinephrine (nor″ep-ĭ-nef′rin) one of the naturally occurring catecholamines; a neurohormone and a major neurotransmitter. It is also secreted by the adrenal medulla and is released predominantly in response to hypotension and stress. 571

normocyte (nor′mo-sīt) a normal-sized red blood cell. 158

normocytic (nor″mo-sit′ik) relating to an erythrocyte that is normal in size, shape, and color. 158

nosocomial (nos″o-ko′me-əl) pertaining to or originating in a hospital. 82

    n. infection, an infection acquired while one is hospitalized. 82

nucleoid (noo′kle-oid) resembling a nucleus. 153

nucleoprotein (noo″kle-o-pro′tēn) a protein found in the nuclei of cells. 153

nullipara (nə-lip′ə-rə) a female individual who has never borne a child. 405

nurse (ners) one who makes a profession of caring for the sick or disabled or of aiding in the maintenance of health; to care for the sick; to nourish at the breast. 30

    licensed practical n., one who is a graduate of a school of practical nursing and who performs certain services to the sick under the supervision of a registered nurse. 30

    licensed vocational n., a graduate of a school of practical nursing who has been legally authorized to practice. 30

    n. midwife, an individual educated in the two disciplines of nursing and midwifery. 23

    registered n., a graduate nurse who is registered and licensed to practice by a state board of nurse examiners or other state authority. 30

nutrition (noo-trĭ′shən) the sum of the processes involved in taking in nutrients and assimilating and using them; nutriment. 266

    total parenteral n., the intravenous administration of the total nutrient requirements of a patient with gastrointestinal dysfunction. 301

nycturia (nik-tu′re-ə) frequent urination during the night, especially the passage of more urine at night than during the day. 336

obesity (o-bēs′ĭ-te) an increase in body weight beyond the limitation of skeletal and physical requirements, as the result of an excessive accumulation of fat in the body. 287

    endogenous o., obesity resulting from the dysfunction of the endocrine or metabolic function. 287

    exogenous o., obesity caused by a caloric intake greater than needed. 287

obsession (ob-sesh′ən) a recurrent, persistent thought, image, or impulse that is unwanted and comes involuntarily. 515

obstetric, obstetrical (ob-stet′rik, ob-stet′rĭ-kəl) pertaining to obstetrics. 23

obstetrician (ob″stə-trĭ′shən) a physician who specializes in the treatment of pregnancy, labor, and delivery. 23, 402

obstetrics (ob-stet′riks) a branch of surgery that deals with the management of pregnancy and delivery. 23, 407

occipital (ok-sip′ĭ-təl) pertaining to the occiput, the posterior part of the head; located near the occipital bone, as the occipital lobe of the brain. 435f, 489

    o. lobe, one of the five lobes of each cerebral hemisphere. 489, 489f

occlusion (o-kloo′zhən) the act of closing or state of being closed; the relation of the teeth of both jaws during mandibular activity; an obstruction. 199, 289f

ocular (ok′u-lər) of, pertaining to, or affecting the eye. 493

ointment (oint′mənt) a medication that contains fat and is of such consistency that it melts when applied to the skin. 551

olfaction (ol-fak′shən) the sense of smell; the act of smelling. 229, 495

olfactory (ol-fak′tə-re) pertaining to the sense of smell. 229, 495

oligospermia (ol″ĭ-go-spur′me-ə) deficiency in the number of spermatozoa in the semen. 384

oliguria (ol″ĭ-gu′re-ə) excretion of a diminished amount of urine in relation to the fluid intake, usually defined as less than 500 mL per 24 hours. 335

omphalic (om-fal′ik) pertaining to the navel. 133

omphalitis (om″fə-li′tis) inflammation of the navel. 134

omphalocele (om′fə-lo-sēl″) hernia of the navel. 133

omphaloma (om″fə-lo′mə) tumor of the navel. 134

omphalorrhagia (om″fə-lo-ra′jə) hemorrhage from the umbilicus. 134

omphalorrhexis (om″fə-lo-rek′sis) rupture of the umbilicus. 134

omphalus (om′fə-ləs) the navel. 134

oncologist (ong-kol′ə-jist) a specialist in the study and treatment of tumors. 23

oncology (ong-kol′ə-je) study of tumors. 23

    radiation o., the medical specialty that treats cancer with ionizing radiation. 55

onychectomy (on″ĭ-kek′tə-me) excision of a nail or nail bed; removal of the claws of an animal. 551

onychomalacia (on″ĭ-ko-mə-la′shə) softening of the nails. 548

onychomycosis (on″ĭ-ko-mi-ko′sis) a disease of the nails caused by a fungus. 548, 549f

onychopathy (on″ĭ-kop′ə-the) any disease of the nails. 548

onychophagia (on″ĭ-ko-fa′jə) habit of biting the nails. 535

onychophagist (on″ĭ-kof′ə-jist) one who has the habit of nail biting. 535

onychosis (on″ĭ-ko′sis) a condition of atrophy or dystrophy of the nails. 548

ooblast (o′o-blast) an embryonic egg. 401

oogenesis (o″o-jen′ə-sis) the origin and formation of eggs in the female sex. 366

oophoralgia (o″of-ər-al′jə) ovarian pain. 371

oophorectomy (o″of-ə-rek′tə-me) the removal of an ovary or ovaries. 376

    laparoscopic o., minimally invasive removal of an ovary by laparoscopic surgery. 376

oophoritis (o″of-ə-ri′tis) inflammation of an ovary. 371

oophoropathy (o-of′ə-rop′ə-the) any disease of the ovaries. 371

oophoropexy (o-of′ə-ro-pek″se) surgical fixation of the ovary. 376

oophorosalpingectomy (o-of′ə-ro-sal″pin-jek′tə-me) surgical removal of an ovary and uterine tube. 377

oophorosalpingitis (o-of′ə-ro-sal″pin-ji′tis) inflammation of an ovary and uterine tube. 371

ophthalmalgia (of″thəl-mal′jə) pain in the eye. 45, 511

ophthalmic (of-thal′mik) pertaining to the eye. 21, 493

ophthalmitis (of″thəl-mi′tis) inflammation of the eye. 70

ophthalmodynia (of-thal″mo-din′e-ə) pain in the eye. 45

ophthalmologic, ophthalmological (of″thəl-mə-loj′ik, of″thəl-mə-loj′ik-əl) pertaining to ophthalmology. 21

ophthalmologist (of″thəl-mol′ə-jist) a physician who specializes in the diagnosis and treatment of eye disease. 21

ophthalmology (of″thəl-mol′ə-je) the study of the eye and its diseases. 21

ophthalmomalacia (of-thal″mo-mə-la′shə) abnormal softness of the eye. 45, 511

ophthalmometer (of″thəl-mom′ə-tər) an instrument for measuring the eye. 498

ophthalmopathy (of″thəl-mop′ə-the) any disease of the eye. 71

ophthalmoplasty (of-thal′mo-plas″te) plastic surgery of the eye or its appendages. 58

ophthalmoplegia (of-thal″mo-ple′jə) paralysis of the eye muscles. 511

ophthalmorrhagia (of-thal″mo-ra′jə) hemorrhage from the eye. 511

ophthalmoscope (of-thal′mə-skōp) an instrument used to examine the interior of the eye. 46, 498

ophthalmoscopy (of″thəl-mos′kə-pe) examination of the eye using an ophthalmoscope. 46, 46f, 498

ophthalmotomy (of″thəl-mot′ə-me) incision of the eyeball. 58

opioid (o′pe-oid) any synthetic narcotic that has opiate-like activities but is not derived from opium; any of a group of naturally occurring peptides that bind at or otherwise influence opiate receptors of cell membranes. 519

    o. analgesics, a class of compounds that block the perception of pain or affect the emotional response to pain. 519

optic nerve (op′tik) a cranial nerve that transmits visual impulses. 494, 494f

optical (op′tĭ-kəl) pertaining to vision. 31

optometrist (op-tom′ə-trist) a specialist in optometry. 31

optometry (op-tom′ə-tre) the professional practice of primary eye and vision care for the diagnosis, treatment, and prevention of associated disorders and for the improvement of vision by the prescription of spectacles and by use of other functional, optical, and pharmaceutical means regulated by state law. 31

oral (or′əl) pertaining to the oral cavity or mouth. 31, 228, 270

    o. surgeon, a physician specialized in oral surgery. 31

    o. thermometer, an instrument designed for measuring temperature by mouth. 49

orchialgia (or″ke-al′jə) pain in a testis. 385

orchidalgia (or″kĭ-dal′jə) pain in a testis. 385

orchiditis (or″kĭ-di′tis) inflammation of a testicle. 385

Papanicolaou test, Pap smear, Pap test (pap″ə-nik´o-la-oo) collection of material from areas of the body that shed cells, especially the cervix and the vagina, followed by microscopic study of the cells for diagnosing cancer. 366, 367*f*

papule (pap´ūl) a red, elevated, solid, and circumscribed area of the skin. 541, 541*f*

paralysis (pə-ral´ĭ-sis) loss or impairment of motor function caused by neural or muscular lesions. 505

paranoia (par″ə-noi´ah) behavior characterized by well-systematized delusions of persecution, delusions of grandeur, or a combination of the two. 516

paraphilia (par″ə-fil´e-ə) a psychosexual disorder characterized by recurrent intense sexual disorders. 516

paraplegia (par″ə-ple´jə) paralysis of the legs and lower part of the body, often caused by disease or injury to the spine. 505

parasympathetic (par″ə-sim″pə-thet´ik) referring to the nerves that are part of the autonomic system and work against the sympathetic nerves. 492

parathormone (par″ə-thor´mōn) parathyroid hormone. 573

paraurethral (par″ə-u-re´thrəl) near the urethra. 360
   p. gland, a gland of the female urethra. 360, 360*f*

parenteral (pə-ren´tər-əl) injection into the body, not through the alimentary canal. 301

paresthesia (par″əs-the´zhə) an abnormal touch sensation, such as burning or prickling, often in the absence of an external stimulus. 500, 509

parietal (pə-ri´ə-təl) pertaining to the walls of a cavity; pertaining to or located near the parietal bone. 127, 231
   p. lobe, a portion of each cerebral hemisphere that is covered by the parietal bone. 489, 489*f*

Parkinson disease (pahr´kin-sən dĭ-zēz´) a chronic nervous disease characterized by a fine, slowly spreading tremor; muscular weakness and rigidity; and a peculiar gait. 509

parotitis (par″o-ti´tis) inflammation of the parotid gland. 290
   epidemic p., mumps. 290

parous (par´əs) having borne one or more offspring. 405

paroxysmal (par″ok-siz´məl) occurring in sudden, periodic attacks or recurrence of symptoms of a disease. 196, 245

parturition (pahr″tu-ri´shən) childbirth. 402

patella (pə-tel´ə) the kneecap, a lens-shaped bone situated in front of the knee. 433*f*, 442, 442*f*

patellar response (pə-tel´ər) a deep tendon reflex elicited by a sharp tap on the tendon just distal to the patella. 487

patellofemoral (pə-tel″o-fem´ə-rəl) pertaining to the kneecap and the femur. 442

patent (pa´tənt) open, unobstructed, or not closed. 250
   p. ductus arteriosus, an abnormal opening between the pulmonary artery and the aorta. 195

pathogen (path´o-jən) any disease-producing agent or microorganism. 76, 164

pathogenic (path-o-jen´ik) disease causing. 76, 151

pathologic, pathological (path″o-loj´ik, path″o-loj´ĭ-kəl) indicating or caused by some morbid process. 22

pathologist (pə-thol´ə-jist) a physician who specializes in the study of the essential nature of disease. 22
   clinical p., a physician specialized in the branch of pathology that is applied to the solution of clinical problems, especially the use of laboratory methods in clinical diagnosis. 22
   surgical p., a physician specialized in the study of disease processes that are surgically accessible for diagnosis or treatment. 22

pathology (pə-thol´ə-je) the study of the changes caused by disease in the structure or functions of the body. 21, 70
   clinical p., the study of disease by the use of laboratory tests and methods. 22

pediatric (pe″de-at´rik) pertaining to pediatrics. 23

pediatrician (pe″de-ə-trĭ´shən) a physician who specializes in the treatment of children's diseases. 23

pediatrics (pe″de-at´riks) the branch of medicine that is devoted to the study of children's diseases. 23

pediculosis (pə-dik″u-lo´sis) infestation with lice of the family Pediculidae. 538

pedodontics (pe-do-don´tiks) the branch of dentistry that deals with the teeth and mouth conditions of children. 275

pedodontist (pe-do-don´tist) a dentist who specializes in the teeth and mouth conditions of children. 275

pelvic (pel´vik) pertaining to the pelvis. 126
   p. cavity, the space within the walls of the pelvis, forming the inferior and lesser part of the abdominopelvic cavity. 126, 126*f*

pelvic—cont'd
   p. exteneration, the surgical removal of all reproductive organs and their lymph nodes, as well as most pelvic organs. 377
   p. girdle, a bony ring formed by the hip bones, the sacrum, and the coccyx. 439, 440
   p. inflammatory disease, an ascending pelvic infection involving the genital tract beyond the cervix uteri. 372

pelvimetry (pel-vim´ə-tre) the measurement of the dimensions and capacity of the pelvis. 407

pelvis (pel´vis) the lower portion of the trunk. The word also means any basin-like structure. 126
   renal p. (re´nəl), in the kidney, the funnel-shaped structure at the upper end of the ureter. 323

penile (pe´nīl) pertaining to or affecting the penis. 380
   p. prosthesis, a device that can be surgically implanted in the penis to treat erectile dysfunction. 388, 388*f*

penis (pe´nis) the male organ of urination and copulation. 380

pepsin (pep´sin) any of several enzymes of gastric juice that break down proteins. 573

percussion (pər-kŭ´shən) the act of striking a part with short, sharp blows as an aid in diagnosing the condition of the underlying parts by the sound obtained. 50, 50*f*
   abdominal p., assessing the organs of the abdomen by percussion. 283

pericardial (per″e-kahr´de-əl) around the heart. 183
   p. cavity, the space between the two pericardial layers. 183

pericardiocentesis (per″e-kahr″de-o-sen-te´sis) surgical puncture of the pericardial cavity for the aspiration of fluid. 203

pericarditis (per″e-kahr-di´tis) inflammation of the pericardium. 198

pericardium (per″e-kahr´de-əm) the sac enclosing the heart and the roots of the great vessels. 182
   parietal p., the outer layer of the double membrane that surrounds the heart. 182, 183*f*
   visceral p., the inner layer of the double membrane that surrounds the heart. 182, 183*f*

perichondrial (per″ĭ-kon´dre-əl) pertaining to or composed of perichondrium. 445

perichondrium (per″ĭ-kon´dre-əm) the layer of fibrous connective tissue that invests all cartilage except the articular cartilage of synovial joints. 445

pericolic (per″e-kol´ik) around the colon. 279

perimetrium (per″ĭ-me´tre-əm) the serous coat of the uterus. 363

perineal (per″ĭ-ne´əl) pertaining to the perineum. 332, 360
   p. muscles, the muscles that form the perineum. 332

perineum (per″ĭ-ne´əm) the pelvic floor and the associated structures occupying the pelvic outlet; it is bounded anteriorly by the pubic symphysis, laterally by the ischial tuberosities, and posteriorly by the coccyx; the region between the thighs, bounded in the male sex by the scrotum and anus and in the female sex by the vulva and anus. 360

periodontal (per″e-o-don´təl) around a tooth; pertaining to the periodontium. 274

periodontics (per″e-o-don´tiks) the branch of dentistry that deals with the study and treatment of the periodontium. 274

periodontist (per″e-o-don´tist) a dentist who specializes in periodontics. 274

periodontitis (per″e-o-don-ti´tis) inflammation of the periodontium, caused by residual food, bacteria, and tartar that collect in the spaces between the gum and the lower part of the tooth crown. 289

periodontium (per″e-o-don´she-əm) the tissues investing and supporting the teeth. 274

periosteum (per″e-os´te-əm) a tough fibrous membrane that surrounds a bone. 431, 431*f*

peripheral (pə-rif´ər-əl) pertaining to the outside, surface, or surrounding areas of a structure or field of vision. 485, 491
   p. nervous system, the various nerve processes that connect the brain and the spinal cord with receptors, muscles, and glands. 485, 486*f*, 492*f*
   p. vascular disease, any abnormal condition that affects the blood vessels and lymphatic vessels, except those that supply the heart. 200, 583

peristalsis (per″ĭ-stawl´sis) movement by which the alimentary canal propels its contents. It consists of a wave of contraction passing along the tube for variable distances. 266

peritoneal (per″ĭ-to-ne´əl) pertaining to the peritoneum. 127
   p. cavity, the potential space between the parietal and visceral layers of the peritoneum. 127

salmonellosis (sal″mo-nəl-o´sis) any disease caused by infection with a species of *Salmonella*. 295

salpingectomy (sal″pin-jek´tə-me) excision of a uterine tube. 378

salpingitis (sal″pin-ji´tis) inflammation of a fallopian tube. 371

salpingocele (sal-ping´go-sēl) hernial protrusion of a uterine tube. 371

salpingo-oophorectomy (sal-ping″go-o-of″ə-rek´tə-me) surgical removal of a uterine tube and ovary. 377, 377*f*

salpingopexy (sal-ping´go-pek″se) surgical fixation of a uterine tube. 378

salpingorrhaphy (sal″ping-gor´ə-fe) suture of the uterine tube. 378

salpingostomy (sal″ping-gos´tə-me) formation of an opening into a uterine tube for the purpose of drainage; surgical restoration of the patency of a uterine tube. 378

sanguinous (sang´gwi-nəs) pertaining to blood. 147

scabies (ska´bēz) a contagious dermatitis of humans and various wild and domestic animals caused by the itch mite. 539

scales (skāls) bits of dry, horny epidermis, usually ready to be sloughed. 542, 543*f*

scapula (skap´u-lə) the shoulder blade, the flat triangular bone in the back of the shoulder. 433*f*, 439

scapular (skap´u-lər) of or pertaining to the scapula. 440

scapuloclavicular (skap″u-lo-klə-vik´u-lər) pertaining to the scapula and the clavicle. 440

schizophrenia (skit″so-fre´ne-ə, skiz″o-fre´ne-ə) a mental disorder or group of disorders consisting of most major psychotic disorders and characterized by disturbances in form and content of thought, mood, and sense of self and relationship to the external world and behavior. 516

sciatic nerve (si-at´ik nərv) the largest nerve in the body, arising in the pelvis and passing down the back of the leg. 491

sciatica (si-at´ĭ-kə) a syndrome characterized by pain radiating from the back into the buttock and into the lower extremity along its posterior or lateral aspect; pain anywhere along the course of the sciatic nerve. 501

sclera (sklēr´ə) the tough, white, outer coat of the eyeball. 494, 494*f*

scleroderma (sklēr″o-dur´mə) chronic hardening and thickening of the skin. 465, 538

scleroprotein (sklēr″o-pro´tēn) a protein that is characterized by its insolubility and fibrous structure. 532

sclerosis (sklə-ro´sis) hardening, chiefly applied to hardening of the nervous system or to hardening of the blood vessels. 77

    multiple s., a chronic disease of the central nervous system in which disseminated glial patches called plaques develop. 509

    systemic s., a systemic disorder of the connective tissue characterized by induration and thickening of the skin, by abnormalities involving both the microvasculature (telangiectasia) and larger vessels (Raynaud phenomenon), and by fibrotic degenerative changes in various body organs, including the heart, lungs, kidneys, and gastrointestinal tract. 465

sclerotherapy (sklēr″o-ther´ə-pe) the injection of a chemical irritant into a vein to produce eventual fibrosis and obliteration of the lumen. 206

scoliosis (sko″le-o´sis) lateral curvature of the vertebral column. 462, 462*f*

scrotal (skro´təl) pertaining to the scrotum. 380

scrotum (skro´təm) the pouch that contains the testes and their accessory organs. 380

sebaceous (sə-ba´shəs) pertaining to sebum or secreting sebum. 534

    s. gland, oil-secreting gland of the skin. 534

seborrhea (seb″o-re´ə) excessive secretion of sebum; seborrheic dermatitis. 539

seborrheic (seb″o-re´ik) affected with seborrhea. 539

    s. dermatitis, an inflammatory skin condition caused by overactive sebaceous glands. 539

sebum (se´bəm) the oily material secreted by a sebaceous gland. 534

secretion (se-kre´shən) the process of elaborating a specific product as a result of the activity of a gland; material that is secreted. 146

secundipara (se″kən-dip´ə-rə) a woman who has had two pregnancies that resulted in viable offspring. 405

seizure (se´zhər) a single episode of epilepsy, represented as a sudden attack. 508

semen (se´mən) fluid consisting of gland secretions and sperm, discharged at ejaculation. 381, 383

semicircular canals (sem″e-sər´kyə-lər kə-nals´) the bony fluid-filled loops in the internal ear that are associated with balance. 495, 494*f*

semicoma (sem″e-ko´mə) a stupor from which the patient may be aroused. 502

semiconscious (sem″e-kon´shəs) only partially aware of one´s surroundings. 502

semilunar (sem″e-loo´nər) resembling a half-moon. 185

    s. valve, a valve with half-moon-shaped cusps, such as the aortic valve and the pulmonary valve. 185, 184*f*

seminal (sem´ĭ-nəl) pertaining to semen. 381, 383

    s. fluid, semen; the fluid discharged from the penis at the height of sexual excitement. 383

    s. vesicles, paired saclike glandular structures in the male sex that produce a fluid that is added to the secretion of the testes and other glands to form the semen. 381, 383

seminiferous tubules (sem″ĭ-nif´ər-əs too´būls) channels in the testis in which the spermatozoa develop. 381, 381*f*, 382

semipermeable (sem″e-pur´me-ə-bəl) permitting the passage of certain molecules and hindering that of others. 99

sensory (sen´sə-re) pertaining to sensation. 485

    s. neurons, cells of the afferent nervous system that pick up stimuli. 487, 488*f*

sepsis (sep´sis) the presence in the blood or other tissues of pathogenic microorganisms or their toxins. 155, 547

septal (sep´təl) pertaining to a septum. 183

    s. deviation, a deviation in a normally straight septum, such as the nasal septum. 232, 233*f*

septicemia (sep″tĭ-se´me-ə) a morbid condition caused by the presence of bacteria or their toxins in the blood. 155, 338, 372

septoplasty (sep´to-plas″te) surgical reconstruction of the nasal septum. 253

septorhinoplasty (sep″to-ri´no-plas″te) plastic surgery of the nasal septum and the external nose. 253

septum (sep´təm) a dividing wall or partition. 183

    cardiac s., the membranous partition that divides the heart's left and right sides. 183

    nasal s., the partition between the two nasal cavities. 228

serosa (sēr-o´sə, sēr-o´zə) any serous membrane; the chorion. 277, 278

serotonin (ser″o-to´nin) a vasoconstrictor, found in various animals, in bacteria, and in many plants. It has many physiologic properties. 487

sexually transmitted disease (sek´shoo-əl-le trans-mit´əd dĭ-zēz´) a contagious disease usually acquired by sexual intercourse or genital contact. 342

shingles (shing´gəlz) herpes zoster. 540, 540*f*

shock (shok) a sudden disturbance of mental equilibrium; a condition of profound hemodynamic and metabolic disturbance characterized by failure of the circulatory system to maintain adequate perfusion of vital organs. 198

shoulder girdle (shōl´dər gər´dəl) a partial arch at the top of the trunk formed by the scapula and clavicle. 439, 440

shunt (shunt) to turn to one side, divert, or bypass; a passage or anastomosis between two natural channels, especially between blood vessels. 144, 203

    ventriculoperitoneal s., a surgically created passageway between a cerebral ventricle and peritoneum for draining of excess CSF. 517*t*, 518, 518*f*

sialadenitis (si″əl-ad″ə-ni´tis) inflammation of a salivary gland. 299

sialography (si″ə-log´rə-fe) radiographic demonstration of the salivary glands after injection of radiopaque substances. 284

sialolith (si-al´o-lith) a chalky concretion or calculus in the salivary ducts or glands. 284

sialolithiasis (si″ə-lo-lĭ-thi´ə-sis) a condition characterized by the presence of stones in the salivary ducts or glands. 299

sickle cell (sik´əl sel) abnormal red blood cell that has a crescent shape. 159

sigmoidoscope (sig-moi´do-skōp) a rigid or flexible endoscope with appropriate illumination for examining the sigmoid colon. 285

sigmoidoscopy (sig″moi-dos´kə-pe) inspection of the sigmoid colon through a sigmoidoscope. 285

sign (sīn) an indication of the existence of something as opposed to the subjective sensations (symptoms) of the patient. 44

silicosis (sil″ĭ-ko´sis) pneumoconiosis caused by inhalation of the dust of stone, sand, or flint containing silicon dioxide, with formation of generalized nodular fibrotic changes in both lungs. 247

sinoatrial (si″no-a´tre-əl) pertaining to the sinus venosus and the atrium of the heart. 186

    s. node, a node in the wall of the right atrium that is the source of impulses that initiate the heartbeat. 186, 186*f*

sinus (si´nəs) a recess, cavity, or channel. 186

    paranasal s., one of several cavities that communicate with the nasal cavity and are lined with a mucous membrane. 228, 228*f*

sinusitis (si″nes-i´tis) inflammation of a sinus. 240

Sjögren syndrome (shur´gren sin´drōm) a symptom complex of unknown cause, usually occurring in middle-aged or older women, marked by keratoconjunctivitis, xerostomia, and the presence of a connective tissue disease, usually rheumatoid arthritis but sometimes systemic lupus erythematosus, scleroderma, or polymyositis. 465

skeleton (skel´ə-tən) the hard framework of the animal body. 432
    appendicular s., the bones of the upper and lower limbs. 433, 433*f*
    axial s., the bones of the cranium, vertebral column, ribs, and sternum. 433, 433*f*
skin flap a layer of skin, usually separated by dissection from a deeper layer of tissue. 550
somatic (so-mat´ik) pertaining to the body. 115, 492
    s. cell, all of the body cells that have the diploid number of chromosomes. 115
    s. death, absence of electrical activity of the brain for a specified period of time under rigidly defined circumstances. 132
somatogenic (so˝mə-to-jen´ik) originating in the cells of the body. 132
somatopsychic (so˝mə-to-si´kik) pertaining to both body and mind, denoting a physical disorder that produces mental symptoms. 132
somatotropic (so˝mə-to-tro´pik) having an affinity for or stimulating the body or the body cells; having a stimulating effect on body nutrition and growth; having the properties of somatotropin. 568
somatotropin (so´mə-to-tro˝pin) growth hormone. 568
somesthetic (so˝mes-thet´ik) pertaining to body feeling or sensation. 132
sonography (sə-nog´rə-fe) the process of using sound waves bouncing off body tissue to form a picture of an internal organ; ultrasonography. 53, 285
spasm (spaz´əm) a sudden, violent, involuntary contraction of a muscle or a group of muscles, attended by pain and interference with function, producing involuntary movement and distortion; a sudden but transitory constriction of a passage, canal, or orifice. 45
specific gravity (spə-sif´ik grav´ĭ-te) the ratio of the density of a substance to the density of another substance accepted as a standard, water often being the standard for liquids or solids. 327
speculum (spek´u-ləm) an instrument used to examine a body orifice or cavity. 366
    vaginal s., an instrument used to hold open the vaginal opening for inspection of the vaginal cavity. 366
spermatic (spər-mat´ik) pertaining to spermatozoa. 380
spermatoblast (sper´mə-to-blast˝) embryonic form of a sperm. 401
spermatocele (sper´mə-to-sēl˝) a swelling of the epididymis or of the rete testis containing spermatozoa. 386, 386*f*
spermatogenesis (sper˝mə-to-jen´ə-sis) the process of formation of sperm. 381
spermatozoon (sper˝mə-to-zo´on) a mature male sperm cell, which serves to fertilize the ovum; the plural is spermatozoa. 382, 382*f*
spermicide (sper´mĭ-sīd) an agent that destroys spermatozoa. 412, 413*t*
spherocyte (sfēr´o-sīt) an abnormally round red blood cell. 158
spherocytosis (sfēr˝o-si-to´sis) the presence of spherocytes in the blood. 158
sphincter (sfingk´tər) a ringlike band of muscle fibers that constricts a passage or closes a natural opening. 276
spina bifida (spi´nə bif´ĭ-də, bi´fə-də) a developmental abnormality marked by defective closure of the bony encasement of the spinal cord. 462
spinal (spi´nəl) pertaining to the vertebral column. 436
    s. cavity, a bone cavity formed by the vertebrae of the backbone and containing the spinal cord and the beginnings of spinal nerves. 127
    s. cord, a long, nearly cylindric structure located in the vertebral canal, and part of the central nervous system. 488, 490
    s. fluid, the fluid that flows through and protects the brain and spinal cord; cerebrospinal fluid. 491
    s. fusion, the fixation of an unstable segment of the spine. 469
    s. puncture, insertion of a needle into the lumbar region of the spine for the purpose of removing spinal fluid or introducing substances; lumbar puncture. 497, 452*f*
spirochete (spi´ro-kēt) a spiral bacterium. 86, 87*f*
spirometer (spi-rom´ə-tər) the instrument used in spirometry. 234, 234*f*
    incentive s., an instrument used to encourage voluntary deep breathing by providing visual feedback about inspiratory volume. 254, 254*f*
spirometry (spi-rom´ə-tre) a measurement of the breathing capacity of the lungs. 234
spleen (splēn) a large, glandlike organ situated in the upper left part of the abdominal cavity, which destroys erythrocytes at the end of their usefulness and serves as a blood reservoir. 209*f*, 210
splenectomy (sple-nek´tə-me) removal of the spleen. 214
splenic (splen´ik) pertaining to the spleen. 210
splenolymphatic (sple˝no-lim-fat´ik) pertaining to the spleen and the lymph nodes. 211
splenomegaly (sple˝no-meg´ə-le) enlargement of the spleen. 213
splenopathy (sple-nop´ə-the) any disease of the spleen. 213
splenopexy (sple´no-pek˝se) surgical fixation of the spleen. 214
splenoptosis (sple˝nop-to´sis) downward displacement of the spleen. 213, 214

splenorrhagia (sple˝no-ra´jə) hemorrhage from the spleen. 213
splenorrhaphy (sple-nor´ə-fe) suture of the spleen. 214
splint (splint) to fasten; an appliance used to hold in position a displaced or movable part. 468
spondylalgia (spon˝dĭ-lal´jə) a painful vertebra. 457
spondylarthritis (spon˝dəl-ahr-thri´tis) inflammation of joints between vertebrae. 464
spondylarthropathy (spon˝dəl-ahr-throp´ə-the) any disease of the joints and spine. 465
spondylosyndesis (spon˝də-lo-sin-de´sis) surgical immobilization or ankylosis of the spine; spinal fusion. 469
sprain (sprān) a joint injury in which some of the fibers of a supporting ligament are ruptured but the continuity of the ligament remains intact. 454
sputum (spu´təm) material ejected from the trachea, bronchi, and lungs through the mouth. 235
staphylococcemia (staf˝ə-lo-kok-se´me-ə) a condition in which staphylococci are present in the blood; septicemia caused by staphylococci. 154
staphylococci (staf˝ə-lo-kok´si) plural of staphylococcus. *Staphylococcus* is a genus of gram-positive bacteria consisting of cocci, usually unencapsulated, 0.5 to 1.5 microns in diameter. The organisms occur singly, in pairs, and in irregular clusters. 85, 85*f*
stasis (sta´sis) a stoppage or diminution of the flow of blood or other body fluid in any part; a state of equilibrium among opposing forces. 45, 161
stenosis (stə-no´sis) narrowing or stricture of a duct or canal. 197, 200, 341
    valvular s., a narrowing or stricture of any of the heart valves. 197
stent (stent) a mold or slender rodlike or threadlike device used to provide support for tubular structures or to maintain their patency. 205
    intracoronary s., a stent used to provide support for a coronary artery. 205
stereotactic radiosurgery (ster˝e-o-tak´tik ra˝de-o-sur´jər-e) a method of treating tumors by ionizing radiation rather than surgical incision. 518
stereotaxis (ster˝e-o-tak´sis) a type of surgery or radiotherapy characterized by computerized positioning to locate the site. 518
sternal (ster´nəl) pertaining to the breastbone. 437
sternalgia (stər-nal´jə) pain in the breastbone. 457
sternoclavicular (stur˝no-klə-vik´u-lər) pertaining to the breastbone and collarbone. 440
sternocostal (stur˝no-kos´təl) pertaining to the breastbone and ribs. 438
sternoschisis (stər-nos´kĭ-sis) congenital fissure of the sternum. 462
sternotomy (stər-not´ə-me) incision of the sternum. 469
sternovertebral (stur˝no-vur´tə-brəl) pertaining to the sternum and the vertebrae. 438
sternum (stur´nəm) the breastbone, a plate of bone forming the middle anterior wall of the thorax. 433*f*, 434, 437
steroid (ster´oid) any of a large number of hormonal substances with a similar basic chemical structure, produced mainly in the adrenal cortex and gonads. 464
stethoscope (steth´o-skōp) an instrument by which various internal sounds of the body are conveyed to the ear of the listener. 50, 50*f*
stillbirth (stil´birth) the delivery of a dead child; fetal death. 410
stoma (sto´mə) any minute pore, orifice, or opening on a free surface; the opening established in the abdominal wall by colostomy, ileostomy, etc. 59, 59*f*
stomatitis (sto˝mə-ti´tis) inflammation of the mouth. 288
stomatodynia (sto˝mə-to-din´e-ə) painful mouth. 288
stomatomycosis (sto˝mə-to-mi-ko´sis) a mouth disease caused by a fungus. 288
stomatoplasty (sto´mə-to-plas˝te) surgical repair of the mouth. 300
strain (strān) an overstretching or overexertion of some part of the musculature. 454
streptococcal (strep˝to-kok´əl) referring to or caused by a streptococcus. 85
    s. pharyngitis, pharyngitis caused by streptococci; strep throat. 85
streptococcemia (strep˝to-kok-se´me-ə) the presence of streptococci in the blood. 154
streptococci (strep˝to-kok´si) plural of *Streptococcus,* a genus of gram-positive cocci occurring in pairs or chains. 85, 85*f*
stress test (stres test) a method of evaluating cardiovascular fitness. While exercising, the person is subjected to steadily increasing levels of work, and the amount of oxygen consumed and an electrocardiogram are monitored. 192
    thallium s. t., a stress test that measures the response to thallium. 192
    treadmill s. t., a stress test that measures the response to exercise. 192
stricture (strik´chər) decrease in the caliber of a canal, duct, or other passage. 200
stridor (stri´dər) a harsh, high-pitched respiratory sound such as the inspiratory sound often heard in acute laryngeal obstruction. 235

therapist (ther´ə-pist) a person skilled in the treatment of disease or other disorder. 31
  occupational t., an allied health professional who is nationally certified to practice occupational therapy. 31
  physical t., one skilled in the techniques of physical therapy and qualified to administer treatments prescribed by a physician. 31
  respiratory t., one skilled in the techniques of respiratory therapy. 31
therapy (ther´ə-pe) treatment of disease. 25
thermometer (thər-mom´ə-tər) an instrument for determining temperatures. 48, 49f
  oral t., a clinical thermometer that is usually placed under the tongue. 49, 49f
  rectal t., a clinical thermometer that is inserted in the rectum. 49, 49f
  tympanic t., a thermometer designed to measure temperature electronically at the tympanic membrane. 49, 49f
thermoplegia (thər″mo-ple´jə) heatstroke or sunstroke. 549
thermoreceptor (thur″mo-re-sep´tər) a nerve ending, usually in the skin, that is sensitive to a change in temperature. 493
thermotherapy (thur″mo-ther´ə-pe) treatment of disease by the application of heat. 55
thoracentesis (thor″ə-sen-te´sis) surgical puncture of the chest wall into the parietal cavity for aspiration of fluids. 252, 252f
thoracic (thə-ras´ik) pertaining to the chest. 126, 117, 436
  t. cavity, the upper ventral body cavity that contains the lungs and mediastinum. 126, 126f, 182
  t. duct, the common trunk of many lymphatic vessels in the body. 209f, 210
thoracocentesis (thor″ə-ko-sen-te´sis) surgical puncture of the chest wall for the aspiration of fluid. 252, 252f
thoracodynia (thor″ə-ko-din´e-ə) pain in the chest. 118
thoracoplasty (thor´ə-ko-plas″te) surgical removal of ribs, allowing the chest wall to collapse a diseased lung. 253
thoracostomy (thor″ə-kos´tə-me) surgical opening in the wall of the chest. 253
thoracotomy (thor″ə-kot´ə-me) surgical incision of the wall of the chest. 117, 252
thorax (thor´aks) chest; the part of the body that is encased by the ribs and extends from the neck to the respiratory diaphragm. 117
thrombectomy (throm-bek´tə-me) surgical removal of a blood clot. 154, 347
thrombocyte (throm´bo-sīt) a blood platelet. 150, 151
thrombocytopenia (throm″bo-si″to-pe´ne-ə) a decrease in the number of platelets in circulating blood. 154, 162
thrombocytosis (throm″bo-si-to´sis) an increase in the number of platelets in the peripheral blood. 154, 161
thromboembolic (throm″bo-em-bol´ik) pertaining to an embolus that has resulted from detachment of a blood clot from its site of formation. 207, 234
thrombogenesis (throm″bo-jen´ə-sis) origin of a blood clot; clot formation. 154
thrombolymphangitis (throm″bo-lim″fan-ji´tis) inflammation of a lymph vessel caused by a blood clot. 213
thrombolysis (throm-bol´ĭ-sis) dissolution of a blood clot. 154
  intravascular t., use of a thrombolytic agent delivered via a catheter to dissolve an internal blood clot. 206
thrombolytic (throm″bo-lit´ik) dissolving or breaking up a blood clot; an agent that dissolves or breaks up a blood clot. 154, 206, 519
thrombopenia (throm″bo-pe´ne-ə) a deficiency in the number of platelets in circulating blood. 154
thrombophlebitis (throm″bo-flə-bi´tis) inflammation of a vein caused by a blood clot. 201
thromboplastin (throm″bo-plas´tin) coagulation factor III. 161
  partial t. time, a test for detecting coagulation defects. 161
thrombosis (throm-bo´sis) the presence of a blood clot. 154
  venous t., a blood clot occurring in a vein. 201
thrombus (throm´bəs) an aggregation of blood factors, primarily platelets and fibrin with entrapment of cellular elements, frequently causing vascular obstruction at the point of its formation. 151, 154, 206
thymectomy (thi-mek´tə-me) excision of the thymus gland. 214
thymic (thi´mik) pertaining to the thymus. 211
thymoma (thi-mo´mə) tumor derived from elements of the thymus. 213
thymopathy (thi-mop´ə-the) any disease of the thymus. 213
thymosin (thi´mo-sin) a substance secreted by thymic epithelial cells that maintains immune system functions and can restore T-cell function in thymectomized animals. 573
thymus (thi´məs) a glandlike body in the anterior mediastinal cavity that usually reaches its maximum development during childhood and then undergoes involution. 210, 211, 573

thyrocalcitonin (thi″ro-kal″sĭ-to´nin) calcitonin; a hormone produced by the thyroid gland that is concerned with the homeostasis of the blood calcium level. 569
thyroid (thi´roid) the thyroid gland, a highly vascular organ at the front of the neck; pertaining to the thyroid gland. 564, 564f
thyroidectomy (thi″roid-ek´tə-me) surgical removal of the thyroid gland. 585
thyroiditis (thi″roid-i´tis) inflammation of the thyroid gland. 580
thyropathy (thi-rop´ə-the) any disease of the thyroid gland. 579
thyrotoxicosis (thi″ro-tok″sĭ-ko´sis) a morbid condition caused by excessive thyroid secretion. Symptoms are sweating, weight loss, tachycardia, and nervousness. 580
thyrotropin (thi-rot´rə-pin) a hormone of the anterior pituitary that stimulates the thyroid. 569, 572
thyroxine (thi-rok´sin) an iodine-containing hormone secreted by the thyroid gland. Its chief function is to increase cell metabolism. 569
tibia (tib´e-ə) the inner and larger bone of the leg below the knee. 443, 443f
tibialgia (tib″e-al´jə) pain of the tibia. 457
tibiofemoral (tib″e-o-fem´ə-rəl) pertaining to the tibia and the femur. 444
tinea (tin´e-ə) any of various skin disorders popularly called ringworm. 540, 540f
tinnitus (tin´ĭ-təs, tĭ-ni´təs) a noise in the ears, such as ringing, buzzing, or roaring. 156, 513
tissue (tish´oo) an aggregation of similarly specialized cells united in the performance of a particular function. 116, 116f
  connective t., tissue that binds together and provides support for various structures. 116, 116f
  epithelial t., tissue that forms the covering of body surfaces. 116, 116f
  muscle t., tissue that produces movement. 116, 116f
  nervous t., tissue that coordinates and controls many body activities, found in the brain, spinal cord, and nerves. 116, 116f
tomogram (to´mo-gram) a radiogram produced by the process of tomography. 52, 52f, 192
tomography (to-mog´rə-fe) the recording of internal body images at a predetermined plane by means of the tomograph. 52
  computerized transverse axial t., a radiologic technique that uses a narrow beam of x-rays to obtain a three-dimensional view of body parts; also called computerized axial tomography (CAT, CAT scan, CT, or CT scan). 52
  computed t., a radiologic technique in which transmission patterns are recorded by electronic detectors and stored in a computer, which then reconstructs a three-dimensional view of internal structures of the body (CT). 52, 52f
  positron emission t., a computerized radiographic technique that uses radioactive substances to examine the metabolic activity of various body structures. 53, 192, 497
tonsil (ton´sil) a small, rounded mass of tissue, especially of lymphoid tissue; generally used alone to designate the palatine tonsil. 209f, 211
tonsillar (ton´sĭ-lər) of or pertaining to a tonsil. 211
tonsillectomy (ton″sĭ-lek´tə-me) excision of the tonsils. 214
tonsillitis (ton″sĭ-li´tis) inflammation of the tonsils, especially the palatine tonsils. 70, 213
tonsilloadenoidectomy (ton″sĭ-lo-ad″ə-noid-ek´tə-me) excision of lymphoid tissue from the throat and nasopharynx (tonsils and adenoids). 214
topical (top´ĭ-kəl) pertaining to a particular surface area, as a topical antiinfective applied to a certain area of the skin and affecting only the area to which it is applied. 305, 376, 551
  t. anesthetic, a medication that produces superficial analgesia. 305, 551
  t. medication, any drug that is applied to the skin or a mucous membrane. 551
tourniquet (toor´nĭ-kət) a device applied around an extremity to control the circulation and prevent the flow of blood to or from the distal area. 202
toxemia (tok-se´me-ə) the condition resulting from the spread of bacterial products (toxins) by the bloodstream. 155
toxic (tok´sik) poisonous; pertaining to poisoning. 80
  t. shock syndrome, a severe infection with *Staphylococcus aureus* characterized by high fever of sudden onset, vomiting, diarrhea, and myalgia, followed by hypotension and, in severe cases, shock. The syndrome affects almost exclusively menstruating women using tampons, although a few women who do not use tampons and a few male individuals have been affected. 155, 372
toxicity (tok-sis´ĭ-te) the quality of being poisonous, especially the degree of virulence of a toxic microbe or of a poison. 167
toxicologist (tok″sĭ-kol´ə-jist) one who specializes in the study of poisons. 80
toxicology (tok″sĭ-kol´ə-je) the science that deals with poisons. 80

toxin (tok´sin) a substance produced by certain animals, some higher plants, and pathogenic bacteria that is highly poisonous for other living organisms. 80

toxoid (tok´soid) a toxin treated in a way that destroys its deleterious properties without destroying its ability to stimulate antibody production. 167

trabeculae (trə-bek´u-le) plural of trabecula, a supporting or anchoring strand of connective tissue, such as one extending from a capsule into the substance of the enclosed organ. 431

trachea (tra´ke-ə) the windpipe. 61, 227

trachealgia (tra″ke-al´jə) pain in the trachea. 244

tracheomalacia (tra″ke-o-mə-la´shə) softening of the windpipe. 244

tracheoplasty (tra´ke-o-plas″te) plastic surgery of the windpipe. 253

tracheoscopy (tra″ke-os´kə-pe) examination of the interior of the windpipe. 232

tracheostenosis (tra″ke-o-stə-no´sis) narrowing or contraction of the trachea. 244

tracheostomy (tra″ke-os´tə-me) surgical formation of a new opening into the windpipe from the neck. 61, 250, 251*f*

tracheotomy (tra″ke-ot´ə-me) surgically cutting into the windpipe. 61, 250

traction (trak´shən) the act of drawing or exerting a pulling force. 468

tranquilizer (trang″kwĭ-liz´ər) a drug with a calming, soothing effect. 520

transcutaneous electrical nerve stimulation (TENS) (trans″ku-ta´ne-əs e-lek´trə-kəl nərv stim″u-la´shən) a method for relief of pain by placement of electrodes over the painful site and delivery of small amounts of electrical current. 519, 519*f*

transdermal (trans-dur´məl) entering through or passing through the skin. 101, 101*f*

transfusion (trans-fu´zhən) the introduction of blood directly into the bloodstream of a person. 162
t. reaction, an adverse reaction to blood received in a transfusion. 162

transient (tran´shent, tran´se-ənt) pertaining to a condition that is temporary. 237
t. ischemic attack, a brief attack (from a few minutes to an hour) of cerebral dysfunction of vascular origin, with no persistent neurologic deficit. 504

transplant (trans´plant) an organ or tissue used for grafting; the process of removing and grafting such an organ or tissue; (trans-plant´) to transfer tissue from one part to another. 167
autologous t., surgical transplantation of any tissue from one part of the body to another location in the same individual. 163

transthoracic (trans″thə-ras´ik) through the chest cavity or across the chest wall. 118

transtracheal (trans-tra´ke-əl) through the wall of the trachea. 250
t. tube, a tube placed in the trachea through an opening in the neck. 250, 251*f*

transureteroureterostomy (trans″u-re″tər-o-u-re″tər-os´tə-me) surgical connection of one ureter to another. 345, 345*f*

transurethral (trans″u-re´thrəl) performed through the urethra. 348
t. microwave thermotherapy, destruction of prostatic tissue using microwave energy, performed through the urethra. 388
t. needle ablation, destruction of prostatic tissue using low level radiofrequency energy, performed through the urethra. 388
t. resection of the prostate, resection of the prostate by means of a cystoscope passed through the urethra. 348, 388

transverse (trans-vərs´) extending from side to side; at right angles to the long axis. 118
t. plane, an imaginary line that divides the body into upper and lower portions. 118, 119*f*

trauma (traw´mə, trou´mə) an injury or wound, whether physical or psychic. 104

traumatic (trə-mat´ik) pertaining to, occurring as the result of, or causing injury. 104

tremor (trem´ər, tre´mər) an involuntary quivering or trembling. 509

triage (tre-ahzh´, tre´ahzh) the sorting and prioritizing of patients for treatment. 28

Trichomonas (trik″o-mo´nəs) a genus of parasitic flagellated protozoa. 88*f*, 367, 420

trichomoniasis (trik″o-mo-ni´ə-sis) infection with *Trichomonas,* a genus of parasitic protozoa found in the intestinal and genitourinary tracts. 88, 418*t*, 420

trichopathy (trĭ-kop´ə-the) any disease of the hair. 548

trichosis (tri-ko´sis) any disease or abnormal growth of the hair; growth of hair in an unusual place. 548

tricuspid (tri-kus´pid) having three points or cusps; pertaining to the tricuspid valve of the heart. 185
tricuspid v., a valve with three main cusps situated between the right atrium and the right ventricle of the heart. 184*f*, 185

triglyceride (tri-glis´ər-īd) a neutral fat synthesized from carbohydrates for storage in animal adipose cells. 191

triiodothyronine (tri-i″o-do-thi´ro-nēn) one of the thyroid hormones. Its symbol is T₃. 569

trimester (tri-mes´tər) a period of three months. 403

tripara (trip´ə-rə) a female who has borne three children. 405

tropic (tro´pik) to stimulate. 568

tubal ligation (too´bəl li-ga´shən) cauterization or tying off of the uterine tubes to prevent passage of eggs and thus prevent pregnancy. 378, 414

tubal pregnancy (too´bəl preg´nən-se) an ectopic pregnancy in which the product of conception implants in the uterine tube. 372

tubercle (too´bər-kəl) any of the small, rounded, granulomatous lesions produced by infection with *Mycobacterium tuberculosis;* it is the characteristic lesion of tuberculosis. A nodule, or small eminence, such as a rough, rounded eminence on a bone. 249

tuberculosis (too-ber″ku-lo´sis) an infectious bacterial disease caused by species of *Mycobacterium* that is chronic in nature and commonly affects the lungs. 249

tubule (too´būl) a small tube. 323
distal t., the portion of the nephron lying between the descending loop of Henle and the collecting duct in the kidney. 324, 324*f*
proximal t., the portion of the nephron between the glomerulus and the loop of Henle. 324, 324*f*
seminiferous t., one of several small channels of the testes in which spermatozoa develop. 381, 381*f*

tympanic membrane (tim-pan´ik) the thin membranous partition between the external acoustic meatus and the tympanic cavity. 49, 494*f*, 495

ulcer (ul´sər) a local defect or excavation of the surface of an organ or tissue, produced by sloughing of necrotic inflammatory tissue. 84*f*, 288
decubitus u., a sore in the skin over a bony prominence that results from ischemic hypoxia of the tissues caused by prolonged pressure; pressure ulcer. 545

ulna (ul´nə) the inner and larger bone of the forearm. 433*f*, 439, 440

ulnoradial (ul″no-ra´de-əl) pertaining to the ulna and radius, the bones of the lower arm. 440

ultrasonic (ul″trə-son´ik) pertaining to sound waves having a frequency beyond the upper limit of perception by the human ear, that is, beyond about 20,000 cycles per second. 99

ultrasonography (ul″trə-sə-nog´rə-fe) the visualization of deep structures of the body by recording the reflections of pulses of ultrasonic waves directed into the tissues. 52, 99

ultrasound (ul´trə-sound) mechanical radiant energy with a frequency greater than 20,000 cycles per second; ultrasonography. 52, 53, 54*f*

ultraviolet (ul″trə-vi´ə-lət) beyond the violet end of the spectrum. 99, 99*f*

umbilical (əm-bil´ĭ-kəl) pertaining to the umbilicus. 125, 133
u. region, abdominal region in the area of the umbilicus. 125, 125*f*

umbilicus (əm-bil´ĭ-kəs) the navel. 125, 133

ungual (ung´gwəl) pertaining to the nails. 535

unilateral (u″nĭ-lat´ər-əl) pertaining to only one side. 122

urea (u-re´ə) the chief nitrogenous constituent of urine and the major nitrogenous end product of protein metabolism. 327

uremia (u-re´me-ə) an accumulation of toxic products in the blood caused by inadequate functioning of the kidneys. 336

ureter (u-re´tər, u´rə-tər) the tubular organ through which urine passes from the kidney to the bladder. 321

ureteral (u-re´tər-əl) pertaining to or used on the ureter. 322

ureterectomy (u-re″tər-ek´tə-me) surgical removal of all or a part of a ureter. 347

ureteritis (u-re″tər-i´tis) inflammation of a ureter. 338

ureterocele (u-re´tər-o-sēl″) hernia of the ureter. 340

ureterocystoneostomy (u-re″tər-o-sis″to-ne-os´tə-me) surgical transplantation of the ureter to a different site of attachment to the bladder. 347

ureterocystostomy (u-re″tər-o-sis-tos´tə-me) surgical transplantation of a ureter to a different site in the bladder; ureteroneocystostomy. 347

ureterolith (u-re´tər-o-lith) a stone that is lodged or has formed in the ureter. 340

ureterolithiasis (u-re″tər-o-lĭ-thi´ə-sis) formation of stones in a ureter. 340

ureterolithotomy (u-re″tər-o-lĭ-thot´ə-me) the removal of a calculus from the ureter by incision. 347

ureteropathy (u-re″tər-op′ə-the) any disease of the ureter. 338

ureteroplasty (u-re′tər-o-plas″te) surgical repair of the ureter. 347

ureteropyelonephritis (u-re″tər-o-pi-ə-lo-nə-fri′tis) inflammation of the ureter, renal pelvis, and the kidney. 338

ureteroscopy (u-re″tər-os′kə-pe) examination of the ureter by means of a ureteroscope. 334

ureterostenosis (u-re″tər-o-stə-no′sis) stricture of a ureter. 341

ureterostomy (u-re″tər-os′tə-me) surgical formation of a fistula through which a ureter may discharge its contents. 344, 345f

urethra (u-re′thrə) the passage by which urine is discharged from the bladder to the exterior. 321, 321f, 322

urethral (u-re′thrəl) pertaining to the urethra. 322, 383

urethritis (u″rə-thri′tis) inflammation of the urethra. 338, 417
   nongonococcal u., urethritis without evidence of gonococcal infection. 417

urethrocele (u-re′thro-sēl) herniation of the urethra. 340

urethrocystitis (u-re″thro-sis-ti′tis) inflammation of the urethra and the bladder. 338

urethrography (u″rə-throg′rə-fe) roentgenography of the urethra after the injection of a radiopaque medium. 333

urethrorectal (u-re″thro-rek′təl) pertaining to the urethra and the rectum. 326

urethrorrhagia (u-re″thro-ra′jə) hemorrhage from the urethra. 337

urethrorrhea (u″thro-re′ə) discharge from the urethra. 337

urethroscopy (u″rə-thros′kə-pe) inspection of the interior of the urethra with a urethroscope. 334

urethrospasm (u-re′thro-spaz″əm) spasm of the urethral muscular tissue. 349

urethrostenosis (u-re″thro-stə-no′sis) stricture or stenosis of the urethra. 341

urethrotomy (u″rə-throt′ə-me) incision of the urethra. 348

urethrovaginal (u-re″thro-vaj′ĭ-nəl) pertaining to the urethra and the vagina. 326, 374
   urgency (ur′jən-se) *a sudden,* compelling need to do something; a sudden, almost uncontrollable, need to urinate. 335

urinalysis (u″rĭ-nal′ĭ-sis) physical, chemical, or microscopic analysis or examination of urine. 326

urinary (u′rĭ-nar″e) pertaining to urine. 26, 321
   u. cast, cells or particles excreted in the urine having the shape of a renal-collecting tubule. 328, 328f
   u. meatus, the external opening of the urethra. 321
   u. reflux, backward or return flow of urine in the urinary tract. 335
   u. retention, the state in which an individual experiences incomplete emptying of the bladder. 332, 335
   u. tract, all organs and ducts involved in the secretion and elimination of urine. 321

urination (u″rĭ-na′shən) the discharge or passage of urine. 325, 325f

urine (u′rin) the fluid excreted by the kidneys through the ureters. It is stored in the bladder until its discharge through the urethra. 143, 143f, 145, 325

urinometer (u″rĭ-nom′ə-ter) an instrument for determining the specific gravity of urine. 327, 327f

urodynamic studies (u″ro-di-nam′ik stud′ēz) tests that measure various aspects of the process of voiding and are used along with other procedures to evaluate problems with urine flow. 332

urogenital (u″ro-jen′ĭ-təl) pertaining to the urinary and genital apparatus. 326, 359

urogram (u′ro-gram) a radiograph of part of the urinary tract. 333, 333f

urolithiasis (u″ro-lĭ-thi′ə-sis) the presence of urinary calculi. 340

urologic, urological (u″ro-loj′ik, u″ro-loj′ĭ-kəl) pertaining to the urinary system. 26

urologist (u-rol′ə-jist) a physician who specializes in treatment of the urinary tract. 26

urology (u-rol′ə-je) the branch of medicine that deals with the urinary tract. 26, 384

uropathy (u-rop′ə-the) any disease of the urinary system. 335

urticaria (ur″tĭ-kar′e-ə) hives, a vascular reaction of the skin marked by transient appearance of wheals. 541, 541f

uterine (u′tər-in) of or pertaining to the uterus. 362
   u. displacement, any variation in the normal position of the uterus within the pelvis. 372, 373f
   u. tube, formerly called the fallopian tube. One of two small tubes attached to either side of the uterus and leading to an ovary. 360, 361f

uterus (u′tər-əs) the hollow muscular organ in female mammals in which the embryo develops. 359t, 361, 361f

uvula (u′vu-lə) a fleshy mass hanging from the soft palate. 86, 228, 254, 273f

uvulectomy (u″vu-lek′tə-me) excision of the uvula. 254

vaccination (vak″sĭ-na′shən) the introduction of vaccine into the body for the purpose of inducing immunity. 167

vagina (və-ji′nə) the canal in the female that receives the penis in copulation and serves as a birth canal when young are born. 359t, 361, 361f

vaginectomy (vaj″ĭ-nek′tə-me) excision of the vagina. 376

vaginitis (vaj″ĭ-ni′tis) inflammation of the vagina. 370

vagotomy (va-got′ə-me) cutting of the vagus nerve. 303, 520
   selective v., division of the vagal fibers to the stomach with preservation of the hepatic and celiac branches. 303

valval, valvar (val′vəl, val′vər) pertaining to a valve. 185

valvate (val′vāt) pertaining to or having valves. 185

valvula (val′vu-lə) a small valve. 185

valvular (val′vu-lər) pertaining to, affecting, or of the nature of a valve. 185

valvulitis (val″vu-li′tis) inflammation of a valve or valvula, especially a valve of the heart. 197

varicocele (var′ĭ-ko-sēl″) a dilation of the venous complex of the spermatic cord. 386, 386f

varicose (var′ĭ-kōs) unnaturally and permanently distended, said of a vein. 201, 202f
   v. vein, a tortuous, dilated vein with incompetent valves. 201, 202f

vas deferens (vas def′ar-enz) the excretory duct by which sperm leave the testes; also called the ductus deferens. 380, 380f

vascular (vas′ku-lər) pertaining to the blood vessels (sometimes indicating a copious blood supply). 177
   peripheral v. disease, any abnormal condition that affects the blood vessels and lymphatic vessels, except those that supply the heart. 200, 583

vasectomy (və-sek′tə-me) excision of the vas deferens or a portion of it. Bilateral excision results in sterility. 389, 389f, 414

vasoconstriction (vas″o-, va″zo-kən-strik′shən) diminution of the size of a blood vessel. 199

vasodilation (vas″o-, va″zo-di-la′shən) dilation of a vessel, especially dilation of arterioles leading to increased blood flow to a part. 199

vasodilator (vas″o-, va″zo-di′la-tər) causing dilation of the blood vessels; an agent that causes dilation of the blood vessels. 207

vasostomy (va″zos-, vas-os′tə-me) surgical formation of an opening into the vas deferens. 389

vasotomy (va-zot′ə-me) incision into or cutting of the ductus (vas) deferens. 389

vasovasostomy (vas″o-, va″zo-va-zos′tə-me) anastomosis of the ends of the severed ductus deferens, done to restore fertility in vasectomized male individuals. 389, 414

vein (vān) a vessel of the circulatory system in which blood flows toward the heart. 179
   pulmonary v., either of the veins carrying oxygenated blood from the lungs back to the heart. 181, 181f, 185
   varicose v., knotted, distended vein, seen most often in the legs, resulting from the sluggish flow of blood and defective valves in the vein. 201, 202f

vena cava (ve′nə ka′və) two large veins (venae cavae) that carry blood to the right side of the heart. 184f, 185
   inferior v. c., the venous trunk for the lower limbs and for pelvic and abdominal viscera. 184f, 185
   superior v. c., the venous trunk draining blood from the head, neck, upper limbs, and thorax. 184f, 185

venereal (və-nēr′e-əl) caused by or propagated by sexual intercourse. 342
   v. disease, a sexually transmitted disease. 87, 342, 415, 418t

venipuncture (ven′ĭ-punk″chər) puncture of a vein. 180

venous (ve′nəs) pertaining to a vein. 180
   v. thrombosis, blood clot within a vein. 201

ventilation (ven″tĭ-la′shən) in respiratory physiology, the process of air exchange between the lungs and ambient air. 226

ventral (ven′trəl) pertaining to the abdomen; situated on the belly surface; the opposite of dorsal. 120, 126, 126f
   v. cavity, a principal body cavity located on the anterior aspect of the body and composed of the thoracic and abdominopelvic cavities. 126, 126f

ventricle (ven′trĭ-kəl) a small cavity or chamber, as in the brain or heart. 183, 507

ventricular (ven-trik′u-lər) pertaining to a ventricle. 183
   v. septal defect, a cardiac anomaly characterized by one or more abnormal openings in the septum separating the ventricles. 195

ventriculitis (ven-trik″u-li′tis) inflammation of a ventricle, especially a cerebral ventricle. 507

ventromedian (ven″tro-me′de-ən) both ventral and median. 120

Venturi mask (ven-too′re) a respiratory therapy face mask designed to allow inspired air to mix with oxygen, which is supplied. 250, 251f

venular (ven´u-lər) pertaining to a minute vein. 180

venule (ven´ūl) a minute vein; small vessels that collect blood from the capillaries and join to form veins. 180

verruca (və-roo´kə) an epidermal tumor caused by a papillomavirus; wart. 539, 540f

vertebra (vur´tə-brə) any of the 33 bones of the vertebral column. 436, 436f
  cervical v., one of the upper seven segments of the vertebral column. 436, 436f
  coccygeal v., one of the vertebrae that fuse to form the adult coccyx. 436f, 437
  lumbar v., one of the five largest segments of the vertebral column, located in the lower back. 436, 436f
  sacral v., one of the five segments of the vertebral column that fuse in the adult to form the sacrum. 436f, 437
  thoracic v., one of the 12 bony segments of the vertebral column of the upper back. 436, 436f

vertebrectomy (ver″tə-brek´tə-me) excision of a vertebra. 469

vertebrochondral (vur″tə-bro-kon´drəl) pertaining to a vertebra and cartilage. 444

vertebrocostal (vur″tə-bro-kos´təl) pertaining to a vertebra and rib. 438

vertebroplasty (vur´tə-bro-plas″te) plastic repair of a vertebra, especially repair by injection of a cement into a vertebra for spinal stabilization and relief of pain. 469

vertebrosternal (vur″tə-bro-stur´nəl) pertaining to the vertebrae and the sternum. 438

vertigo (vur´tĭ-go) an illustration or sensation of movement as if the external world were revolving or as if the person is revolving in space. 513

vesical (ves´ĭ-kəl) pertaining to the urinary bladder. 322

vesicle (ves´ĭ-kəl) a small bladder or sac containing liquid. 542, 542f
  seminal v., one of a pair of pouches attached to the posterior urinary bladder of male individuals. 380, 380f, 381

vesicovaginal (ves″ĭ-ko-vaj´ĭ-nəl) referring to or connecting with the urinary bladder and vagina. 322, 374

vestibule (ves´tĭ-būl) a space or cavity at the entrance to a canal. 360

vibrio (vib´re-o) an organism of the genus *Vibrio,* a gram-negative straight or curved, rod-shaped bacteria. 87

villi (vil´i) plural of villus, a small vascular process or protrusion, especially such a protrusion from the free surface of a membrane. 278, 278f

virulence (vir´u-ləns) the degree of pathogenicity of a microorganism; the competence of an agent to produce pathologic effects. 83

virus (vi´rəs) one of a group of minute infectious agents, characterized by a lack of independent metabolism and by the ability to replicate only within living host cells. 84

viscera (vis´ər-ə) plural of viscus, any large interior organ in any of the three great body cavities, especially in the abdomen. 127, 231

visceral (vis´ər-əl) pertaining to large internal organs, especially those in the abdomen. 127, 231

vocal cord one of a pair of strong bands of elastic tissue in the larynx. 229

voided specimen (void´əd spes´ĭ-mən) a sample of urine for examination that has been obtained by voiding. 329

voiding (void´ing) emptying or evacuating urine from the bladder by urination. 325
  v. cystourethrogram, a record during radiography of the urethra during voiding. 333

volvulus (vol´vu-ləs) intestinal obstruction caused by a knotting or twisting of the bowel. 296f, 297

vulva (vəl´və) the external genital organs of the female sex. 359, 360f

vulval, vulvar (vul´vəl, vul´vər) pertaining to the vulva. 359

vulvectomy (vəl-vek´tə-me) excision of the vulva. 376

vulvitis (vəl-vi´tis) inflammation of the vulva. 370

vulvovaginitis (vul″vo-vaj″ĭ-ni´tis) inflammation of the vulva and the vagina or of the vulvovaginal glands. 371, 420

wheal (hwēl, wēl) a localized area of edema on the body surface, usually but not always accompanied by severe itching. 542, 542f

wheeze (hwēz) a whistling sound made during respiration. 235, 235f

Wilms tumor (vilms, wilms) a malignant neoplasm of the kidney occurring in young children. 337

wound (wōōnd) an injury or damage, usually restricted to those caused by physical means. 58, 134, 545, 545f
  w. irrigation, flushing of an open wound to cleanse and remove debris and excessive drainage. 550

xanthoderma (zan″tho-der´mə) a yellow coloration of the skin. 79

xeroderma (zēr″o-der´mə) a disease characterized by rough, dry skin. 538

xerosis (zēr-o´sis) any dry condition. 538

xiphoid process (zif´oid, zi´foid pros´es, pro´ses) the pointed process of cartilage connected with the lower end of the body of the sternum. 437, 437f

zoophobia (zo″o-fo´be-ə) irrational fear of animals. 515

zygote (zi´gōt) the fertilized ovum; the cell resulting from union of a male and a female gamete (sperm and ovum). 400, 400f